PSYCHIATRIC NURSING

SECOND EDITION

PSYCHIATRIC NURSING

SECOND EDITION

HOLLY SKODOL WILSON
RN, PhD, FAAN

CAROL REN KNEISL
RN, MS

 ADDISON-WESLEY PUBLISHING COMPANY

Nursing Division, Menlo Park, California

Reading, Massachusetts • London • Amsterdam • Don Mills, Ontario • Sydney

Sponsoring editor: *Deborah Gale*
Special projects manager: *Pat Franklin Waldo*
Production coordinator: *Julie Kranhold, Ex Libris*
Book designer: *Julie Kranhold*
Cover designer: *Michael A. Rogondino*
Manuscript editor: *Loralee Windsor*
Illustrations: *Art by AYXA*

Library of Congress Cataloging in Publication Data

Wilson, Holly Skodol.
  Psychiatric nursing.

  Bibliography: p.
  Includes index.
  1. Psychiatric nursing.   I. Kneisl, Carol Ren,
1938-   . II. Title. [DNLM: 1. Psychiatric nursing.
WY 160 W748p]
RC440.W5 1983   610.73'68   82-22725
ISBN 0-201-11702-9
ABCDEFGHIJ-MU-89876543

The authors and publishers have exerted every effort to ensure that drug selections and dosages set forth in this text are in accord with current recommendations and practice at the time of publication. However, in view of ongoing research, changes in government regulations, and the constant flow of information relating to drug therapy and drug reactions, the reader is urged to check the package insert for each drug for any change in indications of dosage and for added warnings and precautions. This is particularly important where the recommended agent is a new and/or infrequently employed drug.

PHOTO CREDITS
ASPCA Archives: page 284
Bettmann Archive: pages 3, 7, 30, 79, 93, 359, 804
George Fry: pages 271, 296, 336, 457
H. Armstrong Roberts: pages 17, 41, 185, 239, 250, 322, 434, 817, 827
L.A. Takats: pages xxx, 65, 82, 85, 113, 137, 168, 236, 342, 345, 380, 405, 496, 499, 526, 566, 634, 666, 691, 700, 745, 756, 788
Magnum Photo: pages 215, 592, 623, 759
Mark Tuschman: pages 104, 389, 606, 717, 777
The Sophia Smith Collection (Women's History Archive), Smith College: pages 55, 793
Wide World Photo: pages 312, 476, 728

▲▼ **Addison-Wesley Publishing Company**
Nursing Division
2725 Sand Hill Road • Menlo Park, California 94025

PREFACE

The acceptance by our peers of the first edition of *Psychiatric Nursing* has been gratifying. *The American Journal of Nursing* honored this textbook by naming it a "Book of the Year" in 1980. Students who have used *Psychiatric Nursing* have reported high scores on the licensing examination. The text has been translated into other languages, and educators, students, and practitioners throughout the world have offered praise as well as constructive criticisms. The response of these readers has vitalized and inspired us to offer a second edition that continues to reflect the state of the art in psychiatric-mental health nursing.

The first edition presented a new way of viewing psychiatric nursing using a holistic and humanistic framework rather than the traditional medical model. It attempted to motivate psychiatric nurses and students to become client advocates with political power rather than settle for the role of keepers and caretakers. It encouraged the development of autonomy, authority, flexibility, worth, honor, and the conviction that nurses can and do think about the complex and diversified ideas and variables that determine the quality of mental health care in contemporary society.

The second edition continues the attempt to challenge and encourage our readers to reach their professional potential within the context of significant changes that have occurred in psychiatric nursing in the late 1970s and early 1980s.

- The diagnostic classification system and the nomenclature presented in the third edition of the American Psychiatric Association's *Diagnostic and Statistical Manual of Mental Disorders* (or DSM-III) are thoroughly described and integrated in this text. All *five axes* of the DSM-III system are provided in the appendixes for additional reference, and DSM-III categories have been capitalized throughout the text for easy identification.

- The 1982 American Nurses' Association Standards of Psychiatric-Mental Health Nursing Practice provide the basis for the new edition. These standards are reprinted in the appendixes for reference.

- The flexibility and adaptability of the *nursing process* and *nursing theories* in the practice of psychiatric-mental health nursing have been emphasized and demonstrated, using clinical examples, nursing care plans, and other methods.

- An annotated list of *nursing research studies* with implications for psychiatric nursing practice has been provided. We recognize that research findings must influence practice decisions if psychiatric nursing is to attain full professional and scientific status.

- The principle that psychosocial concepts must be integrated in nursing practice regardless of clinical setting or the client's primary health care problem is a primary thesis of the new edition.

NEW FEATURES

To help our readers keep pace with the changes in psychiatric nursing theory and practice, the following features have been incorporated into the new edition:

NEW CONTENT

All the chapters have been updated and revised to reflect the state of the art in psychiatric nursing. Several new chapters have been added, strengthening the nursing focus and responding to the informational needs of our audience. A brief description of these new chapters follows:

- THE NURSING PROCESS AND NURSING THEORIES explores the usefulness of the five-step nursing process to mental health nursing. Well-known nursing theories (including those of Orem, Roy, and Rogers) are examined, and their relevance to psychiatric nursing discussed.

- ETHICAL REFLECTIVENESS examines the general concept of ethics and the specific ethical issues confronting psychiatric nurses, such as the stigma of psychiatric labeling and confidentiality.

- ASSESSING THE INDIVIDUAL CLIENT considers the various assessment techniques used in psychiatric nursing practice, such as history taking, psychological testing, and relevant physical examinations.

- MENTAL HEALTH COUNSELING WITH THE AGED rounds out the life-span approach initiated in the first edition.

- THE CULTURAL CONTEXT OF PSYCHIATRIC NURSING PRACTICE addresses not only the ethnic and folk cultures of black, Asian, Hispanic, and other clients, but also examines the cultural systems arising from social and political forces, such as the feminist movement.

PEDAGOGIC AIDS

Many of the pedagogic tools of the first edition have been retained, including case studies, nursing care plans, references, and further readings at the end of each chapter. Tables have been updated, and more illustrations have been added to enhance text explanations of various concepts.

New to this edition is the list of *Key Nursing Concepts* provided at the end of each chapter, which summarizes succinctly the significant nursing principles dis-

cussed in that chapter. In addition, the inviting format and writing style make this an easily read and understood text.

The supplements to the text include a revised and updated student learning guide entitled *Psychosocial Nursing Concepts: An Activity Book*. This guide is comprised of independent, action-oriented, learning experiences. These activities will be useful in a number of nursing courses because they allow students to practice the various subprocesses that are key to clinical practice, such as communication, decision-making, teaching-learning, group dynamics, and leadership.

The *Instructor's Manual* also has been completely revised, offering educators teaching aids that are useful in developing the psychiatric nursing course content regardless of curriculum design. These include:

- Learning objectives
- Content summaries
- Test questions
- Activity suggestions
- Discussion questions
- Questions directly correlated to the text content
- Annotated audiovisual lists for each chapter

Another feature of the *Instructor's Manual* is the Alternate Course Outline, which identifies chapters in the text and learning activities from the workbook that contain essential knowledge. This list is provided because we realize that curriculum frameworks, program lengths, and student needs vary throughout schools of nursing.

The new edition of *Psychiatric Nursing* is as concise, definitive, and cohesive as the the first edition. It is a comprehensive textbook, containing ideas, theories, and facts necessary for thoughtful holistic nursing.

Holly Skodol Wilson
Carol Ren Kneisl

ACKNOWLEDGMENTS

This second edition of *Psychiatric Nursing* reflects a refinement of our thinking based on our learning and professional experiences. But, even so, it represents the personal transactions and humanity of many other people who have enriched and helped us in our endeavors. We would like to acknowledge and thank these people.

- Carol Bradley, Pam Burton, Priscilla Ebersole, Jo-anne Keglovits, Beth Moscato, Joan Sayre, Andy Skodol, Pat Underwood, and Mary-Eve Mirenda Zangari filled three roles—those of contributors, colleagues, and friends. We are grateful for their dependability, professionalism, and commitment to this project.

- Marilyn Petit, RN, MS, Assistant Professor at the University of Rochester, New York, compiled the glossary for both the first and second editions. She is also the author of the *Instructor's Manual*.

- Janet E. Smith, RN, MSN, developed the patient drug information cards in Chapter 23, "Biological Therapies." Her generosity and expertise are much appreciated.

- The depression algorithm in Chapter 14, "Disturbed Coping Patterns: Nonpsychotic Clinical Syndromes," was developed by Marcia Orsolits, RN, PhD, Assistant Professor, State University of New York at Buffalo.

- Karen O'Conner, RN, MA, Program Coordinator of the ANA Division of Psychiatric and Mental Health Nursing Practice was invaluable in obtaining the newly revised Standards of Psychiatric and Mental Health Nursing Practice, which appear in Appendix A.

- The nursing care plans in Chapter 16, "Disintegrative Life Patterns: Psychotic Conditions," were developed by Ellen Drevers, RN, MS; Cecile Mirand, RN, MS; and the ITRS Unit Staff at the Langley Porter Psychiatric Institute, San Francisco, California. Alex Anagnos, RN, MS, is responsible for the medication teaching care plan.

- The Erie County Mental Health Department, Buffalo, New York, and the Veteran's Administration Medical Center, Buffalo, New York, provided a variety of assessment, contract, and problem-oriented medical and nursing forms.

- The photos introducing the parts and many of the chapters were taken by Lee Takats, a talented photographer from Buffalo, N.Y.

- Phil Lenard gave generously of his time and equipment to make sure we had a photograph he knew was important to us.

- Gina Sutor, RN, Assistant Director of Nursing for Administrative Services, Millard Fillmore Hospital, Buffalo, New York, readily opened doors and provided entrées.

- The staff and administration at Buffalo Psychiatric Center generously provided access to their facility. Many of the sensitive photographs in this book were taken there.

- Jim Grout, Director of the Learning Resource Center, University of California, San Francisco, graciously assisted in the compilation of the nursing research studies presented in Appendix D.

- Karen Babich, RN, PhD, Project Director of WICHE Continuing Education in Mental Health Nursing, generously and willingly shared her resources, reports, and advice.

- Martin Slarke, a friend, was a source of encouragement to both of us.

- The following persons have thoughtfully critiqued the first edition. Their comments have significantly influenced this second edition:

Adelaide Bash, RN, MA
Postmaster's Certificate in Higher-Education
Associate Professor of Nursing
Bergen Community College
Paramus, New Jersey

E. Gail Bentley, RN, MSN
Trainee for Associate Chief of Nursing Education
Veteran's Administration Medical Center
Atlanta, Georgia

Lida G. Chase, RN, MS
Assistant Professor
University of Hawaii at Manoa
School of Nursing
Honolulu, Hawaii

Cynthia Cohen, RN, MS
Psychiatric Nurse
Clinical Center
National Institutes of Health
Bethesda, Maryland

Gwendolyn Smith Cook, RN, MS
Assistant Professor and Coordinator
Undergraduate Mental Health Nursing
University of Michigan
Ann Arbor, Michigan

Karen Lee Fontaine, RN, MSN
Assistant Professor of Nursing
Purdue University
Calumet Campus
Hammond, Indiana

Barbara L. Gano, RNC, BSN
Director of Nursing Education
Cherokee Mental Health Institute
Cherokee, Iowa

Patricia S. Lewis, RN, MS
Instructor of Psychiatric Nursing
Rockford Memorial School of Nursing
Rockford, Illinois

Marcene R. Moran, RN, MA
Program Director
Department of Psychological Mental Health Services
Marian Health Center
Sioux City, Iowa

Daniel Pesut, RN, MSN
Educational Nurse Specialist
Adult-Child Psychiatric Hospital
University of Michigan
Ann Arbor, Michigan

Rita Tadych, RN, MS, MSN
Instructor, University of Missouri School of Nursing
Doctoral Candidate
University of Missouri School of Nursing
Columbia, Missouri

Barbara Van Droof, RN, MSN
Professor of Nursing
Shoreline Community College
Seattle, Washington

Pamela Werstline, RN, MN
Assistant Professor
University of North Carolina
School of Nursing
Greensboro, North Carolina

Margo F. Wilson, RN, MS
Formerly Assistant Professor of Nursing
Point Loma College
San Diego, California

• Over the past four years we have received numerous unsolicited letters from psychiatric nurses, faculty, and students who have used our text. They have validated our belief in the humanistic symbolic interactionist approach advocated in this textbook, and we appreciate their support.

• The staff at Addison-Wesley has provided a nourishing environment that has allowed us to immerse ourselves in the revision of *Psychiatric Nursing:* Wayne Oler, Executive Vice-President of Addison-Wesley Publishing Company, has been gracious and supportive. He created the conditions under which a truly collaborative partnership between author and publisher could occur. Nick Keefe, General Manager of the Medical/Nursing Division, has been enthusiastic from the beginning. He is also a good listener.

   Deborah Gale, our Sponsoring Editor, has a keen intellect and a delightful sense of humor. The combination has helped the book and our own mental health. Pat Waldo, Special Projects Manager, has shared our publishing experience in various capacities, always maintaining her confidence in us.

   Julie Kranhold and her staff have undertaken the herculean task of coordinating the production of this book. She has managed somehow to remain composed while searching for creative solutions to problems of production. Julie is also responsible for the inviting design of the book.

As we reflect on it all, it is so much easier to undertake difficult endeavors when we have been believed in, encouraged, and supported by our publisher, professional colleagues, friends, and family.

H.S.W.
C.R.K.

BIOGRAPHICAL NOTES

ABOUT THE AUTHORS

Holly Skodol Wilson, RN, PhD, FAAN, is a professor in the Department of Mental Health and Community Nursing, School of Nursing, at the University of California, San Francisco. Her area of clinical interest and research is community alternatives for nontraditional care of the severely and chronically mentally disordered. She has authored and coauthored other books in the field of psychiatric nursing and is a frequent contributor to professional journals. She is also active in the Institute of Nursing Consultants, a curriculum consultation firm, and as a national and international speaker on such subjects as the teaching and conduct of research, contemporary developments in psychiatric practice, and nursing professionalism. She serves as an honorary member of the editorial board of the *International Journal of Nursing Studies,* the American Psychiatric Association's *Hospital and Community Psychiatry,* and other nursing publications.

Carol Ren Kneisl, RN, MS, is an associate professor of mental health-psychiatric nursing at State University of New York at Buffalo. Her areas of clinical interest and research are group dynamics, group therapy, and liaison psychiatric nursing. Actively involved in clinical practice issues and in the certification for excellence program in mental health-psychiatric nursing of the New York State Nurses' Association, she is a certified clinical specialist in Adult Mental Health Therapy. She has authored and coauthored five psychiatric nursing books, has three other books in process, and serves on the editorial board of the journal *Perspectives in Psychiatric Care.* She presents papers, workshops, and seminars on both national and international levels in the clinical practice of psychiatric nursing and health communication. Her most recent endeavor is as a consultant and facilitator for groups of nurses and other caregivers concerned with their own personal integration and the stresses of their professional roles.

ABOUT THE CONTRIBUTORS

Carol E. Bradley, RN, MS, a clinical specialist with the Youth Service at Langley Porter Psychiatric Institute in San Francisco, is the author of Chapter 20, "Mental Health Counseling with Adolescents." Her graduate degree is in adolescent psychiatric nursing. She is also an assistant clinical professor at the School of Nursing, University of California, San Francisco.

Pamela Burton, RN, MS, is the author of Chapter 13, "Parenting," and Chapter 19, "Mental Health Counseling with Children." She is an instructor at the Weber State College Nursing Program in Ogden, Utah. Her clinical interests are in parenting and primary prevention in child psychiatric nursing.

Priscilla Ebersole, RN, MS, also holds a certificate in gerontological nursing. In addition to having written Chapter 22, "Mental Health Counseling with the Aged," she is the coauthor of a gerontological nursing textbook. She is presently on leave from her nursing faculty position at San Francisco State University to serve as field director of a geriatric nurse practitioner project in Boise, Idaho.

Joanne Keglovits, RN, MS, is a clinical specialist in psychiatric nursing at the Veterans Administration Medical Center, Buffalo, New York. Her Chapter 27, "Legal Considerations in Psychiatric Nursing," is an outgrowth of her interest in the relationship between madness and the law, a concern that began while she was a graduate student.

Beth Moscato, RN, MS, is the author of Chapter 7, "The One-to-One Relationship: Collaboration and Facilitation." She is a clinical specialist certified in Adult Mental Health Therapy through the New York State Nurses' Association. For three years she has been a psychotherapist and consultant in an interdisciplinary private practice group, the Western New York Institute for the Psychotherapies in Springville, New York.

Her previous publications reflect her interest in sexual stereotyping that perpetuates passive roles for women as clients and as therapists.

Joan Sayre, RN, MA (psychiatric nursing), MA (sociology), is an assistant professor at the Hunter-Bellevue School of Nursing of Hunter College of the City University of New York. Her background in sociology and her interests in deviance, development of the personality, and alternative healing methods are demonstrated in Chapter 10, "Life Theories in Optimal Wellness," and Chapter 25, "Alternative Healing Therapies." She is currently a PhD candidate in sociology at the New School for Social Research and a frequent contributor to the nursing literature.

Andrew E. Skodol, MD, wrote Chapter 17, "Medico-psychiatric Conditions," and Chapter 23, "Biological Therapies." He is an assistant professor of clinical psychiatry at Columbia University, College of Physicians and Surgeons, in New York. He also serves as research psychiatrist for Biometrics Research Department, New York State Psychiatric Institute, and as attending psychiatrist at Columbia Presbyterian Hospital. He has a private practice in Manhattan as well.

Patricia R. Underwood, RN, DNS, authored chapter 16, "Disintegrative Life Patterns: Psychotic Conditions." She is an associate clinical professor in the Department of Mental Health and Community Nursing, School of Nursing, and in the Department of Psychiatry, School of Medicine, at the University of California, San Francisco. She is also a clinical specialist on the Inpatient Unit at the San Francisco Veterans Administration Medical Center. Her major career focus has been nursing care of hospitalized psychiatrically ill adults.

Mary-Eve Mirenda Zangari, RN, MS, wrote Chapter 24. "Psychosocial Concepts in the General Hospital Setting." She is currently a private consultant in Roanoke, Virginia and was previously associated with Cooper School of Nursing, Camden, New Jersey, and Thomas Jefferson University Hospital, Philadelphia, where she provided liaison psychiatric nursing and consultation services. She has been active in developing and refining contract negotiation procedures with clients in general hospital settings and in helping caregivers concerned with persons in pain.

CONTENTS IN BRIEF

1 THEORETICAL BASES FOR PSYCHIATRIC NURSING   1

1   HUMANISTIC AND HISTORICAL PERSPECTIVES   2

2   CONCEPTUAL FRAMEWORKS FOR PSYCHIATRIC NURSING   16

3   THE NURSE'S PERSONAL INTEGRATION AND PROFESSIONAL ROLE   40

4   NURSING PROCESS AND NURSING THEORIES   64

2 THE PROCESSES OF PSYCHIATRIC NURSING PRACTICE   83

5   ETHICAL REFLECTIVENESS   84

6   NURSE-CLIENT COMMUNICATION: THE MUTUAL SEARCH FOR MEANING   103

7   THE ONE-TO-ONE RELATIONSHIP: COLLABORATION AND FACILITATION   136

8   ASSESSING THE INDIVIDUAL CLIENT   184

9   UNDERSTANDING GROUP PROCESSES   214

3 HOLISTIC FRAMEWORK FOR PSYCHIATRIC NURSING   237

10   LIFE THEORIES IN OPTIMAL WELLNESS   238

11   LIFE TURNING POINTS: CRISIS THEORY, ASSESSMENT, AND INTERVENTION   270

12   HUMAN SEXUALITY   295

13   PARENTING   321

4 HUMAN DISTRESS AND DYSFUNCTION   343

14   DISTURBED COPING PATTERNS: NONPSYCHOTIC CLINICAL SYNDROMES   344

15   DISRUPTIVE LIFE-STYLES: PERSONALITY DISORDERS AND SUBSTANCE ABUSE DISORDERS   379

16   DISINTEGRATIVE LIFE PATTERNS: PSYCHOTIC CONDITIONS   404

17   MEDICOPSYCHIATRIC CONDITIONS   456

5 INTERVENTION MODES 497

18 STRATEGIES OF GROUP INTERVENTION 498

19 MENTAL HEALTH COUNSELING WITH CHILDREN 525

20 MENTAL HEALTH COUNSELING WITH ADOLESCENTS 565

21 MENTAL HEALTH COUNSELING WITH FAMILIES 605

22 MENTAL HEALTH COUNSELING WITH THE AGED 623

23 BIOLOGICAL THERAPIES 665

24 PSYCHOSOCIAL CONCEPTS IN THE GENERAL HOSPITAL SETTING 699

25 ALTERNATIVE HEALING THERAPIES 727

6 SOCIAL, POLITICAL, CULTURAL, AND ECONOMIC ISSUES 757

26 THE CULTURAL CONTEXT OF PSYCHIATRIC NURSING PRACTICE 758

27 LEGAL CONSIDERATIONS IN PSYCHIATRIC NURSING PRACTICE 787

28 COMMUNITY MENTAL HEALTH 816

Appendixes

A 1982 ANA STANDARDS OF PSYCHIATRIC AND MENTAL HEALTH NURSING PRACTICE 836

B DSM-III CLASSIFICATION: AXES I-V 838

C COMPREHENSIVE MENTAL HEALTH ASSESSMENT 844

D MENTAL HEALTH RESOURCES 861

E ANNOTATED PSYCHIATRIC NURSING RESEARCH STUDIES 863

Glossary 868

Index 888

CONTENTS IN DETAIL

PART ONE   Theoretical Bases for Psychiatric Nursing   1

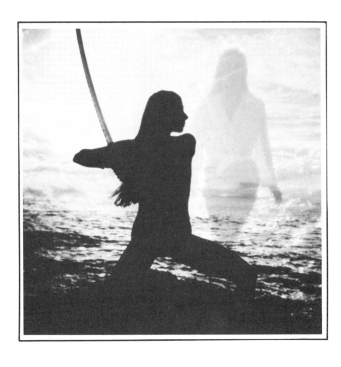

The History of Ideas in Psychiatry   7

Preliterate Times—Era of Magico-Religious Explanations 7, Early Civilization—Era of Organic Explanations 8, The Medieval Period—Era of Alienation 8, End of the Middle Ages—Era of Ritualized Social Exclusion 9, The Classical Age— Era of Confinement 9, The Seventeenth Century— Era of Reason and Observation 9, Late Eighteenth and Early Nineteenth Centuries—Era of Moral Treatment 10, Later Nineteenth and Early Twentieth Centuries 10, The Twentieth Century— Contemporary Developments 12

Emergence of the Discipline of Psychiatric Nursing   13

Key Nursing Concepts   15

References 14, Further Reading 15

CHAPTER 1

HUMANISTIC AND HISTORICAL PERSPECTIVES   2

Philosophical Perspective and Mode of Practice   3

Introduction to Humanistic Symbolic Interactionism   3

Scope of Practice 3, Concepts of "Mental Illness" and "Mental Health" 4, Basic Premises of Symbolic Interactionism 4, Implications of Premises for Psychiatric Nursing 4, Basic Premises of Humanism 5, The Meaning of Humanism for Psychiatric Nursing 6

CHAPTER 2

CONCEPTUAL FRAMEWORKS FOR PSYCHIATRIC NURSING   16

The Medical-Biological Model   18

Assumptions and Key Ideas 18, Implications for Psychiatric Nursing Practice 19, Understanding Medical Nomenclature 19, Critique 21

The Psychoanalytic Model   23

Assumptions and Key Ideas 23, Implications for Psychiatric Nursing Practice 28, Critique 28

The Behaviorist Model   29

Assumptions and Key Ideas 30, Implications for Psychiatric Nursing Practice 31, Critique 32

The Social-Interpersonal Model   **32**
Assumptions and Key Ideas 32, Implications for Psychiatric Nursing Practice 34, Critique 35

The Choice of a Conceptual Framework   **36**

Key Nursing Concepts   **37**
References 38, Further Reading 39

CHAPTER 3

THE NURSE'S PERSONAL INTEGRATION
AND PROFESSIONAL ROLE   **40**

The Emergence of the Self   **42**
Consciousness of Meaning 43, Consciousness and Language 43, Negotiated Reality 43, Feelings: The Affective Self 44, Beliefs and Values 45, A Cognitive Framework for Self-awareness 47

Taking Care of the Self   **49**
Assertiveness 49, Solitude 50, Personal Physical Health 50, Attending to Internal Stress Signals 50

Qualities of Effective Psychiatric Nursing   **51**
Respect for the Client 51, Availability 51, Spontaneity 51, Hope 51, Acceptance 51, Sensitivity 52, Vision 52

Empathy   **52**
The Value of Empathy in Nursing 52, Definition 52, Psychiatric Concepts of Empathy 52, The Therapeutic Use of Empathy 53, Steps in Therapeutic Empathizing 53, Burnout as a Consequence of Empathy 54

The Nurse's Professional Role   **55**

The Members of the Mental Health Team   **55**
The Psychiatric Nursing Clinical Specialist 56, The Registered Nurse Working in a Psychiatric Setting 56, The Psychiatrist 56, The Psychoanalyst 57, The Clinical Psychologist 57, The Psychiatric Social Worker 57, The Mental Health/Human Service Worker, 57, The Psychiatric Aide or Attendant 57, The Occupational Therapist 57, The Recreational Therapist 60, The Creative Arts Therapist 60

Collaborating on the Mental Health Team   **60**
Cooperation versus Competition 60, Respect for the Positions of Others 60, Engaging the Client in Collaboration 61

Key Nursing Concepts   **62**
References 62, Further Reading 63

CHAPTER 4

NURSING PROCESS AND NURSING
THEORIES   **64**

The Nursing Process   **65**
Assessment 66, The Nursing Diagnosis 67, The Nursing Care Plan 70, Implementing the Nursing Care Plan 71, Evaluation 71

Nursing Theory   **75**
Historical Antecedents of Contemporary Theory 75, Overview of Nursing Theories 75, Evaluating Nursing Theories 78, Applying Nursing Theories to Practice 80

Key Nursing Concepts   **80**
References 81, Further Reading 81

PART TWO   The Processes of Psychiatric Nursing Practice   83

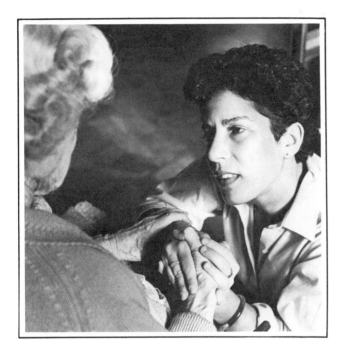

CHAPTER 5

ETHICAL REFLECTIVENESS   84

The Process of Ethical Reflection   85

Analyzing Ethical Issues 85, Dominant Ethical Perspectives 86, Principles of Bioethics 87

Ethical Dilemmas in Psychiatric Nursing   87

The Stigma of Psychiatric Diagnoses 88, Control of Individual Freedom 92, Client Privacy and Confidentiality 95, The Ethics and Politics of Women's Mental Health 98, Political versus Psychiatric Solutions 99, Balancing the Individual and the Social Good 100

Key Nursing Concepts   101

References 102, Further Reading 102

CHAPTER 6

NURSE-CLIENT COMMUNICATION: THE MUTUAL SEARCH FOR MEANING   103

The Process of Human Communication   104

Human Communication Defined 104, Variables that

Influence Communication 104, Levels of Communication 106

Models of Human Communication   107

Communication as an Act 107, Communication as an Interaction 107, Communication as a Transaction 108

Modes of Communication   110

The Spoken Word 110, Nonverbal Messages 110, Relationships between Verbal and Nonverbal Systems 112

Communication in Humanistic Psychiatric Nursing   112

The Theory of Therapeutic Communication 112, The Theory of Pragmatics of Human Communication 115, Ego States as Communication Analysis 116

Facilitative Communication   121

Social Superficiality versus Facilitative Intimacy 121, Essential Ingredients 121, Skills that Foster Effective Communication 125, Ineffective Communication Styles 128

Interaction Process Analysis Case Study (IPA) 129

Key Nursing Concepts   132

References 135, Further Reading 135

CHAPTER 7

THE ONE-TO-ONE RELATIONSHIP: COLLABORATION AND FACILITATION   136

Common Characteristics of One-to-One Relationships   137

Informality or Formality 137, Mutual Definition 138, Mutual Collaboration 139, Goal Direction 139, Professionalism 139

The History of One-to-One Work   140

1940s to 1951: Initial Role Development 140, 1952 to Mid-1960s: Role Clarification 140, Late 1960s to Present: Confirmation of the Specialist Role 141

Philosophical Framework   142

Humanistic Factors 142, Symbolic Interactionist Factors 143

Interpersonal Skills in Therapeutic Relationships   **143**

Therapeutic Effectiveness of Psychiatric Nurses 143, Therapeutic Use of Self 145, Consideration of Client Abilities 145, The Therapeutic Alliance 145

Phases of Therapeutic Relationsips   **145**

Beginning (Orientation) Phase: Establishment of Contact 146, Middle (Working) Phase: Maintenance and Analysis of Contact 148, End (Resolution) Phase: Termination of Contact 156

Processes in Therapeutic Relationships   **157**

Observation 158, Initial Interview 159, Assessment 160, Problem-solving Strategies 161, Transference and Countertransference Phenomena 163, Evaluation 165

The Problems of Resistance in Therapeutic Relationships   **166**

Definition 166, Manifestations 166, Acting Out 166, Acting In 167, General Intervention Strategies for Resistance 168

Specific Nursing Interventions in Common Behavioral Patterns   **168**

Interpersonal Withdrawal 169, Hostility-Aggressivity 170, Manipulation 171, Detachment 172, Excessive Dependence (Learned Helplessness) 172, Transference and Countertransference Phenomena 174

Key Nursing Concepts   **181**

References 182, Further Reading 183

CHAPTER 8

ASSESSING THE INDIVIDUAL CLIENT   184

Collecting, Assessing, and Recording Client Data   **185**

The Psychiatric History 185, The Mental Status Examination 187, Physiological Assessment 190, Psychological Testing 191, Psychiatric Diagnostic Practice According to APA's Criteria (DSM-III) 197, Psychosocial Assessment 204

Systems of Recording   **204**

What to Record 205, Psychiatric Jargon: What to Avoid 205, Source-oriented Recording 206, Problem-oriented Recording 206, Nursing Care Plans 206, Algorithms 207, Psychiatric Audits 207, The Interaction Process Analysis (IPA) 207

Key Nursing Concepts   **212**

References 213, Further Reading 213

CHAPTER 9

UNDERSTANDING GROUP PROCESSES   214

Historical Beginnings of Group Therapy   **215**

Varieties of Groups   **216**

Importance of Group Dynamics   **216**

A Study in Contrast 216, Characteristics of an Effective Group 220

Forces that Modify and Shape Groups   **220**

Physical Environment 220, Leadership 223, Decision-making 224, Trust 227, Cohesion 228, Power and Influence 232

Key Nursing Concepts   **234**

References 235, Further Reading 235

PART THREE Holistic Framework for Psychiatric Nursing   237

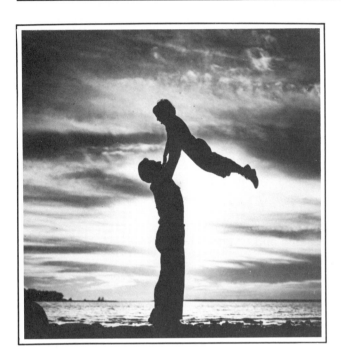

Selye's Stress-adaptation Theory   **257**

The General Adaptation Syndrome 258, The Local Adaptation Syndrome 259, Intervention at Various Levels of Stress 259

Theories of Growth and Development   **260**

The Relativistic Nature of Theories 260, Phases of the Human Life Cycle 260

Critique of the Paradigm of Growth and Development   **265**

The Standard Path of Development 265, The Developmental Model of Behavior 265, The Benefits of a Social Interaction Model 266

The Process of Developing a Deviant Identity   **266**

Deviance as Created by Society 266, Class Differences in Development of Deviant Identity 267

Key Nursing Concepts   **268**

References 269, Further Reading 269

CHAPTER 10

LIFE THEORIES IN OPTIMAL WELLNESS   238

Life Theory as a Holistic Approach   **239**

Historical Perspectives on Human Development   **240**

The Notion of Childhood 240, Erikson's Developmental Life Phases Theory 242, Recent Research 243, The Influence of Symbolic Interactionism 243

The Concept of Development   **245**

Genetic and Environmental Influences 245, The Direction of Development 246, Developmental Stages 246, The Process of Growth 246

Optimal Wellness   **246**

Self-actualization 247, High-level Wellness 247, Health as a Process of Adaptation 248, Characteristics of Optimal Emotional Health 248

Normal Development and Adaptive Difficulties 249

Self-realization 249, Change as Cause of Anxiety 250, Task-oriented and Defense-oriented Reactions 251, Defense Mechanisms 252

CHAPTER 11

LIFE TURNING POINTS: CRISIS THEORY, ASSESSMENT, AND INTERVENTION   270

Crisis Defined   **271**

Stress and Crisis Development   **271**

The Effect of Life Changes 272, Using the Life Change Scale 273

The Emergence of Crisis Theory and Crisis Intervention   **273**

Crisis Intervention as a Therapeutic Strategy   **274**

The Crisis Sequence   **274**

Developmental Crises   **276**

The Mid-life Crisis 276, Retirement 277

Situational Crises   **278**

Death and Loss 278, Body Image Alterations 281

Victim Crises   **283**

Family Violence 284, Natural, Accidental, and Man-made Disasters 285

Suicide as a Coping Mechanism   **288**

*Self-destructive People 289, Social Variables 289,
Demographic Variables 289, Clinical Variables 290,
Suicidal Clues or Cries for Help 290, Assessing
Lethality 290, Intervention with Suicidal Clients 291,
The Victims Left Behind 292*

Crisis Intervention Modes   **292**

*Individual Crisis Counseling 292, Crisis Groups 292,
Family Crisis Counseling 292, Telephone
Counseling 293, Home Crisis Visits 293*

Key Nursing Concepts   **293**

References 293, Further Reading 294

CHAPTER 12

HUMAN SEXUALITY   **295**

Normal and Abnormal Sexuality   **296**

Physiological Sexuality   **297**

*The Female Genitals 297, The Male Genitals 298,
Physiology of Sexual Responses 300, Sexual
Arousal and Intercourse 304, Masturbation 304,
Arousal Techniques 306, Coitus 306, Anal
Intercourse 307*

Psychological Sexuality   **307**

*Gender Identity 307, Theories of Gender
Development 308*

Sociological Sexuality   **308**

Sex Roles 308, Sex and Social Problems 308

Alternative Sexual Patterns   **312**

*Homosexuality 313, Bisexuality 313,
Transsexualism and Transvestism 313, Other
Alternative Sexual Patterns 314*

Sexual Problems and Their Treatment   **314**

*Impairments in Physiological Functioning 315,
Sexual Problems Associated with Other Coping
Problems 315, Therapeutic Counseling 315*

Key Nursing Concepts   **319**

References 319, Further Reading 319

CHAPTER 13

PARENTING   **321**

The Process of Parenting   **322**

*Parenting and Psychiatric Nursing Practice 322,
The Difficulties Inherent in the Parenting Role, 322,
Bonding and Attachment: Beginning of the
Interactive Process 323, Mothering and Fathering
324*

Different Structures of Parenting   **325**

*Single Parents 325, Adoptive, Foster, and
Stepparents 326, Communal Parents 327, Working
Parents 328*

Parents and Children under Stress   **329**

*Poverty and Racism 329, Sexism 330, Adolescent
Parents 331, Battering Parents 332*

Counseling Parents   **334**

*Prenatal Assessment of Parenting Skills, 334,
Working with Parents Postnatally 336, Parent-Child
Fit 338, Intervention Strategies 340*

Key Nursing Concepts   **341**

References 341, Further Reading 341

PART FOUR   Human Distress and Dysfunction   343

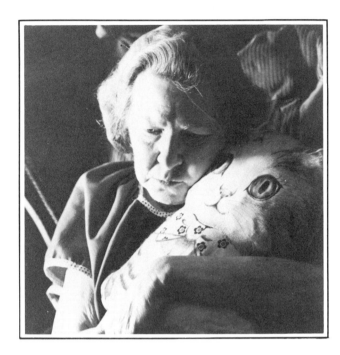

CHAPTER 14

DISTURBED COPING PATTERNS: NONPSYCHOTIC CLINICAL SYNDROMES   344

The Contours of Disturbances   345

The Need for a Holistic View   346

A Humanistic Interactionist Approach   346

Control 347, Balance 347, Stress 348, Anxiety 349, Coping Strategies 352, Inability to Cope Using Everyday Strategies 353

Therapeutic Intervention   355

Specific Patterns Requiring Intervention 356, Anxiety Disorders 356, Dissociative Disorders 363, Somatoform Disorders 364, Affective Disorders 369

Key Nursing Concepts   377

References 378, Further Reading 378

CHAPTER 15

DISRUPTIVE LIFE-STYLES: PERSONALITY DISORDERS AND SUBSTANCE ABUSE DISORDERS   379

The Concept of Life-style   380

Types of Disruptive Life-styles   381

Development of Disruptive Life-styles   382

Styles of Defense and General Life-styles 382, Interaction of Factors in Style Preference 382

Impulsive Life-styles   383

Development of Impulsive Life-styles 383, Common Features 384, Nursing Intervention 385

Addicted Life-styles   386

Alcohol Addiction 386, Drug Dependence 391

Compulsive Life-styles   395

Rigidity 395, Style of Paying Attention 396, General Mode of Activity 397, The Subjective Quality of Trying 397, The Consequences for Quality of Life 397, Nursing Intervention 398

Dependent Life-styles   398

Characteristics 398, Nursing Intervention 398

Eccentric Life-styles   399

Characteristics of a Paranoid Personality 399, Characteristics of Schizoid and Schizotypal Personalities 401

Key Nursing Concepts   402

References 403, Further Reading 403

CHAPTER 16

DISINTEGRATIVE LIFE PATTERNS: PSYCHOTIC CONDITIONS   404

Behavior Associated with Disintegrative Life Patterns   405

Disintegration of Perception 405, Disintegration of Thought 407, Disintegration of Affect 407, Disintegration of Motivation 407

Defining Disintegrative Behavior   **407**

*Personal Definition 407, Social Definition 410,
Legal Definition 411, Statistical Definition 411,
Medical Definition 411*

Examples of Disintegrative Behavior   **414**

**The Study and Treatment of Psychotic
Conditions: 1950–1970**   **415**

*Institutionalization 416, Psychoactive Drugs, 416,
Community Mental Health 417*

**Contemporary Study and Treatment of Psychotic
Conditions: 1970 to Present**   **417**

*Descriptions of Psychotic Conditions 418, Past
History Associated with Psychotic Conditions 419,
Explanations of Psychotic Conditions 423,
Treatment of Psychotic Conditions 427*

Contemporary Nursing Approaches   **429**

*Factors that Influence Care Planning 430, Nursing
Strategies 433, The Nursing Care Plan 445*

Key Nursing Concepts   **453**

References 453, Further Reading 454

CHAPTER 17

MEDICOPSYCHIATRIC CONDITIONS   **456**

Psychophysiological Disorders   **458**

*History 458, Recent Theory 459, Classification 459,
Syndromes 460, Intervention 467*

Mental Retardation   **470**

*Intelligence 470, Definitions of Retardation 471,
Causes of Retardation 471, Problems Encountered
by the Retarded 476, Intervention 477*

Organic Brain Syndromes   **480**

*Myths and Reality about Organic Causes of
Psychiatric Symptoms 481, Assessment 482,
Classification 483, Syndromes, 485, Intervention
491*

Key Nursing Concepts   **493**

References 494, Further Reading 494

PART FIVE   Intervention Modes   497

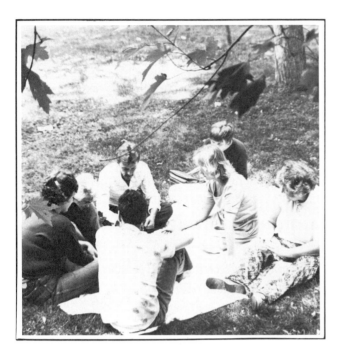

CHAPTER 18

STRATEGIES OF GROUP INTERVENTION   498

Frameworks for Group Analysis   499

*The Johari Awareness Model 499, FIRO: The
Interpersonal Needs Approach 502, The Authority
Relations/Personal Relations Approach 504, The
Therapeutic Problem Approach 507, Small Group
Assessment 510*

Interactional Group Therapy   510

*Advantages of Group over Individual Therapy 511,
Qualified Group Therapists 511, The Curative
Factors 511, Types of Group Leadership 511,
Creating the Group 514, Stages in Therapy Group
Development 516, The Here-and-Now Emphasis
516*

**Other Group Therapies and Therapeutic
Groups**   518

*Analytic Group Psychotherapy 518, Psychodrama
518, Sociodrama 518, Multiple Family Group
Therapy 519, Self-help Groups 519, Remotivation
and Reeducation Groups 519, Client Government
Groups 520, Activity Therapy Groups 521, Groups
of Clients with Pathophysiological Dysfunction and
Families 521, Community Client Groups 522,
Groups with Nurse Colleagues 522*

Key Nursing Concepts   522

References 523, Further Reading 523

CHAPTER 19

MENTAL HEALTH COUNSELING WITH CHILDREN   525

Need for Child Psychiatric Services   526

Levels of Prevention   526

*Basic Prevention 526, Secondary Prevention 527,
Tertiary Prevention 527*

**The Developmental Model as a Basis for
Assessment and Intervention**   527

Emotional Disturbances   527

*Pervasive Developmental Disorders 531, Other
Childhood Disturbances 532, Role of the Nurse in
Residential Treatment 536*

Intervention   540

*Basic Goals of Treatment 540, Assessment 540,
Health Assessment Outline 541, Communication
Skills 544, Conveying Acceptance 545, Setting
Limits 546, Countertransference 547*

Specific Treatment Modes   547

*Treatment Facilities 547, Therapy: An Overview
548, Play Therapy 548, Group Therapy 549, Art
Therapy 551, Brief Therapy 552, Family Therapy
553, Behavior Modification 553, Milieu Therapy
554*

The Hospitalized Child   555

*Anaclitic Depression 555, Separation Anxiety 555,
Castration and Mutilation Fantasies 557,
Psychological Care of the Pediatric Client 557*

Key Nursing Concepts   563

References 563, Further Reading 564

CHAPTER 20

**MENTAL HEALTH COUNSELING
WITH ADOLESCENTS** **565**

The Normative Process of Adolescence **566**
*Physical and Sexual Development 566, Mental
Development 567, Social Development 567,
Emotional Development 568*

Developmental Theories **568**
*Freud and the Reemergence of the Oedipal
Conflict 568, Erikson and the Life Cycle 569,
Sullivan and the Need for Interpersonal Intimacy
571, The Theories in Summary 572*

The Role of the Nurse **572**
*In the Outpatient Setting 572, In the Hospital
Setting 574*

Specific Issues and Problems **579**
*Seduction of the Nurse 579, Communication 580,
Testing and Limit Setting 580, Anxiety and
Resistance 581, Anger and Hostility 583,
Scapegoating 585, Sexual Behavior of the
Adolescent 585, Dietary Problems 589, Drug Use
and Abuse 589, Juvenile Delinquency 591, Suicide
592*

Dealing with Families of Adolescent Clients **601**

Key Nursing Concepts **602**
References 602, Further Reading 603

CHAPTER 21

**MENTAL HEALTH COUNSELING
WITH FAMILIES** **605**

Will the *Real* Family Please Stand Up? **606**
*The Traditional Nuclear Family 606, The Single
Parent Family 607, The Blended Family 607,
Alternative Family Forms 607*

Developmental Tasks Confronting Families **608**

The Family as a System **609**

Family Characteristics and Dynamics **609**
Roles 610, Power 610, Behavior 610

Defining Family Therapy **611**

**The Family Movement in Historical
Perspective** **611**

Approaches to Family Therapy **612**

Qualifications of Family Therapists **612**

**Relational and Communicational Intricacies
in Families** **612**
*The Self-fulfilling Prophecy and Life Scripts 613,
Family Myths, Life-styles, and Themes 613,
Coalitions, Dyads, and Triangles 614,
Pseudomutuality and Pseudohostility 614, Deviations
in the Parental Coalition 615, Scapegoating 615,
Paradoxes and Double Binds 616*

**The Treatment Unit and the Treatment
Setting** **616**

The Components of Family Therapy **617**
*Family Assessment 617, Contract or Goal
Negotiation 620, Intervention 621*

Criteria for Terminating Treatment **623**

The Nursing Process in Family Counseling **623**

**Family-oriented Preventive Psychiatry
Programs** **626**

Couples Therapy **626**
*Developmental Tasks Confronting Couples 628,
Types of Therapy 628, Focus of Therapy 629*

Key Nursing Concepts **630**
References 631, Further Reading 632

CHAPTER 22

**MENTAL HEALTH COUNSELING
WITH THE AGED** **633**

Philosophical Perspective of Aging **634**

Parameters of Old Age and Mental Health **634**

Mental Health in Old Age **635**

Criteria for Mental Health in Old Age **635**
*Understanding the Aged 635, Lifelong Habits and
Strengths 635, Physical and Neural Changes 635,
Needs of the Aged 635, Developmental Tasks of
Aging 636, Nurses' Attitudes toward Aging 638*

Stresses Characteristic of Aging   **640**

Fear of Aging 640, Loneliness 640, Loss 640, Meaninglessness 640, Physical Deterioration 640, Stigma 641, Sexuality 642, Relocation 643, Abuse and Neglect 643

Reactions to Problems of Aging   **644**

Disturbed Behaviors 644, Disruptive Patterns 645, Disintegrative Patterns 646, Cognitive Function 646

Common Evidence of Psychic Distress   **649**

Stress Anxiety 649, Depression 650, Substance Abuse 651, Suicide 651

**Family Reactions to Psychically
Distressed Aged**   **651**

Intervention Strategies   **652**

Family Support Therapy 652, Individual Psychotherapy 653, Brief Psychotherapy 653, Crisis Intervention 653, Psychotropic Drugs 653, Group Work 654, Family Support Groups 654, Networking 655, Confidants 659, Reminiscing 659, Supporting the Dying and the Grieving 660

Key Nursing Concepts   **662**

References 663, Further Reading 664

CHAPTER 23

BIOLOGICAL THERAPIES   **665**

Changing Roles for Nurses   **666**

Negotiating Communication 666, The Nurse as Client Advocate 667

Psychotropic Drugs   **668**

Antipsychotic Drugs 669, Antidepressant Drugs 676, The Antimania Drug (Lithium) 684, Antianxiety Drugs 688, Hypnotic Drugs 690

Electroconvulsive Therapy   **691**

Indications for Use 692, Procedure 692, Course of Treatment 693, Complications 693

Narcotherapy   **694**

Radical Biological Therapies   **694**

Psychosurgery 694, Insulin Coma Treatment 695

Newer Organic Therapies   **695**

Niacin Therapy 696, Electrosleep Therapy 696, Nonconvulsive Electrical Stimulation Therapy 696, Hemodialysis 696

Key Nursing Concepts   **697**

References 697, Further Reading 698

CHAPTER 24

**PSYCHOSOCIAL CONCEPTS IN THE
GENERAL HOSPITAL SETTING**   **699**

**Incorporating Psychosocial Principles in
General Hospital Work**   **700**

A Holistic Concept of Illness 700, Holistic Health Concepts 703, Crisis Theory 704, Preventive Aspects of Consultation 705

**The Role of the Psychiatric
Nursing Consultant**   **706**

History of Consultation in the Hospital Setting 706, Types of Mental Health Consultation 706, Guidelines for Mental Health Consultation 709, Qualifications of the Consultant 709, Building Relationships 710, Negotiating the Consultation Contract 711

Clinical Situations Commonly Encountered   **713**

The Demanding Client 713, The Client in Pain 714, The Dependent Client 715, The Client's Family 717, The Client in the Intensive Care Unit 718, The Client Who Is Sexually Acting Out 720, The Noncompliant Client 721, The Dying Client 723

Key Nursing Concepts   **724**

References 725, Further Reading 725

CHAPTER 25

ALTERNATIVE HEALING THERAPIES   **727**

Historical Roots of the Movement   **728**

Cultural Change 728, Humanistic and Existential Influences 729, Psychotherapies as Social Indices 729, Expanded Definitions of Psychiatric Treatment 730

Basic Premises of the New Therapies   **730**

The Discovery of the Real Self 730, Body-Mind Integration 731, Self-regulation and Responsibility 732

Representative Alternative Healing Therapies 733

Body Discipline and Body-Mind Awareness Therapies 733, Psychological Growth Therapies 737, Consciousness Development Therapies 741

Comparative Analysis   745

General Themes 745, The Therapeutic Problem 748

Relevance for Psychiatric Nursing   749

The Shift from the Medical Model to a Social Model 749, Frameworks for Assessing the New Therapies 750, Applying the New Therapies to Psychiatric Nursing Practice 752

Key Nursing Concepts   753

References 753, Further Reading 754

PART SIX   Social, Political, Cultural, and Economic Issues   757

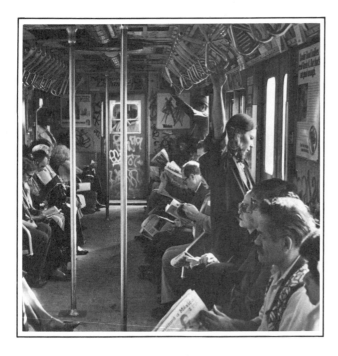

CHAPTER 26

THE CULTURAL CONTEXT OF PSYCHIATRIC NURSING PRACTICE   758

Relevance of Culture for Psychiatric Nursing Practice   759

The Assumptive World 760, When Assumptive Worlds Differ 760, Cultural Complexity and Diversity 761, Dangers in Cultural Stereotyping 761, The YAVIS Syndrome in Mental Health Care 762

Biosocial Factors Influencing Diagnosis and Treatment   762

Ethnicity 763, Socioeconomic Class 763, Religious Beliefs 763, Age 764, Place of Residence 764, Sex and Marital Status 764, Analysis of Biosocial Factors 764, Oppression 765

Contemporary Sociopolitical Influences on Mental Health Care   765

The Feminist Movement 765, The Gay Rights Movement 767, The Gray Panther Movement 768, Religious Cults 768

Folk Beliefs and Healing Practices   771

The Folk Systems of Black Americans 772, The Folk Systems of Hispanic Americans 773, The Folk Systems of Asian Americans 774, The Folk Systems of American Indians 775

Culturally Aware Strategies for Nursing Intervention   776

Understanding Your Own Sociocultural Heritage 776, Incorporating Principles of Effective Communication 777, Becoming Familiar with and Using Folk Beliefs and Healing Practices 777, Using Counseling Techniques Specific to the Client's Distress 777

Key Nursing Concepts   783

References 784, Further Reading 785

CHAPTER 27

LEGAL CONSIDERATIONS IN PSYCHIATRIC NURSING PRACTICE 787

Madness and the Law—A Look at the Past 788
Jewish Law—The Talmud 788, Greek Law 789, Roman Law 789, The Visigothic Code 789, Development of English Law 790, Madness in the New World 791

Twentieth-Century Mental Hygiene Laws 797
Model Legislation—The Draft Act 797, Status of Legislation after the Draft Act 797

Some Recent Court Decisions 798
Right to Treatment 798, Commitment Procedures 799, Civil Rights 800, The Client–Therapist–Public Relationship 800, Right to Refuse Treatment 801

Overview of Mental Hygiene Laws 802
Admission 802, Rights of Clients 805, Participation in Legal Matters 806, Separation from a Mental Institution 807

Two Current Mental Health Laws 808
New York State's Mental Hygiene Law 808, California's Mental Hygiene Law 809

The Implementation of Clients' Rights 811
The Role of Care Givers 811, Staff Knowledge and Attitudes 812

Key Nursing Concepts 813
References 813, Further Reading 814

CHAPTER 28

COMMUNITY MENTAL HEALTH 816

Turning Points in Psychiatric Care 817

Emergence of the Community Mental Health Movement 818
The 1960s: A Bold New Approach 818, The 1970s: Realistic Problems 819, The 1980s: Dismal Prospects 820

Underlying Concepts 822
Systems Perspective 822, Levels of Prevention 822, Interdisciplinary Collaboration 822, Consumer Participation and Control 823, Comprehensive Services 823, Continuity of Care 823

Nursing Roles in Community Mental Health 823
Applying the ANA Standards 824, Levels of Community Mental Health Nursing 824, Primary, Secondary, and Tertiary Prevention 824

Critique of Community Mental Health and the Deinstitutionalization Movement 824
Lack of True Innovation 824, Conceptual Confusion 827

Deinstitutionalized Alternatives 828
The Soteria House Approach 829, Self-care Nursing for True Chronic Clients 830, Emerging Networks 832

Key Nursing Concepts 833
References 834, Further Reading 835

APPENDIXES

A 1982 ANA Standards of Psychiatric and Mental Health Nursing Practice 836

B DSM-III Classification: Axes I-V 838

C Comprehensive Mental Health Assessment 844

D Mental Health Resources 861

E Annotated Psychiatric Nursing Research Studies 863

GLOSSARY 868

INDEX 888

PSYCHIATRIC NURSING

SECOND EDITION

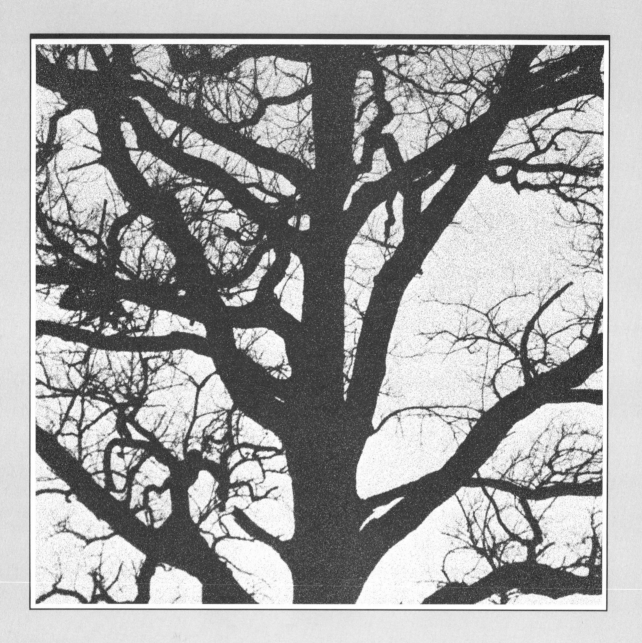

PART ONE

Theoretical Bases
for Psychiatric Nursing

HUMANISTIC PSYCHIATRIC NURSING *practice is enhanced when scientific knowledge is delicately blended with an imagination that is sensitive, aware, and liberally educated. Here, we bring together facts, concepts, theories, issues, and ideas from the sciences and the humanities to form a basis for holistic psychiatric nursing care. Rather than assume an ambiguous and eclectic stance about the conceptual framework suited to psychiatric nursing, we review and critique the major existing psychiatric frameworks and advocate a specific one—humanistic symbolic interactionism. We believe that this perspective, reflected throughout the book, enables nurses to take into account social and cultural factors as well as intrapersonal ones in assessing clients and intervening with them. Through this perspective, nurses function as egalitarian members of the professional psychiatric team; psychiatric and mental health patterns are understood from a nursing rather than an exclusively medical model; and clients are defined as individuals, families, and community groups. Humanistic symbolic interactionism is compared and contrasted with the medical, psychoanalytic, behaviorist, and interpersonal frameworks—all reviewed in the history of psychiatric practice. Nurses always act with either an implicit or an explicit framework for understanding the meanings of interactions with clients and colleagues. Therefore, in Chapters 1 and 2 we urge careful consideration of the theoretical assumptions and principles reflected in their practice decisions. In Chapter 3 we focus on personal and professional integration. In Chapter 4 we evaluate the nursing process and the emerging nursing theories for their usefulness in psychiatric nursing situations according to the 1982 ANA Standards of Mental Health/Psychiatric Nursing Practice and Professional Performance. Part One is a backdrop against which the rest of this book should be viewed. It acquaints the reader with the general problems, issues, debates, and ideas that influence psychiatric care.*

1

Humanistic and Historical Perspectives

CHAPTER OUTLINE

Philosophical Perspective and Mode of Practice

Introduction to Humanistic Symbolic Interactionism

    Scope of Practice

    Concepts of "Mental Illness" and "Mental Health"

    Basic Premises of Symbolic Interactionism

    Implications of Premises for Psychiatric Nursing

    Basic Premises of Humanism

    The Meaning of Humanism for Psychiatric Nursing

The History of Ideas in Psychiatry

    Preliterate Times—Era of Magico-Religious Explanations

    Early Civilization—Era of Organic Explanations

    The Medieval Period—Era of Alienation

    End of the Middle Ages—Era of Ritualized Social Exclusion

    The Classical Age—Era of Confinement

    The Seventeenth Century—Era of Reason and Observation

    Late Eighteenth and Early Nineteenth Centuries—Era of Moral Treatment

    Later Nineteenth and Early Twentieth Centuries

    The Twentieth Century—Contemporary Developments

Emergence of the Discipline of Psychiatric Nursing

Key Nursing Concepts

LEARNING OBJECTIVES

After reading this chapter, students should be able to

- Identify the major ideas of symbolic interactionism
- Identify the major tenets of humanism
- Relate the premises of humanistic interactionism to the psychiatric nursing process
- Describe the history of ideas about madness and psychiatric practice
- Describe the history of psychiatric nursing as a discipline
- Develop a personal philosophical framework for psychiatric nursing practice

CHAPTER 1

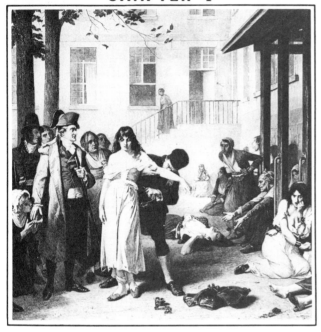

messages to students. They promote a view of human beings based on *humanism* and *existentialism*, which value the individual's freedom of choice and uniqueness. Yet they teach nursing interventions that foster conformity of behavior, of perception, and of life-style.

A psychiatric nurse's philosophical perspective influences the choice of theories and definitions of concepts. Consequently, it influences the nurse's mode of practice. This chapter will introduce readers to a perspective of *humanistic symbolic interactionism*. We feel this perspective integrates most of the variables that contemporary psychiatric nursing needs to address. We hope that readers will be moved to examine some basic philosophical questions and to formulate a philosophy of psychiatric nursing that is useful and meaningful in their own personal and professional lives.

PHILOSOPHICAL PERSPECTIVE AND MODE OF PRACTICE

There are many approaches to understanding people. Each way is a sort of searchlight that elucidates some of the facts while the remainder retreat into the background. The practice of psychiatric nursing proceeds from certain assumptions about human nature, society, and values. It has become a convention in most textbooks to advocate an eclectic philosophical approach to practice on the grounds that psychiatric nursing is still too ill-defined to subscribe to any single perspective, and that multiple perspectives offer psychiatric nurses an array of concepts from which to choose according to the situation or setting. This argument indeed has merit. Yet an unfortunate consequence of such a smorgasbord stance is a tendency to adhere simultaneously to fundamentally contradictory or dramatically opposed points of view. For example, most teachers, writers, and students of psychiatric nursing view people *holistically*—as complex organic wholes with physical, mental, emotional, social, and cultural dimensions inextricably related and linked. Yet, the descriptive, disease-oriented *medical model* of psychiatry continues to dominate psychiatric nursing concepts and philosophies of practice. Teachers may give mixed

INTRODUCTION TO HUMANISTIC SYMBOLIC INTERACTIONISM

Scope of Practice

The quality of human life and its relationship to health are concerns of all nurses. The psychiatric nurse is primarily concerned with the aspects of people's lives that distinguish them as human beings. The ways in which the individual's optimal health is related to feelings of self-worth, personal integrity, self-fulfillment, human rights, comfortable relations with others, basic living needs, and creative expression are particularly central to the practice of the psychiatric nurse. This domain encompasses individual protest, alienation, sudden life changes, mass confrontations, changing identities, family interaction patterns, poverty and affluence, the experiences of birth and death, loss of significant others or body parts, and sustaining and enhancing the individual and the group. This broad-ranging, humanistic, and interactional conceptualization of the scope of psychiatric nursing is dramatically different from the medical and behavioral science orientation of the last three decades. The classic psychiatric and psychological approach (the medical model) has stressed the description and classification of signs and symptoms. Illness is accounted for by individual psychological mechanisms, such as character disorders, weak ego, or failure of defense mechanisms.

Concepts of "Mental Illness" and "Mental Health"

The perspective in this text differs substantially from more traditional modes of psychiatric nursing thought in which a client's "mental illness" or "mental health" is seen as arising from within the individual. We believe these concepts are interactional and derive their meaning from the definitions given to certain acts by certain audiences. We advocate looking at the social conditions under which someone is labeled mentally ill, by whom, and with what consequences. Thus, our *interactionist approach* is inclined to view "mental illness" and "mental health" as outgrowths of interpersonal processes. Examined from this perspective, "mental illness" is not exclusively depicted by particular intrinsic character traits. Nor is it established purely by the nature of certain acts (*symptomatology*). Rather it includes the individual's view of those acts, the reactions of others to them, and the overall cultural context in which they occur. In short, "mental illness" is often a matter of judgment, not a matter of fact. The appropriateness of behavior depends on whether it is judged plausible or not, based on a set of social, ethical, and legal rules that define the limits of appropriate behavior and reality. For example, if a man on a street corner says he is Napoleon, people will not believe him and will consider his statement symptomatic or disturbed. Such a declaration at a masquerade party would hardly merit the same conclusion.

Basic Premises of Symbolic Interactionism

The approach we advocate above has come to be known as *symbolic interactionism,* a term introduced by Herbert Blumer (1969) to describe a relatively distinctive approach to the study of human conduct. It is based on three simple philosophical premises:

1. Human beings act toward things on the basis of the meaning that the things have for them.
2. The meaning of things in life is derived from the social interactions a person has with others.
3. People handle and modify the meanings of the things they encounter through an interpretive process.

Implications of Premises for Psychiatric Nursing

The First Premise   The notion that people's actions in a situation are based on the unique meaning that situation has for them is all but ignored in many approaches to psychiatric nursing. Instead, human conduct is treated as the product of various factors that act on passive human beings—factors such as stimuli, unconscious motives, and character traits. This emphasis on factors alleged to produce "symptoms" neglects the role of individual meaning in the formation of human behavior. We believe that all behavior has meaning and that the psychiatric nurse must be wary of interventions that convey an invalidation of the meaning an experience has for the client in favor of the nurse's own definition of the situation. A corollary is the need for nurses to develop skill in observing, interpreting, and responding to the client's experiences in the hope of arriving at a common ground of negotiated meanings and authentic communication. (See Chapter 6 for general considerations and Chapter 16 for case illustrations of this premise. In Chapter 16 we find the example of Charlene, a twenty-five-year-old hospitalized psychotic client who carried a bag of foul-smelling baby clothes with her at all times. Recognizing that the bag had *special meaning* for the patient, the nurse neither attempted to convince Charlene to part with it, nor tried to take it away from her forceably.)

The Second Premise   As we stated earlier, many conventional approaches in psychiatric nursing account for meanings, such as "normal," "mentally healthy," and "mentally ill," by regarding them as intrinsic to the nature of the behavior, the personality, or the disease. We believe meanings arise in the *process* of interaction with others. Meanings are social products formed in and through interpersonal processes. It is essential, therefore, that psychiatric nurses take into account the social and cultural environment of each client. A holistic assessment of a client accounts for the social psychology of interaction patterns in that person's social world. A Mohawk haircut dyed orange, tight black leather clothing, and grotesque face paint and tattoos may appear bizarre in a milieu of upper-middle-class bankers and businesspeople, yet they represent rather strict adherence to dress and demeanor codes of the punk rock subculture. The group and bisexual patterns of some Americans may be considered immoral and decadent by some cultural segments, but those who choose such values may find them preferable to those of the more traditional nuclear family. Individuals labeled "paranoid" or "neurotic" or "using alcohol or drugs as emotional crutches" cannot be understood outside their unique social context. (See Chapter 26 for a discussion of cultural considerations in mental health care. In Chapter 20, we are reminded that adolescents direct insults and hostile remarks at nurses for many reasons, most of which have little to do with the nurse as a person but a lot to do with the nurse as an adult or authority figure. The social context of an adolescent peer group plays a critical part in determining the meaning of such behavior.) Similarly, it is within interpersonal interaction that clients can learn new definitions for life situations and new repertoires for action. This is the crux of the psychiatric nurse's therapeutic and healing role. The sensitive, intelligent, and humanistic use of self within interpersonal relationships comprises a key dimension of the psychiatric nurse's skill. Nurses have a particular potential for helping clients redefine their experiences in more satisfying ways, learn new patterns of coping with stress, and generally enhance the quality of their lives and social worlds.

The Third Premise   We believe that people handle situations in terms of what they consider vitally important about the situation. They fit their own actions to the actions of others. To understand the actions of people, the psychiatric nurse must become astute at identifying the meanings those actions have for them. This premise needs to be kept in mind when responding to an expression of human distress. A nurse may say, "I wouldn't worry about it," or "don't feel that way," "you are reacting inappropriately," or "it's not so bad." Such clichés are not usually helpful, not because they are in and of themselves "untherapeutic techniques" but because they neglect the basic premise that people interpret the world in their own way in order to act in a specific situation. They deal with what they perceive. This gives their experience some meaning, which in turn becomes a basis for their behavior.

Symbolic interactionism offers psychiatric nursing a perspective of human beings as having purpose and control over their own lives. Symbolic interactionism as interpreted here provides the premises for a philosophy of healing with a strong humanistic cast and a politics of reality. It is clearly different from a position that interprets certain actions as purely medical problems or the result of unconscious drives.

Basic Premises of Humanism

The purpose of this chapter is to specify a synthesized set of premises as a basis for subsequent chapters. The three postulates of symbolic interactionism provide us with a partial orientation. A theory of life centered on human beings, termed *humanism*, rounds out the perspective.

The central proposition of humanism is that the chief end of human life is to work for well-being within the confines of life on this earth. Humanism is a philosophy of service for humanity using reason, science, and democracy.

Psychiatric nurses and students might reasonably ask why issues of philosophy should even be considered. We believe that the guiding pattern in the lives of all psychiatric nurses is their philosophy, even though it may be implicit in actions rather than explicit in the mind. Philosophy teaches people to say what they mean and to mean what they say. It is an attempt to think through the fundamental issues of life and reach reasoned conclusions about society, human nature, action, and values.

Humanism as a philosophical perspective can be clarified in eight central propositions:

1. The human being's mind is indivisibly connected with the body.
2. Human beings have the power or potential to solve their own problems.
3. All theories of universal determinism, fatalism, or predestination are false; human beings, while influenced by the past, possess freedom of creative choice and action and are, within certain limits, masters of their own destinies.
4. Human values are grounded in life experiences and relationships, and our highest goal must be the happiness, freedom, and growth of all people.
5. Individuals attain well-being and a high quality of life by harmoniously combining personal satisfactions with activities that contribute to the welfare of the community.
6. We should develop art and awareness of beauty so that the aesthetic experience becomes a pervasive reality in people's lives.

7. We should apply reason, science, and democratic procedures in all areas of life.

8. We must continually examine our basic convictions—including those of humanism.

See Lamont (1967) for elaboration of these propositions.

The Meaning of Humanism for Psychiatric Nursing

Humanism as a philosophy of psychiatric nursing practice means devotion to the interests of human beings wherever they live and whatever their status. It reaffirms the spirit of compassion and caring toward others. It is a constructive philosophy that wholeheartedly affirms the joys, beauties, and values of human living. The subsequent chapters in this text attempt to operationalize (give specific workable meanings of) these basic premises for psychiatric nursing practice. Among such operationalizations are some fundamental conceptual refinements that are described briefly below.

Holistic View of Mind–Body Relations   There are two basic schools of thought about the relationship of the mind and the body. These two philosophical positions are called *monistic* and *dualistic*. The monistic view asserts that mind and body are one. The dualistic view asserts that mind and body are separate phenomena and may be (1) causally interrelated, (2) parallel but independent, or (3) unrelated. Our humanistic interactionist view is neither monistic nor dualistic. We maintain that physical and mental factors are interrelated and that a change in one may result in a change in another. For example, anger may result in increased blood pressure; an invading organism or toxin or structural change in the body can alter thought processes; and low self-esteem can result in hunched shoulders and severe skeletal muscle contractures. The implications for psychiatric nursing are clear. Healing and caring must be approached holistically. The psychiatric nurse deals with the somatic aspects of a primarily psychological or emotional pattern and the psychological or emotional aspects of physiological experiences. Psychiatric nursing care transcends the bounds of expressly designed "mental hospitals" to include general health care settings and may be directed toward clients whose immediate problems are primarily physical.

Expanded Role for Nurses   The humanistic interactionist perspective on "mental illness," in contrast to the medical model, implies an expanded role for psychiatric nurse practitioners because it enlarges the boundaries of intervention to include political and social dimensions as well as individual client-centered work. When a person's behavior is viewed in terms of psychiatric symptoms, the emphasis is on intrapersonal variables, but we view behavior within an interpersonal field. In our opinion, no one can "have" schizophrenia all alone. We believe that psychiatric nurses should be prepared to work for change within social and political systems. Psychiatric nursing can no longer be limited to client-oriented activities designed exclusively to reduce discomfort and increase the capacity of individuals to adjust satisfactorily to the existing social condition. Instead psychiatric nursing must be involved in social goals that advance health holistically. Because psychiatric nursing has political consequences, it is essential that nurses begin to develop a philosophical and ethical framework to guide and evaluate the political outcome of therapeutic intervention.

Decision-making   A humanistic interactionist perspective suggests a different decision-making format from that of the medical model. The medical model implies that the physician is the chief decision maker. We, on the other hand, do not propose that any particular discipline should provide leadership in psychiatric decision-making. We prefer pragmatic collaboration among interdisciplinary participants to generate effective strategies.

Negotiation and Advocacy   In the humanistic interactionist perspective, the model for intervention and change is one of negotiation and advocacy. The responsibility for change remains with the person who has sought psychiatric help or consultation. Clients are held accountable for their own behavior. They are not passively treated by psychiatric professionals but are supported in the process of developing new perspectives and encouraged to weigh alternatives and make self-directed choices. Psychiatric services in this view are more consultative and advocative than directive. Implied here is a fundamental switch from the approach that upholds the values and life-style of the nurse-therapist as the image of health to an approach that helps clients find a life-style congruent with their own cultures. When translated into practice, this approach is not entirely without conflicts and difficulties.

Critics are quick to point out that California's Charles Manson, convicted of multiple murders, was acting in a manner consistent with his culture. (See Chapter 5 for discussion of ethical issues.)

THE HISTORY OF IDEAS IN PSYCHIATRY

People who have been called "mentally ill" have been with us throughout history—to be feared, marveled at, ignored, banished, sheltered, laughed at, pitied, or tortured. A historical perspective on the place of the "mentally ill," however they have been defined in societies during different periods, brings up several central points:

• Dominant social attitudes and philosophical viewpoints have influenced the understanding and approach to "madness" throughout recorded history and probably before.
• Ideas that may be considered contemporary at one time often have roots centuries earlier.
• The modern medical concept of "madness" as an illness is open to the same scrutiny as other interpretations of the past, such as beliefs about witchcraft, mysticism, or the causality of substances.

We intend to discuss here the specific faces by which madness has been recognized throughout history. Clearly, the meaning assigned to madness has determined whether such persons are perceived as deranged tragic heroes, to be valued and liberated, or as criminals, to be confined and modified. Through a comparative social history we hope to offer perspectives on the odd courses human beings have run in the past and the philosophical, conceptual, and pragmatic positions we are advancing in this volume. In the words of Harley Shands (1971, p. 25):

> When we try to understand human beings, which is to say when we try to understand ourselves, we find it impossible to avoid a series of infinite regressions in circularity. . . . Knowing involves an incessant spiral movement bringing one back again and again to the region of previous knowledge.

Preliterate Times—Era of Magico-Religious Explanations

In preliterate cultures, mental and physical suffering were not distinguished from each other, and both were attributed to forces acting outside the body. Consequently, medicine, magic, and religion were not distinct disciplines. All were variously directed against some mortal or superhuman force that had malevolently inflicted suffering on another. Primitive healers quite logically dealt with the spirits of torment by appeal, reverence, supplication, bribery, intimidation, appeasement, confession, and punishment. These were expressed through exorcism, magical ritual, and incantation. It is possible to perceive some of the rudiments of current psychotherapy in these practices.

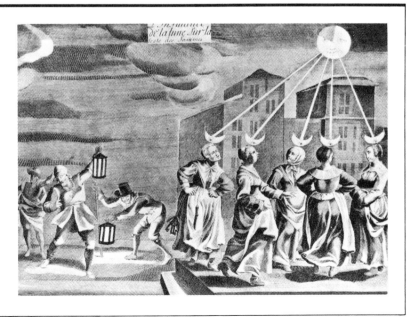

A French engraving of moonstruck women dancing in a seventeenth century town square. This is the source for the word *lunatic*.

Most preliterate cultures believed in:

- The liberation of immaterial (spiritual) forces by divine power or magical arts
- The principle of solidarity or contagion, which implies that human beings are continuous with, not separate from, their surroundings
- Sympathetic, imitative forms of magic occurring by telepathy and other interactions between similar elements
- The symbolism of certain elements such as the purifying role of water

From these beliefs about the nature of suffering there emerged procedures based on the idea of mimetic, or imitative, magic. A medicine man would enact a patient's illness and then slowly recover. This was believed to prompt the patient's own recovery. Based on the principle of continuity—the belief in continued action between things that were once close but now are separated—fingernail parings and afterbirths were seen as devices for influencing the lives of people from whom these things had been removed. An effigy is another example of the continuity notion. Some approaches were based on substitution methods—that is, transferring suffering to a scapegoat. Behavior considered to be "mental illness" by modern Western cultures was attributed in preliterate cultures to the violation of taboos, the neglect of ritual obligations, the loss of a vital substance from the body (such as the soul), the introduction of a foreign and harmful substance into the body (such as evil spirits), or witchcraft. Some of these beliefs remain part of contemporary psychiatry's definition of "mental illness."

Early Civilization— Era of Organic Explanations

There are essentially three sources of the concept of madness in Greek and Roman cultures:

1. Popular opinion continued earlier beliefs in the supernatural causation of mental suffering. This had no prescribed treatment.
2. A medical concept arose, centered on the interaction of four body "humors." It was elaborated in the writings of Hippocrates (fourth century B.C.).
3. The notion developed that violation of moral principles and subsequent punishment by the gods was part of man's destiny. This is evident in the literary and philosophical works of the period.

What might be called the professional opinion on madness was summarized by Hippocrates, who lived from about 460 to 370 B.C. He proposed that psychiatric illnesses were caused mainly by disturbances of body humors—blood, black bile, yellow bile, and phlegm. These four humors resulted from the combination of the four basic qualities in nature—heat, cold, moisture, and dryness. People were classified according to four corresponding temperaments—*sanguine, choleric, melancholic,* and *phlegmatic,* which were supposedly indicative of their prevailing emotional orientation. Personality functioning reached an optimal level when *crasis*—that is, appropriate interaction of internal and external forces—had been achieved. Conflict between the forces indicated an excess of body humor, which then had to be removed by purging. One important consequence of these beliefs was to put psychiatric suffering within the realm of the physician's medical practice.

Three ancient methods of psychotherapeutic intervention stand out because of their widespread use for many centuries in the cultures of the Near East and Mediterranean areas: the interpretation of dreams, ritual purifications, and catharsis. Both words and medicines were used in these methods.

The Medieval Period—Era of Alienation

At the height of their civilization the citizens of ancient Greece found their inner security in knowledge and reason. The Romans adopted the intellectual heritage of Greece but for their peace of mind relied more on their social institutions and the rational organization of society supported by law and military might. When these institutions disintegrated and the empire declined, fear tore apart the fabric of society. The collapse of the Roman security produced a general return to the magic, mysticism, and demonology from which people had retreated during Greek rationality. In the Middle Ages, until the Renaissance, madness was seen as a dramatic encounter with secret powers. Troubled minds were thought to be influenced by the moon (*lunacy* literally means a disorder caused by the lunar body).

Mad people, left wandering on their own, were seen as testimony of the greatness of God and the frailty of humans—a necessary, although sometimes annoying, part of the community. Many participated in religious wars, crusades, and long pilgrimages. Others embraced emotionally charged heretic movements, such as the dance epidemics of the fourteenth century.

By and large, through the thirteenth and fourteenth centuries, the human body and its organic afflictions were dealt with by lay physicians. The problems of the mind, however, remained in the domain of clerical scholars. Two Dominican monks, Johann Sprenger and Heinrich Kraemer, codified the dominant ideology of the times in their book *Malleus Maleficarum (The Witches' Hammer,* 1487), a textbook of both pornography and supposed psychopathology. Witch-hunts became accepted as a system to maintain the status quo. The *Malleus* details the destruction of dissenters, schismatics, and the "mentally ill," most of whom were women and all of whom were labeled *witches*. The favorite way to destroy the devil was to burn his host, the witch. Any unknown disease or illness was thought to be caused by witchcraft. "All witchcraft comes from carnal lust, which is in women insatiable," warned these clerics. Theological rationalizations and magical explanations then served as foundations for burning at the stake thousands of unfortunates. The hangman's noose and the executioner's torch were always in readiness.

End of the Middle Ages—
Era of Ritualized Social Exclusion

A new device appeared in the imaginary landscape at the end of the Middle Ages and the beginning of the Renaissance. It was a "strange drunken boat whose crew of imaginary heroes, ethical models or social types had embarked on a symbolic voyage" (Foucault 1973). The Ships of Fools of the early Renaissance were boatloads of mad people sent out to sea symbolically searching for their reason. In this phase of ritualized social exclusion, social abandonment was viewed as spiritual reintegration. In the image of the Ship of Fools, madness was seen to proceed from a point within reason to a point beyond.

The Classical Age—Era of Confinement

In the era of confinement, the Ship of Fools symbolically docks. It is no longer a ship but a hospital. Tamed, retained (on land), and maintained, madness was reduced to silence through an implicit system of reciprocal obligation between the afflicted and society. Mad persons had the right to be fed but were morally constrained and physically confined. Seventeenth-century society created enormous houses of confinement. In these asylums were gathered the mad, the poor, and various other deviants. A landmark date is 1656, when by decree the Hospital General in Paris

was founded. It was not a medical establishment, but rather a strange implement of power, complete with stakes, irons, prisons, and dungeons that the king established to enforce the law. The "insane" belonged to a world of quasi-absolute sovereignty and jurisdiction without appeal. The Hospital General and others like it had little to do with any medical concept. They were institutions for the maintenance of social order. Michel Foucault (1973, p. 71) describes the conditions in these terms:

> The unfortunate whose entire furniture consisted of a straw pallet, lying with his head, feet and body pressed against the wall, could not enjoy sleep without being soaked by the water that trickled from that mass of stone. . . . In winter the waters of the Seine rose . . . and cells became a refuge for a swarm of huge rats. Madwomen have been found with feet, hands, and faces torn by bites.

Madness thus was given the mask of the beast. Those chained to cell walls were no longer considered people who had lost their reason, but rather beasts seized by a natural frenzy. The animality in madness was seen as evidence that the mad person was not a sick person. Madness was less than ever linked to medicine in this period. It could be mastered only by discipline and brutality.

The Seventeenth Century—
Era of Reason and Observation

During the 1500s, 1600s, and 1700s, some physicians again began to consider psychiatric bases for illness. Johann Weyer (1515–1588), a German physician, believed that "those illnesses whose origins are attributed to witches come from natural causes." He proceeded to explain a variety of so-called supernatural signs on the basis of natural factors. He was a carefully observant clinician and described a wide range of diagnostic categories with associated symptoms, including hysteria, paranoid reactions, toxic organic brain syndrome, epilepsy, folie à deux, depression, and delusions. His position on psychotherapy, however, is considered his most outstanding contribution. He insisted that the needs of individuals rather than the rules of social institutions must be given primary consideration. He recognized the importance of the therapeutic relationship and stressed not only kindness but also a benevolent attitude based on careful observation and scientific principles. His approach was radical and completely alien to the thinking of his time. As a result, his work evoked hostility at first and then was simply ignored.

In retrospect, his contributions are of such importance that he is called "the first psychiatrist."

Late Eighteenth and Early Nineteenth Centuries—Era of Moral Treatment

The continuous development of scientific ideas cannot be neatly divided into centuries. It has simply become a matter of convenience to label the eighteenth century the *epoch of enlightenment.* Enlightenment there was, but the era was full of internal contradictions. Although the insane were unchained, a new threat was invented—the guillotine.

The outstanding characteristic of eighteenth-century psychiatry was that the belief in reason replaced beliefs in faith and tradition. New medical and scientific data had become so overwhelming that synthesis and systematization became necessary. The epoch of enlightenment encompassed a movement from classifying to unchaining the insane.

Eighteenth-century psychiatry typically emphasized the classification of symptoms of mental illness. Even the most sensitive physicians failed to try to understand the sources of mental suffering. Methods of psychiatric treatment were scarcely affected by these classifiers, and, without any means of explanation and understanding, classification became overextended. There was a tendency to dismiss factual data that did not fit, and the system became replete with errors. Among the classifiers was Hermann Boerhaave (1668–1738), a Dutch physician, for whom the practice of psychotherapy consisted of bloodletting, purgatives, dousing patients in ice-cold water, or using other methods to put them in near shock. Boerhaave gave the medical profession one of its first shock instruments, a spinning chair that rendered the patient unconscious. Another was William Cullen (1710–1790), who lectured at Edinburgh and was the first to use the term *neurosis* to denote diseases that are not accompanied by fever or localized pathology. Cullen believed that neurosis was due to decay, either of the intellect or of the involuntary nervous system. By his time psychiatry had discarded the concept that a demon originating outside the patient caused internal disharmony. Physicians now insisted that the evil was disordered physiology.

At the same time, doctors began subscribing to another movement characteristic of the Enlightenment— a zeal for social reform and moral uplift. Rationalism, observation through experimentation, and classification were joined by a fourth approach—reform. In 1793, Philippe Pinel (1745–1826) became superintendent of the French institution Bicêtre for male patients and later of the Salpêtrière for women, where criminals, mentally retarded patients, and the insane were housed. One of his first accomplishments was to release the patients from their chains, open their windows, feed them nourishing food, and treat them with kindness. For this act, he himself was considered mad by his contemporaries.

In 1796, William Tuke (1732–1822), a Quaker tea merchant, founded the York Retreat in England, which sought to reconstruct around madness a milieu resembling the community of Quakers. Tuke's work—liberation of the insane, suppression of constraint, establishment of a humane milieu—substituted the anguish of responsibility for the freedom of madness. With the emergence of moral treatment, the asylum no longer punished the mad person's guilt. It did more, it organized that guilt. By becoming aware of their guilt the mad became aware of themselves as responsible subjects and, consequently, were able to return to reason. At the Retreat the suppression of physical constraint fostered "self-restraint" by patients engaged in work and under the observation of others.

The early treatment of the "mentally ill" at the Pennsylvania Hospital in the United States is closely connected with the work of Benjamin Rush (1746–1813), called "the father of American psychiatry," whose picture is reproduced on the seal of the American Psychiatric Association. Despite his association with humanitarianism and moral treatment, Rush was a major follower of Cullen's ideas in advocating the gyrating chair, bloodletting, and other tricks and inhumane devices.

Later Nineteenth and Early Twentieth Centuries

The Era of Mental Hospitals   Strongly influenced by optimistic and humanitarian beliefs about human nature, some community leaders took the initiative in establishing a few mental hospitals early in the nineteenth century. The most distinguished leader in arousing public interest in building state mental hospitals in the United States was Dorothea L. Dix (1802–1887). Although she was not formally educated as a nurse, she devoted her life to public education concerning the needs of the mentally ill and administered volunteer women nurses during the Civil War. From 1825 to 1865, the number of mental hospitals grew from nine to sixty-two. The first state institution that relied on moral treatment was Worcester State Hospital in Massachusetts.

Toward the end of the nineteenth century, approaches to the "mentally ill" began to change again. Insanity was linked to faulty life habits, and separate hospital facilities were advocated for acute patients. New forms of physical therapy—diet, massage, hydrotherapy, and electroshock therapy—were introduced. Family care and the cottage system were initiated, as were training courses for psychiatric nurses and attendants. As the twentieth century began, a few psychiatrists became interested in research, which led to the founding of the Pathological Institute of New York Hospital in 1895. Adolf Meyer (1866–1950), a Swiss psychiatrist, served on the staff of the institute from 1902 until 1913, when he became director of the newly built clinic at Johns Hopkins University. Meyer dedicated himself to improving the situation for mental patients through any approach that seemed sensible and practical. He was opposed to the dualist philosophy of the separation of mind and body. He regarded each person as a biological unit who experiences unique reactions to social and biological influences. As his realistic, commonsense approach evolved, he became increasingly unwilling to believe that mental illness was the result solely of disorders of the brain or solely of an overwhelming environment. Both had to be taken into account. He introduced the term *ergasia*, meaning integrated mental activity, and even suggested that psychiatry be called *ergasiatry*.

In 1908 another key event occurred in the development of psychiatry. Clifford Beers (1876–1943), a distinguished businessman, published *A Mind that Found Itself*, a book in which he described his intense suffering and mental anguish while receiving custodial care. This book profoundly affected the social consciousness of the nation and led to the organization of spirited groups that Meyer named the *mental hygiene movement*. Public awareness of the needs of the mentally ill was responsible for the development of preventive psychiatry and the formation of child guidance clinics.

Era of Psychoanalysis   The eighteenth-century emphasis on clinical classification peaked in the work of Emil Kraepelin (1856–1926). This physician, like many of his time, was inclined toward an organic, neurophysiological explanation of mental illness. He is best known for bringing the chaotic accumulation of clinical observations into a system of distinct disease entities. His monumental contribution has earned him the title of "the last representative of predynamic psy-

chiatry." He differentiated *manic-depressive psychosis* from *schizophrenia* (which he called *dementia praecox*) and posited that the latter was incurable. Since then, schizophrenia and its treatment have had a fatalistic connotation, although schizophrenia can be—and has been—"cured." A Swiss psychiatrist, Eugene Bleuler (1857–1939), renamed dementia praecox *schizophrenia* and differentiated the disorder into *hebephrenic, catatonic,* and *paranoid* types. Bleuler also expressed a far more optimistic view of the patient's treatment outcome than that held by Kraepelin.

The psychiatric developments of the late nineteenth century formed the background for the work of one of the most influential figures in the history of psychiatry—Sigmund Freud (1856–1939). He succeeded in explaining human behavior in psychological terms and demonstrated that behavior can be changed under carefully constructed circumstances. Freud's contributions to psychiatry per se included his views on the value of catharsis (also recognized in ancient Greek culture), his notion that symptoms represented a compromise between opposing forces (life and death), his interpretations of dreams (also part of ancient traditions), his dynamic explanations of hysteria, and his studies in hypnotism and the character of psychoanalytic technique. For more than 30 years Freud refrained from constructing a comprehensive theory of personality and instead made detailed observations. Finally, in 1929, he published the first in a series of writings compiled in his *New Introductory Lectures on Psychoanalysis*. In these he explained the logic of psychological cause and effect. The specific premises of Freudian psychoanalytic theory are discussed in detail in Chapter 2.

The psychoanalytic concepts of personality and behavior strongly influenced treatment approaches. The aim of therapy became to extend the patient's realm of consciousness to formerly unconscious parts of the personality.

Freud's ideas also profoundly changed people's concepts of themselves. Initially, his concepts provoked a violent and almost universal rejection. But gradually Freud attracted a handful of followers, from Vienna and later from Switzerland, Hungary, and England. This group organized a small professional community devoted to the development of a new discipline—*psychoanalysis.*

- Alfred Adler (1870–1937) is known for his pioneering efforts in psychosomatic medicine, based on a concept of organ inferiority. He held to the notion that the aggressive drive is the strongest influence on personality.

- Carl Jung (1875–1961) developed various original concepts, including the notion of a collective unconscious from which universal archetypes emerge regardless of culture and historical periods. He saw the structure of the human psyche as a composite of persona (social mask), shadow (hidden personal characteristics), anima (feminine identification in man), animus (masculine identification in women), and self (the innermost center of the personality).

- Otto Rank (1884–1939) espoused the view that creativity was a constructive outlet for neurotic conflicts. He was interested in the application of psychoanalysis to literature and art. He later separated from the psychoanalytic movement and minimized the importance of the Oedipus conflict, positing instead that the separation anxiety connected with birth is the most important influence on development and the source of neurosis.

- Ernest Jones (1879–1958) is considered the most faithful pupil of Freud and is best remembered for his biography of Freud (Jones 1953–1957).

- Sandor Ferenczi (1873–1933) was among the first to link homosexuality to paranoia. He also anticipated a later emphasis on ego psychology by advocating active therapy in which patients were encouraged to act and behave to mobilize unconscious material.

- Helene Deutsch, born in 1884, is mainly associated with her two-volume Psychology of Women, in which she described women as essentially passive and masochistic, as making a transition at puberty from a clitoral to a vaginal orientation, and as possessing an inherent maternal role.

- Karen Horney (1885–1952) asserted that cultural factors played a greater part in the development of neurosis than earlier theorists believed. She also anticipated current notions of alienation.

- Anna Freud, the daughter of Sigmund Freud, was born in 1895. She devoted herself to the psychoanalytic study of children and is best known for her refinement of ideas about ego defense mechanisms.

The Twentieth Century— Contemporary Developments

Dealing with contemporary patterns is difficult, since we do not yet have the historian's hindsight to guide our judgments. We offer no final assessment here but merely reiterate the possibility that today's ideas, prac-

tices, and contributions will be subject to reappraisal in the future.

From the mid-1940s to mid-1950s, psychiatric thought in this country was characterized by a strong dichotomy between biological orientation and dynamic orientation. The great number of psychiatric casualties during World War II illuminated the problems of mental and emotional disorders in general. In 1946 the National Institute of Mental Health was opened in Bethesda, Maryland, for the purposes of research, training, and assistance to the states in providing preventive, therapeutic, and rehabilitative psychiatric services.

Dissatisfaction with the theories and methods of psychoanalysis and psychoanalytic ideology has persisted; psychotherapy has become progressively influenced by trends toward both ego psychology and social psychology. Harry Stack Sullivan (1892–1949), the only American-born psychiatrist to found an independent school during this period, was strongly influenced by social scientists such as Ruth Benedict and Margaret Mead. Central to his thinking is an interpersonal theory of psychiatry that is at variance with the strictly individual emphasis of psychoanalysis. His pioneering psychotherapy was aimed at understanding and correcting the patient's disturbed communication process in the context of a patient–therapist relationship based on reciprocal learning.

The American trend emphasizing the social dimension of psychiatry is also seen in the emergence of both group and family psychotherapy. John Bell and Nathan Ackerman were leading proponents of treating a whole family in one place at the same time. Don Jackson, Gregory Bateson, and their colleagues extended this approach to schizophrenic patients and their families. Family therapy by 1960 had become both a diagnostic tool and a mode of treatment. During this period Erik Erikson formulated his psychosocial theory of development, based on the interplay of biological and social factors and encompassing a progressive unfolding of developmental tasks in an entire life span.

During this period of ideological expansion, the issue of mental illness received national attention. With the strong support of the National Institute of Mental Health and many private and professional associations, the Mental Health Study Act was passed in 1955. It established the Joint Commission on Mental Illness and Health to set priorities and define adequate services for the mentally ill throughout the country. After five years of investigation, the commission concluded that psychiatric resources and the network of mental hospitals in this country were totally inadequate. The final report of this commission, *Action for Mental Health* (1961), was essentially a proposal for a concerted attack on mental illness through a better distribution and community orientation of psychiatric services. The commission proposed a massive program of preventive services, a shift of emphasis from institutional to community-based care, and plans for shared federal, state, and local funding of community mental health centers. (See Chapter 28.)

Between 1955 and 1975 the number of resident patients in state mental hospitals decreased from 559,000 to 193,000—almost 66 percent. Proponents of the community mental health and deinstitutionalization movements refer to "a bold new approach," "native caregivers," "crisis-oriented services," "social reform," "civil liberties," "social support," and "social network." Critics use less enthusiastic terms, such as "dumping," "chronicity," "revolving door utilization," and "transinstitutionalization" to characterize modern trends in mental health services (Talbott 1979). In the latter view, the chronically mentally disordered have merely had their locus of care transformed from a single lousy institution to multiple wretched ones.

Some experts conclude that deinstitutionalization and the principles of community psychiatry are a national disgrace and advocate the return of the old state hospital warehouse system. Others, however, prefer to rethink this approach, pointing out that criticism of the deinstitutionalization movement has merely highlighted community psychiatry's lack of true innovation. This group argues not for the desirability of the old state hospital system, but for the development of alternatives to it that emphasize self-care and self-determination for patients, rather than institutionalization (Wilson 1982). In Bachrach's analysis (1978), deinstitutionalization must be viewed in three dimensions:

1. As a fact (the closing of huge single-purpose mental institutions)

2. As a process (processes of care that shift control back to psychiatric clients)

3. As an effect (increased ability for self-determination and self-care among heretofore mentally disabled and disordered people)

One of our needs in the 1980s is for sustained life-support systems for certain chronic client groups, not merely transitional ones. Soteria House in northern California is but one of an expanding network of alternative living situations that balance a client's right to freedom with the community's right to protection. Approaches like Soteria House, however, require sufficient legislation, funding continuity, and coordination to replace the current nonsystem of aftercare left in the wake of closing state mental hospitals.

EMERGENCE OF THE DISCIPLINE OF PSYCHIATRIC NURSING

Although nursing functions have existed since ancient times, the profession of nursing, particularly psychiatric nursing, is a product of the late nineteenth and twentieth centuries. Theodor and Friedericke Fliedner founded the first systematic school of nursing in Germany in 1836. It was this school at Kaiserwerth that Florence Nightingale visited in 1851 before organizing a school to educate nurses in England after the Crimean War. Her school, St. Thomas Hospital in London, stressed cleanliness, good hygiene, and the systematic care of patients. She also emphasized careful observation, a dignified professional status for nurses, and the direction of nursing departments in hospitals by experienced nurses rather than physicians. She was among the first to note that the influence of nurses on their patients went beyond the physical care they provided.

In the early 1870s the first three American nursing schools, organized in the pattern of St. Thomas Hospital, were opened in New York, Boston, and New Haven. Linda Richards, a graduate of the New England Hospital for Women in Boston, spent a significant part of her career developing better nursing care in psychiatric hospitals and is sometimes called "the first American psychiatric nurse." She echoed Nightingale's earlier observation about the nurse's impact on patients. She noted that many a poor woman could date her changed life from a short stay in some hospital ward where trained nurses ministered to her physical needs and with kind and helpful words strengthened her moral character.

In 1880 the first American school for psychiatric nurses was opened at the McLean Hospital in Waverly, Massachusetts, and by 1882, 90 nurses had graduated from its two-year course. By the end of the nineteenth century, trained nurses staffed some mental hospitals in the United States, but they attended mainly to the physical needs of patients and did not pursue systematic interpersonal work with them. Psychiatric theory in this period emphasized providing a physically sound environment that would encourage the recovery of patients. Thus, nurses administered medications such as chloral hydrate and paraldehyde, supervised the use of hydrotherapy, and oversaw the nutritional and physical care of patients. Much of psychiatric nursing practice was custodial, mechanistic, and directed by psychiatrists. A ratio of 1 trained nurse to 140 patients was not unusual, and some large mental hospitals hired no registered nurses at all.

Between 1900 and 1930, psychiatric theory expanded to encompass the interpersonal and emotional dimensions of "mental illness." During these years Sigmund Freud published his works, and Adolf Meyer had his major impact on American and British psychiatry. However, these ideas began to change the nature of psychiatric hospitals and psychiatric nursing only after 1930.

In the late 1920s Harry Stack Sullivan, often called "the founder of interpersonal psychiatry," organized a ward at Sheppard and Enoch Pratt Hospital in Towson, Maryland, where intensive staff–patient relationships were used in the treatment of schizophrenic patients. Sullivan instituted daily conferences in which ward staff members discussed the interpersonal relationships between patients and staff and analyzed their therapeutic and nontherapeutic aspects. Sullivan's concept of *milieu therapy* was a new approach to treating hospitalized patients. During the following decades, it had a discernible impact on psychiatric nursing care. Two of the foremost American hospitals that adopted the milieu therapy model were the Chestnut Lodge in Rockville, Maryland, and the Menninger Clinic in Topeka, Kansas.

Milieu therapy was one of the forces that brought psychiatric nurses into new roles. Their major responsibility shifted from the physical care of patients to the creation of an interpersonal environment that would contribute to the patient's recovery. If patients became emotionally disturbed in the context of unhealthy interpersonal relationships, then healthy relationships logically became important in their care.

Ideological changes clearly contributed to a turn toward more contemporary psychiatric nursing practice but new modes of physical treatment also laid the groundwork for change. Treatments, such as insulin coma, electroshock, and phenothiazine antipsychotic and antidepressant medications provided controls on dramatically bizarre patient behavior and made patients more available for interpersonal interactions.

With the establishment of the National Institute of Mental Health in 1946, psychiatric nursing was added to psychiatry, psychology, and social work as a field in which the highest priority became the preparation of clinically capable persons for positions of leadership. Funds administered by NIMH facilitated advanced education in psychiatric nursing. Before the 1946 act, fewer than a dozen psychiatric nurses held master's degrees in the United States and fewer than 5% of basic nursing education programs were at the baccalaureate level. The psychiatric nursing education given most students consisted of a few weeks of observation on a psychiatric ward. As a result of NIMH funds, nine universities received grants to expand and improve graduate programs in 1948. The number increased gradually and steadily. Beginning in 1956, grants were made available to integrate mental health concepts into the basic nursing curriculum. Traineeships for graduate students increased from 59 in 1948 to 1,012 in 1975. Other grants totaling $185 million were awarded over a 30-year period. Enactment of the Community Mental Health Centers Act in 1963 further motivated a shift in emphasis in graduate psychiatric nursing to include the clinical competence required for community care of patients and for preventive psychiatric programs.

Certain future psychiatric nursing trends seem likely. Increased numbers of psychiatric nurses will pursue advanced degrees for the purpose of systematically defining the scientific nature of the discipline. Undergraduate psychiatric nursing students will continue to expand psychiatric concepts in a more holistic framework, based less on the medical model. In addition, psychiatric nurses will become increasingly political and inclined to widen their scope of practice to include the social problems and issues facing clients. Finally, psychiatric nurses will be required to identify for themselves, their clients, and their colleagues what unique contribution they are able to make on the interdisciplinary mental health team.

References

Bachrach, L. L. "A Conceptual Approach to Deinstitutionalization," *Hospital and Community Psychiatry* 29 (1978): 573–578.

Beers, C. W. *A Mind that Found Itself.* Rev. ed. Garden City, N.Y.: Doubleday, 1948.

Blumer, H. *Symbolic Interaction: Perspective and Method.* Englewood Cliffs, N.J.: Prentice-Hall, 1969.

Deutsch, H. *The Psychology of Women.* 2 vols. New York: Grune and Stratton, 1944–1945.

Fagin, C. "Psychotherapeutic Nursing." *American Journal of Nursing* 67 (1967): 298–304.

Foucault, M. *Madness and Civilization.* New York: Vintage Books, 1973.

Freud, S. *New Introductory Lectures on Psychoanalysis.* Standard ed. Edited and translated by James Strachey. New York: W. W. Norton, 1965.

KEY NURSING CONCEPTS

✔ The humanistic interactionist ideology is one response to a need for a framework of values and concepts in psychiatric nursing that views human beings as having purpose and control over their own lives.

✔ The key premises of symbolic interactionism are that people act toward things on the basis of the meanings those things have for them—that the meanings arise out of social interaction with others and are modified through the process of encountering things.

✔ Implications of symbolic interactionism and humanism for the practice of psychiatric nursing include the importance of finding a common ground of negotiated meaning when dealing with clients, of viewing behavior within its social context, of discovering and respecting each client's individual experience and the meaning attached to it, and of viewing physical and mental factors as interrelated.

✔ The key premises of humanism give rise to a holistic view of mind-body relations, an expanded role for nurses, a collaborative decision-making model, and a general posture of negotiation and advocacy in relation to clients in social, political, and individual arenas.

✔ The meaning of mental illness has differed drastically through history, yet repetition of themes is evident particularly in the issues of biological versus nonbiological causes and the mental patient's responsibility or irresponsibility for actions.

✔ The profession of psychiatric nursing is a product of the late nineteenth and twentieth centuries and was brought about by ideological changes, interest in reform, attention to the importance of milieu, and the introduction of physical modes of treatment.

Joint Commission on Mental Illness and Health. *Action for Mental Health.* New York: Basic Books, 1961.

Jones, E. *The Life and Work of Sigmund Freud.* 3 vols. New York: Basic Books, 1953–1957.

Lamont, C. *The Philosophy of Humanism.* New York: Frederick Ungar Publishing, 1967.

Shands, H. C. *The War with Words.* The Hague: Mouton, 1971.

Talbott, J. "Deinstitutionalization: Avoiding the Disasters of the Past." *Hospital and Community Psychiatry* 30 (1979): 621–624.

Wilson, H. S. *Deinstitutionalized Residential Care for the Severely Mentally Disordered: The Soteria House Approach.* New York: Grune and Stratton, 1982.

Further Reading

Alexander, F. G., and Selesnick, S. T. *The History of Psychiatry: An Evaluation of Psychiatric Thought and Practice from Prehistoric Times to the Present.* New York: Harper and Row, 1966.

Angrist, S. "The Mental Hospital: Its History and Destiny." *Perspectives in Psychiatric Care* 11 (1963): 20.

Berger, P. L., and Luckmann, T. *The Social Construction of Reality.* Garden City, N.Y.: Doubleday Anchor Books, 1967.

Greenblatt, M.; York, R. H.; and Brown, E. L. *From Custodial to Therapeutic Patient Care in the Mental Hospital.* New York: Russell Sage Foundation, 1955.

Leininger, M., ed. *Contemporary Issues in Mental Health Nursing.* Boston: Little, Brown, 1973.

Mead, G. H. *The Philosophy of the Present.* Edited by Arthur E. Murphy. LaSalle, Ill.: Open Court, 1932.

Menninger, W. *Psychiatry—Its Evolution and Present Status.* Ithaca, N.Y.: Cornell University Press, 1948.

Misiak, H., and Saxton, V. S. *Phenomenological, Existential and Humanistic Psychologies: A Historical Survey.* New York: Grune and Stratton, 1973.

Rosen, G. *Madness in Society.* New York: Harper and Row, 1968.

Szasz, T. S. *The Age of Madness: The History of Involuntary Mental Hospitalization Presented in Selected Texts.* Garden City, N.Y.: Doubleday, 1973.

Withington, E. T. "Dr. Johann Weyer and the Witch Mania." In *Studies in the History and Method of Science,* edited by C. Singer. Oxford: Clarendon Press, 1917.

2

Conceptual Frameworks for Psychiatric Nursing

CHAPTER OUTLINE

The Medical–Biological Model
  Assumptions and Key Ideas
  Implications for Psychiatric Nursing Practice
  Understanding Medical Nomenclature
  Critique
The Psychoanalytic Model
  Assumptions and Key Ideas
  Implications for Psychiatric Nursing Practice
  Critique
The Behaviorist Model
  Assumptions and Key Ideas
  Implications for Psychiatric Nursing Practice
  Critique
The Social–Interpersonal Model
  Assumptions and Key Ideas
  Implications for Psychiatric Nursing Practice
  Critique
The Choice of a Conceptual Framework
Key Nursing Concepts

LEARNING OBJECTIVES

After reading this chapter, students should be able to
- Identify the assumptions and key ideas of the medical–biological, the psychoanalytic, the behavioral, and the social–interpersonal frameworks
- Discuss the implications each framework has for psychiatric nursing practice
- Assess the strengths and weaknesses of each of the four frameworks
- Relate their personal framework to the four models presented

CHAPTER 2

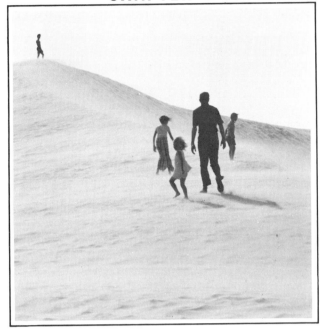

The social-interpersonal framework for psychiatric nursing interrelates clients' social, biological, and psychological interactions, thereby increasing the variables that must be considered to understand them.

The humanistic practice of psychiatric nursing requires that nurses devote themselves to understanding what makes people human, how they express their joy of living, their sadness, their desire to love, their hopes for growth. Understanding these things becomes even more crucial when psychiatric nurses must explain how the joy of living suddenly turns to the desire to die, how love of self and others turns to violence and hate, and how the hope for growth turns to withdrawal and despair.

In Chapter 1 we described one philosophical framework for understanding the human problems and patterns with which psychiatric nurses work. However, what is currently called psychiatric–mental health nursing may undergo far-reaching changes depending on how we define it. The framework presented in Chapter 1 is by no means the dominant conceptual view psychiatric nurses use in caring for clients. In this chapter we offer a comparative analysis of the basic assumptions and implications for practice inherent in four dominant models of psychiatric nursing. These are the *medical–biological* model, the *psychoanalytic* model, the *behaviorist* model, and the *social–interpersonal* model. Either explicitly or implicitly psychiatric nurses choose one or a combination of frameworks from these models in determining what information to seek about clients, what treatment approaches to recommend, and what ultimate goals to set. This chapter approaches the models in critique fashion. By *critique* we mean an

inquiry that reveals the hidden assumptions of a model, that grounds it in history, and that recognizes the subjectivity of the observer. The chapter is written from the humanistic interactionist perspective outlined in Chapter 1, since it is from that perspective that we ourselves view the study and practice of psychiatric nursing.

People base their actions on the meaning they attribute to the behavior and situations they confront. Suppose a twenty-year-old woman hears and uses a private language and relates more to her paintings than to her peers. If nurses view this woman as having an illness called *schizophrenia* with identifiable symptoms such as hallucinations, it is likely that her treatment program will include the use of phenothiazine medications such as Prolixin, Thorazine, or Haldol. The therapeutic emphasis will be on treating and curing a person who has been identified as mentally sick. If, on the other hand, nurses view this woman as "withdrawing into *primary process thinking* to defend against an unconscious conflict rooted in traumatic childhood experiences," the therapeutic approach may emphasize individual psychotherapy designed to bring the conflict to the surface and resolve it. If nurses view this woman's behavior as a learned pattern that has been reinforced by significant others throughout her life, intervention is more likely to follow a learning approach. In this case, the therapist may engage members of the woman's family in planning and learning a new mode of interacting with her, carefully prescribed to extinguish old patterns and to reinforce new, more functional ones. Finally, nurses may not view the young woman as having an illness or an exclusively intrapsychic personal problem at all. Rather, they may view her as one participant in a problematic network of interpersonal relationships that includes her immediate family and extends to her cultural context. In this case the "client" may include the whole constellation of social variables bearing on the young woman's behavior and the meaning assigned to it by significant others. "Therapy" then may include interventions ranging from family counseling to political action.

Consider the different actions that a therapist might recommend to our hypothetical client. She can:

- Take a trip and avoid what is making her anxious
- Take a rest and strengthen her inner defenses
- Yell, scream, cry, and reduce inner pressure
- Have sex if it reassures her
- Avoid having sex if it aggravates her
- Learn sexual techniques that she has avoided out of anxiety, if the sex she is having is unfulfilling and tension-producing
- Breathe deeply or try a massage to loosen up bodily tension
- Work harder and get a reward, if her narcissism is low
- Fail and get punished, if her guilt is high
- Join a religious cult
- Take a drink
- Calm down and try tranquilizers
- Attack the ruling class
- Join the ruling class or work for it
- Be a double agent
- Leave her family
- Make up with her family
- Commit a crime
- Enlighten herself, meditate
- Share her experience with others in a group and try to work out her problem-raising patterns in dealing with others
- Go to an analyst and try to obtain insight into mastery over her unconscious world
- Watch television

If any of these maneuvers tips the balance so that the woman is better able to deal with destructive forces in her life, it may be called *therapeutic*. However, changes cannot be measured by any absolute standard. They can be measured only by the standards of the individual. One person's inner peace is the inertia of a zombie to another. Integrity to one may be rigidity to another.

What, then, are models of therapy? To answer this question, we must begin by noting that a particular strategy is seldom carried out in isolation. A therapeutic model fits therapeutic strategies with an ideology. Each model is based on a certain view of the human

world, a theory of madness and health, a set of practices, qualifications for practitioners, and so forth. Each of the four dominant conceptual models is discussed in detail below. We will present the basic assumptions of each, its implications for psychiatric nursing, and a summary of our critique of it.

THE MEDICAL–BIOLOGICAL MODEL

The medical–biological model in psychiatry originated in the era of classification. The classification of mental disturbances brought the emotional and behavioral aspects of people into the domain of the medical doctor, as we indicated in Chapter 1. This period emphasized the systematic observation, naming, and classification of symptoms. Long-standing and somewhat barbaric treatment approaches were all but overlooked. With the proliferation of diagnostic designations, doctors began to search for the causes of mental illness in an organ or organ system. Emil Kraepelin's monumental descriptive diagnostic classification system is acknowledged as the first comprehensive medical model. It included the notion that the cause of mental illness was organic, that it was located in the central nervous system, that the disease followed a predictable course, and that treatment should be based on accurate diagnosis.

Assumptions and Key Ideas

Proponents of the medical–biological model view emotional and behavioral disturbances in the same way as they view any physical disease. Thus abnormal behavior is directly attributable to a disease process, a lesion, a neural pathological condition, a toxin introduced from outside the human body, or an internally developed toxic biochemical. The medical model position might be summarized as follows:

- The individual suffering from emotional disturbances is sick and has an illness or defect.
- The illness can, at least presumably, be located in some part of the body (usually the central nervous system).
- The illness has characteristic mental symptoms that can be diagnosed, classified, and labeled as an identifiable disease entity.

- Mental diseases run a characteristic course and have a particular prognosis for recovery.
- Mental illnesses are amenable to physical or somatic treatments such as drugs, chemicals, hormones, or surgery.
- The behavioral disorders called mental illnesses are properly within the charge of physicians and should be treated following general medical practice. In other words, take the client's history, give a general physical exam, make a diagnosis, and select a treatment method in keeping with the diagnosis.

Implications for Psychiatric Nursing Practice

Historically, when nurses first became involved in the care of psychiatric clients, they were primarily responsible for the client's physical well-being. Their responsibilities included administering drugs prescribed by the physician and caring for clients undergoing treatments such as insulin shock, electroconvulsive therapy, or hydrotherapy. Although in retrospect the medical model is associated with a comparatively limited view of people and a circumscribed role for nurses, it is still the major mode of naming phenomena, even among nurses in search of more imaginative alternatives. Most psychiatric nursing texts use the nomenclature of disease entities as their organizing structure despite nurses' efforts to apply alternative perspectives, redefine concepts, and realign the boundaries of their practice.

In addition, the medical model provides the conceptual basis for continued use of *somatotherapies* in the care of psychiatric clients, the hospital as the setting for care, research into genetic transmission of mental illness, research on biochemical and metabolic variables among diagnosed psychiatric clients, and dominance of the medical doctor in the psychiatric treatment team.

Understanding Medical Nomenclature

The psychiatric nurse needs to be conversant with current medically oriented nomenclature. Before the publication of the third edition of the Diagnostic and Statistical Manual by the American Psychiatric Association (DSM-III) the rate of agreement about psychiatric diagnoses was amazingly low (five clinicians examining the same client using the medical model approach tended to reach at least three different diagnoses), yet the American Psychiatric Association's nomenclature pre-

dominated. It is still the most frequently used system of classifying behaviorally disturbed people and its validity and reliability statistics have been considerably improved. Therefore even psychiatric nurses who disagree with the disease-oriented approach must be generally familiar with it in order to communicate with peers on the psychiatric team. For this reason the current diagnostic nomenclature is given in Appendix B.

It has been said that neurotics build dream houses, psychotics live in them, and psychiatrists collect the rent. This adage hints at how the diagnostic labeling of clients is done. Minor distortions of reality, such as excessive fantasizing, inability to cope, and worrying, supposedly all lead the diagnostician to consider a broad category of disorders that were called neurotic disorders or *neuroses* before DSM-III. Major alterations in perceptions of reality (such as hallucinations and delusions), massive withdrawal, and major disturbances of affect (feelings), lead to the consideration of psychotic disorders or *psychoses*. The basic difference between neuroses and pychoses presumably depends on how clients perceive the world and how they behave in light of these perceptions. The research of noted social scientists, however, has demonstrated that the distinction may be based on socioeconomic or other factors. In particular, Hollingshead and Redlich (1958) found that neurotic diagnostic labels were applied significantly more often to clients at the higher levels of social class structure and that psychoses were attributed more often to the lower classes.

In his study on diagnostic screening associated with court orders, Thomas Scheff (1966), another sociologist, concluded that mental illness is more a social status than a disease (and an ascribed rather than achieved social status). Problems of definition and diagnosis occur in part because behavior arises in variable social and cultural contexts, and the frames of reference of those making the judgments are not always comparable. Thus, as David Mechanic (1968) points out in his research, the behaviors defined as symptoms of illness may be as much characteristic of some particular situation or group setting as they are enduring attributes of the individual client. Consider the following account of a clinical examination conducted by Emil Kraepelin and described in his own words:

Gentlemen, the cases I have to place before you today are peculiar. First of all, you see a servant-girl, aged twenty-four. In spite of her emaciation the patient is in continual movement. On attempting to stop her movement, we meet with unexpectedly strong resistance; if I place myself in front of her with my arms spread out in order to stop her, she suddenly turns and slips through under my arms so as to continue her way. If one takes firm hold of her, she distorts her face and weeps. She holds a crushed piece of bread in her left hand which she will not allow to be forced from her. If you prick her in the forehead with a needle, she scarcely winces or turns away. To questions she answers almost nothing. . . . [Quoted in Laing 1967, p. 107.]

British psychiatrist R. D. Laing used this illustration to point out that practitioners tend to view such situations primarily from the psychiatrist's point of view. In this context, Kraepelin is sane, and the girl insane; he is rational, she is irrational. This conclusion entails looking at the client's behavior out of the context of the social situation as she experiences it. From the girl's point of view, the psychiatrist's actions are quite extraordinary: he tries to stop her movements by standing in front of her with arms spread out, tries to force a piece of bread out of her hand, sticks a needle in her forehead, and so on.

Psychiatric nurses need to interpret and appraise the contributions of biological sciences to the understanding of human feelings and behavior. Genetics, biochemistry, and biorhythms are prominent areas of current research. Best-known among the studies in psychiatric genetics is Kallmann's (1953) work conducted in Berlin in 1938. His research supports the theory that genetic factors are always at least partially involved in the development (*pathogenesis*) of schizophrenia. Subsequent "twin" studies, which found that schizophrenia is likely to occur in both twins, especially if they were identical, have been cited by proponents of the biological model as evidence of the role of heredity in schizophrenia. Similar family and twin studies were conducted throughout the world in relation to the occurrence of behaviors then labeled *manic-depressive reaction, involutional psychosis, neurosis, male homosexuality, criminal behavior,* and *disorders of aging.*

Biochemistry is another area of active, biologically oriented psychiatric research. In general, the causes and chemical alterations underlying behavioral and emotional disturbances remain an enigma. Certain biochemical changes are demonstrably associated with particular behavior disorders. For example, a defect in the metabolism of *serotonin* is currently being investigated as a possible cause of schizophrenia. Seymour Kety (1959) notes that schizophrenia may result from abnormal transmethylation of catecholamines yielding DMPEA, a compound closely related to mescaline. Wise and Stein (1973) provide evidence that *6-hydrox-

ydopamine* (6HD), an aberrant *dopamine* metabolite, produces schizophrenic symptoms by causing "a prolonged or permanent depletion of brain catecholamine." Evidence of a protein called *taraxein* in the blood of schizophrenics has also been reported. This agent blocks the action of acetylcholine in the limbic system, resulting in the client's inability to experience pleasure or pain. Carlsson and Lindqvist (1973) note that central dopaminergic receptors are blocked by all effective antipsychotic drugs, such as chlorpromazine. In sum, it is hypothesized that biochemical neurotransmission may eventually explain schizophrenia; but as yet most attempts to duplicate these findings have been inconclusive.

Medical–biological research has also found relationships between affective disorders and biochemical changes. Some, if not all, depressions are associated with an absolute or relative deficiency of catecholamines, particularly norepinephrine, at functionally important receptor sites in the brain. Conversely, elation may be associated with an excess of such amines. However, the catecholamines have such complex relationships with other elements of body chemistry that this hypothesis may be an oversimplification.

A relatively new avenue of biological research in psychiatry is the area called *chronopsychophysiology.* Implicit in much of this research is the hypothesis that disturbances in periodic processes (biorhythms) may contribute to psychopathology. These disturbances may not be apparent at the surface level of clinical description and observation. Measurement of such latent periodic processes may therefore be crucial in advancing the psychobiological understanding of psychiatric illness. Rhythms underlie much of the range of homeostasis (the steady state) in people and in the world. A healthy human being's appearance of stability cloaks an inner symphony of biological rhythms ranging from microseconds for biochemical reactions, milliseconds for nerve activity, a second for heart rhythm, the twenty-four-hour rest–activity cycle, and the twenty-seven-day menstrual cycle to the entire life span cycle.

Figure 2–1 provides a schematic spectrum of these rhythms, called *bioperiodicities.* Rhythms that are shorter than 24 hours have been designated *ultradian,* those longer than 24 hours *infradian.* In view of documented *circadian* (daily) fluctuations in human levels of consciousness and liver and kidney function, it is not unreasonable to think that the body also varies cyclically in its ability to tolerate stress or to detoxify and excrete harmful substances. Study of these cycles is

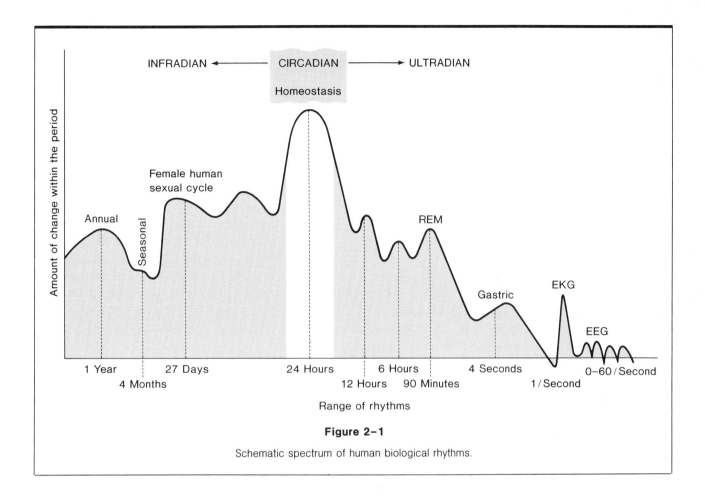

Figure 2–1

Schematic spectrum of human biological rhythms.

the focus of psychophysiological chronotography. If this line of research continues to yield promising findings, it could provide a new precision in preventive psychiatry—perhaps improving on and complementing the traditional retrospective approach of psychoanalysis and the here-and-now emphasis of other techniques.

Catherine Norris's (1975) studies on restlessness represent one example of how human rhythmicity can apply to a client problem. Norris noted that all human life has rhythmicity as a characteristic. While some rhythms are learned and others genetically determined, one of the first indicators of a threat to biological rhythms may be the feeling of restlessness. Her concept of the relationship between rhythmicity and restlessness is portrayed on a continuum between "health" and "illness," as shown in Figure 2–2.

Critique

Perhaps the best known critic of the medical–biological model is psychiatrist Thomas Szasz (1974), who argues that the concept of mental illness or mental disease,

like the explanatory concepts of gods and witches, has outlived its usefulness and now functions merely as a convenient myth. Szasz and others contend that the medical model deals basically with the inner workings of the self, whereas disturbed behavior most often occurs in relationships with others. Since behaviors that are currently referred to as psychiatric symptoms are more likely to be aspects of communication with others, real or illusory, the medical model overlooks half the data. When vocabulary and concepts developed to describe intrapersonal processes are applied to interactional fields the result is strain, ambiguity, and obscurity.

Szasz bases his case against the medical model on several central premises. First, if mental symptoms were manifestations of diseases of the central nervous system, they would correspond more to symptoms that result from diseases of the body, such as blindness or paralysis, rather than problems in living or relating to others.

Second, the medical model's view of mental and physical symptoms is not supported by observations. For example, when practitioners speak of physical

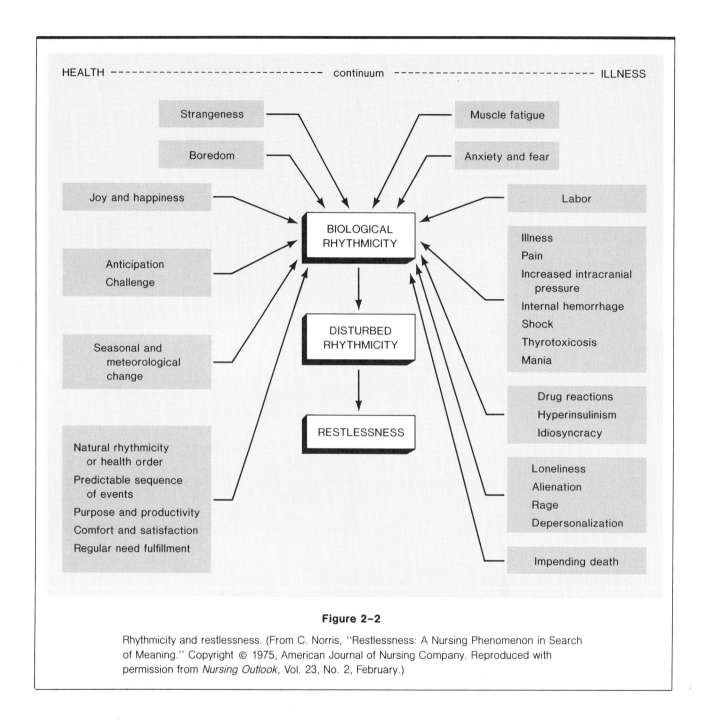

Figure 2-2

Rhythmicity and restlessness. (From C. Norris, "Restlessness: A Nursing Phenomenon in Search of Meaning." Copyright © 1975, American Journal of Nursing Company. Reproduced with permission from *Nursing Outlook*, Vol. 23, No. 2, February.)

symptoms, they mean either signs (such as fever) or symptoms (such as pain). When they speak of mental symptoms, they mean clients' communications about themselves, others, and the world. Practitioners have to judge whether a client's statements correspond with their own and society's ideas, concepts, or beliefs. In short, the notion of a mental symptom is inextricably tied to the social and ethical context in which it occurs. Some studies have shown that knowledge about the orientation and education of the clinician is a bet-

ter predictor of diagnostic outcome than the client's behavior.

A third clear difficulty with the medical model of mental illness concerns the role of illness in excusing conduct. The idea that serious disease is beyond the control and responsibility of the individual has a long-standing history of acceptance. With the emergence of self-healing practices and evidence that life-style choices, such as diet and exercise, affect physical disease, this notion is coming into question. To relieve people of ethical responsibility for their behavior on the ground that they have a disease seems even more questionable. The symptoms of "mental illness" are often behaviors that are associated with the very heart of responsibility—the mind and the character. They are, therefore, quite reasonably beyond excuses.

Szasz's critique of the medical model concludes that mental illness is a name for problems in living according to certain psychosocial, ethical, and legal norms. The idea, for example, that hostility, vengefulness, or divorce is indicative of mental illness is based on the cultural value attached to love, forgiveness, or stable marriage relationships. The irony, then, is that a remedy is sought in terms of medical measures, and even the medical diagnostic labels currently in use provide no indication of the specific treatment that will be tried. A diagnosis of schizophrenia may be followed by any one or a combination of treatments, including drugs, electroconvulsive therapy, psychotherapy, group therapy, milieu therapy, or family therapy. The policies of the clinical setting and the client's age, place within the family structure, socioeconomic status, and (often) sex usually are better predictors of the treatment that will be advised than the diagnosis.

Human behavior is complex. A change in body structure or body chemistry results in a change in function. An organism or a toxin can initiate and ultimately alter thought processes. Similarly, a problem in feelings, such as low self-esteem, can produce structural body changes, such as hunched shoulders or muscle contractions. It is likely that there is no single "cause" of the troubled and troublesome behavior called mental illness and that the medical model's attempt to find one is unnecessarily limiting. It obscures the relevance of interpersonal and cultural factors.

The publication of the American Psychiatric Associations' third edition of the Diagnostic and Statistical Manual of Mental Disorders (DSM-III) in 1980 reflects an effort to respond to these criticisms in several important ways:

- Psychiatric diagnoses according to DSM-III are based on specified, empirical criteria not linked to any particular theory of etiology.
- The diagnostic criteria have been field-tested for reliability and validity, with encouraging results.
- A DSM-III diagnosis is multifaceted in that it assesses the presence or absence of an individual's biological, psychological, and social pathology.

- The diagnosis includes a client's strengths or level of adaptive functioning and contextual stresses.
- The "V" codes allow the clinician to note the presence of a problem in living that does not represent a psychiatric disorder.

(Chapter 8 further discusses this approach to diagnosis.)

THE PSYCHOANALYTIC MODEL

The psychoanalytic model is usually credited to the Viennese physician Sigmund Freud (1962b). Freud's premise was that all psychological and emotional events, however obscure, were understandable. For the meanings behind behavior he looked to childhood experiences that he believed caused adult neuroses. Therapy in this model consists of clarifying the psychological meaning of events, feelings, and behavior and thereby gaining insight about them. Freud's work shifted the focus of psychiatry from classification to a dynamic view of mental phenomena. Psychoanalytic concepts have so widely permeated the education and practice of psychiatric clinicians that they have come to be regarded as a fundamental part of understanding and approaching emotional disorders. Psychoanalysis has emerged as a method of investigation, as a therapeutic technique, and as a body of scientific concepts and propositions.

Assumptions and Key Ideas

Psychic Determinism   A fundamental concept associated with the psychoanalytic model is *psychic determinism*. Psychic determinism posits that no human behavior is accidental. Each psychic event is determined by the ones that preceded it. Events in people's mental lives that seem random or unrelated to what went before are only apparently so. Thus, psychoanalysts never dismiss any mental phenomenon as meaningless or accidental. They always search for what caused it, why it happened. For example, people commonly forget or mislay something. They usually view this as just an accident. Psychoanalysts, on the contrary, seek to demonstrate that the accident was caused by a wish or intent of the person involved. Psychoanalysts also view dreams as subject to the principle of psychic determinism, each dream and each image in each dream bearing some relationship to the rest of the dreamer's life.

Role of the Unconscious A second fundamental concept in the psychoanalytic model is that significant unconscious mental processes occur frequently in normal as well as abnormal mental functioning. These processes are called simply the *unconscious*. The unconscious is so intimately related to the premise of psychic determinism, that it is hard to discuss one without the other. According to psychoanalysts, the fact that much of what goes on in people's minds is unknown to them accounts for the apparent discontinuities in their mental lives. If the unconscious cause or causes of some behavioral symptoms are discovered, then the apparent discontinuities disappear, and the causal sequence becomes clear.

Psychoanalysis The most powerful and reliable method for studying the unconscious is the technique that Freud evolved over several years, called *psychoanalysis*. The basic logic behind psychoanalysis is:

- The client has undergone a *traumatic experience*, that stirred up intense emotion that was painful or disagreeable.
- The traumatic experience represented to the client some ideas that were incompatible with the dominant ideas constituting his or her ego. Thus a *neurotic conflict* was experienced.
- The incompatible idea and the neurotic conflict associated with it force the ego to bring into action *defense mechanisms* that manifest themselves in the client as neurotic symptoms.
- Therapy is directed toward resolving the conflict by uncovering its roots in the unconscious. If the client is able to release the *repressed feelings* associated with the conflict, the symptoms will disappear.

Among the strategies used in psychoanalysis are hypnosis, the interpretation of dreams, and free association, in which the client is encouraged to express every idea that comes to mind—no matter how insignificant, irrelevant, shameful, or embarrassing—ignoring all self-censorship and suspending all judgment.

In the initial phase of psychoanalysis, the analyst's task is to facilitate establishing a *therapeutic alliance*. In the transition to the middle phase of analysis, *transference* occurs and the analyst uses techniques calcu-

lated to induce *regression* in the client. In this stage the analyst remains relatively passive to avoid giving either permissive or authoritarian expressions and to limit observations to interpretations of the client's mental dynamics as heard in the free associations. In the long-range course of analysis, the client undergoes two basic processes—remembering and reliving. *Remembering* refers to the gradual extension of consciousness back to early childhood, when the core of the neurosis was formed. *Reliving* refers to the actual reexperiencing of past events and feelings in the context of the client's relationship with the analyst. The alleviation of symptoms is not usually regarded as the most significant factor for evaluating therapeutic change. Instead the chief basis of evaluation is the client's capacity to attain reasonable happiness, to contribute to the happiness of others, and to deal adequately with the stresses of life. In short, the most important criterion for successful analysis is the extent to which it releases the client's normal potential, which had been blocked by neurotic conflicts.

Topography of the Mind Freud classified mental operations according to regions or systems of the mind in a body of thought now referred to as *topographic theory*. Any mental event that occurred outside of conscious awareness represented the *unconscious region*. Mental events that could be brought into conscious awareness through an act of attention were said to be *preconscious*. Those that occurred in conscious awareness were regarded as the *conscious surface* of the mind. This topographic model, although still used to classify mental events in terms of the quality and degree of awareness, has been supplanted by the structural model.

Structure of the Mind Freud abandoned the topographic model of the mind for the structural model with the publication of *The Ego and the Id* (1962a) in 1923. The structural model of the mind contends that there are three distinct entities—the id, the ego, and the superego. The *id* was seen as a completely unorganized reservoir of energy derived from drives and instincts. The *ego* controls action and perception, controls contact with reality, and, through the defense mechanisms, inhibits primary instinctual drives. One of its fundamental functions is also the capacity for developing mutually satisfying relationships with others. The *superego* is concerned with moral behavior. Frequently, the superego allies itself with the ego against the id, imposing demands in the form of conscience or guilt feelings. The id in a child operates according to what Freud called the *pleasure principle*—the tendency to seek pleasure and avoid pain. This is not always possible, so the demands of the pleasure principle have to be modified by the *reality principle.* The reality principle is largely a learned ego function by which people develop the capacity to delay the immediate release of tension or achievement of pleasure.

Drives Freud believed that psychic energy was derived from *drives.* Instincts or drives were genetically determined psychic constituents. He used the word *cathexis* to refer to the attachment of psychic energy to a person or a thing. The greater the cathexis, the more important the person or object was, psychologically speaking. Initially Freud postulated a life and death instinct, but by 1920, in *Beyond the Pleasure Principle* (1975), he had revised these ideas to accord with the theory of drives accepted by or modified by analysts today. In the later formulation, Freud accounted for the instinctual aspects of people's mental lives by assuming the existence of two drives—the sexual drive and the aggressive drive. The former gives rise to the erotic component of mental activity while the latter gives rise to the destructive component. The two drives can be fused, for example, when an act of intentional cruelty also has some unconscious sexual meaning for the actor and provides a degree of unconscious gratification. The sexual drive has come to be known as the *libido.*

Phases of Psychosexual Development

THE ORAL STAGE The importance of a baby's mouth is obvious to even the most casual observer. Babies suck their thumbs, mouth toys and blankets, gurgle, and blow bubbles. Such oral activities among babies are no longer considered to be exclusively related to hunger. Instead, as Freud pointed out, the mouth is also an organ associated with the infant's pleasure and self-expression. In fact, Freud proposed that, until a child attains the age of 18 months, the mouth is the most important factor in the development of the psyche. The early part of the oral stage of development is dominated by pleasure. A baby feels frustration, eats, relaxes, and goes to sleep. The infant's attitude in this early oral stage is frequently termed *passive* and *receptive.* However, when teeth erupt, the baby enters on the *oral sadistic* or *oral aggressive* part of this phase. Such aggression is usually evidenced by crying, spitting, biting, or chewing. Every child goes through the oral stage. Its duration and course depend on physical

and environmental factors. Either excessive gratification or excessive deprivation can result in fixation or arrested development at this stage.

The developmental goal of this stage is mastery of gratification. Growth toward maturity occurs through gratification of oral needs. The baby learns to deal with anxiety by using the mouth and tongue. According to Freud, orality plays a major role in the early establishment of the ego. The child moves from the biological experience of oral gratification to a rudimentary interpersonal perceptiveness. During this phase babies literally incorporate the objects of pleasure into themselves, and the provider of that pleasure is not clearly distinguished from the self. Ultimately, in later oral stages, it is through delay in gratification that children learn to appreciate the difference between their personal feelings and the objects that bring relief. In this way babies develop the beginnings of independent mastery of their own gratification.

Psychoanalytic theory identifies several problems derived from the oral stage. A child may become an "oral character" throughout life if too severely frustrated in infancy. With undue frustration, the oral dependence is likely to turn either into extreme, effortless pessimism or into a fretful, demanding aggressiveness without constructive effort by the child to meet his or her own needs. Excessively tense or rejecting feeding can spoil or frustrate the oral needs of the baby, which in turn can result in an "oral fixation." Traits associated with oral fixation are narcissism, overoptimism, overpessimism, or the need for excessive attention. Such "oral pathologies" are manifested in the development of an overdependent personality. Orally fixated individuals become dependent on objects for their own view of themselves and thus become envious or jealous. In adulthood, defenses center around the oral experiences of smoking, alcoholism, obesity, nail biting, drug addiction, and general difficulty with trust.

THE ANAL STAGE Anal activity and anal products, according to Freud, are of great emotional import. Like objects that are swallowed, feces are part of the baby. Between the ages of one and three, the child gains more control of the voluntary and semivoluntary muscles, such as the anal sphincter. During this period the baby may experience sexual pleasure and eroticism from anal function. The preoccupation of many young children with anal matters is obvious to the observer of their spontaneous play, if parental taboos have not been too stringent. Furthermore, it appears that retention as well as evacuation is enjoyed for its own sake. The development of knowing control over anal elimination is closely aligned with the shift from the more passive aspects of infancy to the more active aspects of young childhood. The feces can become destructive and potent weapons. Freud refers to this potential as *anal sadism*. Throughout this stage the child seeks to separate self from dependence on and control by the parents. Underretention (messing) and overretention (withholding) are both associated with the child's need to reach an autonomous and independent state, free from shame and doubt over lack of self-control. The ways in which the first important impulses toward control and self-determination are handled are particularly fateful for the development of what is called *character*—those enduring attitudes the individual develops toward the self and the world.

The developmental goal of this stage is self-control of instinctual drives. Growth toward maturity occurs through the resolution of conflict between the emergence of the child's self-control and these drives. Toilet training often becomes the arena for acting out the conflict. The conflict situation that must be resolved has three aspects:

1. Conflict between two instinctual tendencies, elimination and retention
2. Conflict between either one of these tendencies, the child's attempts to control them, and the need to time his or her function
3. Conflict with the external world that has made the structural conflict of timing necessary

Techniques of toilet training and the parents' attitudes are of great importance. The child must learn to give up narcissistic omnipotence. If the child can identify happily with the parents and accept the requirements of others as his or her own, the emerging pride in personal mastery of instinctual impulses can be constructively directed toward social regulation. The child's sense of achievement is enhanced by parental praise. The anal stage thus involves fitting together control of the infant's instinctual drives and the requirements of the outside world. If it is resolved successfully, the individual is personally autonomous, capable of independent action without guilt, capable of self-determination without shame or self-doubt, and able to cooperate with others without being oppressive or defeatist.

Several problems derive from unsuccessful resolution of the anal stage. If the young child is forced to give up any self-determinism out of fear, whether of direct chastisement or loss of love, inner determinism tends to develop in opposition to the external world. The outcome may be either anxious compliance or defiance. The adult anal character is typically lacking in self-confidence, stubbornly self-righteous, and scornful of others, convinced that the only right way of doing things is his or her way. Above all, this person attaches a very special value to possessions. A variation on the parsimonious, obsessively orderly, and obstinate character that is also reflective of anal eroticism or fixation is the person who manifests such character traits as sloppiness, constant fluctuation, contrariness, anger, and sadomasochism.

THE PHALLIC STAGE According to Freud, from approximately three to five years of age the focus of libidinal energy shifts to the genital zone. The child experiences pleasurable sensations in this area, and he or she is said to be in the phallic stage of development. This early bloom of genital sexuality that cannot possibly come to fruition is differentiated from the later genital stage that leads to mature mating and reproduction. Attitudes formed in this stage are purported to be crucial for later heterosexual fulfillment and good relations with people in general. Freud states that the penis is the bodily organ of major stimulation, excitation, and sexual interest for children of both sexes. In little girls, castration fantasies are said to come to the fore, as girls notice their lack of a penis. Guilt about masturbation and sexual longings for the mother can also contribute to the "castration complex" in little boys.

The major developmental goal of this heightened interest in the genitals and genital function is as a basis for the child's development of male or female identity and for transforming previous developmental sexual foci into a generally genital direction. During this stage, erections occur frequently in boys, and masturbation and sex play with other children are virtually universal. The child's attitudes toward spontaneous inquiry are deeply influenced by the adults' reception of the child's strong early interest in body function. Peeping and exploration in company with other children all occur in the interest of clarification and satisfaction of sexual curiosity. Satisfactory resolution of the phallic phase then results in development of awareness of the genital area and learning appropriate sexual identity. More generally speaking, the desired outcome for the phallic stage is the achievement of a sense of initiative without guilt. If the Oedipal or Electra complex (the male child's erotic attachment to the mother, or the female child's erotic attachment to the father, respectively) is resolved successfully, the child will develop personal resources and can regulate his or her own motivation for constructive resolution of everyday problems.

Failure to resolve the phallic stage can produce several problems. Harsh repression of the pleasure children take in looking may have serious consequences for a child's development. Concern with body structure and function is natural at a time when the child knows the world mainly through his or her own bodily feelings. Being punished for this interest rarely helps the child to learn. According to Freud, if curiosity and inquiry meet with too severe a threat, reinforced from within by castration fear, all learning can be inhibited. A wide range of other character traits, including most of the adult disturbed coping patterns, is associated with excessive phallic-Oepidal involvement. Basic issues are said to be penis envy in the female and castration anxiety in the male, both accompanied by their subsequent defenses. The resolution of the Oepidal orientation is another source of distortions in development often associated with this phase. Difficulties with sexual identity, transsexuality, difficulty with authority, homosexuality, and fixation of the Oedipus or Electra complex are considered indicators of problems stemming from poor adjustment to the phallic stage.

THE LATENCY STAGE   Freud was deeply convinced of the dual-phase quality of human sexual development. The settling of the Oedipus or Electra complex, from the fifth or sixth year until the onset of puberty (at eleven to thirteen years of age), is marked by a biological lessening of sexual urges and virtual inactivity of sexual impulses. The growth of ego functions in this period yields an increased amount of control over instinctual drives and sublimation of these aggressive and libidinal urges into creative play and learning. The child's affiliations established in this period are primarily homosexual for both boys and girls. The ability to function effectively with all people in both social and physical terms is developing and important to the child's self-confidence and continued growth. This period has enormous functional importance, preparing the child for his or her later contributions to society and the area of work.

The developmental goal of the latency period is mastery of skills through sexual sublimation. During this period of relative inactivity of the sexual drives, the child learns to use his or her energies to create, develop, and manipulate industriously. The formation of sex roles and identities and the integration of Oedi-

pal identifications are consolidated. Through development of skills and mastery of surrounding objects and concepts, the child becomes self-directed in work and achievements without feelings of defeat, failure, or inferiority. Continued integration of these latency accomplishments is essential for a mature adult life of personal satisfaction and pleasure in love and work.

Several problems may derive from unsuccessful resolution of the latency stage. If early family life has not prepared the child for confidence in school life, if school experiences fail to sustain the initiative and confidence of the child, if the child's constitutional endowment makes it impossible for him or her to keep pace with other children in learning tasks and skills, then the child is likely to develop a sense of inadequacy and inferiority. The youngster's ability to identify with others on the basis of common goals of industry does not develop, and he or she is often led back to the more isolated, less conscious rivalry of the Oedipal phase. In short, very harsh experiences during this period promote regression to earlier patterns. Consequently, the child may shy away from industry, feeling inadequate to the task. Adult behaviors indicative of problems rooted in latency include constricted development of personality or character and an intensely obsessive nature.

THE GENITAL STAGE   The classical Freudian position emphasized the reinstatement of early attitudes and quasi-solutions of the Oedipus or Electra complex during the genital period. This stage, beginning with pubescence and lasting until the attainment of young adulthood, is sometimes also called the *adolescent* or *pubertal* stage of psychosexual development. It is characterized by maturation of hormonal and genital systems. Libidinal drives, along with other drives and motivations, are expressed in increasingly physical ways. Heightened sexual activity and motivation often pose conflicts for the individual. Incompletely or unsuccessfully resolved conflicts from preceding phases of development surface with renewed emphasis.

This stage has two major developmental goals:

1. The creation of nonincestuous, heterosexual, mature relationships.
2. The final separation from libidinal attachment to and dependence on the parents.

According to Freud, successful resolution of the genital stage paves the way for a mature personality capable of full genital satisfaction and potency. Individuals thus can participate freely in both love and work in ways that are personally gratifying and creative and that reflect a strong sense of personal identity.

Unsuccessful resolution of issues in the genital stage results in serious problems that, according to Freud, encompass a vast array of conflicts, fixations, serious character dysfunctions, and pathological traits. The adolescent unable to integrate this stage into a coherent sense of self feels lost and confused.

Other writers, including Erikson, have extended the stages of growth and development throughout the rest of the life span (see Chapter 10).

Implications for Psychiatric Nursing Practice

The psychoanalytic model has historically provided a very limited treatment role for the nurse. Psychoanalytic clients are usually seen in the analyst's office as private clients. With the emergence of psychoanalytically oriented settings such as Chestnut Lodge in Rockville, Maryland, nurses became somewhat more involved, sharing at least in the psychoanalytic language, concepts, and speculations about client dynamics. In the United States a nurse needs a medical degree as well as psychoanalytic training in order to practice as a psychoanalyst. Some nurses have sought preparation as lay analysts at settings such as the William Alanson White Institute and the Chicago Psychoanalytic Institute. However, the nurse has served more frequently as an adjunct therapist focusing on here-and-now issues with clients undergoing psychoanalysis or in a supportive role to family members.

Acknowledging that the psychoanalytic model has provided few clear-cut therapeutic roles for nurses does not suggest that nurses have failed to do useful work with clients undergoing psychoanalytic treatment or that knowledge of psychoanalytic theory is irrelevant to psychiatric nurses. Concepts derived from the psychoanalytic model, such as the unconscious, pervade not only the field of psychiatry but also the entire culture. These concepts are understood by the educated public and are useful in comprehending fields of human endeavor ranging from public relations to art and literature. The psychoanalytic vocabulary has crept into everyday speech through college courses in psychology, personal therapy, and pervasive use in the popular culture. Ordinary people think about being neurotic, check their ids periodically for death wishes and their egos for weaknesses. People who are rejecting are considered egocentric. Castration complexes, sibling rivalry, and phallic symbols are recognized everywhere. Marital and divorce court proceedings are

conducted in "psychoanalese." Certainly if nurses are to participate as equal members of the pysychiatric team, and if they are to be valued as theorists, they must learn the language that dominates the common heritage of psychiatric professionals.

Critique

We criticize Freudian psychoanalysis somewhat uneasily. As one authority put it, "Who knows, they might be right. All of us hardy souls who persist in our skepticism might be 'resisting'—the very evidence of our sickness." Yet some critical analyses of the psychoanalytic movement have emerged. Several differ with small sections of Freud's work (Adler and Horney, for example, disapproved of psychic determinism, the instinct theory, and the structural approach of id, ego, and superego). Others go so far as to found a whole empirical school of behaviorism in opposition to Freudianism, attacking the "absurdities" of the whole.

Perhaps the most compelling synthesis of critical arguments launched against the psychoanalytic model can be found in the literature of feminism. Feminists have pointed out that (a) psychoanalytic theory's emphasis on early childhood determinism underrates the effects of environmental systems on dynamic processes in people; (b) the psychoanalytic model tends to accept as immutable the social context in which repression and resulting neurosis must develop; and (c) Freud's ideas were rooted in the social and political culture of his time (that is, early twentieth-century Viennese society). These critics have noted further that the psychoanalytic framework is blatantly antifemale. Shulamith Firestone (1971), for instance, comments that Freud's theory about women is limited to analyzing them only as negative males (e.g., the Electra complex is an inverse Oedipus complex). His concept of two types of female orgasms, clitoral and vaginal, was refuted as myth in the research of Masters and Johnson. Widespread acceptance of Freudian theory has promoted social adjustment for women instead of feminist revolt, contends Firestone. In short, she sees psychoanalysis as patching up with Band-Aids casualties of the immense social unrest and role confusion associated with the modern, rigid, patriarchal, nuclear family. As evidence of psychoanalytic insensitivity to the objective difference in women's and men's social situations, Firestone cites some of the work of the neo-Freudians. The attitude that almost all women are afraid that the man they love will leave them, but hardly any man is afraid that a woman will leave him, is apparent as a consistent theme. Other examples are the beliefs that girls find their own genitals ugly compared to those of boys, that women devote great effort to adorning their bodies in order to compensate for this physical deficiency, and that women are insecure and self-conscious because they lack penises. Firestone notes examples of such analysts' misinterpretations of client interactions based on these notions.

Helene Deutsch, trained in psychoanalysis by Freud and author of a monumental two-volume work on women (1944–1945), expounded the following ideas in her theories of "normal femininity":

- Preadolescent girls have masochistic longings to be raped.
- Women find enjoyment through childbirth, forced intercourse, and lost causes.
- Women with "masculinity complexes," whom Deutsch "unmasked" in therapy, were cases of thwarted femininity, since women cannot compete successfully with men.
- Motherhood is the only true fulfillment for all women.

Deutsch describes truly "feminine" women as the loveliest and most unaggressive of helpmates, women who do not insist on their own rights but are easy to handle in every way if one just loves them. Most critics view such theories of "normal femininity" as representing a male perspective.

Psychoanalytic thought as developed by Freud, Deutsch, Erikson, and Reik views the difference in genital apparatus between the sexes as the critical variable affecting personality development in men and women. These theorists posit a separate psychology of women linking all traits, interests, attitudes, emotions, and neuroses to an anatomic "defect." Erik Erikson (1968) makes a valiant attempt to wed cultural relativity to innate biological differences, but he still ends up with the advocates of "anatomy as destiny." Most feminists argue that, even if an anatomical theory did explain human behavior, birth and breast envy ought to be given equal time with the penis envy so dominant in Freud's essays.

Other feminists writing about psychoanalysis point out that, although adult mental health in American society is masculine-centered, most psychoanalytic theory has been written about women. Phyllis Chesler (1972) criticizes Freud's vision of women as essentially "breeders and bearers," potentially warmhearted crea-

tures, but cranky children with uteruses, forever mourning the loss of male organs and male identity. The headaches, fatigue, chronic depression, frigidity, paranoia, and overwhelming sense of inferiority that Freud noted in so many of his female clients were never viewed by him as the indirect communications characteristic of slave psychologies. Instead, such symptoms were viewed as hysterical and neurotic productions manufactured by spiteful, self-pitying, and generally unpleasant women. Their inability to be happy as women, Freud concluded, stemmed from unresolved penis envy, unresolved Electra complexes, or general mysterious female stubbornness.

Freud's views about women have been extensively reviewed, criticized, and rejected wholly or partially by such female theoreticians as Karen Horney, Clara Thompson, Margaret Mead, Eva Figes, Simone de Beauvoir, Betty Friedan, Kate Millett, and Germaine Greer. Male theoreticians such as Bronislav Malinowski, Alfred Adler, Harry Stack Sullivan, Wilhelm Reich, Ronald Laing, David Cooper, and Thomas Szasz have also refuted Freudian theory but not necessarily or primarily because of its premises about women.

Those who do emphasize Freud's psychology of women as the basis for their critique argue that biological differences between the sexes have been overemphasized and that all mammals show a vast array of bisexual or unisex behaviors. These theorists modify Freud's libido concept to refer to forces in both sexes that lead to experimentation and growth. They conclude that curiosity, aggressiveness, dependence, expressiveness, interest in the body, self-esteem, and the need for growth, security, and creativity are all part of a common human repertoire that transcends anatomy. These givens, however, can be elaborated, drastically altered, or suppressed as each individual comes into contact with his or her immediate family environment and total culture.

THE BEHAVIORIST MODEL

The behaviorist model in psychiatry has its roots in psychology and neurophysiology. To the behaviorist, symptoms associated with neuroses and psychoses are clusters of learned behaviors that persist because they are somehow rewarding to the individual. One of the most important conceptual contributions to this framework was made by Pavlov (1849–1936), who in 1902

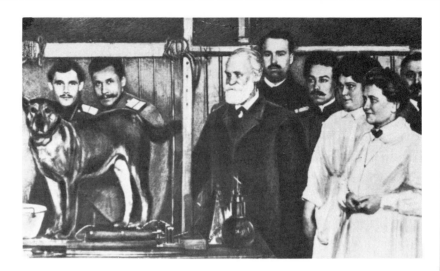

Pavlov and his staff demonstrate the conditioned reflex phenomenon with a dog in his laboratory.

discovered a phenomenon he called the *conditioned reflex* in a famous experiment with a dog and a bell. The basic principle of the conditioned reflex is this:

- A response is a reaction to a stimulus.
- If a new and different stimulus is presented with or just before the original stimulating event, the same response reaction can be obtained.
- Eventually the new stimulus can replace the original one, so that the response occurs to the new stimulus alone.

The conditioned or learned response has come to be viewed as the basic unit of all learning, the unit on which more complex behavioral patterns are constructed. Such construction occurs through a process called *reinforcement,* in which behaviors are rewarded and persist. Pavlov's theories have continued into the present, valued for their simplicity, concreteness, and objectivity. Some behaviorists see them as the key to comprehension and control of the whole range of problematic human behavior.

Assumptions and Key Ideas

The fundamental premises of the behaviorist perspective can be summarized as follows:

- Human beings are merely complex animals. The difference between human and animal is one of *degree* and not kind. Human powers of conceptual thought, propositional language, and abstraction are fully at-

tributable to physiologic complexity rather than some nonmaterial source. Thus the use of animal experience as an analogue to human experience is clearly justifiable.

- The self in humans is the sum or repository of past conditionings or simply the behavioral repertoire. Therapists can know clients only by the clients' behavior. The concepts of consciousness and self and the belief in subjective reality are products of human pride rather than scientific discovery. If they are real, they can be inferred only from observable behavior.

- Behavior is what the organism does. It can be observed, described, and recorded.

- There is, properly speaking, no autonomous person. People are what they do and what they are reinforced for doing by conditions in their environment.

- The self is a structure of stimulus–response chains or hierarchies of habit. It is possible to know and predict conditions under which behavior will occur.

- The symptoms of a person's disorders are, in fact, the substance of that person's troubles. There is no hidden motive, no underlying cause, no internal pathogenic process. There is only the symptom or the behavior, and the aim of behaviorist therapy is to change the behavior.

- The classification of mental diseases is meaningful only to provide legal labels. It provides little or no assistance in prescribing a treatment program.

- People can control others whether others want to be controlled or not. Control is neither good nor bad in and of itself.

• The therapist determines what behavior should be changed and what plan should be followed. Change is effected by identifying events in the client's life that have been critical stimuli for the behavior and then arranging interventions for *extinguishing* those behaviors. A changed way of acting precedes a changed way of thinking, according to behaviorist theory.

Both Joseph Wolpe (1956) and B. F. Skinner (1953, 1971) are associated with psychiatric treatment approaches that represent one form of *conditioning* and reflect the above assumptions. Wolpe defined *neurotic behavior* as unadaptive learned behavior acquired in anxiety-generating situations. He based his therapeutics on the introduction of a response that inhibits anxiety when situations occur that ordinarily evoke anxiety. Relaxation, for example, was considered incompatible with anxiety and, therefore, effective in inhibiting it. Thus, Wolpe would direct his intervention to a counter-conditioning technique, usually putting the client under hypnosis and using various techniques for gradual *desensitization*. For example, a man with a fear of dying might gradually attempt to overcome his anxiety at the sight of a coffin, the attendance of a funeral, and so on, by trying to relax in the face of these situations.

Skinner's approach, called *operant conditioning*, emphasizes discovering why the behavioral response was elicited in the first place and what current variables actively reinforce it. The key concept in operant conditioning is reinforcement. The term *positive reinforcement* is used to describe an event that increases the probability that the response will recur. A *negative reinforcement* is an event likely to decrease the probability of recurrence of that response. The frequency with which a response is given is a clear, observable measure of behavior. Most people exhibit aggressive behavior at some time. To say that a client is hostile suggests that this class of response occurs with a higher frequency than is usually expected. The term given to an intervention designed to change the behavior emitted by a client is *shaping*. It is a procedure of manipulating reinforcement to bring the person closer to the chosen behavior. There are, according to Skinner, times in a client's life when responses are accidentally reinforced by a coincidental pairing of response and reinforcement. This accidental pairing may play a role in the development of phobias (irrational fears) and other so-called neurotic behaviors.

Implications for Psychiatric Nursing Practice

Most psychiatric nurses acknowledge that the application of principles of behavior modification to clients is quite complex, since such interventions are powerful tools with a heavy philosophical overlay. The use of this approach raises issues of control, responsibility for behavior, and the morality of using negative or punitive stimuli in a therapeutic context, to name only a few. Therapists who successfully resolve such basic philosophical issues have designed and implemented behavior modification plans with disturbed, overtly aggressive children, developmentally disabled clients, and violent self-destructive people.

In many institutional environments, clients follow prescribed schedules for daily living that include a token economy. Clients are rewarded for desired behavior by token reinforcers, such as food, candy, and verbal approval. The movement toward community-based psychiatric treatment has illuminated some of the shortcomings of therapies aimed toward resolving everyone's intrapsychic conflicts. The movement has instead attempted to replace maladaptive behavior with behavior that will enable people to function effectively within their natural environment. When parents or others in the client's environment are taught to implement the behavior change procedures, therapy moves away from the partial and artificial situation of the therapist's office into the client's total environment. It no longer requires the presence of highly trained, often expensive experts and thus brings treatment within the grasp of those who are not members of the economic elite.

Some behaviorists envision a future in which behavior therapy based on learning theory will become the dominant mode of psychiatric intervention. This would move psychiatry out of the hospitals and the medical profession and into the practice of teachers in learning centers.

Psychiatric nurses have had a special role in teaching behaviorist principles to people with little training so that they can act as change agents. Nonprofessional staff on psychiatric wards can be taught effective use of behaviorist principles to eliminate chronic, maladaptive behavior by long-term mental clients. Hyperactive children or children with borderline intelligence can be treated in the home by their parents when nurses teach the parents to use approaches such as frequency counts on specific behaviors to be modified, time-outs (short periods of isolation) for undesired behavior, and the bestowal of attention, praise, and affectionate physical contact as rewards.

In general, behavior modification offers a rapid, efficient, and effective system of intervention congruent both with psychiatric nurses' conventional roles as planners and teachers and with trends in community psychiatry. However, it may not accord with a nurse's personal philosophy.

Critique

Intervention based on the behaviorist model has proved effective in the treatment of persons so alienated from society and functionally incapacitated that they are unable to interact with or respond to others. Nonetheless, a very strong line of criticism has been leveled against this model. The criticism fundamentally rests on ethical concerns about people's rights, dignity, and freedom; on the model's simplistic explanation of human feelings and behavior; and on its authoritarian therapist–client relationship.

Advocates of behaviorism contend that without a strict, logical, reductionist methodology, psychiatric practice will be plagued with all sorts of methodological and logical improprieties. Without a strict reduction to empirical or observable content, they assert, therapists are left with a discipline based on emotions, introspection, and subjective feelings.

Humanistic social scientists, on the other hand, contend that ignoring emotions, introspection, and subjective feelings distorts the creative role of people in shaping their environments instead of merely adapting to them. Humanists further argue that these qualities differentiate humans from animals. People are self-aware. They can step outside themselves and reflect on their subjective inner lives. It is their ability to think about themselves that enables them to talk about themselves and to contemplate their future possibilities. Such self-consciousness is the genius of human individuality. No other animal is burdened with this gift. Crucial to this quality, of course, are the abilities to comprehend meaning and to use language.

If Freud's theories challenged the rationality of human beings, many critics find that behaviorist learning theories reduce humans to little more than cogs in a machine that can be conditioned to take almost any form. Such a conception of human beings ignores the ability to be self-conscious, to act intentionally; to experience reality differently from each other; and to create images, dreams, fantasies, and a private inner life. Many clinicians value certain interventions generated

according to principles of stimulus–response learning, but the behaviorists' most basic assumptions about people and their environments contrast harshly with the image of humans and society offered by other theoretical schools.

THE SOCIAL–INTERPERSONAL MODEL

The social–interpersonal model of psychiatry grew out of a general dissatisfaction with approaches that account for "mental illness" in terms of either intrapersonal mechanisms such as the symptoms of a disease or individual personality dynamics such as anxiety, ego strength, and libido. Advocates of this model assert that other models neglect the crucial social processes involved in the development and resolution of disturbed behavior. The social–interpersonal perspective is advanced as more logical, more appropriate, more encompassing of the issues involved, and more readily substantiated by research. It focuses on the larger and more general context of deviant behavior and on the processes by which an individual comes to be labeled or identified as deviant. The humanistic interactionist philosophic base for this text represents an extension and refinement of the social–interpersonal model. It is a synthesis particularly of the sociological and social interpersonal models.

Assumptions and Key Ideas

Three somewhat separate schools of thought that are philosophically congruent make up the social–interpersonal model. These are the sociological, the interpersonal-psychiatric, and the general systems approaches. The assumptions and key ideas of each are discussed below.

The Sociological School of Thought   The sociological approach is summarized partially by sociologist Kai Erikson (1962), who stated: "Deviance is not a property inherent in certain forms of behavior; it is a property conferred upon these forms by audiences which directly or indirectly witness them." A similar view is proposed by Howard Becker (1963, p. 9): "Deviance is not a quality of the act a person commits, but a consequence of the application by others of rules and sanctions to an 'offender.'"

Thus, mental illness is a *label* earned by certain behaviors that violate the rules of conduct imposed by various significant others. The focus for psychiatry is on the interplay between the deviant and the audience—the person and the social context. Sociologically, the critical variable in the study of the forms of deviance labeled *mental illness* is the social audience, rather than the individual person, since it is the audience that eventually decides whether any given action will be labeled a case of deviation. Included in the study of "mental illness," then, are various aspects of audience reactions to behavior, the labeling process, the criteria used in labeling, the extent of consensus on such criteria, the consequences for an individual so labeled, etc.

A well-known example of this approach is the research of Thomas Scheff (1966), who concludes that mental illness is a label given to diverse forms of deviance that do not fit under any other explicit label, such as delinquency. In this regard, he views mental illness as a form of *residual deviance*—a label given to nonconforming behavior. The label reinforces and stabilizes that behavior and enters the labeled patient into a deviant role of "mental patient." Once a person has been labeled deviant and societal reactions have become organized, Scheff argues, the deviant may incorporate the definitions of others into his or her own self-concept.

Scheff's research confirms many of the ideas of sociologist Edwin Lemert (1951), who proposed that mental illness bears a greater similarity to other forms of social deviance than it does to medical disease. Lemert introduced the ideas of primary and secondary deviation to differentiate between occasional or situational lapses from normal behavior and deviation that becomes a life-style or established social role. Lemert went on to argue that, when society becomes the active labeler, occasionally nonconforming primary deviants are cut off from their nondeviant status and begin life as full-time secondary deviants. Hospitalization, commitment, and psychiatric diagnostic classifications are all ways of forbidding the temporarily lapsed person (such as the daydreamer or the person who goes on a bender but is not yet an alcoholic) from reentering the community with "normal" status intact. When the individual begins to develop behavior that fits the new status and finds the new role gratifying, he or she adopts a deviant life-style.

In the sociological school's view then, behaviors that are often called symptoms acquire meaning only when considered within their social context. This view emphasizes the social system consisting of the client, others reacting to the client, and the official agencies of

psychiatric control and treatment. It de-emphasizes individual personal dynamics.

The Interpersonal Psychiatric School of Thought   Significant contributions were made to the social–interpersonal model by psychiatrists Adolf Meyer (1948–1952) and Harry Stack Sullivan (1953) in the first half of the twentieth century. Sullivan trained with William Alanson White and Adolf Meyer rather than Freud. He is viewed as the least reductionist of psychiatric theorists and emphasizes modes of interaction as the real focus of psychiatric inquiry. Sullivan argues that psychiatry should renounce the futile attempt to define isolated individuals and instead define the significant interpersonal aspects of situations. His main theoretical concern is with the integration of organism and milieu. Sullivan became the theoretical and ideological leader of the interpersonal school of psychiatry often associated with the William Alanson White Foundation, which sponsors the well-known journal *Psychiatry*. Although the sociological theorists differ on some points with the interpersonal school of psychiatry (for example, on the relative importance of the self and individual psychology), they are bound together by a number of fundamentally compatible ideas.

One concept that plays a crucial role in the organization of behavior, according to Sullivan, is the *self-system* or *self-dynamism*. The self is a construct built from the child's experience. It is made up of *reflected appraisals* the person learns in contacts with other significant people. The self develops in the process of seeking physical satisfaction of bodily needs and security. To feel secure, the self essentially requires feelings of approval and prestige as protection against anxiety. In summary, Sullivan emphasizes the pervasive interaction between organism and personal environment. He objects in principle to the concept of organized psychological impulses, drives and goals, belonging to the person as an individual and feels instead that the person cannot be distinguished from the person-in-the-interpersonal-situation.

Despite the environmentalist phrasing of many of his key concepts and a certain emphasis on the effects of cultural configurations on the development and functioning of the personality, Sullivan has comparatively little to say about the impact on behavior of specific variations in the social or cultural scene. Other advocates of the interpersonal school of psychiatry, such as Karen Horney (1950) and Erich Fromm (1941), like Sullivan, stress the general climate in the immediate family. Alfred Adler (1971), is one, however, who attempts to understand more of the social and cultural conditions influencing behavior. The interpersonal school of psychiatry in general focuses less on social context than the sociological perspective and takes basically a developmental–interpersonal view of the self.

The General Systems Theory School of Thought General systems theory, when applied to living systems (people), provides a conceptual framework within which the content of the biological and social sciences can be logically integrated with that of the physical sciences. In psychiatry it offers a new resolution of the mind–matter dichotomy, a new integration of biological and social approaches to the nature of human beings, and a new approach to psychopathology, diagnosis, and therapy.

The personality theory proposed by Karl Menninger (1963) presents normal personality functioning and psychopathology in general systems theory terms. His theory deals with four major issues:

1. Adjustment or individual–environment interaction
2. The organization of living systems
3. Psychological regulation and control, known as *ego theory* in psychoanalysis
4. Motivation, which is often called *instinct* or *drive* in the psychoanalytic framework

A salient point of Menninger's theory is the idea of *homeostasis* (human balance). He asserts further that the greater the threat or stress on a system, the greater the number of system components involved in coping with or adapting to it. Therefore pathology can exist at various levels, from the cell and organ level to the group and community level. An example of the former might be the behavioral changes that follow cellular alterations due to addictive drugs such as heroin, to a blood clot, or to a tumor. Examples of pathology at the group level include family conflicts. At the community level, overpopulation, pollution, and poverty are instances of pathology. In systems theory terms, all represent abnormalities or stresses on matter–energy processes and would be included within the domain of psychiatric professionals.

In Menninger's view, then, a system's well-being depends on the amount of stress on it and the effectiveness of its coping mechanisms. He asserts that "mental illness" is an impairment of self-regulation in which comfort, growth, and production are surrendered for the sake of survival at the best level possible but at the

sacrifice of emergency coping devices (1963, pp. 526–527). Mental clients are described as "obliged to make awkward and expensive maneuvers to maintain themselves, somewhat isolated from their fellows, harassed by faulty techniques of living, uncomfortable themselves and often to others" (Menninger 1963, p. 5). Emphasis in therapy according to the general systems approach is on current conflicts, restoration of impaired systems to functioning, and subsequent reintegration of the restored function into future coping strategies.

Implications for Psychiatric Nursing Practice

The social–interpersonal framework gives independent and collaborative psychiatric nursing clear theoretical direction and support. Nursing roles are associated with shifts in the delivery of psychiatric services variously termed *social psychiatry, community psychiatry,* and *milieu therapy.* These methods of delivery are taken up in detail in Chapters 18 and 28. All are associated with efforts to provide psychiatric services more efficiently to large groups of people, particularly those previously neglected, and attempts to counteract the debilitating effects of long-term institutionalization. All are also associated with a political and ideological movement to address the client's social context in providing psychiatric care. According to these orientations, all social, psychological, and biological activity affecting the mental health of the population is of interest to professionals in community psychiatry. Therapeutic interventions may include programs for social change, political involvement, community organization, and social planning. The implications for practice derived from this theoretical model are many:

- Clients are approached in a holistic way, recognizing the interrelatedness and interaction of the biophysical, psychological, and socioeconomic–cultural dimensions of human life. This increases the number of factors that must be evaluated when caring for a client.

- The increased number and diversity of variables to be considered require graduate and undergraduate content in psychiatric nursing education to be revised. Curricula must include concepts, theories, and research findings to support extended and new thinking about mental health, culture, social systems, ethnicity, deviant behavior, and the human condition. These new content areas drawn from the social sciences must then be integrated with conventional psychiatric nursing content to form an internal coherent knowledge base.

- Definitions of the client expand to include the concept of client system. A family, a couple, or even a community may be the focus for help.

- Intervention strategies include primary prevention roles of teacher, social change agent, and researcher. The goals are to help individuals cope with stresses in their environment, alter environments that contribute to pathology, and conduct research to establish the logical basis for preventive measures.

- The yardsticks for measuring "normality" are revised to reflect the notions that some deviant behaviors resemble physical illness and others do not, that applying psychiatric labels on the basis of selective and flimsy evidence often has destructive consequences, and that goals for therapy or treatment should not be set without first investigating the client's interpersonal situation.

- Therapy focuses on helping troubled persons to gain a useful perspective on their life-styles and social environments, rather than on repressing and controlling symptoms. Psychiatric nurses need to acknowledge the political and moral implications of involuntary drug therapy and behavior modification therapy.

- The psychiatric nurse must be prepared to function as an autonomous member of the psychiatric team and to assume more responsibilities. There is a shift away from the dominance of the physician in decision making and toward diffusion of roles. Practitioners' roles are based less on background discipline than on availability and interest in helping the client.

In short, once clients are viewed as becoming disturbed in the context of unhealthy or problematic interpersonal relationships, establishing healthy, constructive interpersonal relationships becomes important in their care. The roles of psychiatric nurses in milieu therapy, primary prevention, social psychiatry, and community psychiatry implement this fundamental idea. To illustrate, let us explore the following case example:

Mrs. S is a 67-year-old, upper-middle-class woman in good physical health. She has become increasingly untidy, forgetful, seclusive, sad, and suspicious since the death of her aggressive, bank president husband from a heart attack six months ago. She recently sold the large

tudor house where she had lived for the past 45 years, and she moved into a two-bedroom apartment in a nearby town. Because of apartment rules, she was unable to take her 12-year-old cat. She sold the house because her husband had told his lawyers that she should do so. (He had made all the family decisions while he lived.) Mrs. S has taken to skipping meals except for candy bars, since she must rely on a friend to drive her to the grocery store. (Her husband never felt she needed to learn to drive.) Her younger sister (age 59), seeking advice about Mrs. S's behavior, phoned the community mental health center on the suggestion of the family physician.

The social–interpersonal psychiatric nurse assessing Mrs. S's situation would tend not to focus on her symptoms as psychological conflicts due to ambivalence toward her dead husband or as manifestations of a psychiatric disease such as major, single-episode depression. Such a nurse would instead focus on the way Mrs. S is functioning in her current interpersonal situation. In this analysis Mrs. S is not seen as diseased and therefore in need of a somatic treatment such as medication. Instead treatment consists of helping Mrs. S to develop strategies for coping with her new situation and satisfying her needs. The nurse will want to see the younger sister and other family members in an attempt to enhance Mrs. S's context or relationships. Efforts may be directed toward mobilizing environmental forces to provide company, stimulation, and proper nutrition for Mrs. S, since the absence of all three contributes to her symptoms and discomfort. A clinical example such as Mrs. S's will undoubtedly reinforce the psychiatric nurse's political efforts to point out the potential consequences of lifelong passive dependence for adult women. The nurse may also become involved in community organizations working for better services for the elderly.

Critique

The social–interpersonal model has been criticized on three major fronts: conceptual, philosophical, and practical. Conceptual criticisms are brought most squarely to bear on Sullivan's interpersonal psychiatric theory. Writers such as Ruth Munroe (1955) view interpersonal psychiatric formulations as *word-building*—thinking up new names for old psychoanalytic concepts. Sullivan's theory is perceived as "losing a lot" when contrasted with the richness of Freudian analysis. Sullivan and the other interpersonal theorists, such as Adler, Horney, and Fromm, underplay the role of the biological demands of the organism and tend to limit social psychiatry to the immediate family of significant others, neglecting the impact of culture and social structure. Furthermore, according to the critics, if the Freudians have neglected the dynamic importance of the self system, the self theories have given the concept too global a role. In sum, the concept does not usually add much to the clinical understanding of any living client. Finally, Munroe proposes that Sullivan's neglect and repudiation of the sexual systems are more a reflection of his era, a reaction against narrow Freudianism, than an intrinsic part of the interpersonal theoretical approach.

Thomas Szasz (1971) emerges as both a partial proponent and a partial critic of the social–interpersonal model, at least on a philosophical level. He argues that this model in community psychiatry looks to public health and preventive medicine for both its theoretical model and its moral justification for using the control power of the state. This is an error, says Szasz. If preventive psychiatry is a logical extension of traditional medical practice, psychiatric professionals can justify promoting their own business. Community psychiatry extends the control and power of mental health workers by asserting that psychiatric professionals have responsibility not only for persons who come for help but also for those who do not. Szasz goes on to point out the political implications of looking to public health medicine as the model for community psychiatry. Hypothetically, laws could be passed enacting compulsory mental health measures supposedly designed to protect the community "from psychological contamination." Like public health laws concerning control of communicable disease, these mental health laws would be presented as value-free and nonpolitical. Szasz concludes that once community psychiatric practice is commissioned and paid for by the state, the crusading psychiatric professional will owe the same unswerving loyalty to the government that the priest owed to the medieval church during the witch-hunts. Through crisis intervention and other methods of environmental manipulation, community mental health programs aim to eliminate known producers of stress. These include urban slums, rural depressed areas, and all other potential breeding grounds for mental disturbance. According to Szasz, preoccupation with "mental health" has the potential of victimizing individuals or groups who may be identified as "producers of stress" for the majority culture. In summary, Szasz attacks the model for its inclusiveness, its posture of condescending benevolence and righteous paternalism, and its covert potential for political repression.

Finally, criticism is brought to bear on the social–interpersonal model from real-world mental health workers who must cope with the window smashing, verbal abuse, and self-destructiveness of a young man brought to the psychiatric ward for threatening to assassinate the governor, or the incoherent bizarre ravings of a vagrant, drunk on cheap wine, brought to the psychiatric emergency room of a New York City hospital from the snowy doorways of Broadway, or the mute, motionless living death of a catatonic woman found hidden away in an attic. For these critics, the social–interpersonal model is impractical, idealistic, and ill-suited to the realities of psychiatric care—where time is limited, money and supplies are even more so, and immediate problems of symptom control must be solved.

THE CHOICE OF A CONCEPTUAL FRAMEWORK

Psychiatric nurses use one or a combination of theoretical frameworks, either implicitly or explicitly, to guide their practice. We have chosen the humanistic interactionist approach elaborated in Chapter 1 as the basis for subsequent ideas in this text. As acknowledged earlier, it represents a synthesis of strengths derived primarily from the social–interpersonal model. In clinical work, however, the selection of a conceptual framework may be influenced by various factors. Among them are the practitioner's education, the philosophy of the setting in which clients are treated, the nature of the client's present problem, the available treatment, the need to be efficient and practical, and even client attributes such as social class and gender. For example, in most cases physicians are inclined to view clients according to the medical model, the approach stressed in their education. This is particularly likely when the client's problem is identified as one of the syndromes for which somatic treatment is readily available and effective in symptom control, such as Major Depression or Bipolar Affective Disorder, Manic Type. The former syndrome has been shown to respond to antidepressant medication and electroconvulsive therapy, and the latter to lithium carbonate. The choice of a biological–medical model is even more likely when the client is from a lower or lower-middle-class background, or elderly, or not highly intelligent or verbal.

Table 2-1 A COMPARATIVE ANALYSIS OF MAJOR FEATURES OF FOUR CONCEPTUAL FRAMEWORKS				
Conceptual Framework	Assessment Base	Problem Statement	Goal	Dominant Intervention
Medical–biological	Individual client symptoms	Disease	Symptom control Cure	Somatotherapies
Psychoanalytic	Intrapsychic Unconscious	Conflict	Insight	Psychoanalysis
Behavioristic	Behavior	Learning deficit	Behavior change	Behavior modification or conditioning
Social–interpersonal	Interactions of individual and social context	Dysfunction	Enhanced awareness and quality of interactions	Group and milieu therapies

These characteristics are often used to rule out candidacy for psychotherapy. If the setting must respond to large numbers of clients on a short-term basis, the decision to label, sort, patch up with medicines, and dispatch back into the community often seems the only realistic alternative.

If, however, the clinician is a psychiatric nurse or social worker; the problem one of relating to others or adjusting to a situation in life; the client relatively verbal, intelligent, young, motivated, and from an upper-middle-class background; and the setting one in which long-term residential milieu therapy or group or individual psychotherapy is possible, the social–interpersonal framework is more likely to be chosen as a basis for assessment and planning of client care.

The failure of any model to "cure" a client may induce clinicians to recast the problem in a different framework with different treatment options. For example, a psychotic client who does not respond to medication may respond to a well-planned behavior modification program. Approaches associated with two or more different models are often used in combination. For example, bizarre, self-destructive behavior may be controlled with medications in order to make the client more available for group or individual therapy. Such a combined or *eclectic approach* demands that a clinician be capable of functioning within any and all models of care, depending on which is best for the client and fits the resources and limitations of the situation. Yet conceptual models often remain implicit and unacknowledged, rather than being knowledgeably, explicitly, and systematically employed. If nurses give adequate consideration to the conceptual framework of their psychiatric nursing, they will foster practice-oriented research and clinical judgments that can be articulated and taught to others. Table 2–1 summarizes the major features of each of the conceptual frameworks discussed in this chapter.

KEY NURSING CONCEPTS

✔ The choice of a conceptual framework for psychiatric nursing treatment determines information sought, approaches recommended, and goals set.

✔ Therapeutic models for mental health practice traditionally include the medical–biological model, the psychoanalytic model, the behaviorist model, and the social–interpersonal model.

✔ The medical–biological model views emotional and behavioral disturbances as diseases and limits the nurse's role to administering somatic treatments and observation.

✔ Critics of the medical model of mental illness suggest that (a) social, ethical, interpersonal, and cultural factors are overlooked or obscured; (b) labeling behavior or "illness" relieves people of responsibility for their behavior; (c) mental symptoms correspond more to problems in living and relating to others than to diseases of the body.

✔ Psychoanalytic theory developed by Freud purports that all psychological events have meaning and are understandable.

✔ Psychoanalytic theory states that much of what goes on in people's minds is unknown to them, or unconscious, and accounts for apparent discontinuities in their lives that are due to unresolved conflicts in oral, anal, phallic, latency, or genital stages of psychosexual development.

✔ In the psychoanalytic model the nurse usually functions in a supportive therapeutic role.

✔ Criticism of Freudian psychoanalytic theory has come from feminists, behaviorists, and ego psychologists.

✔ The behaviorist model views the self and mental symptoms as learned behaviors that persist because they are rewarding to the individual.

✔ In the behaviorist model the nurse's role is expanded to planner, counselor, and educator, but therapeutic goals are limited to symptom control through behavior modification techniques that raise ethical issues.

✔ Criticism of the behaviorist model centers on ethical concerns, on a reductionist explanation of human feelings and behavior, and on a controlling, authoritarian therapist–client relationship.

✔ In the social–interpersonal model, (a) treatment occurs within an interpersonal context; (b) social processes (e.g., labeling by those involved in disturbed behavior) are assessed; (c) the focus is on the broader context of deviant behavior and integrates biological and social sciences through a general systems perspective.

✔ In the social–interpersonal framework treatment is likely to include helping clients develop strategies for coping, mobilizing environmental resources, and therapist involvement in community organization and planning.

✔ The psychiatric nurse's role in the social–interpersonal framework is expanded to include social and political action and community intervention as well as direct intervention with individuals, families, and groups.

References

Adler, A. *The Practice and Theory of Individual Psychology*. Translated by P. Radin. 1929; reprint edition, New York: Humanities Press, 1971.

Becker, H. S. *Outsiders: Studies in the Sociology of Deviance*. New York: Free Press, 1963.

Carlsson, A., and Lindqvist, M. "Effects of Chlorpromazine or Haloperidol on Formation of 3-Methoxytyramine and Normetanephrine in Mouse Brain." *Acta Pharmacological Toxicology* 20 (1973): 140.

Chesler, P. *Women and Madness*. Garden City, N.Y.: Doubleday, 1972.

Deutsch, H. *Psychology of Women*. 2 vols. New York: Grune and Stratton, 1944-1945.

Erikson, E. N. *Identity, Youth and Crisis*. New York: W. W. Norton, 1968.

Erikson, K. "Notes on the Sociology of Deviance." *Social Problems* 9 (1962): 308.

Firestone, S. *The Dialectic of Sex*. New York: William Morrow, 1971.

Freud, S. *The Ego and the Id*. Edited by James Strachey, translated by Joan Riviere. New York: W. W. Norton, 1962 (a).

————. *The Standard Edition of the Complete Psychological Works of Sigmund Freud*. Translated under the general editorship of James Strachey in collaboration with Anna Freud with the assistance of Alix Strachey and Alan Tyson. 24 vols. London: Hogarth Press, 1962 (b).

————. *Beyond the Pleasure Principle*. Edited and translated by James Strachey. New York: W. W. Norton, 1975.

Fromm, E. *Escape from Freedom*. New York: Irvington Publishers, 1941.

Hollingshead, A. B., and Redlich, F. C. *Social Class and Mental Illness*. New York: John Wiley, 1958.

Horney, K. *Neurosis and Human Growth*. New York: W. W. Norton, 1950.

Kallman, F. G. *Heredity in Health and Mental Disorder.* New York: W. W. Norton, 1953.

Kety, S. S. "Biochemical Theories of Schizophrenia." *Science* 129 (1959): 1528, 1590.

Laing, R. D. *The Politics of Experience.* New York: Ballantine Books, 1967.

Lemert, E. *Social Pathology.* New York: McGraw-Hill, 1951.

Mechanic, D. "Some Factors in Identifying and Defining Mental Illness." In *The Mental Patient: Studies in the Sociology of Deviance,* edited by S. Spitzer and N. K. Denzin. New York: McGraw-Hill, 1968.

Menninger, K. *The Vital Balance.* New York: Viking Press, 1963.

Meyer, A. *Collected Papers of Adolf Meyer.* 4 vols. Baltimore: Johns Hopkins University Press, 1948–1952.

Munroe, R. L. *Schools of Psychoanalytic Thought.* New York: Holt, Rinehart and Winston, 1955.

Norris, C. "Restlessness: A Nursing Phenomenon in Search of Meaning." *Nursing Outlook* 23 (1975): 74–78.

Scheff, T. *Being Mentally Ill: A Sociological Theory.* Chicago: Aldine, 1966.

Skinner, B. F. *Science and Human Behavior.* New York: Macmillan, 1953.

————. *Beyond Freedom and Dignity.* New York: Knopf, 1971.

Sullivan, H. S. *The Interpersonal Theory of Psychiatry.* Edited by H. S. Perry and M. L. Gawel. New York: W. W. Norton, 1953.

Szasz, T. S. *The Myth of Mental Illness: Foundations of a Theory of Personal Conduct.* New York: Harper and Row, 1974.

————, ed. *The Manufacture of Madness.* New York: Dell Publishing, 1971.

Williams, J. B. W., and Wilson, H. S. "A Psychiatric Nursing Perspective on DSM-III." *Journal of Psychosocial Nursing* 20 (1982): 14–20.

Wise, C. D., and Stein, L. "L. Dopamine Beta-Hydroxylase Deficits in the Brains of Schizophrenic Patients." *Science* 181 (1973): 384.

Wolpe, J. "Learning versus Lesions as the Basis of Neurotic Behavior." *American Journal of Psychiatry* 112 (1956): 923–31.

Further Reading

Boyers, R., ed. *R. D. Laing and Anti-Psychiatry.* New York: Harper and Row, 1971.

Gornick, V., and Morans, B. K., eds. *Woman in a Sexist Society: Studies in Power and Powerlessness.* New York: Basic Books, 1971.

Hilgard, R. R. *Theories of Learning.* New York: Appleton-Century-Crofts, 1956.

Kaufman, M. R. "Psychiatry: Why 'Medical' or 'Social' Model?" *AMA General Psychiatry* 17 (1967): 347–360.

Kosinski, J. *The Painted Bird.* Boston: Houghton Mifflin, 1965.

Krasner, L., and Ullmann, L. P., eds. *Research in Behavior Modification.* New York: Holt, Rinehart and Winston, 1965.

Milford, N. *Zelda: A Biography.* New York: Harper and Row, 1970.

Pothier, P. C. "Sensory Integration Therapy." In *Current Perspectives in Psychiatric Nursing: Issues and Trends,* vol. 2, edited by C. R. Kneisl and H. S. Wilson, pp. 4–13. St. Louis: C. V. Mosby, 1978.

Spitzer, S., and Denzin, N. K., eds. *The Mental Patient: Studies in the Sociology of Deviance.* New York: McGraw-Hill, 1968.

The Nurse's Personal Integration and Professional Role

CHAPTER OUTLINE

The Emergence of the Self
Consciousness of Meaning
Consciousness and Language
Negotiated Reality
Feelings: The Affective Self
Beliefs and Values
A Cognitive Framework for Self-Awareness
Taking Care of the Self
Assertiveness
Solitude
Personal Physical Health
Attending to Internal Stress Signals
Qualities of Effective Psychiatric Nursing
Respect for the Client
Availability
Spontaneity
Hope
Acceptance
Sensitivity
Vision
Empathy
The Value of Empathy in Nursing
Definition
Psychiatric Concepts of Empathy
The Therapeutic Use of Empathy
Steps in Therapeutic Empathizing
Burnout as a Consequence of Empathy

The Nurse's Professional Role
The Members of the Mental Health Team
The Psychiatric Nursing Clinical Specialist
The Registered Nurse Working in a Psychiatric Setting
The Psychiatrist
The Psychoanalyst
The Clinical Psychologist
The Psychiatric Social Worker
The Mental Health-Human Service Worker
The Psychiatric Aide or Attendant
The Occupational Therapist
The Recreational Therapist
The Creative Arts Therapist
Collaborating on the Mental Health Team
Cooperation versus Competition
Respect for the Positions of Others
Engaging the Client in Collaboration
Key Nursing Concepts

LEARNING OBJECTIVES

After reading this chapter, students should be able to
- Explore the concept of personal integration as it relates to the self and to psychiatric nursing practice
- Identify problems that influence personal integration

CHAPTER 3

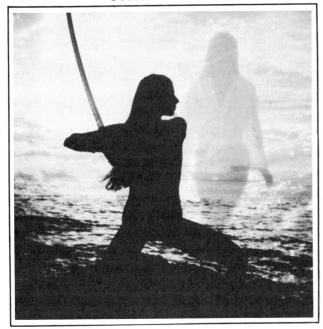

The quality and nature of a nurse's relationships are strongly influenced by the nurse's sense of personal integrity, self-awareness, self-image, and self-respect.

I hated psych—it just didn't seem like nursing to me. I really like to keep busy. When you change someone's dressing, you really feel like you've helped them. Here it's all so uncertain.

All I kept thinking about was that a lot of the patients had done really weird things. This one guy had lived in an apartment with his dead mother's body for three months before they brought him in. Another had tried to shoot the governor. I never felt safe even turning my back on them.

Many students and practitioners faced with relating to people whose behavior they view as offensive, frightening, curious, or socially inappropriate find that their personal attitudes, expectations, myths, and values make it difficult for them to fulfill their professional roles. This was the case in the following example.

* Relate these problems to some strategies for coping
* Describe the roles of members of the mental health team
* Identify the means by which collaboration on the mental health team is achieved

Penny, a baccalaureate nursing student, had selected a clinical placement at a methadone clinic in the community. Despite her initial interest, she developed a pattern of absences from clinical time. When her faculty adviser discussed this observation with her, she blurted out that, much to her surprise, she was unable to assist with the group meetings for pregnant heroin addicts. The thought of addicting babies before their births—babies who would ultimately suffer because of their mothers' self-indulgence—was totally despicable to Penny. She found herself judging their choices constantly and avoiding interaction with them. "I feel like they should be shot instead of given all this free support and sympathy."

The value of self-knowledge among psychiatric professionals is a recurring theme from the current and popular *human potential movement* to the sophisticated and esoteric discussions of *countertransference* in psychoanalytic circles. Libraries are stocked with volumes dealing with the undiscovered self, expanding human awareness, values clarification, strategies for self-realization, and the like. Common to all these references is the idea that the quality and nature of a practitioner's relationships with others are strongly influenced by the ways in which those interactions fit with the practitioner's self view. Consider the following comments made by students in their psychiatric nursing clinical experience.

This chapter will help nursing students and practitioners explore some dimensions of self-knowledge through an examination of the concepts of personal integration and professional role. Specifically, we will examine recurring problems that intersect with the nurse's identity and some strategies for coping with them. Our goal is to enhance the nurse's interactions with clients who may be labeled psychiatric patients.

I just can't take it. . . . I feel myself getting confused about who is the crazy one. There's such a fine line. Sometimes I think I'll be a patient here.

For many nurses, confrontation with deviance reinforces a personal sense of stability. Others are threatened by such confrontation.

One middle-aged psychiatric nurse, in recalling her childhood experiences with community deviants, commented on the intense and sometimes morbid excitement that she and her friends found in taunting "Crazy Helen" to run out on her porch and shout incoherently at the neighborhood children or in telling bizarre stories about a grotesque old man called "Charlie-No-Face," who walked along a road late at night chain smoking from the gaping hole that had once been a mouth.

The interest these characters held for the children, along with "Vince-the-Window-Peeper," "Red-the-Bum," and the other small-town deviants, was reawakened in her as she approached her first psychiatric nursing experience. It was all very frightening, yet seductive and stimulating at the same time. The nursing students gossiped about the bizarre histories of their assigned patients as if to reaffirm their separateness from them— their sense of being normal and okay.

Somehow dealing with people whose personal integration is fragmented, dissolving, divided, or alienated puts the nurse's own identity on the line as well. To respond with both compassion and the critical distance necessary to be effective, psychiatric professionals must confront their own identity; be able to separate it from another's identity, which may indeed be dissolving; and finally be able to integrate different values and behaviors comfortably in the therapeutic relationships they develop with clients.

This personal quality has been called *detached concern*—the ability to distance oneself in order to help others. It is an essential quality not only in avoiding *burnout*, a problem discussed later in this chapter, but also in *values clarification*, in ethical dilemmas, in using appropriate *assertiveness* when collaborating with colleagues, and in maintaining *empathic abilities* in highly stressful situations.

In the conventional focus on the patient or client, the nurse is regarded as the care giver, the provider of services, the therapist. Little attention is paid to the stresses experienced by psychiatric nurses attempting to relate fully to clients while maintaining their own personal integration. This chapter is an attempt to explore that aspect of psychiatric nursing.

THE EMERGENCE OF THE SELF

The concept of self is as elusive as a person's sense of true identity. Whatever else it is, however, it is clearly connected with people's appraisals of themselves and the appraisals others make of them. All social life is conducted in groups in which each member is guessing, assuming, inferring, believing, trusting, suspecting, pleased with, or tormented by the others' experiences, motives, and intentions as each interprets them. Like the images in a kaleidoscope, individual selves make up and are defined by the whole. There is individuality in the colors and shapes of the parts, yet there is order in the whole, and change is ever altering the form. In short, the self both emerges in interactions with others and influences those social interactions.

Human beings, by virtue of having selves, are not ruled by the stimulation of the environment or their biological drives. They can bring their personal behavior under conscious control, because they have the capacity to communicate with themselves, in other words, to think. Thus they can alter their own behavior, exercising guidance and control over it. Individuals are able to internalize the processes of interaction and communication with others in their world. The approaches and responses of others become incorporated into the self and influence the kind of communication people have with themselves. We need only observe a four-year-old talking to herself about cleaning up her room to see this phenomenon in action.

The way in which individuals view themselves depends to a large extent on the kinds of interactions they have had with *significant others*. The self emerges as two parts: an "I" and a "me," a "self for self" and a "self for others." The me or self for others arises in interactions with others in the social environment. This occurs in a process of role taking and rule following— interactions that acquaint the self with the expectations and reflections of others. It is by developing the me, however, that a person can begin to be aware of a subjective I. In being an object for others, the self develops as an entity reflecting the attitudes of significant others.

The appraisals of significant others and the individual's ways of relating to personal experiences are taken in and become part of the self-view. It does not take long for people to adopt qualities that are repeatedly attributed to them. When others treat a boy as if he were vain or self-indulgent, their message can evoke those very qualities in him through an intricate interplay with his own psychology. The treatment becomes a self-fulfilling prophecy. Significant others thus both prophesy and mirror the self. This notion does not suggest the individual self is utterly determined by others in the environment. A person *may* respond to well-organized cues with well-formed habits, but it is equally possible to reconstruct habits by making new interpretations of the situation. For example, the vain, self-indulgent boy who is nagged by others to be more responsible may view their comments as expectations that the old pattern will persist and continue his selfishness, or he may learn to reinterpret feedback from others as encouragement to grow and change.

Consciousness of Meaning

A unique feature of human integration is the ability to develop consciousness of meaning, that is, recognition of one's own attitudes and responses and the ability to interpret the gestures of others. Achievement of such a state requires perception of current sensory stimuli and imagery from past experiences in both memory and fantasy. Thus an individual's interpretation of the meaning of a situation cannot be separated from the person's history.

The ability to use language holds a central position in the ability to define, evaluate, and redefine situations. The ability to reappraise the meaning of situations allows people to change their courses and abandon old paths.

A young woman student dreaded the psychiatric nursing experience because "being around people who can't cope reminds me of my father." The possibility of reframing this understanding of past experiences enabled her to face the present more comfortably and to move beyond the here-and-now into the future.

Individuals who develop a satisfactory consciousness of self are said to have attained a state of *ontological security* or personal integrity. They view themselves as real, alive, and whole; as clearly differentiated from the rest of the world; as a continuum in time; as having an inner consistency, substantiality, genuineness, and worth; as spatially coextensive with their bodies; and as having begun at or around birth and being subject to extinction at death. All these qualities comprise the general notion of personal integration that is taken up in detail in the following pages. One of the most im-

portant tasks in life is identifying one's own sense of self. A concept of self does not form once and for all. Each experience challenges the individual's view of self, demands defenses of it, or permits further development of it.

Consciousness and Language

Consciousness necessitates the possibility of description. Description requires more than a series of unconnected words. It demands a series of sentences with internal organization. Helen Keller's (1902) experience emphasizes this difference. She first learned the use of words at the sign level, and only later grasped the use of language as symbolization, in a dramatic dawning of consciousness. Once Keller recognized that language could order her world, she passionately reviewed and regrasped every object of which she had been mutely aware.

Consciousness, depending as it does on language and the ability to describe, has the function of taking human thinking out of the here-and-now. Words have the magic power of enabling human beings to live in the mind. One logical extension of this idea is that reality becomes the inner, symbolic universe rather than the external, observable universe. To each person reality is something experienced, at least initially, as personal and subjective.

Negotiated Reality

Nurses often find that encounters with psychiatric clients are distancing experiences. The nurses become acutely aware of their difference and separateness from clients. They reaffirm their own subjective rendition of reality and rationalize their actions to keep these actions consistent with their sense of self as healthy, normal people.

Since people are all constantly building and protecting their own self-images, they try to get others to see their image of themselves. However, it is impossible to see another's self-image or world view exactly as it is being experienced by that person. Despite this fact, psychiatry has traditionally attempted to get certain people, labeled *crazy*, to assume the perspective of certain other people, called *therapists*.

A more acceptable alternative seems to lie in the creation of some common ground, a mutually understood, *negotiated reality*. Even to this common ground the nurse and the client bring their own conceptions, feelings, and attitudes toward and images of each other and themselves. In many instances the nurse's image of the client—how the nurse expects the client to act or feel—is not the same as the client's self-image. This causes a lot of confusion and hinders the establishment of therapeutic relationships and effective communication.

Feelings: The Affective Self

The ultimate effectiveness of efforts to relate to and communicate with others depends on how well people know themselves and develop the capacity for empathy. Self-awareness and empathic caring seem to go hand in hand. The fact that human beings are capable of empathizing with each other and trying to understand each other's attitudes and feelings makes social life possible. The fact that each human being is unique makes empathizing a difficult and challenging task. One of the ways to develop this ability is to practice it. Learning to be aware of one's responses to expression of feelings from another person is a starting point.

Josh is a middle-aged man who sought out nursing as a career. Although he is highly proficient in technical skills and charming and engaging in relationships with most clients, he discovers a surprising intolerance for some of the tears, complaints, and self-preoccupation of depressed clients. He finds himself responding with admonitions to stop it, to bite the bullet, to grow up. He personally has seldom allowed himself to experience his own sadnesses but jokingly characterizes himself as a firm believer in repression and denial. The need to empathize with people unable to control their feelings evoked such discomfort that he found himself unable to work with such clients.

Self-Awareness of Feelings Feelings seem like icebergs—only the tips stick up into consciousness, while the deeper parts are submerged. One such feeling is fear (see Figure 3–1). The conscious part may be experienced as dislike, avoidance, reluctance, etc. At a deeper level, the feeling will be reported as anxiety. Even deeper, the person may acknowledge, "I feel scared." Deeper yet, the person may experience genuine panic. Such an iceberg may well explain Josh's attitude toward tearful, depressed clients. His annoyance, irritation, sarcasm, and disdain may represent the tip of the iceberg of Josh's fear of depression.

Other feelings, such as love, hurt, and guilt, also occur in iceberg depths. A person feeling love may be aware only of a liking or attraction for another. Beneath the tip of that iceberg are feelings of warmth and affection. Deeper are feelings of love, and at the deepest level may be feelings of fusion or ecstasy.

Problems with Submerged Feelings One characteristic of icebergs of feeling is that at the tip the feelings lose their experiential quality and become translated into impulses to act. For example, a person with a lot of submerged guilt may express it by doing a lot of worrying and explaining and may be completely unaware of the underlying feelings. The behavior is the only outward manifestation. Being out of touch

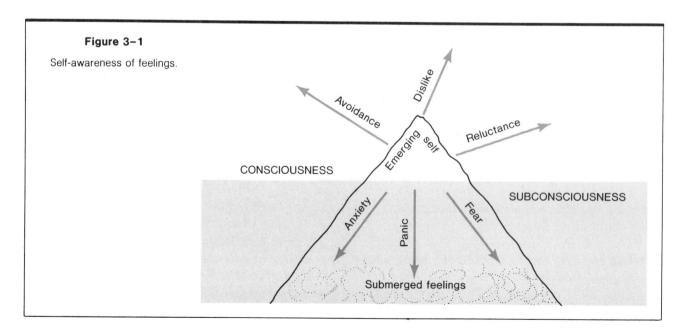

Figure 3–1

Self-awareness of feelings.

with their feelings lessens people's control over some of their behavior.

People lose touch with their feelings over time as they shape their sense of self. They hear messages saying "boys don't cry" or "girls are too sensitive," and they incorporate these injunctions into their emerging self system—especially into the "me" or "self for others." Not being sufficiently aware of one's feelings has several disadvantages:

- What people don't know *can* hurt them. Repressed feelings may reappear in behaviors that are harder to alter. For example, hidden anger may emerge in migraine headaches or a tendency to use sarcasm that alienates other people.
- When people are not aware of their feelings, it is more difficult for them to make decisions. It is hard to tell a "should" from a "wish." Without some awareness of their real wants, they may have trouble saying "no" or requesting something they need. They are more likely to rely on others—experts, authorities, rules and regulations, and so forth—for guidance.
- When people are "out of touch with" or unaware of their feelings, they, like Josh, the nurse in the example, may find it difficult to be really close and empathic toward others. Intimacy and empathy demand the expression of here-and-now feelings, whether positive or negative.

Most people realize the value of thinking clearly. They understand that it is a learned ability and takes practice. Feeling clearly (authentically) can also be practiced and learned. Most writers acknowledge that feelings are as important as facts, because they shape people's versions of reality as much as facts do. Becoming more aware of feelings begins with the search for one's dominant emotional themes.

Dominant Emotional Themes   Nurses need to ask themselves what are the dominant emotional themes in their personalities. If they find that they respond to many situations with the same feelings, they are probably narrowing their range of potential feelings.

Whatever the occasion, Marge used it to be tired or bored. Fatigue and chronically depressed states were ubiquitous in her personality. Holidays, vacations, dinner engagements all evoked the same predictable response.

Joan was afraid of everything. When she met me at the plane, her first question was, "Aren't you afraid of flying?" She was afraid driving home from the airport. The prospect of starting back to school scared her. She was even fearful about wearing a bikini to the swimming club.

When people feel the same way in a variety of situations, they may be missing a lot of what is happening in those situations. They look for and perceive only what will fit a narrowed range of feelings. Becoming aware of limited emotional themes is a way to begin to widen the range of feelings.

Acceptance of Disapproved Feelings   Most people have been taught to block off their awareness and expression of certain feelings. Children are taught that being rude or ungrateful or cranky is rarely acceptable to significant others. In order to retain love and approval, they usually comply, not by stopping the feelings but by acting as if they didn't have them. Nursing students often get similar messages from teachers. It is not acceptable to find a client repulsive, to dislike someone who is sick and dependent, to express anger at or criticism of physicians. Positive feelings of attraction and love may also seem unacceptable. Failure to recognize these feelings can interfere with interactions.

Recognizing and accepting their own feelings makes nurses less vulnerable to other people's ideas about how they should feel. Instead of feeling guilty when they don't feel what others imply they should feel, nurses come to realize that others merely disapprove of the way they do feel. When nurses can allow themselves the right to their own feelings more fully, they can allow clients the right to have and express their own feelings as well.

Beliefs and Values

Beliefs and values take three major forms.

1. Rational beliefs are beliefs supported by available evidence.
2. Blind belief is belief in the absence of evidence.
3. Irrational belief is belief held despite available evidence to the contrary.

Dogmatism includes both blind and irrational belief. Dogmatically held beliefs are not based on personal experience.

Ann argues that a client should be given electroshock treatment "because the client is depressed and the book says electroshock is beneficial in treating depression."

Operating on the basis of dogmatically held beliefs often causes nurses to distort their personal experiences of the world to fit their preconceptions. The following are examples of strongly held beliefs about behaviors that are labeled *mental illness* and about the people who do and don't engage in those behaviors:

- Most clients in mental hospitals are dangerous.
- People who are mentally ill let their emotions control them.
- Normal people think things out.
- If parents loved their children more, there would be less mental illness.
- When a person has a worry, it is best not to think about it.
- Many people become mentally ill just to avoid the problems of life.
- Most mental clients are lazy.
- People would not become mentally ill if they avoided bad thoughts.
- A woman would be foolish to marry a man who has had a mental illness.
- Anyone who is in a hospital for a mental illness should not be allowed to vote.
- To become a mental client is to become a failure in life.
- If a man in a mental hospital attacks someone, he should be punished so he doesn't do it again.
- Most clients in mental hospitals don't care how they look.
- One of the main causes of mental illness is a lack of moral strength.

Most research on strongly held beliefs indicates that people usually know more about the statements they believe than about those they don't believe. The process works like this: If people let themselves find out about those things they don't believe, they might find some validity in the statements. Then they would have to question the beliefs and disbeliefs they already hold.

By staying ignorant about anything they don't already agree with, they can avoid changing. This posture cuts off personal growth and learning that could be derived from the unknown. In *The Teachings of Don Juan: A Yaqui Way of Knowledge* (1968), the sorcerer Don Juan tells author Carlos Castaneda that reality is merely one of many descriptions of the way things are. People take this reality so much for granted that they hardly ever question it.

Feelings, Attitudes, and Opinions   A feeling is a transitory experience. When people feel a certain way toward something or someone over a period of time, it is called an attitude. When an attitude is linked to an idea or belief, it becomes an opinion. An opinion, then, involves both thinking and feeling. Research in this area has shown that people are more comfortable when their beliefs and attitudes are consistent with each other. There are several things people do to keep their attitudes and beliefs consistent:

- They repress the belief or attitude that seems inconsistent.
- They distract their awareness from conflict either physically (e.g., by leaving the room) or psychologically (e.g., by daydreaming).
- They distort their perceptions to fit an existing attitude or belief.

Similar maneuvers take place to keep actions consistent with attitudes or beliefs. Nurses often justify treating psychiatric clients inhumanely or unkindly by arguing that the clients deserved it or were asking for it.

Nurses need to be careful that their self-image—as people who act intelligently—does not keep them from seeing the world clearly. Some attitudes are inconsistent with beliefs or actions. It is probably preferable to acknowledge this point than to engage in the elaborate self-deceptions necessary to avoid it.

Arriving at Values   Every day, each person meets life situations that call for thought, opinion forming, decision-making, and action. At every turn in their personal and professional lives nurses are faced with choices. Their choices are based on the values they hold, but often those values are not really clear. People actively value something to the degree that they are willing to put energy into doing something about it. Their values are shown in their interests, preferences, decisions, and actions.

In talking with colleagues, Susan, a psychiatric nurse, claims to value interacting with clients more than doing paperwork. Yet a quick assessment of how she spends her time—all excuses taken into account—reveals that she acts on other values.

Mel, a nurse working in a state hospital ward for profoundly retarded children, claims that he believes these clients are human beings, despite their uncommunicative, immobile forms. He demonstrates this value in the hours he spends trying to communicate his presence and concern for them, using acupressure, touch, and physical ministrations performed slowly and with genuine feeling.

Table 3–1 SUBPROCESSES OF VALUING	
Subprocess	**Indicator**
Choosing beliefs and behaviors	Choosing from alternatives
	Choosing after considering consequences
	Choosing freely
Prizing beliefs and behaviors	Cherishing
	Publicly affirming
Acting on beliefs	Taking action
	Demonstrating a pattern of action that is consistent and repetitive

Source: Adapted from L. Raths, M. Harmin, and S. Simon, *Values and Teaching* (Columbus, Ohio: Charles E. Merrill Publishing Co., 1966), pp. 3–17.

The distinction in the above examples is between *cognitive* and *active values*. Susan verbally subscribed to values but failed to act on them. These were cognitive values. Mel's actions demonstrated more than lip service for his respect for the dignity of all living beings. He was following active values.

Valuing, according to most authorities, is composed of several hierarchically ordered subprocesses. These are presented, along with their behavioral indicators, in Table 3–1. The behavioral indicators in the phases move from those reflecting moderately held values to those that represent internalized philosophical commitments.

People may learn values in a number of ways:

- Moralizing is a direct, although sometimes subtle, method of inculcating desired values in someone else.
- The laissez-faire approach leaves people alone to forge their own set of values. This may create unnecessary frustration, conflict, and confusion, especially in young people or people being socialized into a profession such as nursing.
- Modeling, in which actions follow professed values, transmits values by setting a living example for a learner to follow.
- Values clarification is a systematic, widely applicable method of teaching the *process of valuing* rather than the content of any specific values. It uses strategies and exercises to engage learners in becoming aware of their beliefs and values, choosing among alternatives, and matching stated beliefs with actions.

The small amount of research comparing these four methods of learning values highlights the advantages of the fourth method. People who engage in values clarification are more zestful and energetic, more critical in their thinking, and more likely to follow through on their decisions than those who learn values in other ways. However, values clarification must be undertaken in circumstances that allow for sufficient follow-up with students who may uncover uncomfortable or disturbing values. A sample values clarification strategy is the individual integrity shield presented in Figure 3–2.

A Cognitive Framework for Self-awareness

There are many ways to think about self-awareness. Some theorists have used the image of multiple masks that people wear under various circumstances, others have written about the "true self" versus "the false self" or the "good me," the "bad me," and the "real me." Common to all these concepts is the idea that self-awareness is a complex, multidimensional phenomenon, often contradictory and partly undiscovered. One relatively clear and graphic interpretation of general self-awareness is the Johari Window (see Figure 3–3). Its name comes from the first names of the men who originated it—Joseph Luft and Harry Ingham (1963). The model delineates the types of self-awareness found in interpersonal relations.

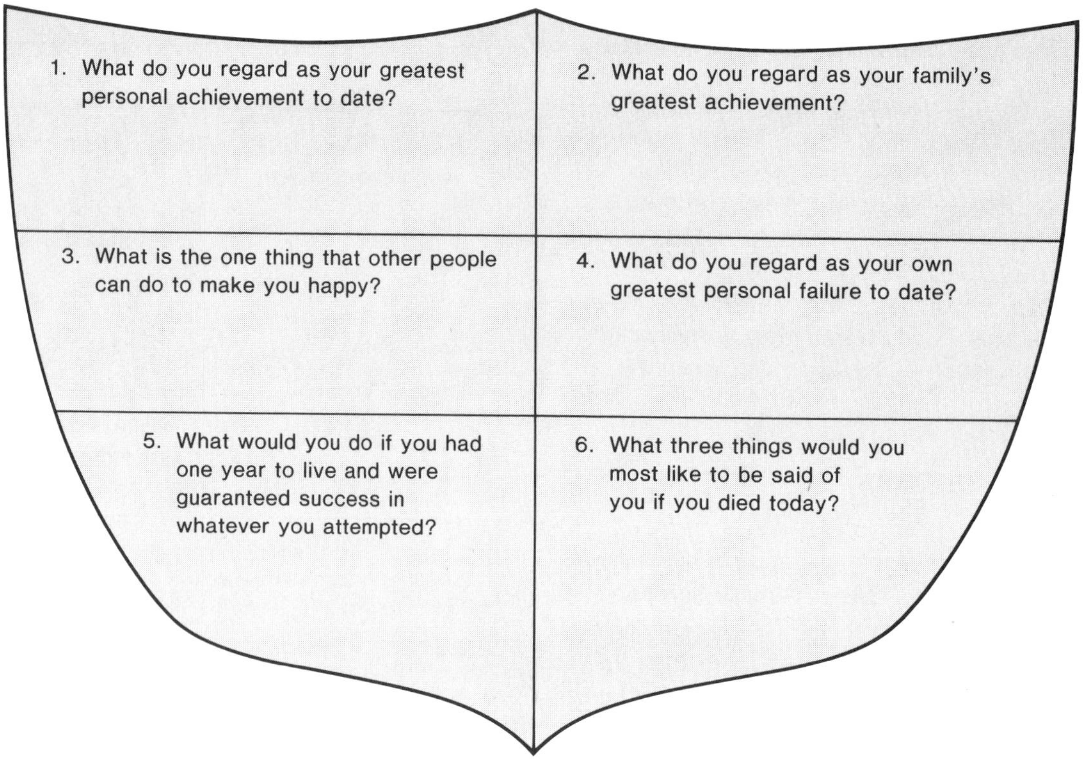

1. What do you regard as your greatest personal achievement to date?

2. What do you regard as your family's greatest achievement?

3. What is the one thing that other people can do to make you happy?

4. What do you regard as your own greatest personal failure to date?

5. What would you do if you had one year to live and were guaranteed success in whatever you attempted?

6. What three things would you most like to be said of you if you died today?

Procedure: Give the students a facsimile of the coat of arms or have them copy this coat of arms.

Students are to answer each of the following questions by drawing, in the appropriate area on their coat of arms, a picture, design or symbol. They are not to use words except in area 6.

Art-work doesn't count. The drawings can be simple, incomplete, and even unintelligible to others, as long as the student knows what they express.

Other questions may be substituted for these; for example:

1. What is something about which you would never budge?

2. What is something you are striving to become? Or to be?

3. What one thing would you want to accomplish by the time you are 65?

4. Draw three things you are good at.

5. What is a personal motto you live by?

Students may then share, in small groups, the drawings on their coats of arms, explaining the significance of the symbols. They may cover any drawing they would rather not share.

Posting the coats of arms and holding a gallery walk is another alternative.

Figure 3–2

Individual integrity shield: a sample values clarification exercise. (Adapted from Sidney B. Simon, Leland W. Howe, and Howard Kirschenbaum, *Values Clarification: A Handbook of Practical Strategies for Teachers and Students.* Copyright 1972, Hart Publishing Company, Inc. Acknowledgment is given to Sister Louise, former principal at the St. Juliana School of Chicago.)

Johari Window Quadrant 1—Open Activity
The first quadrant of the window represents aspects of the self known about oneself and readily available or known to others as well. This is the part of the self that engages in daily social conversation.

Johari Window Quadrant 2—Risk   Quadrant 2 contains characteristics known to others but not to oneself. In this quadrant is information about how the person affects others intentionally or unintentionally. It is an aspect of self about which a person may get honest, genuine, uncensored feedback from others. It is also an area that influences reactions from others that may surprise and shock the individual.

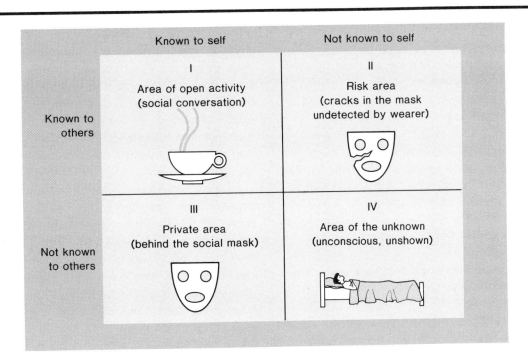

Figure 3-3

A model for self-awareness. (Adapted from Joseph Luft, *Group Process: An Introduction to Group Dynamics* by permission of Mayfield Publishing Company, formerly National Press Books. Copyright 1963, 1970 by Joseph Luft.)

Johari Window Quadrant 3—Private Life Space   Quadrant 3 represents the knowledge one has about oneself that is not known to others. These are the secrets, the personal and private feelings.

Johari Window Quadrant 4—the Unknown   Quadrant 4 contains knowledge about the self that is unconscious for the individual and unknown to others. This quadrant may be brought into awareness through free association, hypnosis, or dream analysis with special guidance.

The Johari Window, like the other ideas and exercises in this chapter, is designed to help explore images of the self. It is applied to the study of self-awareness in small group interaction in Chapter 18.

TAKING CARE OF THE SELF

Knowing who they are is just a beginning for nurses. Taking care of others requires that nurses respect and care for themselves. Assertiveness, solitude, physical health, and attending to personal stress are crucial to preserving the nurse's personal integration.

Assertiveness

"Do you ask for what you want? Or do you sit around hoping others will know what you want and give it to you? If you are not willing to ask for what you want directly, the odds are that you won't get it. When you ask, you may get it or you may not; but you've established your strength and caring for yourself and others by asking. It's never too late to begin asking for what you want."

This speech is paraphrased from an assertiveness training workshop for nurses. This workshop and others like it help nurses learn how to express themselves more effectively. Often people are either so timid that they do not get what they want or so aggressive and belligerent that they offend and alienate others. Assertiveness is asking for what one wants or acting to get it in a way that respects other people. It is the middle way between timid holding back and inconsiderate, offensive aggression. Assertiveness training exercises are designed to teach people to ask for what they want and also to refuse someone without feeling guilty. Following is a sample exercise:

Person A sits facing person B.

A asks B for something or to do something. It can be as simple as asking for a glass of water, or it can involve something that is more important.

When A has asked, B says "no."

A asks again in any way that A thinks might get a positive response.

B must refuse the request at least three times and may then continue to refuse for as long as he or she cares to. B doesn't ever have to give what A is asking for unless A puts it in a way that makes B feel like saying "yes."

A should pay attention to how he or she tries to get B to say "yes." How does A feel while asking? How does A feel when refused?

Then A and B switch roles and repeat the process. How does B try to get A to say "yes"? How does A refuse? How does A feel in doing it?

When both have finished, they talk with each other about what happened between them.

Solitude

Most people need time to be alone to assimilate what has happened in time spent with other people. They also need it for relief from responding to the demands of others. Aloneness need not mean physical distance. People can be alone in a crowded library. What is crucial is that they are making no demands on others and no one is making demands on them. Most people return to their relationships, work, and usual circumstances refreshed from a sanctioned time-out. Planning for time alone is highly preferable to reaching a breaking point and then aggressively and irresponsibly running away from others.

Personal Physical Health

An important way in which nurses take care of themselves is by providing for the physical health of their bodies. A proper diet, adequate rest, and exercise rejuvenate and restore the body. All these activities potentially make nurses more alive and better able to share this quality of aliveness with their clients.

Attending to Internal Stress Signals

Nursing students encountering emotionally disturbed clients commonly begin seeing in themselves all the "symptoms" about which they are learning. This is probably due more to heightened awareness of and attention to emotional aspects of their lives than to anything else. However, it is important for nurses to learn to recognize and respond to their own genuine stress signals. All people have times in their lives when they feel a little crazy. They may become very upset at small disturbances or see things out of proportion to their ultimate importance. These feelings are significant warning signals that the person is not coping adequately with stress.

"Crazy" times can be important turning points in people's lives. They are strong messages that change is needed. It is foolish to ignore these messages. British psychiatrist R. D. Laing has found that if people who have "gone crazy" are given supportive and nurturing conditions, they can often work through important matters while they are in this altered state of consciousness. According to Laing, these individuals emerge "saner than sane" and resume functioning at a higher level than people who are given heavy doses of suppressive drugs.

In their daily lives, nurses are often tempted to handle their own symptoms of stress by suppressing them with tranquilizers or other drugs. They could serve themselves better by really experiencing their feelings and attending to what the signals are saying.

Pain and suffering are sources of some of the most intensely experienced stresses in life. Events such as death of loved ones, divorce, illness, separation from loved ones, and failure are all part of the cycle of life's experience. Being told that they deserve it, or that they really don't have it so bad and therefore have no right to feel the way they feel does not help people cope with pain and suffering. They need to find ways of handling their suffering without being destroyed by it.

There is an old Buddhist teaching that a third of people's suffering is inevitable but they themselves create the rest of it. Realizing that pain and hardship are part of what it is to be a human being makes the pain a bit gentler. Frequently pain centers around losing or being afraid of losing something or someone valued—a job, mate, money, self-respect, etc. People want to continue what was instead of living with what is. It is important to attend to genuine feelings about the loss or prospective loss. They hold messages about what the sufferer needs to do. Some people need to replace what they have lost with something similar. Others need to explore a new dimension in their lives.

The alternative to experiencing pain is to live on the surface, out of touch with the real peak experiences in life as well as the painful ones. A more life-enhancing approach is to experience the whole thing.

QUALITIES OF
EFFECTIVE PSYCHIATRIC NURSING

Psychiatric nursing, according to the A.N.A.'s Congress for Nursing Practice, is "a specialized area of nursing emphasizing theories of human behavior as its scientific aspect and purposeful use of self as its art." Self-awareness, empathy, and moral integrity are all qualities that enable psychiatric nurses to practice the use of self artfully in therapeutic relationships. Some of the characteristics of artful therapeutic practice are: respect for the client, availability, spontaneity, hope, acceptance, sensitivity, and vision. Some of the most widely agreed upon standards are presented in Appendix A.

Respect for the Client

Many psychiatric clients behave in ways that indicate their loss of self-respect. Some may appear dirty and disheveled. Others may plead, beg, cry. Still others may try to do themselves physical harm. A relationship in which they experience a sense of dignity and receive messages that they are valued by the nurse is of inestimable value. The nurse can convey respect in relationships with clients by:

- Taking the time and energy to listen
- Not invalidating their experience of their world with comments such as, "It's not so bad," "Don't be that way," "Time heals all wounds," or "Keep a stiff upper lip"
- Giving clients as much privacy as possible during examinations or treatments or when they are upset
- Minimizing experiences that mortify clients and strip them of identity—allowing them to make as many of their own choices and be in control of as much of their own lives as possible
- Being honest with clients about medicines, privileges, length of stay, etc., even when the truth may be difficult to handle

Availability

Of all the members of the psychiatric team, the nurse has the richest opportunity to be available to clients when needed, at any time of day or night. Being with clients on a relatively constant basis places responsibility in the nurse's hands for:

- Creating a nurturing, healing milieu in the unit
- Assisting suffering clients to meet their basic human needs
- Collecting and conveying crucial data about clients that will influence decisions about them

Spontaneity

Many nurses have come to believe that therapeutic relationships with psychiatric clients require them to be stiff, stilted robots uttering clichés from a list of unnatural-sounding communication "techniques." Nurses who are comfortable with themselves, aware of therapeutic goals, and flexible about using a repertoire of possible interventions for any particular clinical problem will find that being natural and spontaneous is their most effective "technique." Clients experience such nurses as authentic. Each nurse is unique and will necessarily bring a different personal style to practice. We have different ways of putting the words together to convey to clients that we accept and care about them. Sometimes we say it with nonverbal behavior: keeping promises, coming on time, touching, and staying with a client who needs someone. We need to trust our own natural styles in working toward therapeutic goals.

Hope

Effective psychiatric nursing practice is characterized by hope and optimism that all clients, no matter how debilitated, have the capacity for growth and change. Even clients whose most marked attributes are chronicity and deterioration can be helped to some optimal level of well-being by a nurse who believes in their possibilities and is willing to search for some strengths to build on. In one locked ward of a huge government psychiatric hospital, a chronic client joined in a partnership with a creative nurse to assist less able clients toward self-care. It is not unusual in such a situation for the healing to become a source of help to the healer-client.

Acceptance

There is a distinction between acceptance and approval. Acceptance means refraining from judging and rejecting a client who may behave in a way the nurse dislikes. Therapeutic work requires that clients be able to examine, explore, and understand their coping mechanisms without feeling the need to cover up or disguise them in order to avoid negative judgments or punishments from the therapist. Nurses who tell clients that they should say or do or feel a certain thing deny these clients the acceptance they need to explore their problems.

Sensitivity

Genuine interest and concern provide the basis for a therapeutic alliance. Clients will recognize the falseness of memorized phrases and assumed postures considered indicative of sensitive behavior. The nurse conveys general interest and concern by trying to understand the client's perspective, working with the client on mutually formulated goals, and persisting even when breakthroughs and improvements are subtle and slow instead of dramatic and quick.

Vision

Because psychiatric nurses focus their work on enhancing the quality of life for all human beings, they must come to terms with a personal and professional vision of what quality means. Conditions of life associated by some writers with high quality are: influence or power, freedom and accountability—self-determinism, openness to gratifying experience, action, mastery, a sense of purpose or meaning, privacy, hope, stability, nonviolence, and intimacy.

EMPATHY

The Value of Empathy in Nursing

Psychiatric nurses are instructed to engage in "therapeutic use of self." They are told that their "relationship" with a client is the primary therapeutic tool, that they should demonstrate qualities of sensitivity and caring. For many beginning students, these instructions are mysterious jargon quite unlike the clear-cut step-by-step procedures they learn for some physical treatments.

I found myself watching the nurses on the unit and my instructors closely when they talked with the clients. Somehow I thought maybe by imitating things that they did or said I'd figure out what "being therapeutic" was supposed to mean. I knew it had something to do with things the nurse said or didn't say when she talked with

the clients. But it all got very fuzzy to me beyond that very elementary grasp of it. I used to latch onto ideas like "Agreeing is untherapeutic. So is giving advice or opinions." The only entries I felt safe in putting down in my process-recording were stiff-sounding reflections, like "You sound angry."

Telling nurses to use themselves as therapeutic tools when relating to psychiatric clients can be meaningless unless faculty members are clearer and more specific about it. Comprehension of and ability to use the process of empathy gives the nurse one strategy for responding to the feelings of aloneness often experienced by persons labeled psychiatric clients. Nurses are taught skills of active listening. But listening is not enough without empathy. Empathic understanding not only increases the nurse's grasp of the client's difficulties but also provides a basis for offering feedback on how the client affects others. Perhaps its most important function is to enable the nurse to give the client the very precious feeling of being understood and cared about.

Definition

Empathy is a pervasive phenomenon in the life experience of all people. It allows people to feel the feelings of another and respond to and understand that person's experience on his or her terms. A nurse empathizing with a client momentarily abandons the personal self and relives the emotions and responses of someone else. People in everyday life tend to empathize most with those to whom they feel closest. In psychiatric practice, nurses often seek to empathize with persons from whom they feel most separate or whose closeness threatens their own sense of integration.

Empathy has been defined as a subtle imitation through which people assume an alien personality. They become aware of how it feels to behave in a certain way and then feed back into the other person's consciousness this awareness and sensitivity to what the behavior feels like (Ehmann 1971). Empathy characteristically develops early in an infant's pattern of relating to its parents. Tension or anxiety in the parent, for example, induces anxiety in the baby.

Psychiatric Concepts of Empathy

Intimacy is closely related to empathy. Psychoanalytic theory postulates the development of empathy as a process of "mutual incorporation." The mother compensates for her loss of biological oneness with the infant at birth by establishing a primitive unity with the child during the first weeks and months of life—an emotional bonding. The child likewise views the mothering parent as incorporated into its sense of self. Once the child begins to see the mothering parent as a being separate from itself, identification replaces incorporation, and the child experiences the mother as one to imitate in order to secure love and comfort. From identification comes the capacity for empathy. Identification enables human beings to achieve a clearer sense of self, to gain another person's point of view, and to establish an intimate association with others.

People have the capacity to identify not only with contemporaries but also with those who have been significant in the past. Adults can empathize through past, present, and future identifications. Psychiatric nurses must be able to shift from one identity to another without losing their own sense of integration.

Social interactionists discuss empathy as *role taking,* a process through which people feel with one another. They are able to sense the feelings of another because they have aroused in themselves the attitude of the person to whom they are relating. George Herbert Mead, the best-known articulator of the symbolic interactionist perspective, sees role taking among children as a necessary part of social life. It is a means for developing the sense of self and of learning methods for adjusting to society. Mead likens role taking to learning to play games, in which children not only learn to enact their own roles but also become fully aware of the roles of others.

People form an image of themselves because they have learned to assume the roles of others and have developed the ability to see themselves as others see them. The other then is like a mirror in which they see themselves, and that mirror becomes the source of their own image of themselves as persons. According to Mead, faulty ability to take roles is the result of limited opportunity for role experimentation. Individuals who have not experimented enough fail to develop a clear sense of their own integration and thus cannot shift from the role of participant to that of observer.

The capacity for empathy relies on personal integration. Whether problems with empathy are seen as the atrophy of primitive instincts for imitation in the psychoanalytic framework or as the result of inadequate opportunities for role experimentation in the social psychologist's view, the conclusion is the same. A firm sense of self is necessary for a person to be a good empathizer. As people continue to interact with others, they learn to be sensitive to others without losing their own integration.

The Therapeutic Use of Empathy

From time to time we hear accounts of dramatic and surprising breakthroughs with psychiatric clients. There are instances in which the usual tools of systematic, logical problem solving and the application of theory seem to be getting nowhere. Instead therapists fall back for a moment on their empathic sensitivity and get an inside comprehension of some complex emotion. This empathic understanding may be a key to establishing trust with a sullen, withdrawn, suspicious adolescent, or beginning verbal interaction with a chronically mute institutionalized person, or controlling the violent flailing rage of an emotionally disturbed child. In all these instances, empathy is used as a therapeutic tool.

The term *empathy* is often mistakenly used synonymously with *sympathy,* and this confusion is misleading. Empathy contains no elements of condolence, agreement, or pity. When nurses sympathize, they assume that there is a parallel between their feelings and those of the client. The analogy between them makes good judgment and objectivity difficult. Empathy also should be differentiated from *identification.* Identification is generally thought to be an unconscious process and only the initial phase of the empathizing process.

Steps in Therapeutic Empathizing

The process of empathic understanding has four phases:

1. *Identification:* Through relaxation of conscious controls, we allow ourselves to become absorbed in contemplating the client and the client's experiences.

2. *Incorporation:* We take in the experiences of the client rather than attribute our own experiences and feelings to the client.

3. *Reverberation:* We interplay the internalized feelings of the client and our own experiences or fantasies. While fully absorbed in the identity of the client, we still experience ourselves as separate personalities.

4. *Detachment:* We withdraw from subjective involvement and totally resume our own identity. We use the insight gained from the reverberation phase as well as reason and objectivity to offer responses that are useful to the client.

Burnout as a Consequence of Empathy

After hours, days, and months of listening to other people's problems, something inside you can go dead and you don't care anymore. That's when you'd rather sit at the desk and do the paperwork than be out talking to clients on the floor.

The nurse speaking illustrates one of the possible consequences of using empathy when working intensely with troubled people. *Burnout* is the name given this phenomenon, and it happens to poverty lawyers, social workers, clinical psychologists, child-care workers, prison personnel, and others who struggle to retain both their objectivity and their empathic concern for the disturbed people with whom they work.

Burnout is a condition in which health professionals lose their concern and feelings for their clients and come to treat them in detached or even dehumanized ways. It is an attempt to cope with the stresses of intense interpersonal work by a form of distancing. It hurts not only clients but also psychiatric professionals, in that they become ineffective and dissatisfied.

One nurse noted that her emotions shifted dramatically, first toward cynical feelings, then negative ones about her clients. "I began to despise every one of them and couldn't conceal my contempt for them." Another reported, "I found myself caring less and less and feeling really negative about the clients here." In many cases, burning out involves not only thinking in derogatory terms about the clients but also believing that somehow they deserve any problem they have.

There is little doubt that burnout plays a major role in the poor delivery of psychiatric care. It is also a key factor in low staff morale, absenteeism, and high job turnover.

Cues to Burnout   Cues to burnout can be found in the language used to depict clients. Burnout victims may refer to their clients as "crocks," "vegetables," "wackos," "brown baggers," and so forth, or they may become highly analytic and abstract: "That's just a manifestation of his primary process thinking."

Another cue is lack of involvement with clients. Some nurses "hide" in the nurses' station or staff conference room to avoid interacting. Some openly reject bids for human contact.

A newly admitted client tearfully pleads at the nurses' desk. "Will you listen to me! Can't you come down to my room to sit with me? I want to lie down. I need somebody." The nurse replies, "No, I'm not going to send somebody to babysit you and hold your hand. Are you an infant?" The client replies, "No, I'm just scared." The nurse retorts, "Then stay out of your room. Doesn't that make sense?"

Another withdrawal technique involves "going by the book" rather than considering the unique factors in a situation. It is a way of minimizing personal involvement with the client. By rigidly applying the rules, the nurse can avoid having to think about the client's specific problems. Burnout can transform an original and creative nurse into a mechanical bureaucrat.

Another cue to burnout is derogatory joking among staff members, which makes their work less frightening and overwhelming.

When the nurse is asked where Mr. G is, she laughingly reports that he's taking a shower in preparation for his MMPI test. Everyone in the nurses' station breaks up in gales of laughter.

Staff members on one psychiatric ward referred to their morning meeting as the "laugh-in" show and their discussions of the clients as their sociopathy.

In a discharge conference, the psychiatrist says he'd like to discharge E, a young male client with a history of violent outbursts. The nurse replies, "With or without baseball bat?" and everyone chuckles.

Reducing Burnout   Most research indicates that the causes of professional burnout are rooted not in the permanent psychological characteristics of individuals but rather in the social context of their work (Maslach 1976). A number of strategies can therefore be used to reduce and modify its occurrence:

• Keep staff–client ratios low. Staff members can then give more attention to each client and have time to focus on the positive, nonproblem aspects of the client's life.

• Provide for sanctioned breaks rather than guilt-arousing escapes from the work situation for staff members.

• Provide some relief from prolonged direct client contact, through shorter work shifts, or rotating work responsibilities, so that certain staff members are not always working directly with clients.

• Set up formal or informal programs in which staff members can talk over their problems to get advice and support when they need it.

• Encourage staff members to express, analyze, and share their feelings about burning out. Not only does this allow them to get things off their chests, but also it gives them the chance to get constructive feedback from others and perhaps a new perspective as well.

• Encourage staff members to understand their own motivations in pursuing a psychiatric career and to recognize their expectations for work with clients. Nurses can be on a variety of "ego trips," in which their primary purpose is to deal with their own personal problems, not those of the clients.

Empathic involvement with troubled clients can have a number of stressful consequences for the nurse in addition to burnout. Problems can arise at any phase in the empathy process. The nurse may overidentify and lapse into sympathy for the client. The nurse may fail to incorporate the client's feelings and instead project personal ones. The nurse may bypass the reverberation phase, and substitute gut-level intuitions for rational problem solving. At the detachment phase, the nurse may experience overdistancing or burnout. Each of the common obstacles to achieving an empathic concern for clients can be understood as a failure to cope with one of the four phases of achieving empathy. Burning out has been given particular attention here because it is common and is less psychological than circumstantial. It therefore is not inevitable and can be prevented with thoughtful planning.

THE NURSE'S PROFESSIONAL ROLE

The nurse is only one of many persons who works with clients in mental health settings. The American Nurses' Association Standards for Psychiatric–Mental Health Nursing Practice (see Appendix A) recognizes that activities such as assessing, planning, implementing, and evaluating programs are interdisciplinary. They need to be coordinated to meet the mental health needs of clients. This section addresses the coordination of mental health activities; identifies the members of the health team and the nature of their relationships; and discusses how, why, and what they communicate.

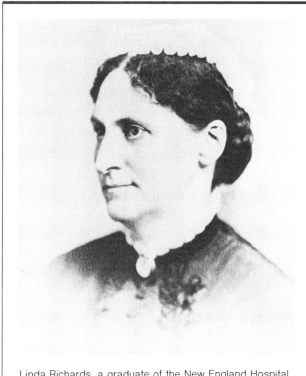

Linda Richards, a graduate of the New England Hospital for Women in Boston, is often considered "the first American psychiatric nurse."

THE MEMBERS OF THE MENTAL HEALTH TEAM

Role definitions have become increasingly blurred among mental health workers as various members of the mental health team have taken on tasks traditionally assigned to other disciplines. This role blurring is perceived as having positive consequences at times and negative ones at others. It has increased the quantity and raised the quality of one-to-one care in mental health settings. It has also increased the anxiety and sense of personal threat experienced by professionals whose comfortable, safe niches have been invaded. Some of the role changes have created anxiety among nurses who have become more interpersonally involved, more autonomous, and more responsible for the quality of mental health services delivered to the consumer. Psychiatrists, the traditional heads of mental health teams, have suffered some anxiety as other mental health workers and clients have sought to share in decision making and as other capable professionals have assumed administrative functions. In many settings, clinical nurse specialists, social workers, and psychologists, among others, have more direct influence than ever before. Roles are less specifically defined, and mental health professionals take on whichever functions they do best.

The descriptions below of the education and tasks of mental health team members reflect more traditional lines. Students should keep in mind that many of the functions are now shared across disciplines when the team member has been educated for the task and when laws permit the sharing of functions.

The Psychiatric Nursing Clinical Specialist

The clinical specialist in psychiatric nursing is a graduate of a master's program providing specialization in the clinical area. A number of colleges and universities provide graduate study in adult, child, adolescent, and family psychiatric nursing and in community mental health liaison psychiatric nursing as well. Nurses may also pursue a doctoral degree in two to four more years of study. A list and description of accredited programs at the master's and doctoral levels is available from the National League for Nursing, 10 Columbus Circle, New York, New York 10019. The National Institute of Mental Health funds some programs, providing stipends and tuition-free study for qualified full-time students. However, federal funding for graduate study in psychiatric nursing has recently been reduced.

Clinical specialists may also seek certification by a professional nursing body. This attests to advanced level competence, and is a means of protecting consumers. Certification programs at the advanced level exist in the states of New York and New Jersey and nationally through the American Nurses Association divisions on nursing practice. Although other mental health professions, such as psychiatry, psychology, and social work, have well-established certification programs, certification for psychiatric nurses is a relatively recent phenomenon.

Clinical specialists in psychiatric settings provide individual, family, and group psychotherapy in inpatient, outpatient, community mental health, and private practice milieus. They also provide indirect services, teach, consult, administer, and do research. The liaison psychiatric nurse provides these services in general hospital settings. The specific role of the liaison psychiatric nurse is considered in Chapter 24. The questions and answers in the chart on pp. 58–59 summarize the information a nurse might provide to a client or community group about the clinical specialist role in the state of New Jersey.

The Registered Nurse Working in a Psychiatric Setting

The *registered nurse in a psychiatric setting* may have received basic nursing preparation in a diploma, associate degree, or baccalaureate program. (According to the A.N.A. the only registered nurse eligible to use the title *psychiatric nurse* is one who is a graduate of a baccalaureate program in nursing.) Basically a generalist who works in a specialized setting, this nurse provides the bulk of the nursing care to clients in inpatient settings. Registered nurses offer direct and indirect care through the nurse–client relationship, although they are not prepared at the psychotherapy level. They have major responsibility for the milieu and have contact with clients at all stages of daily life.

Continuing education programs, in-service programs, and workshops are available to registered nurses who wish to become more proficient but are not engaged in a program of formal study at the master's level. Colleagues who are clinical nursing specialists may provide supervision of and consultation in the registered nurse's therapeutic work.

Nurses at this level may be certified as generalists through the A.N.A. rather than as clinical specialists as described earlier.

The Psychiatrist

The psychiatrist is a physician whose specialty area is mental disorders or mental diseases. Certification in psychiatry by the American Board of Psychiatry and Neurology requires that the physician serve a three-year approved psychiatric residency, engage in two years of clinical psychiatric practice, and successfully complete an examination. Certification in neurology requires further preparation through a two-year neurology residency and an additional examination.

Psychiatrists are responsible for diagnosis and treatment. They are the only members of the mental health team who are allowed by law to prescribe medications and somatic treatments. Some are oriented primarily toward biological therapies, others are psychotherapeutically inclined, and a few are chiefly interested in community psychiatry. In traditional medical model settings and in most inpatient settings, the psychiatrist is usually the team leader or administrator. This is not so in milieus where role distinctions are less clearly defined.

The Psychoanalyst

In the United States, a person must be a physician in order to become a *psychoanalyst.* Analysts are trained at psychoanalytic institutes that provide training programs in psychoanalysis only. The majority of psychoanalysts are in private practice in large urban settings. They may also be certified in the practice of psychiatry, neurology, and/or psychoanalysis. There are non-physician analysts, called *lay analysts,* who are also trained at psychoanalytic institutes. Some nurses have become lay analysts.

The Clinical Psychologist

The *clinical psychologist* is a psychologist specially educated and trained in the area of mental health. In order to be certified, the clinical psychologist must hold a doctoral degree from a program approved by the American Psychological Association and must have completed a one-year psychology internship at an approved clinical facility.

Clinical psychologists perform psychotherapy; plan and implement programs of behavior modification; select, administer, and interpret psychological tests in various mental health settings, including private practice; and carry out research. Their contribution to psychological testing and evaluation is unique.

The Psychiatric Social Worker

The *psychiatric social worker* is a graduate of a two-year master's program in social work with an emphasis in the field of psychiatry. Social workers deal with the full range of social problems that confront clients and their families. Their goal is to help clients and their families cope more effectively. The social worker may also help identify appropriate community resources for clients.

Traditionally, the social worker has helped the hospitalized person maintain relationships with family, friends, and the community and has facilitated the client's return to the community. With the blurring of traditional mental health roles, social workers have undertaken counseling and psychotherapeutic roles in various settings, including private practice.

The Mental Health/Human Service Worker

The newest addition to the roster of persons on the psychiatric team is the *mental health/human service worker.* These "indigenous nonprofessionals" were initially recruited into the mental health delivery system to bridge the gap between middle-class-oriented professionals and clients from lower socioeconomic or otherwise disadvantaged populations: drug-addicts, alcoholics, the aged, the chronically mentally ill, and rural communities.

The growing need for mental health services, the manpower crisis, the widespread popularity and economy of community college programs, and the documented effectiveness of these workers are responsible for the emergence of more than 400 mental health/human service training programs at the certificate, associate, and baccalaureate levels. The Council for Standards in Human Service Education, Inc. of the Southern Regional Educational Board establishes standards for, and reviews and approves these programs.

The Psychiatric Aide or Attendant

Paraprofessionals provide much of the direct service to hospitalized persons, particularly in large public facilities. These nonprofessional workers are known by a variety of titles, including *psychiatric aide, psychiatric technician,* and *psychiatric attendant.* Most agencies that employ psychiatric aides provide in-service training programs to help them use their interpersonal potential. Because a large number of the personnel who work in inpatient settings are psychiatric aides, it is extremely important that they maintain a therapeutic milieu under the supervision of professional nurses.

The Occupational Therapist

Occupational therapists in mental health settings use manual and creative techniques to elicit desired interpersonal and intrapsychic responses. They focus on the psychological aspects of rehabilitation through arts and crafts. In some settings they may participate in preparing clients for return to community living by teaching self-help activities or, in sheltered workshop settings, help clients prepare to seek employment. Occupational therapists prepare for their careers in college and university programs. The Occupational Therapist, Registered (OTR) has completed a baccalaureate degree in occupational therapy or a master's degree in occupational therapy after receiving a baccalaureate in another field. The OTR may also participate in research and administration, and supervises Certified Occupational Therapy Assistants (COTA). A COTA is a graduate of an associate degree program and helps clients follow treatment plans.

MENTAL HEALTH SERVICES PROVIDED BY
CLINICAL SPECIALISTS IN PSYCHIATRIC NURSING

WHAT is a *clinical specialist in psychiatric nursing?*

. . . a registered professional nurse, licensed to practice in N.J.

. . . an R.N. with at least a master's degree plus a wide variety of experience working with many patients in hospitals, clinics, private offices, in communities

. . . an R.N. who is a *specialist* in *clinical* psychiatric nursing, i.e., this person was first a general nurse who went on to specialize in the psychiatric nursing field becoming expert in working directly with patients (versus being a nurse administrator, educator, or researcher).

WHAT can a clinical specialist in psychiatric nursing do for me or my family?

. . . provide consultation about emotional difficulties or distress just for you alone, or for you and your family together—for young children, teenagers, and adults

. . . help you, your family, or your spouse cope better with crises, stress, or those unexpected shattering episodes in life, e.g., unusual prolonged grief in death of a loved one, divorce, or other stressful separations, a severe loss, depression that's worse than the "blues," those feelings of being "mixed up" which continue no matter what you try to do, those nagging fears that something is wrong with you, continued feelings that you just can't mobilize yourself to do what you have to do, anger that often just "gets the best" of you no matter how hard you try to control it, a drinking or drug problem, physical abuse, or those feelings deep inside that things just don't go well enough for you most of the time, leaving you very troubled

. . . do individual psychotherapy

. . . do group psychotherapy

. . . do family therapy, crisis therapy

. . . may direct you to other resource people in the health field

WHERE do I locate a clinical specialist in psychiatric nursing?

. . . write to or call The New Jersey State Nurses' Association, ask for a Directory of Certified Clinical Specialists in Psychiatric Nursing in N.J.

. . . inquire at your local community mental health center

. . . call your local hospital; ask if clinical specialists in psychiatric nursing work there

. . . ask your local clergyman or family physician if they know a clinical specialist in psychiatric nursing

. . . inquire from a clinical psychologist, psychiatrist, psychiatric social worker or from other registered nurses whom you might know.

HOW will I know if the clinical specialist I contact is really professionally competent?

. . . this specialist is a licensed registered professional nurse

. . . this specialist has a bachelor's degree (probably 4 years of college) and a master's degree in the specialty area of clinical psychiatric nursing (probably 2 years of post-graduate study)

. . . this specialist has had a lot of well supervised clinical experience during and after getting a master's or doctoral degree

. . . this specialist is *certified* by The Society of Certified Clinical Specialists in Psychiatric Nursing of the New Jersey State Nurses' Association and/or by The American Nurses' Association

. . . these specialists must continually subject their qualifications for professional approval; they must keep up to date on the latest knowledge and methods of help available in the psychiatric field

. . . they are responsible, professional, accountable— and they do care about you!

WHAT can a clinical specialist do that a psychiatrist, clinical psychologist or psychiatric social worker can't do for me?

ALL of these professionals work clinically to help people with emotional or psychological difficulties or problems.

. . . the clinical specialist in psychiatric nursing brings one unique asset to the health care given, i.e., as registered nurses who have become specialists in their field, they bring with them the total background of day-to-day and hour-to-hour, ripened and complete humanitarian caring for people. They not only give the medication prescribed by the physician, but they have been there to tell the patient about it, to be with the patient, and to observe for signs of improvement—they have been directly and interpersonally *there.* This strong background in the total on-going care of people helps them to know physical needs (what's normal or what's a problem) as well as to know psychological or emotional needs (again, what's usual or what's a real difficulty for you). They've learned a lot about normal growth and how people develop from birth through all the ages of living. From this, the clinical specialist can tell if what's happening with you is to be expected and therefore something you'll adjust to with time. The specialist can tell if there is a problem that you really could use some sound professional help in solving. Nurse specialists have always been closely involved with their patients through counseling, teaching, guiding, and instructing. Some go into the home of the patient when needed, some see you in clinics, hospitals, out-patient departments, community health centers, schools, and in industry.

WHAT are some things that a clinical specialist cannot do?

. . . they can't prescribe medications. Instead, if you do need medicine, they will suggest you see a medical doctor or your own family physician whom you already know. They might suggest why you might need medication and will explain it to you. They will be there during your therapy to oversee your response to the medicine and to answer any questions you might have then or later

. . . they do not do psychological testing

. . . they do not have professional rights to admit you to a hospital.

WHAT do clinical specialists charge for their professional services?

. . . their fees vary and are fairly comparable to those of other professional mental health workers, e.g., those of psychiatrists, of clinical psychologists, of psychiatric social workers

. . . most clinical specialists will consider your ability to pay; they take your own financial situation into account when the fee is determined

. . . some specialists have a standard fee for the initial consultation you will seek; some have a standard fee for service regardless of circumstance

. . . a good guess is this: the clinical specialist in psychiatric nursing might be more accessible for you. While they are busy professionals, you usually do not have to wait months for an appointment.

HOW LONG is an appointment with a clinical specialist?

. . . this depends on whether the specialist works in a clinic, hospital, community mental health center, or private office; it depends on the specialist's own particular way of practicing; and it depends on your particular needs

. . . individual therapy sessions or consultation sessions vary in length from usually 30 minutes to 60 minutes; group or family therapy sessions average about an hour and a half

. . . you might see a clinical specialist just once for consultation or you might want or need continuing therapy—maybe on a weekly basis, or less often or more often.

This all depends on what YOU need and on YOUR motivation as well as on just what the specialist's practice involves. Ultimately, a joint acceptable decision is made by you and the specialist in terms of health care.

HOW LONG does psychiatric help from a clinical specialist take?

. . . this depends on what your needs or problems are; it depends on your motivation and what you desire in your living

. . . therapy, if you need it, can be short term (maybe once a week for 11 or 12 times) or long term (once or twice a week for several months or longer). Long-term therapy doesn't mean you're severely disturbed at all— perhaps you really want to understand yourself or perhaps you want to really change some of the major ways you cope with certain situations

. . . the method of therapy, whether it is counseling, individual therapy, group therapy, family therapy, crisis therapy, will also influence the length of care

. . . YOU have something to say about this, too. You are the consumer of the health services provided by the specialist. You have a right to your own assessment and the specialist has professional opinions and standards to uphold in providing care.

Your own life experiences have made you into the unique and special human being that you are. The health care and time needed for it may be just as individualized as you are!

WHAT special kind of theory, formula, or system do clinical specialists use in the mental health care services they provide?

. . . all kinds that are professionally acceptable

. . . some use a particular theory or approach while others may use a variety of theories or methods; some are Freudian or analytic; some work mainly with communication problems; others work mainly with crisis situations; some work with groups or with families; some deal with the framework or situation in which your problems arise

. . . YOU simply ask the clinical specialist what she or he does.

WHERE do clinical specialists work?

. . . many specialists have private offices and private practices of psychotherapy

. . . other specialists might work with a psychiatrist, clinical psychologist, psychiatric social worker or with other nurse specialists—a specialist might be a member of a health care team

. . . some specialists work in hospitals, clinics, centers, and other community agencies concerned with mental health.

Making good use of professional psychiatric help requires your hard work. If you want it, the help *is* available—not only from clinical specialists in psychiatric nursing but from other professionals in mental health as well.

Prepared by the Society of Certified Clinical Specialists in Psychiatric Nursing of the New Jersey State Nurses Association, May 1980. Reprinted by permission.

The Recreational Therapist

The *recreational therapist* plans and guides recreational activities to provide not only socialization and healthful recreation but also desirable interpersonal and intrapsychic experiences. Recreational activities are based on the therapeutic needs of clients. With increasing frequency recreational therapists are being prepared in university physical education and health education programs.

The Creative Arts Therapist

Creative arts therapists use art, music, dance, and poetry to facilitate personal experiences and increase social responses and self-esteem. Although creative arts therapists are not found in all settings, they are becoming valued and recognized members of the mental health team. Programs of study are available in universities to prepare art, music, dance, or poetry therapists. Creative arts therapists have their own professional organizations, such as the American Art Therapy Association, the American Dance Therapy Association, and the National Association for Music Therapy. Chapter 18 discusses art, music, dance, and poetry therapy groups.

COLLABORATING ON THE MENTAL HEALTH TEAM

Mental health personnel should seldom function totally autonomously. Psychiatric nursing practice, whether in institutions or in private practice settings, requires planning and sharing with others to deliver maximum mental health services to clients. The purpose of collaboration is to use the different abilities of mental health team members to give the client the most effective service available. Relationship problems among mental health team members must be worked through to avoid distorting the team's efforts in behalf of the client.

Cooperation versus Competition

Working together on a common problem for a common purpose is best facilitated by cooperation rather than competition. Cooperation ensures movement toward the common goal, while inappropriate competi-

tion hinders goal achievement and may be destructive to the competing individuals.

Most of the present understanding of cooperative and competitive behavior has come from the efforts of game theorists, who have researched player behavior. Players have been categorized as:

- Maximizers—those interested only in their own gain
- Rivalists—those interested only in defeating their partners
- Cooperators—those interested in helping both themselves and their partners.

Maximizers and rivalists jeopardize the client's welfare because they put themselves first and the client last. Rivalists direct their energies toward being "one up" through putdowns of others. They are concerned not with the client but with the process of winning. Cooperators are interested in helping both themselves and their colleagues to aid the client. Participants who actively recognize the importance of each individual member of the mental health team can influence maximizers and rivalists to become cooperators.

Respect for the Positions of Others

Most nursing textbooks and nursing instructors emphasize the need to respect and accept the client and to act in ways that demonstrate personal trustworthiness. They seldom consider the need to respect, accept, and demonstrate trust in one's colleagues. Yet effective collaboration is based on respect for the position from which another participant acts. Our values and our culture direct our beliefs and the climate in which we operate. Knowing this, we can become aware of the values and culture of others and, in turn, respect them.

Unfortunately, the process of socialization into a profession may make it difficult for a person to respect, accept, and trust the position of another. As students become committed to a profession through the process of socialization they tend to view members of other disciplines with suspicion. Nursing is particularly susceptible in this regard, because nurses have had to struggle to become colleagues with other health professionals. They may not yet have gained the degree of comfort and professional self-esteem that permits nonthreatened respect, acceptance, and trust of others. Of course, the same holds true for other members of the mental health team. As lines become blurred and once-sacred tasks and functions are shared, other colleagues may experience anxiety about respecting, accepting, and trusting the psychiatric nurse.

Another factor also makes it harder for health professionals to respect, accept, and trust the positions of others. Traditional roles may make collegial interaction tortuous and unrewarding. Stein (1967) has described a Doctor–Nurse game that supports their traditional roles. In this game, the nurse paradoxically assumes the initiative and makes significant recommendations, but carefully appears passive so that the physician can seem to be the decision maker. The following example, given by Stein (1967, pp. 699–700), is common in interactions between nurses and physicians:

The medical resident on hospital call is awakened by telephone at 1 A.M. because a patient on the ward, not his own, has not been able to fall asleep. Dr. Jones answers the telephone and the dialogue goes like this:

"This is Dr. Jones."

(An open and direct communication.)

"Dr. Jones, this is Miss Smith on 2W—Mrs. Brown, who learned today of her father's death, is unable to fall asleep."

(This message has two levels. Openly, it describes a set of circumstances; a woman who is unable to sleep and who that morning received word of her father's death. Less openly, but just as directly it is a diagnostic and recommendation statement; i.e., Mrs. Brown is unable to sleep because of her grief, and she should be given a sedative. Dr. Jones, accepting the diagnostic statement and replying to the recommendation statement, answers.)

"What sleeping medication has been helpful to Mrs. Brown in the past?"

(Dr. Jones, not knowing the patient, is asking for a recommendation from the nurse, who does know the patient, about what sleeping medication should be prescribed. Note, however, his question does not appear to be asking for her recommendation. Miss Smith replies.)

"Pentobarbital mg 100 was quite effective night before last." (A disguised recommendation statement. Dr. Jones replies with a note of authority in his voice.)

"Pentobarbital mg 100 before bedtime as needed for sleep, got it?"

(Miss Smith ends the conversation with the tone of a grateful supplicant.)

"Yes, I have, and thank you very much doctor."

Moscato (1976) contends that male and female stereotypes operate explicitly in the traditional nurse–physician relationship. In her view, the Doctor–Nurse Game reflects the stereotypic sex roles of the male physician as dominant decision maker and the female nurse as passive caretaker. While on the surface the participants appear to respect one another's positions, they have essentially denied themselves and each other the opportunity to function to their fullest capacities. Such alliances inhibit open dialogue and reinforce the stereotypes. By cooperating in this game, nurses lose personal, assertive power and are prevented from sharing their expert knowledge and problem-solving skills. Physicians are locked into appearing omnipotent without the freedom to take on learner or collaborative roles. All participants function at less than optimal level, and interdisciplinary cooperation becomes ineffectual.

Supervision, support, and self-exploration are recommended for the expansion of nursing roles within and beyond traditional relationships (Moscato 1976). Clinical supervision of nurses by nurses can help pinpoint times when traditional caretaking roles are appropriate and when they are growth inhibiting. Administrative and peer support for an atmosphere in which nurses are free to share their knowledge, skills, and evolving ideas will increase creativity, depth, and perspective in nursing. Self-exploration and self-assessment, through reading, dialogue with other males and females, and consciousness-raising groups, can help nurses to consider alternatives to traditional stereotypic roles.

Engaging the Client in Collaboration

It is best to include clients in the collaboration of the mental health team whenever possible. This allows clients to participate in their health care and assures nurses that their clients are informed consumers of mental health services.

Clients can also be invited to participate in case conferences. These conferences often have an important place in the functioning of mental health agencies and may have a number of purposes. The client should be invited to participate in case conferences that involve collaboration among a number of agencies or a number of mental health workers moving toward similar goals with the client.

The client should be consulted about the information the nurse shares with other members of the mental health team. Exactly how much should be shared and with whom are not always clear. When the question of confidentiality is not clear, the nurse should also confer with the supervisor or a colleague to determine what should be shared. Decisions should take into consideration the agreement between nurse and client about sharing information and how the person or agency receiving information will use that information in the client's best interests.

KEY NURSING CONCEPTS

✔ The psychiatric nurse's capacity for empathy and ability to collaborate on the mental health team are related to his or her consciousness of meaning, use of language, willingness to negotiate, definitions of reality, awareness of feelings, ability to take care of self, and own self view.

✔ Psychiatric nurses experience significant stresses in attempting to relate fully to clients and still maintain their own personal integration.

✔ Burning out is an attempt to cope with the stresses of intense interpersonal work by a form of distancing.

✔ The causes of professional burnout are most likely rooted in the social context of the individual's work situation, not in his or her permanent psychological characteristics.

✔ Methods the nurse may use to preserve personal integration include development of assertiveness, recognizing and planning for some time alone, maintaining personal physical health, and attending to cues of personal stress.

✔ Characteristics of artful therapeutic practice include respect for the client, availability, spontaneity, hope, acceptance, sensitivity, vision, and empathy.

✔ Phases in the development of empathic understanding are identification, incorporation, reverberation, and detachment.

✔ Quality of mental health services depends on cooperation among health team members and across disciplines, knowledge about each member's contribution, inclusion of the client in decision making, and respect for the position of others.

✔ Members of the mental health team frequently practicing in contemporary United States settings include the psychiatric nursing clinical specialist, the registered nurse working in a psychiatric setting, the psychiatrist, the psychoanalyst, the clinical psychologist, the psychiatric social worker, the mental health/human service worker, the psychiatric aide or attendant, the occupational therapist, and the creative arts therapist.

✔ The clinical specialist in psychiatric nursing is educated at the graduate level and may seek certification by a professional nursing body to attest to advanced competence.

References

Castaneda, C. *The Teachings of Don Juan: A Yaqui Way of Knowledge.* Berkeley: University of California Press, 1968.

Ehmann, V. E. "Empathy: Its Origin, Characteristics, and Process." *Perspectives in Psychiatric Care* 9 (1971): 72–80.

Keller, H. *The Story of My Life.* New York: Doubleday, 1902.

Luft, J., and Ingham, H. "The Johari Window, a Graphic Model of Awareness in Interpersonal Relations." In *Group Processes: An Introduction to Group Dynamics,* by J. Luft, pp. 10–12. Palo Alto, Calif.: National Press, 1963.

Maslach, C. "Burned Out." *Human Behavior,* September 1976, pp. 16–21.

Moscato, B. "The Traditional Nurse–Physician Relationship: A Perpetuation of Sexual Stereotyping." In *Current Perspectives in Psychiatric Nursing: Issues and Trends,* vol. 1, edited by C. R. Kneisl and H. S. Wilson, pp. 3–13. St. Louis: C. V. Mosby, 1976.

Raths, L., Harmin, M., and Simon, S. *Values and Teaching,* Columbus, Ohio: Merrill Publishing, 1966.

Simon, S., Howe, L., and Kirschenbaum, H. *Values Clarification—a Handbook of Practical Strategies for Teachers and Students.* New York: Hart Publishing, 1972.

Society of Certified Clinical Specialists in Psychiatric Nursing. *Mental Health Services Provided by Clinical Specialists in Psychiatric Nursing.* Trenton: New Jersey State Nurses Association, 1980.

Stein, L. "The Doctor–Nurse Game." *Archives of General Psychiatry* 16 (1967): 699–700.

Wilson, H. S., and Kneisl, C. R. *Learning Activities in Psy-*

chiatric Nursing. Menlo Park, Calif.: Addison-Wesley, 1983.

Further Reading

Bates, B. "Doctor and Nurse: Changing Roles and Relations." *New England Journal of Medicine* 283 (1970): 129-134.

Becker, E. *The Revolution in Psychiatry: The New Understanding of Man.* New York: Free Press, 1974.

Cohen, H. *The Nurse's Quest for a Professional Identity.* Menlo Park, Calif.: Addison-Wesley, 1981.

Combs, B. J., et al. *An Invitation to Health.* Menlo Park, Calif.: Benjamin/Cummings, 1980.

Haller, L. L., "Clinical Psychiatric Supervision: Process and Problems." In *Current Perspectives in Psychiatric Nursing: Issues and Trends,* vol. 1, edited by C. R. Kneisl and H. S. Wilson, pp. 36-43. St. Louis: C. V. Mosby, 1976.

Harris, F. G. "What Is Psychiatric Nursing?" *Proceedings of Fourth National Conference on Graduate Education in Psychiatric and Mental Health Nursing* (April, 1979). Pittsburgh, Pa., pp. 20-23.

James, M., and Jongeward, D. *Born To Win: Transactional Analysis with Gestalt Experiments.* Reading, Mass.: Addison-Wesley, 1977.

Keenan, T., et al. *Nurses and Doctors.* Cambridge, Mass.: Oelgeschlager, Gunn and Hain, 1981.

Koldjeski, D. "Mental Health and Psychiatric Nursing and Primary Health Care: Issues and Prospects." *Proceedings of Fourth National Conference on Graduate Education in Psychiatric and Mental Health Nursing* (April 1979). Pittsburgh, Pa., pp. 30-34.

Martin, E. J. "The Psychiatric-Mental Health Nurse Specialist: Scope of Responsibility." *Proceedings of Fourth National Conference on Graduate Education in Psychiatric and Mental Health Nursing* (April 1979). Pittsburgh, Pa., pp. 39-41.

Morrison, E. G. "Aspects of Supervision in Psychiatric Nursing." In *Current Perspectives in Psychiatric Nursing: Issues and Trends,* vol. 1, edited by C. R. Kneisl and H. S. Wilson, pp. 26-35. St. Louis: C. V. Mosby, 1976.

Poland, R. G. *Human Experience: A Psychology of Growth.* St. Louis: C. V. Mosby, 1974.

Sills, G. "Some Dimensions of Professionalism." *Proceedings of Fourth National Conference on Graduate Education in Psychiatric and Mental Health Nursing* (April 1979). Pittsburgh, Pa., pp. 13-16.

Stevens, B. J. *The Nurse as Executive.* Wakefield, Mass.: Contemporary Publishing, 1975.

4

Nursing Process and Nursing Theories

CHAPTER OUTLINE

The Nursing Process
    Assessment
    The Nursing Diagnosis
    The Nursing Care Plan
    Implementing the Nursing Care Plan
    Evaluation
Nursing Theory
    Historical Antecedents of Contemporary Theory
    Overview of Nursing Theories
    Evaluating Nursing Theories
    Applying Nursing Theories to Practice
Key Nursing Concepts

LEARNING OBJECTIVES

After reading this chapter, the student should be able to

- Discuss the steps of the nursing process in relation to the 1982 Standards of Psychiatric–Mental Health Nursing Practice
- Comprehend key concepts in selected contemporary nursing theories
- Evaluate the usefulness of selected contemporary nursing theories for organizing data and guiding the practice of psychiatric nursing
- Apply the nursing process to situations involving clients with psychiatric/mental health problems

CHAPTER 4

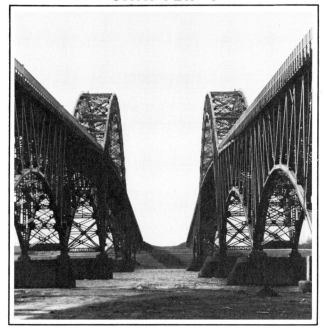

A nurse is asked to assess and implement quality nursing care for the following clients:

Diane S., a twenty-three-year-old woman, is admitted to a medical unit with severe anorexia nervosa and thoughts of suicide. She is agitated and tearful and says life looks so bad that she just wants to get out of it.

B.J. is a twenty-seven-year-old man who walked into the hospital emergency room because he sees the walls sparkling and weaving around, he feels like people are laughing at him, and he tastes petroleum in his mouth, which he describes as the "taste of afterbirth." He was on his way to jump off the George Washington Bridge when he saw the hospital and decided to come in for help.

The client is a fifty-two-year-old, disheveled woman dressed in ragged street clothes and wearing a turban on her head. She believes that there are radio waves in her teeth reporting of a plot to have her committed to mental hospitals. She has lived on the streets of Berkeley for the past two years with all her possessions and clothing in four large brown paper bags. She speaks in an uninterrupted monotone and is hostile toward the nurse.

How does a nurse approach the clinical problems suggested in the case excerpts above? Obviously no quick

and easy cookbook formulas are adequate for responding to such genuine human complexities. The 1982 American Nurses' Association Standards of Psychiatric and Mental Health Nursing Practice reflect the current state of knowledge in the field and offer some guidance in providing nursing care to clients like those described above.

The six standards selected from Appendix A and presented in Table 4–1 are the focus of this chapter. Together, they represent the use of nursing theory and process (data collection, diagnosis, planning, intervention, and evaluation) in the practice of psychiatric–mental health nursing and in so doing offer direction to the nurse. Each of the six standards is taken up in detail in the sections that follow.

THE NURSING PROCESS

Process by its very nature suggests movement toward a goal in phases or stages. The movement may be automatic and mechanical, random and chaotic, or planned and deliberate. The nursing process is the third sort. It is the conscious, systematic set of cognitive and behavioral steps that comprise the clinical act in nursing practice. The steps include:

- Assessment of the client's health status
- Formulation of a nursing diagnosis
- Development of a plan for nursing action
- Implementation of the plan
- Evaluation of the nursing care

This chapter describes the ways in which the nursing process approach is applied to psychiatric nursing practice and urges that the nursing process become the way in which nurses think about clients with the problems taken up in other chapters of this text. It must be recognized, however, that human beings are

Table 4-1   1982 A.N.A. STANDARDS OF PSYCHIATRIC MENTAL HEALTH NURSING
Professional Practice Standards
Standard 1—Theory
The nurse applies appropriate theory that is scientifically sound as a basis for decisions regarding nursing practice.
Standard 2—Data Collection
The nurse continuously collects data that is comprehensive, accurate, and systematic.
Standard 3—Diagnosis
The nurse utilizes nursing diagnoses and standard psychiatric diagnoses to express conclusions supported by recorded assessment data and current scientific premises.
Standard 4—Planning
The nurse develops a nursing care plan with specific goals and interventions delineating nursing actions unique to each client's needs.
Standard 5—Intervention
The nurse intervenes as guided by the nursing care plan to implement nursing actions that promote, maintain, or restore physical and mental health, prevent illness, and rehabilitate.
Standard 6—Evaluation
The nurse evaluates client responses to nursing actions in order to revise the data base, nursing diagnoses, and nursing care plan.

complex. Because psychiatric clients rarely present themselves neatly packaged in the framework of the nursing process, the nurse must adapt the process discussed in this chapter to each client's unique circumstances. There is no single correct method of proceeding through the phases of the nursing process, nor is there a definite pattern to follow in moving from phase to phase. The nursing process is flexible and adaptable. It can be applied in a variety of settings with individual clients, families, groups, and aggregates. It requires that the nurse use judgment and creativity in caring for clients in an organized and systematic way.

Assessment

Standard 2 of the 1982 Standards of Psychiatric and Mental Health Nursing Practice states that

> The nurse continuously collects data that is comprehensive, accurate, and systematic.

The rationale for including assessment among the standards of quality in nursing derives from a belief that effective nursing depends on a comprehensive, accurate, systematic, and continuous data collection process that enables the nurse to reach sound conclusions about the client's problems and needs and plan fitting interventions. Structural and process criteria indicative of appropriate assessment activities include:

1. The nurse informs the clients that data collection is their mutual responsibility.
2. The practice setting provides a method for recording and retrieving client data that protects confidentiality.
3. The nurse seeks at least the following categories of health data:
   - Biophysical, developmental, emotional, and mental status
   - Spiritual resources
   - Family, social, cultural, and community systems
   - Daily activities, interactions with others, and coping patterns
   - Economic, environmental, and political factors affecting the client's health
   - Personally significant support systems including those that are available in the community but not yet used
   - Knowledge, satisfaction, and motivation for change of health practices and status
   - Strengths that can be used in reaching health goals
   - Knowledge pertinent to legal rights
   - Secondary data from the family, significant others, and members of the mental health care team

When clients and their significant others affirm that the data-gathering process was beneficial to them, the nurse has met the outcome criterion for Standard 2.

Data collection involves astute observation, purposeful listening, broad knowledge of human behavior, and understanding of what needs to be known and where to obtain the information. The specific tools used in psychiatric assessment of individual clients—including psychiatric history, mental status examination, psychosocial assessment, neurological assessment, and psychological testing—are discussed in detail in Chapter 8. Assessment strategies for groups and families can be found in Chapters 18 and 21.

The nursing history is the foremost method of collecting data from the primary source (the client). Nursing histories summarize pertinent information about clients that can be used by the nurse to individualize care. They differ from medical or psychiatric histories, which are records of previous diseases, in that they focus on the clients' perception and expectations related to their illness, hospitalization, and care. A sample outline for a nursing history is offered on pp. 68–70.

The data collected from the client as well as from secondary sources like laboratory and psychological test results, family members, and other members of the mental health team ultimately provide a rationale for determining the client's nursing needs, and a basis for planning and evaluating nursing therapy, writing nursing orders, and guiding nursing activities. The assessment phase of the nursing process culminates in the formulation of a nursing diagnosis.

The Nursing Diagnosis

Standard 3 of the 1982 Standards of Psychiatric and Mental Health Nursing Practice states that

> The nurse utilizes nursing diagnoses and standard psychiatric diagnoses to express conclusions supported by recorded assessment data and current scientific premises.

The rationale for inclusion of Standard 3 is that nursing's logical basis for providing care rests on recognition and identification of actual or potential health problems within the scope of nursing practice. In other words, formulation of nursing diagnoses makes it possible to identify the specific contribution of nursing to the health team. A diagnostic classification system for psychiatric nursing practice that applies diagnoses specific to nursing interventions would enhance our ability

---

Table 4–2   CATEGORIES OF NURSING DIAGNOSES FOR PSYCHIATRIC CLIENTS

- Self-care limitations or impaired functioning with general etiologies, such as mental and emotional distress, deficits in the ways significant systems are functioning, and internal psychic or developmental issues relevant to health
- Emotional stress or crisis components of illness, pain, self-concept changes, and life process changes
- Emotional problems related to daily experiences such as anxiety, aggression, loss, loneliness, and grief
- Physical symptoms, such as altered intestinal functioning or anorexia, which occur simultaneously with altered psychic functioning
- Alterations in thinking, perceiving, symbolizing, communication, and decision-making abilities
- Behaviors and mental states that indicate that the client is a danger to self or others or is gravely disabled

---

to define the scope of nursing and answer the question, "What do psychiatric nurses do that's different from what social workers, psychologists, and psychiatrists do?" Structural criteria that reflect achievement of Standard 3 include:

- Peer validation of nursing diagnoses
- Peer exchange, education, and research regarding the scientific and humanistic premises underlying nursing diagnoses

The process criteria for meeting this standard are nursing diagnoses for psychiatric clients that identify actual or potential health problems in respect to the categories outlined in Table 4–2.

The outcome criterion for meeting this standard is that nursing diagnoses are validated by the client or the client's significant others.

Guidelines recommended by members of the First National Conference on the Classification of Nursing Diagnoses (Gebbie and Lavin, 1975) further guide the nurse in this process. They include the following:

- People should be viewed as whole, worthwhile, dignified beings regardless of their degree of dysfunction or level of competence.

NURSING HISTORY GUIDE

A. General Information
  1. Date of interview:
  2. Date of admission:
  3. Hours of time elapsed from admission to first interview:
  4. Client's name:
  5. Client's age:
  6. Diagnosis (medical):
  7. Occupation:
     a. Client's occupation:
     b. Spouse's occupation:
  8. Religion:
  9. Educational level:
  10. Residence (city and state):
  11. Marital status:
B. Guide Questions
  1. Family situation
     a. With whom do you live?
     b. How many children do you have, if any?
     c. Who is caring for them while you are here?
     d. How many brothers and sisters do you have?
     e. Do your parents live nearby?
     f. Was there anything that happened to you or your family in the past year other than this illness that was upsetting to you?
  2. Work situation (including financial aspect)
     a. What type of work do you do?
     b. How long have you done this type of work?
     c. Are you on sick leave from work?
     d. Do you think your illness will interfere with your work?
     e. Do you have health insurance?
  3. Client's activities
     a. What kind of environment and pace are you used to?
     b. What are your feelings concerning your activity schedule in the hospital?
     c. Do you have any special interests or hobbies that you would like to pursue, if feasible, while you are here?
     d. What habits have you had to change here?
  4. Eating habits
     a. Are you on a restricted diet?
     b. Are you allergic to any foods?
     c. Are there any particular foods you like or dislike?
     d. Do you eat breakfast?
     e. Do you need an early morning cup of coffee or the like?
     f. How many times do you eat each day?
     g. When do you usually eat your meals?
     h. Has being sick affected your eating habits? How?
     i. Do you foresee any difficulty with hospital food?
     j. Do you prefer plain or ice water?
     k. Are you accustomed to eating snacks? At regular times?
  5. Sleeping habits
     a. How long do you usually sleep? Between what hours?
     b. Do you sleep well at home?
     c. Do you nap? Occasionally? Regularly? Rarely?
     d. Are you an early riser?
     e. Do you need medication to sleep?
     f. Do you get up at intervals?
     g. Does light or noise disturb you?
     h. If you are awakened at night, can you go back to sleep?
     i. Do you sleep with a night light on?
     j. Do you like an extra blanket at night?
     k. Do you usually sleep with a window closed or open?
     l. Have you found that strange surroundings decrease your ability to sleep soundly?
     m. How many pillows do you use?
  6. Elimination habits
     a. What are your elimination habits at home?
     b. Do you have any difficulty with elimination?
     c. Do you take laxatives? If so, how often?
     d. Do you take any special foods to aid in elimination?
  7. Allergies
     a. Do you have any allergies to drugs, food, adhesive tape, etc.?
  8. Drugs or special diets
     a. Were you on any medications before you came to the hospital?
     b. Do you routinely take any nonprescription medicines?
     c. Did you bring any of these medications with you?

9. Previous illnesses or hospitalizations
   a. Have you had other experiences when you or members of your family were ill?
      1) What kind of experience was it— good, bad, indifferent?
      2) What problems, if any, did you or they encounter?
   b. Have you ever been sick before?
      1) What was wrong?
      2) Were you in the hospital?
      3) How long were you sick?
      4) What do you remember most about being hospitalized?
      5) What did you like most about the hospital care, routines, etc.?
   c. Do you have any disability, other than your present illness, that may restrict your normal activity?
   d. Who cares for you when you are sick at home?
   e. What can you do when you are sick at home that makes you feel better.

10. Current illness
    a. Why are you in the hospital?
    b. What do you think made you ill?
    c. How long have you been ill?
    d. Can you tell me what you feel about your illness?
    e. What kinds of things usually make you feel better when you are sick?
    f. Were there other things that happened when you first became ill?
    g. What do you feel about the outcome of your illness?
    h. What is causing you the most discomfort at this time?

11. Current hospitalization
    a. What do you think you need done for you while you are here?
    b. What do you feel about being here in the hospital?
    c. What do you miss most by being in this hospital?
    d. Are there some things at home that you would like to have here with you? If so, what?
    e. Are there things at home that might bother or worry you while you are here?

12. Personal preferences regarding visitors— family and friends
    a. If feasible, would you prefer to be alone or with other clients during the day?
    b. Would you like to have visitors?
       1) Just family?
       2) Just friends?
       3) Both family and friends?
       4) Just certain individuals? Who?
    c. How many visitors would you like at one time and how frequently?
    d. Is it possible for your family or friends to visit you if you so desire?
    e. Has anyone visited you yet, or did anyone come with you when you were admitted?
    f. (For persons with serious illness, or as hospital policy allows) Would you feel better if it was possible for some of your family to stay here with you overnight?

13. Expectations of hospital personnel and physician by client
    a. Would you like your doctor and nurses to explain everything that is going on with you?
    b. Would you be comfortable enough to ask them questions if they do not explain?
    c. Would you like someone to come in frequently during the day just to talk or be with you?
    d. Is there anything special you expect or would like me to do for you or see that it gets done, if feasible, while you are here?
    e. What do you expect from nurses?
    g. What has your doctor told you about your illness and what to expect while you are in the hospital?
    h. What do you expect from your doctor?
    i. What do you expect from the hospital?
    j. What do you expect from hospital policy or routine?
    k. Would you like a minister to visit with you, if possible?
    i. How best can we help you while you are in the hospital?

C. Visual Observation on General Appearance
   1. Immediate general impression of appearance:
   2. Overall physical appearance:
   3. Motor activity/posture:
   4. Build and weight:

5. Prosthesis / limitations / debilitations:
6. Complexion and appearance of skin:
   a. Color
   b. Lesions
   c. Abrasions
   d. Rash
7. Subjective symptoms:
   a. Watery eyes
   b. Running nose
   c. Cough
8. Mouth:
   a. Oral hygiene
   b. Dentures
9. Eyes:
   a. Eye glasses
   b. Contact lenses
10. Age group:

11. Clothing:
12. Belongings and objects in environment:
13. Speech:
14. Apparent cultural, educational, and intellectual levels:
15. Other pertinent factors:
D. Nonverbal Behavior Observations
   1. Emotional tone, facial expression, attitude:
   2. Gestures, movements, or activities during interview:
   3. Main theme of client's conversation and behavior:
   4. Topics the client seemed to avoid:
   5. Client's response to inverviewer:
   6. Interviewer's response to client:
   7. Other pertinent factors:
E. Summary

From Elaine L. Lamonica, *The Nursing Process: A Humanistic Approach*, pp. 7–11. Copyright © 1979 by Addison-Wesley Publishing Co., Inc., Menlo Park, California.

- Nursing diagnoses should involve the client and should be validated with the client.

- Nursing diagnoses should be stated in terms of concerns and levels of competence or dysfunction.

- Nursing diagnoses should always be referred to as "nursing" diagnoses to avoid confusion with medical diagnoses.

The psychiatric diagnosis discussed at length in Chapter 8 is the mental health team's way of labeling a client's psychiatric disorder. A nursing diagnosis with a psychiatric client is the conceptualization of a client's problem, need, or situation from the unique perspective of the theoretical constructs in the discipline of nursing. Such conceptualizations are abstractions or concepts either generated by the clinician or imported from existing theory to organize, categorize, and ultimately make sense of the data collected during the assessment phase of the nursing process. Selected nursing theories are discussed later in this chapter. Psychiatric nurses must be knowledgeable about both psychiatric diagnostic nomenclature (see Chapter 8 for presentation of the American Psychiatric Association's nomenclature for mental disorders DSM-III) as well as the expanding efforts of nurses to develop their own diagnostic nomenclature. Both are essential for communication with colleagues and for developing an individualized nursing care plan.

The Nursing Care Plan

Standard 4 states that

The nurse develops a nursing care plan with specific goals and interventions delineating nursing actions unique to each client's needs.

The rationale for inclusion of this standard is that the nursing care plan is used to guide therapeutic intervention and to achieve desired goals or outcomes effectively and affirmatively. Structural criteria that reflect the presence of nursing care planning include:

- Tools and mechanisms for communicating nursing diagnoses and nursing care plans, progress, and evaluation to colleagues and to the client

- Evidence of a collaborative team effort to plan care so that the client's needs are addressed in a consistent way

The well-developed nursing care plan conforms to the qualities outlined in Table 4–3.
Nursing care plans have various formats depending on the resources and constraints of a setting and the operating conceptual framework or philosophy for practice. Many of the formats for nursing care plans have been incorporated into subsequent chapters of this text. One of them is illustrated in Table 4–4.

Table 4–3   PROPERTIES OF AN EFFECTIVE NURSING CARE PLAN

1. Identifies priorities of care
2. States realistic goals in measurable terms with an expected date of accomplishment
3. Is based on identifiable psychotherapeutic principles
4. Indicates which client needs are the primary responsibility of the psychiatric nurse and which will be referred to others with appropriate expertise
5. Reflects mutual goal setting and shared responsibility for goal attainment at the level of the client's abilities
6. Forms the basis for client care activities done by others under the nurse's supervision

---

The ultimate outcome criterion for this standard is evidence that regardless what format is used for the care plan, it is revised as goals are achieved, changed, or updated.

Planning nursing care requires that both short- and long-term goals be set for the client. Such goals, however, must reflect the client's own goals, and when the two sets of goals are not compatible, negotiation should occur.

The first step in determining whether to try to convince the client that the nurse's goals are the right goals or to alter the nurse's goals is to ask clients what their goals are and how the psychiatric professional can help them achieve their goals. Some clients will respond that they just came along to appease a significant other who is the one with the real problem. Others believe they are there for a "rest" or a "checkup." Some want to be taken care of and protected, and some believe they have been tricked or betrayed and locked up against their will. Having asked, the nurse must *listen*. Sometimes the simple experience of being heard and understood without being invalidated and dismissed out of hand becomes the ground for subsequent negotiations and eventual agreement about mutually determined goals.

Once a nursing diagnosis has been identified and clear, unambiguous, goals have been set and listed in order of priority, the nurse can consider possible solutions by using what are known as "predictive principles." Bower (1977, p. 101) calls predictive principles "guides for developing realistic alternatives of action or action hypotheses that tell the nurse what will pro-

mote or inhibit progress toward a desired goal." The nurse selects one intervention from many choices based on a prediction of the likely or probable consequences of each option. The use of predictive principles cuts down on trial-and-error and the rigid use of standard operating procedures. Figure 4–1 illustrates the sequences of decision-making process for a depressed client.

Implementing the Nursing Care Plan

The following topics outline the major categories of nursing intervention with psychiatric clients (see Appendix A).

- Psychotherapeutic interventions
- Health teaching
- Self-care activities
- Somatic therapies
- Therapeutic environment
- Psychotherapy

Each of these areas is taken up specifically in a subsequent chapter of this text.

Yura and Walsh (1978) characterize the implementation phase of the nursing process as a time when the nurse continues to collect data about the client's condition, problems, reactions, and feelings. The plan is not carried out blindly as if all decision-making phases have been completed. Changes in identified goals will alter the effectiveness of intervention strategies. Therefore, the nurse must be alert, observant, attentive, thoughtful, and caring, continually using decision-making skills to evaluate and modify intervention strategies and use of available resources.

Evaluation

Standard 6 states that

The nurse evaluates client responses to nursing actions in order to revise the data base, nursing diagnoses, and nursing care plan.

The rationale for inclusion of this standard is that psychotherapeutic nursing care is a dynamic process with events that sometimes alter data, diagnoses, or plans previously made.

Structural criteria that facilitate achievement of Standard 6 include supervision or consultation with colleagues that assists the nurse in analyzing the effec-

	Table 4-4 NURSING CARE PLAN	
Problem	**Outcome**	**Nursing Orders**
1. Air, Food, Fluids No problem 2. Elimination No problem 3. Personal Hygiene No problem	Will maintain independent self-care in problem areas 1,2, and 3.	1. Assess problem areas 1,2, and 3 for health teaching needs.
4. Rest/Activity Frank has difficulty regulating his daily schedule to attend all required meetings and get to meals. He becomes frustrated, then angry, and often acts out destructively when he is reminded of his schedule.	Frank will be able to regulate his activities better and to discuss his frustrations without "exploding." He will be able to verbalize anger rather than act out in destructive ways.	1. Following angry exchanges between others, explore how he is reacting: first, what he is thinking; later, how he is feeling. 2. Encourage him to voice complaints or anger directly rather than attempting to "ignore" it. 3. Allow him distance if he feels overwhelmed rather than pushing him to discuss feelings when he cannot; encourage him to acknowledge his feelings without the expectation that he must explore them at the moment. 4. Do not rescue him in frustrating circumstances; allow him to wrestle with problems. Provide positive feedback for successful solutions.
5. Solitude and Social/ Interaction a. Frank has difficulty forming meaningful relationships with others including peers.	Frank will begin to establish trusting relationships with peers and with staff on the unit.	Confront him in a nonpunitive manner when he is being evasive or charming in lieu of a direct expression of feeling or thought. Encourage his creative skills and talents (e.g., his interest in guitar) and creative opportunities for productive activities with peers. Approach him to establish rapport and allow him to know you; do not interact *only* when problem arises or if limit-setting is necessary. Be honest and direct with him and expect the same in return.

Table continues on next page

tivess of care given. Two process criteria reflect achievement of this standard:

1. The nurse pursues validation, suggestions, and new information that is subsequently discussed with colleagues.

2. The nurse documents results of the evaluation of nursing care.

The outcome criterion for this standard is that clients or those acting on behalf of clients indicate that their evaluations of the nursing process have been sought and validated.

Evaluation is a judgment of merit or worth. It is the natural intellectual activity to complete the phases of the nursing process, because it indicates the degree to which the nursing diagnosis and nursing actions have been correct. As in all other phases, clients and their significant others are involved in evaluation.

Since Isobel Stewart first developed guidelines in 1919 to measure the quality of nursing care, numerous others have been tested. Methods for monitoring the

Table 4–4 continued		
Problem	**Outcome**	**Nursing Orders**
b. Frank has an unrealistic view of behavior and consequences. For example, he rationalizes that some of his difficulties are due to the school system.	Frank will obtain a more realistic view of his behavior and its consequences, including the feelings of others in response to it. He will assume more responsibility for his actions and behavior.	Suggest other reasons for difficulties, when appropriate. Offer your reactions to his behavior, both positive and negative. Encourage him to check out with his peers how they felt about certain negative behaviors or statements. Expect that he will assume responsibility for his actions. Do not be "taken in" by guilt-inducing accusations.
c. Frank has a tendency to use a charming or seductive manner in attempt to manipulate environment. For example, he uses seductive behavior with female staff to get his way, and bribes his roommate to do undesirable tasks for him (e.g., wash clothes).	Frank will learn to accept responsibility for his behavior and its consequences. He will begin to use more direct means of expression in meeting his needs.	Do not respond favorably to manipulations; confront him with his intentions in as nonpunitive a way as possible. Encourage his peers to explore their behavior in relation to him and to express their reactions openly. Encourage him to ask more directly for things.

Source: Patricia Underwood and Associates, Inpatient Treatment and Research Services, Langley Porter Psychiatric Institute, San Francisco, Calif.

quality of nursing care have been developed that simultaneously consider people, activities, and environmental elements, as well as the administrative and organizational structure for delivery of care. Instruments to evaluate care received by clients while the care is in process have been developed and tested. Periodic nursing audits are used increasingly by nurses to inspect or review records and other accounts of nursing transactions. Betts (1978) has related the psychiatric audit to a model for quality assurance in nursing.

Bower (1977) urges nurses to recognize the importance and necessity of structuring evaluation outcome criteria in client-centered behavioral terms. Nurses may have to discard the attitude that nursing care is composed of ethereal, well-meaning qualities or that certain aspects of the clinical act and its art just "can't be evaluated." The 1980s represent an era of resource retrenchment and accountability among consumers of health care, and psychiatric nurses are experiencing the challenges of this era. We are challenged to provide cost and quality accountability for our practice

and to demonstrate that nursing is a profession capable of in-depth self-study sufficient to prove quality performance by its practitioners. If we do not maintain the confidence of the public we will soon cease to be a social force.

Professional Service Review Organizations (PSRO), mandated by Congress in 1972, require that professionals and health care delivery systems implement quality control methods if they wish to maintain professional autonomy. This legislation was the source of evaluation by peer review. The A.N.A. has defined peer review as evaluation against the stated norms or standards of the profession. These standards have been presented as a framework for relating the nursing process to practice with psychiatric clients. The first of these standards, however, requires that

Nurses base practice decisions on the application of theory to clinical phenomena.

Standard 1 is the focus for the remainder of this chapter.

NURSING PROBLEM	PREDICTIVE PRINCIPLES (guides to action)	ALTERNATIVES	CONSEQUENCES	PROBABILITY	VALUE	RISK	NURSING DECISION
How to increase Mr. Fox's sense of self-esteem, self-respect, and self-worth. How to get Mr. Fox to take fluids and food.	• The level of depression determines the type of nursing action. • An open and accepting attitude facilitates a development of trust.	1. Sit next to Mr. Fox and try to get him to verbalize his feelings.	He will verbalize his feelings. He will not verbalize his feelings.	0.2 0.8	+ –	Low High	...
	• The outward expression of aggression and hostile feelings decreases the possibility that these feelings will be turned inward and thus lower self-esteem. • Believing someone cares promotes feelings of worth.	2. Say, "You must feel very uncomfortable in those wet clothes, come with me and let's get you more comfortable." Get a *male nurse* or orderly if necessary.	He will know you care. He will feel cleaner. His dignity will have been preserved. His skin will be clean and less liable to breakdown.	0.8 0.9 0.9 0.8	+ + + +	Low Low Low Low	Alternative 2
	• Nursing interventions that encourage severely depressed persons toward acts of daily care protect that person from further deterioration. • Feelings of self-esteem, self-respect, and acceptance enhance a positive and realistic self-concept, thus lifting feelings of depression.	3. In the privacy of his room, offer Mr. Fox sips of fruit juice and selections of food.	He will take juice and food. He will not take juice and food. His dignity and self-respect will be preserved since he has privacy.	0.7 0.3 0.8	+ – +	Low Moderate Low	Alternative 3

Figure 4–1

Decision-making sequence for a depressed client. (From Fay Louise Bower. *The Process of Planning Nursing Care*, 2 ed. St. Louis: The C.V. Mosby Company, 1977.)

NURSING THEORY

Professional nursing knowledge consists of three elements:

1. Basic natural, social, and behavioral sciences (see Chapter 2)
2. The tools, skills, and attitudes that comprise the clinical act in nursing, such as communication, assessment, and ethical reflectiveness
3. The theories for and of nursing

A *theory of nursing* refers to a grand general theory that addresses the definition of the domain and scope of nursing. A *theory for practice* consists of a set of interrelated propositions that specify actions and intended consequences in a situation. In other words, it guides the clinician in deciding what to do to achieve certain results.

Historical Antecedents of Contemporary Theory

Our first era might well be described as the *magico-religious era*. Nursing took place within the confines of huge institutions where nursing practice was shaped by values of self-sacrifice and dedication. Nursing ceremonies formalized these values and attitudes, and remnants of these ceremonies, such as capping rituals, are still familiar to us today. Educational programs for nurses were based on assumptions of passivity and sameness among nursing students.

With the publication of the Sue Barton and Cherry Ames books, nursing moved into another phase in relation to its guiding perspective, a perspective termed *romanticism* by some. The image of the nurse was idealized, open, simplistic, and glamorous but nursing was seen as a temporary job en route to *every woman's* true goal: marriage and motherhood.

As a result of the two world wars nursing moved into an era of *pragmatism*. The emphasis was on tools, tasks, and procedures; the goal was efficiency. Hospital geography dominated the organization of nursing knowledge. In our educational programs we rotated through ER, OR, the nursery, the clinics, central supply, and even formula lab, which was thought to be essential learning experiences in every student's curriculum. Watered-down medicine, modeled after the disease and body systems paradigms used by physicians,

organized both the curriculum and the practice of nursing. We learned and delivered diabetes nursing, cancer nursing, ENT nursing, rare tropical disease nursing, and so on.

Since approximately the early 1950s, however, nursing has moved away from such dualistic approaches. Contemporary conceptual schemes are more *holistic and humanistic*. Changes in technology, other disciplines, and health care needs have all contributed to this development. Even the image of the nurse has undergone some revision.

The concept of nursing as primarily technological (e.g., hypodermics, bedpans and other tools of the trade) has been replaced by the idea that nursing is theory based. Still, nursing remains more divergent than convergent when it comes to identifying the theories to be applied. Most authorities concur that *theoretical pluralism*—that is the simultaneous refinement and testing of numerous contenders for nursing's dominant theory—is highly appropriate for the present early phase in nursing's scientific and intellectual history. Let's briefly examine a few of the best known contenders and attempt to identify the concepts and principles most relevant to psychiatric nursing.

Overview of Nursing Theories

In the early fifties Lydia Hall, Virginia Henderson, and Hildegard Peplau had already published precursors to contemporary nursing theories, and Faye Abdellah had begun empirical observations that led to the formulation of her theory by 1955. Lydia Hall's theory is best represented by three interlocking circles depicting what she called the "aspects of nursing." Hall's three aspects of nursing were The Person (the Core), The Disease (the Cure), and The Body (the Care). She developed her theory at the Loeb Center for Rehabilitation primarily for the adult client recuperating from a physical illness in a residential treatment center. She showed relationships among the three concepts by varying the size of the three circles to represent the amount or proportion of nursing time focused on each. See Figure 4–2. Most psychiatric nursing practice would focus on the Core component of her model.

Virginia Henderson contributed the now famous definition of nursing:

> Nursing is primarily assisting the individual (sick or well) in the performance of those activities contributing to health or its recovery (or a peaceful death) that he would perform unaided if he had the necessary strength, will, or knowledge.

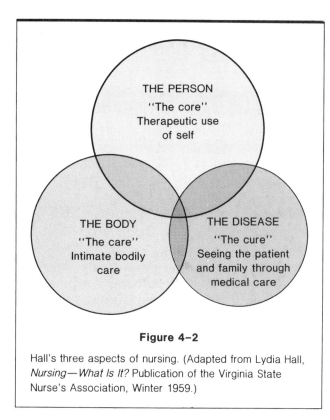

Figure 4–2

Hall's three aspects of nursing. (Adapted from Lydia Hall, *Nursing—What Is It?* Publication of the Virginia State Nurse's Association, Winter 1959.)

Henderson went on to identify a list of fourteen components of basic nursing care with the notion that nurses either helped the patient with the activities or provided conditions under which the patient would perform them unaided. The categories are:

1. Breathe normally.
2. Eat and drink adequately.
3. Eliminate body wastes.
4. Move and maintain desirable postures.
5. Sleep and rest.
6. Select suitable clothing—dress and undress.
7. Maintain body temperature within normal range by adjusting clothing and modifying the environment.
8. Keep the body clean and well-groomed and protect the integument.
9. Avoid dangers in the environment and avoid injuring others.
10. Communicate with others in expressing emotions, needs, fears, or opinions.
11. Worship according to one's faith.
12. Work in such a way that there is a sense of accomplishment.

13. Play or participate in various forms of recreation.
14. Learn, discover, or satisfy the curiosity that leads to normal development and health and use of the available health facilities.

The first nine activities encompass a version of basic physiological human needs. The remaining five include needs for communication, spirituality, work, play, and learning—the categories that are emphasized by psychiatric nurses.

Hildegard Peplau published her nursing theory in the classic book *Interpersonal Relations in Nursing* (1952). She defined nursing as a significant therapeutic interpersonal process, and the core concepts of her theory were the four phases of the nurse–client relationship.

1. Orientation
2. Identification
3. Exploitation
4. Resolution

Some say that these phases are ancestors of the phases of the nursing process. Psychiatric nurses continue to use Peplau's theory to understand and guide decisions in the one-to-one relationship. (See Chapter 7.)

Faye Abdellah presented a list of twenty-one nursing problems that she developed over a five-year period in the late fifties. The list, presented in Table 4–5, includes physiological as well as sociopsychological needs and resembles both Henderson's fourteen nursing care components and Maslow's hierarchy of needs.

Dorothea Orem's theory of self-care was originally introduced around 1959 and identified ten Universal Self-care Requisites, which are divided into six categories that encompass both physical and psychosocial human needs. Orem also introduced a second order of concepts originally called Health Deviation Self-care Demands to refer to care required in the event of illness, injury, or disease. Nursing, a second key component of her scheme, was divided into Wholly Compensatory, Partially Compensatory, and Supportive-Educational Systems of Care that could be matched to the client's assessed level of self-care functioning in each area (see Figure 4–3). This theory firmly established the notion of a goal of self-care as integral to the discipline of nursing's perspective on the meaning of health and has been particularly well adapted to meet-

Table 4-5   THE TWENTY-ONE NURSING PROBLEMS
1. To maintain good hygiene and physical comfort
2. To promote optimal activity: exercise, rest, and sleep
3. To promote safety through the prevention of accidents, injury or other trauma, and infection
4. To maintain good body mechanics and prevent and correct deformities
5. To maintain a supply of oxygen to all body cells
6. To maintain nutrition of all body cells
7. To facilitate elimination
8. To maintain fluid and electrolyte balance
9. To recognize the pathological, physiological, and compensatory responses of the body to disease conditions
10. To maintain regulatory mechanisms and functions
11. To maintain sensory function
12. To identify and accept positive and negative expressions, feelings, and reactions
13. To identify and accept the interrelatedness of emotions and organic illness
14. To maintain effective verbal and nonverbal communication
15. To promote the development of productive interpersonal relationships
16. To facilitate progress toward achievement of personal spiritual goals
17. To create or maintain a therapeutic environment
18. To facilitate awareness of self as an individual with varying physical, emotional, and developmental needs
19. To accept the optimum possible goals in the light of physical and emotional limitations
20. To use community resources in resolving problems arising from illness
21. To understand the role of social problems as influencing factors in the cause of illness.

Source: Reprinted with permission of Macmillan Publishing Co., Inc., from Patient-Centered Approaches to Nursing by Faye G. Abdellah, Almeda Martin, Irene L. Beland, and Ruth V. Matheney. © Copyright, Macmillan Publishing Co., Inc., 1960

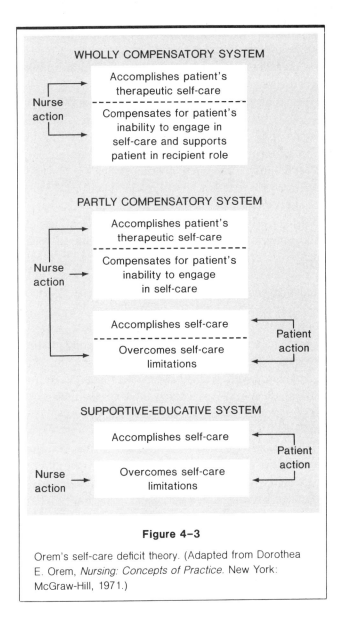

Figure 4-3

Orem's self-care deficit theory. (Adapted from Dorothea E. Orem, *Nursing: Concepts of Practice*. New York: McGraw-Hill, 1971.)

ing nursing care needs of the severely and chronically mentally disordered. (See Chapter 16.)

Martha Rogers drew on knowledge from anthropology, sociology, religion, philosophy, mythology, and general systems theory to define nursing as a wholistic science of human nature and development. Rogers's key nursing principles are called the Principles of Homeodynamics. Subprinciples of homeodynamics are:

- The principle of complementarity, which refers to the continuous, simultaneous interaction process between human and environmental fields

- The principle of resonancy, which refers to the tendency of humans to function according to patterns that can be studied

- The principle of helicy, which states that the nature and direction of human and environmental change are continuous, innovative, probabilistic, and diverse but also evolutionary and goal directed

These three principles are ways of viewing human beings holistically. Changes in life processes are irreversible, nonrepeatable, and rhythmic, and indicate patterns of increasing complexity and organization. Most of her concepts have counterparts in general systems theory, but she has added the notions of life processes, change, and human-environmental interaction to the concepts central to nursing. Rogers requires that psychiatric nurses use such holistic principles to guide their practice and consider physical as well as psychosocial problems and needs.

Sister Callista Roy's adaptation theory views people as constantly faced with the need to adapt to focal, contextual, and residual stimuli. She goes on to identify four modes of human adapting: (1) *physiological needs*, (2) *self-concept*, (3) *role function*, and (4) *interdependence*. Obviously these adaptive modes again include physiological, psychological, and social aspects of people and the notion of coping or adapting to stimuli again relates nursing to people in interaction with their environment. Self-concept, role function, and interdependent areas of coping all lend themselves to the conceptualization of the practice of psychiatric nursing.

The sample of theories presented in the past few pages in no way represents the entire universe of contenders. Ida Jean Orlando stresses the interaction of meanings between nurse and client. Ernestine Wiedenbach's work presents an example of a "situation-producing" theory that conceptualizes a goal and a nursing prescription for fulfilling the goal. Myra Levine uses four Conservation Principles to conceptualize nursing interventions: (1) *conservation of energy*, (2) *conservation of structural integrity*, (3) *conservation of personal integrity*, and (4) *conservation of social integrity*. Imogene King discusses concepts of social systems, perceptions, interpersonal relations, and health and their impact on people.

A review of these theories indicates some clear differences in emphasis and perspective and some intriguing similarities. From these theories are emerging the parameters of our discipline. Such parameters provide the beginnings for directing practice, focusing nursing research, and providing a framework of concepts integral to the teaching of professional students.

Evaluating Nursing Theories

Although it is premature to close the question of which among the array of contending paradigms will dominate the discipline of nursing and which is best suited to psychiatric nursing, we can and should assess each according to a framework of questions derived from *metatheory*. Problems of metatheory raise general issues, provide criteria of choice or standards, and should be discussed in any serious consideration of the construction of theory and its proper application. Three metatheoretical questions are used to assess the value of nursing theories for psychiatric nursing practice.

- Is it a theory?
  What definition of theory should prevail in our shared understanding?

- Is it a nursing theory?
  What, if any, theoretical orientations comprise and inform nursing's unique body of knowledge?

- Is it any good?
  What standards might we select to evaluate a theory or a fragment of a theory?

There seem to be almost as many definitions of what a theory should be as there are contemporary theorists in nursing. However, most authorities agree that it is the business of a theory to describe, explain, and predict truths about the world or that part of the world on which the theory focuses. Furthermore, most theorists accept the focal concepts for nursing as *people*, *nursing*, *health*, and *society*.

A theory can be defined as "a system of propositions containing interrelated concepts." A nursing theory must include the concept of nursing and explain and predict how nursing actions affect or interrelate with the person and environment to produce a desired health-related outcome.

Practically, a theory is considered fairly complete if it contains:

- Concepts to describe and classify empirical facts
- Definitions that allow for consensual meaning and potential measurement
- Propositions that connect two or more concepts and allow for beginning explanations and predictions
- Linkages between the propositions forming a system or scheme

The ordering of these propositions into some specific inductive or deductive arrangement is an elegance achieved slowly, and it characterizes only mature sciences. A final point bearing on our definition of a theory is its distinction from a model. A *model* is a concrete rendition of the theory that can be used to help

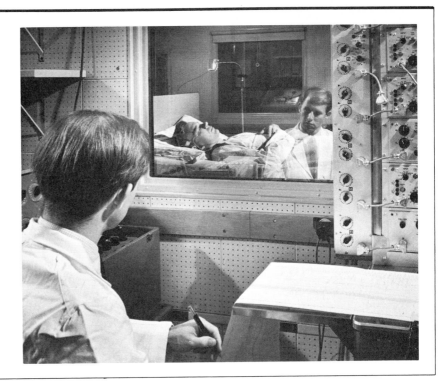

A psychiatric nurse conducting research on dream patterns at the National Institute of Mental Health.

visualize and understand the abstraction that cannot be directly observed. Models may be replicas, analogies, or symbols.

Our second metatheoretical problem concerns the debate about the existence of any unique nursing theory. In science there are often boundary disputes about the proper focus for a discipline that claims to be a science. Many humanists and philosophers of science are opposed to what they call "disciplinary territorialism" and urge that alert and industrious scholars can acquire the skills to investigate any question that arouses their curiosity. Yet an admonition from Immanuel Kant (1900) suggests a contrasting point of view. He wrote:

> To yield to every whim of curiosity and to allow our passions for inquiry to be restrained by nothing but the limits of our ability shows an eagerness of mind not unbecoming to scholarship. But it is wisdom that has the merit of selecting from among the innumerable problems which present themselves, those whose solution is important to mankind.

In the view of many nurses, it is on such wisdom that the definition, refinement, and growth of nursing theory will depend.

The debate boils down to one question. Can and should we develop nursing theories? Those opposed base their opposition on the contention that there are no phenomena unique to nursing and therefore nurses

have nothing about which to develop theories. Those who believe that nurses should develop nursing theories base their argument on the need for a systemically organized body of knowledge on which to base practice. A related assertion is that nurses have a great need for knowledge that scientists in other fields may not be interested in developing, and therefore nurses must take responsibility for developing the knowledge themselves.

Our final question is: On what bases can we judge or evaluate a theory or theory fragment? Nine conventional standards used for this purpose are:

1. Clarity. Is the theory presented in such a way that it can be understood? Are the key concepts and propositions clear in both their connotative and denotative meanings?

2. Consistency. Is the theory internally consistent in the meanings of terms, interpretations of concepts, inclusion of principles, implications for method, and basic assumptions?

3. Logical development. Is the conclusion logically warranted based on its premise? In other words does the theory's development follow the rules of logic?

4. Utility. Is the theory useful in education, research, or practice? Can the concepts of the theory be

operationalized in ways that allow for application and testing?

5. **Significance.** Does the theory address essential issues and genuinely contribute to the development of the knowledge base in the discipline?

6. **Scope.** How many of the basic problems in a discipline or specialty can be handled by the theory?

7. **Parsimony.** Does the theory explain as much as possible with the fewest possible variables?

8. **Precision of prediction.** Does the theory provide reasonable, precise prediction of outcomes?

9. **Accurate explanation.** Is the theory right or true? Obviously, this is a place where empirical verification through research plays a vital role.

Applying Nursing Theories to Practice

We have discussed the question: What is a good theory? Selma Fraiberg (1959) asks: What good is a theory? She challenges us to explain what practical use all this research and theorizing has. To do so we must consider the application of theory to clinical practice in psychiatric nursing.

There are many ways of knowing what to do in the clinical act. Some of us rely on authority, others on past experience. Trial and error is a time-tested epistemology, and some of us yearn for divine inspiration. Scientists, however, are governed by canons of empirical research methodology either for deductively testing and confirming or refuting theories or inductively generating them from data.

Most nurses acknowledge that principles govern their actions regardless of how practical the nurse's orientation. Without the concepts and propositions of nursing theory we cannot categorize data acquired through assessment, formulate nursing rather than medical diagnoses, and select from possible nursing actions those with the greatest probability of achieving the desired goal. Appendix E summarizes selected contemporary nursing research related to practice with psychiatric clients.

Some of our colleagues challenge us to demonstrate the ways in which what is emerging as uniquely nursing theory is more than mere restatement of well-known psychological, physiological, systems, or medical principles in a special jargon. If all nursing theory exists ultimately for the sake of practice, the theory developed to guide psychiatric nursing practice ought to be clearly distinguishable from mental health prac-

tice based on borrowed theories in other disciplines. Colleagues in other disciplines cannot be expected to learn and apply new terms to describe familiar phenomena just because we in nursing choose to use them. Nursing theories must have both intellectual and practical coherence if they are to achieve a foothold in the knowledge base of the mental health team.

References

Abdellah, F. G. *Patient-Centered Approaches to Nursing.* New York: Macmillan, 1960, pp. 24–25.

American Nurses' Association. *Standards of Psychiatric and Mental Health Nursing Practice.* Kansas City, Mo.: American Nurses' Association, 1982.

Betts, V. "Using Psychiatric Audit as One Aspect of a Quality Assurance Program." In *Current Perspectives in Psychiatric Nursing,* vol. 2, edited by C. R. Kneisl and H. S. Wilson, pp. 202–208. St. Louis: C.V. Mosby, 1978.

Bower, F. *The Process of Planning Nursing Care.* 2d ed. St. Louis: C.V. Mosby, 1977.

Bussman, J. W., and Davidson, S. V. *P.S.R.O.: The Promise, Perspective, and Potential.* Menlo Park, Ca.: Addison-Wesley, 1981.

Fitzpatrick, J.; Whall, A.; Johnston, R.; and Floyd, J. *Nursing Models and Their Psychiatric Mental Health Applications.* Englewood Cliffs, N.J.: Prentice-Hall, 1982.

Fraiberg, S. *The Magic Years.* New York: Charles Scribners', 1959.

Gebbie, K. M., and Lavin, M. A., eds. *Classification of Nursing Diagnoses.* St. Louis: C.V. Mosby, 1975, p. 39.

Hall, L. *Nursing–What Is It?* Publication of the Virginia State Nurse's Association, Winter 1959.

Henderson, V. *The Nature of Nursing.* New York: Macmillan, 1966, p. 1.

Kant, I. *Dreams of a Ghost Seer.* New York: Macmillan, 1900.

King, I. M. *Toward a Theory of Nursing: General Concepts of Human Behavior.* New York: John Wiley, 1971.

Lamonica, E. *The Nursing Process: A Humanistic Approach.* Menlo Park, Calif.: Addison-Wesley, 1979.

Levine, M. E. "The Four Conservation Principles of Nursing," *Nursing Forum* VI (1967): 45–59.

Orem, D. E. *Nursing: Concepts of Practice.* New York: McGraw-Hill, 1971, p. 48.

Orlando, I. J. *The Dynamic Nurse-Patient Relationship: Function, Process and Principles.* New York: G.P. Putnam, 1961.

Peplau, H. E. *Interpersonal Relations in Nursing.* New York: G.P. Putnam, 1952.

KEY NURSING CONCEPTS

✔ The nursing process and contemporary nursing theories based on research organize knowledge and provide a scientific way of knowing what to do with psychiatric clients.

✔ Phases of the nursing process include assessment, nursing diagnosis, planning, intervention, and evaluation.

✔ The 1982 American Nurses' Association Standards for Psychiatric and Mental Health Nursing Practice reflect the current state of knowledge and base practice on theory.

✔ The nursing process is a conscious, deliberate, yet flexible and adaptable systematic set of cognitive and behavioral steps that describe the clinical act in nursing practice with individuals, families, groups, and aggregates.

✔ Effective nursing depends on accurate, systematic, and continuous data collection.

✔ Nursing diagnoses express conclusions about client problems supported by recorded assessment data, current scientific premises, and humanistic principles.

✔ The nursing care plan is used to guide therapeutic intervention, achieve desired goals; it should reflect agreement between client and professional on short and long-term goals.

✔ The implementation phase of nursing process is characterized by continued data collection and observation as well as modification in intervention strategy and timing, if necessary.

✔ Evaluation completes the phases of the nursing process and occurs in order to revise the data base, nursing diagnosis, and nursing care plan.

✔ Concepts serving as focus for contemporary nursing theories are man, society, health, and nursing.

✔ Contemporary debate in nursing theory includes questions as to what a theory of nursing should be, whether any unique nursing theory exists, and how it might be evaluated.

Rogers, M. E. *The Theoretical Basis of Nursing.* Philadelphia: F.A. Davis, 1970, pp. 4–10.

Roy, C. *Introduction to Nursing: An Adaptation Model.* Englewood Cliffs, N.J.: Prentice-Hall, 1976, pp. 11–13.

Wiedenbach, E. *Clinical Nursing, A Helping Art.* New York: Springer Publishing, 1964.

Yura, H., and Walsh, M. *The Nursing Process.* New York; Appleton-Century-Crofts, 1978.

Further Reading

Chinn, P. L., ed. "Nursing Theories and Models." *Advances in Nursing Science* 3 (1980).

Dickoff, J.; James, P. A.; and Wiedenbach, E. "Theory in a Practice Discipline II. Practice-Orientated Research," *Nursing Research* 17 (1968): 545–554.

Donaldson, S., and Crowley, D. "The Discipline of Nursing." *Nursing Outlook* 26 (1978): 113–120.

Kim, M. J., and Moritz, D. A. *Classification of Nursing Diagnoses: Proceedings of the Third and Fourth National Conferences.* New York: McGraw-Hill, 1982.

Kuhn, T. *The Structure of Scientific Revolutions.* 2d ed. Chicago: University of Chicago Press, 1970.

Meleis, A., Wilson, H., and Chater, S. "Toward Scholarliness in Doctoral Dissertations: An Analytical Model." *Research in Nursing and Health* 3 (1980): 115–124.

Nursing Theories Conference Group. *Nursing Theories: The Base for Professional Nursing Practice.* Englewood Cliffs, N.J.: Prentice-Hall, 1980.

Reihl, J., and Roy, C. *Conceptual Models for Nursing Practice.* 2d ed. New York: Appleton-Century-Crofts, 1980.

Schwab, J. *The Teaching of Science as Inquiry.* Cambridge, Mass.: Harvard University Press, 1962.

Sills, G. "Research in the Field of Psychiatric Nursing, 1952–1977." *Nursing Research* 26 (1977): 201–207.

Stevens, B. *Nursing Theory: Analysis, Application, Evaluation.* Boston: Little, Brown, 1979.

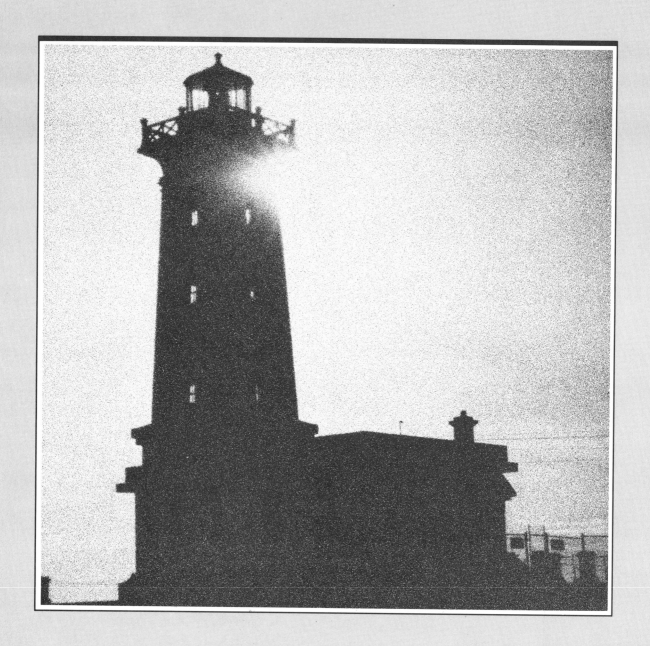

PART TWO

The Processes of
Psychiatric Nursing Practice

IN THIS SECTION WE PRESENT *the essential psychiatric nursing processes—ethical reflection; communication; interpersonal relationships; and assessment of individuals and groups. Processes traditionally considered to be mental health nursing content are also covered. Decisions not grounded in theory are often philosophical and ethical ones. Nurses must turn to their sense of right and wrong, to personal and professional values, to their inner resources and to their own unique personalities for guidance. In Chapter 5 we are directed toward this goal.*

There was a time in the not too distant past when therapeutic nursing care was viewed and taught as a list of "dos" and "don'ts." Well-meaning nurses struggled to avoid the evils of "social relationships" with clients, and at all costs nodded and "mirror-reflected" the standard phrases designated by some authority as therapeutic responses. Communication as a mutual search for meaning is our basis for Chapter 6.

Genuinely effective psychiatric nursing intervention is quite different from overworked scripts or routine approaches. Instead, it requires nurses to carry out processes of assessment, decision making, and problem solving. We believe that interpersonal skills are crucial to the practice of all nurses, regardless of a client's setting or health problem. In Chapters 7 and 8 we focus on collaboration, facilitation, and assessment in the nurse-client relationship. Of particular interest in Chapter 8 is our complete introduction, overview, and explanation of DSM-III, the American Psychiatric Association's new nomenclature for diagnosis of mental disorders. We explore the basis for assessing and understanding group processes in Chapter 9.

5

Ethical Reflectiveness

CHAPTER OUTLINE

The Process of Ethical Reflection
    Analyzing Ethical Issues
    Dominant Ethical Perspectives
    Principles of Bioethics
Ethical Dilemmas in Psychiatric Nursing
    The Stigma of Psychiatric Diagnoses
    Control of Individual Freedom
    Client Privacy and Confidentiality
    The Ethics and Politics of Women's Mental Health
    Political versus Psychological Solutions
    Balancing the Individual and the Social Good
Key Nursing Concepts

LEARNING OBJECTIVES

After reading this chapter, students should be able to
- Discuss the process of ethical reflection used in analyzing an ethical issue
- Compare and contrast dominant ethical perspectives
- Define the six major principles of bioethics
- Identify and discuss ethical dilemmas in psychiatric nursing
- Formulate a personal stand on the ethics and politics of psychiatric nursing practice

CHAPTER 5

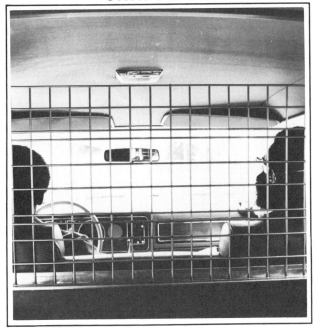

> *Ethical dilemmas in psychiatric care often revolve around the balance between individual rights and social control.*

THE PROCESS OF ETHICAL REFLECTION

A young teacher of nursing bioethics and philosophy once wrote, "Reasoning in ethics means bringing all one's faculties in a balanced way to bear on the sincere concern for human well-being in general and the meaning of human experience. Being reasonable in ethics is more like having integrity than like being smart." (Jameton in press.) This chapter describes a process of ethical reflection to be used as a framework for analyzing ethical issues and resolving ethical dilemmas in psychiatric nursing. Reason and reflection have always held an important place in the study of ethics, for ethics is more than a personal or inspirational enterprise used to answer moral questions. Moral judgments are most highly developed when the *process of arriving at them* and the *reasons for believing in them* are clear and convincing. At the heart of ethical judgments are the reasons for them. The process of applying ethical reflection to concerns in psychiatric nursing can improve the quality of our professional decisions, raise the level of our ability to communicate with others, increase our sensitivity to others, and perhaps offer a sense of moral clarity and enlightenment about our work.

Throughout the history of nursing education, teachers and students alike have professed a concern with ethical matters. A closer look, however, reveals that the concern has been less with moral principles and ethical dilemmas and more with legal aspects of practice and what psychiatric nurse–bioethicist Anne Davis refers to as "the etiquette of the profession." (Davis and Aroskar 1978.) With nursing's notable advances toward professional autonomy in recent years, however, has come the need and responsibility to account for and accept the consequences of professional decisions and actions. Autonomy, according to Aroskar (1980) has to do with the right of self-determination, governance without outside control, and the capability of existing independently. Professionals do this by: developing codes of ethics, which provide guidelines for defining professional responsibility; setting rigorous qualifications for entry into the profession; establishing peer review procedures; and setting standards for practice, such as the *A.N.A. Standards of Practice* (see Appendix A). These mechanisms attempt to balance the goal of more autonomy in nursing with efforts to achieve what providers and consumers determine is the common and the individual "good" in health care.

On a personal level, however, each reader begins a chapter on ethical concerns with the hope of finding an uplifting code or credo of beliefs that can provide us all with a standard against which to judge the rightness or wrongness of our thinking and practice . . . an elevated and elevating declaration of noble ethical imperatives from which to derive positive, inspired answers to difficult, perplexing questions. Such a hope—easy and comforting though it may be—is somewhat short-sighted. In the words of Alfred North Whitehead, "The single-minded use of the notions of right or wrong is one of the chief obstacles to the progress of understanding." The goal of this chapter is not to preach right and wrong but to help students develop a way of thinking about complex ethical issues and dilemmas.

Analyzing Ethical Issues

One of the major difficulties in ethical analysis is that there are no definite, clear-cut solutions to ethical dilemmas. For centuries moral philosophers—beginning

---

Table 5-1 FRAMEWORK OF QUESTIONS FOR ANALYZING AN ETHICAL ISSUE

1. Who are the relevant actors in the situation?
2. What is the required action?
3. What are the probable and possible consequences of the action?
4. What is the range of alternative actions or choices?
5. What is the intent or purpose of the action?
6. What is the context of the action?

---

with Socrates, Plato, and Aristotle—have struggled with two main ethical questions: (1) What is the meaning of right or good? and (2) What should I do? In order to identify, clarify, define, and defend a stand on an ethical issue, we must engage in a process of reflective thinking about data that can be gathered by using the framework of six critical questions set out in Table 5-1.

Psychiatric nurses must often identify alternative courses of action and decide what to do when there is a conflict of rights and obligations between clients and families, between themselves and other mental health workers, or between the clients' good and the community or social good. For example, if a woman's disturbed functioning or distress is in part a reaction to aspects of her social context, a therapist can alleviate the disturbance either by helping the person adjust to her situation as it is or by helping her to change her situation. In a sense a psychiatric nurse becomes both an ethicist and a political agent in resolving this choice. Consider the ethical threads in this excerpt from a letter written by an American psychiatric nurse who spent the summer of 1981 in England.

On the south-west coast of England, near toy town villages like Penzance, Fowey, St. Austel and Newquay, noted for pirates, pubs and Cornish clotted cream, Sylvia Plath wrote a bitter, but remorseless novel about one young woman's vulnerability and personal experience with madness. She left us all with the poignant and eerie image of a bell jar, something she described as "descending upon her with its stifling distortions." As you know, on February 11, 1963, Sylvia Plath ultimately took her own life and passed into myth in her cold English flat at about four in the morning . . . "that still, blue almost eternal hour before the baby's cry, before the glassy music of the milkman settling his bottles."

Yet, twenty years after Sylvia Plath created the metaphor of a bell jar to express a view of herself as "stopped and black as a dead baby" and of the world itself as "a bad dream," I met a young woman also living on the Cornish coast and still stuck within the bell jar's frightening and distorting lens. Living in quiet desperation with a five-year-old wisp of a son and an A-type personality husband, she describes herself as "a nothing, a nobody" and wonders why her husband puts up with her weeping, her fatigue, her trembling anxiety attacks. Her husband chooses to ignore his wife's inability to get out of bed in the morning to face the day for the two years that have passed since her miscarriage. He somehow believes that refusing to confront his wife's problem will make it go away. To her physician she is a "silly girl" who should snap out of it and appreciate all that she has. To the psychiatric consult, she is a ten-minute interview for whom Librium, Tofranil, and Dalmane were prescribed with unlimited refills. To her parents, she is a puzzle that can be solved with a friendly visit and a nice spot of tea. To me, she has been the reason for a sometimes obsessive and usually upsetting voyage of reflections on the ethical and political issues surrounding the topic of women's mental health, and her figure looms like a specter in my memory asking me as a woman and a mental health professional, "What is there beyond the bell jar?"

(Anonymous)

Dominant Ethical Perspectives

Various ethical positions or perspectives provide different ways of structuring the answers to the framework of questions identified in Table 5-1, thus leading to different decisions about what is the right action. The dominant ethical perspectives include the following traditions.*

- *Egoism.* The egoist answers questions about the morally right thing to do by saying that something is good because "I desire it." The right act, then, is the one that maximizes the pleasure of the person asking the question.

- *Deontology.* The deontologic or formalist approach suggests that rightness or wrongness depends on the nature or form of the action for moral significance. In this tradition there are both *act deontologists* and *rule deontologists*—that is, rightness may be based on performing certain morally significant acts properly or adhering to certain preestablished rules or principles. This position requires a commit-

---

*Adapted from Anne J. Davis and Mila A. Aroskar. *Ethical Dilemmas and Nursing Practice*. Norwalk, Connecticut: Appleton-Century Crofts, 1978.

ment to the *principle of universality*—that is, one will make the same moral judgment in any similar situation regardless of time, place, or persons involved. Many rule deontologists believe in the Divine Command Theory—an act is wrong because it is forbidden by God. The difficulty for both believers and nonbelievers with this position is that sometimes the rules conflict. In an attempt to get out of the conflicting rules problem, Immanuel Kant, writing in the late eighteenth century, stated that you should act only on a maxim that you can simultaneously will to be a universal law. Unfortunately, Kant's position doesn't help with moral *conflict.* For example, if returning the institutionalized mentally disturbed to the community was identified as a morally good action, Kant would have us ignore any specifics of a particular situation, even though an individual might end up living in a dingy stairwell and stealing food.

- *Utilitarianism.* The theory of utility defines good as "happiness or pleasure," and right as "the greatest good for the greatest number of people." Implicit in this position is the assumption that one can weigh and measure harm and benefit and come out with the best possible balance of good over evil. Among the questions raised by this position is what happens to individual justice in the emphasis on general welfare.

- *Theory of Obligation.* The basic principles of the theory of obligation are: (a) the principle of beneficence that asks us not just to *want* good but to *do* good rather than evil, and (b) the principle of justice meaning equal treatment designed to distribute benefits and burdens equally through society. What to do when the two principles conflict at the public policy or individual action level is a residual problem with this position.

- *Ideal Observer Theory.* This perspective outlines the characteristics of ethical reason as consistency, disinterest, dispassion, omnipresence, and omniscience, and states that these are the qualities of an *ideal observer* or *moral judge.* The ideal observer has only general interests, such as the welfare of all, and does not make decisions on practical or emotional grounds. Needless to say, the questions of who should be the moral judge and where the development of this moral consciousness will occur are left unanswered.

- *Justice as Fairness.* The principles of justice as fairness are: (a) each person is to have an equal right

to the most extensive liberty for all, and (b) social and economic inequities are to be arranged so that they most benefit the least advantaged. In this system, the first principle of maximizing liberty for all has absolute priority. Five criteria emerge from this position for judging the rightness of any ethical principles:

1. Universality. The same principles hold for everyone.
2. Generality. They must not be geared to specific people or situations.
3. Publicity. They must be known and recognized by all.
4. Ordering. They must order conflicting claims.
5. Finality. They may override the demands of law or custom.

Principles of Bioethics

The preceding ethical traditions or a combination of them operate when nurses reflect on ethical dilemmas. Bioethics is a recently developed field that applies ethical reasoning to issues and dilemmas in the area of health care.

Taking a stand on an ethical issue involves much more than merely accepting the moral position or personal values of another. Bioethicists (Davis 1981) offer the six principles in Table 5–2 as important guidelines.

ETHICAL DILEMMAS IN PSYCHIATRIC NURSING

The conceptual and philosophical orientation of this book represents a shift in perspective from the past. The traditional framework for psychiatric nursing was dominated by ideas associated with medical practice. Although much of psychiatric nursing continues to take place in settings with a disease orientation, the knowledge base of the nursing discipline is in a state of transition. Psychiatric nursing is in effect being redefined to emphasize enhancing the quality of life for clients, who are seen in a holistic view. The focus of psychiatric nursing is widening to deal with the place clients hold in the collective, historical experience of their society. Nurses no longer view people as totally propelled by instinctual drives and partially restrained

---

Table 5-2   PRINCIPLES OF BIOETHICS

1. Autonomy—the right to make one's own decisions
2. Nonmaleficence—the intention to do no wrong
3. Beneficence—the principle of attempting to do things that benefit others
4. Justice—the distribution, as fairly as possible, of benefits and burdens
5. Veracity—the intention to tell the truth
6. Confidentiality—the social contract guaranteeing another's privacy

Source: From A. J. Davis, "Ethical Dilemmas in Nursing." Recorded at JONA and Nurse Educator's 1981 Joint Leadership Conference. Available from Teach'em Inc., 160 East Illinois St., Chicago, Ill.

---

by defense mechanisms such as repression. Rather they take the more phenomenological view that people construct their actions based on the images and meanings that their particular circumstances hold for them. People who are labeled psychiatric clients are no longer excused for their actions by virtue of having an illness over which they have no control. It is thus no longer easy to justify nursing interventions such as seclusion, involuntary intramuscular medication, and restraint on the ground that the client's behavior is crying out for others to control it.

The nurse must protect the rights of the individual client yet mediate between these rights and the interests of the social group. Sometimes the two are in conflict. To complicate the situation, Kai Erikson (1962) and Thomas Szasz (1974) argue that deviance can sometimes help stabilize society and therefore actually makes a valuable contribution to social life. According to these authors, only by public displays of rule-breaking behavior can the group learn its tolerance ranges for acceptable behavior. This position is a far cry from a traditional view of the psychiatric client as a dangerous enemy of society—an actual or potential aggressor to be controlled by society's designated keepers. The new ideology implies that practices accepted as standard under the traditional theories must change. Ultimately nurses must reconcile a number of crucial ethical dilemmas with their personal and professional values. Among these issues are:

- The potential stigma of psychiatric diagnostic labels
- Psychiatry's right to control individual freedom
- The justification for involuntary confinement

- The use of repressive treatment interventions
- The client's right to suicide
- The client's right to privacy
- The politics and ethics of women's mental health
- Psychiatry's responsibility in defending society's dominant life-style
- The psychiatric professional's role in social and political reform

To practice psychiatric nursing requires ethical responsibility. The quality of a nurse's moral commitment is a measure of professional excellence. Psychiatric nursing is practiced at the intersection of people and rules. If rules are shared and understood, deviance exists only as a potential, and the psychiatric nurse's role is clearer. However, when there is conflict about the ground rules for behavior, whether the conflict is between client and social group, nurse and profession, or nurse and agency, problems emerge phrased in the ethical language of right and wrong. Circumstances likely to give rise to such problems include the following:

- The professional and the client are from different social classes and have different statuses or cultural values.
- The voluntary nature of the client is compromised.
- The client's competence to enter into an agreement about intervention is questionable, or clients are subjected to interventions they do not realize are in effect.

Every nursing relationship begins with an unusual burden of ethical responsibility, yet there is little in nursing education that prepares the nurse for the moral issues that arise in practice. The following pages explore some of these moral issues.

The Stigma of Psychiatric Diagnoses

The list of stereotypes associated with diagnostic categories is well known to most nurses. Equally familiar are the consequences to people on whom these diagnoses are conferred in the interest of "helping" them. Psychiatric diagnoses may have fateful consequences for clients and their families. Evidence that they have lacked credibility, reliability, and validity should continue to prompt refinements and research among psychiatric professionals on this topic.

Diagnostic labels can come to have a life of their own. People with records labeling them as drug addicts, alcoholics, homosexuals, convicts, paranoids, etc. acquire a discredited social identity because of the character flaws often associated with these categories. To much of society, the labels used in psychiatry suggest decadence, immorality, and wanton disregard for society's values. Sociologist Erving Goffman subtitles his monograph on stigma, *Notes on the Management of Spoiled Identity* (1963). It is important to consider how and when psychiatric nurses, while advocating humane treatment for clients, indirectly contribute to their spoiled identities by participating in the use of oppressive labels.

The Need to Label   Diagnosis has considerable value in ordinary medical practice. Putting clients into diagnostic categories makes it easy for health professionals to communicate with each other about the client. Occasionally the diagnosis dictates a particular course of treatment and enables the health team to prognosticate about a client's recovery. Diagnostic categories enable nurses to plan comprehensively for client care.

Before the publication of the third edition of American Psychiatric Association's Diagnostic and Statistical Manual of Mental Disorders (DSM–III), diagnostic categories such as schizophrenia, paranoia, or sociopathy were not sufficiently precise to give a clear idea of desirable treatment. A person labeled schizophrenic can be treated with phenothiazines, milieu therapy, or behavior modification techniques. All of these could be justified by one theoretical orientation or another. Nonetheless, the diagnostic label was felt to be the key to subsequent decisions about a client, especially the choice of medication. In most cases when clients failed to respond favorably to the medication indicated by their diagnosis, the diagnosis was changed.

We missed the diagnosis initially. We focused on the paranoid schizophrenic elements and missed the cycles. We need to take him off the Prolixin and consider Lithium for his manic depression.

Advocates for the criteria-based DSM–III believe that its use will greatly improve diagnostic practices. (See Chapter 8.)

The Labeling Process   A substantial proportion of "treatment time" in any modern inpatient setting is devoted to piecing together stories about the clients in order to sort them into diagnostic or legal categories. Intelligence-gathering tactics consume staff attention and energy during the early days of a client's confinement, if not longer. Staff members trying to uncover information about a client interact with clients trying to hide what they believe are damaging data about themselves. One staff member comments to another, "Have you picked up a little paranoia in David or is it only guardedness?" Clients often sense that they are being evaluated for fateful decisions. They try to learn the scripts that will produce the most positive fates for them. One client asked the nurse, "Does it go against you to be lying down two hours in a row?"

A highly ritualized example of the process of piecing together a story occurs in group intake interviews in most inpatient settings.

Bianca, a newly admitted client, is confronted by a group of eight staff members in an interview room and questioned in a mildly interrogative style. Because of the need to "get to know the client as quickly as possible," her story does not just unfold. Instead she is frequently faced with a barrage of questions. She is standing, barefoot, in a robe, in front of eight strangers. At one point, she pleads: "I just want to go home. I feel like I'm going to be put away for the rest of my life. I don't like it here. I'm sorry, I'm trying to cooperate. I just don't feel I can be close to any of you." She starts to cry. "I'm confused because you ask so many questions. I just don't trust a group of strangers. I'm sorry, but I just need time to think."

Based on this interview and data in the client's chart, the staff pieces together her "story." One staff member summarizes: "I think we've observed a depressed gal with a history of inadequacy and dependency. The pathology is first and foremost depression with her hysterical personality disorder coming out to cover up."

There is little in the range of human behaviors that cannot at some time or another earn its way into a psychiatric classification. Thomas Szasz likens this observation to the ordeal by water used in seventeenth-century witch-hunts: floating was defined as guilt and drowning as innocence. Szasz notes that in over twenty years of psychiatric work he has never known of a projective psychological test (such as the Rorschach inkblot test; see chapter 8) that reported the subject to be a normal, mentally healthy individual. Szasz offers an anecdote about a psychiatrist devising an assessment tool for psychiatric problems in school-age children. Under "symptomatic" behaviors were listed:

- Academic problems — underachievement, overachievement, erratic performance
- Social problems with peers—the submissive child, the aggressive child, the show-off
- Problems in relations with authority figures—defiant behavior, submissive behavior, ingratiation
- Overt behavioral problems—nail biting, thumb sucking, interests more befitting the opposite sex (a tomboy girl or an effeminate boy)

There seem to be few childhood behaviors that a psychiatric professional could not place in one of these categories. This would be funny if the consequences to the child were not so serious. Professionals joke that the psychiatric client who is early for an appointment is anxious, the one who is late is hostile, and the one who is on time is compulsive. The jokes, however, do not change the "heads I win, tails you lose" nature of some psychiatric diagnoses.

The Self-fulfilling Label   One of the most common characteristics of psychiatric labeling might be called a *correctness assumption*. Frequently, staff members have already decided that a client will be given medication, even though the client has refused it. Before the start of the precertification seventy-two-hour observation period required by California law, staff members may have decided that the client will be certified for fourteen days. Contacts with the client are then used more to justify the decision than to make a decision in the first place.

Another major characteristic of psychiatric diagnosis is the invalidation of the client's point of view. A client's statement that he or she does not want psychiatric help is used as evidence that the person needs it. A client's tears in an interview are viewed as a psychiatric symptom rather than a result of the immediate social context of interrogation, locked ward, involuntary confinement, fatigue, or other stressful circumstances.

Setups—contrived situations—often characterize the information-gathering operations prerequisite to diagnosis. Because diagnostic decisions usually must be made on the basis of limited contacts with clients, setting a situation up to "see how the client reacts" is sometimes used to help establish one diagnosis over

another. The client's response to the setup is considered evidence of illness.

A client's diary had been brought to the hospital by a friend. Some discussion ensued among the psychiatric team members about whether "she knows we have this." The staff members decided to leave the diary on the desk in front of the interviewee to "see how she reacts." Any sign of outrage and anger would be viewed as an indicator of her emotional disorder rather than as a justified response to the circumstances.

It is not unusual for psychiatric labeling to have what might be called a "double whammy" effect. This notion is akin to the self-fulfilling prophecy. Staff members' interventions reinforce and elicit the very behavior that earned the client the label.

One client was reported as very paranoid and very delusional, because he thought the staff was trying to hypnotize him. The therapeutic treatment solution to his problem was to increase his medications.

Another client was described as obsessive–compulsive, because she was preoccupied about whether the staff would label her as crazy. Staff members told her that they only wanted to talk about how to help her stop worrying, but they reminded each other that they needed to get a diagnosis on her immediately.

Sociocultural Influences on Diagnosis   The diagnostic labels used in Western psychiatry are found to be of limited value in cross-cultural comparisons. Observations indicate that the behavior called *schizophrenia* differs from one culture to another. Even in Western society, the diagnostic label given to a particular behavior is related to the client's position in the class structure. Affective disorders predominate among the upper classes and psychoses characterize the lower classes. Repressive attitudes toward women, blacks, and homosexuals influence diagnoses. In sum, more often than we would like, conventional psychiatric diagnoses are more affected by characteristics of the social situation in which the deviant and the labelers interact than by actual characteristics of the deviant. Usually the deviant responds inadequately to the interpersonal demands of someone else in a situation. Factors that influence the outcome of such acts include (a) whether the act is labeled as symptomatic by a professional outsider, (b) how serious the act itself is, (c) how frequently the act has occurred, and (d) the social context. Most of the time families develop elaborate accommodation mechanisms to keep a deviant member within the home setting. These accommodation patterns are disrupted only when the public visibility of deviant behavior is highlighted by a diagnosis. The "V-codes" of DSM–III are intended to improve this situation. The V-codes refer to problems in living that are a focus of attention but do not reflect a mental disorder.

Diagnostic Stereotypes

THE HOMOSEXUAL   Acts of physical love with a member of the same sex often bring harsh or brutal punishment in the United States. Persecution of the homosexual has become quite common, despite the fact that most homosexuals seem to be more discreet, less predatory, and less violent than many heterosexuals. Society's aversion to homosexuality is demonstrated by the fact that it has been considered both a crime and a disease. Oppression of the homosexual today is maintained primarily by the fear that homosexuality threatens the stability of the society and by the irrational belief that homosexuality implies weakness. Even though the label of homosexuality has been replaced in the psychiatric nomenclature by the more limited term *ego-dystonic homosexuality* (meaning that the pattern of homosexual arousal causes distress to the client and is unwanted), psychiatric professionals continue to view this particular life-style as reflecting immaturity, deep-seated psychological problems, emotional disturbances, and severe conflicts.

THE SCHIZOPHRENIC   On the basis of a rather vague concept, thousands of Americans have been labeled and hospitalized as schizophrenics. An individual designated schizophrenic becomes a pariah who is approached with a mixture of distrust and fear. The labeled schizophrenic may be denied employment, particularly in sensitive or important jobs. The pride and self-confidence of diagnosed schizophrenics are often shattered, and they may come to view themselves as incapable of controlling their impulses. Some clients living in agony find reassurance in being told that at least they are not schizophrenic. This diagnosis has become psychiatry's equivalent of cancer in its connotation of hopelessness. Again, advances cited in DSM–III include a considerably narrower concept of schizophrenia.

THE PARANOID   The diagnostic term *paranoid* has taken on an almost totally pejorative meaning. The term is not restricted to those who behave strangely, are overtly suspicious, or tend to blame their failings on others. Professionals apply it to many who take deviant positions on social issues. To accuse an adversary of being paranoid has become a kind of trump card for discrediting any opponent's position.

THE ADDICT   A person who uses alcohol or other drugs to excess may be overwhelmed with all sorts of personal and social difficulties and still maintain a respectable role in society. However, once labeled an alcoholic or addict, this person is cast into a different social role. Addicts elicit pity from some, scorn from others. Under some circumstances they can be imprisoned, even though the substances they use are harmful only to themselves.

The Nurses's Moral Stance on Diagnoses

Does labeling with psychiatric diagnoses merely provide psychiatric professionals with some additional sense of control in their dealings with clients? It is true that a diagnosis gives staff members an increased sense of being able to predict client behavior and a way of viewing calmly what might otherwise be upsetting behavior: "That's just her hysterical personality coming out," or "Those complaints are just paranoid delusions." The consequences of psychiatric labels for clients and their families, however, raise moral questions about the legitimacy of their arbitrary use. Consider the following, adapted from a letter to a newspaper advice columnist.

I am a 12-year-old girl who is left out of all social activities because my father is an alcoholic. I try to be nice and friendly to everyone, but it's no use. The girls at school have told me that their mothers don't want them to associate with me because my father might be dangerous. Is there anything I can do? I am very lonesome because it's no fun to be alone all the time. My mother tries to take me places with her, but I want to be with people my own age. Please give me some advice.

Sincerely,

An Outcast

Nurses have a moral responsibility to question practices that exact a price from clients far in excess of the benefits. Only through involvement in such issues can nurses create a moral environment for health care in which practices truly respond to clients' needs. Every moment of moral injustice takes its toll on nurses as well as clients. Every moment of moral responsibility strengthens their sense of personal integrity.

Control of Individual Freedom

Psychiatric professionals limit and control the freedom of clients through the subtle process of assigning labels to their behavior that have fateful consequences. They also control individual freedom in more straightforward and direct ways. The most frequent examples of direct controlling interventions are involuntary hospitalization, and use of repressive treatments, usually when a person is judged to constitute a danger to self or others.

Involuntary hospitalization and treatment of psychiatric clients are usually considered humanitarian efforts to help "the mentally ill." Yet any practice that directly and coercively deprives a person of freedom has political implications. In most states a client who is involuntarily committed to a mental hospital has few of the legal protections that even a criminal offender has. In addition, in some states clients have no guarantee that they will ever be released from this hospital unless they alter their behavior sufficiently to please their keepers.

Violence and Social Control

VIOLENCE AGAINST OTHERS   Psychiatric nurses are faced with the dilemma of trying to be both healer–helpers and agents of social control. In dealing with violently destructive clients, and some others, the value of life is being balanced against the value of liberty. Thomas Szasz (1974) argues that there is never adequate justification for involuntary commitment under the guise of medical help. He believes that violence toward others is a crime and should be treated as such, not as a mental disease. Szasz argues that contemporary psychiatry confuses deviance with disease and control with cure, and makes decisions and policies that he believes constitute grave threats to personal freedom and dignity. Seymour Halleck (1971), another politically oriented psychiatrist–writer, suggests that society needs to make distinctions among the kinds of violence to decide which kinds might legitimately be controlled by civil procedures. His intent is to limit severely the instances that justify psychiatric intervention. Like Halleck, psychiatrists Andrew Sko-

dol and T. B. Karasu (1978) contend that psychiatric professionals can do little to help prevent spontaneous violence. So many variables contribute to such behavior that it is practically impossible for anyone to predict its occurrence. Because it is so difficult to know precisely who will be violent, it becomes an unjustifiable infringement of civil liberties to incarcerate someone who behaves peaceably most of the time and has not committed a crime but is only suspected of being prone to impulsive outbursts. In contrast, Halleck identifies a group of people who plan violence and act in irrational, strange, or self-defeating ways even with members of their own subculture. It is reasonable to assume that these people are experiencing emotional difficulty, he feels. In this group would be a woman who talks of killing her children because she is commanded to do so by God, or a person who feels driven to obtain sexual pleasure by mutilating and molesting strangers. These individuals are justifiable candidates for involuntary detention on psychiatric grounds, in Halleck's view. Szasz, on the other hand, prefers the application of legal-criminal controls to this category of people.

SUICIDE   Suicide is a form of violence to oneself and as such represents another point at which the moral issue of balancing liberty and life comes up for psychiatric nurses. The extent to which homicide and suicide are equivalent is another basic ethical question that bears on society's right to control suicide. Szasz views homicide and suicide in the same relation to each other as rape and masturbation. Homicide, according to Szasz, is the gravest crime, while suicide in his opinion is a basic human right.

Traditionally, nurses have felt that they should do everything possible to preserve life. They have relied on this imperative to justify coercive intervention in suicide attempts as well as heroic technical measures to avert impending deaths. Recent reconsideration of euthanasia, however, seems to raise questions about a client's right to suicide. *Euthanasia* has been defined as the intentional termination of a life of such poor quality that it is not worth living. The concept of allowing a person to die without the use of life-prolonging treatment is called *passive euthanasia. Active euthanasia,* on the other hand, is defined as an act that results in the death of a person. The treatment given to dying clients is often in conflict with the treatment they desire. For example, a physician may disregard a client's protests against treatment. The doctor may assert that the client's medical condition is causing the client to behave irrationally. It is no great logical jump from clients dy-

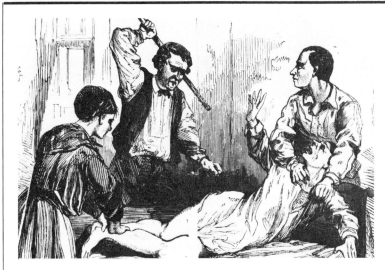

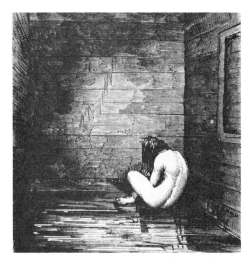

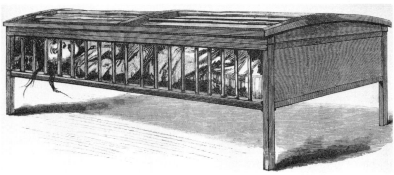

Actual beatings of the "insane," isolation cells, and devices such as the "restraining crib" represent repressive psychiatric treatments from earlier historical eras.

ing of physical deterioration to clients dying of emotional or mental deterioration. Many of the same ethical questions emerge about the suicidal client:

- How is *quality of life* defined?
- Is the definition limited to physical factors?
- Who should have the right to make the definition?
- How is rationality to be measured?
- Are people always in conscious control of their choices?

The following report by Robert Trumbull (1977) suggests that the social mores concerning the right to death are being reexamined in many quarters of society:

The Anglican Synod of Canada has been asked to consider endorsing the termination of life at birth for severely retarded infants as well as the withdrawal of life support for the terminally ill . . . one of the prominent members of the committee who prepared the report endorsed mercy killing of infants born with brain damage that leaves them permanently bereft of all human attri-

butes except that they look human and were born of humans—human vegetables so defective that they have no chance of gaining a modicum of spiritual or intellectual life. . . . Similar thoughts were put forward in relation to passive euthanasia for terminally ill patients where the quality of life is marginal, when the patient is irremediably comatose, or when death is already in sight.

Needless to say, such a formal recommendation meets with considerable dissent and disagreement. Some argue that society never has the right to take anybody's life, because that should be in the hands of God. Other more secular objections are raised by those who cite continual advances in medical science. These advances are potentially capable of improving the lot of both mentally retarded infants and the terminally ill.

An individual's right to choose when and how to die is a complex biomedical issue currently receiving more attention than ever before. It behooves the thoughtful professional nurse to clarify the issues, give them careful consideration, and search for a personal position.

There are many ways in which people can deliberately shorten their own lives. They can destroy themselves quickly with a gun, or slowly through the chronic use of drugs such as tobacco or alcohol. When is coercive intervention by psychiatric practitioners justified? Do professionals have the right to restrain people against their will if those people have not committed an illegal act?

Use of Repressive Treatments   At some time in their lives, all people experience the kind of excessive stress that makes them feel miserable or even desperate. Some people, however, communicate these feelings in ways that are inappropriate, troublesome, unreasonable, or frightening to others. A young woman who in times of stress mutilates her body by burning it repeatedly with cigarettes; a teenager who breaks everything in sight during violent, destructive outbursts; and a belligerent male who initiates physical fights with anyone and everyone without provocation all usually become candidates for *symptomatic treatments*— that is, behavioral control measures often used against the person's will.

PSYCHOSURGERY   The most dramatic of repressive measures is *psychosurgery*, the surgical removal or destruction of brain tissue with the intent of altering behavior even though there may be no direct evidence of structural disease or damage in the brain. (For description and analysis of psychosurgery, see Chapter 23.) Psychosurgery has become the subject of marked controversy on ethical grounds. Advocates claim that it is done to restore rather than destroy individual freedom. They argue that before psychosurgery, the client is crippled by mental illness. Individual autonomy is compromised by the client's bizarre behavior or internal psychological state. After the surgery, clients supposedly are more autonomous than before, by their own and others' criteria. Advocates of selective use of psychosurgery, even when it is against the client's will, outline three conditions that must be met to justifiy it:

1. The illness being treated is seriously disabling and untreatable by nonsurgical means such as medication or therapy.
2. The treatment is undertaken with some sort of systematic investigative protocol—in short, it is accompanied by evaluation research.
3. The treatment occurs in settings with as many safeguards as possible to arrive at informed consent, if possible, perhaps using a client advocate during the procedure.

Thomas Szasz (1963) is the outspoken opponent of this form of "treatment." He does not oppose the surgical procedures themselves, for he is in favor of what he calls "free trade" in psychosurgery between consenting adults. He believes that a person ought to be free to seek a lobotomy. But Szasz condemns the idea that under certain circumstances "psychotics" ought to be lobotomized whether they like it or not. This concept is a menace to medicine, morals, and personal liberty, he argues. What justifies a "therapeutic intervention" such as surgery by an individual called a psychiatric professional against another individual called a client? To the true believer in the medical model of psychiatry, the justification is the client's mental illness. To the medical autocrat, it is the physician's judgment that the client and/or society would benefit from the intervention. To the employee of government-supported care agencies, it is the decision of the government that the operation should be done. To the libertarian, the only justification is the consent of the would-be client. Overlooking or confusing these conflicting moral and political perspectives, says Szasz, is the source of most current problems in the ethics of health care.

PSYCHOTROPIC DRUGS   The discovery that certain drugs can radically alter human emotions has had an enormous impact on psychiatry. Although the number of clients entering mental hospitals has continued to increase, since the advent of tranquilizing drugs, clients are now patched up and discharged more rapidly. The mental hospital is no longer seen as a warehouse for storing society's deviants; it is now a clearinghouse where clients are sorted, renovated, and dispatched back into their communities with symptomatic behavior under control through one or another of the current psychiatric medications.

Psychiatric professionals have associated the advent of psychotropic medications with a new optimism and less fear about working with persons labeled mentally ill. Conceivably, the impact of the drugs on attitudes of nurses may increase the amount of humane contact clients are given while in the hospital. Furthermore it might be argued that the drugs have helped keep people out of the hospital and have decreased the need for other more dramatic treatments, such as electroshock treatment.

On the other hand, drugs that make people feel better can lessen their motivation to confront an oppressive situation. This can have serious implications for the political and moral climate of society. Consider, for example, a common clinical problem:

A woman is married to a domineering and insensitive man. She becomes increasingly unhappy, then intensely anxious. When she is on the verge of fighting back to try to alter her oppressed situation, she becomes more agitated and visits a psychiatric clinic. Her therapist prescribes a medicine that alleviates her tension. As a consequence she has less awareness of her plight and is less inclined to confront her problems. She ultimately continues to submit to her husband's oppressiveness.

It is conceivable that pills could be developed to keep such a woman quietly enslaved throughout her married life. Suppose drugs were coercively given to anyone whose unhappiness was rooted in social oppression. We can even contemplate the possibility that the state might become repressive enough to force all dissidents to take medicine.

Drugs cautiously and judiciously used with the consent of clients can be helpful to people. Used unreflectively, they can close off moral and political confrontations. Decisions about the use of drugs must be made in the context of the social situation and environment.

In the inpatient setting, medications are regularly used to reduce symptoms and increase the manageability of client behavior. Most staff members legitimize their use of chemical controls by defining violent or bizarre behavior as an indirect request for limits. When this kind of meaning is assigned to the use of drugs, practitioners can feel that their actions to suppress symptoms are based on the client's needs rather than on the staff's management motives.

After pacing angrily up and down the hall in front of the nurses' station for twenty minutes or so, Carlotta kicks over some mops in a bucket. A male staff member shouts to the nurse to get her PRN medication ready and strides into the hall telling the client to stop it. She cries and shouts, and they begin struggling. Several other staff members rush over to assist. They drag and carry her into her room, where she gets Haldol (10 mg.). She continues fighting and screaming. The staff members decide to put her in "soft" restraints and continue to wrestle with her in her room. Finally they decide to transfer her to the ward downstairs, where she can be put into a seclusion room. In a report, a staff member describes the incident as, "Carlotta blew up and needed controls." In further discussion of the case, it became apparent that the decision to put her into seclusion was made because restrained clients have to be checked and

released every 10 minutes, which is a lot of work for the staff.

It is possible that all these controls would not have been necessary had a nurse behind the glass windows of the nurses' station responded to the nonverbal cues of mounting tension that the client communicated before kicking over the mops.

Structural Controls   Even the physical characteristics of psychiatric inpatient settings convey the notion that clients are not expected to be capable of self-control and that staff members have the responsibility for providing it. Many clients view these interventions as forms of abuse, while the staff sees them as "helping people who can't take care of themselves." Consider the following directions on use of restraints:

The acutely psychotic client who is delusional, the angry individual who is testing limits, and the intoxicated client are the types of individuals to whom restraints may be applied for their own protection and that of others. These individuals are nonverbally asking for help to control their potentially inappropriate behavior. When all other techniques have failed and it is quite obvious that the client is out of control, the staff must take action and forcibly apply restraints.

All the judgments that must be made about restraints involve moral decisions. What other techniques have been tried? Is the client obviously out of control? How does the nurse decide? What will be the effects on the client of such a dramatic intervention? What are the effects on others in the milieu? In weighing decisions, nurses must keep in mind that any intervention that removes symptoms without simultaneously increasing the client's awareness of the underlying experience is potentially repressive. Clients themselves have begun to guard against repressiveness by issuing a bill of rights.

Client Privacy and Confidentiality

When people seek psychiatric help, they must usually reveal highly personal, possibly embarrassing, and potentially condemnatory information about themselves. Almost all modes of therapeutic intervention rely on the client's willingness to talk openly and honestly about personal concerns, feelings, or problems. The solo therapist in private practice with voluntary clients

MENTAL PATIENT'S BILL OF RIGHTS

We are ex-mental patients. We have been subjected to brutalization in mental hospitals and by the psychiatric profession. In almost every state of the union, a mental patient has fewer de facto rights than a murderer condemned to die or to life imprisonment. As human beings, you are entitled to basic human rights that are taken for granted by the general population. You are entitled to protection by and recourse to the law. The purpose of the Mental Patients' Liberation Project is to help those who are still institutionalized. This Bill of Rights was prepared by those at the first meeting of MPLP held on June 13, 1971, at the Washington Square Methodist Church. If you know someone in a mental hospital, give him/her a copy of these rights. If you are in a hospital and need legal help, try to find someone to call the number listed below.

1. You are a human being and are entitled to be treated as such with as much decency and respect as is accorded to any other human being.
2. You are an American citizen and are entitled to every right established by the Declaration of Independence and guaranteed by the Constitution of the United States of America.
3. You have the right to the integrity of your own mind and the integrity of your own body.
4. Treatment and medication can be administered only with your consent and, in the event you give your consent, you have the right to demand to know all relevant information regarding said treatment and/or medication.
5. You have the right to have access to your own legal and medical counsel.
6. You have the right to refuse to work in a mental hospital and/or to choose what work you shall do and you have the right to receive the minimum wage for such work as is set by the state labor laws.
7. You have the right to decent medical attention when you feel you need it just as any other human being has that right.
8. You have the right to uncensored communication by phone, letter, and in person with whomever you wish and at any time you wish.

9. You have the right not to be treated like a criminal; not to be locked up against your will; not to be committed involuntarily; not to be fingerprinted or "mugged" (photographed).
10. You have the right to decent living conditions. You're paying for it and the taxpayers are paying for it.
11. You have the right to retain your own personal property. No one has the right to confiscate what is legally yours, no matter what reason is given. That is commonly known as theft.
12. You have the right to bring grievance against those who have mistreated you and the right to counsel and a court hearing. You are entitled to protection by the law against retaliation.
13. You have the right to refuse to be a guinea pig for experimental drugs and treatments and to refuse to be used as learning material for students. You have the right to demand reimbursement if you are so used.
14. You have the right not to have your character questioned or defamed.
15. You have the right to request an alternative to legal commitment or incarceration in a mental hospital.

The Mental Patients' Liberation Project plans to set up neighborhood crisis centers as alternatives to incarceration and voluntary and involuntary commitment to hospitals. We plan to set up a legal aid society for those whose rights are taken away and/or abused. Although our immediate aim is to help those currently in hospitals, we are also interested in helping those who are suffering from job discrimination, discriminatory school admissions policies and discrimination and abuse at the hands of the psychiatric professions. Call number listed below if you are interested in our group or if you need assistance.

MPLP
56 East 4th Street
New York, N.Y. 10003
(212) 254-4270

Source: Mental Patients' Liberation Project.

is usually able to avoid compromising the clients' rights to confidentiality. In fact, many private therapists view themselves as vigilant protectors of their clients' privacy. Nurses, however, may encounter a serious ethical conflict in being at the same time the confidant of the client and an employee of the organization. These nurses have dual allegiances—to the client and to the agency. Clients usually assume that health professionals have no other purpose than to help them. They lose sight of the fact that nurses often are asked to collect data about them that might be highly influential in determining their medications, their disposition, and even their civil rights. While it is often the psychiatrist who makes final pronouncements about a client's mental health status, diagnosis, prognosis, and the like, such pronouncements rest on information collected and communicated to the doctor by nurses. This information-gathering process merits serious scrutiny.

It is not unusual for a kind of fiction to develop about a hospitalized client, in the staff's eagerness to gather juicy tidbits of information. Data are passed from one nursing shift to another and written on the chart without thought to their validity or reliability. These are then used to make generalizations about the client. The following are typical entries about clients in nurses' notes:

Little socialization.
Somewhat seclusive.
Superficially appropriate.
Looks flat.
Very poor insight.
High as a kite.
May be hallucinating.

Often the requirement that nurses exchange tidbits such as these with each other becomes the motivation for getting out to talk to the clients so that the nurse will have something to report. Yet it is considered sufficient simply to have a comment to make. Little concern is shown about how representative that comment may be.

The information garnered in this way may be confirmed by repetition in shift reports and daily charting, without additional exploration. This arouses another reaction in some nurses—reluctance to report any observations.

On one occasion a few staff members in an inpatient facility expressed concern about the things people choose to put in reports, because of "the way things get latched onto around here." For example, a client may acquire a reputation as a homosexual or heroin addict because of revealing one experimental experience to a nurse in what the client believed to be a confidential exchange. One nurse said, "Somehow it seems more ethical to write 'I didn't talk to the client today' or 'I don't know what's going on with this person' than to select out of an eight-hour period one or two phrases or behaviors, often expressed in clichés."

Notes are subject to multiple interpretations within the immediate social context. If they are frequently blown out of proportion into a widely accessible portrait of the client, nurses may be unwilling to contribute to the information-gathering process.

Almost all human behavior taken out of context can be construed as pathological. A West Coast psychiatric team recently conducted an experiment in which they posed as clients and had themselves admitted to psychiatric wards. After telling their initial admission story of disturbed behavior, they behaved absolutely normally, except that they openly took notes about the ongoing ward activities. When asked by the staff what they were doing, they responded that they were psychiatric researchers studying the hospital ward. One staff member reported:

> D. R. engages in compulsive writing behavior. Is highly delusional . . . may be dangerous.

Only the other clients began to suspect the truth. They asked the researchers, "What are you doing? Writing a book or something?"

Information gathering and sharing are part of the psychiatric nurse's role. When the employer is a federal- or state-supported agency that might have some investment in quelling deviants, however, the nurse is put in a double-agent role. The client's rights to privacy and confidentiality are increasingly threatened by computerized data banks for information storage, certain medical and other insurance procedures, and even the Professional Standards Review Organization (PSRO) system in clinical agencies. Thoughtful handling of this dilemma is facilitated by two safeguards:

1. Nurses must convey to clients the limit of confidentiality in their exchanges—that is, what the nurses do with the information a client shares.

2. Nurses must attempt to portray accurately to others how reliable, valid, and representative are the data they communicate about a client.

The Ethics and Politics of Women's Mental Health

In the past two decades, nurses have become aware of the impact of feminism on the institution of psychotherapy and the sensibilities of those professionals who concern themselves with a special subsection of the client population—women. Brodsky's (1973) review of a decade of feminist influence on psychotherapy cited changes in theories, treatment techniques, and assessment approaches, all reflecting more enlightened attitudes toward women as therapists and clients. Yet as recently as February 1978, a special populations subpanel on the mental health of women submitted a report to the President's Commission on Mental Health that began:

> American women rank with the racial and ethnic minorities as a segment of the population who are overrepresented among the mentally ill, and underserved by the mental health system. While the numbers place women clearly in a majority position, other data suggest that women continue to be accorded disadvantaged status in all areas of American society. Despite the 1974 amendments to the Civil Rights Act of 1964, discrimination against women continues in all major institutions of this society.

The report further describes the documented social, economic, and psychological status of women as follows:

- More than half the women in the United States are now employed outside the home, but they are clustered in the lowest-paying occupations and at the bottom of the achievement ladder.
- Equal opportunity programs and affirmative action notwithstanding, qualified women employed full-time in 1976 earned less than 56 percent of what men earn.
- One woman in four but one man in eighteen lives on an annual income of less than $4,000.
- Increasing numbers of families are comprised of a mother and her children, and there are few social supports for her outside the immediate family.
- Whether or not women are employed outside the home, housework remains largely women's work. Thus many American women have two full workdays every twenty-four hours.

- Fifty percent more women than men report having used barbiturates.
- Estimates of the proportion of alcoholic women in the population range from 20 percent to 50 percent, but the numbers are increasing.
- Twice as many women as men use the two most popular tranquilizers, Valium and Librium.
- Although exact numbers are not yet available, increasing numbers of women are reporting that they have been beaten, raped, or abused, often in their own homes.
- There are 175 women to every 100 men admitted to hospitals for the treatment of depression (Weissman 1975).
- There are 283 women to every 100 men treated for depression in outpatient services (Weissman 1975).
- More women than men in the general population report that they experience symptoms of depression.
- The highest rate for treatment in public facilities is for nonwhite women and women between twenty-five and forty-four who are separated or divorced.
- Among married women in the general population, symptoms of depression are more common among women whose children are living with them.
- Older women whose children have left home and women who have never married show fewer symptoms of depression (Guttentag 1976).
- The conflict between self-esteem and incongruent role is reported as a source of stress for women.
- Since no evidence suggests that women are innately more vulnerable to mental illness, it must be assumed that social institutions have a different, more stressful impact on women than on men.
- Most mental health professionals are men, and most clients are women.
- Women in therapy comment that many therapists: foster traditional sex roles; have biases and expectations that devalue women; use traditional psychoanalytic concepts in a sexist way; and often respond to women as sex objects.

This rather disconcerting and thought-provoking summary underscores the necessity of viewing women's mental health as a clinical or research area requiring our most responsible and expert ethical and political reflectiveness.

Phyllis Chesler (1972), the outspoken author of *Women and Madness,* analyzes the status of women in our culture in her own unique, rhetorical style.

> Women are submissive. We're altruistic. And especially we're self-sacrificing. Usually our altruism comes from

very low self-esteem. We're always guilty. We're losers—trained to be losers in life. We're also mothers or can be mothers and that's another reason why we might be altruistic.

Chesler goes on to identify four premises that run through all the theories of psychiatry and apply to most clinical practices. These premises, in Chesler's view, reflect how the mental health professions see women and how women have been taught to see themselves.

1. Everybody is crazy.
2. While everybody is crazy, women are crazier. To be mentally healthy is to be male.
3. Male homosexuality is sick, and lesbians don't exist.
4. In order for a woman to be a real woman, she's got to become a mother, and once you've become a mother, everything that goes wrong with your family's mental health is your fault.

Chesler contends that the more than 615,000 women who have gotten themselves involved in careers as hospitalized psychiatric clients are rejecting their sex-role stereotypes. In her view, those women who aren't crazy are unhappily living out their roles. In other words, when a woman is mad in this culture, she's telling us something about the condition of women in general. For those of us in the mental health professions, particularly those of us who are also women, thinking along these lines can be like looking carefully in a mirror for the first time—threatening, somewhat awesome, a little frightening, and not at all easy.

Depression in Women: A Microcosm of the Problem   Perhaps more than any other, the diagnosis of depression illustrates the ethical and political issues of women's mental health practice. Studies of the epidemiology of mental disorders and mental health facility use patterns concur that both treated and untreated depression predominate in women. Some therapists conclude from the prevalence data that women have less coping ability, have a greater tendency to exaggerate perceived stress, are more willing to express psychological symptomatology, and are more willing to remain in dependent roles than men. Scattered throughout the theories accounting for depression are indications of the overriding attitudes toward women who exhibit its symptoms. Psychoanalytic schools of thought have emphasized the importance of

orality, internalized aggression, punitive superegos, and extreme narcissism in determining a person's predisposition to depression. Other widely held views are that depression-prone people are inordinately dependent on others to maintain their self-esteem, that their frustration tolerance is low, and that they employ manipulation, submission, coercion, and pity, and demand to maintain desperately needed but ambivalent relationships with their love objects. Depression, in short, has been a problem of losers and weaklings, and women have slipped into this diagnosis with the ease of donning a custom-made garment.

Only recently, the winds of awareness and change have begun to rattle the doors of the institution of psychiatry and raise questions about the relationship of low social status and legal and economic discrimination to rates of clinical depression. Nurses have a moral responsibility to raise such questions.

Political versus Psychiatric Solutions

The End of Neutrality   For a long time nursing has hidden behind the cloak of political neutrality, arguing that the role of caretakers and healers permits, even demands, a detachment from political, economic, and social issues. Psychiatric nursing services have been defined as client-oriented activities designed to reduce pain and discomfort and to increase the capacity of the individual to adjust satisfactorily. This position was easier to defend when psychiatric problems were viewed in terms of the medical model. As long as nurses saw their psychiatric work as simply treating illnesses of the mind in the same way they treated illnesses of the body, they could accept the notion that psychological illness, like physical illness, indicated a defect in the individual, not in the social milieu. Practitioners tended to search for the causes of emotional suffering in anomalies of the client's biological or psychological past rather than considering factors in the client's environment that might account for strange, troublesome, or irrational behavior. This view of the human condition and the nurse's role avoided any critical examination of society and the nurse's relationship to it.

The medical model is no longer accepted blindly. New conceptual frameworks and nursing theories take into consideration not only internal individual perceptions of stress, but also the immediate and broader social contexts that contribute to an individual's experience of stress (see Chapter 4). Nurses are beginning to realize that a person identified as a client may be miserable and not coping at any given moment not only because of personal perceptions of oppression, but also because they are actually being oppressed. As the saying goes, "Even paranoids have real enemies."

Combating Environmental Stress   In the complex superstructure of global society, environmental stresses may be generated both directly by the selfishness, apathy, or malevolence of those in power and indirectly by subtly imposed prejudices, outmoded and inflexible rules, and an economic system that deprives certain citizens (often the poor and members of minority groups) of basic human needs. Black people directly exposed to humiliation by bigoted whites have a clear idea who their oppressors are. They are aware of their anger and know toward whom it is directed. Black people living in a society where racism is institutionalized but not overt may be exposed to repeated indirect microaggressions that leave them frustrated and angry, but they have difficulty identifying the source of their sense of oppression. Halleck (1971) asserts that any citizens who believe in the basic benevolence of their society but do not partake of its benefits will have similar reactions. It is not unusual for people in these circumstances to express their frustration and anger in alcoholism, drug use, violence, or suicide.

Environmental stress is also generated in the smaller microcosm of immediate families or groups of significant others. A parent may abuse a child. An employer may harass or insult an employee. These are direct sources of stress. Stress generated in immediate social systems also may be indirect, leaving the individual totally or partially unaware of its source. For example, a domineering, chauvinistic husband may send day-to-day demeaning messages that chip away his wife's self-esteem in disguised ways. She may find herself feeling chronically depressed or anxious without knowing why. A domineering wife may do the same to her husband.

The Social Psychiatric Model   A psychiatric nurse who is willing to try to help clients to change the stresses in their environment rather than adapt to them is engaging in an aspect of social psychiatric practice. Halleck (1971), describing a social psychiatric model for practice, urges psychiatric professionals to abandon the hoax of a politically neutral profession and make their personal political positions explicit. He feels that it is illogical to believe that professional activ-

ities designed to change the status quo are political, while those designed to strengthen the status quo are neutral. He emphasizes the important role of psychiatric professionals in social reform. All therapists base their efforts to help clients and society on some idea of the optimum human condition. Therefore, psychiatric professionals must think through the meaning of *optimum human condition* in order to gain insight into their own ideologies and to sharpen their ethical criteria for intervening in social systems or sustaining the status quo.

Thomas Szasz (1970) distinguishes between *institutional psychiatric practice* (unsolicited by clients and practiced by professionals in the employ of the state) and *contractual psychiatry* (practiced with voluntary clients who actively contract for therapy). He believes that the former is a formidable political weapon and the latter is not. Perry London (1970) argues that the methods of behavior control in both kinds of practice have political and moral consequences.

Acting to sustain and preserve a desirable social order is by no means immoral or unethical. Society relies on psychiatric professionals as agents of social control to bring a humane and caring perspective to their often difficult and uncertain work with clients. Many of these clients have engaged in behavior patterns believed to be despicable, destructive, and burdensome to others. As one somewhat hardened nurse put it:

We are the junk pickers of society—picking up society's casualties and trying to rework them into some useful form.

In the novel *One Flew Over the Cuckoo's Nest* (1962), Ken Kesey echoes this in harsher terms. He characterizes Big Nurse as a depersonalized agent of "the Combine" delegated the task of "rewiring" clients brought to her ward so that they will fit in smoothly. The rewiring process, disguised as treatment and therapy, is no less than a complete stripping of the spirit.

Social psychiatry must counteract such approaches while finding a balance point between the conflicting needs of clients and society.

Balancing the Individual and the Social Good

The judgments that label someone's experience as paranoid rather than simply unpopular are frequently based on arbitrary and shifting criteria. Behavior that is considered bizarre or unreasonable in one cultural context may be considered desirable in another (see Chapter 26). The definitions of those who need psychiatric help are constantly changing. Nurses are necessarily guided in therapeutic work by a belief system—by some vision of what kinds of changes would improve a client's life. Nurses are further guided by some moral principles that limit the extent to which they will help a client obtain happiness at the expense of others and the extent to which they will participate in the oppression of an indi-

vidual in the interests of societal control. Laws represent yet another source of limits (see Chapter 27).

Nursing is frequently faced with two goals: (1) to respond to the therapeutic needs of individuals, and (2) to serve society by preserving some degree of social order. Often these two goals are in conflict, and nurses must face the dilemma of placing one above the other. The only way to resolve the conflict is for them to clarify their own goals and values through a process of ethical reflection.

KEY NURSING CONCEPTS

✔ Ethical reflection is an essential process of psychiatric nursing practice for achieving clear and convincing reasons for taking actions or making moral decisions rather than discovering a singular right or wrong situation for ethical dilemmas.

✔ Ethical dilemmas are situations with conflicting moral planes, or a conflict between two obligations.

✔ Nurses move toward professional autonomy through development of codes of ethics, setting qualifications for practitioners, participating in peer review, setting standards, and accepting consequences for professional decisions.

✔ Known dominant ethical perspectives include Egoism, Deontology, Utilitarianism, Theory of Obligation, Ideal Observer Theory, and Justice as Fairness.

✔ Egoism posits that the right act is the one that maximizes the pleasure of the person asking the question.

✔ The Deontologic position suggests that rightness or wrongness depends on the form of the action for moral significance.

✔ The Theory of Utilitariansim defines good as happiness and right as maximizing the greatest good and the least harm for the greatest number of persons.

✔ Theory of Obligation suggests that individuals ought to do good, not just want good, and that benefits and burdens ought to be distributed equally throughout society.

✔ The Ideal Observer Theory suggests that characteristics of ethical reason are consistency, disinterestedness, dispassionateness, omnipresence and omniscience.

✔ Justice as Fairness states that each person is to have maximum liberty, and social and economic inequities are to be arranged so that the greatest benefit goes to the least advantaged.

✔ Principles of bioethics include autonomy, nonmaleficence, beneficence, justice, veracity, and confidentiality.

✔ Contemporary health-related ethical dilemmas include the effects of psychiatric labeling, control of personal freedom, use of repressive treatments, the client's rights, and the ethics and politics of women's mental health.

✔ The nurse must protect the rights of the individual yet mediate between these rights and the interests of the social group.

References

American Psychological Association. Task Force on Sex Bias and Sex Role Stereotyping in Psychotherapeutic Practice. "Guidelines for Therapy with Women." *American Psychologist* 33 (1978): 1122–1123.

Aroskar, M. A. "Establishing Limits to Professional Autonomy: Whose Responsibility?" *Nursing Law and Ethics* 1 (1980).

Brodsky, A. "The Consciousness-raising Group as a Model for Therapy with Women." *Psychotherapy: Theory, Research and Practice* 10 (1973): 24–29.

Chesler, P. *Women and Madness.* New York: Doubleday, 1972.

Davis, A. J. "Ethical Dilemmas in Nursing." Recorded at JONA and Nurse Educator's 1981 Joint Leadership Conference, available from Teach'em Inc., 160 East Illinois Street, Chicago, Illinois.

Davis, A. J., and Aroskar, M. A. *Ethical Dilemmas and Nursing Practice.* New York: Appleton-Century Crofts, 1978.

Erikson, K. "Notes on the Sociology of Deviance." *Social Problems* 9 (1962): 308.

Goffman, E. *Stigma: Notes on the Management of Spoiled Identity.* Englewood Cliffs, N.J.: Prentice-Hall, 1963.

Guttentag, M.; Salasin, S.; and Belle, D. *The Mental Health of Women.* New York: Academic Press, 1980.

Halleck, S. L. "Psychiatry and the Dilemma of Crime." In *Violent Men,* edited by H. Toch. Chicago: Aldine Publishing, 1969.

———. *The Politics of Therapy.* New York: Harper and Row, 1971.

Jameton, A. *Ethics in Nursing.* Englewood Cliffs, N.J.: Prentice-Hall, in press.

Kesey, K. *One Flew Over the Cuckoo's Nest.* New York: Viking Press, 1962.

London, P. *Behavior Control.* New York: Harper and Row, 1970.

Mechanic, D. *Mental Health and Social Policy.* Englewood Cliffs, N.J.: Prentice-Hall, 1969.

Scheff, T. *Being Mentally Ill: A Sociological Theory.* Chicago: Aldine Publishing, 1960.

Skodol, A., and Karasu, T. B. "Emergency Psychiatry and the Assaultive Patient." *American Journal of Psychiatry* 135 (1978): 202–205.

Szasz, T. *Law, Liberty and Psychiatry.* New York: Macmillan, 1963.

———. *The Manufacture of Madness.* New York: Harper and Row, 1970.

———. *The Myth of Mental Illness.* Rev. ed. New York: Harper and Row, 1974.

Task Force on Mental Health of Women. *Report to the President's Commission on Mental Health.* Washington, D.C.: U.S. Government Printing Office, 1978.

Trumbull, R. *New York Times,* July 28, 1977, p. 10.

Further Reading

Brody, E. "Psychiatry and the Social Order." *American Journal of Psychiatry* 12 (1965): 81–87.

Broverman, I. K., et al. "Sex Role Stereotypes and Clinical Judgments of Mental Health." *Journal of Consulting and Clinical Psychology* 34 (1970): 1–7.

Buss, A. R. "The Emerging Field of the Sociology of Psychological Knowledge." *American Psychologist* 30 (1975): 988–1002.

Caplan, G. *Principles of Preventive Psychiatry.* New York: Basic Books, 1964.

Cummings, E., and Cummings, J. H. *Closed Ranks.* Cambridge: Harvard University Press, 1957.

Goffman, E. *Asylums.* Garden City, N.Y.: Doubleday, 1961.

Gove, W. R. "Mental Illness and Psychiatric Treatment Among Women." *Psychology of Women Quarterly* 4 (1980): 345–362.

Grier, W., and Cobbs, P. *Black Rage.* New York: Basic Books, 1968.

Hollingshead, A. B., and Redlich, F. C. *Social Class and Mental Illness.* New York: John Wiley, 1958.

Klerman, G. L., and Weissman, M. *The Mental Health of Women.* New York: Academic Press, 1980.

Lakin, M. "Some Ethical Issues in Sensitivity Training." *American Psychologist* 24 (1969): 923–928.

Rappaport, J. R., ed. *The Clinical Evaluation of the Dangerousness of the Mentally Ill.* Springfield, Ill.: Charles C. Thomas, 1967.

Riesman, D. *Individualism Reconsidered and Other Essays.* New York: Free Press, 1954.

Rogers, C. R., and Skinner, B. F. "Some Issues Concerning Control of Human Behavior: A Symposium." *Science* 124 (1956): 1057–1066.

Stolz, S. B., et al. *Ethical Issues in Behavior Modification.* San Francisco: Jossey-Bass, 1978.

Wilson, H. S., and Kneisl, C. R. *Learning Activities in Psychiatric Nursing.* Menlo Park, Calif.: Addison-Wesley, 1983.

Nurse-Client Communication: The Mutual Search for Meaning

CHAPTER OUTLINE

The Process of Human Communication
  Human Communication Defined
  Variables that Influence Communication
  Levels of Communication
Models of Human Communication
  Communication as an Act
  Communication as an Interaction
  Communication as a Transaction
Modes of Communication
  The Spoken Word
  Nonverbal Messages
  Relationships between Verbal and Nonverbal Systems
Communication in Humanistic Psychiatric Nursing
  The Theory of Therapeutic Communication
  The Theory of Pragmatics of Human Communication
  Ego States as Communication Analysis
Facilitative Communication
  Social Superficiality versus Facilitative Intimacy
  Essential Ingredients
  Skills that Foster Effective Communication
  Ineffective Communication Styles
Interaction Process Analysis Case Study (IPA)
Key Nursing Concepts

LEARNING OBJECTIVES

After reading this chapter, students should be able to
- Describe the process of human communication
- Compare linear, interactional, and transactional models of communication
- Identify the major concepts in a symbolic interactionist approach to communication
- Discuss verbal and nonverbal modes of communication
- Relate three major theories of communication to humanistic psychiatric nursing practice
- Identify concepts of facilitative communication that are essential ingredients of interpersonal relationships
- Apply skills that foster effective communication throughout the nursing process
- Use Interaction Process Analysis to assess nurse–client communication

CHAPTER 6

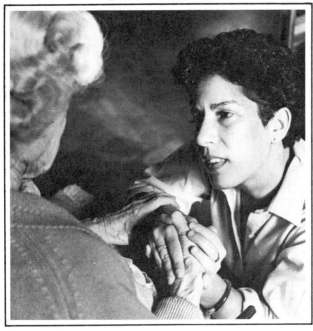

Person-to-person communication is at the heart of humanistic psychiatric nursing. The nurse's body position, eye contact, and facial expression demonstrate her interest in the client.

THE PROCESS OF HUMAN COMMUNICATION

When John Bowlby (1951) discovered that infants in foundling homes were literally dying for lack of human contact and affection, the scientific community began to attach new importance to the old dictum that *people need people*. It is recognized today that the mechanism for establishing, maintaining, and improving human contacts is interpersonal communication. Communication is a very special process and the most significant of human behaviors. Moreover, it is the main method for implementing the nursing process.

The therapeutic interpersonal relationship in humanistic psychiatric nursing practice often develops through a storytelling experience. Telling stories is as natural and human as breathing. When they tell "their story," clients explain themselves, the events of their lives, and the circumstances they face.

The major role of the psychiatric nurse is to help clients tell their stories, explore the circumstances of their lives, and resolve the things that have gone wrong. However, the process of communication is so complex and multidimensional that it cannot be reduced to a few simple steps that nurses can memorize and perform.

Human Communication Defined

Communication is an ongoing, dynamic, and ever-changing series of events, each of which affects and is affected by all the others. The essence of effective communication is *responding with meaning* to the series. Unfortunately, some persons define communication simply as the transfer of information or meaning from one human being to another. This chapter will demonstrate that meaning cannot be transferred from one human being to another but must be mutually negotiated, because meaning is influenced by a number of significant variables.

Variables that Influence Communication

Perception A person's image or perception of the world is an essential element in communicating. The term *perception* refers to the experience of sensing, interpreting, and comprehending the world in which the person lives. This makes perception a highly personal and internal act.

The information that people have of the world around them is processed through their senses. However, seeing is not always believing. Contemporary communication specialists have discovered that because of human physiological limitations, the eye and brain are constantly being tricked into seeing things that are not really what they seem. Figure 6–1 shows an illusion that reflects physiological constraints. Before continuing to read, stare at Figure 6–1 for 20 seconds. The illustration will appear to swing back and forth. Verify that the movement is an illusion by checking the visual perception against tactile sensations.

What people "see" or sense is influenced very strongly by a number of factors. Stop reading here and look at Figure 6–2. Past experiences have prepared us to see things, persons, and events in particular ways. When we read the sayings in Figure 6–2, past experience encourages us to see them inaccurately as the

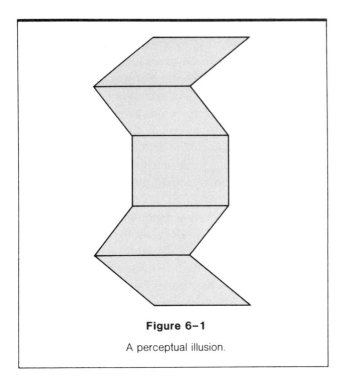

Figure 6–1

A perceptual illusion.

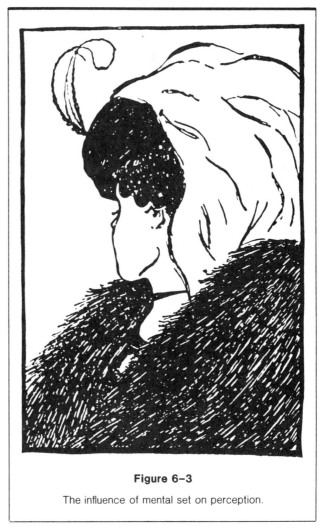

Figure 6–3

The influence of mental set on perception.

familiar sayings "Snake in the grass," "Quick as a flash," and "Paris in the spring." The words actually are "Snake in *the the* grass," "Quick as *a a* flash," and "Paris in *the the* spring."

People tend to observe more carefully when a purpose guides the observation. The purposes or reasons for engaging in an observation also determine what is observed. The nurse in an Intensive Care Unit makes different observations of the cardiac surgery patient from those made by a family member.

Finally, when understandings differ, people can look at the same object and see different things. Mental set helps determine how and what a person perceives. Before you read any further, take a look at the picture of the young woman in Figure 6–3. Do you see the sil-

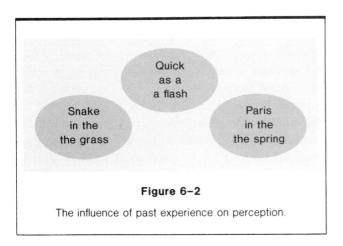

Figure 6–2

The influence of past experience on perception.

houette of a young woman? Do you also see the face of an elderly woman? Our use of the phrase *the picture of the young woman in Figure 6–3* encouraged you to perceive the illustration in a particular way. Now you should also be able to see the elderly woman in the illustration.

As the illustrations demonstrate, the old axiom might be better stated: "Believing is seeing." Because people tend to perceive in terms of past experiences, expectations, and goals, perceptions may be a prime obstacle to communication. No two individuals will perceive the world in exactly the same way, and the meanings of events will differ because people's perceptions of them differ. Perceptions of other human beings are of particular importance since human communication is inevitably affected by participants' perceptions of one another.

In order to see others at all as they are, people need to know themselves and to know how the self affects the perception of others. Reviewing Chapter 3 will help in the self-perception process and the process of perceiving others.

Values   Values are concepts of the desirable. People value what is of worth to them. Values influence the process of communication, because people's values, like their perceptions, differ.

Value systems differ for a number of reasons. Age is one. Children's values shift when they become teenagers. The college or work experience generally influences values in yet other directions. Marrying or being a parent or grandparent may cause other value changes or shifts.

Psychiatric nurses must ultimately come to terms with the problem of values, because conflicting value systems among mental health professionals expose clients to uncertainty and confusion. Consider the following examples:

The parents of a fifteen-year-old girl were upset to find a small plastic bag of marijuana in her dresser drawer. She had been playing hooky from school and wore jeans that her parents considered sloppy. After a series of lengthy, angry discussions with her parents she was confined to her room. During this period she refused to eat or drink.

When the girl was seen by a mental health treatment team, the members' opinions were divided. Some said that her behavior signaled an emotional disturbance and labeled her antisocial, depressed, and anxious. Others believed her parents were too rigid in attempting to force her to accept their values.

In another instance, a thirty-five-year-old man was firmly committed to prayer. Most of his spare time was connected in some way to church-related activities. Staff members at a mental health clinic where he sought counseling told him that he was resorting to an early infantile attitude about God as the magic worker.

Clearly, these staff members were influenced by their own values.

The daily roles people take also influence their values. In any one day a man may be a student, husband, father, nurse, citizen, speaker, artist, son, and teacher. A review of the section on values in Chapter 3 will help in further understanding the role of human values in the communication transaction.

Culture   Each culture provides its members with notions about how the world is structured and what it means. These preconceptions, learned at an early age, are so subtle that they often go unrecognized. They nonetheless set limits on communication and interaction with others. As Chapter 26 describes, relying on culturally determined generalizations or stereotypes can have profound effects on people's relationships with others.

Communication is culture-bound in a wide variety of ways. The culture and the subculture (the culture within the culture) teach people how to communicate through language, hand gestures, clothing, and even in the ways they use the space around them.

The nurse who does not know that "run it by me" means to explain something, that a "close-knuckle drill" is a fistfight, or that "hit on a broad" means to sweet-talk a female may be confused by conversations with members of certain subcultures—adolescents and street people, for example. The nurse who overhears two clients talking about "angel dust" is likely to come to erroneous conclusions if unaware that the term refers not to a Christmas decoration but to PCP—an animal tranquilizer. In some cultures, belching after dinner is a compliment to the host and is considered proper etiquette. In other cultures it may be thought uncouth or an insult. When Americans make a circle with thumb and forefinger and extend the other fingers, they mean "okay." To Brazilians the same gesture is an obscene sign of contempt. These examples make it obvious that communicating with meaning requires that the participants take culture well into account. How people communicate with others who do not share similar histories, heritages, or cultures is of critical importance in humanistic psychiatric nursing practice.

Levels of Communication

Communication takes place on at least three different levels—intrapersonal, interpersonal, and public. *Intrapersonal communication* is what occurs when people communicate within themselves. When a nurse walks into a client's room and thinks, "The first pint of blood is almost finished. I'd better get the next one ready for infusion," the nurse is communicating intrapersonally. The intrapersonal process is primary to the other two levels of communication, because it involves perceptions of self and others, necessary components in all communicative encounters.

Interpersonal communication, which this chapter discusses in depth, is communication that takes place between dyads (groups of two persons) and in small groups. This level of person-to-person communication is at the heart of humanistic psychiatric nursing.

Public communication is communication between a person and several other people. Its most common form is the presentation of a public speech. Communications through the mass media are other forms of public communication.

MODELS OF HUMAN COMMUNICATION

One of the easiest ways to illustrate the nature of human communication and the elements or components that make up the process is through a model, or visual representation.

People use models frequently for many purposes. They might use a map, which is a visual representation of a territory, to find their way to the community mental health center they plan to visit. Health professionals use EEGs to give them a visual representation of the electrical activity in the brain. However, models provide incomplete views—a map does not show all the trees, buildings, or park statues in the territory, and the EEG tracing does not show the color, size, or blood supply of the brain. It is important to keep this in mind when looking at models. They sometimes make a process look simpler than it is.

Communication as an Act

Viewing human communication as an act is a linear concept of communication. It sees communication as a one-way phenomenon: A talks to B. Communicators who follow this concept attempt to transfer the thoughts or ideas in their heads into someone else's head. Communication then becomes something that is done *to* another person. The process is illustrated in Figure 6–4.

Two major assumptions behind this view are that skill is all-important, and that meaning is transferable. Such a model fails to take into account the variables discussed earlier—perception, values, and culture. It suggests that the receiver plays a passive role and does not affect the communicator. It places primary emphasis on the selection of "correct" messages. When misunderstandings occur, either the communicator is faulted for failing to send the correct message or the receiver is faulted for having allowed something to interfere with the transmission of a correct message. Both persons become preoccupied with laying blame and constructing perfect messages to be understood. These implications and assumptions are evidence that the model of communication as an act is inadequate.

Communication as an Interaction

The interactional perspective takes into account the process of mutual or reciprocal influence in communication. Essentially, this view holds that when two people interact, they put themselves into each other's shoes. Each tries to perceive the world as the other perceives it, in order to predict how the other will respond. In other words, communication is two-way, not one-way. It is a circular process in which the participants take turns at being communicator and receiver: A (communicator) talks to B (receiver), and B (communicator) talks to A (receiver). Figure 6–5 illustrates communication as interaction.

Clearly, this view is not as reductionistic as the previous model. However, it still oversimplifies human communication, because it treats it as a series of causes and effects, stimuli and responses.

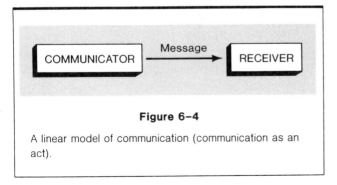

Figure 6–4

A linear model of communication (communication as an act).

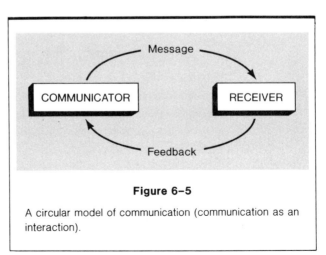

Figure 6–5

A circular model of communication (communication as an interaction).

Communication as a Transaction

Mutual Influence between Communicators   In a transaction, the participants are both communicators. No one is labeled either communicator or receiver. Communication is viewed as a process of simultaneous mutual influence rather than as a turn-taking event.

In a transactional perspective, participants are who they are in relationship to the other person with whom they are communicating. For example, in each dyadic communication event there are at least *six* persons involved: A's A, A's B, A's impression of the way B sees A, B's B, B's A, and B's impression of the way A sees B. Therefore, in addition to the content message, a relationship message also exists. If, when A passes B in the corridor A says "Hi, how are you," and B answers "Just fine, thanks" moving down the corridor and away from A as quickly as possible, B's behavior is a comment on the relationship between A and B. Their subsequent communication will be affected by how A perceives B's response. If A thinks B walked away because B wanted to get home before the thunderstorm that was predicted, A is likely to respond one way to B the next time they meet. If A believes B

is angry with A, A is likely to respond quite differently at the next encounter. The symbolic interactionist model described below helps explain what takes place between A and B.

A Symbolic Interactionist Model of Communication   A symbolic interactionist model is based on a transactional perspective. It views human communication on the social, interpersonal level and accounts for the whole persons involved in the process. The participants are products of their social system and integral parts of it. In the communication, some events take place *within* the participants (they are intrapersonal), and some take place *between* the participants (they are interpersonal).

A model constructed by Hulett (1966, p. 14) according to symbolic interactionist principles, and adapted for this text, is shown in Figure 6–6. It shows five phases in each person's communication sequence: input, covert rehearsal, message generation, environmental event, and goal response.

The phase of *input* is one in which the person is motivated through some stimulus, either external or internal, toward some goal that requires engaging in a social relationship with another. Let us say that Jeff is

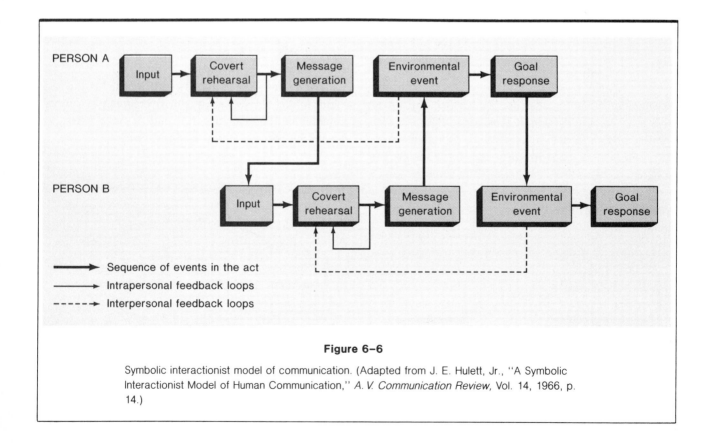

Figure 6–6

Symbolic interactionist model of communication. (Adapted from J. E. Hulett, Jr., "A Symbolic Interactionist Model of Human Communication," *A. V. Communication Review,* Vol. 14, 1966, p. 14.)

attracted to Sarah and would like to get to know her better.

In the *covert rehearsal* phase, the person moves to make sense of the input received and develops and organizes a message *before* generating it. Figure 6–7 represents the symbolic interactionist model of the covert rehearsal. The individual first scans the information about self and others (Jeff enjoys theater and remembers hearing Sarah tell a friend that she'd really like to see the new musical comedy in town) and then rehearses, within his or her own head, possible actions to take (role playing) and possible reactions of the other (role taking). Successive readings of the map of the social structure and the resulting refinements give the person the opportunity to organize the eventual message as closely as possible to that desired. (Jeff thinks of four different ways to approach Sarah.) This process is represented by the intrapersonal feedback loop.

The covert rehearsal phase is really the core of the communication process. In it, Jeff decides what to say, how to say it, and even whether to send the message to Sarah at all.

Message generation, the third phase, is one in which the instrumental act of giving a message is performed.

The message generated by Jeff serves as the input or stimulus for Sarah. Sarah then engages in covert rehearsal, and the message Sarah generates serves as the *environmental event,* the fourth stage in the sequence of Jeff, whose *goal response* serves as the environmental event for Sarah, who then has a goal response as well.

A second, or interpersonal, feedback loop connects the person's environmental event phase to the covert rehearsal stage. It allows the person an opportunity to determine whether he or she has made an error in the approach to the other and to make appropriate corrections by repeating the covert rehearsal and devising an altered message. (Jeff carefully considers Sarah's response. He listens to what she says and watches her behavior toward him. If her response is less than enthusiastic, he will try to determine what went wrong and how it can be corrected.)

In summary, the symbolic interactionist view of communication includes the following concepts:

• People run through a series of internal trials in the process of organizing a message.

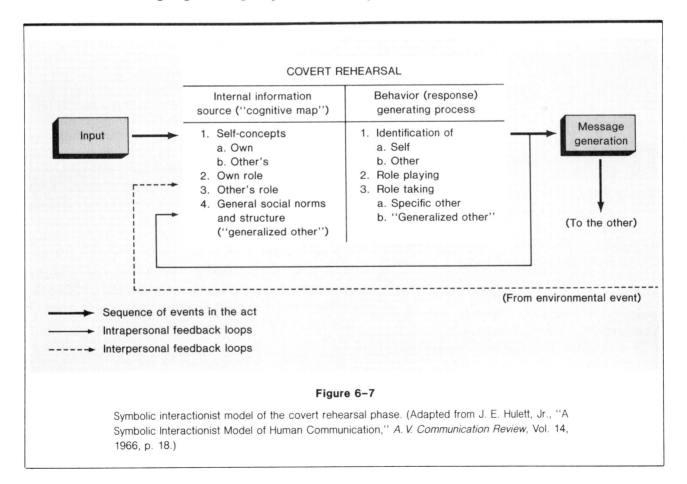

Figure 6–7

Symbolic interactionist model of the covert rehearsal phase. (Adapted from J. E. Hulett, Jr., ''A Symbolic Interactionist Model of Human Communication,'' *A. V. Communication Review,* Vol. 14, 1966, p. 18.)

- People select and transmit the message that will, in their view, have the highest probability of success.
- Success depends on the accuracy and completeness of the cognitive map of the environment and the accuracy and efficiency of the intrapersonal and interpersonal feedback loops.
- Communication is a dynamic (ever-changing) process that is unrepeatable and irreversible.
- Communication is complex.
- The meaning of messages is not transferred, it is mutually negotiated.

MODES OF COMMUNICATION

The Spoken Word

It is verbal language, the ability to utter the spoken word, that makes people human and distinct from other animals. Yet problems arise as humans discover that words mean different things to different people. That is, *words* do not "mean" something, *people* do.

If communication between nurse and client is to be mutually negotiated, the nurse at least must understand the four concepts discussed next.

Denotation and Connotation   A *denotative meaning* is one that is in general use by most persons who share a common language. A *connotative meaning* usually arises from a person's personal experience. While all Americans are likely to share the same general denotative meaning for the word *pig*, the word may have completely different connotations for a farmer, a butcher, a consumer of meat, a person of the Moslem faith, an orthodox Jew, a college student, a prisoner, and a police officer. These positive and negative connotative meanings can arouse powerful emotions.

Private and Shared Meanings   In order for communication to take place, meaning must be shared. What happens when meaning is not shared is illustrated in a bewildering conversation between Alice and Humpty Dumpty:

> ". . . There's glory for you!"
>
> "I don't know what you mean by 'glory,'" Alice said.
>
> Humpty Dumpty smiled contemptuously. "Of course you don't—till I tell you. I meant 'there's a nice knock-down argument for you!'"

> "But 'glory' doesn't mean 'a nice knock-down argument,'" Alice objected.
>
> "When I use a word," Humpty Dumpty said, in rather a scornful tone, "it means just what I choose it to mean—neither more nor less."
>
> (Carroll 1965, p. 93)

By assigning meanings to a word without agreement, Humpty Dumpty essentially created a private language.

Private meanings can be used to communicate with others only when the parties agree about what the word means. The private meaning then becomes a shared meaning. It is common for families, two friends, or members of larger social groups (military personnel, drug users, adolescents, etc.) to use language in highly personal and private ways. Problems arise when assumptions are made that persons outside of the group share these meanings.

People labeled schizophrenic may use language in an idiosyncratic way or may use a private, unshared language referred to as *neologisms*. Such people are unaware that this use of language is not shared with others. They expect to be understood and may become upset when they are not.

A young man who was hospitalized on a psychiatric unit complained to other clients and staff that he had been odenated, and he became increasingly frustrated and anxious when it became apparent that he wasn't being understood. With some help he was able to explain that he was upset about having been moved to a private room. The room was, he said, so dark and dingy that it looked like a cave. Animals live in caves that are called dens. In his view he had been o-den-ated—put in a cave.

In trying to make private meanings shared, the nurse should make an effort to reach mutual understanding of the client's message. It is insufficient, and quite possibly inaccurate, to attach meaning based solely on the nurse's (or the client's) interpretation of an event, a word or phrase, or a nonverbal gesture.

Nonverbal Messages

There are numerous nonverbal communication channels. Most researchers seem to agree that nonverbal channels carry more social meaning than verbal channels. Nonverbal cues help us judge the reliability of verbal messages more readily.

There is a wide variety in nonverbal channels—facial expressions, hand gestures, body movements, use of space, pitch, rate, and volume of the voice, touch, body aromas, and so on. The following categories will be considered here: kinesic behavior (body movement), paralanguage (voice quality and nonlanguage sounds), proxemics (use of personal and social space), touch, and use of cultural artifacts (such as clothing and cosmetics).

Kinesics   The study of body movement as a form of nonverbal communication is called *kinesics*. Facial expressions, gestures, and eye movements are the most commonly used categories.

Facial expressions are the single most important source of nonverbal communication. They generally communicate emotions. The silent film comedians—blank-faced Buster Keaton and comic, endearing Charlie Chaplin—and the great mime Marcel Marceau communicate not only isolated acts but complete sequences of behavior with kinesics alone.

An infinite range of body movements and gestures provide clues about persons and about how they feel toward others. Hand gestures can communicate anxiety, indifference, and impatience, among other things. Foot shuffling and fidgeting may express the desire to escape. Body position gives cues about how open a person is to another person, or how interesting and attractive they appear. People tend to position their bodies according to their feelings about the person with whom they are communicating.

Eye contact is another very important cue in communicating. For example, proper sidewalk behavior among Americans is for passers-by to look at each other until they are about eight feet apart. At this distance, both parties look downward or away so they will not appear to be staring. Erving Goffman (1963, p. 84) has referred to this phenomenon as a "dimming of our lights." Michael Argyle (1967, pp. 105–116) has written of several of the unstated rules about eye contact.

• Interaction is invited by staring at another person on the other side of a room. If the other person returns the gaze it is generally considered that the invitation to interact has been accepted. Averting the eyes signals a rejection of the looker's request.
• A looker's frank gaze is widely interpreted as positive regard.
• Greater mutual eye contact occurs among friends.

• Persons who seek eye contact while speaking are usually perceived as believable and earnest.
• If the usual short, intermittent gazes during a conversation are replaced by gazes of longer duration, the target person is likely to interpret this as meaning that the task is secondary to the relationship between the two persons.

Paralanguage   *Paralinguistics* or *paralanguage* refers to something beyond or in addition to language itself. The two principal components are *voice quality*, such as pitch and range, and *nonlanguage vocalizations*, such as sobbing, laughing, or grunting—noises without linguistic structure.

Vocal cues can differentiate emotions. Who hasn't heard the injunction: "Don't speak to me in that tone of voice!" Sometimes vocal cues are used to make inferences about personality traits. For example, persons who increase the loudness, pitch, timbre, and rate of their speech are often thought to be active and dynamic. Those who use greater intonation and volume and are fluent are thought to be persuasive. Status cues in speech are based on a combination of word choice, pronunciation, grammatical structure, speech fluency, and articulation, among other features.

Proxemics   *Proxemics* is the study of space relationships maintained by persons in social interaction. It includes the dimensions of *territoriality* (fixed and permanent territory that is somehow marked off and defended from intrusion) and *personal space* (a portable territory surrounding the self that others are expected not to invade). Both territoriality and personal space are discussed more thoroughly in Chapter 9.

The intervention of physical objects such as tables also influences social interaction. Furniture and furniture arrangements can be used to increase or decrease interpersonal distance.

Knowing something about proxemics is useful, for example, in planning the physical space in which communication events are going to occur. Mental health workers should be especially sensitive to the constraints imposed on communication by physical objects. Proxemics can also help practitioners decipher verbal communication by paying attention to how others use interpersonal space.

Touch   Touching behaviors, because they tend to personalize communication, are extremely important in emotional situations. In American society the use of touch is governed by strong social norms. Who, when, why, and where people touch are all controlled by unwritten guidelines.

Most of the taboos against touching seem to stem from the sexual implications of touching behavior. However, although touching is a physical act, it may or may not be sexual in nature. A realization of the importance of touch (see Chapter 25 for a discussion of the healing effects of touch) and an understanding that touching is not necessarily a sexual behavior may make this channel of communication available to more people. It is equally important to be sensitive to the other person's disposition toward touching, so as not to alienate another by infringing on the person's right not to be touched.

Cultural Artifacts   Artifacts are items in contact with interacting persons that may act as nonverbal stimuli: clothes, cosmetics, perfume, deodorants, jewelry, eyeglasses, wigs and hairpieces, beards and moustaches, and so on.

Think about what information is communicated through artifacts such as a full-length mink coat, hair that has been dyed purple, a gold band on the third finger of the left hand, a military uniform, or a Phi Beta Kappa key.

Relationships between Verbal and Nonverbal Systems

The verbal and nonverbal elements of human communication are inextricably bound together. Six different ways in which verbal and nonverbal systems interrelate have been identified by Ekman (1965). Each is discussed below.

Repeating   A nonverbal cue may say the same thing as a verbal cue but in a different way. The deep-sea fisherman who tells verbally how big the sailfish that he caught was may also extend both hands to indicate its length. The gesture serves to repeat the idea.

Contradicting   Nonverbal behavior may also contradict verbal behavior. Consider the woman who meets a college roommate she hasn't seen for quite some time. She says, "You haven't changed a bit," but her tone of voice and facial expression convey sarcasm. When verbal and nonverbal cues contradict one another, it is usually safer to put more faith in the nonverbal cues.

Complementing   Nonverbal messages that add to or modify verbal messages are said to be complemen-

tary. When a man says he is a "little" irritated about being kept waiting, his tone of voice and body actions may indicate a more profound anger.

Accenting   There are nonverbal cues that accent or emphasize verbal cues. A woman shrugs her shoulders when she says she doesn't really care which movie she and her companion see. A master of ceremonies holds up his hand when he asks for quiet. These gestures and body movements emphasize the words.

Relating and Regulating   Cues that tell people when to start talking or when to stop talking are usually nonverbal. A woman who keeps opening and closing her mouth briefly while others are talking is indicating that she wants a turn too.

Substituting   Sometimes nonverbal cues are used in place of words. A wave from a friend at a distance says "hello." Applause at the end of a play tells the actors that they have pleased the audience.

COMMUNICATION IN HUMANISTIC PSYCHIATRIC NURSING

The Theory of Therapeutic Communication

A theory of therapeutic communication has been developed by the psychiatrist Jurgen Ruesch (1961). In his view, communication includes all the processes by which one human being influences another human being. Ruesch's theory applies to the symbolic interactionist view because it takes into account the perceptions and interpretations that influence one person's view of the other. Further, Ruesch assumes that in order to survive, the individual must communicate successfully.

Basic Concepts   The basic concepts of this theory are:

- Communication occurs in four different settings—intrapersonal, interpersonal, group, and societal.
- The ability to receive, evaluate, and transmit messages is influenced by perception, evaluation (which involves memory, past experiences, and value systems), and transmission quality of messages (amount, speed, efficacy, and distinctiveness).

- Communication occurs in five systems of codification:
  1. Somatic language—statements mediated through the autonomic nervous system.
  2. Sign language—gestures.
  3. Action language—movements as statements mediated primarily through the central nervous system.
  4. Object language—intentional and nonintentional display of material things, such as clothing and jewelry, art objects, and footprints.
  5. Digital language—verbal or discursive language, spoken words.
- Messages achieve meaning when they are consensually validated or verified between the two parties. (In Ruesch's view, however, it is the psychiatrist's reality that verifies a message. A symbolic interactionist works toward a definition mutually agreed on by client and therapist. Agreement is reached by moving to make the private shared rather than by assuming that the private must necessarily be altered.)
- Metacommunicative messages contain instructions on interpretation of messages by both sender and receiver on the levels of denotation and connotation.
- Correction through feedback is basic to adaptive, healthy behavior and successful communication.

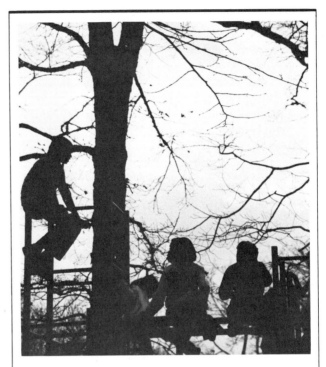

An important developmental task is learning to communicate with groups of people.

Growth and Development in Communication

According to Ruesch, communication is one of the hardest human functions to master. It takes a long time to learn because it occurs in a series of steps, each built from the previous one. Effective communication requires decades of continuous practice. It is believed that interference at an early age leaves an indelible mark. These notions are fully detailed in Table 6–1.

Characteristics of Successful and Disturbed Communication

The four formal criteria for successful communication are efficiency, appropriateness, flexibility, and feedback. When these criteria are not met, communication is disturbed.

EFFICIENCY Simplicity, clarity, and timing are all components of efficient messages. Nurses frequently find themselves using complex and scientific words or professional mental health jargon (known as "psychobabble"—see Chapter 8) to convey messages. If a person said: "Coruscate, coruscate diminutive stellar orb, how

inexplicable is your existence," would anyone know that this meant: "Twinkle, twinkle, little star, how I wonder what you are"? Obtuse or clumsy language and introduction of irrelevant or useless information may prevent others from understanding a message.

Clear messages have a sense of order or structure and reduce ambiguity by narrowing the number of possible interpretations or meanings. Emphasizing the important ideas helps.

Proper timing also is important. It is best to give messages when the other person is available to "hear" them, when there are no intervening noises or inputs, and when the other person can interpret them without undue haste. Problems occur if the time interval between the messages of two people is either too short or too long.

APPROPRIATENESS Messages are appropriate when they are relevant to the situation at hand and when there is mutual fit of overall patterns and constituent parts. When communication does not fit the circumstance, is irrelevant, or is misconstrued, it is said to be inappropriate.

Communication can also be inappropriate in amount. Since every individual has both high and low tolerance levels for stimulation, a person's ability to cope with ideas, make decisions, and act is affected by the amount and rate of sensory input received. Ex-

	Table 6-1 PATHOLOGY OF COMMUNICATION BY DEVELOPMENTAL AGE LEVEL	
Age Level	**Salient Features of Development**	**Age-specific Interference with Communicative Behavior**
Intrauterine period (forty weeks)	Organism responds to thermal, mechanical, and chemical stimuli.	Toxic, infectious, vascular, hormonal, and mechanical interference with communication apparatus of fetus.
Neonatal period (first twelve weeks)	Infant learns to respond to tactile, auditory, and visual stimuli.	Stimulation exceeding tolerance limits of baby, including neglect and erroneous timing.
Infancy (three to twenty-four months)	Mastery of head, eye, and hand movements (second quarter); trunk and fingers (third quarter); legs and feet (fourth quarter); speech (second year).	Interference with muscular system and locomotion. Premature training, insufficient exercise, absence of nonverbal exchange, particularly in terms of action, may prevent establishment of feedback processes.
Early childhood (two to five years)	Interpersonal communication with one person at a time (mother, father, sibling, other relative, or friend).	Interference with speech and social action; selective and tangential responses; separation from mother; and interference with perception.
Later childhood (six to twelve years)	Group communication with several persons at a time. Learning communication with children of same age, with emphasis on members of same sex.	Interference with group behavior; broken families, nonparticipation in school; separation from father; erroneous setting of limitations; lack of transmission of skills at home; lack of responsiveness of parents in verbal terms.
Adolescence (twelve to eighteen years)	Interpersonal communication with members of opposite sex resumed; growing attempts to communicate with members of outgroups.	Interference with participation in autonomous groups, with premating behavior, with attempts to make decisions and to be independent; inadequate provisions for athletic activities and acquisition of information.

Table continues on next page

ceeding a tolerance level is called *overload*. A person who is overloaded by too many messages, or because messages come too fast, cannot handle incoming messages. *Underload* occurs when delay or lack of information interferes with the person's ability to comprehend the message of another. The infants in foundling homes that John Bowlby (1951) studied were subjected to underload both verbally and emotionally.

The tangential reply is another example of inappropriateness. A tangential reply to a statement disregards the content of the message and is directed toward either an incidental aspect of the intitial statement, the type of language used, the emotions of the sender, or another facet of the same topic.

FLEXIBILITY People cannot always be sure how a message will be received, because each person with whom they communicate is unique and changing.

Since they cannot expect constancy from others, people need to be flexible. In communication, lack of flexibility manifests itself as either exaggerated control or exaggerated permissiveness. Both extremes increase the likelihood of frustrating, ungratifying, or disturbed communication.

It is occasionally difficult to maintain flexibility when it requires a person to desert or temporarily lay aside a carefully planned goal. To be flexible, a person must have the ability to set new priorities and to move to meet immediate goals. Humanistic psychiatric nursing practice asks that nurses work to achieve flexibility in their relationships with clients and colleagues.

FEEDBACK Feedback is the process by which performance is checked and malfunctions corrected. It performs a regulatory function in the communication process. Feedback enables people to decide which

	Table 6–1 continued	
Age Level	**Salient Features of Development**	**Age-specific Interference with Communicative Behavior**
Young adulthood (nineteen to late twenties)	Mastery of complexity and heterogeneity of adult communication, multiplicity of roles, and diversity of rules. Communication with age superiors. Young adult is occupationally placed in a position of subservience; observes and follows orders.	Interference with mating behavior, acquisition of skills, and learning of multiple roles. Changeover from family system of communication to other systems may be interfered with by relatives; nonconformance to group practices may jeopardize support from group.
Middle adulthood (thirty to middle forties)	Peak of communication with age inferiors and children. Switch from role of perceiver and transmitter to position of greater responsibility.	Interference with communication vis-à-vis youngsters. Position between two generations is delicate and ill-defined when pull from either side is too strong.
Later adulthood (forty-five to sixty-five)	Intake of information and learning now displaced in favor of output of information, teaching, governing, and ruling. Participation in decision-making groups.	Interference with independence and decision-making. Realization of failure to implement self-chosen ideals; collapse of wishful thinking; interference with identification with younger generation.
Age of retirement (sixty-five to eighty)	Preparation for relinquishment of power and gradual retirement from decision-making. Philosophical considerations after completion of life cycle. Symbolic and global treatment of events.	Inactivity. Sudden withdrawal from participation in communication networks. Lack of stimulation.
Old age (eighty and older)	Life in retrospect, with emphasis on early memories.	Interference with equilibrium. Tolerance limits for over- and understimulation and over- and underactivity quickly reached.

Source: From *Disturbed Communication* by Jurgen Ruesch, M.D., with the permission of W. W. Norton & Company, Inc. Copyright © 1972, 1957 by W. W. Norton & Company, Inc.

messages have been understood as intended. It requires the cooperation of two persons—one to give it, and one to receive it.

Under certain circumstances of disturbed communication, feedback either fails to function or functions poorly. When messages do not get through or are mutilated, appropriate replies cannot be obtained and corrective feedback does not occur. If content elicits anxiety, fear, shame, or any of several other strong emotions, feedback is likely to be hampered. Feedback is discussed in greater depth later in this chapter.

The Theory of Pragmatics of Human Communication

A theory of the pragmatics of human communication was developed by Watzlawick, Beavin, and Jackson (1967), based on the assumption that communication is synonymous with interaction. These authors maintain that, in the presence of another, all behavior is com-

municative. This theory is concerned with the pragmatics, or the behavioral effects, of human interaction. The term *pragmatics* is intended to refer to the interpersonal relation between communicators. What makes this theory particularly useful for this book is its conception of human communication as a reciprocal process.

Some Axioms of the Theory   According to this theory, one cannot *not* communicate. Message value is found in both activity and inactivity, verbalizations and silences. This communication occurs on two levels. The *content level* of a communication is the report aspect, in which information is conveyed. The *relationship level* is communication about a communication, a *metacommunication*, which says something about the relationship between the participants.

All interchanges can be viewed as either *symmetrical* (based on equality) or *complementary* (based on difference). In symmetrical relationships the partners usually mirror each other's behavior, thus minimizing difference. Complementary relationships, on the other hand, are characterized by the maximization of difference.

Disturbances in Human Communication   Watzlawick, Beavin, and Jackson (1967) identified the disturbances in human communication. Communication can be disturbed when a person attempts *not* to communicate. In this framework, the basic dilemma in schizophrenia is considered the schizophrenic person's attempt not to communicate. However, since it is impossible not to communicate, the person is faced with the need to deny that he or she is communicating while denying that this denial is a communication.

Another disturbance occurs when a person communicates in a way that invalidates the messages sent to or received from the other person. Such communications, called *disqualifications,* include a wide range of behavior: self-contradictions, inconsistencies, subject switches, incomplete sentences, misunderstandings, obscurities in style, interpreting a metaphor literally, and interpreting a literal statement metaphorically.

A person may communicate in a way that confirms, rejects, or disconfirms the other person's view of self. Confirmation of one person's self-view by another is thought to be the greatest single factor ensuring mental development and stability. Rejection of the other's definition of self essentially says "You're wrong." Disconfirmation, on the other hand, says "You don't exist"—it questions the other's authenticity. Disconfirmation leads to alienation and has been found to occur with some regularity in interactions between persons labeled schizophrenic and the members of their families.

Although all relationships are necessarily either symmetrical or complementary, runaways (exaggerations to the point of disturbance) may occur in either of the patterns. For example, the danger of competitiveness is ever-present in symmetrical relationships. Symmetrical interactions that lose their stability may enter a spiral in which each individual attempts to be just a little bit "more equal" than the other. Runaways are seen in quarrels between people or wars between nations, behaviors that are relatively open. Rejection of the other's self is generally observed when a symmetrical relationship breaks down.

Breakdowns in complementary relationships, however, are generally characterized by disconfirmations of the other. For this reason they are usually viewed as more pathological.

Ego States as Communication Analysis

Eric Berne's (1960) *transactional analysis* is a model of communication analysis proposing that a person may display the self from different psychological positions. Transactional analysis (T.A.) is a method of therapy as well as a method of communication analysis and is discussed as such in Chapter 25. Transactional analysis theory is appropriate to this chapter because it is concerned with the changes in a person's posture, verbalization, voice, attitude, and feeling. Transactional analysis is both quick and easily understood. It is useful in brief contacts with clients or colleagues when there is little time to establish a rewarding relationship. Nurses can use T.A. concepts in understanding their own behavior as well.

Structural Analysis   Each person has three main sources of behavior, or ego states—the Parent, the Adult, and the Child as illustrated in Figure 6–8. The Child is manifested through archaic modes of communication and relationship as well as by childlike behavior similar to that of an actual child less than seven years old. Giggling, coyness, naiveté, charm, boisterousness, and whining are characteristics of the Child ego state. So are "I want"; "gosh"; "golly"; "me"; "mine"; "I dunno."

By the time children become adults they learn that the spontaneous and free expression of feelings in

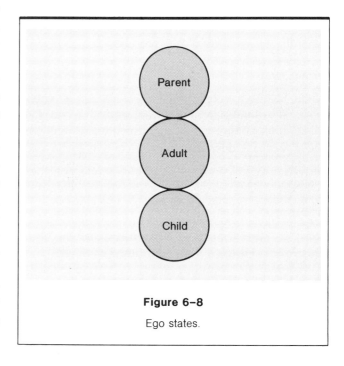

Figure 6–8

Ego states.

their natural state must be adapted to meet the demands and expectations of parents and the culture in which they live. Their adaptive behavior results in the Adapted Child ego state, which has two common manifestations: compliance with parents or other authority figures or rebellion and refusal to follow orders. Most people's Child falls somewhere between the two extremes.

Objective appraisal of reality and the capacity to process data are the domain of the Adult. The Adult is manifested in accomplishments beyond those of children, such as accurate analysis of complex realities and realistic manipulation of concepts. Perceptive skill, data processing, sociability, and communicativeness are attributed to the Adult. So are "it appears"; "I think"; "why"; "what"; "where"; "when"; "how."

The Parent incorporates the feelings and behaviors learned from parents or authority figures. A Parent ego state can be identified when the person's behavior includes the language, intonations, attitudes, postures, and mannerisms of one or both parents. All-wise, all-knowing, benevolent, prim, critical, or righteous attitudes are some examples. So are "if I were you"; "how many times have I told you"; "poor dear"; "disgusting"; "now what"; "do it this way." The Nurturing Parent ego state cuddles, protects, and cares for, while the Critical Parent ego state corrects or condemns.

Berne postulated that an individual exhibits a Parent or an Adult or a Child ego state, and that shifts can occur from one ego state to another. A nursing student, new to an inpatient unit of a community mental health center, reported her ego state switches in the following situation.

When I walked into the TV room to pick up my pen that I had left there, I saw a man pacing the floor; he was angrily muttering a string of obscenities. (Adult ego state) I don't mind telling you that I was plenty scared. I was afraid that he might hurt me. (Child ego state) I told myself that I should do something about reducing his anxiety and distress. (Parent ego state) But, I felt so helpless and dumb. (Child ego state) Then I decided that I really didn't know how to handle this situation and remembered something you said in class—that it's okay to ask for help—and I didn't feel scared or dumb any more. This has really turned into a good learning situation for me. (Adult ego state)

Structural analysis includes the determination of which ego state controls the executive power at a particular

time. Spontaneity, charm, creativity, and enjoyment reside in the Child, while the Adult not only is necessary for survival in dealing effectively with the outside world but also regulates and mediates the activities of the Parent and the Child. The Parent enables an individual to act effectively as a parent and makes many automatic responses that free the Adult from routine, trivial decisions. Each of the three ego states serves vital functions.

Ego States in Wellness/Illness   Most of the time, persons who are ill or hospitalized are in a Child ego state. In the general hospital setting, one often hears of the "problem client" who is demanding, extremely dependent, or refusing to follow a prescribed medical regimen. That problem client is using his or her Adapted Child in unfamiliar or frightening situations. On the other hand, the overly cheerful, overly friendly, or overly helpful client is less often identified as a problem, but is also using the Adapted Child ego state to cope with the stress of hospitalization. The Child ego state may also be seen in the client who is confused, disoriented, screaming, enraged, striking out at others, or withholding information because of fear of retaliation.

Sick people in their Parent ego state may be critical of hospital staff, or suspicious of their intentions. Sometimes they nurture and protect other clients or even the staff. A person in a Parent ego state is critical of himself for being ill, or for being unable to cope with the stresses of life. Such people berate themselves for bothering the staff, family, and friends. Some persons even hallucinate figures or voices that criticize them for their real or imagined transgressions.

The client who is able to decide when to sleep or rest, whether to visit with friends or family, and what steps to take to decrease stress contributes to wellness in the Adult ego state. People in this ego state are able to accept the temporary limitations imposed by illness or stress, to care for themselves within the confines of the limitations imposed, and to seek partnership in decisions about the directions of health care.

Obviously, the sick person in the Adult ego state is in the best possible situation under the circumstances. However, other ego states can also contribute to both illness and wellness. For example, persons in the Nurturing Parent ego state can allow themselves to be taken care of by others and may give themselves "permission" to be sick or to feel depressed. A quicker return to a state of well-being is more likely for these people than for those who are constantly berating themselves

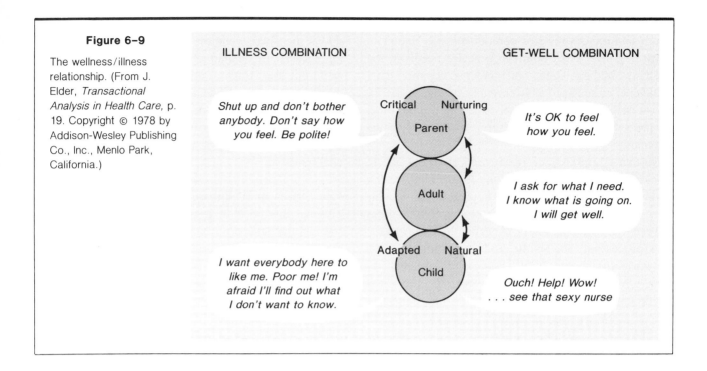

Figure 6–9

The wellness/illness relationship. (From J. Elder, *Transactional Analysis in Health Care*, p. 19. Copyright © 1978 by Addison-Wesley Publishing Co., Inc., Menlo Park, California.)

ILLNESS COMBINATION

Shut up and don't bother anybody. Don't say how you feel. Be polite!

I want everybody here to like me. Poor me! I'm afraid I'll find out what I don't want to know.

Critical   Nurturing
Parent

Adult

Adapted   Natural
Child

GET-WELL COMBINATION

It's OK to feel how you feel.

I ask for what I need. I know what is going on. I will get well.

Ouch! Help! Wow! . . . see that sexy nurse

for being ill or succumbing to life's stresses. The Child ego state is helpful in achieving wellness, because it allows for the natural expression of feelings that can then be handled. These ego states in a wellness/illness relationship are illustrated in Figure 6–9.

Transactional Analysis   While structural analysis is directed more toward the analysis of the individual's personality, transactional analysis is broadened to focus on what occurs between two or more persons.

COMPLEMENTARY TRANSACTIONS   Complementary transactions are those in which the transactional stimulus and the transactional response occur on identical ego levels. Transactions are complementary when a message sent to an ego state is responded to from that ego state. Consider two possible interactions between a nurse and a client, as illustrated in Figure 6–10. Complementary transactions such as these can go on uninterruptedly until one or the other of the participants changes ego state. Most of the time, productive communication occurs in complementary transactions, because the participants behave according to the perceived and predicted ego states of one another. However, continuing, or locked, complementary transactions—as from Critical Parent to Adapted Child—result in uninterrupted but uncomfortable, nonfacilitative communication. The Parent–Child transaction of nurse and client in Figure 6–10 limits the client's growth. It encourages dependency and discourages responsibility.

CROSSED TRANSACTIONS   Crossed transactions result from changes in ego states that terminate the complementary relationship. As Figure 6–11 illustrates, the lines of transaction intersect in crossed transactions, and the predicted response is not forthcoming.

A crossed transaction will occur if the client tries to relate to the nurse on an Adult to Adult level but the nurse responds on a Parent to Child level. In instances of crossed transactions, communication is usually not smooth or satisfactory and will soon be terminated. When complementary transactions have become locked (and interpersonally uncomfortable), it may be useful to cross ego states in order to move the communication forward. For example, if a nurse is aware of having behaved like a Critical Parent to a client who responds from the Adapted Child state, the nurse can alter communication behavior by switching to Adult ego state. The client will probably follow this lead, leaving client and nurse better able to work together effectively.

ULTERIOR TRANSACTIONS   Ulterior transactions are complex phenomena that occur on two levels—social (the surface, or overt one) and psychological (the hidden, or covert one). *Games* are series of ulterior transactions with concealed motivations. Figure 6–12 shows an ulterior transaction as it occurs in the "Why don't you . . . Yes, but . . ." game. In this game, one person presents a problem to another person or to members of a group, who offer solutions to the problem. All solutions, however, are rejected by the first player.

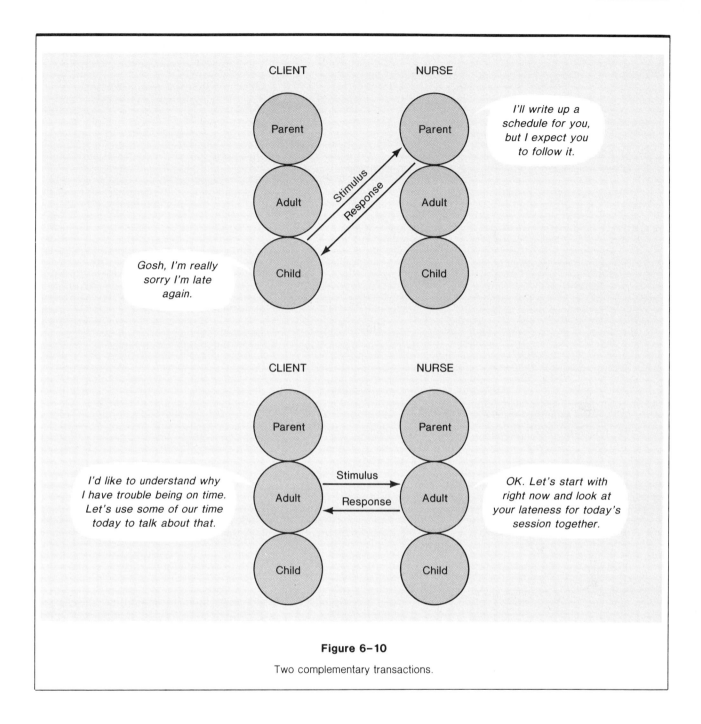

Figure 6–10

Two complementary transactions.

The gimmick, or concealed motivation, is that, although this is supposedly an Adult request for information, the psychological level is Child to Parent. The Child always wins, as the supposedly "wise" Parents are confounded and confused one by one.

Since the interactions are complementary at both social and psychological levels, the game can be played indefinitely until the Parents give up or a more sophisticated person who recognizes what is happening breaks it up. "Why don't you . . . Yes, but . . ." can also be played in one-to-one relationships, particularly when the client has had years of experience in playing

the game and the nurse is unaware of the psychological level. The following interaction is typical of such a client–nurse situation. The client has been discussing her view of the problems she has experienced since her mother-in-law moved in.

NURSE: *The problem seems to be that you give in to your mother-in-law all the time. How about trying to talk to her?*

CLIENT: *If I talk to her, it won't do any good. She'll just continue to act the same way.*

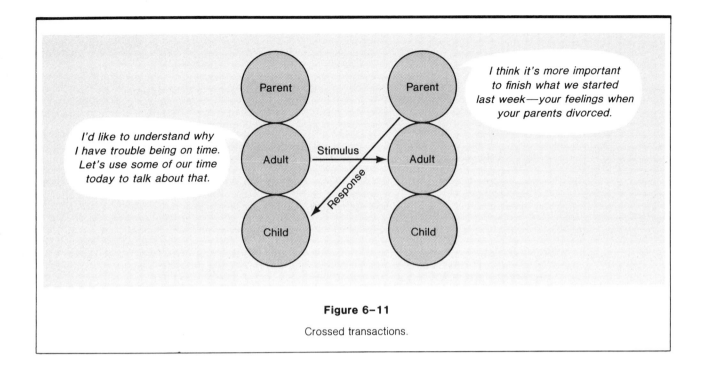

Figure 6–11

Crossed transactions.

NURSE: *How about getting your husband to help?*

CLIENT: *I'd ask him to talk to her, but he says that it's my house, so I should give the orders and there should be no problem.*

NURSE: *You mentioned that she has another son. Do you think that you could talk to him and work out some plan to have her live by herself?*

CLIENT: *No. We haven't talked to him in a long while, and anyway she doesn't have enough money to live on her own.*

NURSE: *How about a nursing home?*

CLIENT: *We can't afford to send her to a nursing home.*

Apparently giving up on finding a solution for the client's "mother-in-law problem," the nurse begins to

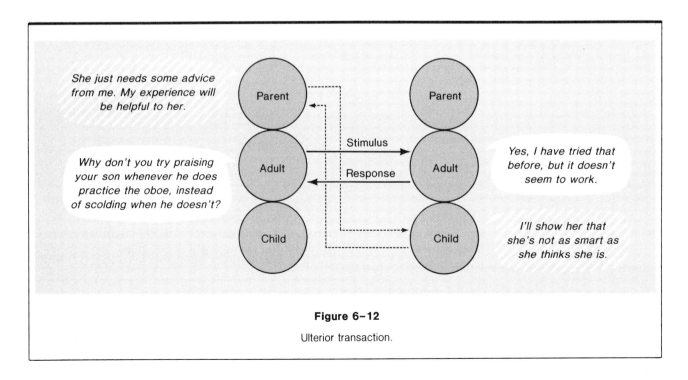

Figure 6–12

Ulterior transaction.

work on other tangentially related household problems.

NURSE: *You said that taking care of six children is quite a job. Do you think you could hire a baby-sitter to watch them in the afternoon?*

CLIENT: *There's nobody in the neighborhood who I can get to sit. Either they're too young or they don't want to.*

NURSE: *Do you think you could hire someone to clean the house one day a week?*

CLIENT: *Well, we could afford it, but my husband says that I don't need anyone to help me and that I could do everything by myself.*

The game was broken up, and the participants moved on to more productive communication after the nurse assessed her own and her client's ego states. She was able to do so by moving into her Adult ego state, figuring out the dynamics and her contributions to them, and then changing her responses.

TRANSITIONAL TRANSACTIONS Transitional transactions are bargaining sessions that bridge the gap between crossed or ulterior transactions and complementary transactions. The interactions between a staff nurse and a head nurse are illustrated in Figure 6–13 and demonstrate how the gap may be bridged. Transitional transactions signal the willingness of a communicator to change the self-in-process—to accommodate the other's view of self and other. Although the head nurse did not immediately recognize the staff nurse's ego state switch, a complementary set was achieved by the third exchange.

Analysis of Ego States in Clinical Practice

The transactional analysis of ego states in a communication setting helps nurses gain a better understanding of the processes and behaviors that take place. It is a way of viewing the self-in-process—that is, the self changing in response to interaction with another self—a way of understanding a person in the process of becoming. It can be used to understand how ego states of participants—nurses as well as clients—help or hinder communication efforts. Transactional analysis theory has been liberally illustrated, with clinical examples, by Elder (1978).

FACILITATIVE COMMUNICATION

Facilitative communication aims at initiating, building, and maintaining fulfilling and trusting relationships with other people. Being able to communicate ideas and feelings with clarity, efficiency, and appropriateness helps a person be interpersonally effective. In reading the rest of this chapter, try to relate the therapeutic communication principles and practices discussed earlier to these ideas about facilitative communication.

Social Superficiality versus Facilitative Intimacy

Most relationships between people begin at the level of social superficiality. In a client–nurse relationship, we try to develop facilitative intimacy, which differs from social intimacy. For example, the interdependence that characterizes the social relationship is greatly reduced. In social relationships participants may "tell their stories" to one another. In facilitative relationships that have therapeutic goals, only one—the client—is engaged in storytelling with the nurse. The process is specifically focused. Clients not only explain themselves, the events of their lives, and the circumstances they face but also do so with a purpose in mind—understanding the circumstances through exploring them and moving to improve the circumstances of their lives. Table 6–2 and Figure 6–14 further compare and contrast social and therapeutic relationships.

The movement toward therapeutic intimacy may be difficult at first. For one thing, such intimacy violates certain social taboos. For example, at a cocktail party it may be socially incorrect to comment on a person's anxiety, stuttering, or facial tic. In the practice of facilitative and therapeutic communication, all messages, including these nonverbal ones, are heeded and may be discussed.

Therapeutic intimacy also requires that the participants move beyond social chitchat into meaningful areas of concern for the client. Therapeutic intimacy requires high involvement and commitment.

Essential Ingredients

Several communication principles and practices are essential to the achievement of facilitative intimacy.

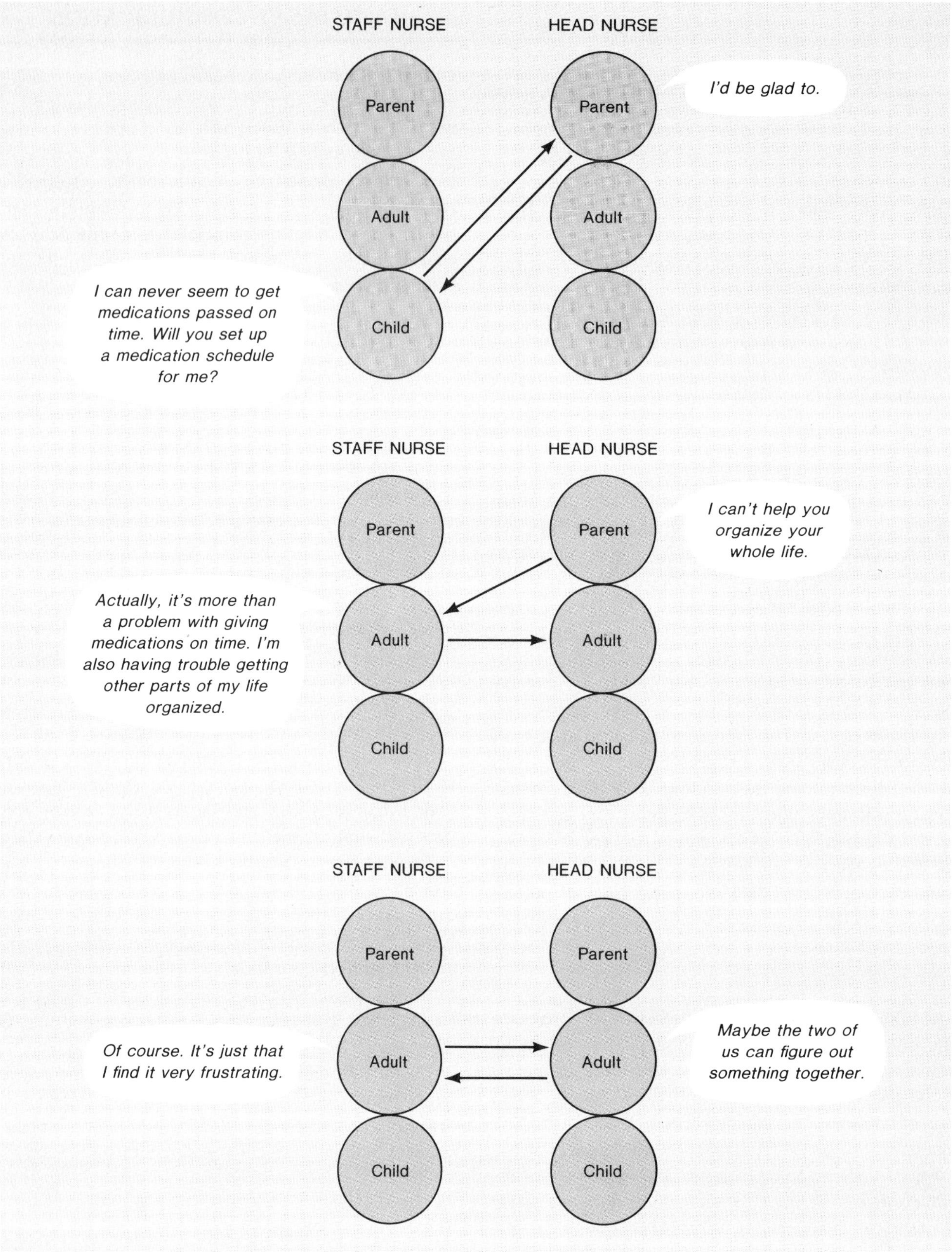

Figure 6–13

Transition from one transactional set to another.

Table 6-2 SOCIAL AND THERAPEUTIC RELATIONSHIPS CONTRASTED		
Components of Relationship	**Social (Superficial)**	**Therapeutic (Intimate)**
Mutual self-disclosure	Variable	Client: self-disclosure; nurse: self-disclosure in terms of response to patient only
Focus of conversation	Unknown to participants	Known to nurse and client
Pertinence of topic	Social, business, generalized, impersonal	Personal and relavant to nurse and client
Relationship of experiences to topic	Sense of uninvolvement and use of indirect knowledge	Sense of involvement and use of direct knowledge
Time orientation	Past and future	Present
Use of feelings	Sharing of feelings discouraged	Sharing of feelings encouraged by nurse
Recognition of individual worth	Not acknowledged	Fully acknowledged

Source: Adapted from A. Coad Denton, "Therapeutic Superficiality and Intimacy," in *Clinical Practice in Psychosocial Nursing: Assessment and Intervention*, edited by D. C. Longo and R. A. Williams (New York: Appleton-Century-Crofts, 1978), p. 26.

Responding with Feedback   Feedback helps others become aware of how their behavior affects us and how we perceive their actions. Responding with feedback can be therapeutic self-disclosure. It allows the nurse to offer clients constructive information to help them become more aware of their impact on others. Total self-disclosure by the nurse is inappropriate in the nurse–client relationship. It would place a burden of interdependence on the client and limit the time and energy available to work on the client's concerns. Reciprocal self-disclosure is more appropriate in friend and colleague relationships.

It is important to give feedback in a way that will not be threatening to the client and increase defensiveness. The more defensive the client, the less likely it is that she or he will hear and understand the feedback. Some characteristics of helpful, nonthreatening feedback are listed in Table 6–3.

Responding with Confrontation   Productive change often results from constructive confrontations. A *confrontation* is a deliberate invitation to another to examine some aspect of personal behavior in which there is a discrepancy between what the person says and what he or she does. Confrontation requires careful attention to nonverbal communication and the discrepancies between nonverbal and verbal messages.

Confrontations may be informational or interpretive, and they may be directed toward both the resources and the limitations of the client. An *informational confrontation* describes the visible behavior of another person. An *interpretive confrontation* expresses thoughts and feelings about the other's behavior and includes drawing inferences about the meaning of the behavior.

Responding with Empathy   "Putting oneself in someone else's shoes" is a way of describing empathy. Most theorists believe that this is the most important dimension in the helping process. Without a high level of empathic understanding, there is no real basis for helping. Empathy facilitates interpersonal exploration. An in-depth discussion of empathy is included in Chapter 3.

Responding with Respect   Responding with respect demonstrates that the nurse values the integrity of the client and has faith in the client's ability to solve the presenting problems, given appropriate facilitation. By encouraging the client to put forward possible plans of action, the nurse conveys respect for the client's ability to take charge of his or her destiny. On the other hand, giving advice conveys a directly opposite message.

Responding with Genuineness   Genuineness refers to the ability to be real or honest with another. To be effective, genuineness must be timed properly and based on a solid relationship. Honesty is not always the best policy, especially if it is brutal or if the client is not capable of dealing with it.

To the extent the client can experience the authen-

Therapeutic Intimacy Depends on:					
Focus of Conversation	Focuses on people or events not personally known to nurse and client	Focuses on people or events known to either nurse or client	Focuses on people or events known to both client and nurse	Focuses on client's concerns and self-disclosures or on nurse's concerns re client	Focuses on mutually shared aspects and concerns of therapeutic relationship
Pertinence of Topic	Topicis not pertinent or important to nurse or client		Topic is important to nurse or client		Topic is of concern and importance to both nurse and client
Time Orientation	Past or future orientation that does not clarify or relate to present time			Focus on present time; any discussion of people or events that helps to clarify the present	
Relationship of Experiences to Topic	Abstractions and vague reports of events or interactions; no supportive, illustrative examples; sense of uninvolvement			Sense of involvement in interaction or event; supported with specific, concrete examples and observations; recognition that distortion occurs with indirect knowledge	
Use of Feelings	Sharing of feelings is avoided and is considered disruptive and meaningless; indirect reflection of feelings is common; generalizations, judgments, intellectualizations about events and people			Sharing of feelings is considered beneficial; feelings are considered natural and acceptable by nurse and client; initially, feelings are shared from client to nurse, but as therapeutic relationship develops the nurse shares feelings re present time and therapeutic relationship	
Recognition of Individual Worth and Autonomy	Lack of acknowledgment of individual worth and autonomy; client or nurse may strive to convince the other to be like him or her, to do as he or she does			Fundamental integrity and worth of individual is acknowledged; respect for personal autonomy. This concept is valued by nurse and client	

(left margin: SUPERFICIALITY) (right margin: INTIMACY)

Figure 6–14

Continuum of therapeutic intimacy. Adapted from A. Coad-Denton, ''Therapeutic Superficiality and Intimacy,'' in *Clinical Practice in Psychosocial Nursing: Assessment and Intervention,* edited by D. C. Longo and R. A. Williams. New York: Appleton-Century-Crofts, 1978, p. 27.

ticity of the nurse, the client can risk greater genuineness and authenticity herself or himself. The nurse who is genuine is more likely to deal with and eventually help the client resolve real problems rather than just those that are safe or socially acceptable.

Responding with Immediacy Responding with immediacy means responding to what is happening between the client and the nurse in the here-and-now. Because this dimension may involve the feelings of the client toward the nurse, it can be one of the most difficult to achieve. For example, the client may confront the nurse with overt or implied criticism of the nurse's role or competence. If the nurse responds in a defensive or evasive way, the relationship may be threatened. If the nurse is open, reasonable, and concerned, the relationship may be strengthened. However, if the nurse focuses attention on the relationship too early, the formation of an adequate base may be impaired.

Table 6-3   CHARACTERISTICS OF HELPFUL, NONTHREATENING FEEDBACK

Strategy	Rationale	Strategy	Rationale
Focus feedback on behavior rather than on client	Refer to what client actually does rather than on how nurse imagines client to be	Focus feedback on exploration of alternatives rather than answers or solutions	Focusing on variety of alternatives for accomplishing a particular goal prevents premature acceptance of answers or solutions that may not be appropriate
Focus feedback on observations rather than inferences	Refer to what nurse actually sees or hears client do; inferences refer to conclusions or assumptions nurse makes about client	Focus feedback on its value to client rather than on catharsis it provides nurse	Feedback should serve needs of client not needs of nurse
Focus feedback on description rather than judgment	Report what occurred rather than evaluating it in terms of good or bad, right or wrong	Limit feedback to amount of information client is able to use rather than amount nurse has available to give	Overloading will decrease effectiveness of feedback
Focus feedback on "more or less" rather than "either/or" descriptions of behavior	"More or less" descriptions stress quantity rather than quality (which may be value-laden)	Limit feedback to appropriate time and place	Excellent feedback presented at an inappropriate time may be ineffective or harmful
Focus feedback on here-and-now behavior rather than there-and-then behavior	The most meaningful feedback is given as soon as it is appropriate to do so	Focus feedback on what is said rather than why it is said	Focusing on why things are said or done moves away from observations and toward motive or intent (which can only be assumed, unless verified)
Focus feedback on sharing of information and ideas rather than advice	Sharing ideas and information helps client make decisions about own well-being; giving advice takes away client's freedom to be self-determining		

Responding with Warmth   Warmth is so closely linked with empathy and respect that it is seldom communicated as an independent dimension. It is important, however, to note some additional points about the expression of warmth. Effusive, chatty, "buddy-buddy" behavior should not be confused with warmth. Warmth is most often conveyed in communications of respect and empathy.

The nurse should be aware of and accept the client's right to maintain distance in the relationship, particularly in the early phases. Warmth and intimacy cannot be forced. Initially high levels of warmth can be counterproductive for clients who have received little warmth from others in their lives or have been taken advantage of by others. Warmth alone is insufficient for building a relationship and solving problems.

High initial levels of warmth from certain nurses may indicate their limitation in clinical practice. The nurse should try to understand the need to express warmth. Is the nurse trying to buy the respect of the client through expressions of warmth?

Skills that Foster Effective Communication

The presentation of a how-to manual or cookbook of communication skills is antithetical to most of the concerns of this chapter and this book. A set of communication skills employed rigidly as a sort of relationship "magic" is antihumanistic in many ways. Relationships, and the people within them, are much too complex and unique to depend on a set of directions for being facilitative. The following skills are therefore presented with some reluctance and many misgivings. It is important for students to remember that a holistic approach essentially militates against the rigid, inflexible application of communication techniques. Those presented here should be viewed as having the potential to foster effective communication. They must be adapted individually for each human encounter.

Reflecting   Reflecting can respond to two dimensions of communication—content and feelings. In reflecting the *content* of the message, the nurse repeats basically the same statement as the client. This gives the client the opportunity to hear and mull over what he or she has said:

- "You believe things will be better soon."
- "You think it would be better to take a part-time job."

Content reflection is perhaps one of the most misused and overused methods in mental health counseling. It loses its effectiveness when used for lack of other choices.

Reflecting *feelings* consists of verbalizing what seems to be implied about feelings in the client's comment.

- "Sounds like you're really angry at your brother."
- "You're feeling uncomfortable about being discharged from the hospital."

In reflecting feelings, the nurse attempts to identify latent and connotative meanings that may either further clarify or distort the content. Reflection is useful because it encourages the client to make additional clarifying comments.

Imparting Information   Statements that give information help the client by supplying additional data. They therefore encourage further clarification based on new or additional input.

- "Group therapy will be held on Tuesday evening from 6:30 until 8:00."
- "I am a nursing student."

It is not constructive to withhold helpful or useful information from the client or to reply "What do you think?" to a straightforward information-seeking question. However, the nurse must be careful not to distort the giving of information into advice or use it to avoid an area of interpersonal difficulty. If the nurse gives

personal social information, the conversation may move out of the realm of therapeutic intervention.

Clarifying   Clarifying is an attempt to understand the basic nature of a client's statement.

- "I'm confused about . . . Could you go over that again, please."
- "You say you're feeling anxious now. What's that like for you?"

Asking the client to give an example to clarify a meaning helps the nurse to understand the client's intended message better. A person who describes a concrete incident is more likely to be able to see the connections between it and similar occurrences. Illustrations are very useful qualifiers.

Paraphrasing   In paraphrasing, the nurse restates what she or he has heard the client communicating.

- "In other words, you're fed up with being treated like a child."
- "I hear you saying that when people compliment you, you feel embarrassed. If they knew the real you, they'd stay away."

Paraphrasing offers the opportunity to test the nurse's understanding of what the client is attempting to communicate. It is reflective in nature, in that it lets the client know how another person is understanding the message.

Checking Perceptions   The nurse who shares how she or he perceives and hears the client is engaged in the process of checking perceptions. After sharing perceptions of the client's behaviors, thoughts, and feelings, the nurse asks the client to verify the perception.

- "Let me know if this is how you see it too."
- "I get the feeling that you're uncomfortable when we're silent. Does that seem to fit?"

A perception check is used to make sure that the nurse understands the client. An effective perception check conveys the message "I want to understand. . . ." It allows the other person the opportunity to correct inaccurate perceptions. It also allows the nurse to avoid actions based on false assumptions about the client.

Processing Processing is the most complex and sophisticated technique used by the nurse. Process comments are those that direct attention to the interpersonal dynamics of the nurse–client experience. These dynamics are illustrated in the content, feelings, and behavior expressed.

- "It seems that important things that need to be taken care of come up in the last five minutes we have together in our session."
- "Today is the first day our session has started out with silence. Last week it seemed there wouldn't be enough time."

Processing is most useful when therapeutic intimacy has been achieved. For a more comprehensive discussion, see Chapter 18.

Structuring Structuring is an attempt to create order or evolve guidelines. The nurse helps the client to become aware of problems and the order in which they might be dealt with.

- "You've mentioned that you want to improve your relationships with your wife, your sister, and your boss. Let's put them in order of priority."
- "No, I won't be giving you advice, but we can discuss the possible solutions together."

Structuring is particularly useful when clients introduce a number of concerns in a brief period of time with little idea of which to begin work on. In addition to structuring content, nurses use structuring to delimit the parameters of the nurse–client relationship and identify how the nurse will participate with the client in the problem-solving process.

Pinpointing Pinpointing calls attention to certain kinds of statements and relationships. For example, the nurse may point to inconsistencies among statements or to similarities and differences in the points of view, feelings, or actions of two or more persons, or between what one says and what one does.

- "So, you and your wife don't agree about how many children you want."
- "You say you're sad, but you're smiling."

Linking In linking, the nurse responds to the client in a way that ties together two events, experiences, feelings, or persons. Linking may be used to connect past experiences with current behaviors. Another example is linking the tension between two persons with current life stress.

- "You felt depressed after the birth of both your children."
- "Do you think the trouble is more with him or with you, since you both have been under increased job strain?"

Questioning Questioning is a very direct way of speaking with clients. But when used to excess, questioning controls the nature and range of the client's responses. Questions can be useful when the nurse is seeking specific information. When the nurse's intent is to engage the client in meaningful dialogue, however, questions should be limited.

When the nurse is using questions, it is best to make them open-ended rather than closed. An *open-ended question* focuses the topic but allows freedom of response.

- "How were you feeling when your mother said that to you?"
- "What's your opinion about. . . ?"

The *closed question* limits the client's choice of responses generally to "yes" or "no" ("Were you feeling angry when your mother said that?"). Closed questions limit therapeutic exploration.

"Why" questions usually have the same effect. They often are impossible to answer and rarely lead to a clearer understanding of the situation. However, "who," "what," "when," and "how" questions may be helpful when used judiciously.

Confronting The main concepts behind constructive confrontation were discussed earlier. There are six skills to þe incorporated in constructive confrontations. They are:

1. Use of personal statements with the words *I, my,* and *me*
2. Use of relationship statements in which the nurse expresses what he or she thinks or feels about the client in the interaction
3. Use of behavior descriptions (statements describing the visible behavior of the client)

4. Use of description of personal feelings, specifying the feeling by name

5. Use of responses aimed at understanding, such as paraphrasing and perception checking

6. Use of constructive feedback skills (see Table 6–3)
- "When you wring your hands I feel anxious."
- "Sometimes when you turn your head away from me I think you're angry."

Summarizing Summarizing is a way of highlighting the main ideas that have been discussed. It reviews for the client and the nurse what the main themes of the conversation were. Summarizing is also useful in focusing the client's thinking and aiding conscious learning.

- "The last time we were together you were concerned about...."
- "You had three main concerns today...."

This technique can be used appropriately at different times in the client–nurse interaction. For example, summarizing the previous interaction is useful in the first few minutes of the time the nurse and the client spend together. When summarization occurs early, it helps the client recall the areas discussed and also provides the client with the opportunity to see how the nurse has synthesized the content of a previous session. Summarizing is useful because it keeps the participants directed toward a goal.

The most frequent error with this technique is injudicious use. A nurse may rush to summarize despite other, more pressing and immediate concerns of the client. In this instance, summarizing is likely to meet the nurse's need for structure while disregarding the client's here-and-now concerns.

Ineffective Communication Styles

Three clinical situations are presented below to give examples of some ways of responding to clients that are generally not helpful and may even be harmful (adapted from Gazda 1973, pp. 62–65). They illustrate a few of the common response styles that are not facilitative. An example of a helpful response is given at the end of each of the situations.

Situation 1

CLIENT: "They wouldn't let me join their pinochle game!"

Responses that are not helpful:

DETECTIVE: Who wouldn't?

Detectives are eager to track down the facts of the case. They grill the client about the details of what happened and respond to this factual content instead of giving attention to feelings. Detectives control the flow of the conversation, and this often puts the client on the defensive.

MAGICIAN: It's time to eat dinner, so it doesn't matter now, does it?

Magicians try to make the problem disappear by telling the client it isn't there. This illusion is not lasting. Denying the existence of a problem denies the validity of the client's own experience and perception.

MANAGER: Would you help me get everyone together for the picnic?

Managers believe that if the client can be kept too busy to think about the problem, there will be no problem. Doing this has the effect of saying that the task assigned to the client by the manager is more important than the client's problem. An effective nurse communicates awareness of the magnitude of any particular problem to the client.

JUDGE: Remember yesterday when you didn't play fair? Of course they wouldn't want to play with you today!

Judges give rational explanations to show that the client's past actions have caused the present situation— that the client is the guilty party. Although such responses may be accurate, they are rarely helpful, because they are premature—they are being given before the client is ready to accept and use them.

Responses that are helpful:

"It hurts to be turned down!" or "That hurt!"

Situation 2

CLIENT: "You asked me to chair the community meeting next week, but I can't do that. Please get somebody else. Anybody would be better than me."

Responses that are not helpful:

DRILL SERGEANT: Later tonight figure out what each person should do. Give them assignments and make sure they work on it some each day. Get organized now and it will come out fine.

Drill sergeants give orders and expect them to be obeyed. Because they know just what the client should do, they see no need to give explanations, listen to the client's feelings, or explain their commands to the client.

GURU: You won't find out what you can do, if you don't try new things. It's better to try and fail than not to try at all.

Gurus dispense proverbs and clichés on every occasion, as though they were the sole possessors of the accumulated wisdom of the ages. Unfortunately, their words are too impersonal and general to apply to any individual's situation with force or accuracy, and often the sayings are too trite to be noticed at all.

MAGICIAN: You don't *really* mean that do you?

Responses that are helpful:

"You're sort of afraid to accept this responsibility. It looks like more than you can handle."

Situation 3

CLIENT: "I don't know what to do with my kids! They won't listen!"

Responses that are not helpful:

DETECTIVE: What's causing the problem?

FLORIST: With all your ability? I can't believe that! Why, you're such a good parent.

Florists are uncomfortable talking about anything unpleasant, so they gush flowery phrases to keep the client's problem at a safe distance. Florists mistakenly think that the way to be helpful is to hide the problem under bouquets of optimism.

JUDGE: You know, you got off to a bad start with your kids. You are going to have a hard time changing them.

SIGN PAINTER: You're a born pessimist!

Sign painters think a problem can be solved by being named. They have an unlimited inventory of labels to affix to persons and their problems.

DRILL SERGEANT: First get them all tested psychologically. Then write up some behavior contracts. Keep your kids busy with simple projects. Then . . .

GURU: Things always look the worst before they get better.

PROPHET: If you don't get some results with them pretty soon there will be trouble!

Prophets know and predict exactly what is going to happen. By declaring the forecast, prophets relieve themselves of responsibility. They sit back to let the prophecy come true.

MAGICIAN: You're imagining things. They're good kids, and you know it. They're a lot better than you give them credit for!

Responses that are helpful:

"I guess it gets you down when you do all you know how to do and then don't get results."

INTERACTION PROCESS ANALYSIS CASE STUDY (IPA)

The following clinical data and its analysis are presented to give nurses a start in analyzing the interpersonal communication between therapist and client. The IPA format is given in Chapter 8.

Environment

The following two interactions take place on one of the twenty-bed units of a large public psychiatric hospital. The client, Mr. M, and the nurse, Ms. S, are seated facing each other in one corner of the dayroom. Other clients are milling about or seated around the room. Occasionally clients and staff play Ping-Pong at a table in the dayroom. The emotional tone of the unit is one of aimlessness with the exception of a few extremely disturbed clients who periodically display obvious anxiety and out-of-control behavior. The general attitude of the milieu appears to be custodial. There are few staff members for the number of clients. Staff contacts with clients, when they do take place, are around activities of living, such as meals and medications.

Mr. M seems to be quite anxious and urgent in his interactions with the nurse. The nurse is also anxious, mostly about "saying the right thing." At times her anxiety prevents her from really "hearing" the client. These interactions take place during the second week of their relationship and represent sessions 3 and 4. The nurse and the client had agreed to spend a half hour together talking twice a week.

Description of Client

Mr. M is a twenty-five-year-old, single male who displays an obvious amount of anxiety. At times he has been overtly flirtatious with staff members.

Goals

Nurse-centered goals are (1) to encourage Mr. M's verbalization in order to collect data; and (2) to handle the nurse's own anxiety so that it does not interfere with her effectiveness.

Client-centered goals are (1) to offer Mr. M an opportunity to verbalize his feelings; (2) to help Mr. M learn new ways of handling his anxiety; (3) to assist Mr. M in staying with the nurse and using the help she can offer; and (4) to aid Mr. M in beginning to solve his problems—specifically, to help him see that a problem indeed exists and to help him identify it.

Session 3

The interactions of session 3 are presented with an analysis of each in Table 6-4, which follows the IPA format described in Chapter 8.

Evaluation in Light of Current Goals

In terms of the nurse-centered goals, the nurse's anxiety interfered with her perception of covert themes. In terms of the client-centered goals, the nurse at times cut off or shifted from a focus on Mr. M's feelings and failed to focus on Mr. M's feeling tone. She did, however, communicate the expectation that Mr. M stay with her and talk, thus partially meeting her goal of assisting him to use her help.

		Table 6–4 INTERACTIONS AND ANALYSIS OF CASE STUDY SESSION 3	
Nurse	**Client**	**Nurse-centered Analysis**	**Client-centered Analysis**
	I want to have things more or less . . . I just want to relax . . .		Mr. M exhibits his high anxiety here by being unable to finish his sentence. Essentially he is saying: "I don't know what I want. I feel so anxious."
Relax?		The nurse uses reflection of the client's last word to encourage him to go on. She feels anxious here, because she does not understand what he's trying to say. As an alternative, she might have said: "Tell me more about what it is that you want," or "Are you feeling anxious right now?"	
	Yes, not work very much for the rest of my life, but work some.		Mr. M perceived the nurse's response as being accusatory, so he felt compelled to assure the nurse that he would work, not simply loaf. He is trying to avoid her disapproval. Also he seems to intend to keep the conversation on neutral ground, away from feelings.
These are things you want in the future?		The nurse is again repeating the content of the client's words in the form of an indirect question. She is responding to the obvious content level of this interaction and failing to look for the covert meaning. She doesn't understand what the client is trying to say. An alternative would be: "I'm not sure I follow what you're trying to tell me."	
	Yeah. I want my ideas heard. I want my side heard. I don't want to be domineered.		Mr. M senses that he's not "being heard" and indirectly communicates this feeling to the nurse. This seems to be a very significant piece of data, since it is repeated by the client.
Just now I told you I wanted to see you.		The nurse feels concerned that she offended the client in the past. Instead of asking if he's feeling "not heard" right now, she shifts the focus to something about which she feels guilty. She moves out of her professional role when she asks the client for reassurance.	
	Yes.		
Did I domineer you?			

Table continues on next page

		Table 6–4 continued	
Nurse	**Client**	**Nurse-centered Analysis**	**Client-centered Analysis**
	No, no, you didn't (Pause.) I don't want to say my feelings, because I might be hurt. I don't know if I should be talking to you.		Mr. M reassures the nurse and then tries to focus back on *his* feelings (something the nurse should have done). He tells her essentially that he fears the closeness of a relationship, because it can be painful. He also alludes to concerns about confidentiality. These concerns are consistent with the fact that this interaction takes place in the early phase of their relationship.
You don't?		By reflecting the client's words, she fails to communicate that she is genuinely interested in the *specifics* of the client's concerns. She also fails to get them clarified.	
	No, I don't think I should. (Moves toward edge of seat.) I'd like to go and play Ping-Pong now. I want to play with that gal. She's my idea of the kind of woman I like.		He senses that the nurse is not understanding him and tries to withdraw from the situation. He attempts to ''hurt the nurse back'' by referring to ''that gal.'' He says something about his possible expectations of his relationship with the nurse when he uses the word ''play.''
Well, 8:30 to 9:00 is the time we can spend together. You could play Ping-Pong after that.		The nurse feels very anxious here because she perceives herself as failing. But she still does not pick up on any of the covert messages of the client directly, for example, ''I wonder if you feel it would be easier for us to play instead of work on problems?'' Nor does she pick up on his remark about ''his kind of woman'' with the goal of defining her role with him. Instead she repeats the structure of their relationship and essentially gives her permission for him to play later.	
	Oh, I think you're fooling me.		
Fooling you?			
	Yeah.		

Table continues on next page

Table 6–4 continued			
Nurse	**Client**	**Nurse-centered Analysis**	**Client-centered Analysis**
I don't understand. Can you tell me what you mean?			
	I don't know. I think you're fooling me.		
I'm fooling you. . . . I'd like to know what you mean but I don't.			
	Well, I'm going to go watch her play Ping-Pong now. Is it all right?		The client withdraws both physically and psychologically in response.
I'll be free until 9:00 if you want to see me.			
	(He leaves.)		

Future Goals

A nurse-centered future goal is to define the nurse's role. A client-centered future goal is to deal with Mr. M's concerns about confidentiality in the client–nurse relationship.

Session 4

The data from the next meeting between Mr. M and the nurse are presented in Table 6–5 to offer an opportunity for readers to do a similar analysis. At this session, the nurse is seated in the dayroom, watching staff and clients play cards, when Mr. M comes over.

Table 6–5 INTERACTIONS OF CASE STUDY SESSION 4 FOR ANALYSIS			
Nurse	**Client**	**Nurse-centered Analysis**	**Client-centered Analysis**
	Can I talk to you?		
Yes, where do you want to talk?	(He goes to library and looks in. It's occupied. Nurse and Mr. M sit on chairs in the dayroom.)		
	I like you. That's hard to say, but I like you.		

Table continues on next page

Table 6–5 continued			
Nurse	**Client**	**Nurse-centered Analysis**	**Client-centered Analysis**
Yes, it can be hard to tell someone you like them.			
	I think you're very attractive.		
Thank you, Mr. M. (Pause.) Then it's the way I look that you like?	Sort of. What I want is a woman who will admire me . . . who will talk to me in the morning and the night.		
Well, I will be here in the morning on Tuesday and Thursday for the next three months. I'll be happy to talk with you then.			
	Three months? Will I be here that long?		
I don't know, Mr. M. You'll be here until you're ready to go out. (Pause.) What I meant was that I'll be here three months. If you are here, I'll be glad to talk with you.			
	(Silence.)		
We were talking yesterday about playing Ping-Pong. Shall we play a game now?			
	Sure, if no one is using it.		
(Nurse and Mr. M play Ping-Pong. Mr. M wins.)			

KEY NURSING CONCEPTS

✔ Communication is an ongoing, dynamic, and everchanging series of events, each of which affects all others; it is the mechanism by which people establish, maintain, and improve their human contacts.

✔ Meaning cannot be transferred from one human being to another but must be mutually negotiated between persons. Words and gestures do not "mean" something, people do.

✔ Communication takes place on intrapersonal, interpersonal, and public levels and includes nonverbal messages that are interrelated with the spoken word.

✔ Relationships with clients are initiated, built, and maintained through the vehicle of interpersonal communication.

✔ Variables that influence the meaning of communication include perception, values, and culture.

✔ In order to help clients deal with problems, nurses need to be aware of how their own perceptions, values, and culture influence the way they process information about the world.

✔ Various models of human communication present communication as an act, as an interaction, and as a transaction.

✔ The symbolic-interactionist model of communication is transactional in perspective and views communication as a social and interpersonal process.

✔ The symbolic-interactionist view of human communication posits that (a) after a series of internal trails people reflect and transmit the message they believe has the highest chance of success; (b) success depends upon the accuracy and completeness of the person's "cognitive map" of the environment and of the intrapersonal and interpersonal feedback loops; (c) communication is a complex, dynamic process in which the meaning of messages is mutually negotiated, not merely transferred.

✔ Nonverbal communication channels that help us judge the reliability of a message include facial expressions, hand gestures, body movements, use of space, voice, touch, and body aroma.

✔ Theories of communication useful for the practice of humanistic psychiatric nursing include the theory of therapeutic communication, the theory of pragmatics of human communication, and transactional analysis theory.

✔ In the development of the client-nurse relationship, a major focus is the development of facilitative intimacy.

✔ Facilitative intimacy is enhanced when nurses respond with feedback, constructive confrontation, empathy, respect, genuineness, immediacy, and warmth.

✔ Relationships are too complex and unique for a set of rigid, inflexible communication techniques to be consistent with humanistic psychiatric nursing practice.

✔ Communication skills that may foster effective communication include reflecting, imparting information, requesting illustrations, paraphrasing, checking perceptions, processing, structuring, pointing, linking, questioning, and summarizing.

References

Argyle, M. *The Psychology of Interpersonal Behavior.* Baltimore: Penguin, 1967.

Berne, E. *Games People Play.* New York: Grove Press, 1964.

————. *Transactional Analysis in Psychotherapy.* New York: Grove Press, 1960.

Bowlby, J. *Maternal Care and Mental Health.* 2d ed. Geneva: World Health Organization, 1951.

Carroll, L. *Through the Looking Glass and What Alice Found There.* New York: Random House, 1965.

Ekman, P. "Communication Through Nonverbal Behavior: A Source of Information about an Interpersonal Relationship." In *Affect, Cognition and Personality,* edited by S. S. Tomkins and C. E. Izard. New York: Springer, 1965.

Elder, J. *Transactional Analysis in Health Care.* Menlo Park, Calif.: Addison-Wesley, 1978.

Gazda, G. M. *Human Relations Development.* Boston: Allyn and Bacon, 1973.

Goffman, E. *Behavior in Public Places.* New York: Free Press, 1963.

Hulett, J. E., Jr. "A Symbolic Interactionist Model of Human Communication." *A. V. Communication Review* 14 (1966): 5–33.

Ruesch, J. *Therapeutic Communication.* New York: W. W. Norton, 1961.

Watzlawick, P.; Beavin, J.; and Jackson, D. *The Pragmatics of Human Communication.* New York: W. W. Norton, 1967.

Further Reading

Blondis, M. N., and Jackson, B. E. *Nonverbal Communication with Patients.* New York: John Wiley, 1977.

Faules, D. F., and Alexander, D. C. *Communication and Social Behavior: A Symbolic Interaction Perspective.* Reading, Mass.: Addison-Wesley, 1978.

Hall, E. T. *The Silent Language.* New York: Fawcett World Library, 1959.

————. *The Hidden Dimension.* Garden City, N.Y.: Doubleday, 1969.

Hastorf, A.; Schneider, D.; and Polefka, J. *Person Perception.* Reading, Mass.: Addison-Wesley, 1970.

Knapp, M. *Nonverbal Communication in Human Interaction.* New York: Holt, Rinehart and Winston, 1972.

Long, L., and Prophit, P. *Understanding/Responding: A Communication Manual for Nurses.* Monterey, Calif.: Wadsworth, 1981.

Miller, G., and Steinberg, M. *Between People.* Chicago: Science Research Associates, 1975.

Montagu, A. *Touching: The Human Significance of the Skin.* New York: Harper and Row, 1971.

Okun, B. F. *Effective Helping: Interviewing and Counseling Techniques.* North Scituate, Mass.: Duxbury Press, 1976.

Pluckhan, M. *Human Communication: The Matrix of Nursing.* New York: McGraw-Hill, 1978.

Ruesch, J. *Disturbed Communication.* New York: W. W. Norton, 1957.

Ruesch, J., and Bateson, G. *Communication: The Social Matrix of Psychiatry.* New York: W. W. Norton, 1968.

Smith, A. L. *Transracial Communication.* Englewood Cliffs, N.J.: Prentice-Hall, 1973.

Sommer, R. *Personal Space: The Behavioral Basis of Design.* Englewood Cliffs, N.J.: Prentice-Hall, 1969.

Wilmot, W. W. *Dyadic Communication: A Transactional Perspective.* Reading, Mass.: Addison-Wesley, 1975.

7

The One-to-One Relationship: Collaboration and Facilitation

by Beth Moscato

CHAPTER OUTLINE

Common Characteristics of
One-to-One Relationships
  Informality or Formality
  Mutual Definition
  Mutual Collaboration
  Goal Direction
  Professionalism
The History of One-to-One Work
  1940s to 1951: Initial Role Development
  1952 to Mid-1960s: Role Clarification
  Late 1960s to Present: Confirmation of the
  Specialist Role
Philosophical Framework
  Humanistic Factors
  Symbolic Interactionist Factors
Interpersonal Skills in Therapeutic Relationships
  Therapeutic Effectiveness of Psychiatric Nurses
  Therapeutic Use of Self
  Consideration of Client Abilities
  The Therapeutic Alliance
Phases of Therapeutic Relationships
  Beginning (Orientation) Phase: Establishment of
  Contact
  Middle (Working) Phase: Maintenance and
  Analysis of Contact
  End (Resolution) Phase: Termination of Contact

Processes in Therapeutic Relationships
  Observation
  Initial Interview
  Assessment
  Problem-solving Strategies
  Transference and Countertransference Phe-
  nomena
  Evaluation
The Problems of Resistance in Therapeutic
Relationships
  Definition
  Manifestations
  Acting Out
  Acting In
  General Intervention Strategies for Resistance
Specific Nursing Interventions in Common
Behavioral Patterns
  Interpersonal Withdrawal
  Hostility–Aggressivity
  Manipulation
  Detachment
  Excessive Dependence (Learned Helplesness)
  Transference and Countertransference Phe-
  nomena
Key Nursing Concepts

CHAPTER 7

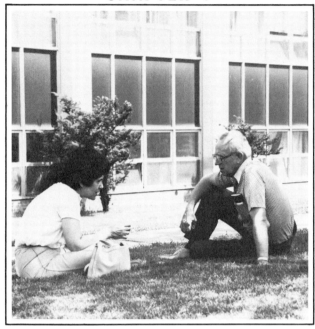

The essence of the one-to-one client-nurse relationship is mutual collaboration. In this interaction the nurse is attending to both content and process.

LEARNING OBJECTIVES

After reading this chapter, students should be able to

- Identify humanistic and symbolic interactionist aspects of the one-to-one relationship
- Identify the phases, processes, and problems of individual relationship work
- Discuss the interpersonal skills of the nurse that facilitate one-to-one relationships, including therapeutic use of self
- Describe the client abilities and behaviors most often associated with growth-producing outcomes
- Apply specific intervention strategies in establishing and maintaining one-to-one relationships

The psychiatric nurse who enters into a one-to-one relationship with a client finds that the invitation to any individual relationship is at once intriguing, challenging, and anxiety-provoking.

A one-to-one relationship may evolve in any nursing situation: between the nurse who makes home visits and the debilitated client; or the nurse in a hospital and the child intermittently hospitalized with leukemia; or the nurse–counselor and the high-risk pregnant woman. Of particular relevance is the one-to-one rela-

tionship that evolves between the psychiatric nurse and the client in medical facilities, psychiatric institutions, community mental health centers, and private practice settings. This individual psychiatric nurse–client relationship traditionally serves as the cornerstone of psychiatric nursing theory and practice.

How is it possible to define, initiate, and use effectively a one-to-one relationship where outcomes are unpredictable and depend on the skills of the psychiatric nurse and the capabilities of the client? This chapter demystifies the characteristics, phases, processes, and problems of one-to-one relationship work, so that psychiatric nurses will approach these relationships with increased awareness of their own interpersonal effectiveness and with practical guidelines on how to facilitate interpersonal effectiveness with clients. In addition, psychiatric nurses who participate in one-to-one relationship work will learn principles, phases, and processes applicable to group, family, and community interventions or therapies.

COMMON CHARACTERISTICS OF ONE-TO-ONE RELATIONSHIPS

The one-to-one relationship between psychiatric nurse and client is a mutually defined, mutually collaborative, goal-oriented professional relationship. It may involve informal relationships or more formal relationship work, including crisis intervention, counseling, or individual psychotherapy.

Informality or Formality

A one-to-one relationship can be either informal or formal. Spontaneous, informal nurse–client relationships may occur at one end of the continuum, with more formalized relationships in individual counseling or psychotherapy at the other end.

Informal nurse–client relationships may be prearranged and planned, but more often they occur

Table 7-1   SIMILARITIES AND DIFFERENCES OF INFORMAL AND FORMAL ONE-TO-ONE RELATIONSHIPS

Characteristic	Nature of Relationship	
	Informal	*Formal*
Setting	Varied	Generally psychiatric settings
Frequency and Duration of Contact	Flexible depending on client need or tolerance. Example: short, frequent intervals on daily basis	Structured. Example: once weekly, with possible crisis sessions. Duration usually set at 30 minutes or one hour
Duration of Relationship	May or may not involve time commitment. Generally a few days to a few weeks	Involves time commitment Weeks to months, for short-term work Months to years, for long-term work
Type of Dysfunction	In general, more effective with severe dysfunction	In severe dysfunction, may be useful after client is stabilized on medication
Use of Therapeutic Contract	May involve simple therapeutic contract	Utilizes therapeutic contract; the more specific, the better
Fees	Usually not relevant	Relevant. Usually part of therapeutic contract
Degree of Skill Required	Nursing student or psychiatric nurse	Advanced degree beneficial
Degree of Supervision	May or may not be necessary, depending on practitioner's effectiveness	Consistent supervision or consultation necessary
Degree of Effectiveness	For both, depends on client's level of functioning, skills of the psychiatric nurse, and time allotment	

spontaneously. They consist of a set of interactions limited in time. There is minimum structure and a sense of immediacy. These relationships occur in numerous medical and nonmedical settings and are particularly common in psychiatric institutions and community mental health settings.

The more formalized one-to-one relationship is used in counseling or individual psychotherapy. It generally requires more planning, structure, consistency, nursing expertise, and time. It occurs in various psychiatric settings, including psychiatric institutions, community mental health centers, and private practice.

The choice of informal or formal relationship work, and its effectiveness, depends on the client's level of functioning; the psychiatric nurse's current abilities and skills; and, to some degree, the length of time available to both participants. It is crucial to note that the principles, phases, processes, and problems of an informal relationship parallel those of a formal one. Thus, a comprehensive overview of all aspects of relationship work may offer beginning practitioners who are not involved in individual psychotherapy, per se, much to

apply to their practice. Table 7-1 highlights the similarities and differences of informal and formal relationship work. The differences between informal and formal relationships are discussed throughout this chapter.

Mutual Definition

A one-to-one relationship is mutually defined by the two participants. Both psychiatric nurse and client voluntarily enter the relationship and specify the conditions under which it is to evolve. For example, the client may seek immediate alleviation of symptoms rather than long-term individual psychotherapy. Nurse and client identify together where and when they will meet and other conditions of their participation. This contractual aspect of the one-to-one relationship is explored further in the discussion of the beginning (orientation) phase of therapy later in this chapter. Once the relationship is established, its maintenance depends on the commitment of both participants.

Table 7–2 DIFFERENCES BETWEEN PROFESSIONAL AND SOCIAL RELATIONSHIPS		
Characteristic	**Professional Relationship**	**Social Relationship**
Purpose	Systematic working-through of problematic thoughts, feelings, and behaviors	Companionship, pleasure
Role delineation	Roles for psychiatric nurse and client with explicit use of psychiatric nursing skills and interventions	Generally not present
Satisfaction of needs	Client is encouraged to identify, develop, and assess ways to meet own needs more effectively	Mutual sharing and satisfaction of personal and interpersonal needs
	Does not address personal needs of psychiatric nurse	

Mutual Collaboration

A third common characteristic in one-to-one relationship work is mutual collaboration between the two participants. Both participants enter a relationship in which goals, strategies, and outcomes evolve within the context of the therapeutic work together. Mutual collaboration implies that each participant brings personal abilities, capabilities, and power to the relationship. Thus, the psychiatric nurse does not assume responsibility for client behaviors but actively works with the client to assess the self-defeating and growth-promoting aspects of specific behaviors. Mutual collaboration also means that the psychiatric nurse assesses and is accountable for her or his own behavior with the client. Ongoing supervision often helps the nurse meet these particular goals.

Goal Direction

One-to-one relationship work is always goal-directed. The client is expected to identify and achieve specific physical, emotional, and social goals within the context of the relationship. Client goals may have a broad range in type and depth. For example, in informal relationship work, a client's goal may be to initiate one peer relationship within an inpatient psychiatric unit. Other examples include resolution of a divorce involving children and shared personal possessions, or coming to terms with the client's impending death from acute, terminal physical illness. Often the client's initial goal is to solve an immediate problem, and this serves as a basis for establishing more extensive psychosocial

goals. The psychiatric nurse also formulates personal therapeutic goals to enhance the growth-producing elements of the relationship.

Professionalism

One-to-one relationships reflect a professional, rather than social, relationship. Psychiatric nurses enter the relationship intending to use their personalities, interpersonal skills and techniques, and theoretical knowledge of psychiatric nursing practice in a purposeful, goal-directed manner based on what may be useful to their clients. This professional relationship differs from a social relationship in several significant ways. A social relationship is generally structured for companionship and pleasure, while a one-to-one relationship generally involves the systematic working through of specific problematic thoughts, feelings, or behaviors. A social relationship does not usually involve a delineation of roles, while the one-to-one relationship between psychiatric nurse and client carries the implication that the nurse will play a specific role, using professional psychiatric nursing skills and interventions. The focus of the one-to-one relationship is on the client's identifying, developing, and assessing ways to meet personal needs effectively, rather than on meeting the personal needs of the nurse. Table 7–2 summarizes the major differences between professional and social relationships.

The one-to-one relationship may also be differentiated from the nurse–client interaction. An interaction is some segment of actual behavior that takes place between the psychiatric nurse and the client. The one-to-one relationship may be viewed as a series of sequential nurse–client interactions with the following additional elements:

- The interactions occur over a designated period of time (daily, weekly, monthly).
- The interactions take place within a structure in which specific phases, processes, and problems evolve that are unique to the developing relationship between psychiatric nurse and client.
- The interactions occur in a designated setting that tends to remain stable over time (home, private-practice office, mental health clinic, inpatient psychiatric unit, medical unit).

THE HISTORY OF ONE-TO-ONE WORK

The one-to-one relationship between psychiatric nurse and client has evolved as the cornerstone of psychiatric nursing theory and practice. Before the 1940s, the therapeutic role of the nurse was to provide custodial care. Nurses also performed specific medical-surgical procedures as psychiatry developed somatic therapies for the treatment of specific disorders. These included deep sleep therapy in 1930, insulin shock therapy in 1935, psychosurgery in 1935–1936, and electroshock therapy in 1937. Thus, it was through the use of medical-surgical skills that psychiatric nurses gained recognition as significant participants in psychiatric treatment. Although nurse–client relationships were used intermittently as therapeutic tools, it was not until 1946, with passage of the National Mental Health Act, that any systematic development of relationship work began.

1940s to 1951: Initial Role Development

Enactment of the National Mental Health Act was the government's response to growing recognition of mental illness as a national health problem. During World War II, 43 percent of all army discharges were classified as psychiatric disabilities. This created a sharp increase in the demand for psychiatric services. The National Mental Health Act provided for:

1. Establishment of the National Institute of Mental Health

2. Development of programs to train professional psychiatric personnel, including psychiatric nurses

3. Support for psychiatric research

4. Aid in developing mental health programs

Eight graduate programs were initiated in 1947 for the advanced preparation of psychiatric nurses. These programs prepared many of the nursing leaders who later developed theoretical frameworks for one-to-one relationship work.

Until the early 1950s, psychiatric nurses formulated only vague concepts about how nurses might participate in one-to-one relationships with clients. Some pressed for trained postgraduate nurses to provide psychotherapy and become functioning members of an interdisciplinary treatment team that would include psychologists and social workers. Ambiguity about professional psychiatric nursing roles characterized this period.

1952 to Mid-1960s: Role Clarification

A period of role clarification was initiated in 1952 by Dr. Hildegard Peplau's publication of *Interpersonal Relations in Nursing*, the first systematic theoretical framework in psychiatric nursing. Peplau's framework represents a cornerstone in the development of psychiatric nursing theory and practice. She has had greater impact than any other nursing theoretician to date. The roots of her ideas lie in the interpersonal theory of Harry Stack Sullivan, supplemented by learning theory. Lego (1975, p. 6) summarizes Peplau's framework as follows:

> Briefly described, it provides a system within which the nurse helps the patient to examine carefully his current interpersonal experiences in order to improve them through the development of interpersonal competences which have been either lost or never learned. The emphasis is on the nurse helping the patient to observe his behavior; describe it in detail to the nurse; analyze it with the nurse; formulate, in a clear way, the connections resulting from the analysis; validate this formulation with others; test new behavior, integrate this learning into new, more satisfying behavior; and, finally, use these new behaviors in many situations.

Peplau continued to enrich her formulations of nursing theory regarding one-to-one relationship work for the next twenty years.

Frances Sleeper's address to the American Psychiatric Association in 1952 advocating the use of psychiatric nurses as psychotherapists heralded another major new trend in psychiatric nursing. Her advocacy ushered in a heated, ten-year controversy over caretaker versus psychotherapist roles for psychiatric nurses. The literature from 1946 to 1958 reveals that paramount attention was given to psychiatric nursing functions that primarily reflect the caretaker role: ward staffing and management, assistance with physical care and medical therapies, observation and recording of client behaviors, and client supervision. Advocates of the caretaker role stressed nurses' unique function in management and supervision of the client's environment. They also viewed the nurse as coordinator of care, ward organizer, mother surrogate, treatment facilitator, and leader of ward activities. In contrast, others urged that psychiatric nurses be practitioners of intensive psychotherapy. However, even these proponents limited the nurses' psychotherapeutic role to collaborative work with a psychiatrist or as the second member of the psychiatric team. The nurse was to be a psychotherapist for only certain clients, usually those selected by the psychiatric staff as candidates for supportive therapy.

A milestone report, ignored by most of the psychiatric nurses involved in the controversy, was published in 1956 by the National Working Conference on Graduate Education in Psychiatric Nursing (see Lego 1975, p. 3). It introduced the concept of the psychiatric clinical nurse specialist, and theoreticians began to differentiate functions based on master's level preparation of psychiatric nurses.

In 1957, June Mellow introduced the second major theoretical framework in psychiatric nursing, resulting from her intensive one-to-one relationship work with schizophrenic clients. Again, Lego (1975, p. 6) summarizes the crucial elements of Mellow's concept:

It is called nursing therapy and draws on psychoanalytic theory in the sense that an intensive, symbiotic relationship is developed between the nurse and patient. The emphasis is on providing a corrective emotional experience rather than on investigation of pathological process or of the interpersonal developmental process. Unlike the strict psychoanalytic mode, emotional closeness is manifested through such physical intimacy as bathing, feeding, and clothing the patient and recreation with him.

Mellow's formulations, like Peplau's, center on the development of a one-to-one nurse–client relationship.

Other developments strengthened the psychotherapist role for psychiatric nurses. First, psychiatric nurses were given encouragement from the Joint Commission

on Mental Illness and Health in the publication *Action for Mental Health* to develop therapeutic effectiveness in individual as well as group and milieu therapy. Second, in 1962, Peplau wrote that the primary role of the psychiatric nurse was as psychotherapist or counselor, rather than as mother, socializer, or manager. Others agreed (see Bueker and Churchill reported in Lego 1975; Fagin 1967; Mellow 1968). Peplau predicted that nurses would be functioning in private practice within a decade. Nursing roles emphasized in the literature of the time included the nurse as consultant, casefinder, diagnostician, therapist, and cotherapist.

The Comprehensive Community Mental Health Act was passed in 1963, giving impetus for nurses to move from hospital to community settings. The following year, Orlando's generalized theoretical framework for all nurse–client relationships was applied by some practitioners in psychiatric settings. This theory briefly sees the nurse as observing the client's distress or need, assisting the client in ascertaining the meaning of behaviors in relation to the distress, and finally assisting the client to explore what help is required to alleviate the distress. It is interesting to note that the three major theoretical frameworks for one-to-one relationship work all use a medical model approach to psychiatric nursing intervention.

The launching in 1963 of *Perspectives in Psychiatric Care*, a journal for psychiatric nurses, was a significant event in psychiatric nursing history. It provided a forum for airing issues and sharing professional psychiatric nursing theories. The *Journal of Psychosocial Nursing* (formerly called the *Journal of Psychiatric Nursing* and the *Journal of Psychiatric Nursing and Mental Health Services*) also began in 1963. These publications further established the one-to-one relationship as the basis of psychiatric nursing, whether it was defined as psychotherapy or not. Thus, controversial role clarification and refinement characterized this period of psychiatric nursing.

Late 1960s to Present: Confirmation of the Specialist Role

The period since the mid-1960s has been characterized by confirmation of the psychiatric clinical nurse specialist as a viable role in psychiatric nursing practice. The clinical specialist received professional endorsement to assume the role of therapist in individual, group, family, and milieu work in a 1967 American Nurses' Association *Position Paper on Psychiatric Nursing* (see Lego 1975, p. 5). Two years later, the reality of nurse psychotherapists moving into the realm of private practice was reported by Meldman and her associates (1969). The clinical specialist role received additional confirmation with the initiation of a certifying body for psychiatric clinical nurse specialists by the state nurses' associations in New Jersey (1972) and New York (1975). For a further historical overview and detailed discussion of the psychiatric clinical nurse specialist role and the development of the certification process, see Chapter 3.

PHILOSOPHICAL FRAMEWORK

Humanistic Factors

Humanistic philosophy in one-to-one relationship work involves viewing humanness not as a static condition, but as an evolving, active process unique to each person. Traditional psychoanalysis incorporated some initial humanistic considerations. Freud and his colleagues stressed the importance of the therapist. The psychoanalyst enters the drama of the client's life and facilitates the client's achievement of greater personal freedom through the use of transference and interpretation. In contrast, behaviorist psychology is generally viewed as discounting personal freedom. Behaviorism appears to reduce the individual to a reactor to environmental stimuli, rather than an actor spontaneously affecting an optimistic world.

Openness   Humanism stresses openness and honesty in human relations. Within a humanistic framework, the one-to-one relationship between nurse and client may be viewed as an experience in *shared dignity*. The psychiatric nurse adapts to the client to allow the client to reveal his or her humanness freely and openly to the nurse. Each aspect of the nurse's verbal and nonverbal behavior encourages or inhibits the client from further revealing humanness.

Negotiation   Humanism views the client as exercising free will, as an active decision maker. In addition, humanism stresses the client's uniqueness and the subjectiveness of the experiences underlying personal actions. The one-to-one relationship relies on the client to determine the type and length of involvement in one-to-one work and to be personally accountable for the work. The atmosphere of give and take within the rela-

tionship emphasizes mutuality, reciprocity, and interpersonal fairness. Establishment of a clearly defined, mutually agreed-on therapeutic contract represents a prime example of negotiation in one-to-one work. (The therapeutic contract is covered in the discussion of the beginning phase of therapy later in this chapter.)

Commitment   Commitment is based on the therapeutic contract between nurse and client. The contract establishes the limits of the relationship, as well as the time and energy that will be allotted to it. At some point in relationship work, the psychiatric nurse may be confronted by the reality of the client's dysfunction. The beginning psychiatric nurse may respond by actively colluding with the client to deny or ignore the dysfunction and remain on a superficial, social level of communication. This protects the nurse from having to address the client's exposure of helplessness, desperation, hostility, or raw grief. The nurse who does not allow such exposure and deal with it is not sufficiently committed to the client. The antithesis is also problematic. The overcommitted psychiatric nurse may assume an omnipotent role to "cure" the client. This robs the client of active decision-making power and accountability. The nurse's degree of commitment will be tested by the client in some phase of relationship work, and this needs to be dealt with explicitly on verbal and nonverbal levels by both nurse and client.

Responsibility   Personal responsibility for the one-to-one relationship is also based on the therapeutic contract between nurse and client, and it, too, will be tested by the client in some phase of the work. Beginning psychiatric nurses usually encounter responsibility problems as they begin to perceive unattractive, dysfunctional, or blatantly offending interpersonal behavioral patterns or habits in their clients. Both nurse and client must deal explicitly with "who is responsible for what." In addition, the nurse should avoid making any agreements with a client that the nurse may be unable to fulfill.

Authenticity   The appreciation of spontaneity and authenticity is another aspect of humanistic philosophy that appears particularly pertinent to one-to-one relationship work. Psychiatric nurses need to create an atmosphere that conveys permission to express pain and pleasure. Expressions of joy and assessments of client abilities, talents, and capabilities are an often-neglected, yet essential, aspect of relationship work. Cronbach (1975, p. 125) stresses the need for "an open-eyed, open-minded appreciation of the surprises" that often emerge spontaneously in relationship work.

Humanistic Nursing Education   The main purpose of any humanistic psychiatric nursing education program is the growth and creative development of the individual student. Each student is viewed as a unique being encouraged to nurture and test out personal values, strengths, and talents, rather than as a receptacle for learning. In addition, students are urged to develop and refine their personal sensitivity rather than suppress their awareness of their personal feeling states. Nursing educators need to recognize that a chief hazard to humanistic learning may be the student's immature emotional involvement with clients. The educational program should provide experiences to facilitate student maturity and therapeutic effectiveness. One innovative approach is for psychiatric nursing students to do student consultation with fellow students on medical-surgical rotations. This enables students to apply psychiatric theory outside psychiatric settings and forges a link between psychiatric and medical services for client benefit (Jansson 1979). Finally, humanistic nursing education needs to consider the rights of the clients used for teaching purposes and protect them from unnecessary exposure or exploitation.

Symbolic Interactionist Factors

A symbolic interactionistic framework in one-to-one relationship work focuses on the trend from psychiatric to psychosocial nursing, and consideration of the significance of meaning between nurse and client.

The development of psychosocial nursing, with emphasis on preventing emotional dysfunction, received impetus with the shift to community-based programs in the 1960s. Psychosocial nursing expanded traditional psychiatric nursing approaches to include family, economic, political, and cultural influences in the client's environment among the major areas subject to nursing assessment and intervention. Thus, the scope of nursing intervention moves well beyond the confines of the client's intrapersonal experiences.

Personal identity is not considered a fixed product but something constantly confirmed through interaction with others. The nurse–client interaction is subject to continuous reassessment of the client by the nurse and the nurse by the client in a process called *identity confirmation*. Meanings of individual words, gestures, events, and situations must be explored to determine

the exact significance assigned to them by the client. The therapeutic contract itself provides initial meaning to nurse–client interactions.

In a more general way, psychiatric nurses are working with clients in a search for meaning in their lives. It is essential that nurses establish their own personal meaning and integration of self, for these are key resources in treatment. For psychiatric nurses to be effective, they must already possess the personal skills necessary to deal with the client's symptomatology, or must have personally worked through any problems they had that resembled those of the client. For example, a nurse who cannot cope with her own depressed feelings will not be effective with a severely depressed client.

INTERPERSONAL SKILLS IN THERAPEUTIC RELATIONSHIPS

Therapeutic Effectiveness of Psychiatric Nurses

The effectiveness of psychiatric nurses has often been subjectively assumed, unquestioned, or discounted without a scientific data base for evaluation. Our consideration here of their therapeutic effectiveness will include a brief exploration of past research, exploration of the conflict between caretaker and therapist roles, and delineation of personal characteristics known to facilitate therapeutic effectiveness.

Summary of Past Research   In 1969, Griffith and Trogdon studied self-expressive styles among college students, including those preparing for careers in nursing. Nurses scored high on humanistic scales (which measured preference for nurturing, helping, supporting, comforting, and assisting), and low on promotional scales (which measured preference for organizing, planning, administering, and managing). This evidence supports nurses' preference for a professional caretaker role.

Additional studies focus exclusively on the psychiatric nurse. The Hargreaves and Runyon (1969) study of interactional patterns of nursing staff and inpatients showed differences in their roles, following traditional patterns: the nurse offers directions or suggestions to the client, but the reverse is not true. Hargreaves and Runyon also discovered that, while nurses often seek information about clients, they rarely reveal any information about themselves. Altshul (1970) further studied nurse–client interactions in hospitalized settings, with the following findings:

- Clients with organic brain disorders received far more interactions, depressed clients far fewer, and neurotic clients minimal interactions from nurses.
- Clients hospitalized more than eight weeks interacted very little with nurses, and interactions were always on the clients' initiative.

Data from this study imply that the neediest clients receive the least treatment from psychiatric nurses. One client reported:

> I never have any rapport with the nurses. I think I should have benefited, but because I read they don't think I need anyone. I am more apart than the people who just sit and stare. Someone goes and talks to them! [Altschul 1970, p. 38.]

In 1972, Munsadis studied psychiatric nurses as one-to-one leaders in small ward groups of acutely disturbed hospitalized clients. More frequent and longer-lasting individual contact with the nurse achieved the following results in clients: improvement in personal hygienic habits, improvement in work performance, and increased use of passes. Peitchinis (1972), reviewing the literature, reported that registered nurses rate low in the following qualities associated with therapeutic effectiveness: empathy, warmth, and genuineness. Her sample is significant in that it includes nurses in a variety of settings and nursing students in diploma, associate degree, and baccalaureate programs. She does, however, point to evidence that nurses may be realizing their limitations and attempting to overcome them. Finally, Reich and Geller (1977) studied self-images of psychiatric nurses and found that they identified with traits of achievement, self-assertiveness, and self-control to a greater degree than a general nursing group. Psychiatric nurses in this sample saw themselves as cautious, serious, cooperative, methodical, and able to work well with others.

Conflict between Caretaker and Therapist Roles   The traditional nursing education may hamper the psychiatric nurse in developing therapeutic effectiveness because it stresses both the denial of personal feelings and the need to continue a caretaker role. Nurses may erect rigid defenses aimed at denying their feelings because of the emotional demands of nursing. For example, some procedures actually require the nurse to violate a client's emotional or physical state (injections, dressings). Defending against feelings becomes one way for the nurse to cope with inflicting pain on another person. Yet psychiatric nurses can deal effectively with the feelings of clients only to the extent that they explore their own personal feelings.

Continued assumption of the caretaker role also hampers psychiatric nurses in developing therapeutic effectiveness. One-to-one relationship work requires the psychiatric nurse to help the client actively explore the meaning underlying the client's personal pain, distress, or discomfort. Nurses must avoid the caretaker role in which they alleviate pain rather than encouraging clients to develop ways to do so for themselves. Similarly, the caretaker role requires nurses to make decisions for clients. It does not encourage clients to be accountable for their own decisions.

Facilitative Personal Characteristics   Psychiatric nurses may increase their therapeutic effectiveness by knowledge and practice of specific interpersonal skills in therapeutic relationships. Truax and Carkhuff (1967) first emphasized the need for certain core facilitative conditions to enhance any therapeutic relationship. Schuable and Pierce (1974) demonstrated that clients who were successful in therapy had therapists who functioned at higher levels of empathy, warmth, genuineness, and concreteness than the therapists of clients who were unsuccessful in therapy. Chapters 3 and 6 discuss these facilitative conditions. However, studies suggest no more than a weak relationship between these characteristics and client improvement. Shapiro (1976) has questioned the adequacy of original studies by stressing the need for a methodologically sound, experimental study to more definitively demonstrate the effectiveness of these facilitative characteristics.

Research repeatedly indicates that interpersonal skills may be acquired, increased, and refined through educative experiences, workshops, and human relations laboratories. Nursing research has begun to evaluate the effectiveness of training programs to teach interpersonal skills to nursing personnel. For example, Miller and Orsolits (1978) developed and researched the effectiveness of a didactic-experiential program to train nurses as primary counselors engaged in one-to-one work on an acute psychiatric inpatient service. Results include a significant improvement in use of supportive skills to clients. The one-to-one relationship was viewed as a critical factor in enhancing the quality of care extended to clients.

Therapeutic Use of Self

Therapeutic use of self involves a pulling together of several important personal elements to bring to any one-to-one relationship work. Students must first develop a healthy self-awareness. Psychiatric nursing students are often bombarded with numerous and varied inputs, including unfamiliar psychiatric jargon, policies, and settings; the experience of being supervised; dysfunctional client behaviors; and the whole new role as change agent in the mental health field. All this may be stressful and emotionally draining. Students may fear client exploitation and question what they could possibly offer in one-to-one relationship work. To develop healthy self-awareness, students might start by identifying and labeling their feelings as they perceive them (see Chapter 3).

It is essential for students to see themselves holistically if they are to develop a holistic approach to others. This involves increasing awareness of their personal impact on others. It includes learning about current abilities and skills, as well as personal limitations, and attending to personal internal stress signals as identified in Chapter 3.

Students also need to develop a comprehensive theoretical and experiential knowledge base. Reliance on sound mental health theory is not only in the best interests of the client, but also enhances the self-confidence of the beginning psychiatric nurse.

In summary, therapeutic use of self orchestrates three major aspects of self:

- Development of healthy self-awareness
- Exploration of the growth-facilitating, humanistic self
- Thorough use of theoretical and experiential knowledge in mental health

Thus, Lego's definition of a psychotherapist might also be used to describe the therapeutic use of self by one who "... is self-aware, humanistic, knowledgeable theoretically, and who has had good supervision" (Lego 1980, p. 39).

Consideration of Client Abilities

The psychiatric nurse may increase the success of the therapeutic outcome by knowledge of specific client abilities. Schuable and Pierce (1974) have demonstrated that the following characteristics of clients are conducive to effective relationship work: awareness of in-

ternal feeling states; ownership of feelings; desire to change; and ability to differentiate feelings, concerns, and problems. These characteristics warrant further exploration.

First, the nurse–client relationship will be more effective if clients are aware of and show willingness to assume responsibility for his or her feelings and actions. In contrast, some clients act as if their problems are entirely external and beyond their control. Second, clients must admit their feelings and show awareness that the feelings are tied to specific behaviors. This contrasts with clients who avoid accepting their personal feelings and view them as belonging to others or as situational and outside themselves. Third, clients need to express a clear desire to change and cooperate with the nurse as opposed to resisting involvement. Finally, clients have to be able or show willingness to learn how to differentiate feelings, concerns, and problems and must recognize their unique reactions and individuality.

The Therapeutic Alliance

The facilitative personal characteristics of the psychiatric nurse, the nurse's therapeutic use of self, and the client's abilities form a therapeutic alliance in one-to-one relationship work. In therapeutic alliances, psychiatric nurses present themselves as real persons who strive to truly encounter clients. In so doing, nurses work to form a mature alliance with the conscious adult ego of their clients. More specifically, the psychiatric nurse identifies and provides feedback regarding the client's patterns of reaction, assets, and potentials. The client can use these assets and potentials to handle unresolved problems constructively. While the establishment of the therapeutic alliance enhances informal one-to-one relationships, it is essential in formal one-to-one relationship work. This binding alliance between psychiatric nurse and client allows for the continuation of psychotherapy, especially when the client experiences increased anxiety and resistance to interpersonal change.

PHASES OF THERAPEUTIC RELATIONSHIPS

One-to-one relationship work has three distinct phases:

1. The beginning (orientation) phase, characterized by the establishment of contact with the client

2. The middle (working) phase, characterized by maintenance and analysis of contact

3. The end (resolution) phase, characterized by the termination of contact with the client

Each phase of relationship work is distinguished by specific therapeutic objectives, therapeutic tasks, client behaviors, and psychiatric nurse behaviors.

The specific length of time required for each phase depends on the severity of client dysfunction, the psychiatric nurse's skills, the number and types of problems surfacing during treatment, and the type of therapeutic contract negotiated between psychiatric nurse and client. It is essential to note that while these phases are presented here in their entirety to develop a comprehensive theoretical framework, nurses rarely experience them in such detail and sequence. Nurses are more likely to experience the development of one or two therapeutic tasks, and to experiment with several subsequent approaches in any phase of relationship work. Nevertheless, an exploration of each phase will increase the nurse's familiarity with the flow—that is, "what comes next"—and provide a framework in which the psychiatric nurse can see client and nurse behaviors as partial expressions of a specific phase.

Beginning (Orientation) Phase: Establishment of Contact

An exploration of the beginning (orientation) phase of one-to-one relationships necessitates a brief review of nursing literature, delineation of the therapeutic objectives of the phase, and exploration of the therapeutic task of this phase, which includes negotiation of the therapeutic contract. Establishment of contact refers to the manner in which both psychiatric nurse and client approach and deal with each other initially, verbally and nonverbally. In informal relationship work, contact usually begins with the psychiatric nurse seeking out the client in an inpatient psychiatric setting. In formal relationship work, contact begins with the client's inquiry about services, or contact of the client by the psychiatric nurse following referral. This phase of the therapeutic relationship concludes with mutual agreement to a therapeutic contract, making explicit the client's goals for treatment and the nurse's professional responsibilities.

There has been little nursing research addressing the beginning phase of relationship work. Studies generally involve long-term, hospitalized, middle-aged

Table 7–3   SIGNS OF A WORKING RELATIONSHIP

For Nurse	For Client
Sense of making contact with the client	Nonverbal and verbal evidences of liking the nurse
Sense that client is responding well to the relationship	Sense of relaxation with nurse
Sense that nurse can facilitate client growth regardless of severity of client dysfunction	Sense of confidence in nurse

schizophrenic clients. Stastny (1965) reported a case study on how nurses develop trust among clients by listening attentively to client feelings, including repetitive and negativistic ones, responding to client feelings rather than emphasizing logic and actions, and exhibiting therapist consistency, especially regarding appointment times. McArdle (1974) reported a case study on humane and therapeutic use of self in long-term individual relationship work that emphasized the nurse's need to view situations from the client's world view. For the most part, however, psychiatric nurses have left research on the beginning phase of one-to-one relationships to others.

Objective of the Phase   The primary objective of the beginning phase is to establish contact, or a working relationship with the client. In informal relationships, establishment of contact may involve developing client awareness of the nurse's presence, followed by working to communicate with the client on a verbal level. In formal relationship work, it is the sense of working together in the therapeutic alliance that enables the client to endure anxiety and deal with resistance to change, both of which inevitably surface in the course of individual psychotherapy. The working relationship in this initial phase is the framework on which the client constructs behavioral change in the next phase. Table 7–3 highlights common signs of a working relationship as viewed by Wolberg (1977).

The term *establishment of contact* refers to the nurse's perception of having a personal impact or effect on the client, and the nurse's acknowledgment of the client's personal impact as a unique individual on the nurse. This contrasts with *physical contact*, which is used cautiously in therapeutic work. Nurses general-

Table 7–4 SUMMARY OF BEGINNING (ORIENTATION) PHASE		
Objective	Therapeutic Tasks	Nursing Approaches
Establishment of contact in the form of a working relationship with the client	Clarification of purpose of relationship work, role of nurse, and responsibilities of client	Educative Provide information regarding purpose, roles, and responsibilities in relationship work to alleviate initial client anxiety Immediately and explicitly address any misconceptions, fantasies, and fears regarding relationship work and/or nurse.
	Addressing client suffering directly, and offering to work with the client toward its alleviation	Use facilitative characteristics, especially empathic understanding Avoid premature reassurance (allow trust to evolve) Be explicit about who has access to client's revelations (degree of confidentiality)
	Negotiation of therapeutic contract (client's definition of personal goals for treatment and nurse's professional responsibilities)	Whenever possible, encourage delineation of goals that: • Are specific • Address intrapersonal and interpersonal behavioral patterns • Designate degree of change necessary for client self satisfaction In informal relationship work, contract generally includes determination of time and place for working together to the extent that client function permits. In formal relationship work, the contract generally includes: • Place, duration, and time of therapy • Fees and payment intervals, if any • Optional referral sources

ly avoid unplanned physical contact without a therapeutic rationale.

Therapeutic Tasks   Three therapeutic tasks are important in the beginning phase of relationship work. The goal is to enhance the development of a working relationship between psychiatric nurse and client. Table 7–4 summarizes the therapeutic tasks and offers specific nursing approaches to establishing the working relationship. Concerns about trust, confidentiality, and negotiation of the therapeutic contract deserve special consideration.

TRUST   Concerns about trust come to the surface in this first phase of the relationship. Trust between psy-

chiatric nurse and client evolves over time as the client tests the emotional climate of sessions, risks self-disclosure, and observes nurse follow-through on responsibilities delineated in the therapeutic contract. The nurse's response to all the client's feeling states without evaluation or attempts to control emotive expression is of prime importance in facilitating the development of trust. Self-awareness of personal feeling states on the part of the nurse also enhances trust. It allows the client to disclose uncomfortable, even forbidden, feelings in safety. A common failing among those learning relationship skills is focusing on technique. This produces mechanical, unfeeling responses. It is also important to avoid giving premature reassurances about trust, which may inhibit exploration of this vital therapeutic issue and create distance between therapist and client. The verbatim example in Table 7–5 illustrates the emergence of trust as an initial therapeutic issue.

CONFIDENTIALITY Client concerns about the level of confidentiality also surface in this first phase of the therapeutic relationship. Like the issue of trust, the issue of confidentiality must be explicitly addressed when the client makes even vague reference to it. The psychiatric nurse should state explicitly which persons will have access to client revelations (clinical instructor, case supervisor, consultant, colleague) and explore how the client feels in response to this information.

THERAPEUTIC CONTRACT The therapeutic contract, which is used in all relationship work, consists of an initial definition of client goals and nurse responsibilities. In informal relationship work, the therapeutic contract may be brief and simple. It may simply involve the client's definition of goals to work on (however simplistic), some determination of time and place for meeting together, and delineation of the nurse's responsibilities. Even a simple therapeutic contract may take several meetings to formulate. For example, an elderly inpatient with organic mental disorder agrees to meet with a nursing student every Wednesday when she visits his unit. He wishes to anticipate ways to deal with isolation following eventual discharge. The nursing student agrees to contact the client via phone in the event that she is unable to meet with him on any specific Wednesday.

In formal relationship work, as in individual psychotherapy, the therapeutic contract is more detailed, more elaborate, and generally includes three practical matters:

1. Determination of the place, duration, and time of therapy
2. Establishment of fees and payment intervals, if any
3. Consideration of optional referral sources, should the client seek psychotherapy but be unable to negotiate an agreement on the first two matters

The most essential aspect of the therapeutic contract is the client's definition of goals for treatment. Client goals most often contribute to the establishment of a working relationship when they are specific, address intrapersonal or interpersonal behavior patterns, and delineate the degree of change necessary for client self-satisfaction.

Nurses need to develop a working knowledge of therapeutic contracts and to learn appreciation for their versatility. Two different samples of therapeutic contracts illustrate how a contract can be designed to meet specific client needs. Figure 7–1 shows a sample mental health contract suggested by Ralph Nader's health research group. This contract addresses three important areas: specific practical arrangements for meetings, intrapersonal and interpersonal behavioral patterns, and degree of confidentiality. Figure 7–2 shows a therapeutic contract used by the Mental Health Corporations of the Erie County Department of Mental Health in New York State. This second contract is very specific in addressing intrapersonal and interpersonal behavioral patterns, and the degree of change necessary for client self-satisfaction. It is vague regarding the nurse's responsibilities within the working relationship. Note that this second contract shows evidence of the middle (working) phase of relationship work, where analysis of behavioral patterns and institution of behavioral change take place. The middle phase of relationship work will be discussed in the next section.

Middle (Working) Phase: Maintenance and Analysis of Contact

Once contact is established, attention turns to maintenance and analysis of contact in the middle or working phase of one-to-one relationships. This contact allows for the behavioral analysis that leads to growth-producing change in the client. Literature regarding the middle phase of therapeutic relationships is sparse and primarily considers long-term schizophrenic clients. The issue of resistance is addressed generally without any systematic working through of major aspects of psychotherapy. Of particular note is Cloud's (1972) consideration of the plateau in nurse–client relationships, when the client typically uses some type of resistance—such as denial, avoidance, hostility, and rejection—to avoid the anxiety associated with change. Cloud described two therapeutic shifts in orientation to counteract client resistance: use of recreation, and playback of tapes from recorded sessions.

Initial Objective and Therapeutic Tasks The initial objective of the middle (working) phase of one-to-one relationships is the mutual determination of the dynamics of the client's behavioral patterns, especially those considered to be dysfunctional. This objective

Table 7–5 VERBATIM EXAMPLE, ORIENTATION PHASE		
Verbatim Interaction	**Nursing Intervention**	**Rationale**
Client: It's so difficult for me to talk . . . to let you know about me.		
(Thirty-second pause.)	None	To allow client space to proceed at own pace; if silence is uncomfortably long to client in first few contacts, nurse may use reflection, e.g.: "I sense how difficult talking is for you."
Client: Every time I start to tell anybody about myself, they usually end up laughing at me.		
Nurse: Can you give an example of this?	Encourage elaboration	To explore meaning of this statement to client
Client: Well, just last week I started talking to my neighbor. I told him that I was laid off from work again. Next thing you know, he's laughing, slapping my back, and saying "Hey, hard times, eh?"		
(Shifts in chair, poor eye contact.)		
Nurse: What was this like for you?	Explore client's personal reaction, expecially accompanying feelings	To further explore meaning of this specific incident as perceived by the client
Client: Awful . . . lousy . . . that's all.		
(Pause.)		
Nurse: I wonder if you're concerned that the same might happen here—that you'll be laughed at?	To apply concern regarding "external" issue to here-and-now, i.e., one-to-one relationship	Issues concerning client's immediate life situations often reflect parallel issues in nurse–client relationship
Client: Well, maybe. . . . I don't know you, so how do I know what you might do? You don't look like the type, but then again—how do I know?		
Nurse: It sounds like you're wondering if it's safe to trust me.	Move to what appears to be the *metamessage* or underlying central concern (theme)	Reflection of what appears to be the central concern (theme) encourages client assessment by validation or correction
Client: Yeah . . . no offense, though.		
Nurse: Let's talk about how safe you feel today and as we continue to work together.	Underline trust as an issue for further exploration; stress evolving working relationship	Avoid premature reassurances so that trust can evolve and be assessed periodically

ELEMENTS OF A CONTRACT

A contract cannot by itself guarantee results. It does represent an attempt to define the nature of services to be provided by the mental health professional and fosters accountability on the parts of both the therapist and the patient while providing ongoing documentation of those services. To give the consumer an idea of what a contract might look like, a sample follows. This form should not be considered definitive or restrictive—indeed, the flexibility of the contract is one of its most valuable characteristics. It is intended only as a fictitious example.

1. Name of each party
2. Date of beginning and end of agreement
3. Length of each session
4. Goals of sessions stated as specifically as possible
5. Cost per session and when payable
6. Definition of services provided by psychotherapist stated as clearly as possible

7. Provisions for cancellation:
   a. no penalty for termination
   b. amount of time necessary for warning doctor of cancellation
   c. protection for doctor against willful no-show on part of patient
   d. provision for unavoidable and unforeseen events causing patient to be unable to meet session
8. Renegotiation at end of stipulated period
9. Allowance for changing goals within stipulated period
10. Definition of nature of services; no guaranteed results; guarantee of intention and good faith
11. Establishment of access by patient and doctor to document which becomes part of medical record; guarantee of confidentiality and control by patient over medical record and its contents and use of any information therein.

Figure 7–1

Mental health contract, Public Citizen's Health Research Group. *Continues on next page.*

flows from the therapeutic contract in which the client identified specific goals for the therapy experience.

There are several therapeutic tasks involved in the exploration of the client's dynamics. First, the psychiatric nurse collaborates with the client in identifying important behavioral trends and patterns. Once a pattern is identified, it is explored in elaborate detail to determine its origin, causes, operation, and effects on the client and those who populate his or her world. Environmental factors (familial, political, economic, or cultural) are separated from intrapersonal factors contributing to the pattern. The client figuratively holds the pattern to the light to look at, examine, and make sense of its every aspect. The elements of one pattern will inevitably link with others, so that the major life patterns gradually unfold. The verbatim example in Table 7–6 from the middle (working) phase demonstrates how elements of one behavioral pattern are linked to others and gradually reveal central life patterns. In this case the client's initial anger in reaction to concerned relatives led to awareness of the need to

shun contact in several additional situations. The nurse may now help the client explore what appears to be a central life pattern of interpersonal isolation devoid of intimacy. The first part of Table 7–7 summarizes the therapeutic tasks undertaken to achieve this objective and offers specific nursing approaches to helping the client.

There are two noteworthy considerations regarding therapeutic tasks of the first objective:

1. As clients begin to describe and reexperience conflict, they will consciously or unconsciously use defenses to ward off the anxiety this awakens (see Chapter 10). The development of a good working relationship enables clients to tolerate increased anxiety in the working phase of the one-to-one relationship.
2. As clients become familiar with self-assessment, they may modify original personal goals, or develop additional goals, in keeping with what has been learned.

SAMPLE CONTRACT

[1] I, *Mr. Client,* agree to join with *Ms. Therapist* each Thursday afternoon from May 1, 1975,

[2] until June 5, 1975, at 3 p.m. until 3:50 p.m.

[3] During these six 50-minute sessions we will direct our mutual efforts towards three goals:

[4] 1. Enabling me to fly in airplanes without fear
2. Explaining to my satisfaction why I always lose my temper when I visit my parents
3. Discussing whether it would be better for me to give up my full-time job and start working part-time

[5] I agree to pay $30 per session for the use of her resources, training and experience as a

[6] psychotherapist. This amount is payable within 30 days of the session.

[7] If I am not satisfied with the progress made on the goals here set forth, I may cancel any and all subsequent appointments for these sessions, provided that I give Ms. Therapist 3 days warning of my intention to cancel. In that event I am not required to pay for sessions not met. However, in the event that I miss a session without forewarning, I am financially responsible for that missed session. The one exception to this arrangement being unforeseen and unavoidable accident or illness.

[8] At the end of the six sessions Ms. Therapist and I agree to renegotiate this contract. We include the possibility that the stated

[9] goals will have changed during the six-week period. I understand that this agreement does

[10] not guarantee that I will have attained those goals; however, it does constitute an offer on my part to pay Ms. Therapist for access to her resources as a psychotherapist and her acceptance to apply all those resources as a psychotherapist in good faith.

I further stipulate that this agreement become a part of the medical record which is accessible to both parties at will, but to no other person without my written consent. The therapist will respect my right to maintain the

[11] confidentiality of any information communicated by me to the therapist during the course of therapy. In particular, the therapist will not publish, communicate, or otherwise disclose, without my written consent, any such information which, if disclosed, would injure me in any way.

_____

Date

_____

Name

_____

Name of Professional

Figure 7–1 continued

The initial objective of determining the dynamics of the client's behavioral patterns continues throughout the working phase. The objective is achieved when the client has awareness of, understanding of, and insight into the causes and manifestations of patterns in his or her current personality structure and can assess these major trends.

Second Objective and Therapeutic Task   The second objective of the middle phase is initiation of behavioral change, particularly in self-defeating,

growth-inhibiting patterns. Establishing behavioral change flows from the first objective. The objectives are interrelated and essential for successful psychotherapeutic work. Understanding and insight need to be complemented by behavioral implementation. This statement deserves much attention, since particular clients may consistently generate and thrive on sophisticated insights while continuing to assume a powerless stance about implementing constructive change in their condition.

The beginning nurse must learn the value of active

SERVICE CONTRACT

Name _Terry Harris_   ID# _120005_

Significant Other _Kim Harris_

Case Manager _Janice Smith, R.N._

Supervisor _Kelly Ray, R.N., M.S._

Physician _Joan Oster, M.D._

(Client is a 21-year-old single female living at home with parents.)

Code

1. Physical	6. Residential
2. Self-Acceptance	7. Financial
3. Vocational	8. Decision Making
4. Immediate Family	9. Life Philosophy
5. Intimate Relationship(s)	10. Leisure Time / Community Involvement

	11. Feeling Management
	12. Lethality (self)
	13. Lethality (other)
	14. Substance Use
	15. Legal
	16. Agency Use

S=Satisfied   U=Unsatisfied

Code #	Date	Problem Statement	Date	Method/Technique/Tasks for achieving goals (include review date)	Expected Outcome (include date)	Goal Achieved S or U	Date
11	2/9/81	Moderate depression, manifested by feelings of helplessness and inability to complete task	2/9/81	Agrees to meet once weekly for 30-minute sessions to work on identified problems (see problem statements)	2/18/81 Antidepressant prescribed—Elavil b.i.d. May bring depression to more workable level	S	3/9/81
	2/16/81	Avoids any personal accountability for depression—blames mother	2/18/81	Initial medication assessment. Medication supervision within sessions			
			2/23/81	Decides to keep daily diary, noting any awareness regarding depressed feelings (time, place, situation, people involved, how depressed feelings are perceived, results, etc.)	3/9/81 Useful tool. Likes writing. Awareness of depression associated with: Mother's domination, Boredom, Loneliness		
					3/30/81 Continues to be useful tool. Less subjective complaints of depression. Has instituted behavioral changes regarding mother and boredom	S	3/30
4 and 8 (combined)		Relationship with mother characterized by excessive dependence. "She treats me like a baby. Does everything for me." Delegates decision making to others, esp. mother	2/25/81	Wants autonomy in activities of daily living			
			3/2/81	Will do own laundry.		S	3/16
			3/9/81	Does dinner dishes	Improved.	S	3/23
			3/16/81	Walks to sessions alone rather than mother driving	Improved, despite mother's attempts to do tasks. Depends on weather	U to S	4/13

No.	Date	Problem	Plan / Action	Evaluation	V/S	Date
5	2/16/81	Avoids all peer relationships	Wants autonomy regarding use of leisure time. Chooses to go for a walk outside home on daily basis / Sets no goals. Does not see as a problem / 4/6 Locates a pen-pal. Begins writing on a monthly basis	Gets discouraged easily, esp. if weather is slightly unpleasant / No behavioral change	V & S / U	4/6 / 3/30
10	3/2/81	Boredom	3/23 Volunteers to work at library three times weekly / 4/13 Auditions and is accepted into church choir	Likes writing, so may use this skill to establish contact with peer, indirectly / Enjoys this. May revert to increase social system / Beneficial. Confirms vocal talent	S / S / S	4/27 / 4/6 / 4/6
3	3/2/81	Unemployed for two years. (Has high school diploma)	3/2 Will write to local community colleges for course offerings	No follow-through. "I'm not interested in a career of any kind. I don't like any of the jobs that are available."	U	to date
1	3/2/81	Obesity (Weighs 175 lbs — 51 lbs. over desired weight)	3/9 Obtains 1,200-calorie/day diet from family physician. Negotiates to lose 1½ lbs. weekly	4/6 Lost 5 lbs. in one month / 4/27 Lost 11 lbs. total / Continues to modify eating patterns to lose weight	S	4/27

Figure 7–2

Sample service contract. From L. A. Hoff, *People in Crisis* (Menlo Park, Calif.: Addison-Wesley Publishing Co. 1978), p. 326. Reproduced by permission of the Erie County Department of Mental Health: Mental Health Services, Erie County, Corporation IV, South East Corporation V, and Lakeshore Corporation VI.

The form was developed by a Task Force of workers representing Corporation IV, South East Corporation V, Lakeshore Corporation VI, and the Erie County Department of Mental Health. Members: Marsha Aitken, Maureen Becker (Chairperson), Barbara Bernardis, George Deitz, Lee Ann Hoff, Elizabeth Keller.

For samples of forms not included here and for complete specifications for use of these forms, the reader is referred to Erie County Department of Mental Health, 95 Franklin Street, Buffalo, New York 14202.

Table 7-6 VERBATIM EXAMPLE, WORKING PHASE		
Verbatim Interaction	Nursing Intervention	Rationale
Client: My nosy relatives are at it again. Since my mother died and I'm living alone, they keep phoning me to see if I'm all right.		
Nurse: You sound irritated. . . .	Reflection of feeling tone to explore client's reaction to this situation	Reflection of feeling tone encourages client to validate or clarify emotive response to situation
Client: Not irritated—mad! Those phonies don't care about me. Why should they? Why should they?!? They don't.		
Nurse: What motivates them to call?	Seeking clarification about how client perceives the immediate situation	Clarifying statements help explore the meaning of this specific situation as perceived by the client
Client: To pester me. People do it all the time. That one woman at work that I told you about last week—she does the same thing. She smiles and says good morning. She's concerned . . . but I don't want anything to do with her either.		
Nurse: You're talking about two situations where you don't want to deal with people: your relatives and the woman at work. I remember your description of how you wanted to avoid an old classmate last month. Is there something common to all these situations?	Actively linking elements of several behavioral patterns accumulated over time (current session, last session, last month) to search for commonality	Elements of one pattern may link to others with a gradual unfolding of central life patterns
Client: I can't see anything— except that I go out of my way to avoid people. I avoid everyone. I live alone and want to stay alone.		

experimentation to test the effect of new behaviors. The introverted male client who resolved to establish relationships with women may assume various postures (cavaliering, paternalism, sexual seduction, etc.) with a female psychiatric nurse to determine the appropriateness of these behaviors before displaying

them outside of sessions. Permission to "try on" behaviors must also include freedom to make mistakes. Errors and blunders are rich sources of additional learning and occasional fun. A client who is able to see humor in errors in a nondefeatist manner has acquired a new skill. The client can be encouraged to apply this

Table 7-7   SUMMARY OF MIDDLE (WORKING) PHASE

Objectives	Therapeutic Tasks	Nursing Approaches
Maintenance and analysis of contact Consists of: Mutual determination of dynamics of client's behavior patterns, especially those considered dysfunctional	Identification and detailed exploration of important behavior patterns	Explore behavior pattern in depth, including origin, causes, operation, and effect of pattern (intrapersonally and interpersonally)
		Separate environmental factors (familial, political, economic, cultural) from intrapersonal factors
		Link elements of one behavior pattern to other patterns as appropriate, for a gradual unfolding of central life patterns
	Analysis of client's mode of conflict resolution	Encourage detailed exploration of how client reacts to reduce anxiety associated with conflict
		Increase awareness of defenses employed to ward off anxiety awakened by such exploration
	Facilitation of client self-assessment of growth-producing and growth-inhibiting behavior patterns	Encourage client to evaluate each behavior pattern to determine which are self-defeating and/or thwart gratification of basic needs
Institution of behavioral change, especially in dysfunctional behavior patterns	Address forces that inhibit desired change (problematic thoughts, feelings, and behaviors)	Assist client in challenging client's personal resistance to change
		Use problem-solving strategies, active decision making, and personal accountability
		Encourage client to assert own needs when external environmental conditions (group, agency, institution) are an inhibiting force
	Create an atmosphere offering permission for active experimentation to test and assess effectiveness of new behaviors	Allow freedom to make and assess mistakes and blunders
		Avoid parental judgment of any behavioral experimentation— encourage client self-assessment instead
	Facilitate development of coping skills to deal with anxiety associated with behavioral change	Address, rather than avoid, anxiety and its manifestations
		Strengthen existing growth-promoting coping skills, especially regarding unalterable conditions (e.g., terminal illness, physical deformity, loss of significant other by death)
		Encourage development of new coping skills and their application to actual life experiences

skill, and any other coping skills learned in relationship work, to normal maturational and situational crises encountered throughout life.

Nursing responsibilities in the working phase of relationship work include: making arrangements for professional supervision or consultation (especially about new, difficult, or anxiety-provoking behavior patterns); active intervention in severe self-defeating behavior patterns (suicide, homicide, starvation, self-mutilation); and endorsement of growth-producing behaviors.

The psychiatric nurse and the client have moved through the first two phases of therapeutic relationships when they have established a working relationship, and analyzed the dynamics of the client's behavioral patterns, and the client has effectively instituted behavioral changes in keeping with the therapeutic contract. In informal relationship work, the nurse may only touch upon one or two aspects of the middle (working) phase of one-to-one relationship work. Even the advanced psychiatric nurse rarely addresses all therapeutic tasks in this phase of relationship work. Nevertheless, presentation of the entire middle (working) phase may provide a type of road map to designate "where one can go," should the immediate situation, client ability, and time permit. The latter part of Table 7–7 summarizes the therapeutic tasks to achieve the second objective of the working phase and again offers specific nursing approaches.

There are two major categories of forces that inhibit desired change:

1. Intrapersonal forces, which may arise from problematic thoughts, feelings, or behaviors. Examples include: thoughts that hamper the client's sense of worth; the client's inability to control and express emotion appropriately; or the client's inability to relate to others in a meaningful manner.

2. The client's personal resistance to change, which is the greatest inhibiting force. In fact, it is the client's challenge to these resistances that constitutes the major work in one-to-one relationships.

Discussion of specific types of resistance and appropriate nursing interventions appears in a later section of this chapter.

End (Resolution) Phase: Termination of Contact

The end (resolution) phase of one-to-one relationships is characterized by termination of contact between psychiatric nurse and client. This phase is as important as the previous two, although it is frequently avoided by nurse and client alike.

The resolution phase is the phase most often described by nurses. A number of nurse–authors have offered clinical examples of how to handle termination, reviewed the problems encountered at termination, and proposed nursing interventions. Perhaps Vennen (1970) offers the most humanistic approach to termination, viewing it as a painful, difficult process characterized by melancholy, denial, and finally solitary grief. She views termination as a separation of what was unique to the nurse, unique to the client, and temporarily shared in the one-to-one relationship. More recently, McCann (1979) skillfully reviews the significance, dynamics, and theories regarding termination in an expert and humanistic manner.

Objective of the Phase   The objective of the end phase of one-to-one relationships is termination of therapy in a mutually planned, satisfying manner. A smooth and complete termination sometimes occurs in actual practice. In informal relationship work in inpatient settings, termination more often occurs with the client's abrupt departure or planned medical discharge. Even in formal relationship work in community settings, contact often ceases without explanation after a series of missed appointments, or with a phone call by the client to inform the therapist of the client's decision to terminate, or with the client abruptly leaving a session and failing to resume subsequent contact. In these instances, follow-up contact by the nurse is advisable, by letter or telephone, to encourage an additional session to deal with either the therapeutic good-bye or a willingness to continue the relationship work. Termination requires careful preparation, adequate time for the client to work through the feelings about ending, and an opportunity for the psychiatric nurse to explore personal reactions with a clinical instructor, colleague, supervisor, or consultant.

The psychiatric nurse must be alert to the surfacing of any behavior on termination. Any of a number of client responses—repression, regression, anger, denial, sadness, acceptance, and joy, among others—may surface. When repressing, the client gives no evidence of any emotional response. The psychiatric nurse may respond by repeatedly observing that the client is not addressing the issue of impending separation and may move to explore this avoidance. The client who reverts to a previously abandoned behavior pattern with a message of "I can't make it without you" demonstrates regression. The psychiatric nurse may move to address possible underlying fears of abandonment, while also stressing the reality of termination. The acting-out client may protest termination in numerous ways (suicide gestures or attempts, psychiatric hospitalization, terminating employment, rejection of therapist, etc.) before the termination date. In general, the underlying feelings, fears, and fantasies need ventilation, exploration, and working through. The client reactions of anger, depression, or grief require the same. An exception to this general guideline occurs when the client uses distraction maneuvers, such as the introduction of explosive new material in final sessions. The following clinical example illustrates a client's manipulative attempts to prevent termination by using acting-out behaviors. Limit setting, rather than exploration, was used by the psychiatric nurse because of time constraints specific to this one-to-one work. The example also illustrates that there may be "unfinished business" despite planning and effort.

Kim was a nineteen-year-old, single female who was self-referred to a local university student counseling center. Her chief complaint was an inability to maintain relationships with both female and male peers. History included excessive drug experimentation and frequent superficial sexual encounters with males who subsequently mistreated and left her. Kim negotiated for two semesters of individual psychotherapy and was informed that the psychiatric nurse was not available beyond this time framework due to relocation. Behavior in sessions was characterized by attempts to trap the nurse, displacement and projection of anger onto others, and avoidance of accountability for her presenting problem. Although termination was carefully planned and referral sources considered, Kim resisted by offering money, crying, and leaving sessions early. She resisted exploration of any thoughts or feelings regarding termination and refused consideration of alternate referral sources. During the last session, she eagerly reported having her first homosexual experience with a woman who resembled the nurse. She then asked how the one-to-one relationship could end without exploring this new behavior. The nurse was aware of the far-reaching implications of this final issue in terms of Kim's psychodynamics as well as its impact on the one-to-one work. The nurse was also aware of Kim's challenging attitude associated with another attempt, this time regarding sexual acting out, to prolong sessions. In this instance, the nurse underlined this explosive issue as needing further exploration, again discussed and encouraged use of referral sources, and addressed the issue of goodbye. Both nurse and client were dissatisfied with the immutable time limitation in this case. A sense of mutual termination was not realized.

Nursing responsibilities in this final phase of one-to-one relationship work include anticipation of the nurse's personal reaction to separation and an optional expression of this reaction in a manner that does not burden the client. In addition, the nurse may share a special wish for the client, based on the client's particular assets within the therapeutic relationship. A sense of freedom to move on to other relationships also accompanies a therapeutic good-bye. The end phase may take from one meeting to several months of meetings, depending on the duration of the one-to-one relationship. In general, the longer the duration of the relationship, the longer the time needed to deal explicitly with termination of contact. Table 7–8 summarizes the objective, therapeutic tasks, and specific nursing approaches to the end (resolution) phase of one-to-one relationship work. Ideally, the client can completely work through feelings regarding separation so that there is no unfinished business between the psychiatric nurse and client. The nurse–client relationship has given the client the opportunity to depend on another in a realistic and mature manner. Assessment of the experience helps the client practice self-assessment skills, and may help set the stage should the client desire additional relationship work at a future date. Participating in a direct, explicit goodbye is frequently the first such experience for the client. It is usually a moment of unique humanness for both the psychiatric nurse and client.

PROCESSES IN
THERAPEUTIC RELATIONSHIPS

In addition to familiarity with significant phases of one-to-one relationships, the psychiatric nurse needs to develop awareness of and effectiveness in using numerous processes that occur in any one-to-one relationship work. This section highlights the following essential processes: observation, interviewing, assessment, problem-solving strategies, transference and countertransference phenomena, and evaluation. The beginning nurse often attends carefully to the *content* of the client sessions—that is, "what the client says"—and only after considerable experience becomes actively attuned to *processes*. The experienced practitioner is simultaneously aware of both content and process, interweaving both for maximum therapeutic effectiveness.

Table 7-8 SUMMARY OF END (RESOLUTION) PHASE

Objective	Therapeutic Tasks	Nursing Approaches
Termination of contact in a mutually planned, satisfying manner	Assist client evaluation of therapeutic contract and of psychotherapeutic experience in general	Encourage client's realistic appraisal of personal therapeutic goals (motivation, effort, progress, outcome) as these evolved in treatment
		Provide appropriate feedback regarding appraisal of goals
		Underline client's assets and therapeutic gains
		Underline areas for further therapeutic work
	Encourage transference of dependence to other support systems	Encourage client to develop reliance on others in client's immediate environment (spouse, relative, employer, neighbor, friend) for empathic, emotional support
	Participate in explicit therapeutic good-bye with client	Be alert to surfacing of any behavior arising on termination (repression, regression, acting out, anger, withdrawal, acceptance, etc.)
		Assist client in working through feelings associated with these behaviors
		Anticipate own reaction to separation and share in a manner that does not burden client
		Allow "time" and "space" for termination; the longer the duration of the one-to-one relationship, the more time is needed for the resolution phase

Observation

Observation, a process long regarded as essential to clinical nursing practice, is of particular importance in one-to-one relationship work. Peplau (1952, p. 263) emphasizes the interpersonal function of observation in the following assertion:

> The aim in observation in nursing, when it is viewed as an interpersonal process, is the identification, clarification, and verification of impressions about the interactive drama, of the pushes and pulls in the relationship between nurse and patient, as they occur.

Peplau maps out the following steps in the process of observation:

- Observation generally begins on a subjective, sensory level.

- The observer conceives of a generalization or "hunch" about what is occurring in a particular situation. This observation is accurate when the psychiatric nurse attends only to what is observable in the situation.

- The observer collects data to analyze whether personal observations are accurate in this particular setting.

- The observer elaborates on the first whole impression. The psychiatric nurse must note many minute details to gain an overview of what is occurring.

- The observer, as participant in the observing process, refines the intuitive abilities that can then be applied to other situations.

Observation is an intensive process requiring concentration and practice to gather data through the use of all the senses. The observer strives to develop simultaneous sensitivity to vision, hearing, smell, taste, and touch in nurse–client interactions. The observer also needs to check out personal distortions, biases, or unreality. In addition to observing what elements are present, the nurse notes elements in the nurse–client interaction that are missing, distorted, or imbalanced.

Observation Concerning Critical Distance

Observations are made of the manner in which the client uses physical space in the course of one-to-one relationship work. Hall (1966) asserts that people require a *critical distance* from others to maintain their well-being and that the specific distance depends on the relationship between the individuals involved. Parks (1966) advocates use of physical distance as a nursing approach in the beginning phase of therapy to facilitate communication at a verbal level and to keep the client's anxiety and/or hostility at a workable level. Moving rapidly toward closeness, especially in establishing the nurse–client relationship, may overwhelm the client and increase anxiety.

The amount of physical distance between the psychiatric nurse and the client can be indicative of other therapeutic processes. For example, a client may sit in a chair at the greatest distance from the nurse during initial meetings but move closer and closer as the working relationship becomes established. The psychiatric nurse needs to assess the possible interpersonal implications of proximity for each client, and to assess whether physical distance or proximity reduces client anxiety, particularly when intervening at panic or near panic levels.

Initial Interview

Interviewing is a process that generally occurs in the beginning (orientation) phase of one-to-one relationship work. While the structured initial interview may be used by the advanced psychiatric nurse in formal one-to-one work, it is rarely used in informal relationship work. Nevertheless, it is important to consider so that beginning nurses can familiarize themselves with the kinds of background data collection useful in mental health work and can incorporate various elements of the initial interview as appropriate for specific clients over an extended time span. The initial interview has the following purposes:

- To establish rapport with the client
- To obtain pertinent client data
- To initiate client assessment
- To make practical arrangements for treatment

The initial interview is crucial in that it sets the stage for subsequent therapeutic contact.

Amount of Structuring   The psychiatric nurse must structure the initial interview to establish rapport and convey an active willingness to address the client's suffering. The initial interview may begin with the psychiatric nurse's personal introduction, an invitation for the client to be seated, and a statement concerning information thus far known about the client's seeking of services. An open-ended question, such as "How is it that you are here today?" provides an opportunity for initial client revelations. The psychiatric nurse may explicitly inform the client that the initial interview is structured to give an overview of the client's current situation to determine the availability of appropriate services. Dillon (1971) elaborates on the deleterious effect that lack of structuring may have on the nurse–client relationship.

Collection of Essential Data   One primary purpose of structuring the initial interview is to collect essential data. The presenting problem or chief complaint constitutes a concise statement of the most distressing current problem, recorded in the client's own words. After gathering the client's personal, descriptive account, the practitioner moves to obtain specific information about the presenting problem in a directive manner: its history, development, manifestation, effect on present physical functioning (appetite, sleep, sexual expression), and effect on present social functioning (family, employment, friends). It is important to pinpoint the event that caused the client to seek services. The client should also describe any other current problems. Additional areas of brief exploration at the initial interview include: family constellation, physical health status, psychosocial development, history of previous emotional difficulties, history of therapy, drug and alcohol use/abuse, coping skills and methods of resolving conflict, and present level of motivation. One final relevant area of data collection involves the client's identifying characteristics: name, age, sex, address, telephone number, marital status, education, occupation, employment record, and cultural and ethnic origins. The Initial Contact Sheet used by the Erie County Department of Mental Health at Buffalo, New York, shows the data collected in the initial interview process (see Chapter 8).

It is important for the psychiatric nurse to address client resistance if it should surface during the initial interview. This may occur when the client has initiated services at someone else's request or insistence, has fears and misconceptions about therapy, or has had an unsatisfactory therapeutic experience in the past. Nursing intervention calls for explicit exploration of the specific resistance before further data collection. The client's initial confusion about or misinterpretation of information given during the initial interview may be a function of moderate to high anxiety levels that most clients experience at onset of therapy. Manifestations of anxiety must be differentiated from manifestations of resistance, and information may need to be repeated several times or in subsequent meetings. The major tasks of the initial interview are:

1. Structure interview to
   a. Establish rapport
   b. Convey an active willingness to address the client's suffering
2. Collect pertinent data, including
   a. Presenting problem
      (1) History
      (2) Development
      (3) Manifestations
      (4) Effect on psychosocial functioning
   b. Event causing client to seek services at this time
   c. Description of other problems in client's current life situation
   d. Psychosocial functioning and development
      (1) Family constellation
      (2) Physical health status
      (3) History of previous emotional difficulties
      (4) History of any therapy
      (5) History of drug use/abuse
      (6) Coping skills and methods of resolving conflict
   e. Present level of motivation
   f. Identifying characteristics
      (1) Name
      (2) Age
      (3) Sex
      (4) Address
      (5) Telephone number
      (6) Marital status
      (7) Occupation
      (8) Employment record
      (9) Cultural and ethnic origins
3. Initiate client assessment
4. Address any initial client resistances
5. Make practical arrangements for treatment

Wolberg (1977, pp. 455–457) offers the following list of practices for the psychiatric nurse to avoid during the initial interview. These apply to informal, as well as more formal, one-to-one relationships.

- Do not argue with, minimize, or challenge the client
- Do not praise the client or give false reassurance
- Do not make false promises
- Do not interpret to the client or speculate on the dynamics of the client's problem
- Do not offer the client a diagnosis even if he or she insists on it
- Do not question the client on sensitive areas
- Do not try to "sell" the client on accepting treatment
- Do not join in attacks the client launches on parents, mate, friends, or associates
- Do not participate in criticism of another therapist

Chapter 6 discusses specific aspects of communication that are important to the interviewing process.

Assessment

Client assessment begins at the first moment of contact. The process continues throughout the relationship, but it is of particular significance in the beginning phase. Assessment involves nonverbal, verbal, and environmental observations, in addition to consideration of the emotive, cognitive, and behavioral aspects of the client. Psychosocial assessment is considered in depth in Chapter 8.

Emotive Assessment Assessment of the client's *affect*, or emotional state, is based on the observable manifestations of emotional reactions and the client's description of the subjective experience. In emotive assessment, the therapist notes such characteristics of the client's affect as degree of spontaneity, appropriateness, flatness, existence of ambivalence, and mood swings. The client's predominant affective reactions are noted and described as euphoric, resigned, anxious, depressed, resentful, irritable, and so forth. In addition, the psychiatric nurse assesses whether the client's emotional state is appropriate to his or her speech, behavior, and immediate situation.

Cognitive Assessment   Cognitive assessment includes evaluation of *thought content, sensorium,* and *intelligence.* Thought content is evidenced by the client's trend of speech, association of ideas, preoccupations, and concerns. Examples of disturbances in thought content include delusional ideas, obsessions, phobias, compulsions, serious considerations of suicide, and ideas of reference (see Chapters 14–16). Assessment of sensorium includes considerations of degree of consciousness, past and present memory, and orientation to time, place, and person. Assessment of intelligence reveals limited or appropriate functioning.

Behavioral Assessment   Behavioral assessment reflects the client's general attitude or manner. The client's presenting attitudes may be described as confident, friendly, fearful, evasive, demanding, distrustful, passive, sullen, or dependent. In addition to interpersonal attitudes, behavioral assessment involves overt manifestations of the client's interpersonal relationships. The client's behaviors toward those who populate his or her world may be described as asocial, conforming, aggressive, narcissistic, submissive, or appropriate, for example. Finally, the client's ability to meet sociocultural needs through family, friends, and community groups (religious, social, recreational, and rehabilitative) needs exploration to determine the adequacy of these support systems.

Problem-solving Strategies

Problem solving is a crucial process of particular significance in the middle (working) phase of one-to-one relationships. Problem-solving strategies are essential after the identification, detailed exploration, and client assessment of important behavioral patterns. As the client addresses the forces that inhibit desired changes, the psychiatric nurse can help the client use the sequential problem-solving strategies discussed below.

Observation   Observation as a problem-solving strategy involves gathering and analyzing facts about a

potential problem area. It eliminates opinions and impressions and emphasizes facts.

Definition   Definition is perhaps the most significant and far-reaching problem-solving strategy. It involves an initial specification of a problem, followed by a question. Starting a problem-solving exploration with the word "How" (for example, How is it? How does it manifest itself? How has this come about?) focuses on the process regarding a specific problem. It is generally more useful than asking "Why," which emphasizes rationale. For example, an adolescent girl finds herself repeatedly tense in the presence of her middle-aged male employer despite his kind manner. The question "How is it?" is asked to determine if the problem has been defined in its most basic form. The answer may be that the client senses tension because her employer is a middle-aged male, and she usually experiences anxiety with this age group. As the same inquiry is repeated, this second definition may appear as a subproblem in a more basic definition of the problem. Thus, the client may redefine her problem: "In what ways can I deal with the anxiety associated with paternal figures?" Note that the statement of the problem begins with "in what ways," rather than "how," to allow for numerous approaches.

Next, it is helpful to determine whether the problem involves fact-finding (calling for data answers), judgment or decision, or creative exploration. In dealing with problems requiring creative exploration, all the ideas that imagination can produce may be helpful. Thus, evaluation is temporarily deferred or suspended to allow for the consideration of numerous alternatives.

The following clinical material illustrates definition of the most basic form of a problem:

Fern is a nineteen-year-old, single female seeking individual counseling at a local university counseling center. She was referred because she felt depressed following a split with her boyfriend over the summer. Emotional concerns included a marked feeling of depression, plus verbalized feelings of guilt, loneliness, and confusion. Physical concerns involved sleep disturbance (difficulty falling asleep with resultant sense of fatigue), eating disturbance (increased compulsive eating when under stress, with subsequent sudden weight gain), and minor self-mutilative gestures (picking skin around fingernails and scratching face). Fern denied suicidal ideation and appeared to be a minimal suicide risk. She showed a general flatness of affect, characterized by very slow, monotonous speech accompanied by minimal facial or body gestures, and occasioned by periodic silences and quiet weeping. She resides in an apartment shared by three female roommates, and maintains a 3.8 academic average as a junior student majoring in biology. She negotiated for weekly one-hour sessions of individual psychotherapy for the duration of the school year. The following exchanges occurred in the final ten minutes of the third session:

FERN: *This weekend will be a long weekend. I don't know what to do.*

NURSE: *I'd like to hear more about this long weekend.*

FERN: *Well, Marc might want to go out with someone else, so I don't want to take up his time. My three roommates are busy. . . . I don't want to call Marty. . . . My friend Judy won't be home. . . .*

NURSE: *Which of these is most troublesome for you?*

FERN: *Well, I don't care about Marc anymore. . . . My roommates are always busy. . . . Sometimes Judy gets on my nerves. . . .*

NURSE: *What do you suppose is the problem about all this?*

FERN: *I feel that I'm not going to have a good time. I won't study. Usually no one is home . . . and I'll be lonely. Yeah, . . . I'll be lonely again.*

NURSE: *The problem with this long weekend seems to be more loneliness for you.*

FERN *(Sighs): That sums it up.*

In the above verbatim example, the client moved from identifying several subproblems to the more basic problem of loneliness. The nurse assisted the client by encouraging definition and reflecting the probable central theme back to the client.

Preparation   Preparation involves collecting additional pertinent data related to the basic problem that may prove useful in later stages of problem-solving strategies.

Analysis   Analysis as a problem-solving strategy involves breaking down the relevant material into subproblems so that each subproblem may be assessed separately.

Ideation   Ideation involves accumulating alternative ideas on how to resolve the basic problem. The following clinical material illustrates Fern's initial use of ideation as a problem-solving strategy in the beginning of the fourth session:

FERN: *My weekend wasn't that bad. (Laughs mildly.)*

NURSE: *Let's hear about it.*

FERN: *Well, Saturday night I went out to dinner with my roommate, and Friday night I went to the movies.*

NURSE: *I wonder what were the "good" and "bad" parts of this.*

FERN: *Well, I can honestly say that I enjoyed the movie, and dinner with Sara [roommate] was okay, too.*

NURSE: *What did you do to make your weekend "not that bad"?*

FERN: *Well, I planned my time, so I wasn't always alone. I had some studying to do for one exam.*

Fern changed the topic to discuss one teacher who added requirements to his course. When she mentioned the weekend again, the nurse tried to refocus.

NURSE: *Fern, are you aware of any steps involved in dealing with loneliness over the weekend?*

FERN: *Yeah. I actively sought out doing things. I made sure that I was doing things.*

NURSE: *Can you be more specific?*

FERN: *I kept busy. I had to study. I went to the library on Saturday so I wasn't home alone. I told you about going out to dinner and the movie.*

Incubation   Incubation is used when the problem-solving process or one aspect of it is set aside for a period of time to allow for illumination.

Synthesis   Synthesis as a problem-solving strategy involves putting all elements of the basic problem, subproblems, and possible alternatives together.

Evaluation   Evaluation consists of making judgments about the resultant ideas.

Development   Development as a final problem-solving strategy involves planning the implementation of these ideas.

Problem-solving abilities may improve with time and experience. During the eighth session, Fern and the nurse were skilled enough to piece together the "map" in Figure 7–3. It concerns Fern's definition of her current problem: how to handle angry feelings without feeling trapped by them. The map is not complete, but it represents a sorting of the known dynamics in that particular instance.

The specific situation precipitating that exploration was that Fern's roommate repeatedly left dishes in the sink for days, after having agreed to clean them night-

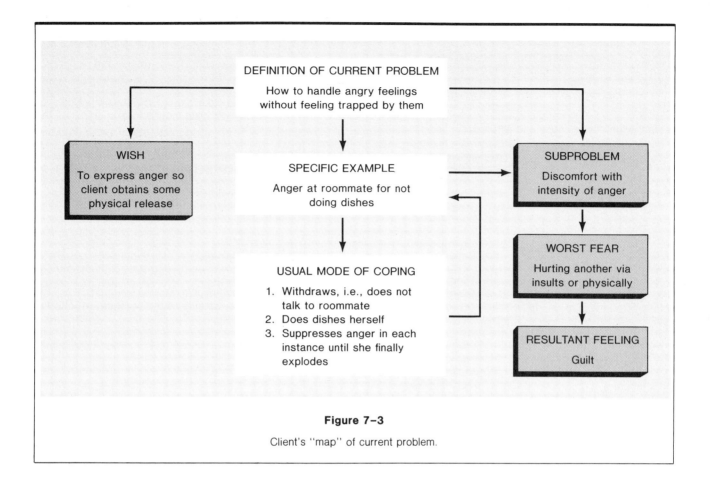

Figure 7–3

Client's "map" of current problem.

ly. Fern identified two problem-solving alternatives in this session. First, Fern could set the dirty dishes aside for her roommate to see. She evaluated this to be a less satisfactory solution, since her roommate might then avoid the kitchen area. Secondly, Fern might directly share her anger with the roommate. Fern had never before risked sharing anger directly with anyone. She anticipated that she could maintain her assertive position by justifying that everyone has to assist in housework. Fern judged that if the actual task was accomplished by the roommate, then the outcome would be satisfactory for her. Table 7–9 summarizes Fern's possible problem-solving outcomes.

Preparation and incubation had been used as problem-solving strategies, since Fern had determined many pieces of the "map" in the interim between the seventh and eighth sessions. Synthesis was apparent in Fern's integration of known subproblems of an identified problem and active seeking of alternatives. Ideation and evaluation were used in her identification of problem-solving alternatives and evaluation of the potential outcome of each. In informal relationship work, some or all elements may be used in a similar manner.

Transference and Countertransference Phenomena

Consideration of nursing processes would be incomplete without attending to transference and countertransference phenomena. These are normal phenomena that may surface and inhibit effectiveness in any phase of one-to-one relationship work. Fenichel (1943, p. 29) offers the following basic definition of the transference process:

> The patient misunderstands the present in terms of the past; and then instead of remembering the past, he strives, without recognizing the nature of his action, to relive the past and to live it more satisfactorily than he did in childhood. He "transfers" past attitudes to the present.

Transference is viewed as a form of resistance in which the client defends against recollection of childhood conflicts. Instead, the client transfers these conflicts to the present therapeutic relationship.

A social interactionist may view transference phenomena as distortions of meaning between psychiatric

Table 7-9 EVALUATION OF CLIENT'S PROBLEM-SOLVING ALTERNATIVES	
Alternative	**Evaluation**
Set aside dirty dishes for roommate to see	Anticipates that roommate might avoid kitchen area
	Probable unsatisfactory outcome
Tell roommate directly about anger regarding dirty dishes	Never shared anger with anyone
	Anticipates following sequence:
	Shares anger regarding dirty dishes
	Roommate gives excuses
	Maintains assertive position that everyone assists with housework
	Roommate agrees to do task
	Outcome judged satisfactory if task is done by roommate

nurse and client in one-to-one relationship work. The therapist may suspect that a client is in transference when the client repeatedly assigns meaning to the nurse–client relationship that belongs to one or more of the client's past relationships. It is as if the client's ability to assess the nurse–client interactions becomes confused and/or thwarted by the unfinished conflicts belonging to past interactions with significant others. Thus, the psychiatric nurse may be viewed as parent, sibling, lover, or friend.

The development of transference offers the psychiatric nurse an opportunity, by direct observation, to understand the development of the client's past conflicts. The appearance of highly emotional responses that do not "fit" the current therapeutic situation may indicate client transference. In traditional psychoanalytic work, handling the transference becomes the core of treatment. In the social interactionist approach to transference the psychiatric nurse explores the meaning of individual words, gestures, events, and situations in the current one-to-one relationship to determine how these reflect or replay distortions in past

relationships. The therapeutic task is to separate feelings, thoughts, and behaviors that belong to the current one-to-one relationship from those that represent unfinished conflicts in past relationships. Increasing awareness of the transference process often frees the client to work through past conflicts and explore the more creative, self-actualizing aspects of personal identity as they evolve in the current relationship. The psychiatric nurse must not behave as the client's parent or other transference figure has behaved. Rather, the nurse may use the technique of interpretation in which the nurse helps the client bring an unconscious event into consciousness, to examine its cause and meaning. Chessick (1974) elaborates on the significance of transference and the use of interpretation as a delicate art and skill. Two clinical examples of hospitalized clients illustrate how transference may surface in clinical settings:

Conrad Wilson is a forty-year-old married man hospitalized with moderate depression, which is manifested by restless agitation, inability to complete tasks, and subjective feelings of hopelessness. Conrad was assigned to a primary counselor, a male psychiatric nurse, in keeping with the unit's treatment regime. Over the course of several meetings with his counselor, Conrad assumed a cowering, ingratiating manner. He seemed to resemble a little boy awaiting punishment from an intimidating, punitive father. This interpersonal orientation was observed by other male staff who informally initiated interaction with Conrad on the unit. In this instance, the transference figure appeared to be a parental father figure.

The counselor chose not to explore Conrad's past relationships. The aim of short-term work was to focus on concrete ways to decrease depressed feelings in Conrad's present life situation—that is, in the "here-and-now." The counselor addressed ingratiating behaviors in the nurse–client relationship only when they appeared to have an adverse effect on their short-term work together.

Corrine Travers is a thirty-year-old, married woman admitted to the same inpatient unit due to an acute psychotic episode. She appeared intensely competitive on the ward and strived for absolute supremacy in any interpersonal situation involving a female. A young female nursing student tried repeatedly, but unsuccessfully, to involve Corrine in informal one-to-one relationship work. Each attempt was met with accelerating hostility and verbal threats. After guidance from her clinical instructor, the student chose to work with another client who requested increased staff involvement. It was unknown by ward staff at that time that Corrine's childhood history included a violently competitive relationship with her younger sister to win parental affections. In this instance, the sibling relationship seems to be the basis of the transference phenomena.

It is important to note that negative transference responses that seem related to deep-seated depression or paranoia are usually not dealt with in relationship work. The reason is that exploration may stir up issues and intense emotions that cannot be dealt with in a limited time span (Areiti 1975).

While transference involves client reactions to the psychiatric nurse, countertransference involves the nurse's reactions to the client. The psychiatric nurse may develop powerful counterproductive fantasies, feelings, and attitudes in response to the client's transference or general personality structure. A social interactionist may also view countertransference as a distortion of meaning between psychiatric nurse and client in one-to-one relationship work. A clinical instructor or supervisor may suspect countertransference when the psychiatric nurse repeatedly assigns meaning to the nurse–client relationship that belongs to the nurse's other past relationships. In countertransference the psychiatric nurse's ability to assess the nurse–client interactions becomes confused or thwarted by unfinished conflicts of the past. Thus, the nurse may unconsciously employ behaviors (as parent, sibling, lover, or friend) that attempt to replay in the current situation some past identity with significant others. Countertransference indicates unresolved conflict in the psychiatric nurse, which may be expressed in acts of omission or commission, in irrational friendliness or annoyance, in a covert or an overt manner.

Countertransference is a normal occurrence, requiring supervision or consultation to prevent any inhibitory effect on the one-to-one relationship. Supervision may enable the psychiatric nurse to separate feelings, thoughts, and behaviors that belong to the current relationship from those that represent unfinished conflicts in past relationships. Awareness of the existence of countertransference is crucial, since unrecognized countertransference may be acted out and may inhibit client understanding. This can undermine the entire psychotherapeutic process. A later section of this chapter briefly explores specific problems and appropriate interventions in troublesome cases of transference and countertransference.

Evaluation

Evaluation is an ongoing nursing process in several aspects of one-to-one relationship work:

- The psychiatric nurse's continuous evaluation of client behaviors
- Development of client self-evaluation
- Mutual evaluation of the one-to-one relationship, especially during the end (resolution) phase of relationship work
- The psychiatric nurse's self-evaluation in each one-to-one relationship

The first three types of evaluation have been discussed previously. The nurse's personal ongoing self-evaluation warrants emphasis here. It is essential that the psychiatric nurse continuously evaluates which personal behaviors consciously or unconsciously promote, inhibit, and actively block growth-producing client abilities. This evaluation ideally occurs in a formal supervision arrangement, regardless of the practitioner's degree of therapeutic skill and expertise.

Supervision is essential if psychotherapy is to be effective. Professional supervision helps the psychiatric nurse use transference effectively and recognize countertransference phenomena. Mellow (1968) has identified the following functions of a supervisor in relation to the supervised psychiatric nurse:

- A teaching function for the transmission of learnable techniques and attitudes.
- A supportive function for difficulties that are inherent in or imposed on the therapeutic relationship.
- An analytic function to increase the awareness of how he or she affects the therapeutic relationship and outcome.

More recently, Benfer (1979) used the supportive function of supervision to monitor the personal needs of the nurse and decrease the likelihood of severe clinical stress and burnout. There are various methods of evaluation: interpersonal process recordings, videotapes, audiotapes, didactic instruction, and referral to specific clinical readings. These methods of evaluation are discussed in Chapter 3. There are several kinds of supervision available, such as intradisciplinary supervision with a clinical instructor or psychiatric clinical nurse specialist, or interdisciplinary supervision by another mental health professional (psychologist, psychiatrist, psychiatric social worker). All can be helpful, depending on the skills and availability of supervisors/ consultants. Supervision helps the psychiatric nurse effectively define, initiate, use, and evaluate client and self in any therapeutic relationship.

THE PROBLEMS OF RESISTANCE IN THERAPEUTIC RELATIONSHIPS

A comprehensive overview of one-to-one work must consider problems that frequently occur in therapeutic relationships. Under the general concept of resistance, are included withdrawal, hostility-aggressivity, manipulation, detachment, excessive dependence, and transference and countertransference phenomena.

Definition

Resistance inevitably surfaces in the course of one-to-one work as the client begins to address self-defeating, nonintegrated aspects of self. Resistance refers to all the phenomena that interfere with and disrupt the smooth flow of feelings, memories, and thoughts. Resistance in the traditional psychoanalytic sense means anything that inhibits the client from producing material from the unconscious. Conscious phenomena (feelings, memories, thoughts) may be forceful or weak, significant or unimportant. The same is true of unconscious material. However, in the psychoanalytic view, some unconscious productions may be intense forces under high pressure to be discharged (archaic sexual and aggressive impulses), regardless of whether they are unrealistic, inappropriately timed, or illogical. These intense forces can be controlled only by another force equal in strength, which is labeled *resistance*.

Resistance is often mistakenly seen as the client's struggle against the nurse. Instead, the client is struggling against change, against modifying behavior patterns. Although the client's behavior patterns may have self-defeating aspects, they have also provided some satisfaction or prevented some discomfort. The client may also resist giving up a defense that offered protection from the anxiety associated with unbearable thoughts and impulses.

Manifestations

In general, the therapist may suspect resistance when the client's behavior appears to impede the progress of therapy. There are innumerable ways to express re-

sistance, including forgetting events; focusing on the past to avoid talking about the present (or vice versa); consistent avoidance of certain topics or inquiries; antagonism toward, or falling in love with, the therapist; acting out; and acting in. (The last two are discussed later in this chapter.)

Some manifestations of resistance may be more subtle. For example, a client may introduce an abrupt crisis, an alarming childhood memory, or an intense new relationship whenever a certain topic is approached. Likewise, a client may use flirtatious or seductive behaviors that embarrass the nurse to avoid accountability for problem resolution. Silence may indicate resistance, and so may an invigorating clinical discussion intended as a filibuster or "smoke screen" to avoid emotive expression or problem resolution.

The nurse must exercise caution in evaluating a client's behavior as resistive. The client's silence may indicate pensiveness, a pause before emotive expression, or a sense of completion. The client who is habitually late may have real difficulties adjusting a full personal schedule to accommodate the sessions. Resistance to specific topics or concerns may indicate that the client is not ready for investigative work at this time. Likewise, the client may resist giving up a defense that is desperately needed in order to keep anxiety about a present situation at manageable levels. Thus, in short-term one-to-one work, it is generally advisable to go around the suspected resistance rather than to expose it directly.

The humanistic stance is that the client has a right to assume a genuine and legitimate position of resisting one aspect of or the entire therapeutic process, as a matter of choice. The humanistic therapist views the client as exercising free will, an active decision-maker in all that shapes the client's well-being, including the one-to-one relationship.

Acting Out

Acting out is a particularly destructive form of resistance in which the client puts into action (that is, "acts out") a memory that has been forgotten or repressed. Thus, the client's conflict is externalized, always involving other people in the environment. In acting out, the client acts toward a mate, friend, relative, or other person those feelings and attitudes that he or she does not express toward the nurse. An example of acting-out behavior is the development of third-person relationships to absorb the emotions and fantasies that belong within the therapeutic relationship. Exaggerated feelings of intense hostility toward the nurse may lead to violence or physical harm to the third person, or intense feelings of love for the therapist may precipitate an affair or marriage with the third person.

Acting out is difficult to deal with, because the client does not talk about the feelings that precipitate the behavior and later tends to conceal or rationalize the behavior. Acting out can abruptly break up treatment, unless it is identified and dealt with explicitly. Specific nursing interventions regarding acting-out behaviors include:

- Bring acting out to the attention of the client.
- Encourage the client to *talk about* impulses rather than to act them out.
- Encourage identification of feelings *before* putting them into action.
- Increase frequency of contact.
- Look for evidence of transference phenomena toward the nurse.
- With repeated dangerous acting out, consider withdrawing from the relationship unless the client sets limits on these personal behaviors.

The following clinical example illustrates acting out in a clinical setting:

Sharon is a fifteen-year-old adolescent female with a history of self-abusive behavior. She had been the victim of repeated incestuous experiences with her stepfather over several years, despite her mother's knowledge of such activity. On an inpatient adolescent evaluation unit, she met daily in informal relationship work with a nursing student, of whom she seemed fond. One day she received a message from the team leader stating that the student had the flu and was unable to meet with Sharon that day but planned to meet again the following day. When the team leader asked Sharon's reaction to this, Sharon refused to speak. She rushed out of the dayroom area, ran to her room, and pounded her fist into the cement wall numerous times, fracturing her right hand in two places.

The next day, the nursing student approached Sharon. Sharon offered no comment. The student's inquiry regarding the previous day's message also met with no comment. The student stated her concern for Sharon's welfare and her confusion regarding Sharon's injury. Sharon remained silent. The student stated her wish to sort things out together as they had done in the past and then sat quietly with Sharon. After two minutes, Sharon began crying, and talked about feeling alone.

Acting In

Acting in may be viewed as a more subtle form of resistance occurring directly within a meeting. In acting in, like acting out, the unconscious impulse is not verbalized or remembered. The behavior puts into action in the therapeutic relationship a memory that has been forgotten or repressed. It may be a cue that transference has occurred.

While gross acting out is obvious and blatantly interrupts therapy, acting in is far more subtle. It is difficult but essential to recognize it. Acting-in behaviors include postural acts and body movements. For example, the client may turn his or her back to the therapist or pose seductively. Acting in may also occur when the client's behavior during the session can be demonstrated to be in response to an original transference figure.

It is possible for the nurse–client interactions to address therapeutic issues even while a significant amount of acting in is going on during a session. The psychiatric nurse must recognize acting-in behaviors, however, since these reflect client conflicts without the client's conscious awareness. Acting in is a behavioral comment on the current psychiatric nurse–client relationship and can move to destructive acting-out behaviors if not dealt with immediately and explicitly.

Specific nursing interventions regarding suspected acting-in behaviors include:

- Specifically explore the meaning of these behaviors with the client
- Specifically explore how the client views the nurse and the nurse–client relationship at that instant
- Encourage identification of feelings associated with these behaviors

The following clinical material exemplifies acting-in behaviors and subsequent nursing interventions.

Gary Moore is a twenty-four-year-old single male who negotiated an initial therapeutic contract for six weeks of one-to-one work with a female psychiatric nurse at a community mental health center. His prime goal was to explore why he was unable to maintain employment. Despite a college degree and a history of academic excellence, he was fired from three jobs within one year due to his inability to deal with anyone in authority. In the first two sessions, he appeared to avoid or talk around employment issues. The following occurred in the middle of the third session:

CLIENT: *I don't think that I'm any further ahead today figuring out why I'm unemployed than I was the day I met you.*

NURSE: *How come?*

CLIENT *(pauses . . . looks away, rubbing fingers through hair, smiling slightly)*: *You know, you're a real sweetheart to spend this time with me . . . trying to help me out. I really appreciate that. (Smiles and winks.)*

NURSE: *And what does your winking mean?*

CLIENT: *You know . . . that you're OK in my book. I really mean it. (Raises eyebrows and breaks into a wide grin.)*

NURSE: *Let's talk about how you see me and how you are using this session.*

In this case, the nurse picked up and asked for clarification of subtle, nonverbal behavior. She suspected this as a seductive maneuver and collected additional verbal and nonverbal cues regarding the client's acting-in behaviors. She immediately and explicitly moved to explore the current nurse–client relationship. The nurse also underlined the client's use of the session as an area for exploration, since the seductive behaviors began when the client spoke about an apparent lack of progress.

It is important to note that acting in can also be demonstrated by the psychiatric nurse who manifests maternal, paternal, erotic, sexual, or hostile behaviors. This behavior by the psychiatric nurse encourages gross acting out by the client. Maternal and paternal, or caretaker, behaviors are the most common among beginning practitioners. They express the nurse's need to nurture and feed the client. This may indicate a countertransference problem for the nurse, and it discounts the client's ability to assure his or her own well-being. Recognition of acting in by the psychiatric nurse is essential. This is another reason why practitioners should have formal supervision or consultation.

General Intervention Strategies for Resistance

Several consecutive approaches are used as general nursing intervention strategies for resistance. They begin with the psychiatric nurse's awareness of the resistance. This is followed by labeling the resistive behavior with the client. The psychiatric nurse may allow the resistance to occur several times to demonstrate its presence to the client. It is as if the psychiatric nurse were holding up a mirror for the client, reflecting and clarifying the specific resistive behavior. The nurse may then explore the accompanying emotion and the

history of its development. Finally, the psychiatric nurse facilitates working through the resistance by fully understanding and appreciating its implications in the client's life. This sequence may occur repeatedly before adequate resolution of a specific resistance takes place.

SPECIFIC NURSING INTERVENTIONS IN COMMON BEHAVIORAL PATTERNS

The middle (working) phase of the one-to-one relationship involves two primary objectives: (1) determination of the dynamics of the client's behavioral patterns, and (2) the establishment of behavioral change, particularly in self-defeating, growth-inhibiting behavior patterns. Effective intervention depends on the psychiatric nurse's unique skills, the unique manner in which the client's behavior pattern manifests itself, and a determination of what appears most effective (that is, what "fits") in the specific one-to-one relationship. Recognizing the individuality of each situation, only brief strategies are suggested here for several common behavior patterns, to give the psychiatric nurse some direction

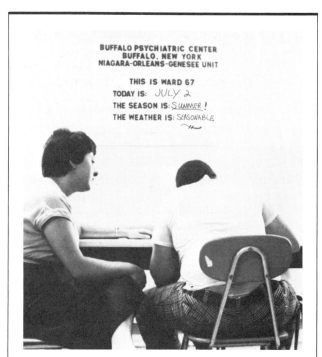

Interpersonal withdrawal from the threat that a one-to-one relationship may bring is an often temporary, but important coping method, for clients with lowered self-esteem.

for intervening. The behavior patterns discussed are a sampling of behaviors that may confront the beginning practitioner.

Interpersonal Withdrawal

Withdrawal is the behavior pattern characterized by avoidance of contact. Clients may avoid interpersonal relationships and/or a sense of reality. Withdrawal as a behavior pattern may be functional or dysfunctional. Temporary withdrawal as a response to crisis is an important coping skill for particular individuals. Severe or permanent withdrawal from interpersonal or reality-based contact is dysfunctional and requires nursing intervention. The primary goal in nursing intervention is to enhance the client's self-esteem and therefore increase the client's willingness to satisfy emotional needs through interpersonal contact.

Physical Withdrawal   Physical withdrawal, in its extreme form, is manifested by suicide attempts, gestures, or threats. Suggested interventions include:

- Avoid punishment of the client.
- Encourage ventilation of feelings.
- Accept any expressions of anger.
- Explore the source of present distress and the history of past distressful experiences.
- Decrease isolation.
- Provide crisis contact with the therapist or a crisis service.
- Assess what the client values.

In inpatient settings, the client may manifest physical withdrawal by sitting or standing apart from others, retreating to another room, purposely hiding, indicating psychomotor retardation, or assuming catatonic postures. In severe withdrawal, the emphasis is on the establishment of contact through physical proximity. Suggestions for the practitioner include:

- Move into the client's visual field (same eye level).
- Identify self.
- Make a general introductory inquiry.
- Invite the client to speak.
- State the amount of time you are willing to stay with the client whether the client chooses to speak or not.

Attention to physical needs may be an effective intervention to establish some initial bond of contact. Withdrawal by preoccupation with hallucinations, ritualistic compulsions, obsessional thinking, and the like is discussed in Chapters 14 and 16.

When avoidance of sessions surfaces in inpatient, one-to-one relationship work, the nurse may use the following strategies:

- Follow through by locating the patient.
- Explore the absence in a concerned manner.
- State availability to discuss the absences.
- Stress the necessity for the patient to share responsibility for the continuance of the relationship.
- Change the context of the contact (for example, go for a walk together).

The following clinical example shows how one psychiatric nurse intervened when the client physically withdrew in an inpatient setting.

Jason is a forty-year-old, single male who was hospitalized following his second suicide attempt with a drug overdose. In both instances, attempts were preceded by gradual social isolation, i.e., withdrawal from friends and neighbors. In addition, Jason lived alone in a small rented apartment. He hesitantly negotiated for daily one-to-one relationship work with a female psychiatric nurse. The first two sessions were characterized by silence and a few superficial interactions. He did not attend the third session. The psychiatric nurse waited the thirty minutes, then sought Jason out on the ward. The following exchanges occurred:

NURSE: *(sitting in chair to be at eye level with client):* Hi, Jason. I'd like to talk with you for a few minutes, if it's okay with you.

JASON: *(forty-five-second silence)*

NURSE: *I'm not sure what your silence means.*

JASON *(after thirty-second silence):* Go ahead. . . . *(Gestures in what appears to be an agreeable manner, as if to indicate to continue.)*

NURSE: *I waited for you in the conference room today and was concerned when you didn't come.*

JASON *(winces eyes in what appears to be a questioning manner, after twenty-second silence):* I didn't want to.

NURSE: *I respect your choice not to meet together today. Can you fill me in on how it was that you chose not to come?*

JASON *(in monotone voice seemingly devoid of feeling):* I don't want to talk anymore now.

NURSE: *I hear you. I'll be available between 4 and 5 p.m. today, and I'll be in the conference room tomorrow at the time that we agreed on together. I'll see you tomorrow, Jason.*

In this example, the psychiatric nurse used the following intervention techniques: she sought to explore the meaning of the client's silence; she stated her concern; she underlined Jason's option not to participate, yet sought out his rationale; she stressed her availability; and she underlined her expectation of mutual continued contact rather than engaging in mutual withdrawal.

In outpatient settings, physical withdrawal may necessitate outreach by telephone and changing the environmental structure of the setting in terms of time, place, or persons. For example, the client may respond better to home visits than having to contend with a crowded waiting room. One client brought his dog to initial sessions since he viewed the dog as his only support system and contact.

Verbal Withdrawal   Verbal withdrawal represents avoidance of contact through silence or, in its extreme form, mutism. When periodic silence occurs in the therapeutic relationship, it is important to explore its significance. But the beginning practitioner must learn to tolerate silences without verbalizing unnecessarily. Silence may indicate resistance, a pensive moment, or simply that a discussion has concluded with nothing more to say. Strategies for intervention include:

- Explore "what is said" by silence.
- Take an attitude of continued interest.
- Accept the client's self-expression at present through silence.

In cases of mutism, Gruber (1977) recommends the no-demand, third-person interview in which the client is referred to in the third person, yet given the freedom to comment. Altering communication techniques may provide an outlet for various forms of nonverbal communication, as shown in the following case.

Karen is a fourteen-year-old, single female referred by her parents to an outpatient adolescent unit because of gradual withdrawal from family and peers during the past six months. She has refused to go to school, staying in her bedroom for the last two weeks. Although Karen was mute during the entire initial interview, she consented (by shaking her head) to meet with a psychiatric nurse for one-hour sessions weekly. During the initial two sessions, Karen sat in a chair, avoided eye contact, and said nothing. Two strategies for the third session were: (1) to decrease sessions to a half hour to decrease discomfort, and (2) to invite the client to use the available blackboard, paper and pencil, or sketch pad if she chose. Although Karen remained motionless during the session, a handwritten note was found on the nurse's desk that same day. It read: "I don't want to talk right now, but I like you." Similar notes continued until the ninth session, when Karen began talking.

Hostility-Aggressivity

Hostility is the behavioral pattern characterized by actual or threatened aggressive contact. Hostility is differentiated from anger in that anger may be constructive, whereas hostility is destructive in intent. Moore (1968, p. 58) offers the following definition:

> Hostility is an emotional reaction to a personal threat or frustration wherein either verbal and/or motor aggressive action offers relief, or ego defense mechanisms are called into operation to cope with the anxiety and tensions involved.

The operational steps in direct expression of hostility are:

- The client experiences a frustration or threat.
- Anxiety surfaces, associated with feelings of helplessness and inadequacy.
- Verbal or motor aggressive action alleviates the increased anxiety.

The aggressive action in this case is directed toward destruction of the object perceived as the source of the frustration or threat. This object may be self, others, or an inanimate object. When forces inhibit the direct expression of hostility, the client may cope with the hostility by using various defense mechanisms. Examples include displacement and projection (see Chapter 10).

Basque and Merhige (1980) researched the type and frequency of dangerous behaviors encountered in psychiatric facilities. The following findings from their sample are based on a frequency of at least once a week.

- Three-fourths of the nurses encountered verbally abusive clients.
- One-third of the nurses encountered clients who were physically abusive to other clients.
- One-fifth of the nurses encountered clients who physically abused staff.
- One-third of the nurses encountered clients who endangered themselves.

Although Lathrop (1978) asserts that prevention is the most successful form of intervention when dealing with aggressive behaviors, three-fourths of the nurses in the Basque and Merhige study reported no training in the prevention and management of aggressive behaviors.

VERBAL THREATS The psychiatric nurse may be the recipient of the client's hostile threats, comments, or insults. When any of these occur, suggested strategies for intervention include the following:

- Continue client contact rather than avoid it.
- Explore the threat or frustration that preceded the indication of hostility.
- Allow the client to verbalize feelings associated with the threat or frustration (helplessness, inadequacy, anger, etc.).
- Encourage the client to make the connection between the specific threat or frustration, the subsequent feelings, and the specific manifestation of hostility.

A further possible intervention for hostile threats is to explore the client's need for extreme controls. These may consist of medication, exercise, and assessment of the degree of closeness tolerated by the client. In addition, the nurse may provide a consistent set of expectations and guidance toward client self-control. These latter strategies are used in the following dialogue:

CLIENT: *Look out for me today.*
NURSE: *How come?*
CLIENT: *I feel like breaking bones. (Moves closer.)*
NURSE: *You and I can talk about this feeling "like breaking bones."*

In this dialogue, the psychiatric nurse demonstrates regard for the client while verbalizing the clear expecta-

tion that further self-expression will be verbal rather than physical.

PHYSICAL AGGRESSIVITY The nurse may also be the recipient of the client's physical aggressivity. Physical aggressivity may vary in degree (from irritation to global rage) and target (inanimate objects, self, others). For example, the client may break his or her cigarette, a chair, or another client's nose. In addition to the intervention strategies described above for verbal threats, the following may prove helpful:

- Address, rather than avoid, the client and the specific behavior.
- Avoid any retaliatory actions.
- Approach the client in a calm, firm manner.
- Attempt to talk with the client.
- Convey acceptance of the client, but not of the aggressive behavior.
- Encourage an alternative expression of aggression, such as use of Bataccas (cylindrical clubs of a soft, padded material so that injury is avoided), pillows, or paper or foam balls.
- Intervene early when the client first gives verbal and nonverbal signs of aggression (frowns, threats, clenching of fists).
- Remove the client from the immediate environment when necessary, to help reestablish self-control.

Lenefsky (1978) elaborates on safe intervention of violent behaviors via physical restraint. Steward (1978) illustrates specific physical techniques to restrain a weapon-wielding client. He emphasizes, however, that other approaches, plus an increased number of visible staff, usually suffice to maintain control and prevent injury.

Manipulation

Manipulation is characterized by attempts to exploit, or actual exploitation of, interpersonal contact. Manipulation occurs in one-to-one relationship work when the client maneuvers to have the therapist meet the client's immediate needs. Manipulative methods may be exhibitionistic, seductive, or masochistic, and they are always immature in nature. When the manipulation is successful, the client's experience is not a constructive one. Nurses who cooperate to meet the client's need reinforce the client's use of the existing dysfunctional behavior pattern, and allow themselves to be used in a mutually maladaptive relationship. A common manipulative maneuver is one in which the client makes the nurse feel successful by giving flattery if the nurse carries out the client's demands. Conversely, the nurse may be treated as an ineffective nurse if client demands are not met. Failure to recognize manipulative behavior will delay client progress.

Intervention Strategies The primary intervention strategy in a manipulative behavior pattern is to provide clear, firm, and consistent expectations in which the therapeutic interests of the client are foremost. The manipulative client will test the consistency and extent of the limits and will maneuver to reestablish previous interpersonal patterns to obtain immediate gratification of needs. Table 7-10 analyzes examples of manipulative maneuvers used by a client to avoid accountability for personal problems, create nurse discomfort, and control interactions. This table also illustrates how the nurse may move interactions from an emphasis on content (what is said) to an emphasis on process (what is happening in the nurse–client relationship at that moment). This is particularly useful when the client uses behaviors intended to disturb, confuse, or anger the nurse.

Dealing with Seductive Behavior Seduction is characterized by verbal or physical advances toward sexual contact. Seductive behaviors (comments, suggestions, or physical contact) from clients of the same or opposite sex may cause discomfort to the beginning practitioner. Seductive behavior needs to be explicitly discussed rather than avoided, by client and nurse together. The following clinical material illustrates this point:

Sandra began employment as a psychiatric nurse in an institution for the treatment of drug abuse. The female patients could opt for a daily walk outside if accompanied by staff. Sandra saw this as an opportunity to establish client rapport. While she was walking with five female clients, one walked very close to her and started to stroke Sandra's arm in a consistently teasing, sexual manner. The following interaction occurred:

SANDRA *(in a very firm voice): I'm uncomfortable with you stroking my arm. I want you to stop.*

PATIENT *(discontinuing stroking): Simmer down, sweetheart. You have no idea what it's like here without men!*

Table 7-10 ANALYSIS OF VERBATIM EXAMPLE OF MANIPULATION	
Verbatim Interaction	**Analysis of Responses**
Client: Sometimes I feel uncomfortable about you. You meet with me every week and listen to my problems. I wonder if you're bored sometimes	Manipulative maneuver: suggests that therapist has a problem regarding boredom
Nurse: I don't know how to respond. Has this happened before— that someone listens to you and you wonder if they're bored?	Nursing interventions: avoids angry or defensive response; suspects projection, and gives client option to work on boredom as client's own problem
Client: Once in a while, but not here. It's probably not boredom—maybe you're just nervous. Sometimes I see you shifting back and forth in your chair. Maybe you're new at this and not sure of yourself yet	Manipulative maneuvers: discounts boredom as own problem; abruptly switches to other problems—suggests therapist has problems with nervousness and inexperience
Nurse: You seem to have a lot of questions about me today	Nursing interventions: avoids angry or defensive responses; moves to focus on *process* rather than *content* of session, i.e., client's focus on therapist's behavior

SANDRA: *I'd like you to tell me about your predicament in words, and I'll listen.*

Detachment

Detachment is the behavioral pattern characterized by a generalized aloofness in interpersonal contact. Detachment, as a form of resistance, can retard relationship work and discourage the practitioner. Manifestations of detachment include intellectualization, denial, and superficiality.

Intellectualization   Intellectualization is a defense mechanism excessively employed by particular clients to avoid emotional awareness and its concomitant physiological reactions. The client may be particularly adept at delving into behavioral dynamics and developing insights about the causes of personal problems. This inhibits therapy in two ways. First, the client may consistently seek explanations and reasons in order to avoid actual behavioral change. Secondly, the client usually does not address the emotive aspects of the self. The client may present an always reasonable self and refuse to develop an understanding of emotions. For further discussion, see Chapter 10.

Denial   Denial consists of refusal to acknowledge personal displeasure, painful sensations, or facts—the client need not address whatever is denied. Denial may be used temporarily to avoid the anxiety associated with new awarenesses in therapeutic work, or it may be used extensively and permanently to inhibit psychotherapeutic endeavors. Denial as a defense is explored in depth in Chapter 10.

Superficiality   Superficiality is a form of resistance characterized by shallowness of contact. It is used by clients to avoid interpersonal intimacy. The client may be superficial in the definition and exploration of problem areas, and/or in the implementation of behavioral change.

Specific Nursing Intervention Strategies   Interventions for detachment and any of its manifestations (intellectualization, denial, superficiality) emphasize establishing awareness of the process of detachment—that is, what the client does to detach from or remain aloof in interpersonal contact. The psychiatric nurse may encourage client assessment of how this serves the client, including delineating any self-defeating aspects. Finally, the nurse may explore any fears and fantasies inhibiting emotional expression and actively emphasize emotive content in subsequent psychotherapeutic work. The following verbatim exchange illustrates how a problematic behavior pattern of detachment was handled:

CLIENT: *I keep exploring this inner realm of my consciousness between sessions, in an effort to determine the type of existence I'm seeking.*

NURSE: *I don't understand. Can you be more specific about what you want for yourself?*

CLIENT: *Oh, it's an existential dilemma of sorts. I'm searching, constantly searching. . . .*

NURSE: *And how do you feel as you search?*

CLIENT: *Feel? Unsettled? Is it unsettled? I guess so.*

NURSE: *Can you describe how "unsettled" feels to you?*

CLIENT: *Sort of sad. . . .*

The nursing interventions used included seeking clarification of unclear responses, encouraging the client to move from global generalities to specific personal comments, and active emphasis on awareness and exploration of feelings.

Excessive Dependence (Learned Helplessness)

Excessive dependence is characterized by attempts to establish and maintain contact by adopting a helpless, powerless stance. Diener and Dweck (1978) studied patterns of learned helplessness in children. They found that mastery-oriented children focused on remedies when they failed, while helpless children focused on causes of failure.

Specific nursing interventions regarding excessive dependence include the following:

- Set clear, firm, and consistent limits on the various forms of excessive dependency.
- Avoid any retaliatory actions, including withdrawal.
- Emphasize the client's determination of and accountability for personal feelings, thoughts, and behaviors.
- Avoid making decisions about, guiding, or otherwise assuming responsibility for the client's behavior.
- Give positive reinforcement for development of more independent, growth-facilitating behaviors over time.

The client attempts to involve the nurse in a dominance–submission relationship, in which the client does everything to placate the nurse (being helpful, using flattery, giving gifts). Helplessness may be expressed by maneuvers to have the practitioner make decisions about, guide, or otherwise assume responsibility for the client's behavior. Exclusiveness may also characterize this behavior pattern, manifested by the message "No one understands me but you." Thus, the client uses a stance of helplessness that was learned in previous relationships, and avoids growth toward self-awareness, mutuality, and autonomy. This common manipulative behavior pattern deserves emphasis, since clients who adopt it frequently view nurses as mother substitutes and the nurse may readily assume a caretaker role.

The following clinical material illustrates an intervention:

Terry is a twenty-seven-year-old, single female with an extensive history of psychotherapy and one psychiatric hospitalization. The precipitating event for hospitalization was a suicide gesture by overdose. The result was that Terry's mother slept by her bedside for several subsequent months. Presenting problems at the initial interview were depression, boredom, obesity, and an inability to initiate peer relationships. Terry was unemployed and lived at home with her mother but did not participate in any household tasks. Terry's mother drove her two blocks to attend sessions, regardless of weather conditions.

Terry negotiated for weekly half-hour sessions of individual psychotherapy. Her behavior in the sessions was characterized by emphasis on the exclusivity of the therapeutic relationship, thus attempting to duplicate this element in the mother–daughter relationship. After several sessions, Terry began requesting, and later demanding, that the nurse physically hug her several times during the course of each session. At the close of one session, Terry took out a bottle of tranquilizers screaming, "If you don't hug me, I'll take these! Here! Keep these from me!" She threw herself on the floor and sobbed. The nurse verbally reflected Terry's apparent desperateness and discomfort, acknowledged that Terry had the power to make a choice regarding the tranquilizers, and reinforced the use of crisis contact by phone. Terry chose not to take the pills and continued with individual psychotherapy.

Transference and Countertransference Phenomena

Consideration of the problems in therapeutic relationships would be incomplete without a brief reference to transference and countertransference phenomena. Although there are many aspects of transference, negative and psychotic transference warrant particular attention.

Negative Transference In negative transference, the client shows a number of reactions based on forms of hate (hostility, loathing, bitterness, contempt, annoyance, etc.). Although there are both positive and nega-

tive aspects to every transference, a predominately negative transference is uncomfortable for client and practitioner alike. The client does not like to be aware of and express this hate, and the practitioner does not like to be the target of it. When negative transference appears unresolvable, it may be advisable to terminate relationship work rather than run the risk of further client dysfunction.

Psychotic Transference In psychotic transference, or transference psychosis, the relationship with the psychiatric nurse supersedes all other relationships, although the client has no insight into the existence of the transference and denies its presence. Psychotic transference requires repetitive, concrete reality testing to separate the nurse from significant others in the client's life. The following clinical example illustrates how psychotic transference may be manifested. Concrete reality testing is the primary intervention strategy.

Jean is a forty-two-year-old, married female who was hospitalized twice for acute psychotic episodes in which she believed she was the female counterpart of Jesus Christ. She negotiated for a half hour of individual psychotherapy every other week and subsequently developed extreme dependence on her female therapist. Psychotic transference first became apparent when the therapist took a one-week vacation. Jean's tenuous adjustment became disorganized to a point at which rehospitalization was considered. In subsequent treatment, Jean found it difficult to separate the identity of the therapist from her mother, her sister, and her girlfriend, all of whom she perceived as having abandoned her in some way.

During the course of two years of therapy, the therapist became pregnant and needed to take a temporary maternity leave. Jean had trouble dealing with this, despite extensive planning on the part of the therapist, which included introducing her to a client-selected second therapist who would work with her in the interim. Approximately two months before the temporary separation, Jean ended one session showing marked anxiety. The following interaction occurred:

JEAN: *I can't believe you're leaving me! I know that you're not doing this on purpose. You'll have a baby to take care of, but I don't know if I can make it. I'm afraid of what might happen. I was always close to my sister, Sally, and when she got married and had a baby, she moved away! We were never close after that. And my mother left. She went into the hospital and never came back! She died! They both left me! And now you are!*

THERAPIST: *Jean, we'll continue to talk about Sally, and your mother, and how you felt "left" by them. We also need to talk about me and my plans. I'm not Sally. I'm not your mother. I'm your therapist. I'll be taking a temporary leave of absence for three months and will then continue to work with you as I am now.*

JEAN *(sighing): It's so hard for me to remember that.*

In addition to repetitive, concrete reality testing, psychotic transference may be minimized by decreasing the frequency and/or duration of contact with the client. This latter strategy is contraindicated in the above situation, since it would only increase Jean's fears of abandonment. Both negative transference and psychotic transference problems require consistent supervision and cautious management by every practitioner regardless of expertise.

Unanalyzed Countertransference   Unanalyzed countertransference is almost always a problem, because it inhibits client understanding and may be acted out. One purpose of supervision is to help the beginning therapist develop awareness of individual countertransference reactions. Chessick (1974) highlights the following signs of countertransference in waking life or while dreaming:

• Anxiety reactions
• Reactions of irrational concern about and irrational kindness toward the client
• Reactions of irrational hostility toward the client

More specific signals that countertransference may be a problem include:

• Uneasy feelings during or after meetings
• Being late or extending the agreed-upon duration of meetings for no apparent reason
• Dreaming about the client
• Preoccupation with the client during the therapist's leisure time

This fourth signal is further explored by Geach and White (1974) in their description of the process of *empathic resonance* with the client's feeling state. In this process, feelings that clients were unable to control or communicate were also experienced by student therapists as they developed closeness with their clients. A similar process occurs in the *blotting paper syndrome* described by Johnson (1967). The syndrome arises in psychiatric inpatient settings, when a client experiences an intense feeling but is unable to express, or even to experience, that particular feeling: staff members unconsciously begin to act out the feeling that the client is unable to express or experience. This syndrome occurs especially in relation to symptomatology.

It is reassuring that most countertransference problems can be resolved by self-assessment with professional supervision. In rare instances, however, referral to another nurse is appropriate when the first nurse remains unable to control his or her disturbed attitudes and emotions.

Once the countertransference process is identified, the nurse can consciously develop therapeutic, goal-directed responses. The existence of countertransference reactions confirms the necessity of ongoing supervision or consultation for all psychiatric nurses engaged in one-to-one relationship work. Table 7–11 summarizes common behavior patterns, their identifying characteristics, and suggested nursing interventions.

Table 7–11   SUMMARY OF INTERVENTIONS IN COMMON BEHAVIOR PATTERNS

Behavior Pattern	Identifying Characteristic	Suggested Nursing Interventions	Rationale
Withdrawal	Avoidance of contact (interpersonal relationships and/or sense of reality)		
Physical	Avoidance of physical contact through missed sessions, hiding, sitting far away, etc.	In severe withdrawal, establish contact through physical proximity: Move into client's visual field (or at client's eye level)	Encourages orientation to current external reality, the ''here-and-now,'' despite client's possible internal preoccupation
		Identify self	
		Make introductory inquiry	
		State invitation to hear from client	
		State amount of time willing to stay regardless of whether client chooses to verbalize	
		Give attention to client's physical needs	May establish initial physical bond of contact. Enhances client self-esteem
		In inpatient relationship work: Follow through by locating client	Interrupts dyfunctional behavioral pattern of avoidance via physical withdrawal. Gives message that there are other behavioral patterns
		Explore absence from session in a concerned manner	
		State availablity to discuss absence, where realistic	
		Stress necessity that client share responsibility for continuance of relationship	
		Change context of contact (for example, go for walk together)	
		In outpatient relationship work: Follow through with outreach by phone	Interrupts dysfunctional behavioral pattern
		Consider changing environmental structure in terms of time, place, or persons (e.g., home visits)	External environmental conditions, rather than client conditions, may be an inhibiting force

Table continues on next page

Table 7–11 continued

Behavior Pattern	Identifying Characteristic	Suggested Nursing Interventions	Rationale
Verbal	Avoidance of contact through silence or, in its extreme form, mutism	Explore "what is said" by silence	Silence may have numerous meanings (resistant, pause before emotive content, etc.)
		Maintain attitude of continued interest	Avoids rejection or punitive maneuvers that client may typically experience from others because of silence
		Show acceptance of client's self-expression presently through silence	Silence is nonverbal communication, i.e., "I don't choose to talk now"
		Alter communication techniques (e.g., use painting, music, letter writing)	Opens up communication through nonverbal channels, where verbal skills are not required
		Consider no-demand, third-person interview in cases of mutism	Empathic approach to say "I'm with you." Underlines client's free choice to speak or remain mute
Hostility-aggressivity	Actual or threatened aggressive contact		
Verbal threats		Continue, rather than avoid, client contact	Interrupts dysfunctional behavioral pattern
		Explore threat or frustration that preceded indication of hostility	Focuses on thinking, rather than action, regarding threat and encourages identification of feelings
		Allow time/space for client to verbalize feelings associated with threat or frustration (helplessness, inadequacy, anger, etc.)	New experience may be laden with anxiety
		Encourage client to make connections between specific threat or frustration, subsequent feelings, and specific manifestation of hostility	Analysis of client's mode of conflict resolution
		Explore client's possible need for external controls (medication, exercise, assessment of degree of closeness tolerated by client)	Sets limits regarding threatened aggressive contact
		Provide consistent set of expectations about and guidance toward self-control	Respects personal choice, yet emphasizes expectation for self-control
Physical aggressivity		Address, rather than avoid, client and specific behavior	Interrupts dysfunctional behavioral pattern

Table continues on next page

Table 7–11 continued

Behavior Pattern	Identifying Characteristic	Suggested Nursing Interventions	Rationale
		Avoid retaliatory actions	Retaliatory actions do not meet client's needs in growth-facilitating manner
		Approach client in a calm, firm manner	Provides role model of appropriate self-control
		Attempt to talk with client, conveying acceptance of client, but not of aggressive behavior	Emphasizes need to change behavioral pattern, while maintaining positive regard for client
		Encourage alternative expressions of aggression (use of Bataccas, pillows, paper balls, etc.)	Constructive channeling of energies teaches coping skills
		Intervene early, when client first gives verbal and nonverbal signs of aggression (frowns, threats, clenching of fists)	Most successful form of intervention in physical aggressivity
		When necessary, remove client from immediate environment to help reestablish self-control	Sets external limits until client can assume responsibility for self-control
Manipulation (including seduction)	Attempted or actual exploitation of interpersonal contact	Address, rather than avoid, client and specific behavior	Interrupts dysfunctional behavioral pattern
		Avoid colluding to meet client's immediate needs when manipulative maneuvers are used	Avoids reinforcement of dysfunctional behavioral pattern
		Provide clear, firm, and consistent expectations in which therapeutic interests of client are foremost	Sets limits, yet emphasizes growth-facilitating behaviors
		Avoid any retaliatory actions	Retaliatory actions do not meet client's needs in growth-facilitating manner
Detachment (including intellectualization, denial, and superficiality)	General aloofness in interpersonal contact	Establish awareness of process of detachment, i.e., what client does to remain aloof in interpersonal contact	Focuses on dysfunctional behavioral pattern and encourages self-awareness
		Encourage client assessment of how this serves client, including delineation of any self-defeating aspects	Encourages client to evaluate behavioral pattern to determine which parts are self-defeating and/or thwart gratification of basic needs
		Explore any fears and fantasies inhibiting emotional expression	Links thought processes to emotive expression

Table continues on next page

Table 7–11 continued

Behavior Pattern	Identifying Characteristic	Suggested Nursing Interventions	Rationale
Excessive dependence (learned helplessness)	Attempts to establish and maintain contact by taking a helpless, powerless stance	Actively emphasize emotive content	Interrupts dysfunctional behavioral pattern
		Set clear, firm, and consistent limits regarding various forms of excessive dependence	Sets limits to avoid reinforcement of dysfunctional behavioral pattern
		Avoid any retaliatory actions, including withdrawal	Retaliatory actions do not meet client's needs in growth-facilitating manner
		Emphasize client determination of and accountability for own feelings, thoughts, and behaviors	Reverses helpless, powerless stance and stresses development of autonomy
		Avoid making decisions about, guiding, or otherwise assuming responsibility for client's behavior	Interrupts dysfunctional behavioral pattern
		Give positive reinforcement for development of more independent growth-faciliatating behaviors over time	Endorses a more growth-facilitating behavioral pattern
Transference	Distortion in interpersonal contact based on unresolved conflict from client's past relationships		
Negative transference	Occurs when the client generally reacts to the nurse with reactions based on hate, without awareness of the source of these reactions	Accept client's reactions	Maintains contact in the best therapeutic interests of the client
		Encourage client to develop awareness of source of hate	May free client to deal with nurse as individual separate from original transference figure
		Consider termination of relationship work if negative transference appears unresolvable and client risks further dysfunction	Termination preferable to escalating dysfunction
Psychotic transference	Occurs when the client's relationship with the nurse supersedes all other relationships, without insight into the existence of the transference and while denying its presence	Use repetitive, concrete reality testing to separate nurse from significant others in client's life	Helps prevent further distortion in a client with poor reality-testing ability

Table continues on next page

Table 7–11 continued			
Behavior Pattern	**Identifying Characteristic**	**Suggested Nursing Interventions**	**Rationale**
		Decrease frequency and/or duration of contact	May decrease emotional intensity of the relationship to a more workable level
		Secure consistent supervision and cautious management to prevent further client dysfunction	Helps avoid detrimental, even dangerous behaviors that may surface to dissipate highly charged emotional relationship
Countertransference	Distortion in interpersonal contact based on unresolved conflict from therapist's past relationships	Develop awareness of individual countertransference reactions: Anxiety reactions by therapist in relation to client Reactions of irrational concern and kindness toward client Reactions of irrational hostility toward client	Helps avoid unrecognized countertransference reactions not in the best interests of the client
		Once countertransference is identified, consciously develop therapeutic, goal-directed responses	Focus on "here-and-now" may protect client from the nurse's unfinished business of the past
		Secure consistent supervision to increase awareness of and develop intervention strategy for countertransference phenomena	Minimizes harmful effects of countertransference phenomena
		In rare instance, consider referral to another nurse should the first nurse remain unable to control disturbed attitudes and emotions	

KEY NURSING CONCEPTS

✔ A therapeutic one-to-one relationship may evolve in any nursing situation.

✔ The one-to-one relationship between psychiatric nurse and client is a mutually defined, mutually collaborative, goal-oriented professional relationship.

✔ Characteristics of a humanistic one-to-one relationship include openness, negotiation, commitment, responsibility, and authenticity.

✔ The social-interactionist framework in one-to-one relationship work emphasizes the significance of meaning between nurse and client.

✔ Facilitative personal characteristics of the nurse that may increase therapeutic effectiveness include empathy, warmth, genuineness, concreteness, and active listening.

✔ Client abilities that tend toward successful therapy outcomes include awareness and ownership of feelings, desire to change, and ability to differentiate feelings, concerns, and problems.

✔ The establishment of a therapeutic alliance is an essential ingredient of formal one-to-one relationship work.

✔ Phases of a therapeutic relationship include the beginning (orientation), middle (working), and end (resolution).

✔ The beginning phase of the relationship is characterized by the establishment of contact and the formation of a working relationship.

✔ The beginning phase of one-to-one relationship work focuses on establishing rapport, obtaining pertinent information, initiating client assessment, and making practical arrangements for treatment.

✔ The middle phase of the relationship is characterized by mutual determination of the dynamics of the client's behavioral patterns, and initiation of behavioral change.

✔ The problem-solving process generally occurs in the middle phase of a one-to-one relationship and includes strategies of observation, definition, preparation, analysis, ideation, incubation, synthesis, evaluation, and development.

✔ The end phase of the therapeutic relationship is characterized by the termination of therapy in a mutually planned, satisfying manner.

✔ Evaluation is an ongoing psychotherapeutic process and includes continuous evaluation of client behaviors, development of client self-evaluation, mutual evaluation of the relationship, and the nurse's self-evaluation in each one-to-one relationship.

✔ Psychiatric nurses need to be aware of both content and process in a one-to-one relationship.

✔ Resistance in psychotherapy is best understood as the client's struggle against change.

✔ The humanistic stance is that the client has a right to resist the therapeutic process.

✔ Problematic behavioral patterns frequently occurring in therapeutic relationships include interpersonal withdrawal, hostility-aggressivity, manipulation, detachment, excessive dependence, and problematic transference and countertransference phenomena.

✔ The social-interactionist may view transference phenomena as distortions of meaning between nurse and client.

✔ In order to deal effectively with countertransference phenomena, it is important that psychiatric nurses engaging in formal one-to-one work have clinical supervision or consultation.

References

Altschul, A. "Patient-Nurse Interaction in the Psychiatric Scene." *Nursing Mirror* (April 1970): 37-41.

Arieti, S., Ed. *American Handbook of Psychiatry.* 2d ed. Vol. V. New York: Basic Books, 1975.

Basque, L., and Merhige, J. "Nurses' Experiences with Dangerous Behavior: Implications for Training." *Journal of Continuing Education in Nursing* 11 (September-October 1980): 47-51.

Benfer, B. "Clinical Supervision as a Support System for the Care-Giver." *Perspectives in Psychiatric Care* (January-February 1979): 13-17.

Carter, F. *Psychosocial Nursing: Theory and Practice in Hospital and Community Mental Health.* 2d ed. New York: Macmillan, 1976.

Chessick, R. *The Technique and Practice of Intensive Psychotherapy.* New York: Jason Aronson, 1974.

Cloud, E. "The Plateau in Therapist-Patient Relationships." *Perspectives in Psychiatric Care* (July-September 1972): 112-121.

Cronbach, L. "Beyond Two Disciplines of Scientific Psychology." *American Psychologist* 30 (1975): 116-127.

Diener, C., and Dweck, C. "An Analysis of Learned Helplessness: Continuous Changes in Performance, Strategy, and Achievement Cognitions Following Failure." *Journal of Personality and Social Psychology* 36 (1978): 451-462.

Dillon, K. "A Patient-structured Relationship." *Perspectives in Psychiatric Care* (July-August 1971): 167-172.

Fagin, C. "Psychotherapeutic Nursing." *American Journal of Nursing* 67 (1967): 298-304.

Fenichel, O. *The Psychoanalytic Theory of Neurosis.* New York: W. W. Norton, 1943.

Geach, B., and White, J. "Empathic Resonance: A Countertransference Phenomenon." *American Journal of Nursing* 74 (1974): 1282-1285.

Griffith, A., and Trogdon, K. "Self-expressive Styles among College Students Preparing for Careers in Nursing and Music." *Journal of Counseling Psychology* 16 (1969): 275-277.

Gruber, L. "The No-Demand, Third Person Interview of the Non-verbal Patient." *Perspectives in Psychiatric Care* (January-March 1977): 38-39.

Hall, E. *The Hidden Dimension.* Garden City, N.Y.: Doubleday Anchor Books, 1966.

Hargreaves, W., and Runyon, N. "Patterns of Psychiatric Nursing: Role Differences in Nurse-Patient Interaction." *Nursing Research* 18 (1969): 300-307.

Jansson, D. "Student Consultation: A Liaison Psychiatric Experience for Nursing Students." *Perspectives in Psychiatric Care* 17 (1979): 77-82, 94.

Johnson, B. "The Blotting Paper Syndrome: A Countertransference Phenomenon." *Perspectives in Psychiatric Care* (September-October 1967): 228-230.

Jourard, S. *The Transparent Self.* Princeton, N.J.: D. Van Nostrand, 1964.

Lathrop, V. "Aggression as a Response." *Psychiatric Care* 16 (1978): 202-205.

Lego, S. "The One-to-One Nurse-Patient Relationship." In *Psychiatric Nursing 1946-1974: A Report on the State of the Art,* edited by F. Huey. New York: American Journal of Nursing, 1975.

————. "Point/Counterpoint: A Psychotherapist Is a Psychotherapist . . ." *Perspectives in Psychiatric Care* 18 (1980): 27 and 39.

Lenefsky, B., de Palma, T., and Locicero, D. "Management of Violent Behaviors." *Perspectives in Psychiatric Care* 16 (1978): 212-217.

McArdle, K. "Dialogue in Thought." *American Journal of Nursing* 74 (1974): 1075-1077.

McCann, J. "Termination of the Psychotherapeutic Relationship." *Journal of Psychiatric Nursing and Mental Health Services* 17 (October 1979): 37-39, 45-46.

Marshall, K. "Empathy, Genuineness, and Regard: Determinants of Successful Therapy with Schizophrenics? A Critical Review." *Psychotherapy: Theory, Research and Practice* 14 (1977): 57-64.

Mellow, J. "Nursing Therapy." *American Journal of Nursing* 68 (1968): 2365-2369.

Miller, T., and Orsolits, M. "A Model for Training Nursing Staff as Primary Counselors for Psychiatric Service." *Journal of Psychiatric Nursing and Mental Health Services* 16 (1978): 28-33.

Moore, J. "Encountering Hostility during Psychotherapy Sessions." *Perspectives in Psychiatric Care* (March-April 1968): 58-65.

Munsadis, I. "Therapeutic Effects of Nurse-Patient Relationships." *British Journal of Social Psychiatry and Community Health* 6 (1972): 134-140.

Peitchinis, J. "Therapeutic Effectiveness of Counseling by Nursing Personnel: Review of the Literature." *Nursing Research* 21 (1972): 138-148.

Peplau, H. *Interpersonal Relations in Nursing.* New York: G. P. Putnam, 1952.

————. "Interpersonal Techniques: The Crux of Psychiatric Nursing." *American Journal of Nursing* 62 (1962): 50-54.

Reich, S., and Geller, A. "The Self-Image of Nurses Employed in a Psychiatric Hospital." *Perspectives in Psychiatric Care,* 15 (1977): 126-128.

Schuable, P., and Pierce, R. "Client In-Therapy Behavior:

A Therapist Guide to Progress." *Psychotherapy: Theory, Research, and Practice* 11 (1974): 229-234.

Shapiro, D. "The Effects of Therapeutic Conditions: Positive Results Revisited." *British Journal of Medical Psychology* 49 (1976): 315-323.

Stastny, J. "Helping a Patient Learn to Trust." *Perspectives in Psychiatric Care* 3 (1965): 16-28.

Steward, A. "Handling the Aggressive Patient." *Perspectives in Psychiatric Care* 16 (1978): 228-232.

Truax, C., and Carkhuff, R. *Toward Effective Counseling and Psyshotherapy.* Chicago: Aldine, 1967.

Vennen, M. "Notes on Termination." *Perspectives in Psychiatric Care* (September-October 1970): 218-221.

Wolberg, L. *The Technique of Psychotherapy.* Volumes 1 and 2. New York: Grune and Stratton, 1977.

Further Reading

Albeiz, A. "Reflecting on the Development of a Relationship." *Journal of Psychiatric Nursing,* (November-December 1970): 25-27.

Anchor, K., and Sandler, H. "Psychotherapy Sabotage Revisited: The Better Half of Individual Psychotherapy." *Journal of Clinical Psychology* 32 (1976): 146-148.

Bolzoni, N. "Premature Reassurance: A Distancing Maneuver." *Nursing Outlook* 23 (1975): 49-51.

Buckles, J.; Cashar, L.; and Olson, L. "Learning Purposeful Nursing Intervention." *American Journal of Nursing* 68 (1968): 2578-2580.

Burd, S. "The Application of Theoretical Knowledge in Nurse-Patient Relationships." *Nursing Clinics of North America* 1 (1966): 187-195.

Caldwell, J. "Community Psychiatric Nursing: Working from a Health Centre." *Nursing Times* 76 (1980): 1066.

Campbell, W. "Psychotherapy. The Therapeutic Community: Problems Encountered by Nurses. *Nursing Times* 75 (1979): 2038-2040.

Davis, R., and Woodcock, E. "The Nursing Contract: An Alternative in Care." *Journal of Psychiatric Nursing* (May-June 1971): 26-27.

Feather, R., and Bissell, B. "Clinical Supervision vs. Psychotherapy: The Psychiatric/Mental Health Supervisory Process." *Perspectives in Psychiatric Care* 17 (1979): 266-272.

Finkelman, A. "Commitment and Responsibility in the Therapeutic Relationship." *Journal of Psychiatric Nursing* (January-February 1975): 10-14.

Fulton, J. "Nurse-Patient Relationship Therapy." *Nursing Mirror* (December 1976): 51-52.

Geach, B. "The Problem-solving Technique as Taught to Psychiatric Students." *Perspectives in Psychiatric Care* (January-March 1974): 9-12.

Hartigan del Campo, E. "Psychiatric Nursing Therapy: Philosophy and Methods." *Journal of Psychiatric Nursing and Mental Health Services* 16 (1978): 34-37.

Hicks, C. "Taking the Lid Off . . . Sexuality and the Nurse." *Nursing Times* 76 (1980): 1681-1682.

Kaplan, H., and Sadock, B. *Modern Synopsis of Comprehensive Textbook of Psychiatry/III.* 3d ed. Baltimore: Williams and Wilkins, 1981.

Larson, M. "From Psychiatric to Psychosocial Nursing." *Nursing Outlook* 21 (1973): 520-523.

Leonard, C. "Patient Attitudes toward Nursing Intervention." *Nursing Research* 24 (1975): 335-339.

Melat, S. "The Development of Trust." *Perspectives in Psychiatric Care,* 3 (1965): 28-35.

Nurse, G. "Education. Counseling and Helping Skills: How Can They Be Learned?—1." *Nursing Times* 76 (1980): 737-738.

———. "Education. Counseling and Helping Skills: How Can They Be Learned?—2." *Nursing Times* 76 (1980): 789-790.

Okkenhaug, L. "Manipulation in a Nurse-Patient Relationship." *Canadian Nurse* (August 1967): 46-47.

Park, J. "A Study of Nurse-Patient Relationships." *New Zealand Nursing Forum* 8 (1980): 8-9.

Parks, S. "Allowing Physical Distance as a Nursing Approach." *Perspectives in Psychiatric Care* (November-December 1966): 31-35.

Peplau, H. "Psychotherapeutic Strategies." *Perspectives in Psychiatric Care* (November-December 1968): 264-270.

Ross, T. "Psychiatric Emergency Clinic: In Time of Trouble." *Nursing Mirror* 151 (1980): 22-23.

Stewart, W. "Nursing and Counseling—a Conflict of Roles?" *Nursing Mirror* (February 1975): 71-73.

Story, B. "The Catatonic Schizophrenic and Relationship Therapy." *Journal of Psychiatric Nursing and Mental Health Services* 16 (1978): 46-50.

Walt, A., and Gillis, L. "Factors that Influence Nurses' Attitudes Toward Psychiatric Patients." *Journal of Clinical Psychology* 35 (1979): 410-414.

8

Assessing the Individual Client

CHAPTER OUTLINE

Collecting, Assessing, and Recording Client Data
    The Psychiatric History
    The Mental Status Examination
    Physiological Assessment
    Psychological Testing
    Psychiatric Diagnostic Practice According to APA's Criteria (DSM-III)
    Psychosocial Assessment
Systems of Recording
    What to Record
    Psychiatric Jargon: What to Avoid
    Source-oriented Recording
    Problem-oriented Recording
    Nursing Care Plans
    Algorithms
    Psychiatric Audits
    The Interaction Process Analysis (IPA)
Key Nursing Concepts

LEARNING OBJECTIVES

After reading this chapter, students should be able to

- Describe the processes of psychiatric history taking, mental status examination, neurological assessment, and physiological and psychological testing

- Discuss the DSM-III's multiaxial system for making a psychiatric diagnosis

- Evaluate the DSM-III's congruence with psychiatric nursing's perspective

- Describe the process of individual psychosocial assessment

- Discuss the differences between processes of source-oriented and problem-oriented systems of recording

- Identify methods for recording verbatim nurse–client interactions

- Comprehend the organization and function of the Interaction Process Analysis (IPA)

CHAPTER 8

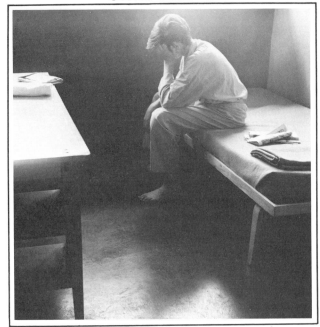

Psychiatric clients can be hidden and obscure making problem identification and nursing diagnosis challenging and difficult. Each nurse must utilize the multiple and complex skills and processes of assessment to plan, collaborate, and communicate with others about a client's mental health problems.

COLLECTING, ASSESSING, AND RECORDING CLIENT DATA

The systematic scientific approach known among nurses as *the nursing process* has evolved as the cornerstone of clinical practice. The nursing process begins with processes of assessment designed to collect and analyze data about the clients with whom nurses work. The primary resources for client data in most instances are the clients themselves. Other resources, such as psychological tests, nurses' notes, and physicians' orders, are secondary data sources that can enlarge, clarify, and substantiate data obtained directly from the client.

Systems of collection and assessment vary among mental health agencies. In some agencies observation and assessment commonly occur during the traditional psychiatric examination. The examination consists of two parts: history and mental status. It is most often done during initial or early interactions with a client and in traditional settings. It is often seen as a function of the psychiatrist, because a major goal of the examination is making a psychiatric diagnosis, although in some agencies it has become the responsibility of the intake worker. The traditional psychiatric examination is discussed in this chapter because it is still used in settings in which psychiatric nurses work.

In less traditional settings, the psychiatric history and the mental status examination have given way to

the *psychosocial assessment*. This assesses the social and psychological data gathered from interaction with the client. The primary goal of a psychosocial assessment is not a psychiatric diagnosis but an assessment of the client's difficulties in living. A psychosocial assessment form is given in Appendix C.

The following Initial Contact form (Figure 8–1) precedes the history and mental status exam and is intended to provide basic demographic and problem information at the time the client requests service or is presented for service by another person or agency. This information should provide the clinician with enough data to make some early key decisions:

- How urgent is the situation?
- Who is to be assigned responsibility for proceeding with the next step?
- What type of response is indicated as "the next step"?

This form is used chiefly by the member of the mental health team designated to handle all incoming calls and requests for service during a specified period of time.

The Psychiatric History

The information gathered during psychiatric history-taking can be obtained from multiple sources. Family, friends, police, mental health personnel, and others may contribute data to the psychiatric history. Not all data are provided by the client. When the sources are varied, the psychiatric history focuses on the perceptions of others, how they see the client and the circumstances of the client's life. It is necessary to include the perceptions of the client if the data are to be meaningful from that person's viewpoint. The sources of the psychiatric history and their relationship to the client should always be clearly indicated. Information given by these sources should be reviewed and understood in terms of their relationship.

The psychiatric history generally includes the following information:

INITIAL CONTACT SHEET

Today's Date _12-4-82_

Time ___9___ AM
          PM

Walk-in _____
Phone ___✓___
Outreach _____
Written _____

ID # _____
SS # _123-45-6789_
Welfare /
Medicaid # _____

SERVICE REQUESTED FOR
Client's NAME _____Mary_____ _____Jane_____ | _____Smith_____
                  First   Middle   Last

Address _1 Success Drive_   _West Egg, N.Y. 10101_ _____
           Street   City/Town   Zip   County

Permanent ___✓___
Temporary _____

Catchment Area _____

Phone # _666-1234_ Means of Transportation _Auto_
Directions to home _____
   (if outreach) _____
Sex __ Male _____ Date of Birth _1-14-43_ Age _39 yrs_ _____
      Female _✓_

SERVICE REQUESTED BY
☐ AGENCY   Name _____   Phone # _____
☐ OTHER   Address _____   Time(s) seen by _____
☑ SELF   If Agency-Contact Person _____   the agency _____

PRESENTING SITUATION / PROBLEM - What made you decide to seek help today?
   (use other side if needed)

   Feeling depressed about relationship with husband and life in general. Difficulty sleeping, low energy level, "I need to get help."

Have you talked with anyone about this?   Yes _____ Who? _____
Address _____   No _✓_   Phone # _____
                     Date of last contact _____
Are you taking ANY medication now?   Yes _✓_   What? 1. _Valium_
   (If more than 3 begin list on MH-2) No _____   2. _Dalamane_
                                                          3. _Aspirin_

CRISIS RATING How urgent is your need for help?
☐ Immediate (within minutes)
☐ Within a few hours
☐ Within 24 hours
☐ Within a few days
☑ Within a week or two

Comments
Intelligent housewife with marital problems — would probably benefit from counseling and perhaps couples group later

DISPOSITION (Check all that apply)
☐ Crisis
☐ Medical Emergency
☐ Assessment (specify) _____
☐ Discharge Planning
☐ Expediting / Advocacy
☐ Other (explain) _____
☑ Referral made to _Individual Counseling_ _____ Confirmed—Yes _✓_ No _____ Date _12-14-82_
Date of Next Contact _12-15-82_ _____ Assigned to _____
Date of Assignment _____ Request taken by _____

MH-1

Figure 8–1

Initial contact sheet. From L. A. Hoff, *People in Crisis* (Menlo Park, Calif.: Addison-Wesley Publishing Co., 1978), pp. 294–95, 319. Reproduced by permission of the Erie County Department of Mental Health; Mental Health Services, Erie County, Corporation IV, South East Corporation V, and Lakeshore Corporation VI.

   The form and specifications were developed by a Task Force of workers representing Corporation IV, South East Corporation V, Lakeshore Corporation VI, and the Erie County Department of Mental Health. Members: Marsha Aitken, Maureen Becker (Chairperson), Barbara Bernardis, George Deitz, Lee Ann Hoff, Elizabeth Keller.

   For samples of forms not included here and for complete specifications for use of these forms, the reader is referred to Erie County Department of Mental Health, 95 Franklin Street, Buffalo, New York 14202.

CRISIS RATING: HOW URGENT IS YOUR NEED FOR HELP?

- *Very Urgent:* Service request requires an immediate response within minutes; e.g., crisis outreach; medical emergency—requiring an ambulance to be called (overdoses); severe drug reaction; police contacted if situation involves extreme danger or weapons.
- *Urgent:* Response requires rapid but not necessarily immediate response, within a few hours. Example: low/moderate risk of suicide, mild drug reaction.
- *Somewhat Urgent:* Response should be made within a day (approximately 24 hours). Example: planning conference in which key persons are not available until the following evening.
- *Slightly Urgent:* A response is required within a few days. Example: client's funding runs out within a week and needs public assistance.
- *Not Urgent:* When a situation has existed for a long time and does not warrant immediate intervention, a week or two is unlikely to cause any significant difference. Example: child with a learning disability, certain types of marital counseling.

- *Complaint*—the main reason the client is having a psychiatric examination. The client may have personally initiated the psychiatric examination, or it may have been initiated by others (courts, hospital staff, family, referral from school or industry).
- *Present symptoms*—the nature of the onset and the development of symptoms.
- *Previous hospitalizations and mental health treatment.*
- *Family history*—generally, whether any family members have ever sought or received mental health treatment.
- *Personal history*—the person's birth and development; past and recent illnesses; schooling and educational problems; occupation; sexual development, interests, and practices; marital history; use of alcohol, drugs, and tobacco; and religious practices.
- *Personality*—the client's relationships with others, moods, feelings, interests, and leisure time activities.

The traditional history-taking process is most concerned with gathering information. Its medical model orientation is evident.

The Mental Status Examination*

The mental status examination is usually a standardized procedure in agencies that use it. Its primary purpose is to gather data to be used in determining etiology, diagnosis, prognosis, and treatment. The sections of the mental status examination that deal with *sensorium* and *intellect* are particularly important in sorting out the existence of organic brain disease. The purpose of this examination differs from that of psychiatric history in that it is used to identify the person's *present* mental status.

The mental status examiner generally seeks the following information not necessarily in the sequence presented here.

1. *General behavior and appearance*—a complete and accurate description of the client's physical characteristics, apparent age, manner of dress, use of cosmetics, personal hygiene, and responses to the examiner. Postures, gait, gestures, facial expression, and mannerisms are included in the description. The examiner also notes the client's general activity level.

   A thirty-five-year-old, white male, dressed in torn, disheveled jeans. Presented a blank facial expression, slouched posture, shuffling gait, generally low activity level, and sullen behavior.

2. *Characteristics of talk*—the form, rather than the content, of the client's speech. The speech is described in terms of loudness, flow, speed, quantity, level of coherence, and logic. A sample of the client's conversation with the examiner may be included. The following patterns, if present, should be particularly noted.

   a. *Mutism*—no verbal response from the client despite indications that he or she is aware of the examiner's questions.

   b. *Circumstantiality*—cumbersome and convoluted detail volunteered by the client but unnecessary to answer the interviewer's questions.

   c. *Perseveration*—a pattern of repeating the same words or movements despite apparent efforts to make a new response.

   d. *Flight of ideas*—rapid, overly productive responses to questions that seem related only by chance associations between one sentence fragment and another. Associated with flight of ideas might be rhyming, clang associations, punning, and evidence of distractibility.

   e. *Blocking*—a pattern of sudden silence in the

*Reprinted with permission of Sandoz Pharmaceuticals, Division of Sandoz, Inc. From S. M. Small, *Outline for Psychiatric Examination*, 1980.

stream of conversation for no obvious reason but often thought to be associated with intrusion on the client of delusional thoughts or hallucinations.

3. *Emotional state*—the person's mood or affective reaction. Both subjective and objective data are included. Subjective data are obtained through the use of nonleading questions such as: "How are you feeling?" If the client replies by using such general terms as "nervous," he or she should be asked to describe how the nervousness shows itself and its effect, since such words may mean different things to different individuals. Objectively, the examiner should observe facial expression, motor behavior, the presence of tears, flushing, sweating, tachycardia, tremors, respiratory irregularities, states of excitement, fear, and depression. Much valuable information may be obtained by noting the relationship between the client and the examiner. Attitudes of hostility, suspiciousness or flirtatiousness, a desire for bodily contact, or outspoken criticisms should be noted.

The psychiatric client is apt to have a persistent emotional trend based on a particular emotional disorder such as depression. If this is true, further inquiry should attempt to reveal the intensity and persistence of this reaction.

It is desirable to record a verbatim reply to questions concerning the client's mood. The relationship between mood and the content of thought is particularly significant. There may be a wide divergence between what the client says or does and his emotional state as expressed by attitudes or facial expressions.

Note whether intense emotional responses accompany discussion of specific topics. *Shallowness or flattening of the affect* is indicated by an insufficiently intense emotional display in association with ideas or situations that ordinarily would call for a more adequate response.

Dissociation or *disharmony* is often indicated by an inappropriate emotional response, such as smiling or silly behavior, when the attitude should be one of concern, anxiety, or sadness.

Evaluation of emotional reactions may be even more difficult because some clients may use *simulation* or play-acting. Clients who are trying to cover up a deep depression may feign cheerfulness and good spirits. The reverse may also be true.

The client's emotional reactions may be constant or may fluctuate during the examination. Try to specify the ease or readiness with which such changes occur in response to pleasant or unpleasant stimuli. Use such terms as the following to indicate intensity of response:

- Composed, complacent, frank, friendly, playful, teasing, silly, cheerful, boastful, elated, grandiose, ecstatic.
- Tense, worried, anxious, pessimistic, sad, perplexed, bewildered, gloomy, depressed, frightened.
- Aloof, superior, disdainful, distant, defensive, suspicious.
- Irritable, resentful, hostile, sarcastic, angry, furious.
- Indifferent, resigned, apathetic, dull, affectless.

The relationship of affect to content should be noted in terms of the influence of content on affect and disharmony between affect and content or thought. Constancy and change in the emotional state should be noted.

4. *Special preoccupations and experiences*—delusions, illusions, or hallucinations, depersonalizations, obsessions or compulsions, phobias, fantasies, and daydreams. (These terms are defined in the Glossary and discussed in Chapters 14–16.) These data may be elicited by asking the client questions, such as "Do you have any difficulties you complain of?" or "Have you been troubled or ill in any way?"

If the client has delusions of being the object of environmental attention some of the following questions might reveal them: "Do people like you?" "Have you ever been watched or spied upon or singled out for special attention?" "Do others have it in for you?"

Delusions of *alien control* (passivity) are feelings of being controlled or guided by external forces. If these delusions are suspected, ask the client such questions as "Do you ever feel your thoughts or actions are under any outside influences or control?" "Is your mind controlled by thought-waves, electricity, or radio-waves?" "Are you able to influence others, to read their minds, or to put thoughts in their minds?"

Nihilistic delusions are those in which the client more or less completely denies reality and existence. The client states that nothing exists, or everything is lost. He or she may say such things as "I have no head, no stomach," "I cannot die," or "I will live to eternity."

Delusions of *self-depreciation* are often seen in connection with severe depressions. The client describes feelings of unworthiness, sinfulness, ugliness, or emitting obnoxious odors.

Delusions of *grandeur* are associated with elated states, such as great wealth, strength, power, sexual potency, or identification with a famous person—even God.

Somatic delusions are focused on having cancer, obstructed bowels, leprosy, or some horrible disease. This is to be distinguished from a preoccupation with normal, visceral, or peripheral sensations.

Hallucinations are false sensory impressions without any external basis in fact. Try to elicit the clearness of the projection to the outside world (e.g., whether the client hears voices from outside or inside his or her head, the clarity and distinctness of the perception, and the intensity). Be tactful in approaching the client for evidences of hallucinatory phenomena, unless he or she is obviously hallucinating.

Obsessions are insistent thoughts recognized as arising from the self usually regarded by the client as absurd and relatively meaningless, yet they persist despite endeavors to get rid of them.

Compulsions are repetitive acts performed through some inner need or drive and are supposed to arrive against the subject's wishes and yet produce feelings of tension and anxiety if omitted.

Fantasies and *daydreams* are preoccupations that are often difficult to elicit from the client. The difficulty may be due to a lack of understanding on the part of the client of what the examiner wants, but he or she is often ashamed to talk about them because of their content.

5. *Sensorium or orientation*—orientation in terms of time, place, person, and self to determine the presence of confusion or clouding of consciousness. One may introduce such questions by asking "Have you kept track of the time?" If so, "What is today's date?" If the client says he or she does not know, he or she should be asked to estimate approximately or to guess at an answer. Many clinicians begin the mental status exam with these questions since the validity and reliability of subse-

quent data require that the client be reasonably oriented.

6. *Memory*—the person's attention span and ability to retain or recall past experiences in both the recent and the remote past. If memory loss exists, the examiner should determine whether it is constant or variable and whether the loss is limited to a certain time period. The examiner should be alert to the client's confabulations or attempts to devise memories to take the place of those he or she cannot recall. It is useful to introduce questions relating to memory by some general statement such as "Has your memory been good?" or "Have you had difficulty remembering telephone numbers or appointments?"

   a. *Recall of remote past experiences.* The person can be asked to review the important chronological facts of his or her life. The information given can be compared with information obtained from other sources during the history-taking process.

   b. *Recall of recent past experiences*—such as the events leading to the present seeking of treatment.

   c. *Retention and recall of immediate impressions.* The examiner might ask the client to repeat a name, address, and color immediately and again after three to five minutes, or to repeat three-digit numbers at a rate of one per second, or to repeat a complicated sentence.

   d. *General grasp and recall.* The person might be asked to read a story and then repeat the gist of it with as many details as possible. "The Cowboy Story" is an example suggested for this purpose in a concise guide for conducting a psychiatric examination developed by S. M. Small (1980).

The Cowboy Story

A cowboy from Arizona went to San Francisco with his dog, which he left at a friend's while he purchased a new suit of clothes. Dressed in the new suit, he went back to the dog, whistled to him, called him by name and patted him. The dog would have nothing to do with him in his new hat and coat, but gave a mournful howl. Coaxing had no effect, so the cowboy went away and donned his old garments. Then the dog immediately showed his wild joy on seeing his master as he thought he ought to be.

7. *General intellectual level*—a nonstandardized evaluation of intelligence. The examiner looks for the person's ability to use factual knowledge in a comprehensive way.

   a. *General grasp of information.* The person may be asked to name the five largest cities of the United States, the last four presidents, or the governor of the state.

   b. *Ability to calculate.* Tests of simple multiplication and addition may be given. Another test consists of subtracting from one hundred by sevens until the person can go no farther (Serial Seven's).

   c. *Reasoning and judgment.* Clients are commonly asked what they might do with $10,000 if it were given to them. Examiners must be particularly careful to correct for their own biases and values in assessing each client's answer.

8. *Abstract thinking*—the distinctions between such abstractions as poverty and misery or idleness and laziness. It is common to ask the client to interpret simple fables or proverbs, such as "Don't cry over spilled milk."

9. *Insight evaluation*—whether the client recognizes the significance of the present situation, whether the client feels the need of treatment, and the cli-

ent's own explanation of the symptoms. Often it is helpful to ask the client for suggestions for his or her own treatment.

10. *Summary*—the important psychopathological findings and a tentative diagnosis. Any pertinent facts from the medical history and/or physical examination should be added to the summary.

Table 8–1 differentiates some of the mental status examination findings in organic brain syndromes, mental retardation, disintegrative life patterns, and disturbed personal coping patterns.

Physiological Assessment

As the summary of the mental status examination and Table 8–1 suggest, nurses must carefully consider the possibility that a client's symptoms may have a physiological, particularly neurological, basis. In some reported instances, clients with brain tumors or bromide intoxication have been hospitalized on psychiatric units and treated exclusively for their seemingly psychiatric symptoms. Such a critical oversight obviously delays and seriously hampers appropriate treatment of an organic or neurological problem. The value of careful screening for physiological disorders cannot be overemphasized in the assessement of an individual client.

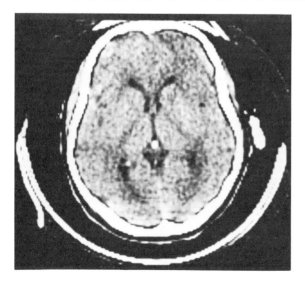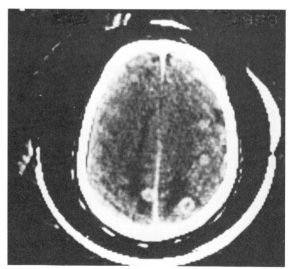

CT (computed tomography) brain scans were used in the trial of John Hinckley, Jr. to attempt to support the claim that Hinckley was suffering from schizophrenia when he shot President Reagan on March 30, 1981. Recent research shows that while the CT scan remains an imperfect tool for studying mental conditions, it is valuable in diagnosing tumors, strokes, or structural defects. The normal brain of a twenty-eight-year-old man is on the left. The photo on the right shows the presence of tumors in the brain of a fifty-five-year-old man.

In many community settings in which psychiatric nurses practice, these nurses are the only mental health care providers prepared to undertake a physiological and neurological assessment and interpret the results. The objectives of these assessments include:

- Detection of underlying and perhaps unsuspected organic pathology that may be responsible for psychiatric symptoms
- Understanding of disease as a factor in the overall psychiatric disability
- Appreciation of somatic symptoms that reflect primarily psychological rather than organic problems

History Taking   Of several procedures that enlighten the nurse who is attempting to rule out organic causes of psychiatric symptoms, the client's history is certainly a major one. The nurse should inquire into two primary aspects of physiological history: (1) facts about known physical diseases and dysfunction, and (2) information about specific physical complaints. Information about previous illnesses may provide essential clues. If the presenting symptoms include paranoid delusions and the client has a history of similar episodes, each of which responded to diverse forms of treatment and left no residual symptoms, there is a strong possibility of amphetamine- or other drug-related psychosis, and a drug screen may be indicated. An occupational history may provide information about exposure to inorganic mercury that has led to symptoms of psychosis or exposure to lead that has produced an Organic Mental Disorder. Organic Mental Disorders are discussed in detail in Chapter 17.

The second emphasis in history taking is eliciting information from the client about any specific physical complaints that may be present. Again, it is crucial that the nurse be aware of symptoms in terms of not only assessing psychiatric conditions, but also detecting physical diseases. Symptoms that are atypical for psychiatric disorders are particularly effective clues. For example, if a client with hallucinations and delusions also complains of a severe headache at the onset of the symptoms, the symptoms together suggest possible brain pathology and call for careful and repeated neurological assessment. History taking should also include information about medications currently being taken by the client. Digitalis intoxication may result in impairment. Reserpine may produce symptoms generally considered psychiatric in nature (Kaplan and Sadock 1981).

Observation   The nurse's powers of observation also yield important data bearing on the possible presence of organic disorders. An unsteady gait may suggest diffuse brain disease or alcohol or drug intoxication. Asymmetry—dragging a leg or not swinging one arm—might be a sign of a focal brain lesion. While inattention to proper dress and hygiene is common in emotional disorders, it is also a hallmark of organic brain disease, particularly lapses such as mismatching socks or shoes. Frequent, quick, purposeless movements are characteristic of anxiety, but they are equally characteristic of chorea or hyperthyroidism. Tremors accompanied by anxiety may point to Parkinson's disease. The status of a client's nutrition may also be significant. Recent weight loss, although often encountered in depression and schizophrenia, may be due to gastrointestinal disease, carcinomatosis, Addison's disease, and many other physical disorders. The nurse should observe the color of the skin, pupillary changes, alertness and responsiveness, and quality of speech and word production, keeping in mind the possibility of organic brain dysfunction, substance intoxication, or other diseases.

Neurological Assessment   A careful neurological examination is mandatory for each client suspected of having organic brain dysfunction. Its goal is to discover signs pointing to circumscribed, focal cerebral dysfunction or diffuse, bilateral cerebral disease. A guide for evaluating the presence of signs of central nervous system disorders or "neurological soft signs" is presented in the chart on pages 194 and 195.

Authorities in mental health practice consistently remind clinicians of the need for thorough physiological assessment of clients seen in psychiatric settings. The psychiatric literature abounds with stories of clients whose symptoms were initially considered exclusively psychiatric but ultimately were proved to be organic, especially neurological. Assessment errors occurred not because there were no features to suggest organicity, but because such features were accorded too little weight or were misinterpreted by the evaluator.

Psychological Testing

Clinical psychologists administer and interpret a wide variety of psychological tests. There are two types of psychological tests: those concerned with intelligence, and those concerned with personality. Both kinds are included in a comprehensive psychological evaluation.

Table 8–1 DIFFERENTIATION OF MENTAL STATUS EXAMINATION FINDINGS

	Organic Brain Syndrome		Mental Retardation	Disintegrative Life Patterns (Psychotic Conditions)		Disturbed Personal Coping Patterns (Affective Disorders)
	Acute (Delirium)	Chronic (Dementia)		Manic Episode	Schizophrenic Disorders	Depression
Appearance and Behavior	Fluctuating impairment of consciousness, restlessness	May show deterioration of personal habits but state of consciousness not clouded		Hyperactive, elated, assertive, boistrous, with rapid emphatic speech; may become suddenly angry or argumentative	Variable	Dejected, slowed, slumped, troubled
Mood	Anxiety, fear, lability	Irritability, lability		Elation, sometimes anger and irritability	Blandness, impoverishment or inappropriateness of affect	Depression, hopelessness
Thought Processes and Perceptions						
Coherence and relevance	May be confused, incoherent	May become confused		Rapid association of ideas that may seem illogical	Often incoherent, disorganized	
Thought content	May have delusions			May have delusions and feelings of persecution	May have feelings of unreality, depersonalization, persecution, influence and reference; delusions that are bizarre and symbolic	May have delusions, often involving guilt, self-depreciation, somatic complaints
Perceptions	May have illusions, hallucinations			May have illusions, rarely hallucinations	May have hallucinations and illusions, often bizarre and symbolic	May have illusions, rarely hallucinations

Cognitive Functions					
Orientation	May be disoriented	May be disoriented	Depends on severity of deficiency	Well-oriented	Usually but not always well-oriented
Attention and concentration	Poor	Poor	Limited	Distractable	
Recent memory	Poor	Poor	May be poor		Usually well-preserved but may be difficult to test because of inattentiveness and indifference
Remote memory	May become poor	May become poor	May be poor		Usually well-preserved but may be difficult to test because of inattentiveness and indifference
Information	Preserved until late	Preserved until late	Limited		
Vocabulary	Preserved until late	Preserved until late	Limited		
Abstract reasoning	Concrete	Concrete	Concrete		Concrete, may be bizarre
Judgment	Poor	Poor	May be poor		
Perception and coordination	May be poor	May be poor	May be poor		

Source: Adapted from B. Bates, A Guide to Physical Examination (Philadelphia, J. B. Lippincott Co., 1974), pp. 312-313.

NEUROLOGICAL ASSESSMENT GUIDE

| TIME & DATE | PUPILS | | | L.O.C. | S-R | T.R. | MOTOR | | | | TOTAL |
	R	 = >	L				RUE	RLE	LUE	LLE	MAX. 25

Explanation of Codes

Pupils

Reaction time, right (R) and left (L)

(2) Reacts briskly

(1) Reacts slowly

(0) No reaction

Size

(=) Equal

(<) Right lesser than left

(>) Right greater than left

Level of Consciousness (L.O.C.)

(5) Alert and oriented x 3 = awakens easily; oriented to person, place, time

(4) Alert and partially oriented = awakens easily but oriented in only one or two of the three spheres

(3) Lethargic but oriented = slow to arouse, possibly slurred speech, but oriented x 3

(2) Lethargic and disoriented = slow to arouse, oriented in only one or two spheres or completely disoriented

Chart continues on next page

Intelligence Tests   Intelligence tests may be useful particularly in evaluating the presence and degree of mental retardation. Commonly used intelligence tests are the Stanford–Binet Test, the Wechsler Adult Intelligence Scale, the Wechsler Intelligence Scale for Children, the Gesell Developmental Schedules, and the Vineland Social Maturity Scale. These intelligence tests and the limitations of intelligence tests for prediction and evaluation are discussed in Chapter 17.

Personality Tests   Personality tests are also called *projective tests* because they evoke projection in the responses of the person being tested.

THE RORSCHACH TEST   Hermann Rorschach, a Swiss psychiatrist, developed the Rorschach test in 1921. It consists of ten standardized inkblots in black and white or color on separate cards, displayed one by one, to which clients are asked to respond in terms of their

OR

(2) Restless/combative (confused) = spontaneously thrashing about in bed; striking out at others; inattentive to commands

(1) Responds to stimulation only = exhibits only some type of withdrawal or posturing in response to stimulation

(0) Unresponsive = gives no response of any kind

Stimulus–Response (S–R)

(5) Responds to commands = gives appropriate responses to orientation questions, complies with instructions on hand grasp, toe wiggling, etc.

(4) Responds to name = opens eyes to name or gives some indication that he or she hears (nods, moves, etc.), but does not follow all commands

(3) Responds to shaking = responds only to vigorous physical stimulation

(2) Responds to pinprick = responds to light pain applied with pin to trunk or extremities to elicit either withdrawal or posturing

(1) Responds to deep pain = responds only to mandibular pressure, periorbital rub, sternal rub, or pinch

(0) Unresponsive = gives no response to any stimulus

Type of Response (T.R.)

(3) Complex withdrawal = withdrawal and attempt to remove stimulus

(2) Simple withdrawal = withdrawal from stimulus alone

(1) Posturing = decorticate—head, arms, and hands flexed; decerebrate—head extended, arms extended and pronated, back arched

(0) Flaccid = no response

Motor

Right Upper Extremity (RUE)

Right Lower Extremity (RLE)

Left Upper Extremity (LUE)

Left Lower Extremity (LLE)

(2) Full spontaneous use = moves designated extremity or extremities with or *without* any stimulus

(1) Moves to stimulus only = responds only to touch, pin, or deep pain

(0) No movement = does not respond to any stimulus

Weakness of an extremity is indicated by writing "weaker" under the appropriate column.

associations, thoughts, and impressions (see Figure 8–2). Since each card contains only inkblots, clients responses are *projected,* that is, they come from within the clients themselves. People may see persons, animals, insects, objects, anatomical parts, or other things. For example, popular responses to card I in Figure 8–2 are "a bat" and "a butterfly." The examiner scores the response using a system of symbols in relation to the following:

• *Location.* Where on the blot area was the response seen?

• *Content.* What did the client see?

• *Determinant.* What characteristic of the blot prompted the response?

• *Form–level.* How closely did the response correspond to the contour of the blot area used?

• *Originality.* How common a response is it?

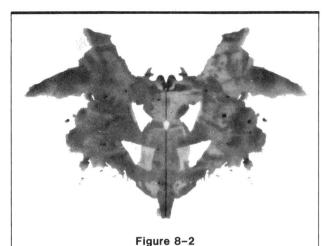

Figure 8–2

Card I of the Rorschach test. (Reprinted by permission, Hans Huber Medical Publisher, Berne.)

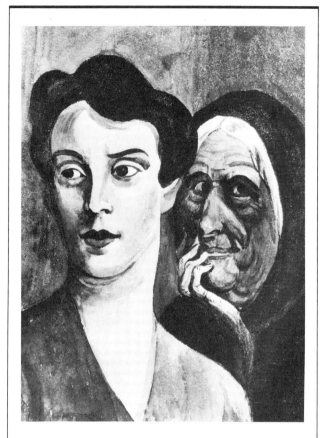

Figure 8–3

Card 12 GF of the Thematic Apperception Test. (Reprinted from H. A. Murray, *Thematic Apperception Test* (Cambridge: Harvard University Press, 1943. Copyright © 1943 by the President and Fellows of Harvard College: 1971 by Henry A. Murray.)

Interpretation is based on a complicated system of scoring symbols and analyzing content. The Rorschach is the most highly developed of all the projective tests used to evaluate the personality.

THE THEMATIC APPERCEPTION TEST (TAT)   The TAT also consists of a series of cards shown one by one. However, TAT cards are pictures of people in various emotional situations (see Figure 8–3). Clients are asked to describe what seems to be happening in the picture or to tell a story about it. The pictures themselves are quite ambiguous, so that what clients choose to say reveals aspects of their own emotional lives. The psychologist who interprets and scores the TAT looks for themes, threads, and patterns in the responses to the cards. Some adaptations of the TAT for use with children are available.

THE MINNESOTA MULTIPHASIC PERSONALITY INVENTORY (MMPI)   The MMPI is a complex and lengthy test consisting of 550 questions asked of the client. Scoring is done in relation to nine areas: preoccupation about body diseases; depression; hysteria; antisocial personality; masculine or feminine features; paranoid qualities; anxiety, phobias, and psychogenic fatigue states; schizophrenic features; and manic features. (These terms are described in Chapters 14–16.) A clinical profile of personality structure is drawn from the client's responses in these areas.

Since the MMPI is largely self-administered and can be scored quickly on computers, it has been advocated as a screening measure for colleges and universities, industrial and business settings, and government agencies, among others. The large-scale collection and use of such information is alarming because of the pejorative labeling that may derive from such psychological testing.

THE DRAW-A-PERSON TEST   In the Draw-a-Person Test, clients are asked first to draw a human figure and then, usually, to draw a figure of a member of the opposite sex (see Figure 8–4). The drawings may be interpreted to give information about clients' concepts of their own bodies and personality structures; their relationships with persons of the opposite sex, the same sex, and parents; and their views of the roles of men and women.

THE SENTENCE COMPLETION TEST   The Sentence Completion Test presents an extensive series of incomplete sentences to clients, who are asked to complete the sentences with the first thoughts that come to mind. The sentences are designed to elicit responses concern-

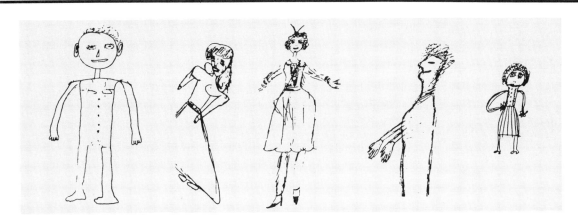

Figure 8-4

Examples of the Draw-a-Person Test done by five women who had been hospitalized for two years. (From R. H. Spire, "An Experimental Study of the Use of Photographic Self-Image Confrontation as a Nursing Procedure in the Care of Chronically Ill Schizophrenic Female Patients" [project in partial fulfillment of M.S. degree, State University of New York at Buffalo, 1967] pp. 243, 248, 249, 251, 256.)

ing fantasies, fears, daydreams, and aspirations, among other things.

THE BENDER–GESTALT TEST   The Bender–Gestalt Test asks clients to reproduce, as best they can, nine geometric designs that are printed on separate cards. Because this test can be used to evaluate memory, it is believed to be particularly helpful in identifying organic brain damage. It is also used to evaluate the maturation level of children in the coordination of visual, motor, and intellectual functions. For an example of a Bender–Gestalt design series, see Figure 17–5.

These and other instruments commonly used by clinical psychologists are briefly discussed in Table 8–2.

Psychiatric Diagnostic Practice According to APA's Criteria (DSM-III)*

The American Psychiatric Association published a third edition of the Diagnostic and Statistical Manual of Mental Disorders in the summer of 1980. (See Appendix B for an outline of categories for diagnosis and numerical codes.) Important features distinguish DSM-III from its predecessors. It uses specified diagnostic criteria to improve the reliability of diagnostic judgments and offers a multiaxial or multidimensional ap-

*This section is based on a previously published article co-authored by Janet B. W. Williams and Holly Skodol Wilson, "A Psychiatric Nursing Perspective on DSM-III," Journal of Psychosocial Nursing 20 (1982): 14–20.

proach to clinical assessment of psychiatric clients in which five different classes of data are collected and assessed.

The first edition of the Diagnostic and Statistical Manual of Mental Disorders was published by the APA in 1952. In 1968 the main achievement of the second edition was to move into compatibility with the International Classification of Diseases, Injuries and Causes of Death (ICD-9) published by the World Health Organization. The DSM-II was widely criticized for its low reliability and tendency to reflect an individual psychiatrist's philosophy or such client characteristics as social class rather than actual clinical data. In the first edition of this text, we charged that most psychiatric diagnostic practice had been subject to speculation about unconscious dynamics, was limited to intrapsychic variables, and represented a reductionistic and dualistic approach to human beings.

The DSM-III represents the current state of knowledge about diagnosing mental disorders. It is composed of a list of all the official numerical codes and terms for all recognized mental disorders, along with a comprehensive description of each and specified diagnostic criteria that must be present in order to make each diagnosis.

Nurses have historically avoided instruments and tools for client assessment that: ignore stressors in a person's social context; emphasize symptoms, pathology, and illness to the exclusion of strengths, capabilities, and areas of adaptive functioning; and are, in short, exclusively "medical model approaches." Many

Table 8–2	COMMON PSYCHOLOGICAL TESTS IN CLINICAL USE	
Name of Test	**Description**	**Method**
Bender–Gestalt test	A test of visual–motor coordination that is most useful with adults as a screening device to detect the presence of organic impairment. It may also be used to evaluate the level of maturation in the coordination of intellectual, muscular, and visual functions in children	The client is asked to copy nine separate geometric designs onto plain white paper, one at a time. Sometimes the client is asked to draw the design from memory after an interval of forty-five to sixty seconds.
Blacky test	A projective test used most frequently with children (although it is also designed for adults) to determine the level of psychosexual development.	The client is shown various cartoons about a dog (who may be identified as male or female) and the dog's family and is asked to make up a story about each cartoon.
Draw-a-Person test	A projective test used with both adults and children to elicit information on the client's body image or perception of self and the client's relationship to the environment. It is also used as a screening device to detect the presence of organic impairment. With children it may be used to compare the age level of expression with the child's chronological age for a rough approximation of intelligence.	The client is asked first to draw a human figure and later to draw a person of the opposite sex. The test may be expanded by asking the client to draw a picture of a house and a tree as well (called the House–Tree–Person test), an animal, or a family.
Minnesota Multiphasic Personality Inventory (MMPI)	A self-administered objective (as opposed to projective) personality test designed to yield a broad examination of personality functioning that is amenable to statistical interpretation—such as self-attitudes, certain aspects of ego functioning, and profiles of symptoms or psychopathology.	The client responds to 550 statements, by indicating either "true," "false," or "cannot say." The client's personality profile is sketched in terms of: • Preoccupation with body diseases • Depression • Hysteria • Antisocial personality • Masculine or feminine features • Paranoid qualities • Anxiety, phobias, and psychogenic fatigue • Schizophrenic features • Manic features
Rorschach test	A projective test that is the most highly developed of the personality tests. It reveals personality features and symptoms and is commonly used as a diagnostic tool.	The client responds to ten cards, one at a time, consisting of black and white or colored, standardized inkblots. Responses include the impressions, thoughts, and associations that come to mind while the client looks at the inkblot.
Sentence Completion test	A projective test designed to elicit conscious associations to specific areas of functioning to illustrate the fears, preoccupations, ambitions, and idiosyncrasies of the client.	The client is asked to complete spontaneously sentences such as: "I feel guilty about. . . ," "Sex is. . . ," "My mother. . . ," "Sometimes I wish. . . ," Both mood and content are noted.

Table continues on next page

	Table 8–2 continued	
Name of Test	**Description**	**Method**
Stanford-Binet Intelligence test	A general intelligence test based on an age-level concept from two years to about fifteen years. It is particularly useful to test children and to evaluate mental retardation.	The client is asked to do a graded series of tasks designed to correlate with the abilities of children of a particular age group. Each set is more difficult than the one before it.
Thematic Apperception Test (TAT)	A projective test offering a standardized set of stimuli for exploring the client's emotional life. Themes and interpersonal problems emerge in the client's responses.	The client is shown a series of ambiguous pictures of people in various emotionally significant situations and is asked to respond by describing what is happening in the picture and telling a story about it. Adaptations have been designed for use with children. In these, the central figure is a child or the pictures are cartoons of animals.
Wechsler Adult Intelligence Scale (WAIS)	A general intelligence test for persons sixteen years of age and older. It is the most widely used and best standardized intelligence test.	The client completes eleven subtests, which yield both verbal and performance scores as well as full-scale IQs. Subtest raw scores may also be compared to reveal variability in functioning. The subtests are: information, comprehension, arithmetic, similarities, memory for digits, vocabulary, digit symbol, picture completion, block design, picture arrangement, and object assembly.
Wechsler Intelligence Scale for Children (WISC)	A general intelligence test for children from five through fifteen years of age.	Similar to the Wechsler test for adults, this test asks the client to complete ten subtests, which yield separate verbal, performance, and full-scale scores.
Wechsler Memory Scale	A psychological test for immediate, short-term, and long-term memory.	The client is asked to do seven memory tests, including current information, orientation, mental control, logical memory, digits forward and backward, visual reproduction, and associate learning. A memory quotient (MQ) score is useful in the determination of organic mental syndrome.
Word Association Test	A projective test similar in form and organization to the Sentence Completion test. It is designed to elicit associations to areas of conflict.	The client is asked to respond spontaneously to a series of fifty or more words, presented one at a time. Words presumed to be related to the conflicts of the specific client are mixed with words that generally produce an emotional reaction.

of our colleagues believe that the new DSM-III, while not entirely free of controversy, represents the state-of-the-art in the field of psychiatric diagnosis. According to Spitzer, Williams, and Skodol (1980), it has been adopted for use in most facilities throughout the United States.

Basic Principles of the Multiaxial System   The

multiaxial framework for client assessment provided by DSM-III is congruent with holistic views of people, recognizes the role of environmental stress in influencing behavior, and requires that the clinician collect data about client adaptive strengths as well as about symptoms or problems. One of DSM-III's most important features is its increased interclinician reliability due to the use of specified observable criteria rather than diverse theories of etiology for mental disorders (Spitzer and Forman 1979). Its multiaxial approach is undoubtedly of equal significance to psychiatric nursing (Williams and Wilson 1982).

The principle behind a multiaxial system is illustrated in the following example.

A thirty-five-year-old man came to an outpatient mental health clinic for evaluation. This young man came in for treatment of a severe fear and avoidance of flying that amounted to a phobia. However, he also had a long-term personality disturbance, and suffered from eczema. If three different clinicians were asked to evaluate this man, a clinician who was particularly biologically oriented would certainly diagnose the eczema, but might fail to notice the personality disturbance and make little of the phobia. A more psychodynamically oriented clinician would be sure to diagnose the personality disorder but might overlook the eczema and the phobia, considering them to be merely manifestations of the underlying personality disturbance. Finally, a clinician who was more behaviorally oriented would notice the phobia, but might fail to diagnose the personality disturbance and the eczema. It is clear, then, that due to their differing theoretical orientations these clinicians have a rather high likelihood of diagnostic disagreement.

This same man was presented to the same three colleagues, and this time each of the clinicians was required to evaluate him in each of three different areas of functioning: (1) behavioral or psychological, (2) personality, and (3) physical functioning. In this case, all three clinicians would be much more likely to diagnose all three conditions and thus agree on the total evaluation of the individual.

In the DSM-III multiaxial system, each individual is evaluated on five axes, each dealing with a different class of information about the client. A multiaxial evaluation system provides a much more comprehensive evaluation of an individual, and increases the likelihood that clinicians will agree among themselves about the condition of the individual being evaluated.

The DSM-III multiaxial system includes the five axes presented in Table 8-3 (see also Appendix B).

Table 8-3   DSM-III AXES

Axis I:	Clinical Syndromes
	Conditions Not Attributable to a Mental Disorder That Are a Focus of Attention or Treatment (V Codes)
	Additional Codes
Axis II:	Personality Disorders
	Specific Developmental Disorders
Axis III:	Physical Disorders
Axis IV:	Severity of Psychosocial Stressors
Axis V:	Highest Level of Adaptive Functioning Past Year

Axes I and II include all the mental disorders in DSM-III, and so might be said to represent the intrapersonal or *psychological* area of functioning. Axis III is for recording physical disorders and conditions that are related to the understanding or management of the individual, and thus represents the area of *physical* functioning. Axes IV and V, for psychosocial stressors and highest adaptive functioning, might be said to represent an evaluation of the individual's *social* functioning. In this sense, the multiaxial system provides a more comprehensive biopsychosocial approach to assessment.

Description of the Axes   It is essential that nurses have a thorough understanding of the components of the multiaxial system in order for it to be used most effectively. What follows is a brief description of each of the axes; more details are given in Chapter 2 of *DSM-III* (1980). Nurses are encouraged to read this chapter early in their use of DSM-III.

AXES I AND II   Axes I and II comprise all the Mental Disorders and Conditions Not Attributable to a Mental Disorder That Are a Focus of Attention or Treatment (called "V" Codes). The easiest way to differentiate between these first two axes is to deal first with Axis II. On Axis II are personality disorders, usually diagnosed in adults, and specific developmental disorders, usually diagnosed in children and adolescents. The remaining mental disorders and associated conditions are recorded on Axis I. The two classes of disorders on Axis II were given their own axis because their usually mild and chronic symptomatology is often overshadowed by a more florid Axis I condition. If a person appears in an emergency room with a floridly psychotic major depression, for example, that person's under-

Table 8–4 EXAMPLES OF DSM-III MULTIAXIAL EVALUATION ON AXES I AND II		
Example 1		
Axis I:	303.93	Alcohol Dependence, in Remission
Axis II:	301.70	Antisocial Personality Disorder
Example 2		
Axis I:	V71.09	No diagnosis
Axis II:	301.22	Schizotypal Personality Disorder

Table 8–5 EXAMPLES OF DSM-III MULTIAXIAL EVALUATION ON AXES I, II, AND III		
Example		
Axis I:	312.23	Conduct Disorder, Socialized, Aggressive
Axis II:	V71.09	No diagnosis
Axis III:		Diabetes

lying personality disorder may well be missed. Listing personality disorders on a separate axis reduces the likelihood that they will be overlooked.

In addition to the other mental disorders, Axis I includes the V Codes. The V Codes include such conditions as Marital Problems, Occupational Problems, and Parent–child Problems, in which the problem being evaluated or for which clinical care is sought is not due to a mental disorder. A mental disorder is differentiated from other problems in living as a clinically significant behavioral pattern that occurs and is associated with either a painful sympton (distress) or impairment in functioning (disability). Further, the distress or disability do not primarily reflect a conflict between an individual and society.

If a person with Bipolar Disorder, a mental disorder that has been in remission for many years, now develops marital difficulties for reasons unrelated to that person's psychiatric history or condition (perhaps, for example, a conflict has arisen because that person's wife wants to resume a career), both Marital Problem and Bipolar Disorder in Remission could be recorded on Axis I. If, however, the Bipolar Disorder was not in complete remission, and marital conflict develops as a result of the person's changeable moods and other symptoms associated with the mental disorder, the marital problem would not be recorded in addition to Bipolar Disorder, since the marital problem in this case is due to the person's mental disorder.

Axis I also includes a code for "Unspecified Mental Disorder (Non-psychotic)," which indicates that the cli-

nician has determined that there is some (nonpsychotic) Axis I mental disorder but, perhaps due to lack of information, cannot yet be more specific. Finally, there are codes for indicating that a diagnosis or condition is deferred on either Axis I or Axis II, or that there is no mental disorder. Examples of evaluations of individuals, using only Axes I and II are present in Table 8–4.

AXIS III Axis III is for recording physical disorders and conditions that are important to take into account in planning treatment or are relevant to understanding the etiology or exacerbation of the mental disorder. A clinician might also want to record other significant physical findings, such as soft neurological signs, or even a single symptom (e.g., vomiting). An example of an evaluation done through Axis III is presented in Table 8–5.

In this example, in addition to the fact that diabetes is a major physical disorder and should probably always be noted, the child will probably not be very compliant with treatment, due in large part to his psychological problems (Conduct Disorder, as the mental disorder, being noted on Axis I).

In the event of lack of information on Axis III, that fact should be stated: "No information" or "Diagnosis deferred—not evaluated" or "Referred to Dr. Smith for evaluation." In any event, *something* should be noted on this axis, omitting it for lack of information undermines the purpose of a holistic multiaxial system.

AXIS IV Axis IV provides the seven-point rating scale shown in Table 8–6.

This scale rates the severity of the psychosocial stressors that in the nurse's judgment contributed to the initiation or exacerbation of the mental disorder. In making this judgment, the nurse should generally take into account only stressors that occurred in the year preceding the mental disorder.

In order to standardize the severity ratings across stressors, and to avoid rating an individual's idiosyncratic vulnerabilities, the severity rating of the stress-

Table 8-6   AXIS IV: SEVERITY OF PSYCHOSOCIAL STRESSORS

Code	Term	Adult Examples	Child or Adolescent Examples
1	None	No apparent psychosocial stressor	No apparent psychosocial stressor
2	Minimal	Minor violation of the law; small bank loan	Vacation with the family
3	Mild	Argument with neighbor; change in work hours	Change in schoolteacher; new school year
4	Moderate	New career; death of close friend; pregnancy	Chronic parental fighting; change to new school; illness of close relative; birth of sibling
5	Severe	Serious illness in self or family; major financial loss; marital separation; birth of child	Death of peer, divorce of parents; arrest; hospitalization; persistent and harsh parental discipline
6	Extreme	Death of close relative; divorce	Death of parent or sibling; repeated physical or sexual abuse
7	Catastrophic	Concentration camp experience; devastating natural disaster	Multiple family deaths
0	Unspecified	No information, or not applicable	No information or not applicable

Source: American Psychiatric Association, *Diagnostic and Statistical Manual* of *Mental Disorders (DSM-III)*, (Washington, D.C.: 1980), pp. 20-30.

ors should be made with an "average" person in mind. The nurse should take into account the individual client's circumstances and sociocultural background, and rate the severity of the stressors as experienced by the "average" person within these constrictions. In this way, an abortion would probably be more stressful for a Catholic than for an atheist.

The nurse should also take into account the total number of stressors the client recently experienced, how desirable they were, to what extent they were under the client's control (e.g., whether the individual quit a job or was fired), and the amount of change they caused in the individual's life (e.g., the development of a serious chronic physical illness could be expected to cause a great deal of change in the "average" person's life).

The extensive field trials of DSM-III were efforts to ascertain the reliability with which ratings could be made on Axis IV by clinicians with no special training in the use of the multiaxial system. In evaluations of 601 adults, the correlation of interrater agreement was .63; in evaluations of 122 children and adolescents, it was .68. Perfect agreement would be 1.0 and no agreement, .0. These results indicate that clinicians can agree on the severity of the psychosocial stressors that their clients have recently experienced.

In addition to rating the severity of the stressors, evaluators should also note in their own words the specific stressors that they consider pertinent. Thus a multiaxial evaluation, up through Axis IV, might look like the example presented in Table 8-7.

In this example, the client developed Panic Disorder (a condition in which there are recurrent panic attacks) as she began classes in college.

AXIS V   This axis provides the seven-point rating scale shown in Table 8-8. One of the most accurate indicators of clinical outcome is the level of premorbid functioning that an individual sustained. For this reason, Axis V provides a scale to rate the highest level of adaptive functioning that an individual was able to sustain for at least a few months during the past year.

Table 8-7   EXAMPLE OF A DSM-III MULTIAXIAL EVALUATION ON AXES I, II, III, AND IV

Axis I:	300.01	Panic Disorder
Axis II:	301.83	Borderline Personality Disorder
Axis III:		No Diagnosis
Axis IV:		3—Mild (began college)

Table 8–8 AXIS V: HIGHEST LEVEL OF ADAPTIVE FUNCTIONING PAST YEAR		
Levels	**Adult Examples**	**Child or Adolescent Examples**
1. Superior—unusually effective functioning in social relations, occupational functioning, and use of leisure time.	Single parent living in deteriorating neighborhood takes excellent care of children and home, has warm relations with friends, and finds time for pursuit of hobby.	A twelve-year-old girl gets superior grades in school, is extremely popular among her peers, and excels in many sports. She does all of this with apparent ease and comfort.
2. Very good—better than average functioning in social relations, occupational functioning, and use of leisure time.	A sixty-five-year-old retired widower does some volunteer work, often sees old friends, and pursues hobbies.	An adolescent boy gets excellent grades, works part-time, has several close friends, and plays banjo in a jazz band. He admits to some distress in "keeping up with everything."
3. Good—no more than slight impairment in either social or occupational functioning.	A woman with many friends functions extremely well at a difficult job, but says "the strain is too much."	An eight-year-old boy does well in school, has several friends, but bullies younger children.
4. Fair—moderate impairment in either social relations or occupational functioning; or some impairment in both.	A lawyer has trouble carrying through assignments; has several acquaintances, but hardly any close friends.	A ten-year-old girl does poorly in school, but has adequate peer and family relations.
5. Poor—marked impairment in either social relations or occupational functioning, or moderate impairment in both.	A man with one or two friends has trouble keeping a job for more than a few weeks.	A fourteen-year-old boy almost fails in school and has trouble getting along with his peers.
6. Very poor—marked impairment in both social relations and occupational functioning.	A woman is unable to do any of her housework and has violent outbursts toward family and neighbors.	A six-year-old girl needs special help in all subjects and has virtually no peer relationships.
7. Grossly impaired—gross impairment in virtually all areas of functioning.	An elderly man needs supervision to maintain minimal personal hygiene and is usually incoherent.	A four-year-old boy needs constant restraint to avoid hurting himself and is almost totally lacking in skills.
0. Unspecified.	No information.	No information.

Source: American Psychiatric Association, *Diagnostic and Statistical Manual of Mental Disorders (DSM-III)* (Washington, D.C.: 1980), pp. 29–30.

Overall adaptive functioning is defined by three areas of functioning: (1) social relations; (2) occupational functioning; and (3) use of leisure time. The quality of the client's functioning in each of these three areas should be considered, with the breadth and quality of social relationships being given the greatest weight because of their high prognostic value. Use of leisure time is a serious consideration only in those individuals who have been functioning on a very high level.

The judgment on Axis V is also a reliable one. In the reliability study of 637 adults, the correlation obtained was .77; in the study of 120 children and adolescents, it was .65 again based on a 1.0 for perfect correlation and .0 for no correlation between diagnoses of two clinicians.

DSM-III's Usefulness to Psychiatric–Mental Health Nursing   From the perspective of psychiatric nursing, the DSM-III represents some progress toward values that mental health nurses have espoused for decades. For example, as Williams and Wilson have stated (1982), DSM-III:

- Provides a framework for interdisciplinary communication
- Based revisions on a series of formative evaluations
- Represents a collaborative achievement
- Represents progress toward a more holistic view of mind–body relations
- Provides for diagnostic uncertainty
- Incorporates, at least in part, biological, psychological, and social variables
- Has achieved positive results of extensive field testing for validity and reliability
- Considers adaptive strength as well as problems
- Reflects a descriptive, phenomenological perspective rather than any psychiatric theoretical orientation

Of all the axes represented in DSM-III, Axis IV and V, Psychosocial Stressors and Adaptive Functioning, best represent the practice of nursing rather than medicine. These are the areas in which nursing's greatest contribution may be.

Psychosocial Assessment

The psychosocial assessment is a dynamic process. While it is begun in the initial contact with the client, it continues throughout the nurse–client experience. Psychosocial assessments may be made of an individual, a family, or a group. In any case, they begin with the identifying characteristics, such as name, sex, age, marital status, and ethnic and cultural origins. Problem identification and definition are also necessary phases in the assessment process. The method for assessment described below has been adapted from the problem-solving model of Compton and Galaway (1979, pp. 250–251).

Individual Assessment   The individual assessment should consider the following factors:

1. *Physical and intellectual*
   a. Presence of physical illness and/or disability
   b. Appearance and energy level
   c. Current and potential levels of intellectual functioning
   d. How client sees personal world, translates events around self; client's perceptual abilities
   e. Cause and effect reasoning, ability to focus

2. *Socioeconomic factors*
   a. Economic factors—level of income, adequacy of subsistence; how this affects life-style, sense of adequacy, self-worth
   b. Employment and attitudes about it
   c. Racial, cultural, and ethnic identification; sense of identity and belonging
   d. Religious identification and link to significant value systems, norms, and practices

3. *Personal values and goals*
   a. Presence or absence of congruence between values and their expression in action; meaning of values to individual
   b. Congruence between individual's values and goals and the immediate systems with which client interacts
   c. Congruence between individual's values and assessor's values; meaning of this for intervention process

4. *Adaptive functioning and response to present involvement*
   a. Manner in which individual presents self to others—grooming, appearance, posture
   b. Emotional tone and change or constancy of levels
   c. Style of communication—verbal and nonverbal; ability to express appropriate emotion, follow train of thought; factors of dissonance, confusion, uncertainty
   d. Symptoms or symptomatic behavior
   e. Quality of relationship individual seeks to establish—direction, purposes, and uses of such relationships for individual
   f. Perception of self
   g. Social roles that are assumed or ascribed; competence in fulfilling these roles
   h. Relational behavior
      (1) Capacity for intimacy
      (2) Dependence–independence balance
      (3) Power and control conflicts
      (4) Exploitiveness
      (5) Openness

5. *Developmental factors*
   a. Role performance equated with life stage
   b. How developmental experiences have been interpreted and used

c. How individual has dealt with past conflicts, tasks, and problems

d. Uniqueness of present problem in life experience

The Place of Assessment in Practice Assessment is essential in clinical practice and serves several purposes:

- Identifying problems
- Identifying client motivations, strengths, and resources
- Identifying forces that may hinder the therapeutic plan (forces both internal and external to the client)
- Setting reasonable goals
- Determining appropriate intervention strategies
- Providing continuous evaluation of the process and indicating when the therapeutic plan should be changed

Although the individual assessment has been presented in linear form, it would be a mistake for nurses to make assessments in this structured way. Assessment is an ongoing, continually changing, dynamic process that Compton and Galaway (1979, p. 287) describe as a "squirming, wriggling, alive business." It provides an opportunity for nurse and client to engage in a partnership based on mutual definition of problems and goals. One example of a mental health assessment form in current use is the Erie County, New York, Comprehensive Mental Health Assessment reprinted in Appendix C.

Group and family assessment methods are discussed in Chapters 18 and 21, respectively.

SYSTEMS OF RECORDING

It is necesssary to communicate adequately in writing to inform mental health team members of the client's patterns of interaction. Recording is an important process; it often provides the basis for alterations in a treatment plan, for determining appropriate intervention strategies, for connecting members of the mental health team or mental health agencies with each other, for providing around-the-clock data on hospitalized clients, for evidence in court, and for research. An often unrecognized or disregarded purpose of recording is to provide quality accountability of psychiatric nursing practice. Recorded data can be used to give nurses feedback about their practice, through processes such

as the *psychiatric audit* (discussed later in this chapter). Exactly what system of recording is used depends on the agency.

What to Record

The most significant events the nurse records are the behavior patterns and interpersonal interactions of the client. It may also be important to record other significant happenings—the client's sleeping, eating, and elimination patterns, physical appearance, somatic treatments and medications, and so on.

The following types of notes should be made:

- *Progress over time.* Mental health agencies may require that notes be entered at specific times, such as at the end of each eight-hour shift or at the end of each twenty-four-hour period. When events of special significance occur, they should be recorded as soon after the event as possible, not held until the eight or twenty-four hours have elapsed.
- *Nurse-client relationship.* Notes are often made after each session with the client in individual, group, or family therapy. These notes summarize what occurred during the experience.
- *Summary report.* Summary reports are usually made at the termination of contact with the client—that is, when individual, group, or family therapy has ended. The summary report presents a clear and concise picture of the highlights of the experience.

Behavior and interaction notes should include examples rather than interpretations. Instead of writing "Ms. W. is hallucinating," it is preferable to write "Ms. W. states she hears Moses telling her not to get dressed today or leave her room."

Psychiatric Jargon: What to Avoid

The mental health field is rich in terms that nurses must learn if they are to speak the language in which mental health professionals converse. However, a heavy dose of jargon may cloud meaning and be counterproductive. The language of mental health, which relies heavily on words and phrases from psychology, has also borrowed from public health, sociology, anthropology, philosophy, and the federal bureaucracy. As Morgan and Moreno have put it (1973, p. 2): "In staff meetings of some centers, English is hardly spoken at all."

One journalist has labeled this psychological patter *psychobabble,* and he dubs the person using it "Psychobabbler"—"the victim of his own inability to describe human behavior with anything but platitudes" (Rosen 1975, p. 45). The roots of the old psychobabble, Rosen says, were really in the wholesale use of Freudian terms. It was a sort of intellectual one-upmanship.

Today, however, repetitive verbal formalities reduce psychological growth and therapeutic processes to a collection of standardized insights inadequate for the infinite variety of human problems. Unremitting use of jargon simplifies problems until it is difficult to see any depth in them. These terms are of very little help in understanding what is going on with a client. Nurses should, therefore, use jargon sparingly. The glossary at the end of this book may be particularly useful not only in defining the terms that mental health professionals use but also in identifying the point of view or perspective from which the terms have come into popular use.

Source-oriented Recording

Source-oriented records are becoming less common, as more agencies institute problem-oriented methods of recording. Source-oriented recording usually consists of a clinical record or chart that includes unassembled chronological notations made by individual health team members. Physicians write orders and progress notes in one place, and nurses chart their notes in another. Other members of the team may not contribute in writing at all. Laboratory findings are kept in a third isolated section of the chart. Close communication among mental health team members is hindered by source-oriented recording. Such systems often duplicate efforts and fail to pull information about the client into a logical whole.

Problem-oriented Recording

The problem-oriented system of recording is a major improvement over the source-oriented form. It is a way of organizing the same raw data into a comprehensive whole that can be used for assessment, planning, evaluation, research, and health care audits. The process stimulates mental health team members to gather, document, and describe data.

There are four necessary elements in problem-oriented recording systems:

1. *Data base.* The data base consists of all the information gathered at the initial contact with the client. It includes psychiatric history, psychosocial assessment, laboratory and physical findings, and the results of mental status examinations and psychological tests. The mental health supplement to the standard defined data base that is used in one mental health facility is presented in Figure 8–5.

2. *Problem list.* The problem list emerges from the data base and summarizes the problems of the client. It should also include the client's assets. It is continually updated in order to present an accurate picture of the client's current situation.

3. *Initial plans.* A section of the record delineates the therapeutic plans for the client. Plans are formulated in terms of the problems to which they relate.

4. *Progress notes.* Progress notes parallel items in the problem list. They are used to monitor the plans, identify the need for modification, and provide a follow-up. The progress notes include narrative notes, flow sheets, and a discharge summary.

   a. Narrative notes are written in SOAP style, an acronym for *subjective* (the problem as perceived by the client), *objective* (clinical findings or observations), *assessment* (what is suggested by an analysis and synthesis of the subjective and objective data), and *plan* (proposed solutions for the identified problems).

   b. Flow sheets are used to tabulate information in graphic form. They are useful when some factor must be monitored frequently.

   c. The discharge summary is a summary of each problem area and the level of resolution reached. It provides the essential data for community follow-up services.

Figure 8–6 demonstrates how one mental health facility uses problem-oriented progress notes.

Nursing Care Plans

Nursing care plans are a means of providing nursing personnel with information about the needs and therapeutic plans for each client. They are of major importance when an agency uses source-oriented recording methods, because they provide an ongoing, up-to-date record of goal-directed, individualized nursing care. When problem-oriented recording methods are used, nursing care plans may be an outgrowth of the record. Examples of nursing care plans appear in Chapters 14, 16, and 19, among others.

Algorithms

Algorithms are behavioral steps, or step-by-step procedures, for the management of common problems. Algorithms have proved useful protocols, particularly in settings that employ large numbers of paraprofessionals. At intake points in community mental health settings, such as walk-in neighborhood clinics, mental health workers often make the initial psychosocial assessment and may plan and implement treatment strategies. Clinical algorithms for common mental health problems would provide the nonprofessional with structured, standardized guidelines for decision-making.

Professional nurses in nonpsychiatric settings find clinical algorithms particularly useful in their front-line assessment as the primary care giver. Algorithms for depression and suicidal lethality have been found to be reliable and valid in these circumstances. See Figure 14–4 which presents this particular clinical algorithm.

Psychiatric Audits

The psychiatric audit is one means by which the quality of mental health services received by consumers can be appraised. The client's chart is reviewed to compare criteria for quality care with actual practice. Problem-oriented recording systems provide the descriptive documentation necessary for such a program. Although documentation may not always accurately indicate the quality of the care given, it is an important part of the process of keeping mental health workers accountable to consumers of their services.

The Interaction Process Analysis (IPA)

The Interaction Process Analysis is a verbatim and progressive recording of the verbal and nonverbal interactions that ensue between client and nurse within a given period of time. It is an important means of communication between nurses or nursing students and their clinical supervisors, consultants, or instructors about their client relationships. If nurses are to learn the function of therapeutic intervention—the process of the therapeutic client–nurse relationship—they must be able to study and review with objectivity the verbal and nonverbal components of the interaction to learn their potential significance. These components may express the existence of problems or attempts at resolution of these problems.

Purposes   The IPA serves a number of purposes:

- It helps nurses sharpen their skills of observation and listening by providing an opportunity to find clues that were not recognized during the face-to-face encounter.

- It improves the communication skills of nurses. When nurses examine their words, gestures, and nonverbal communication, they can reduce their use of clichés, double messages, and stereotyped, automatic comments.

- It gives the nurse a tool for assessing nurse–client interactions and gives the instructor, clinical supervisor, or consultant a tool for assessing and guiding the nurse in clinical work. It supplements memory, facilitates evaluation, and acquaints the student with rudimentary applied research skills. It also asks the nurse to produce written comments grounded in theory.

- It provides data from which nurses can assess their own behavior in interactions with clients. By encouraging nurses to examine their personal reactions to client behavior, the IPA enriches their self-understanding and experience. An added advantage of the IPA is that it allows nurses to look at the dynamics of nurse–client behavior when they are away from the interpersonal situation. They can often gain some objectivity through distance.

- It helps nurses plan nursing interventions. By evaluating the effectiveness of therapeutic strategies in actual clinical situations, and linking their observations to theory, nurses can identify additional or alternative nursing interventions.

Methods   There are a number of ways in which IPAs can be structured. Two-, three-, or four-column styles may be used. Regardless of the organizational style, however, the IPA should include these components:

- The verbal and nonverbal communication of the client

- The verbal and nonverbal communication of the nurse

- Analysis or interpretation of the possible significance of the communication

MEDICAL RECORD	SUPPLEMENT DEFINED DATA BASE

SUPPLEMENT TO *(Check only one)* PART ☑ I ☐ II ☐ III ☐ IV ☐ V ☐ VI

PREPARED BY *(Signature & Title)*	SERVICE	DATE
T. Knight, R.N. Clinical Specialist	Emergency	12-23-82

CHIEF COMPLAINT: In patient's own words and your impressions.

Gaunt, disheveled man in mid-thirties complains, "I have no purpose in life."

HISTORY AND DEVELOPMENT OF COMPLAINT

A. Date of onset and circumstances under which complaint developed.

Since resigning responsible position as electronics engineer 10 years ago, client has been drifting aimlessly, living at minimal level of subsistence. Brought in by police who found him living in his car in a school parking lot.

B. Previous hospitalizations and treatment-response to psychotropic drugs.

Unkown

C. Previous history of violent behavior, suicidal behavior, alcohol and drug abuse, previous arrests, and treatment by alcohol, drug and forensic program.

Experimentation with LSD and marijuana for 10 years at least 3x per week ... often once per day, with related impairment of social & occupational function. (No job, no dating relationships or social life)

MENTAL STATUS EXAMINATION

A. Overall general appearance. *Thin, unshaven dirty man in mid-thirties with poor nutrition, hygiene and tearful expression.*

B. Attitude and degree of cooperativeness.

Generally despondent but passively cooperative

C. Thought content and process—what patient thinks about—how patient thinks over and underproductive, spontaneous, circumstantial.

Thought content focuses on discovering solution to life's mysteries ... finding the key or answer.

Thought processes are vague and disconnected. Long periods of silence between verbalizations.

SUPPLEMENT

DEFINED

DATA BASE

VA FORM 10-7978g

D. Motoric behavior—overactive, underactive, inappropriate.

Slow, underactive bordering on catatonic low energy level

AFFECT

A. How the patient feels—shallow, anxious, depressed appropriate, inappropriate.

Depressed and discouraged — feelings of inadequacy

SENSORIUM MENTAL GRASP AND CAPACITY

A. Orientation/memory

Oriented to time, place + person

B. Abstract thinking

Can interpret proverbs but ponderously

C. Judgment/insight, adequate, complete, incomplete, distorted

Questionable

D. Cognitive disorder—hallucinations and delusions

No data available at this time

E. Estimate of intelligence

Average or above

DIAGNOSTIC IMPRESSION

Substance use disorder, Dysthymic Disorder (or Depressive Neurosis), Possible Avoidant Personality

TREATMENT PLAN

PROBLEMS	GOALS	TREATMENT
Poor nutritional status	*Improve status*	*Offer balanced, high cal diet suited to his vegetarian preference.*
Poor hygeine status	*Improve status*	*Encourage daily bathing. Refer to Dentist*
Dependence on Cannabis	*Decrease usage*	*Refer to Group Therapy*
Depression	*Control Sx*	*Prescribe anti-depress. medication. Refer to Psych. Therapist for individual counseling*

Figure 8–5

Example of supplement to data base. (From Veterans Administration Hospital, Buffalo, N.Y.)

MEDICAL RECORD	PROBLEM-ORIENTED PROGRESS NOTES

PROBLEM	Format—Problem title (Do not abbreviate) S-Subjective O-Objective A-Assessment P-Plans. (All notes must have signature and title
DATE / NO.	of person making entry.) Continue on reverse.

12-4-82 / 3

Problem Title: Angry and agitated.

Subjective: "I can't take anymore of this — I have to get out!"

Objective: Client is pacing, crying, waving his hands, yelling at nursing staff and other patients. Looks very upset.

Assessment: Client has just completed interview with his private therapist, who told him his wife has filed for divorce, and won't talk to him about it.

Plan:
1. *Give client time and space to decrease agitation*
2. *Offer him use of quiet room*
3. *Keep him in eye contact but do not engage him at this time*
4. *If he is not quieter in 1 hr offer PRN medication.*

T. Knight, RN
Clinical Specialist

PROBLEM-ORIENTED
PROGRESS NOTES

EXISTING STOCK OF VA FORM 10-7978i,
OCT 1974, WILL BE USED.

VA FORM 10-7978i

Figure 8-6

Sample form for problem-oriented progress notes. (From Veterans Administration Hospital, Buffalo, N.Y.)

- Identification of the nurse's own feelings
- Identification of the possible intent of the nurse's own communication
- Identification of the nurse's perception of the client's emotions and the intent of the client's communication
- Evaluation of the effectiveness of the approach, based on the above data
- The nursing alternatives used and the rationale for their use

The raw data or verbatim recording can be obtained in a number of ways.

ON-THE-SPOT RECORDING   The nurse may make brief notes on the spot, often using some type of shorthand code consisting of symbols and abbreviations, in a stenographer's notebook. There are several advantages to this form of recording. Notes on verbal communication can be made easily, it is a more accurate technique than attempting to recall after the experience, and it prevents the nurse from unwittingly editing out important material. It also demonstrates that the nurse is paying close attention to what the client says and does. However, the nurse usually interacts less freely and becomes less spontaneous when recording on the spot, because of the need to attend to the note-taking task. It may also limit observation of the nonverbal components of the client's communication.

AFTER-THE-FACT RECORDING   When gathering data by recall, it is important to record them as soon as possible after the interaction with the client. The most successful method is for nurses to structure their time so that they can begin writing in a quiet area immediately. The longer the time between interaction and recording, the less able nurses are to remember words and actions and their sequence. If it is difficult to set aside enough time, raw data alone should be recorded at once, and analysis of the data may be delayed. A delay may actually be helpful. It may allow a more objective interpretation, as time and distance make nurses less protective of their original behavior.

This method of recording is advantageous in that it does not require the nurse to take notes while paying close attention to the client. It thus does not curtail the nurse's spontaneity. The major disadvantage is that distortion may occur in the nurse's attempt to recall the interaction. Nurses using this method of recording tend to edit out or shorten important details.

TAPE-RECORDING   The most common form of mechanical recording is by audiotape. Tape recorders are now smaller, less expensive, and less obtrusive than earlier models were. Videotape recordings may also be used. Although now available in portable form, they are costly and are less commonly used.

Tape-recorded data can be transcribed at the nurse's leisure and provide a more accurate record of verbal interactions than notes. The recording avoids unintentional editing or condensation of important content. Nurses who use a tape recorder can reexperience tones of voice, pauses, silences, speaking rates, actual words, and sequences of responses. Because tapes force nurses to listen to themselves as they actually are rather than as they would like to be, using a tape recorder may cause anxiety. Clients may fear being "on tape" and refuse to give the nurse permission to tape the session. Other disadvantages to tape-recording are that it does not pick up visual cues, and transcribing the tape can be costly and/or time-consuming.

Confidentiality and Comprehensiveness of IPAs

The nurse who records client data has the responsibility to protect the client from unwarranted exposure. The client's name should not appear on the IPA, and the record should not be treated cavalierly or left lying about. The nurse's respect for the client's self-disclosures is one means by which the client can gauge the nurse's trustworthiness.

Cutting corners in preparing an IPA is inadvisable, because meaningful exchanges may be bypassed. In order to be an effective learning tool, the IPA should be comprehensive in its data collection. (See Chapter 6 for an example.)

KEY NURSING CONCEPTS

✔ The nursing process begins with assessment, and the primary resource for client data in most instances is the client.

✔ Correct problem identification and intervention strategies often depend on the quality of information sharing.

✔ Psychiatric client information is gathered and assessed through psychiatric history taking, mental status examination, psychological testing, psychosocial assessments, and interaction process analysis.

✔ The traditional history-taking process has a medical model orientation and is most concerned with gathering information about a client's psychiatric problem.

✔ The mental status examination is used to identify a person's general behavior and appearance, characteristics of talk, emotional state, special preoccupations and experiences, sensorium or orientation, memory, general intelligence, abstract thinking, and insight; its primary purpose is to gather data to formulate a psychiatric diagnosis, prognosis, and treatment plan.

✔ Psychological tests are tests concerned with measuring intelligence or personality.

✔ It is particularly important for the nurse to rule out a physiological or neurological basis for mental symptoms by conducting a thorough history, directly observing the client, and completing a neurological assessment.

✔ The *Diagnostic and Statistical Manual of Mental Disorders* (DSM-III) represents the American Psychiatric Association's most contemporary system for diagnosing and classifying mental disorders and is more congruent with holistic views of people than were DSM-II or DSM-I.

✔ Axes IV (Severity of Psychosocial Stressors) and V (Highest Level of Adaptive Functioning in the past year) of DSM-III best represent the practice domain of nursing and are the areas in which nursing's greatest contribution may lie.

✔ In conducting a psychosocial assessment to determine a client's problems include physical, intellectual, socioeconomic and developmental factors, personal values and goals, adaptive functioning, and response to present involvements.

✔ Recording provides the basis for alterations in treatment plan, determining intervention, linking health team members, round-the-clock data on hospitalized clients, evidence in court, and research.

✔ The most significant events the psychiatric nurse records are the behavior patterns and interpersonal interactions of the client.

✔ The psychosocial nurse uses psychiatric jargon sparingly, recognizing its inadequacies for understanding the depth and variety of human problems.

✔ Problem-oriented systems of recording are comprehensive in nature, logical in structure, and can be used in the psychiatric audit, to develop nursing care plans, and devise algorithms.

References

Compton, B. R., and Galaway, B. *Social Work Processes.* 2d. ed. Homewood, Ill.: Dorsey Press, 1979.

Diagnostic and Statistical Manual of Mental Disorders. 3d ed. Washington, D.C.: American Psychiatric Association, 1980.

Kaplan, H. I., and Sadock, B. J. *Modern Synopsis of Comprehensive Textbook of Psychiatry.* 3rd ed. Baltimore: Williams and Wilkins, 1981.

Morgan, A. J., and Moreno, J. W. *The Practice of Mental Health Nursing: A Community Approach.* Philadelphia: Lippincott, 1973.

Rosen, R. D. "Psychobabble." *New Times,* October 31, 1975, pp. 44–49.

Small, S. M. *Outline for Psychiatric Examination.* East Hanover, N.J.: Sandoz, 1980.

Spitzer, R. L., and Forman, J. B. W. "DSM-III Field Trials: II. Initial Experience with the Multiaxial System." *American Journal of Psychiatry* 136 (1979): 818–820.

Spitzer, R. L., Williams, J. B. W., Skodol, A. E. "DSM-III: The Major Achievements and an Overview." *American Journal of Psychiatry* 137 (1980): 151–164.

Williams, J. B. W., and Wilson, H. S. "A Psychiatric Nursing Perspective on DSM-III." *Journal of Psychosocial Nursing* 20 (1982): 14–20.

Further Reading

Alston, J., and Levet, J. "What's Happening? Practical Applications of the Mental Status Exam." *Nurse Practitioner Journal,* July–August (1977): 37–44.

Atwood, J.; Mitchell, P.; and Yarnall, S. "The POR: A System for Communication." *Nursing Clinics of North America* 9 (1974): 229.

Becknell, E., and Smith, D. *System of Nursing Practice: A Clinical Nursing Assessment Tool.* Philadelphia: Davis, 1975.

Berger, M. M., ed. *Videotape Techniques in Psychiatric Training and Treatment.* New York: Brunner/Mazel, 1970.

Berni, R., and Readey, H. *Problem-oriented Medical Record Implementation: Allied Health Peer Review.* St. Louis: C. V. Mosby, 1974.

Betts, V. T. "Using Psychiatric Audit as One Aspect of a Quality Assurance Program." In *Current Perspectives in Psychiatric Nursing: Issues and Trends,* vol. 2, edited by C. R. Kneisl and H. S. Wilson, pp. 202–208. St. Louis: C. V. Mosby, 1978.

Dodd, J. "Assessing Mental Status." *American Journal of Nursing* 78 (1978): 1501–1503.

Francis, G. M., and Munjas, B. A. *Manual of Socialpsychologic Assessment.* New York: Appleton-Century-Crofts, 1976.

Gahan, K. A. "Using Problem-oriented Records in Psychiatric Nursing." In *Current Perspectives in Psychiatric Nursing: Issues and Trends,* vol. 1, edited by C. R. Kneisl and H. S. Wilson, pp. 117–134. St. Louis: C. V. Mosby, 1976.

Hershey, N., and Laurence, R. "The Influence of Charting upon Liability Determinations." *Journal of Nursing Administration,* March–April (1976): 35.

Krall, M. L. "Guidelines for Writing Health Treatment Plans." *American Journal of Nursing* 76 (1976): 236.

Megahed, M. S., and Rosendahl, P. R. "Brain Tumors— an Assessment for Nursing Practitioners." *Nurse Practitioner Journal,* July–August (1977): 9–16.

"Patient Assessment: Neurological Examination" (Programmed Instruction). *American Journal of Nursing 75* (1975): Part I, September 1975, P.I. pp. 1–24; Part II, November 1975, P.I. pp. 1–24; and 76 (1976): Part III, April 1976, P.I. pp. 1–25.

Witt, R., and Mitchell, P. H. "Psychosocial and Mental-Emotional Status." In *Concepts Basic to Nursing,* 2d ed., edited by P. H. Mitchell, pp. 189–241. New York: McGraw-Hill, 1977.

Understanding Group Processes

CHAPTER OUTLINE

Historical Beginnings of Group Therapy

Varieties of Groups

Importance of Group Dynamics

    A Study in Contrast

    Characteristics of an Effective Group

Forces that Modify and Shape Groups

    Physical Environment

    Leadership

    Decision-making

    Trust

    Cohesion

    Power and Influence

Key Nursing Concepts

LEARNING OBJECTIVES

After reading this chapter, students should be able to

- Develop an appreciation for the influence of group dynamics in the lives of people
- Discuss the influence of the physical environment on a group
- Discuss the influence of the leadership approach on a group
- Discuss the process of decision making and the various decision-making methods
- Discuss the importance of trust in group functioning
- Discuss the importance of cohesion to effective group functioning
- Describe how power influences the nature, operation, and interpersonal patterns in groups

CHAPTER 9

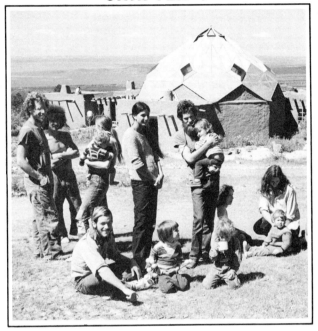

At the Lama Foundation in New Mexico, a communal, spiritual training center, the members share similar beliefs and attitudes. They achieve their goals and improve the quality of their lives through maximizing the forces that shape and modify enduring and effective groups.

destructive cults, a social phenomenon that is growing rapidly.

Much of the nurse's professional life is spent in groups—groups of clients and groups of colleagues with whom the nurse plans and implements the delivery of health care services. These groups can be more satisfying and rewarding if the nurse understands their dynamics. The goal of this chapter is to help the nurse understand group process and to lay the foundation for understanding Chapter 18, which deals with group therapy.

HISTORICAL BEGINNINGS OF GROUP THERAPY

Joseph Hersey Pratt, a Boston physician, began to work with tubercular clients in groups in the United States in 1906. His didactic groups of clients were organized as weekly classes of twenty to twenty-five members to whom he lectured on the importance of strict hygiene, diet, and rest in the treatment of tuberculosis. Pratt also offered support and encouragement to his clients, whose lengthy course of illness was discouraging at best. By 1930 he had established a clinic at the Boston Dispensary in which the group method was the central therapeutic focus. His writings throughout more than fifty years of work with groups of tubercular clients demonstrate his increasing awareness of the individual and group dynamics of this style of treatment. He is usually credited with being the founder of group psychotherapy.

Just before World War I, some physicians in the United States began to use group approaches in the treatment of psychiatric clients. E. W. Lazell, one of the better-known physicians, published the first contribution to the literature on use of group treatment with psychotic (specifically schizophrenic) individuals (1921). Like Pratt, he used the didactic lecture method. During this period, the emphasis was on encouraging, in-

People live most of their lives in groups. They depend on others for much of their sense of personal fulfillment and achievement. The activities they undertake toward personal fulfillment are, more often than not, activities that are carried out in the company of others.

Why are groups so important? Human beings are born into a group—the family—and their survival from the moment of birth depends on relationships formed with other human beings. The sense of self, of being, of personal identity derives from the ways in which people are perceived and responded to by the other members of the groups to which they belong. The self, according to the symbolic interactionist George Herbert Mead (1934), is essentially a social structure that arises from social experience. People interact with others at all stages of their lives in various groups—family groups, peer groups, work groups, play groups, worship groups.

Many of the goals people set for themselves cannot be achieved without membership in groups. Other people are important to each of us, just as we are important to others. Through cooperation and coordination in groups, we are able to achieve objectives and reach goals that would be unreachable through individual effort alone. In this way groups help us improve the quality of our lives. In certain circumstances, however, the effects of group membership may be disastrous. Chapter 26 details the effects of membership in

spiring, and persuading group members, while providing information designed to educate and influence them. At about the same time, a minister named L. C. Marsh, who became a psychiatrist, began to use other techniques in his work with groups. He had the members participate in art and dance classes, for example (Marsh 1935).

Joshua Bierer (1942) began his work in 1939 in Great Britain, where he established social clubs for the treatment of the mentally ill. His methods included discussion, writing, painting, and entertainment. Bierer believed that it was best to discuss individual problems in an impersonal way. He often disguised the problems for discussion to keep members of the group from realizing that their particular problems were under consideration. Bierer attempted to help persons solve their problems of daily living and change their attitudes toward life to more positive ones. His methods were based on those of Alfred Adler, who was using group psychotherapy in his child guidance work. Adler, a socialist and one of Sigmund Freud's first students, had established clinics to provide a variety of services and resource persons to large groups of working-class people with emotional problems. Social clubs like Bierer's gained importance in the United States over the years. Social clubs for the rehabilitation of "nervous persons" are still popular and can now be found throughout the United States. Perhaps the best known is Recovery, Inc.

A Viennese psychiatrist, Jacob L. Moreno (1946), introduced the term *group psychotherapy* into the clinical literature in 1932. His interest in drama, and particularly in what he called the "theatre of spontaneity," led him to formulate a particular kind of group psychotherapy called *psychodrama*. It uses dramatic techniques and the language and settings of theatrical productions to achieve psychotherapeutic goals. Moreno founded the first professional journal concerned with group psychotherapy and the first professional organization of group psychotherapists—known today as the American Society of Group Psychotherapy and Psychodrama.

During the late 1920s and early 1930s, Trigent Burrows (1927), another pupil of Freud's, became interested in applying psychoanalytic principles of treatment within group settings. An American psychoanalyst, Alexander Wolff (1949, 1950), began to apply these principles in groups. In his psychoanalytic group, he analyzed the individual in interaction with other individuals instead of treating a group. He took the position that it is not valuable, and may be detrimen-

tal, to attend to group dynamics in group analysis. At about the same time that Wolff was establishing psychoanalytic groups in the United States, S. H. Foulkes began a similar practice in Great Britain (see Foulkes and Anthony 1957). Both Wolff and Foulkes implemented their techniques with the armed forces in the United States and Great Britain.

Samuel R. Slavson, who is best known for developing activity group therapy for children, was also active in using psychoanalytic concepts in therapy groups (see Slavson 1947). He was a prime mover in establishing the American Group Psychotherapy Association and was the first editor of the *International Journal of Group Psychotherapy*.

During World War II, group psychotherapy grew extensively in the United States. It was hailed for its economic advantages, since a large number of clients could be treated by the relatively few available psychotherapists. It was also popular among military psychiatric personnel, who found themselves overwhelmed with the number of soldiers experiencing traumatic neuroses and needing some form of psychotherapy.

VARIETIES OF GROUPS

Since World War II there has been a tremendous proliferation of group methods. In addition to the recreational groups, educational groups, and even therapy groups that gained acceptance after the war, growth groups have become popular. These are oriented to understanding the self and the experience of membership by analyzing interactions with others in groups. The similarities and differences of these various groups are identified in Table 9–1.

IMPORTANCE OF GROUP DYNAMICS

A Study in Contrast

The Health Science Student Council at Anomie University held its monthly meeting yesterday. The council is composed of six members, four men and two women, who represent the health science schools on campus. The women represent nursing and occupational therapy, the men medicine, dentistry, pharmacy, and physical therapy. The members arrived out of breath and in

		Self-Awareness/		
Characteristic	**Task Groups**	**Growth Groups**	**Therapy Groups**	**Social Groups**
Purpose, goals	Performance of specific job or task explicitly agreed on by all members at initiation of group. Member participation is determined by task.	Development or use of interpersonal strengths. Broad objectives, such as to study group process, communication patterns, or problem solving are usually apparent at initiation of group.	Clearly defined: to do the work of therapy. Individual works toward self-understanding, more satisfactory ways of relating, handling stress, and so on.	Recreation, relaxation, and comfort promoted through mutual pleasure and enjoyment among friends and acquaintances in a social situation such as a party at someone's home.
Shared aim	To achieve group's task goal.	To improve functioning of group one returns to (job, family, community) through translation of one's own interpersonal strengths or to improve perception of members.	To improve perception of members and to improve individual health.	To experience fun, companionship, and satisfying relationships with friends.
Format	Defined at outset by leader and/or members. Method is specific to task to be performed.	Specific format, if any, and methods defined throughout group process by all members and leader/trainer. Lack of agenda and structure may produce some difficulty.	Defined by therapist within context of some psychotherapeutic orientation. Definition is apparent through implementation of therapeutic principles.	Usually spontaneous. May be defined by members in case of planned recreational activities.
Focus	Completion of specific task.	Interpersonal concerns around current situations.	Member-centered. Past experiences may be just as relevant as current concerns depending on therapist's orientation.	Member-centered toward enjoyment and mutual meeting of needs.

Table 9–1   DIFFERENCES IN CHARACTERISTICS OF TYPES OF GROUPS

Table continues on next page

disarray. The meeting had been called only one hour before by the council president, the representative from the medical school. One member arrived in damp and sweaty clothes directly from the racquetball court; another had been taking a nap and arrived without changing his clothes or washing his face, a third arrived in uniform and breathless, after dashing from the hospital unit to which she was assigned. The meeting was held in the health science library in a cramped and dusty room that stored little-used books from the early 1900s. The vice-president of the council chose to sit at the head of the rectangular table, forcing the president to take a seat on one side.

The meeting, to decide joint projects to be undertaken during the current academic year, got off to a rocky start. The vice-president attempted to open the meeting, until the president reminded him of his subordinate status. The president then reminded the members at length that,

Table 9–1 continued

Characteristic	Task Groups	Self-Awareness/ Growth Groups	Therapy Groups	Social Groups
Role of leader	To establish exchange of information among members and direct group toward task accomplishment, adhering to agenda.	To establish group interaction at emotional level among group members, and to serve as resource person guiding group by calling attention to certain events or processes and facilitating problem solving, mutual understanding, communication.	To establish group interaction between self and individual members and among group members. To facilitate members' interactions in work of therapy.	To meet basic requirements for social companionship, providing place, planning activity, preparing food, drink, etc.
Title of leader	Usually called chairperson.	Usually called trainer.	Usually called therapist.	Usually called host or hostess.
How leader differs from members	Chairperson identifies specific task, clarifies communication, and assists in expressing opinions and offering solutions.	Trainer differs from members by having superior skills in specialized area (understanding and facilitating group process). Trainer's superiority diminishes as group continues and members learn and implement similar skills.	Therapist differs from members by having superior skills in specialized area (group psychotherapy). Therapist never truly becomes member but may at times take on members' roles.	Host or hostess is member of group and works toward own as well as others' pleasure and enjoyment.
Requirements of leader	Qualified background and expertise in area of task emphasis. Must be accepted by members as an appropriate leader.	Sufficient preparation, experience, and skill to maintain effective control of interpersonal tensions.	Sufficient preparation and skill to undertake psychotherapy within context of situation.	Willingness to take steps to initiate social interaction.
Orientation of group work	Reality-oriented in terms of adhering to explicit work goal. If group deviates into interpersonal realm, task is not accomplished most efficiently.	Reality testing with here-and-now emphasis. Assumption is that members can correct inefficient patterns of relating and communicating with each other. Members learn group process experientially through participation and involvement.	Oriented toward having members gain insight as basis for changing patterns of behavior toward health.	Oriented toward having fun, seeking pleasure and relaxation, releasing tension.

Table continues on next page

Table 9-1 continued

Characteristic	Task Groups	Self-Awareness/ Growth Groups	Therapy Groups	Social Groups
Selection of members	Selection made possibly in terms of individual's functional role, not usually in terms of personal characteristics, often in terms of employment status.	Selection criteria range from simply expressed desire to become more self-aware to mixture of criteria based on personality characteristics— Fundamental Interpersonal Relationship Orientation (FIRO) scales (see Chapter 18), defenses, behavior patterns, etc.	Selection usually based on extensive consideration of constellation of personalities, behaviors, and needs and identification of group therapy as treatment of choice.	Selection based on considerations of friendship or social obligation. Host or hostess chooses whom to invite.
Title of members	Known as committee members.	May be called trainees.	Known as clients or, in some settings, patients.	Known as guests.
Interviewing of prospective members	Usually not interviewed before entry into group.	May or may not be interviewed and/or requested to complete questionnaires on personal data and personality characteristics before entry into group.	Extensive selection interview(s) required before entry into group.	Not interviewed. Usually known through prior social acquaintance.
Length of group life	Target date usually set in advance.	Tends to be short-term, with target date set in advance.	Usually not set. Termination date usually determined mutually by therapist and members.	May be set in advance or spontaneously determined.

of all the health science schools on campus, the medical school could provide the largest money grants to the council, because of that school's large alumni contributions and research grants. Most members expressed their unhappiness with the president's lecture. Members then began to debate which school was "better," had greater university and national recognition, had more money, and represented the most prestigious health science profession. Within ten minutes, the vice-president, the secretary, and two members had walked out. The question of which joint projects the council would undertake had not even been raised.

At the same time a group meeting was taking place at Connection College. Six women elected by their classmates represented the freshman, sophomore, junior, senior, first-year graduate, and second-year graduate nursing classes. The members arrived at the meeting ahead of the scheduled time. The chairperson had reserved one of the conference rooms at the Student Union, which are made available to student organizations, clubs, and committees for meetings. It was a comfortable room with bright windows, lounge chairs, and coffee service. The members sat around the circular table to discuss the items on the agenda—the choice of a place, date, and speaker for the commencement banquet.

The hour-long meeting proceeded smoothly. It was opened by the chairperson, who identified the group task and reviewed the experiences of the previous year's committee. She requested the opinions and ideas of each member and paid careful attention to any ideas or *suggestions offered. Each suggestion was discussed and evaluated by the entire group before being either accepted or rejected. Unanimous decisions were reached. After adjournment most members stayed behind to chat about other matters unrelated to the commencement banquet.*

These two group meetings were clearly different experiences for their members. The Health Science Student Council meeting at Anomie University was characterized by dissension, unilateral activity on the part of members, interpersonal conflict, and ineffectiveness. The Commencement Banquet Committee at Connection College was friendly, organized, thorough, and effective. This chapter will demonstrate that the factors that influence the behavior of the members of the Health Science Student Council and the Commencement Banquet Committee are factors that influence all groups in action—nursing teams, therapy groups, or whatever. These are the factors that make the difference between effective and ineffective groups.

Characteristics of an Effective Group

Any group, in order to be effective, has three main functions:

1. Accomplishing its designated goals
2. Maintaining its own cohesion
3. Developing and modifying its structure to improve its effectiveness

Some factors that influence these functions and can be used to evaluate the effectiveness of a given group are detailed in Table 9–2. They constitute the major characteristics generally observable in effective and ineffective groups and illustrate different ways of dealing with the dynamic forces in every group.

FORCES THAT MODIFY AND SHAPE GROUPS

Several forces shape the structure and functioning of groups. The following sections elaborate on factors such as: space and seating arrangements; color, noise level, and decor; leadership styles and roles; methods of decision-making; member trust; risk-taking behavior; cohesion and conformity; interpersonal attraction; and power and influence.

Physical Environment

Groups exist in complex environmental settings that strongly influence the group process. The building, room, and chair and table arrangements are aspects of the environmental setting that influence the operation of the group. Superimposed on the physical structure are the influences of territoriality, personal space, and cultural background. As you read about these influences, try to visualize the specific and peculiar features of hospital units, nurses' stations, and ward versus private accommodations for hospitalized clients.

Territoriality   Most people at some time have experienced violating an unspoken and unwritten rule by sitting in someone else's chosen seat. The violator may be treated to some form of protest—a direct one in which the "proprietor" of the seat points out the transgression, or a less direct one in which the proprietor may complain of the behavior to others and/or send darting glances of hostility in the violator's direction.

This assumption of proprietary rights to space is but one example of the notion of territoriality. *Territoriality* can be defined as the assumption of a proprietary attitude toward a geographical area by a person or a group. People defend their right to the designated territory against invasion by others despite the lack of legal sanction. People do not really "own" their territory but rather occupy it, permanently or intermittently, and act as if the property belonged to them.

Avoidance of intragroup conflict depends in part on the degree to which group members respect one another's territorial rights. Intergroup conflict may result when one group fails to respect the territorial rights of another group. In addition, territoriality provides a modicum of privacy for the individual or the group. It may also serve as a method of dominance by an individual or a group over others. The head nurse's chair, or the unit chief's chair at the head of the conference table, are concrete examples.

Personal Space   Personal space is an invisible bubble of territory around a person's body into which intruders may not come. It differs from territoriality in that it is space maintained and carried around with the person, rather than a specific geographical location.

Factor	Effective Groups	Ineffective Groups
	Table 9–2 COMPARATIVE FEATURES OF EFFECTIVE AND INEFFECTIVE GROUPS	
Atmosphere	Informal, comfortable, and relaxed. It is a working atmosphere in which people demonstrate their interest and involvement.	Obviously tense. Signs of boredom may appear.
Goal setting	Goals, tasks, and objectives are clarified, understood, and modified so that members of the group can commit themselves to cooperatively structured goals.	Unclear, misunderstood, or imposed goals may be accepted by members. The goals are competitively structured.
Leadership and member participation	Shift from time to time, depending on the circumstances. Different members assume leadership at various times, because of their knowledge or experience.	Delegated and based on authority. The chairperson may dominate the group, or the members may defer unduly. Member participation is unequal, with high-authority members dominating.
Goal emphasis	All three functions of groups—goal accomplishment, internal maintenance, and developmental change—are emphasized.	One or more functions may not be emphasized.
Communication	Open and two-way. Ideas and feelings are encouraged, both about the problem and about the group's operation.	Closed or one-way. Only the production of ideas is encouraged. Feelings are ignored or taboo. Members may be tentative or reluctant to be open and have "hidden agendas" (personal goals at cross-purposes with group goals)
Decision-making	By consensus, although various decision-making procedures appropriate to the situation may be instituted.	By the highest authority in the group with minimal involvement by members, or an inflexible style is imposed.
Cohesion	Facilitated through high levels of inclusion, trust, liking, and support.	Either ignored or used as a means of controlling members, thus promoting rigid conformity.
Conflict tolerance	The reasons for disagreements or conflicts are carefully examined and the group seeks to resolve them. The group accepts basic disagreements that cannot be resolved and lives with them.	Attempts may be made to ignore, deny, avoid, suppress, or override controversy by premature group action.
Power	Determined by the members' abilities and the information they possess. Power is shared. The issue is how to get the job done.	Determined by position in the group. Obedience to authority is strong. The issue is who controls.
Problem-solving ability	High. Constructive criticism is frequent, frank, relatively comfortable, and oriented toward removing obstacles to problem solving.	Low. Criticism may be destructive, taking the form of either overt or covert personal attacks. It prevents the group from getting the job done.
Self-evaluation as a group	Frequent. All members participate in evaluation and decisions about how to improve the group's functioning.	Minimal. What little evaluation there is may be done by the highest authority in the group, rather than by the membership as a whole.
Creativity	Encouraged. There is room within the group for members to become self-actualized and interpersonally effective.	Discouraged. People are afraid of appearing foolish if they put forth a creative thought.

Robert Sommer (1969), a psychologist who studied the effects of physical setting on attitudes and behavior, has stated that the best way to learn the location of the invisible boundary of personal space is to keep walking until somebody complains. The "Dear Abby" letter reprinted below offers one example of how unwanted intrusion into an individual's personal space may evoke discomfort, anger, and guilt.

> Dear Abby: I have a pet peeve that sounds so petty and stupid that I'm almost ashamed to mention it. It is people who come and sit down beside me on the piano bench while I'm playing. I don't know why this bothers me so much, but it does. Now you know, Abby, you can't tell someone to get up and go sit somewhere else without hurting their feelings. But it would be a big relief to me if I could get them to move in a nice inoffensive way. . . .
>
> Lost Chord

> Dear Lost: People want to sit beside you while you're playing because they are fascinated. Change your attitude and regard their presence as a compliment, and it might be easier to bear. P.S. You might also change your piano bench for a piano stool. [Abigail Van Buren, "Dear Abby," *San Franciso Chronicle,* May 25, 1965.]

Abigail Van Buren's piano stool suggestion illustrates a common defensive response to unwanted intrusion: selecting a position that is as inaccessible as possible. Another common response is flight. The need to defend personal space may also interfere with group functioning. Unwanted intrusion of one member into another's personal space evokes discomfort, unease, and other negative feelings. These feelings are revealed in the group dynamics and interfere with group progress.

The Influence of Cultural Background   Cultural background has been identified by the anthropologist Edward T. Hall (1969) as a strong influence on territoriality and personal space. An American who wants to be alone goes into a room and shuts the door, relying on architectural features for screening. English people have never developed the habit of using space to protect themselves from others. They use other barriers, such as "the silent treatment," which they expect others to recognize and respect. When an Englishman becomes silent in the company of an American man, the American is likely to expend extra effort to break through the barrier to assure himself that all is well.

Americans believe that propinquity (geographical nearness) is an acceptable basis for interaction. Living next door to a family entitles a neighbor family to socialize with the members, borrow a cup of flour from them, and have its children play with theirs. To the English, propinquity is not enough. Their relationships are patterned around social status rather than space.

English people and Americans vary in their use of the voice as well. Most English people and Europeans perceive Americans as loud. They believe this to be an intrusive trait, for being overheard interferes with the privacy of others. On the other hand, Americans perceive their "loudness" as an expression of openness, of having nothing to hide. They perceive the quiet or hushed conversations of others as sly or secretive.

Conditions that people in the United States perceive as crowded, others (Latin Americans and those from Mediterranean cultures) may perceive as spacious. A North American in Latin America or the Middle East is likely to feel crowded and hemmed in. People come too close and touch too much. The Middle Eastern or Latin American may experience the North American as cold. In English and Scandinavian cultures, it is the North American who perceives the others as aloof.

Subcultures as well as the major culture influence territoriality and personal space. For example, an English Canadian teacher in the province of Quebec may feel uncomfortable with the close presence of French Canadian students and colleagues of that subculture. Midwesterners may feel that the Jewish child from New York's Lower East Side is too personal and intrusive. The child might view the Midwesterner as cold and distant.

Influences from the various cultures carry over from generation to generation. For satisfactory functioning, a group must pay attention to the cultural factors that influence the individual member. In the large hospital or metropolitan mental health center where members of many cultures come together, these differences may promote misunderstandings and thwart effective group functioning. Special attention is paid to sociocultural considerations in Chapter 26.

Material Aspects of the Setting   The material aspects of the physical environment influence the functioning of groups in interesting ways. Students in social science courses are generally told of the well-known studies of worker productivity conducted at Western Electric Company (Roethlisberger and Dickson 1939). The investigators found that workers at first were more productive when the intensity of lighting was increased. However, after a period of weeks, production fell. This time the researchers decreased the lighting intensity and found the same effect—productivity increased again—even though this environmental change was directly opposite to the first one. This phenomenon, called the *Hawthorne effect,* spurred a host of other studies. Similar results were reported in studies that introduced music, coffee breaks, and so on. The primary variable seemed to be the workers' perception of the situation; if they believed that someone cared enough about them to be concerned about the conditions under which they worked, they responded by working harder and/or more effectively than when they believed no one cared about them.

Color and noise have been found to influence people's perceptions and performance. In one work situation, women workers complained of feeling uncomfortably cold with the thermostat at seventy-five degrees when the room was painted a cool blue (Seghers 1948). The same women complained of feeling too warm at the same temperature, when the room was painted in warm yellows and restful greens. Recent research indicates that a specific shade of pink initially decreases aggressive behavior. In response, some prisons have painted their jail cells pink. Unpredictable noise has been found to evoke feelings of frustration and lead to a decrease in performance. Sound conditioning of work areas has been found to reduce worker discomfort and annoyance.

Other studies have been done on the effects of "beautiful" rooms versus "ugly" rooms. The beautiful room was an attractively decorated, comfortable study. The ugly room was a dissheveled, unkempt, and unsightly storeroom. Participants in the ugly room reported more headaches, monotony, fatigue, hostility, discontent, and room avoidance than did participants in the beautiful room (Mintz 1956).

These studies about the material aspects of a setting indicate that elements of the environment are important in determining group and individual behavior. Productivity, interpersonal behavior, and intrapsychic experiences are all affected.

Spatial Arrangements   Seating arrangements have been methodically studied since Bernard Steinzor first wrote about the face-to-face discussion groups he was conducting in 1950. His interest was piqued by the behavior of one of his group members—a man who changed his seat in order to sit directly opposite another man with whom he had previously had an argument. Since that time, researchers have found that adults prefer a side-by-side arrangement for cooperation and a direct face-to-face arrangement for competi-

tion. This knowledge can be helpful in understanding the interaction among members of a psychotherapy group, a nursing team conference, or an interdisciplinary clinical conference at a community mental health agency.

People also select positions according to their perceived status in the group. Studies of twelve-person jury tables have demonstrated that jurors holding managerial or professional status frequently select the chair at the head of the table. Jurors seated at the end positions of the rectangular jury table tended to be more influential and to participate more than persons who chose side positions (Strodtbeck and Hook 1961).

There is also a relationship between spatial arrangement and leadership. Since the person who sits at the head of the table is usually perceived as the leader, the spatial position a person occupies in a group has important consequences for that person's chances of emerging as a group leader or for undertaking significant leadership responsibilities. Round tables tend to enhance the development of leadership traits among the membership rather than to invest certain members with authority because of their spatial position.

There are many other fascinating facets to the influence of space and environment on groups and individuals. This presentation provides only a starting point for further study by interested readers.

Leadership

Leadership functions within a group are executed under two general conditions: (1) by the person designated as the leader, and (2) by members who engage in leadership behavior. This distinction is an important one for understanding the emergence of leadership within groups.

The process of leadership is an influence relationship that occurs among mutually dependent group members in their attempts to achieve the group's goals. Because all group members influence other members, at times, each member will exert leadership at some time in the group's life. This approach to understanding leadership behavior is called the *distributed functions approach.* Other approaches will also be considered in this section.

Trait Approach   The trait approach is essentially a "great person" theory. It is based on the belief that a leader is a charismatic person who possesses unique, inborn leadership traits. Its central thesis is that leaders are born, not made; discovered, not trained.

However, researchers have found similar traits both in leaders and in followers, so this theory does not explain what makes one person assume a leadership role while another does not. The assumption can be made, however, that people who are energetic, self-confident, determined, and motivated to succeed will become leaders, because they work hard to reach positions of leadership.

Position Approach   The position approach defines leadership as a position of authority in the formal role system that defines the authority hierarchy. While this approach can certainly explain who has the designated title of leader, at a drug-abuse outreach center, for example, it does not take into account the fact that other members beside the designated leader influence the group's activities.

Style Approach   This classic theory of leadership behavior developed in 1939 by Lewin, Lippitt, and White identified three leadership styles: democratic, autocratic, and laissez faire. In the *democratic* style, the leader functions as a facilitator who encourages group discussion in decision-making. The *autocratic* leader is one who determines policies unilaterally and gives orders and directions to the group members. The *laissez faire* condition is characterized by a "hands off" style in which the leader participates at a minimal level.

The democratic style has proved the most effective. However, there are conditions under which each of the other two styles seems to be the most effective. For example, when an urgent decision is necessary, the autocratic style may be the most effective. A laissez faire style facilitates group functioning best when a group has made an effective decision, is committed to it, and is able to implement it.

Popularity of the style approach has now waned in favor of the more comprehensive distributed functions theory of leadership.

Distributed Functions Approach   The functional approach to group leadership is based on two major beliefs:

1. Any member of a group may become a leader by taking actions that serve group functions.
2. Different members may fulfill various functions.

Each member may enact more than one role during a meeting of the group and a wide range of roles in successive participations. Any or all of the roles may be played by any member. The various functional roles may be grouped in two categories:

1. *Task roles* are related to the task of the group. Their purpose is to facilitate and coordinate group efforts in the selection, definition, and solution of a group problem. Examples of task roles are *information seeker, information giver, elaborator, procedural technician, coordinator, opinion seeker,* and *opinion giver* among others.
2. *Maintenance roles* are oriented toward building group-centered attitudes among the members and maintaining and perpetuating group-centered behavior. Members who function as *encourager, compromiser, standard setter, follower, group observer,* or *harmonizer* carry out some of the maintenance roles possible in groups.

Sometimes members of a group behave in ways designed to satisfy individual needs that are irrelevant to the group task. These *self-serving roles* (the *recognition seeker, blocker, aggressor, dominator, self-confessor,* and *playboy* for example) may also be negatively oriented to group maintenance functions. If a group is to function effectively, it must perform a self-diagnosis to determine what the needs of the group are, and how they can be met, so that the self-serving roles no longer present obstacles to effective functioning.

The functional theory of group leadership emphasizes the importance of distributing leadership functions among the group members. Distributed leadership is believed to be the most effective approach, because it teaches people the diagnostic skills and behaviors needed to accomplish the group task and maintain good interpersonal relationships. The distributed functions approach can be best described through its main assumption: Responsible membership is the same thing as responsible leadership. Of course, in psychotherapy groups, there may be some functions or activities that are largely, or even solely, the province of the therapist.

Decision-making

A group that makes sound decisions is a group that functions effectively. The purpose of group decision-making is to construct well-conceived, well-understood, and well-accepted realistic actions toward the goals agreed on by the group.

Effective Decisions

Five major characteristics of effective decisions are:

1. The resources of the group members are well used. The group listens to all members who have ideas or input helpful to the decision-making process.
2. The group's time is well used. The group concentrates on the task at hand and keeps interruptions and sidetracks to a minimum.
3. The decision is correct or of high quality. The alternative the group picks to execute is appropriate, reasonable, and error-free.
4. The decision is put into effect fully by group members. Members feel committed to the decision and responsible for its implementation.
5. The problem-solving ability of the group is enhanced. Members feel satisfied with their participation, and the positive group atmosphere increases the members' perception of themselves as adequate problem solvers.

Decision Methods

There are several ways in which decisions can be made by a group.

- Decisions by *consensus* are reached when a group arrives at a collective opinion after each member has had a fair chance to exert influence. Unanimity is not always present in consensus decisions. However, members support the decision and are willing to give it a try.
- Sometimes group decisions are made by the person selected as the *group expert.*
- *Averaging members' opinions* is another method for arriving at decisions. It means that the most popular opinion becomes the group decision. It may nonetheless be held by fewer than half the members.
- *Decision by majority vote,* 51 percent or more of the members, is the most common method used.
- Decisions can be made through *minority control* of a group. Executive committees of groups with many members exercise minority control of the whole group. A small minority may also quickly and forcefully "railroad" decisions (force the group to accept them by exerting intense pressure).

- In decision-making by an *authority after discussion* with the members, the designated leader makes the final decision but first discusses the issue with the members to get their ideas and views.
- In decisions by *authority rule without discussion,* the designated leader makes decisions without consulting the group.

Each of these decision-making methods is appropriate at certain times. In psychotherapy groups, certain decisions (such as whether to add a new member, for example) should be made by the group expert—in this instance the group therapist—who has the clinical expertise. These are further discussed in Chapter 18. A group that has to make a decision must take several factors into account before selecting a method. Questions such as these should be raised: What type of decision has to be made? How much time can be spent in the decision-making process? What resources are available to the group? What is the past history of the group? What is the task to be worked on? How does the setting influence the method that should be chosen? What are the consequences of the particular method for the group's future operation? These questions are answered for each of the seven decision-making methods in Table 9–3.

Risk Taking in Group Decisions

An interesting phenomenon, the *risky shift,* occurs in the decision-making process of groups. Social psychologists Kogan and Wallach (1964) have observed that, when individuals who had previously made private decisions engaged in group discussion, the group reached riskier decisions than the members' private decisions. A risky shift has profound implications, particularly when the decision of a group may involve a large number of people.

Three major explanations for the risky shift have been given. The first is that high risk takers are more influential and persuasive than low risk takers. Thus, in a group decision the high risk takers' position will tend to win out over less risky alternatives. The second hypothesis is that in group decision-making, responsibility is diffused. Any cost or imagined loss that might result from a risky decision is shared by all rather than placed at the feet of just one individual. The final explanation is that information about peer norms is received by group members through decision-making.

Table 9–3   STRENGTHS AND LIMITATIONS OF DECISION-MAKING METHODS

Method	Strengths	Limitations
Consensus	Produces innovative, creative, and high-quality decision Elicits commitment by all members to implement decision Uses the resources of all members Enhances future decision-making ability of group Is useful in making serious, important, and complex decisions requiring commitment from all members	Takes great deal of time and psychological energy and high level of member skill Can be used only when time pressure is minimal and no emergency is in progress
Expert	Is useful when expertise of one person is so far superior to that of all other group members that little is to be gained by discussion Should be used when need for membership action in implementing decision is slight	Can be ineffective when it is difficult to determine who is expert Does not build commitment for implementing decision Loses advantages of group interaction May result in resentment and disagreement that can sabotage and deteriorate group effectiveness Does not use resources of other members
Average of members' opinions	Is useful when it is difficult to get group members together to talk, when decision is so urgent that there is no time for group discussion, when member commitment is not necessary for implementing decision, and when group members lack skills and information to make decision any other way Is applicable to simple, routine decisions	Does not allow enough interaction among group members for them to gain from each other's resources and to get benefits of group discussion Does not build commitment for implementing decision Leaves unresolved conflict and controversy that may damage future group effectiveness
Majority vote	Can be used when sufficient time is lacking for decision by consensus or when decision is not so important that consensus needs to be used, and when complete member commitment is not necessary for implementing decision Closes discussion on issues that are not highly important for group	Usually leaves an alienated minority, which damages future group effectiveness May lose relevant resources of many group members Does not build total commitment for implementing decision Does not obtain full benefit of group interaction

Table continues on next page

They learn the value attached to being risky in the process. Members then attempt to meet the group norm in relation to both risk and caution.

Indecisiveness   Sometimes a group has a hard time making decisions. Members find themselves unable to agree what the decision should be. Some reasons for indecisiveness are:

- Fear of the consequences of the decision
- Conflicts among members that make cooperative activity difficult
- Choice of a decision-making method inappropriate to the immediate situation
- Member loyalty to other groups that makes it difficult to commit themselves to making good decisions in this group

	Table 9–3 continued	
Method	**Strengths**	**Limitations**
Minority control	Can be used when everyone cannot meet to make decision, when group is under such time pressure that it must delegate responsibility to committee, when only few members have any relevant resources, when broad member commitment is not needed to implement decision Is useful for simple, routine decisions	Does not use resources of many group members Does not establish widespread commitment for implementing decision Can leave unresolved conflict and controversy that may damage future group effectiveness Does not obtain much benefit from group interaction
Authority rule after discussion	Like consensus, uses resources of group members more than other methods Gains some benefits of group discussion	Does not develop commitment for implementing decision Does not resolve controversies and conflicts among group members Tends to create situations in which group members either compete to impress designated leader or tell leader what they think leader wants to hear
Authority rule without discussion	Applies more to administrative needs than to member needs Is useful for simple, routine decisions Should be used when very little time is available to make decision, when group members expect designated leader to make decision, and when group members lack skills and information to make decision any other way	Uses only one person as resource for every decision Loses advantages of group interaction Develops no commitment among other group members for implementing decision Can produce resentment and disagreement that may sabotage and reduce group effectiveness Does not use resources of other members

Source: David W. Johnson and Frank P. Johnson, *Joining Together: Group Theory and Group Skills* © 1975, pp. 80-81. Adapted by permission of Prentice-Hall, Inc., Englewood Cliffs, New Jersey.

Once the reasons for indecisiveness have been identified and put on the table, a group can work to remove the obstacles in its way. It may be necessary for the group to rearrange its membership, redefine its task, select another decision-making method, or work at resolving the conflicts among its members before continuing its work on the identified task.

Trust

The complex phenomenon of trust has been studied by a variety of theorists and researchers. Some of the better-known work has been done by Morton Deutsch (1949, 1958). In his view, trusting behavior consists of the following four steps:

1. A person is in a situation where the decision to trust another may result in either positive or negative consequences for the self. The person realizes the risk involved in trusting another.

2. The person realizes that the future behavior of the other determines whether trusting will bring positive or negative consequences for the self.

3. The person will suffer more if the trust is violated than the person will gain if the trust is fulfilled.

4. The person feels reasonably confident that the other will behave in ways that will bring the beneficial consequences.

The person who decides to have minor elective surgery of little consequence is engaging in trusting behavior. The client recognizes that the choice could lead to either beneficial or harmful consequences, realizes that the consequences of the choice depend on the behavior of the surgeon, would suffer much more if the trust is violated and the surgeon does a bad job, and feels relatively confident that the surgeon will make sure that beneficial consequences result.

Trust within relationships is built when people disclose more and more of their thoughts, perceptions, attitudes, and reactions to one another. The group member who makes a suggestion; discloses an attitude, feeling, experience, or perception; gives feedback; or confronts another also engages in trusting behavior and assumes the risks inherent in trusting. Trusting and being trusted are intimately linked to risk taking. The level of trust among the members of a group determines the extent of risk-taking behavior in the group.

Cohesion

"Hanging together" is the aspect of group life generally referred to as *group cohesiveness*. Groups that hang together or cohere possess a certain spirit of common purpose. The members can be said to have a yen for each other, for mutual association. Groups in which cohesion is minimal are those that seem always on the verge of breaking up or falling apart. Cohesion is the primary factor keeping a group in existence and working effectively.

The Need for Attraction A group is cohesive when its members are attracted to it. People are attracted to a group for a wide variety of reasons. The group may meet their needs for affiliation, interpersonal security, or financial security. It may have admired members who not only are available for human interaction but also share salient attitudes, values, interests, and beliefs. An attractive group has explicit, mutual, and attainable group goals with clear paths to goal attainment. Its members engage in a sort of interdependence that is cooperative rather than competitive. The activities the group undertakes are satisfying and successful, and there is a high degree of member participation in a democratic structure. Communication networks are open, central, and flexible in a warm and friendly atmosphere.

This implies that cohesive groups are not born but developed. While some features of attraction may account for a "love-at-first-sight" phenomenon, others do

not become evident until the group has come together long enough to have shared experiences that provide the basis for attraction.

Evaluating Cohesion What indicates that the "spirit" of cohesion exists in a given group? How do groups with sufficient cohesion differ from groups with minimal cohesion? At the beginning of this section on group dynamics we introduced two groups whose characteristics were radically different. The Health Science Student Council at Anomie University was only minimally cohesive. The more effective group, the Commencement Banquet Committee at Connection College, was "groupier." Table 9–4 identifies the characteristics of highly cohesive groups and compares them to those of minimally cohesive groups.

Building Cohesion How can a group's tendency to cohere be enhanced? Most of the methods have been touched on already in this chapter. They include: increasing the trusting and trustworthy behavior of members; the affection expressed among members; the expressions of inclusion and acceptance among members; and the influence that members have on one another. Two other methods for building cohesion are promoting group norms and structuring cooperative relationships among group members.

PROMOTING GROUP NORMS *Norms* are the set of unwritten rules of conduct or prescriptions of behavior established by members of a group. They derive from the common beliefs of the group about appropriate behavior. In other words, they tell how members are expected to behave. Norms prevent chaos because they lay out the expectations of members. They help members predict the behavior of others and anticipate the actions that they should take themselves.

Norms are evaluative. They tell members what *ought* and *ought not* be done. They represent value judgments that establish accepted standards for behavior. Some of the characteristics of norms that influence group behavior are:

- Norms are developed around situations that are important to the group. Groups do not establish norms for every conceivable situation.

- Norms may apply to every member of a group, or to certain members in specific roles only. For example, skiers are expected to wait their turn in the chair lift line, but a member of the National Ski Patrol may cut in at the head of the line without challenge.

Table 9–4	GROUP COHESION ASSESSMENT		
Characteristics of High Cohesion Groups	**Characteristics of Low Cohesion Groups**	**Characteristics of High Cohesion Groups**	**Characteristics of Low Cohesion Groups**
Members like one another	Members seem uncaring or may actively dislike one another	Group goals are consistent with goals of individuals	Group goals and individual goals are not consistent
Members are friendly and willing to interact	Members seem unfriendly and unwilling to become involved	Group goals can best be handled by group action	Goals can best be handled by individual action
Members enjoy interacting with one another and interact readily	Members gain little pleasure from interaction and interact reluctantly	Group goals difficult to achieve are met by persistent efforts	Group goals difficult to achieve are given up
Members receive support on issues from one another	Members fail to give one another active support	Attendance is high, and members arrive on time	Attendance is low or uneven, and members may arrive late or leave early
Members praise one another for accomplishments	Members fail to acknowledge, or move to denigrate one another's accomplishments	Efforts are directed toward maintaining, strengthening, and regulating group	Efforts are not directed toward maintaining, strengthening, and regulating group
Members share similar opinions and attitudes	Members have dissimilar or mutually exclusive opinions and attitudes	Risk taking is high	Risk taking is low
		Participation is high	Participation is low
Members are likely to influence one another and are willing to be influenced by other members	Members make few influence attempts and are unwilling to be influenced by other members	Commitment to group goals increases	Commitment to group goals is minimal
		Communication is high	Communication is low
		"We" is frequently heard in discussions	"I" is frequently heard in discussions
Members accept assigned tasks and roles readily	Members are reluctant or refuse to accept assigned tasks and roles	Leadership is democratic	Leadership is autocratic
Members trust one another	Members do not trust one another	Group action is interdependent and cooperative	Group action is independent and competitive
Members are loyal to group and defend it against external criticism and attack	Members do not defend group and may criticize it to others	Group output and productivity are high	Group output and productivity are low
		Group norms are adhered to and protected	Group norms are violated
Members stay in group	Members drop out	Members experience increase in security and self-esteem and reduction in anxiety	Members experience decrease in security and self-esteem and increase in anxiety
Group goals are valued	Group goals are not valued	Satisfaction with members and work of group is high	Satisfaction with members and work of group is low

• Norms vary in the degree to which they are accepted by group members. Most persons accept the norm that the driver of a vehicle should not pass a stopped school bus, but many violate the norm that drivers of slow-moving vehicles should stay in the right-hand lane.

- Norms vary in the extent to which people can permissibly deviate from them. Violating a norm that members arrive for meetings on time is a more acceptable transgression than violating the norm against killing another person.
- Norms differ in the sanctions applied for their violation. Members who arrive late may be subjected to mild disapproval, but the member who kills another may be punished with life imprisonment or the death penalty.

The importance of norms in the power, influence, and conformity aspects of group life is discussed more completely later in this chapter.

STRUCTURING COOPERATIVE RELATIONSHIPS All task groups have group goals. Anomie University's Health Science Student Council had the goal of deciding the joint projects to be undertaken during the current academic year. Connection College Commencement Banquet Committee was to decide the place, date, and speaker for the banquet. It takes cooperative action on the part of members to meet group goals.

In addition to group goals, members have individual goals. When the personal or individual goals of group members differ from the group goals, competitive relationships may develop that destroy the effectiveness of group relationships. For example, it is common for members who are in disagreement with the group goals to acquire hidden agendas that interfere with group functioning. A *hidden agenda* may be defined as a personal goal, unknown to the other group members, which is at cross-purposes with the dominant group goals. The vice-president of the Health Science Student Council at Anomie University may have had a hidden agenda (deposing the president, for example) that influenced his selection of a seat at the traditional "head of the table" position and his usurping of the president's privilege of opening the meeting.

In order to structure cooperative relationships around group and individual goals, it is important to review and discuss group goals thoroughly when the group is formed even though goals may have been prescribed for the group by others. Member understanding of the goals and the tasks necessary to reach them will be clarified or corrected through discussion. The group goals should be recognized and rephrased during the discussion, encouraging members to feel a sense of "ownership" toward the goals. Table 9–5 provides suggestions for dealing with hidden agendas.

Cooperative relationships to meet goals are extremely important for group effectiveness. When hidden agendas structure a group competitively, members will strive for individual goal accomplishment in a way that blocks others from obtaining the group goal.

Groupthink: A Special Case of Cohesion The Bay of Pigs incident during the administration of President John F. Kennedy was based on the beliefs of the in-group that the Cuban air force was ineffectual and the army weak, that a small group of Cuban exiles could establish a beachhead, and that Fidel Castro would be unable to suppress an uprising in support of the exiles. All these beliefs proved false, and the invasion of Cuba based on them was a fiasco. Similarly, the in-group around Admiral H. E. Kimmel failed to prepare for the Japanese assault on Pearl Harbor during World War II despite repeated warnings that such an attack was imminent; President Lyndon B. Johnson's "Tuesday Luncheon Group" made a series of grossly miscalculated decisions with scarring effects on the people of Vietnam and the United States; and the inner cabinet of England's Neville Chamberlain turned over Czechoslovakia, Austria, Poland, and other small European countries to the Nazis before World War II.

Groups that "hang together" can sometimes be more easily hanged. Irving Janis (1971a, 1971b) has coined the term *groupthink,* a word reminiscent of George Orwell's *1984* society, as a way to refer to the mode of thinking engaged in by members of a highly cohesive in-group in which uniformity and agreement are given such high priority that critical thinking is impossible or unacceptable. Groups infected with groupthink have developed group norms around the maintenance of unity and loyalty, no matter what the cost. The religious cults discussed in Chapter 26 are examples of groups in which critical thinking is both impossible and unacceptable.

How can one tell if a group is obsessed with the need for concurrence that characterizes groupthink? Janis (1971a, p. 44) lists the following main symptoms of groupthink:

- *Invulnerability.* Most or all members of the in-group share an *illusion* of invulnerability that gives them some degree of reassurance about obvious dangers. It makes them overoptimistic and willing to take extraordinary risks. It also makes them ignore clear warnings of danger.
- *Rationale.* Victims of groupthink collectively construct rationalizations in order to discount warnings and other forms of negative feedback that, taken seriously, might lead the group members to reconsider

Table 9-5 STEPS FOR DEALING WITH HIDDEN AGENDAS	
Suggestion	**Rationale**
Look for the presence of hidden agendas.	The group cannot diagnose or solve a problem until its presence is recognized.
Once the presence of hidden agendas has been pinpointed, judge whether or not they should be brought to the surface and rectified.	Sometimes hidden agendas should be left undisturbed, if the consequences of bringing them to the attention of the entire group may be negative, rather than facilitating the work of the group.
Determine whether group members are willing and able to deal with hidden agendas. Suggest that perhaps not all there is to say has been said, but do not force members to disclose their hidden agendas.	Disclosing hidden agendas may be harmful to group attempts to reach cohesion and may result in the premature ouster of the member with the hidden agenda.
Accept members whose hidden agendas have been revealed, without rejecting or criticizing them.	Hidden agendas are common and legitimate group occurrences. They should be worked on in the same way that group tasks are.
Devote group time to working on the hidden agendas of members.	Hidden agendas impede group progress. The attention given to hidden agendas should be determined by the extent of the effect on group effectiveness.
As a group, evaluate the group's ability to deal with hidden agendas.	Learning better ways of handling agendas more openly will result from evaluation and reduce the need for keeping agendas hidden.

their assumptions each time they recommit themselves to past decisions.

- *Morality.* Victims of groupthink believe unquestioningly in the inherent morality of their group. This belief inclines the members to ignore the ethical or moral consequences of their decisions.

- *Stereotypes.* Victims of groupthink hold stereotyped views of the leaders of enemy groups, considering them either so evil that genuine attempts at negotiating differences with them are unwarranted, or too weak or stupid to deal effectively with the group's attacks. This leads the group to make riskier attempts to defeat the enemy's purposes.

- *Pressure.* Victims of groupthink apply direct pressure to any individual who momentarily expresses doubts about any of the group's shared illusions or questions the validity of the arguments supporting a policy alternative favored by the majority. This gambit reinforces the concurrence-seeking norm that loyal members are expected to maintain.

- *Self-censorship.* Victims of groupthink avoid deviating from what appears to be a group consensus. They keep silent about their misgivings and minimize even to themselves the importance of their doubts.

- *Unanimity.* Victims of groupthink share an *illusion* of unanimity within the group about almost all judgments. This is expressed by members who speak in favor of the majority vote.

- *Mindguards.* Victims of groupthink sometimes appoint themselves as mindguards to protect the leader and fellow members from adverse information that might break the confidence they share in the effectiveness and morality of past decisions.

Members afflicted with groupthink behave in characteristic ways, according to Janis (1971a, p. 75):

- They limit group discussions to a few alternative courses of action (often only two) without an initial survey of all worthwhile alternatives.

- Members fail to reexamine the course of action initially preferred by the majority after they learn of risks and drawbacks they had not considered originally.

- Members spend little or no time discussing whether there are gains they may have overlooked in a rejected alternative or ways of reducing the seemingly prohibitive costs that made a rejected alternative appear undesirable to them.

- Members make little or no attempt to obtain information from experts within their own organizations who might be able to supply more precise estimates of potential losses and gains.

- Members show positive interest in facts and opinions that support their preferred policy. They tend to ignore facts and opinions that do not.

- The group spends little time deliberating about how the chosen policy might be hindered by bureaucratic inertia, sabotaged by political opponents, or temporarily derailed by common accidents. It fails to work out contingency plans to cope with foreseeable setbacks that could endanger the overall success of the chosen course.

How can groupthink be prevented? Table 9–6 identifies goals that prevent or remedy groupthink and suggests constructive behaviors a group may undertake to correct its functioning.

Groupthink has a negative influence on the quality of the decisions made by a group. The groupthink decision is less reliable than decisions by consensus. Too much cohesiveness leads members to pat each other on the back even while headed toward disaster.

Power and Influence

Power is a potent force that explains a good deal about the nature, operation, and patterns of interpersonal behavior. It is clearly impossible to discuss group dynamics without discussing power because it is impossible to interact without influencing, and being influenced by, others. This process constantly occurs within groups, forcing members to adjust to one another and modify their behavior. In some instances, attitudes and beliefs are modified as well. *Power* can be defined as the ability of one person to influence another person in some way. The terms *power* and *influence* are used interchangeably in this chapter.

There is a definite process by which power is mobilized to help in accomplishing goals. Powerful people determine and clarify their personal goals, affirm the resources or informational level they bring to the group (what they can contribute toward the accomplishment of their goals and the goals of group members), determine what coalitions are necessary to secure the information and resources needed to accomplish the goals, develop the necessary coalitions so that the resources can be applied (that is, find out what they want from the others, what the others want

from them, and what they can exchange so that everyone can accomplish the goals), and carry out the necessary activities for reaching the goals.

Some people perceive power and influence as negative forces. These people are frequently unaware of the influence they themselves exert on others, or they confuse the judicious use of power in building effective groups with the use of power to control, manage, and manipulate others. Nurses are only now becoming aware of how they might employ influence in the service of their clients and their profession. Chapter 5 takes up the problem of power phrased in the language of ethics.

Power Sources According to power theorists, there are six possible sources of a person's power:

1. Reward power
2. Coercive power
3. Legitimate power
4. Referent power
5. Expert power
6. Informational power

People have *reward power* if they can deliver positive consequences or remove negative ones in response to the behavior of group members. They have *coercive power* if they can deliver negative consequences or remove positive ones in response to the behavior of group members. When group members believe a person ought to have influence over them because of the person's position in the group or organization, that person can be said to have *legitimate power*. A person has *referent power* when group members identify with or want to be like that person. Members do what that person wants out of liking, respect, and the desire to be liked themselves. The person with *expert power* is seen by the group as trustworthy and having some special knowledge or skill. When a person has *informational power*, group members believe that this person has access to information not available elsewhere that will be useful in accomplishing their goal.

The Problem of Unequal Power A group in which certain members have high power and others have low power is likely to be in trouble. The unequal distribution of power affects both the task and the maintenance functions of a group. When members believe they have little influence within the group they are less likely to feel committed to group goals and to implementation of group decisions. Their dissatisfac-

---

Table 9-6   PREVENTING GROUPTHINK

Goal	Preventive and Remedial Behaviors	Goal	Preventive and Remedial Behaviors
Discouraging members from soft-pedaling their disagreements; not allowing their striving for concurrence to inhibit critical thinking.	Each member should be assigned the role of critical evaluator to encourage the group to assign high priority to open airing of objections and doubts. This practice needs to be reinforced by the leader's acceptance of criticism.	Challenging the majority position.	Whenever the agenda of the group calls for an evaluation of policy alternatives, at least one member should take on the "devil's advocate" role, functioning as a good lawyer would in challenging the testimony of those who favor the majority position.
Encouraging open inquiry and impartial probing of a wide range of policy alternatives.	An impartial stance, rather than a statement of preferences and expectations at the beginning, should be adopted by the key members of a hierarchy when they assign a policy-planning task to any group within their organization.	Discouraging stereotyped views of other groups.	When the issue involves relations with a rival group, the group should devote a sizable block of time to surveying the signals and cues from the other group and writing alternative scenarios on the rivals' intentions.
Preventing the insulation of an in-group.	Several outside policy-planning and evaluation groups with different leaders should be set up to work on the same policy question.	Encouraging alternative plans.	The group should, from time to time, break up into two or more subgroups that meet separately, with different leaders, develop separate plans, and then come back together to negotiate differences.
Preventing the establishment of desire for "unity at all costs."	Each member should be asked at intervals to check out group conclusions with trusted associates and to report their reactions back to the group.	Rethinking the entire issue.	After reaching a preliminary consensus, the group should hold a "second chance" meeting, encouraging each member to express residual doubts before making a final choice.
Discouraging members from accepting unchallenged the views of core members.	One or more outside experts should be invited to each meeting, on a staggered basis, and encouraged to challenge the views of core members.		

Source: Compiled from I. L. Janis, "Groupthink," *Psychology Today*, November 1971, p. 76.

---

tion with the group decreases its attractiveness and reduces its cohesion.

High-power people often are the most popular or have the most authority. Neither circumstance is satisfactory for high-quality decision-making. High-quality decision-making results when power is based on expertise, competence, and relevant information, not on popularity or authority.

Destructive Obedience to Authority   Stanley Milgram (1963, 1964) conducted an absorbing and rather frightening series of social science experiments on obedience to authority. Milgram became interested in the obedience phenomenon that occurred during World War II, which formed the defense of many accused war criminals during the Nuremberg trials. He set up experiments in which subjects were to administer increasingly high doses of electric shocks to others who failed to memorize a given sequence of words. Subjects believed they were administering mild to severe (up to 300-volt) shocks that could have damaging physical consequences. Despite the possible severe consequences, 62 percent of the subjects administered the most extreme level of electrical shock under no compulsion other than the repeated verbal requests of the experimenter. Such unquestioning obedience to au-

thority may prevent rational and humane decision-making behavior. Group members should assess and critique suggestions from the authority to avoid the consequences of uncritical obedience. Because much of the role socialization of the nurse emphasizes "following orders," nurses must be especially critical of an unquestioning tendency to behave in concert with the wishes of persons in authority.

KEY NURSING CONCEPTS

- ✔ Most people's lives are spent interacting with other human beings in groups. An individual's sense of being arises through membership in groups that help achieve goals they set for themselves.

- ✔ Nurses interact with groups of clients and colleagues in a wide variety of settings. In order to use groups rationally and effectively, nurses must understand the forces that underlie small group interactional processes and recognize their own patterns of participation.

- ✔ Varieties of groups, developed since World War II, include recreational groups, educational groups, therapy groups, and growth groups.

- ✔ Effective groups accomplish their goals, maintain cohesion, and develop and modify their structure in ways that improve effectiveness.

- ✔ Regardless of setting or composition, several forces shape and modify the structure and functioning of groups. They include space and seating arrangements, material aspects of the physical environment, leadership styles and roles, methods of decision-making, trust, risk-taking, cohesion and conformity, interpersonal attraction, and power and influence.

- ✔ The most effective group leadership is one based on the assumption that responsible membership is the same thing as responsible leadership. In this distributed-functions approach, both the leader and the members engage in leadership behavior.

- ✔ Groups make decisions by consensus, selection of a group of experts, averaging members' opinions, majority vote, minority control, authority rule after discussion, and authority rule without discussion. Each method is appropriate at certain times.

- ✔ Sound decision-making that constructs well-conceived, well-understood, and well-accepted realistic actions toward the goals agreed on by the group is the hallmark of a group that functions effectively.

- ✔ The existence of trust in groups allows members to make suggestions; disclose attitudes, feelings, experiences, and perceptions; give feedback; and confront one another.

- ✔ Cohesion in groups is the spirit of "we-ness" that develops when a group has had shared experiences that provide a basis for attraction—the primary factor keeping a group in existence and working effectively.

- ✔ Power and influence in groups operates constantly and forces members to adjust to one another and modify their behavior.

- ✔ Too much cohesiveness (groupthink) may have a negative influence on the quality of a group's decisions.

References

Benne, K. B., and Sheats, P. "Functional Roles of Group Members." *Journal of Social Issues* 4 (1948): 41–49.

Bierer, J. "Group Psychotherapy." *British Medical Journal* 1 (1942): 214–217.

Burrows, T. "The Group Method of Analysis." *Psychoanalytic Review* 19 (1927): 268–280.

Deutsch, M. "The Effects of Cooperation and Competition upon Group Process." *Human Relations* 2 (1949): 129–152, 199–231.

———. "Trust and Suspicion." *Journal of Conflict Resolution* 2 (1958): 265–279.

———. "Conflicts: Productive and Destructive." *Journal of Social Issues* 25 (1969): 7–41.

Foulkes, S. H., and Anthony, E. J. *Group Psychotherapy.* London: Penguin Books, 1957.

Haley, J. "The Power Tactics of Jesus Christ." In *The Power Tactics of Jesus Christ and Other Essays,* pp. 19–52. New York: Grossman, 1968.

Hall, E. T. *The Hidden Dimension.* Garden City, N.Y.: Doubleday, 1969.

Janis, I. "Groupthink." *Psychology Today,* November 1971, p. 43. (a)

———. "Groupthink among Policy Makers." In *Sanctions for Evil,* edited by N. Sanford, pp. 71–89. San Francisco: Jossey-Bass, 1971. (b)

Johnson, D. W., and Johnson, F. P. *Joining Together: Group Theory and Group Skills.* Englewood Cliffs, N.J.: Prentice-Hall, 1975.

Kogan, N., and Wallach, M. S. *Risk-taking: A Study in Cognition and Personality.* New York: Holt, Rinehart and Winston, 1964.

Lazell, E. W. "The Group Treatment of Dementia Praecox." *Psychoanalytic Review* 8 (1921): 168–179.

Lewin, K.; Lippitt, R.; and White, R. K. "Patterns of Aggressive Behavior in Experimentally Created Social Climates." *Journal of Social Psychology* 10 (1939): 271–299.

Marsh, L. C. "Group Therapy and the Psychiatric Clinic." *Journal of Nervous and Mental Disorders* 32 (1935): 381–390.

Mead, G. H. *Mind, Self, and Society.* Chicago: University of Chicago Press, 1934.

Milgram, S. "Behavioral Study of Obedience." *Journal of Abnormal and Social Psychology* 67 (1963): 371–378.

———. "Group Pressure and Action against a Person." *Journal of Abnormal and Social Psychology* 69 (1964): 137–143.

Mintz, N. "Effects of Esthetic Surroundings: II. Prolonged and Repeated Experience in a 'Beautiful' and an 'Ugly' Room." *Journal of Psychology* 41 (1956): 459–466.

Moreno, J. L. *Psychodrama.* New York: Beacon Press, 1946.

Roethlisberger, F. J., and Dickson, W. J. *Management and the Worker.* Cambridge: Harvard University Press, 1939.

Seghers, C. E. "Color in the Office." *Management Review* 37 (1948): 452–453.

Slavson, S. R. *The Practice of Group Psychotherapy.* New York: International Universities Press, 1947.

Sommer, R. *Personal Space: The Behavioral Basis of Design.* Englewood Cliffs, N.J.: Prentice-Hall, 1969.

Steinzor, B. "The Spatial Factor in Face-to-Face Discussion Groups." *Journal of Abnormal and Social Psychology* 45 (1950): 552–555.

Strodtbeck, F. L., and Hook, L. H. "The Social Dimensions of a Twelve Man Jury Table." *Sociometry* 24 (1961): 397–415.

Wolff, A. "The Psychoanalysis of Groups." *American Journal of Psychotherapy* 3 (1949): 525–558, and 4 (1950): 16–50.

Further Reading

Berscheid, E., and Walster, E. H. *Interpersonal Attraction.* Reading, Mass.: Addison-Wesley, 1969.

Cartwright, D., and Zander, A. *Group Dynamics: Research and Theory.* New York: Harper and Row, 1968.

Cathcart, R. S., and Samovar, L. A. *Small Group Communication.* Dubuque, Iowa: William C. Brown, 1974.

Davis, J. H. *Group Performance.* Reading, Mass.: Addison-Wesley, 1969.

Fisher, B. A. "Decision Emergence: Phases in Group Decision-making." *Speech Monographs* 37 (1970): 53–66.

Fisher, B. A., and Hawes, L. C. "An Interact System Model: Generating a Grounded Theory of Small Groups." *Quarterly Journal of Speech* 57 (1971): 444–453.

Kiesler, C. A., and Kiesler, S. B. *Conformity.* Reading, Mass.: Addison-Wesley, 1969.

Maier, N. R. F. "Assets and Liabilities in Group Problem-solving: The Need for an Integrative Function." *Psychological Review* 74 (1967): 239–249.

May, R. "The Meaning of Power." In *Power and Innocence,* pp. 99–119. New York: W. W. Norton, 1972.

Taylor, S. E., and Mettee, D. P. "When Similarity Breeds Contempt." *Journal of Personality and Social Psychology* 20 (1971): 75–81.

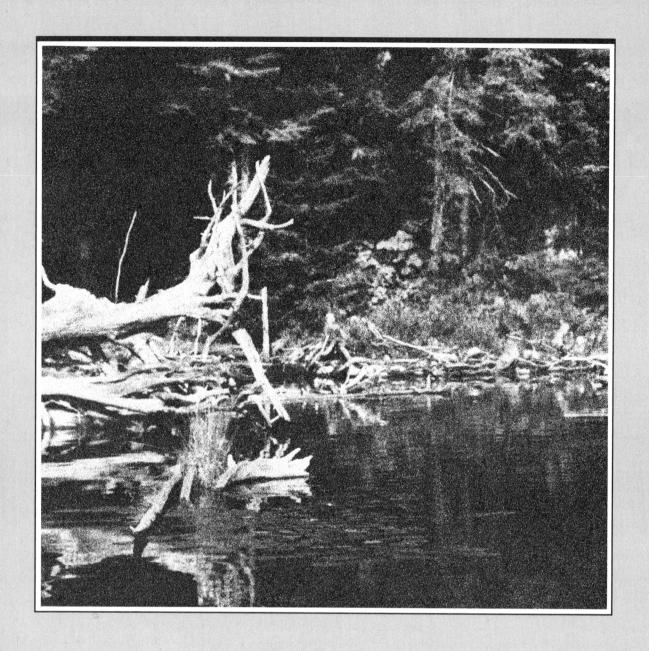

PART THREE

Holistic Framework
for Psychiatric Nursing

DECIDING EXACTLY WHAT *differentiates the interests, concerns, and practice of psychiatric nurses from all other nurses is a topic of debate. Some propose that the domain of psychiatric nurses is defined by the client's psychiatric diagnosis. Others rely on psychiatric nurses practicing in mental health agencies to distinguish their arena. Still others delegate the psychiatric nurse to caring for the mind and emotions separate from caring for the body. Here, we convey our position that the psychiatric nurse is uniquely suited to deal with the whole person at various stages of growth and development, in various role transitions, and at life's major turning points. In dealing with life's stresses, otherwise healthy people may have trouble relying on their characteristic coping patterns. In Chapter 10 we synthesize the major contributions of psychology to psychiatric nursing—including a presentation of stages of growth and development and ego defense mechanisms. The emphasis of this chapter and the ones that follow is on the knowledge nurses need in order to relate to essentially well clients. Developmental and situational crises that serve as turning points and benchmarks in a client's life is our focus in Chapter 11. In Chapter 12 we survey the physiological, psychological, and sociological aspects of human sexuality and the psychiatric nurse's role as a counselor with clients who have problems or concerns about sexuality. One of life's most complex and important social–psychological tasks—parenting—is the topic of Chapter 13. Throughout these chapters, we address problems and patterns of everyday coping styles, across the life span, viewed along a wellness continuum, according to a synthesis of psychological, sociological, and physiological concepts called "life theories." We have sifted through existing bodies of knowledge from the natural and social sciences to select and summarize the theories and data most central to understanding and assisting clients from a holistic framework.*

10

Life Theories in Optimal Wellness

by Joan Sayre

CHAPTER OUTLINE

Life Theory as a Holistic Approach
Historical Perspectives on Human Development
    The Notion of Childhood
    Erikson's Developmental Life Phases Theory
    Recent Research
    The Influence of Symbolic Interactionism
The Concept of Development
    Genetic and Environmental Influences
    The Direction of Development
    Developmental Stages
    The Process of Growth
Optimal Wellness
    Self-actualization
    High-level Wellness
    Health as a Process of Adaptation
    Characteristics of Optimal Emotional Health
Normal Development and Adaptive Difficulties
    Self-realization
    Change as Cause of Anxiety
    Task-oriented and Defense-oriented Reactions
    Defense Mechanisms
Selye's Stress-adaptation Theory
    The General Adaptation Syndrome
    The Local Adaptation Syndrome
    Intervention at Various Levels of Stress
Theories of Growth and Development
    The Relativistic Nature of Theories

Phases of the Human Life Cycle
Critique of the Paradigm of Growth and Development
    The Standard Path of Development
    The Developmental Model of Behavior
    The Benefits of a Social Interaction Model
The Process of Developing a Deviant Identity
    Deviance as Created by Society
    Class Differences in Development of Deviant Identity
Key Nursing Concepts

LEARNING OBJECTIVES

After reading this chapter, students should be able to

- Comprehend the holistic approach to life theories
- Discuss the concepts of optimal wellness, normal development, and adaptive difficulties
- Identity the major defense mechanisms
- Discuss Selye's General Adaptation and Local Adaptation Syndromes
- Describe postadolescence, and the psychosocial moratorium: adulthood and the mid-life crisis and middle age
- Relate the premises of the development of a deviant identity to the psychiatric nursing process
- Develop a personal philosophy about labeling behavior as deviant

CHAPTER 10

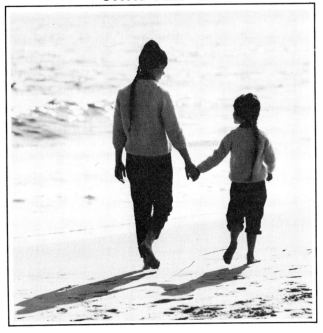

Just as our behavior is a reflection of our experience, this little girl's ability to cope and optimize health reflects her mother's.

The formation of personality is a complex and arduous process. The creation of a self begins at birth and ceases only at death. Although humans are born into an ongoing culture with certain propensities and capacities, it is only through socialization that they learn how to be human. As humans develop, they continually integrate new knowledge about the nature of life into their self-concepts. Thus, one's behavior is a reflection of all one's experience. Self-concept is the most important knowledge a person has, for it regulates interactions with others. The extent to which the crucial qualities of trust, autonomy, initiative, and identity have been developed influences the self-image of the adult. The meanings that people share with others in their culture enable adults to live in a reasonably predictable world and to widen their repertoire of social roles. The holistic approach to life theory helps clarify the process of growth and development in adulthood.

LIFE THEORY AS A HOLISTIC APPROACH

Theories of growth and development, or stress adaptation, emphasize specific perspectives on the life process. For example, Selye's stress-adaptation theory deals mainly with physiological reactions to stressors. Maslow's theory of basic human needs is a framework for viewing physical and emotional needs in a hierar-

chical order. Freud's structural hypothesis is an example of an analytic theory of personality, dealing primarily with intrapersonal processes. It is necessary to know such specific theories in order to understand life theories in optimal wellness. However, these specific theories must be placed in a holistic framework.

A holistic approach to life theory integrates the cognitive, physiological, emotional, social, and spiritual factors that influence the individual. Holistic theory explains the life process as a total field of events. In this field the individual and the individual's environment are engaged in a constantly changing interaction. Theorists who work from this holistic viewpoint can use all available concepts to explain growth and development.

Current approaches to health exemplify holistic theory. These approaches focus not on a specific disease but on the total health of the individual. Their goal is to help the person engage in a healthier life-style so as to enjoy a higher level of wellness. A holistic health program might include a natural food regime, exercise, yoga, and various forms of meditation. When people in this kind of program suffer a disturbance in their health, they tolerate their symptoms until the underlying cause is found. Symptoms are not suppressed with medication. According to holistic theory, the disturbance may be caused by a number of factors. For instance, periods of depression might be caused by high dietary intake of sugar or fat, by current destructive relationships, by environmental toxins, by cultural pressures, or by the feeling that the person's life has no purpose. Once the causes are located, the person provides the necessary conditions for the body to heal itself by eliminating destructive influences.

Holistic theory provides a specific viewpoint of the process of development. Holistic theorists understand that a person participates in an ever-changing field of physical, cultural, and emotional forces, and that his or her behavior is a reflection of this interaction. Holistic theorists are comfortable with a variety of theories, because they understand that a single developmental theory is not adequate to explain the complexities of human behavior. They appreciate the fact that optimal wellness is not a final or ultimate goal, since one's degree of wellness varies continually. Development is a lifelong process. During this process people strive to adapt to and change the varying situations of life and live up to their full capabilities.

HISTORICAL PERSPECTIVES ON HUMAN DEVELOPMENT

Many people assume that the course of development is curvilinear—that is, that growth is characterized by a rapid increase in abilities until the peak of maturity is reached, after which abilities gradually decline until death. According to this view, development is dramatic during the prenatal period, infancy, childhood, and adolescence. During the relatively stable periods of adulthood and middle age, a plateau of consolidation is reached. This consolidation is centered around family life and work. A final period of decline occurs during old age, when people must adapt their goals and behavior to their decreasing abilities. Placing the concept of development in a historical perspective reveals that the concept itself has changed.

The Notion of Childhood

The notion of childhood is relatively recent. The view of the child as a miniature adult has been common throughout history. Until recently it was assumed that the individual's potential was determined by heredity, and that all the skills, knowledge, and ability manifested later in life were present at birth. Socialization was important to fulfill this potential, but socialization in itself could add nothing new to the individual. This view of the child as a miniature adult had important implications for child rearing. Children were treated as rational beings. Their thinking processes were assumed to be the same as those of adults, and children who made errors in judgment according to adult standards were considered stupid or lazy. A child's infringement of moral rules and social standards for behavior was evidence not of immaturity but of the presence of evil. Such transgressions were punished.

This viewpoint was altered through the influence of John Locke (1632–1704). While Locke also believed that children were incomplete adults, he rejected the concept of the genetic determination of development. Locke compared the mind of an infant to a *tabula rasa,* or "blank slate." According to this view, the child's mind is empty at birth and is gradually filled by

knowledge from experience of the world. Simple ideas are formed from direct sensory experience, and more complex ideas develop from associations between these simple ideas. Personality is formed through an accumulation of knowledge. Locke considered the early experiences of childhood crucial to the formation of personality. He believed that infants were significantly influenced by even very small impressions, which might completely alter the direction of their lives. This idea that children are extremely malleable and open to experience is still significant in developmental psychology.

The French philosopher Jean-Jacques Rousseau (1712–1778) was one of the first thinkers to suggest that children were qualitatively as well as quantitatively different from adults. Rousseau rejected the idea that the infant was a formless being created through the accidents of experience. He did not think that the child was an incomplete adult or that the child's reasoning processes were an imitation of adult thinking. Rousseau thought that from the moment of birth the infant was actively engaged in exploring and constructing a personal knowledge of the world. If left to nature, development would occur in an orderly progression, and at each stage the individual would be complete. The implication of this view for child rearing was that the adult should not interfere too much with the spontaneous process of development. The child is a "noble savage," endowed by nature with moral values. Adults who try to alter a child's behavior to conform to their own values will distort the child's development. Rousseau's ideas remain influential today. They account for the emphasis placed on discovery, rather than on didactic education, in the teaching methods of Dewey and Montessori.

Much of the early speculation on the nature of childhood was purely philosophical. It was not based on actual observations of children. The emergence of psychology as a scientific discipline in the nineteenth century focused attention on direct observations of behavior. G. Stanley Hall (1846–1924), influenced by Darwin's evolutionary thesis, adopted a recapitulation theory of growth. He postulated that each individual's development reflected the growth of the species through its various evolutionary stages. Although this theory was later abandoned by developmental psychologists, Hall's systematic method of observing development established him as the founder of developmental psychology in the United States.

Several other psychologists did important work in this field during the nineteenth century. Gesell de-

Table 10-1 COMPARATIVE IDEAS ABOUT CHILDHOOD

Key Idea	Major Theorist	Implications for Child Rearing
Child as miniature adult	—	Punishment for "immature" behavior, which was thought to be caused by the presence of evil
Child as blank slate	Locke	Close attention to guiding early experiences so that the child would develop in the "proper" way
Child in the process of spontaneous development	Rousseau	Noninterference with development
Child as mirroring the growth of the species	Hall, Gesell	Systematic observation of development
Child in interaction between environmental influences and genetically determined attributes	Piaget	Increase in attention to environmental and social factors

scribed in detail the development of children at different ages; Watson attempted to explain the development of behavior through the principles of classical conditioning; and Freud's theory that the experiences of infancy and childhood largely determined the adult personality gradually became very influential.

Piaget's Cognitive Development Theory During the 1950s, developmental psychology underwent a change in focus. Table 10-1 compares these and earlier ideas about childhood. Studies of general behavioral development were abandoned for inquiries into specific developmental problems such as perception, memory, and abstract thinking. Jean Piaget (1952, 1958) viewed development as a constant process of interaction between environmental influences and the innate, genetically determined attributes of the individual. Piaget conducted an extensive investigation of cognitive development that still dominates developmental psychology. His basic theory is that the development of knowledge involves not only learning new things but also replacing paradigms or sets of ideas with more adequate paradigms. Piaget saw the end goal of development as the acquisition of the psychological structure necessary to reason abstractly and think logically. Children inherit a mode of intellectual functioning that remains essentially the same throughout life. Cognitive structures are not inherited; they are formed through intellectual development. According to Piaget, in order to grow, individuals must adapt their cognitive structures to the demands of the environment. Intelligent behavior facilitates this adaptive process.

The structure of the intellect consists of schemata and operations. A *schema* is the internal representa-

tion of some specific action. The infant has a number of innate schemata for sucking, grasping, crying, seeing, and so on. During the course of development these schemata become integrated and further elaborated. They are the fundamental structure of knowing. Operational schemata are mental structures of a higher order. They are not usually acquired until adolescence, when abstract thinking becomes possible.

Another key concept in Piagetian theory is adaptation. *Adaptation* occurs whenever an interchange between the organism and the environment results in a modification of the organism that enhances its capacity for further interchange. Adaptation involves two components—assimilation and accommodation. *Assimilation* means the adjustment of an object to the structure of the organism. *Accommodation* means the adjustment of the organism to an object in the environment. Assimilation and accommodation operate simultaneously in the mutual adaptation between the individual and the environment.

The process of ingesting food offers a prototype of adaptation. Adaptation of the food to the needs of the individual occurs through a mutual transformation. The food is chewed and digested (assimilation). The body makes the necessary adjustments to facilitate the process, such as opening the mouth, secreting gastric juices, and so on (accommodation). If one applies the concept of adaptation to cognitive development, one begins to understand that every cognitive encounter involves a structuring process. This process meshes the individual's particular intellectual organization with the special characteristics of the object that is perceived. For instance, a child playing with a ball will first make a series of exploratory accommodations, such as looking and touching or rolling the ball back and forth. These accommodations are directed by concepts of touching and rolling, which are already part of the child's cognitive organization. These actions with respect to the ball are both accommodations to the roundness and size of the ball and assimilations of the ball to the child's cognitive organization.

Piaget's work in the definition of the fundamental characteristics of intelligence is still being developed. His key concepts are listed below.

1. The concept of development:
   - Developmental processes occur in absolute continuity.
   - This continuity proceeds by a continuous unfolding of capacities.
   - The development of each new capacity has its origins in a previous phase and continues into the next phase.
   - Each developmental phase entails a repetition of the processes of the previous level of development in a different form of organization or schema.
   - The continuous development of more highly differentiated schemata creates a hierarchy of experience and action. Previous behavioral patterns are seen as inferior to present levels of behavior.

2. The process of development occurs through adaptation, or the cognitive striving of the thinking person to find an equilibrium between self and environment. It involves interlocking processes:
   - Assimilation is the adaptation of the environment to oneself, the taking in of as much experience as the individual can integrate.
   - Accommodation is the incorporation of an experience as it actually is—the taking in of the actual impact of the environment.

Erikson's Developmental Life Phases Theory

Erik Erikson's major contribution to developmental theory is his conception of the life cycle as a series of developmental phases. These phases are a universally experienced sequence of biological, social, and psychological events. The individual's personality is constantly redeveloping in response to changing inner and outer requirements. This developmental process is governed by the *epigenetic principle,* a concept Erikson adapted from embryology. According to this prin-

ciple, physical and psychosocial growth are regulated by a plan that is innate in the capacities of the individual on the one hand and arises in relation to others through social expectations on the other. The innate capacity for development of intellectual skills arises during school age. It is also encouraged by parents' and teachers' expectations that children will apply themselves to learning at this age.

Developmental phases are a series of normative conflicts or specific psychosocial tasks with which every person must deal. During each developmental period, two opposing energies—a positive and a negative force—occur together and must be synthesized. For instance, in the first stage of development in infancy, the potential for trust and the potential for mistrust exist side by side. Infants who experience a feeling of physical comfort and minimal fear will jeopardize some of their feeling of safety in order to gain new experience. Each experience of having this sense of trust validated tends to produce positive expectations for new experience. However, in infancy, as in all phases of life, there are physical and psychological hazards. The rapid physical changes in infancy can in themselves foster mistrust as the infant experiences continual change. The infant learns to sit up, crawl, kneel, and walk within a period of months. If he or she has many unsatisfactory physical and psychological experiences, the feeling of mistrust will predominate. This will lead the infant to fear the future. Such infants also find it hard to trust others. If the synthesis between trust and mistrust is basically positive because the mother nurtures the infant, a sense of trust will pervade the individual's life. However, the potential for mistrust will still exist to some degree and must be worked out in future developmental phases. In early childhood, the individual must maintain a sense of trust while dealing with the frustrations of toilet training and parental discipline.

The subjective feeling of having accomplished or failed to accomplish the tasks appropriate to a specific phase influences the progress of development to the next phase. The most crucial factor for the infant, for instance, is the achievement of a sense of trust. However, this achievement must take place during infancy. At the age of 1 to 1½, childhood begins, bringing with it the new task of resolving a sense of autonomy and a sense of shame and doubt. Children who have not already accomplished the earlier task of achieving trust will be handicapped in dealing with the next developmental phase. There is a crucial time when each new function must develop. This principle is obvious in the growth of the fetus. Each organ system must develop during its own crucial time, or defects will result. The same principle applies after birth in the achievement of psychosocial tasks.

Significant others help to resolve developmental crises by satisfying the subject's interpersonal needs and by conveying their interpretations of the meaning of the crisis. People who have enough opportunities to realize their developmental potential during the crucial period grow out of the crisis with important new abilities. If the crisis is not resolved in a constructive way, the person develops attitudes that are not helpful in future developmental tasks.

Bob, who is twenty-two, has not been able to develop a sense of identity. He feels lost and confused. He can't decide on a career, and he is afraid of emotional involvements. He will be handicapped in the next developmental phase, early adulthood, because he will not be able to risk an insecure sense of identity in closeness with others. He will find it equally difficult to commit himself to a career. Retardation or failure in one developmental task will prevent him from achieving personality growth now, and it will endanger his whole hierarchy of development. Bob's inability to formulate a secure identity may prevent him from getting married. Or it may propel him into a relationship with a person as fearful of intimacy as himself. If he has children, he may not be able to develop concern for their needs, because he is still so involved with meeting his own needs. In old age he may feel a sense of bitterness and failure. It is possible that good luck may reverse this process, but according to Erikson, Bob will continue to experience difficulty unless he manages to resolve his problems.

Thus Erikson conceived of the life cycle as a series of building blocks, one influencing the next as the individual grows progressively more or less capable of dealing with life. This progression is depicted in Table 10–2. Developmental phases are a kind of timetable for personality development. Developmental tasks also reflect the structure of the society, since the culture dictates the desirable rate of development and favors certain aspects of development at the expense of others. American culture, for instance, stresses competition and achievement. These are appropriate concerns for young adults. However, American culture devalues the tasks of later years. These include the wisdom and contemplation that characterize the successful resolution of the last phase of life. Therefore, people in this

culture may not experience a sense of achievement in fulfilling their potential in this phase. Although all the people in a given culture face similar developmental tasks, Erikson recognizes that each person resolves these tasks in an individual way. For example, some people may resolve the task of generativity by nurturing children. Others may do so by producing artistic or scientific works.

Erikson uses the concept of life stages in somewhat the same way as Piaget. His unique contribution is his demonstration that development does not end in adulthood but continues until death. He also demonstrates reciprocity of development. For instance, in order to meet her infant's need to develop trust, a mother herself must successfully resolve the dichotomy of adulthood—that of generativity versus stagnation. If she cannot focus on her children's development, she will not be able to provide experiences that allow them to trust the world. Erikson's concepts of development remain very important in explaining personality and are compared with those of Freud and Sullivan in Chapters 19 and 20.

Recent Research

Current investigations in developmental psychology are being carried out in several different directions. New electronic and photographic equipment has made it possible to determine with great precision the specific skills and responses of infants. Studies have been made of auditory and visual abilities, perceptual discrimination, and patterns of interaction. New work in development is also focusing on the previously neglected areas of middle and old age. These investigations indicate that the individual is engaged in a lifelong process of integrating new capacities and experiences.

The Influence of Symbolic Interactionism

As developmental research becomes more diversified and discrete, other, more general theoretical accounts of development are being constructed. These accounts are influenced by the symbolic interactionists and by phenomenology. Theorists today are studying the process of formation of the self through interaction. Symbolic interactionism stresses that the self both influences and is influenced by interpersonal relationships. Social behavior is continually constructed during the process of interaction. Society itself is in a continuous process of creation through the construction of new meanings. The phenomenological approach does not

Table 10-2   ERIKSON'S EIGHT STAGES OF MAN

Age	Stage of Development	Area of Resolution	Basic Attitudes
Birth to eighteen months	Infancy	Trust versus Mistrust	Ability to trust others and a sense of one's own trustworthiness; a sense of hope
			Withdrawal and estrangement
Eighteen months to three years	Early childhood	Autonomy versus Shame and doubt	Self-control without loss of self-esteem; ability to cooperate and to express oneself
			Compulsive self-restraint or compliance; defiance, willfulness
Three to five years	Late childhood	Initiative versus Guilt	Realistic sense of purpose; some ability to evaluate one's own behavior
			Self denial and self-restriction
Six to twelve years	School age	Industry versus Inferiority	Realization of competence, perseverance
			Feeling that one will never be "any good," withdrawal from school and peers
Twelve to twenty years	Adolescence	Identity versus Role diffusion	Coherent sense of self; plans to actualize one's abilities
			Feelings of confusion, indecisiveness, possibly antisocial behavior
Eighteen to twenty-five years	Young adulthood	Intimacy versus Isolation	Capacity for love as mutual devotion; commitment to work and relationships
			Impersonal relationships, prejudice
Twenty-five to sixty-five years	Adulthood	Generativity versus Stagnation	Creativity, productivity, concern for others
			Self-indulgence, impoverishment of self
Sixty-five years to death	Old age	Integrity versus Despair	Acceptance of the worth and uniqueness of one's life
			Sense of loss, contempt for others

assume the existence of society in explaining behavior. It asks a more basic question: How is society made possible in the first place? Society is not considered a natural reality. It exists only insofar as it has meaning for its participants. According to symbolic interactionism, knowledge is invented. It is produced in human interaction, as people decide that various theories about society and behavior are "true."

These ideas have profound implications for the study of development. First, since experience in the world cannot be apprehended in its own right but only through the mind's experience of it, what people experience as development is a very subjective process. There are no fixed standards of development. Also,

since reality is socially constructed, it is continually in the process of negotiation. People agree on the qualities and standards of development. Deviations from these standards are not abnormalities in any absolute sense. They are only abnormal relative to people's decisions about normal development.

The self is developed in children by the process of play. In this process children imagine what others are like by imitating them. They imagine the rules by which others conduct themselves and begin to observe objectively how they themselves behave vis-à-vis the social rules. Thus children define themselves as they learn about society. They begin to play roles properly according to the rules. This process is not merely a matter of conforming to social requirements. Through this play, children develop the ability to see themselves as others see them. Children take on roles in relation to the people they are closest to and whose attitudes are decisive for their conception of themselves. As they grow, children learn to relate to the expectations not only of their parents but of society at large. That is, they find that not only their parents but society as a whole expects them to learn to read, for example. Each social role has a certain identity attached to it. Some roles—such as student or soldier—are temporary. Others—such as sexual identity—are permanent. These identities, which people consider to be their essential selves, have in reality been socially assigned. They are sustained and transformed through cultural processes.

The following are the basic premises of symbolic interactionism and phenomenology (also see Chapter 1):

- The self is produced through interaction with others.
- Social behavior, as well as society itself, is in a continuous process of creation. This creation is achieved by interaction between people.
- Society exists only as far as it has meaning for its participants. It is not a natural phenomenon.
- No theory is true in any absolute sense, since all knowledge is invented.

These basic premises have the following implications for theories of growth and development:

- There can be no definite standards for development.
- All theories of growth and development are constantly changing as people's opinions about them change.
- There can be no such thing as "abnormal" or "normal" development in any absolute sense. Groups of people at any given time decide what is normal and abnormal.

Although there are undoubtedly certain inherited biological characteristics, the extent of genetic inheritance is still unknown. According to symbolic interactionism, there is a very narrow scope for social influence within genetic limits. Although early familial influences cannot be chosen, our freedom to influence our own development increases with age, since as we grow, our potential for social contacts widens.

Every social act entails a choice of identity. The self is a process continuously created anew in each social setting, structured to some extent by memories of the past. This does not necessarily mean that change is easy. We can become very used to a certain identity. When our social circumstances change, we may have difficulty meeting new social expectations. For example, retirement often produces new expectations of behavior that are hard to meet. We are expected not only to adjust quickly to changes in social and economic status but also to behave consistently. Others become alarmed, for example, if a person who is generally aggressive and independent becomes dependent and passive for any length of time.

In the context of symbolic interactionism, developmental stages are socially provided opportunities for identity change. What advantage we take of these opportunities depends on the meaning they hold for us. It also depends on the reciprocity granted us by our intimates. A certain degree of role discrepancy is permitted. But a person who goes beyond society's limits must assume a defective or deviant identity. Thus, though slow changes in behavior are permitted, the results are carefully monitored for social acceptability.

The following discussion of the concept of development and its various stages is influenced by the perspective of symbolic interactionism. It is also influenced by Erikson's conception of developmental tasks and by Piagetian ideas about the growth of thought processes.

THE CONCEPT OF DEVELOPMENT

The concept of development is a very fruitful one, involving as it does the notion of the process of change in a continually shifting social context. Basic to the idea of development is the individual's continual self-modification in response to general cultural expectations and the individual's own expectations. The term *development* generally refers to the series of processes underlying changes in behavior and ability that are associated with increasing age. The mere passage of time does not explain behavioral change. Chronological age is simply a convenient way of measuring the time during which various processes occur.

Genetic and Environmental Influences

Genetic and environmental influences interact in the developmental process. Since the organism needs innate structure in order to act, and since innate structure is hereditary, there is a genetic component in development, though its influence varies. Hereditary influences are most noticeable in physical features, such as body type and hair color. Less obvious are primary reaction tendencies, such as sensitivity to stimuli, adaptability, and activity level. Other abilities are even more difficult to assess. Although IQ may be genetically determined to some extent, it is not genetically fixed. The quality of the environment, the type of interaction with others, and the expectations of others are important determinants in the development of intelligence. Though some constitutional factors are socially influenced, many remain relatively stable throughout life. Differences in constitutional factors may account for the diversity of individual reactions to similar environmental conditions.

The Direction of Development

Development proceeds in a characteristic direction. In the functionalistic evolutionary view, the concept of development implies progression from an earlier mode of behavior. This view suggests that the processes of passing through successive stages of infancy, childhood, and adolescence into adulthood involve increasingly mature levels of functioning. The maturity of adulthood is thus viewed as the goal of the developmental process. A symbolic interactionist perspective may view development as directional in that it involves the sequential acquisition of new abilities. However, there is no single, definite end point, since reality is in a continual process of construction. In fact, since a person's state of behavioral development at any point is a reflection of socially negotiated identities, it follows that there is a variety of end points. Since behaviors differ because life experience varies, it is difficult to arrive at a fixed definition of maturity or at one identity style that is more effective than another.

Developmental Stages

Although the underlying continuity in the life cycle makes it difficult to separate it into components, development can be viewed in terms of interlinking stages of growth. Though developmental stages proceed in an orderly sequence, the rate of growth is not consistent over time. There are periods of rapid growth and other periods of quiescence. Each individual demonstrates the same developmental sequence in general, but great differences occur both in the rate of development and in the new behavior patterns. Each subse-

quent stage of development builds on the events of previous stages and in turn provides the foundation for future developmental events. These stages generally imply an increasing complexity and differentiation of behavior.

The Process of Growth

The process of growth is essentially one of acquiring new functions and abilities. The functions in question are physiological, emotional, and interpersonal. The major focus of psychosocial development is the expansion of the capacity for relatedness and communication within the matrix of societal expectations. Encouraging growth stimulates the integration of new abilities; ignoring or discouraging growth prevents such integration. Children who are not given opportunities to initiate action will not learn to be active on their own behalf.

John, a fourteen-year-old boy, thought he would be interested in a career in engineering. Yet he found it impossible to seek the necessary information from his guidance counselor. John had never been allowed to initiate actions for himself. He knew that he would need certain science courses in high school in order to be accepted at a good college. But rather than actively seek out the information he needed, he told himself that he would wait awhile and see if he changed his mind about engineering.

If a new function does not receive adequate validation from emotionally significant people, it will not be completely consolidated in the self.

People never stop developing. In every individual there is always an area of developing functions. People whose growth is retarded will attempt to accomplish this growth. They are motivated by their own need to develop and by the cultural expectation that people will continually expand their capabilities.

OPTIMAL WELLNESS

Some definitions of optimal wellness rely on the standard of *normality*. According to these definitions, optimal wellness means feeling and functioning as well as most other people. It also means measuring up to the standards of society in work and interpersonal relationships. Thus being mentally well would mean "being adjusted." The adjusted person survives, reproduces, is self-supporting, and is generally successful in seeking pleasure and avoiding pain. An adjusted person may not be creative, stimulating, or productive, however.

Three theories of optimal wellness—those of Abraham Maslow, Halbert Dunn, and Ivan Illich—are discussed below. Other definitions of emotional health have been dominated by a medical framework. This medical framework implies that health is the absence of disease. According to this view, symptoms of disordered functioning, such as irrational fears or depression, are signs of illness. A state of health is thus indicated by the absence of symptoms. This definition has caused its adherents to focus on disorders rather than on the characteristics of healthy emotional functioning.

Self-actualization

Abraham Maslow was one of the first writers to criticize the emphasis on the study of disordered emotional functioning (Maslow 1962). He believed that mental illness cannot be understood without a prior knowledge of mental health. Maslow focused his attention on the positive aspects of human behavior, such as happiness, contentment, and elation. His studies of self-actualizing people—those he considered to be exceptionally healthy and mature—resulted in a more comprehensive, multidisciplinary approach to human problems. He saw mental health as involving *every* aspect of the individual's functioning.

Maslow defined *self-actualizing people* as those who make full use of their talents and potentialities, those who are doing the best they can do. Self-actualizing people are characterized by the ability to see life as it is rather than as they wish it were. Self-actualizing people are less emotional and more objective than those who have not achieved this level of development. They see people clearly, for they do not allow their own hopes and wishes to distort their judgment. Self-actualizing people understand themselves better than other people do. This enables them to consider the opinions of others and to admit their own lack of knowledge. Self-actualizing people are dedicated to some duty or vocation. They are creative, which allows them to be spontaneous, open, and experimental in their work and relationships. They are not in conflict with themselves, for their personalities are integrated around important values and life goals. Though they enjoy relationships with others, they may give the im-

Table 10–3 MASLOW'S HIERARCHY OF NEEDS

Name	Definition
Physiological	Biological needs for food, shelter, water, sleep, oxygen, sexual expression
Safety	Avoiding harm; attaining security, order, and physical safety
Love and belonging	Giving and receiving affection; companionship; and identification with a group
Esteem and recognition	Self-esteem and the respect of others; success in work; prestige
Self-actualization	Fulfillment of unique potential
Aesthetic	Search for beauty and spiritual goals

pression of remoteness, since they rely fully on their own capacities and do not need other people to complete their personalities. They are governed far more by their own nature and goals than by the opinions of others. The basic difference Maslow saw between these people and the average person is that people who are not self-actualizing are motivated by deficiencies. Much of their energy is focused on fulfilling basic needs for safety, belonging, love, respect, and self-esteem. Self-actualizing people have met these security needs. They are motivated primarily by the need to develop and actualize their fullest capacities. Maslow's hierarchy of needs appears in Table 10–3.

High-level Wellness

Halbert Dunn also emphasizes the idea that health is more than the absence of disease (Dunn 1961). He defines health as a state of complete physical, mental, and social well-being. Dunn believes that people are not simply ill or well in general, but that their degree of health fluctuates according to their inner and outer circumstances. Dunn envisions illness and wellness on a graduated scale with death as the ultimate state of illness and high-level wellness as the ultimate state of health.

High-level wellness is characterized by energy, vitality, and zest for life. Mental health is synonymous with physical, spiritual, and social health. Mental health requires a balance between the integrated body, mind, and spirit on the one hand and the environment on the other. To be healthy, we need meaningful work, but we also need periods of rest and sleep. In order to maximize our potential, we must continually provide a balance among various capabilities within the framework of a meaningful life purpose.

Thus Dunn defines health in a positive sense and recognizes that the dichotomy between health and illness is too simplistic. Individuals actually function on various levels of wellness, since intrapsychic and environmental influences are constantly changing. Dunn points out that everyone experiences periods of lassitude. During these times we fulfill our obligations with much effort. At other times we may be charged with the feeling that no task is too difficult to accomplish. Wellness is not achieved once and for all. It is a process of maximizing one's capacities.

Dunn offers various suggestions for achieving high levels of wellness. One is to develop the ability to face inconsistencies in one's thinking. Another is to examine other people's viewpoints and adjust our own views to achieve mutual understanding. Dunn also emphasizes the importance of cherishing important relationships by making time for unhurried interaction with others, giving recognition to people we care about, and being helpful and nonpossessive.

Health as a Process of Adaptation

Ivan Illich defines health as a process of adaptation during which we can actively change our life situation (Illich 1976). His definition encompasses the ability to adapt to changing social environments and to deal with maturation, aging, suffering, and death. Maximizing our potential is a way of developing the ability to function under the great variety of biological and social influences that we experience. Everyone has many desires, which are constantly changing as we age and accumulate more experience. Thus, good health is different for various ages and social groups. The requirements for good health vary for each individual. They change with the shifting importance of family and professional responsibilities and new recreational and social interests. Health as a process of adaptation focuses on a purposefully designed life-style. This life-style enables us to achieve the highest possible levels of health as we progress through the life cycle.

The key ideas in the optimal wellness theories of Maslow, Dunn, and Illich are compared in Table 10–4.

Table 10–4   THEORIES OF OPTIMAL WELLNESS

Key Idea	Theorist
Fully mature persons are motivated by needs for growth and actualization of their abilities	Abraham Maslow
Individuals function on various levels of wellness due to fluctuating internal and external states of well-being	Halbert Dunn
Health is a process of adaptation to ever-changing life circumstances	Ivan Illich

Characteristics of Optimal Emotional Health

These definitions stress that wellness is a process with no definite end. Many writers emphasize the cultural variations in definitions of wellness. There is no global consensus about the characteristics of optimal emotional health. There are, however, some generally agreed-on characteristics. These include self-esteem, self-knowledge, satisfying interpersonal relationships, environmental mastery, and stress management.

Self-esteem and Self-knowledge Emotionally healthy people are relatively free of feelings of inadequacy and inferiority. Their self-confidence is based on an accurate estimation of themselves rather than on denial of their limitations or exaggeration of their abilities. Their self-esteem is based on many values, at least some of which are relatively permanent. Physical attractiveness and strength can be an effective source of self-esteem in youth. But mentally healthy people can relinquish these values as they age and substitute others, such as family relationships or work achievements.

Understanding one's unique personality contributes heavily to self-esteem. Because emotionally healthy people like and accept themselves, they can be aware of many of their feelings and conflicts. In psychodynamic terms, they have less need to repress painful realities. Some degree of repression is necessary to protect the self from unacceptable impulses and painful memories. But too much repression may reduce ability to assess reality logically. It is preferable, in terms of ego strength, to deal with painful experience and learn what we can from it. It is also more effective to reject an unacceptable wish consciously than to repress it, because repression may lead to unintentional, unexpected behavior.

Healthy people can accept their limitations and problems and can deal with them as well as circumstances allow. When their emotions make it hard for them to handle a situation objectively, healthy people can control these emotions to achieve objectivity. A boy who is going away to college, for instance, will accept and endure a certain amount of anxiety about leaving his family to face an uncertain future, because he can understand that his future development depends on experiences that going to college will make possible. Another boy, who is less aware of his anxieties about leaving home, may feel the same reluctance about new experience but may be unable to deal with his feelings. He may express his emotions indirectly by failing his courses or by vacillating from one career choice to another.

Satisfying Interpersonal Relationships   Healthy people do not necessarily need a lot of friends or an extensive social life. But they are able to work with others to meet common or reciprocal needs, such as maintaining a family or collaborating on a work project. Healthy people do require a few intimate and rewarding relationships in which intense emotional needs are met without exploitation, power struggles, or jealousy. The healthier one is, the more one can provide tenderness and validation for the growth of others. Healthy people accept the inherent mutuality of growth in a close relationship. Though they are capable of full commitment to another person, their commitments are based on knowledge of themselves as independent entities free to choose their own associates. Mentally healthy people are autonomous in that they can manage for themselves if necessary. They are independent of social influences to some extent. They can be self-directed in situations where they feel that common social mores are destructive to their own growth. Emotionally healthy people can relate sympathetically to the human community in general. They can find common denominators with people who are apparently quite different from themselves.

Environmental Mastery   Mentally healthy people can meet the situational requirements of life in their relationships and work. They can adapt and adjust to change and can solve problems effectively. They can

make conscious and deliberate decisions. In choosing between two or more alternatives, they recognize that each carries its own consequences, not all of which may be desirable, while not making a decision or postponing one also has predictable consequences. A mentally healthy young woman accepts, for instance, that a decision to further her education may mean a prolonged period of hard work. She accepts the fact that her choice of career may even have to be readjusted as she develops and as the needs of society change.

Healthy people do not act impulsively. They defer a decision long enough to study alternatives or try out a course of action. They make major decisions, such as the choice of a marriage partner or a career, on the basis of conscious determinants, recognized needs, and predicted consequences.

Stress Management   Healthy people can accept and cope with stressful situations, because they can tolerate anxiety without needing to seek immediate relief. When they cannot meet certain needs, they can defer gratification or seek substitutes. When they are frustrated, they recognize that they must satisfy important needs. They do not sublimate desires in a way that conceals their underlying needs and may prevent gratification under more opportune circumstances. For instance, if an important relationship ends, a healthy man does not deny his needs for intimacy and love. Instead, he attempts to satisfy them with a more suitable person. When healthy people encounter stressful situations, they try to define and clarify the problem and then to modify the situation. They work through any tendency to blame others or to dwell on past injustices. In this way they can assume responsibility for themselves. If they cannot modify the situation and ease stress, they either modify their own expectations or find a way to escape from the stressful situation.

NORMAL DEVELOPMENT AND ADAPTIVE DIFFICULTIES

Self-realization

Self-realization is desirable in any developmental stage. Self-realization is the fullest possible expression of the individual's uniqueness. It can be achieved at any time in the life cycle—whether it manifests itself in the forging of a reliable identity in adolescence or in the careful parenting of children in adulthood.

Just as nutrition, rest, and shelter are crucial to biological maintenance, so the fulfillment of certain needs is crucial to psychological maintenance. Psychological needs have been variously defined. One useful formulation specifies a need for close relatedness, a need to feel competent in coping with life, and a need to be approved by and belong to a social group. Other psychological needs include the need for self-esteem and the need for a value system that confers order and predictability on experience. Many obstacles can interfere with the fulfillment of psychological needs. These include developmental expectations, which often create pressures on the individual, and situational crises, such as a sudden illness or an economic reversal. Sudden changes of social roles related to developmental events, such as the birth of a first child or graduation from college, also interfere with needs because they require behavioral change.

Change as Cause of Anxiety

Behavioral change causes stress or anxiety. Stress serves an important purpose. It signals a danger to the integrity of the self and causes the individual to respond in a specific way in order to resolve the problems involved. How we respond to stress depends on many factors. These include the amount of support we receive from others, the number of choices we have in solving the problem, and how we have dealt with stress in the past. The nature of the individual's self-concept is basic to the ability to deal with stress.

Our self-concept depends on the evaluations of others. Once formed, it is continually subject to further social evaluations. Positive and negative evaluations from teachers, parents, siblings, and friends have become organized into the self-concept. Young children have no guide to self-evaluation except what they have learned from adults. They cannot question adult opinions because they dare not risk their own security. So they passively accept adult judgments. This is how children learn who they are. Behaviors that the parents respond to and validate remain in the child's self-awareness. Any new knowledge that may modify the self-concept is controlled by awareness. New situations arouse anxiety, because they threaten the established sense of self. Anxiety and the resulting defense mechanisms tend to control awareness and prevent the self from encountering any new experiences that may contradict the self-system. This is true even of people who feel basically hostile toward themselves. People need consistency even more than they need a positive self-concept. Thus they may misinterpret expressions of positive feelings from others in order to preserve a consistent—if negative—self-concept. Anxiety and defense mechanisms do not preclude change, however, and we can change our self-concept to some extent.

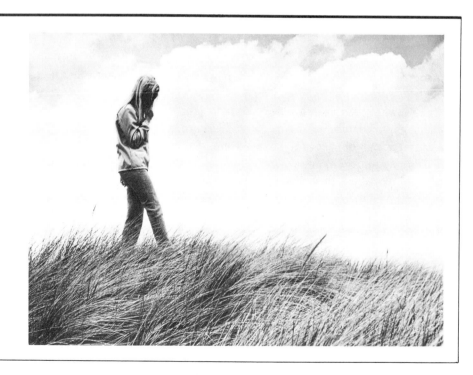

When we feel unable to cope with life's stresses, and situations are threatening to our sense of self, we tend to use defense-oriented mechanisms.

	Table 10-5 DEFENSE MECHANISMS	
Name	**Definition**	**Example**
Repression, dissociation	Unacceptable feelings are unconsciously kept out of awareness	A man is jealous of a good friend's success but is unaware of his feelings.
Suppression	Unacceptable feelings and thoughts are consciously kept out of awareness	A student taking an examination is upset about an argument with her boyfriend but puts it out of her mind so she can finish the test.
Identification	Unconscious assumption of similarity between oneself and another	After hospitalization for minor surgery a girl decides to be a nurse.
Introjection	Acceptance of another's values and opinions as one's own	A woman who prefers a simple life-style assumes the materialistic, prestige-oriented values of her husband.
Projection	One's own unacceptable feelings and thoughts are attributed to others	A man who is quite critical of others thinks that people are joking about his appearance.
Denial	Blocking out painful or anxiety-inducing events or feelings	A boss tells an employee he may have to fire him. On the way home the employee shops for a new car.
Fantasy	Symbolic satisfaction of wishes through nonrational thought	A student struggling through graduate school thinks about a prestigious, high-paying job he wants.
Rationalization	Falsification of experience through the construction of logical or socially approved explanations of behavior	A man cheats on his income tax return and tells himself it's all right because everyone does it.
Reaction formation	Unacceptable feelings disguised by repression of the real feeling and by reinforcement of the opposite feeling	A woman who dislikes her mother-in-law is always very nice to her.
Displacement	Discharging of pent-up feelings on persons less dangerous than those who initially aroused the emotion	A student who has received a low grade on a term paper blows up at his girl friend when she asks about his grade.
Intellectualization	Separating an emotion from an idea or thought because the emotional reaction is too painful to be acknowledged	A man learns from his doctor that he has cancer. He studies the physiology and treatment of cancer without experiencing any emotion.

Task-oriented and Defense-oriented Reactions

Nurses can be more helpful if they understand the specific changes the client is undergoing. Reactions to threatening situations, such as illness and hospitalization, can be divided into two general categories—task-oriented and defense-oriented responses. When we feel competent to deal with stress, and the situation is not too threatening to our sense of self, our behavior tends to be task-oriented. Task-oriented behavior is geared toward problem solving. A student who is majoring in mathematics fails his courses. If he is not too frightened by the possibility that he may not be suited for a

career in this field, he can assess the situation and change his major. This is a task-oriented reaction. It is based on a realistic appraisal of the situation and involves a series of carefully thought-out judgments about what course of behavior would be most effective.

When we feel inadequate to cope with stress, and the situation is extremely threatening to our sense of self, we tend to engage in defense-oriented reactions (see Table 10-5). The diagnosis of a terminal illness, for instance, may be so overwhelming that a person must temporarily defend against acknowledging this reality. Everyone uses defense-oriented behavior from time to time as a protective measure. Such behavior becomes harmful only when it is the predominant means of coping with stress. In such cases, problem-solving and reality-based behavior are continually avoided.

Defense Mechanisms

Defense-oriented behavior is not a specific attempt to solve a problem. It consists of using coping patterns to lessen uncomfortable feelings of anxiety and to prevent pain. These coping patterns are commonly called *defense mechanisms*. They are unconscious. They protect the self by enabling us to deny or distort a stressful event or by restricting awareness and reducing the sense of emotional involvement. But they can also interfere with rational decision-making. People who use defense mechanisms are excluding some information about the situation they are in. They are also denying their own feelings about it.

Because human behavior is so complex and various, any classification of defense mechanisms is necessarily incomplete. Definitions of various defense mechanisms overlap, and the same observed behavior may often be explained by more than one type of defense. People do not use one method of defense at a time. Usually they rely on a combination of defenses. For study purposes, common defense mechanisms may be classified as: repression; dissociation; suppression; identification; introjection; projection; denial; fantasy; rationalization; reaction formation; displacement; and intellectualization.

Repression   Repression is the involuntary exclusion from awareness of a painful or conflictual thought, memory, feeling, or impulse. Repression is the underlying basis of all of the defense mechanisms, and the other defenses reinforce it. It is initiated to bar access to consciousness of feelings and thoughts that would cause anxiety and thus disrupt the self-concept. It also affords protection from sudden, traumatic experience until the individual is able to deal with the shock. From the individual's point of view, a repressed memory is "forgotten" and cannot be deliberately brought to awareness. The repressed feelings remain out of awareness but continue to exert pressure for expression. The self must exert energy to maintain the repression and in instances of extreme stress may not be able to sustain repression. In situations of extreme anxiety and in febrile or toxic states, repression may begin to fail. Clients who are intoxicated by alcohol or drugs or who are emerging from anesthesia may verbalize feelings that they usually repress.

Susan was raped. She was brought to an outpatient clinic by her roommate. Susan said she felt very anxious but could not remember the events of the past few hours. Her use of repression protected her from facing her fears and humiliation.

Nursing intervention in such cases should be supportive and protective of the client's defenses. After the initial shock has lessened and the client's anxiety level has been reduced, the client can be helped to examine the traumatic event.

Dissociation   Dissociation resembles repression, but it has a different origin. The self is formed through the process of disapproval and approval from significant other people. Therefore the self *dissociates* or refuses awareness to the expression of personal qualities and experiences that significant other people disapprove of. These feelings come to exist separately from the person's self-concept. A little girl with latent artistic abilities that are not validated by her parents will not think of herself as artistic. She may deny her abilities even when other people point them out.

People who express dissociated feelings or qualities do not "notice" what they are doing. This limitation of awareness is maintained because the person experiences anxiety whenever permissible levels for the self are trespassed.

Ms. T consciously believes that sexual overtures are wrong, yet she behaves seductively toward men. She cannot understand why men see her behavior as a sexual invitation. The use of repression or dissociation complicates Ms. T's problems. She needs to ignore or deny aspects of her situation in order to feel comfortable in it. Other people notice and point out Ms. T's seductive behavior, but she cannot recognize it because it is not a part of her self-concept. If Ms. T admitted her sexual feelings she would experience severe anxiety and personality disorganization.

Suppression   Suppression is the conscious analog of repression. Because it is conscious, it is not a defense mechanism in the strict sense of the term. Suppression is the intentional exclusion of material from consciousness. For instance, a student who is trying to study finds herself thinking about her weekend plans. These thoughts are interfering with her concentration, so the student consciously decides not to think about her weekend in order to study effectively. A client may refuse to consider his difficulties by saying that he "doesn't want to talk about it" or that he will "think about it some other time." This, too, is suppression.

We can deal with suppression in the same way we deal with repression or dissociation. Suppression is generally easier to deal with because the material remains conscious. We can be somewhat more directive in assessing why the client avoids talking about a situation, and we can structure our expectations of the client. For instance, a client who is suppressing thoughts about his diagnosis of diabetes may respond to the nurse's suggestion that he try to look at his situation because it is important to make future plans. The nurse may begin to deal with suppression in the client by offering him information about diabetes. This may enable him to look at his situation objectively. As he learns more about his condition, it may become less threatening to him.

Identification Identification is the wish to be like another person and to assume the characteristics of that person's personality. It represents an estrangement from our own personality. Identification is unconscious. In this it differs from *imitation,* which is the conscious copying of another person's qualities. Identification with admired persons can serve an important function in maturation by evoking latent qualities. The little girl identifies with her mother and sisters and thus learns the behavioral characteristics of womanhood.

The most primitive type of identification is seen in the infant's relationship with the mother. Infants seem to perceive no difference between their mothers and themselves and only gradually become aware that their mothers exist apart from them. Small children deal with people in terms of how those people meet their needs. They do not see them as separate persons with needs of their own. Such identifications may persist into adult life in people who have not differentiated themselves psychologically from seemingly powerful parents.

One specific manifestation of identification is an attitude of passive receptivity rather than reciprocity in relationships. People who feel they have no resources of their own will overvalue the resources of others and expect to be taken care of. People who are most identified with their parents tend to be people who were not allowed to develop their own individuality. Part of the process of self-realization occurs in adolescence, when we discard, with much anxiety and insecurity, our identification with the parents on whom we have been so dependent. Some clients may not have

achieved a degree of self-identity sufficient to enable them to do this. Continuing the process of identification can inhibit our usefulness, because it prevents us from focusing on our own capacities.

Identification can be seen in clients who rely heavily on the nurse's advice and support. They expect that all their needs will be met and that nothing will be expected of them. Such clients are not interested in dealing with their own problems.

Mr. L is diabetic. He is not interested in learning about the diet he must follow and the medication he must take. He expects the nurse to take the responsibility for seeing that he gets the right food and medicine. Nursing care should be focused on helping Mr. L replace his feelings of powerlessness with confidence in his own productivity. We should recognize that a client who feels completely dependent on us may also resent his apparent helplessness. Mr. L's nurse should clarify with Mr. L what his expectations of her are. She should help him make use of the nurse–client relationship in a way that will increase his own skills. She must correct Mr. L's preconception that she will take care of his diabetes. She can then present the issue of diabetes as her own and Mr. L's joint concern. She can give recognition to any sign that Mr. L is taking some responsibility for his own care. A final step in dealing with identification is to help Mr. L formulate his own medication and diet plan independently of her.

It is important to recognize that identification, which can be seen as an annoying passivity on the part of the client, can be used constructively to teach proper health care. A client can learn to make use of the nurse's skills while respecting the differences between their two roles and perspectives.

Introjection Introjection is closely related to identification. It is the process of accepting another's values and opinions as one's own even if they contradict the values one had previously held. A man whose employer engages in shoddy workmanship may introject his employer's values even though they are contrary to his own moral beliefs, because he is afraid of losing his job. Introjection also occurs in severe depression following the death of a loved person. The depressed person may assume many of the deceased person's characteristics and in so doing lose some self-awareness. The nurse can treat introjection like identification, remembering that introjection is more primitive and more intractable. It originates in our experience of being fed as infants. We incorporated people and objects into ourselves in the same way we swallowed food. We felt a sense of oneness with everything in the external world and could not differentiate ourselves from others. Because thinking processes are not involved in the first experience of introjection, this defense tends to be difficult to explore on the verbal level.

Projection Projection is an unconscious means of dealing with personal difficulties or unacceptable wishes by attributing them to others. We blame other people for our shortcomings or see them as harboring our own unacceptable feelings or thoughts. In the course of development, the child, who needs the parents' approval, will identify with them and will also deny what they seem to condemn or fail to acknowledge. For instance, if her parents do not openly express and recognize angry feelings, a little girl will tend to regard anger as dangerous. She will then deny awareness of her own anger. Anger in others will disturb her, and she will tend to condemn in others the anger she cannot accept in herself. It is common knowledge that people often tend to criticize in others their unacknowledged inferiorities. The person who fears being taken advantage of is often an opportunist.

It is not so generally recognized that more positive qualities may also be projected. Such projected qualities are an important force in personality development. A child commonly idealizes teachers and older children who possess qualities that are undeveloped parts of the child's own personality. Through the emotional contact in the relationship, such children assimilate latent qualities into their own personalities, thus further delineating themselves.

In adult life, projection can be destructive if it interferes with our ability to acknowledge our own feelings. The tendency to attribute our own undesired feelings to others also blurs the boundaries between ourselves and others. This, in turn, makes it difficult to understand other people's feelings. People who make excessive use of projection tend to attribute to others hostile or seductive motives that do not actually exist. This prevents them from forming trusting and reciprocal relationships. A tendency to projection may also interfere with problem solving. A student who believes he is failing a course because of his teacher will not focus his energies on his studies.

Clients who must deal with the stress of serious illness may shift the blame for their condition onto the nurse. They may complain of poor nursing care to a

nurse who is actually very skillful. These clients may actually fear that they have caused their own problems by neglecting their health. They may believe that they are being "paid back" for wrongdoing in the past. If nurses feel that such a client is accusing them falsely, they should not show anger and retaliate but should show, through consistency and attention, that they respect these clients and are concerned about their welfare. As clients feel more secure in the nurse–client relationship, nurses can encourage these clients to explore the realistic aspects of their situation. For example, a client who blames his family for his alcoholism can be helped to explore objectively what is known about the etiology of alcoholism. This may help him come to terms with his feelings of guilt and anger. This type of intervention will help the client to separate his own feelings from the objective facts of the situation.

Denial Denial of reality is one of the simplest of the defense mechanisms. In denial, painful or anxiety-producing aspects of awareness are blocked out of consciousness. The reality of a situation is either completely disregarded or transformed so that it is no longer threatening. Denial is one of the commonest defenses against the stress of diagnosis and illness. It may be helpful as a temporary protection against the full impact of a traumatic event. Denial is typically present in the first few minutes of adjustment to the death of a loved person. The bereaved individual may believe that the death did not really happen, or that some mistake was made in identifying the body.

A client may transform a threatening situation into a nonthreatening one. For instance, a client admitted to a psychiatric hospital for a psychotic episode may say he just "needs a rest."

Mr. S is denying the seriousness of his myocardial infarction. He refuses to remain in bed, and he continues to smoke. Mr. S consciously believes that nothing is wrong with his heart because he cannot deal with the fear of disability and death that recognizing the truth would entail.

Sometimes denial is the best solution for the client. In such situations, the defense should be supported. A terminally ill client who believes she will soon recover, and who cannot think about her illness, should be allowed the protection of denial. Not all clients need to face up to reality. The nurse should recognize that denial may be preventing serious personality disorganization.

Sometimes, however, denial is directly harmful to the client, as when a man refuses to take medication that is crucial to his survival. In such cases, the motivation for the client's behavior should be assessed. Once the particular protective function the denial is serving has been discovered, the nurse can focus attention on helping the client meet these needs in a way that is not self-destructive. A client who behaves like Mr. S may wish to maintain his self-image of physical strength and masculinity. The nurse should be careful not to deprive this client of things he can do for himself. Instead, he can be helped to recognize the strengths he still has as he mourns the loss of his past capacities. He can learn to refocus his source of self-esteem onto other activities and skills. For instance, he may accept the fact that he can never play football again, but he can still write or paint. We can also help him identify with others who have successfully adjusted to heart disease. Helping the client recognize that he has other resources and can still be productive, though in different ways, will decrease the need for denial. The nurse can help by taking care not to reinforce patterns of denial. Instead we should focus on instances when the client seems to be dealing with reality. For example, if the client remarks, "Maybe I should slow down after this heart attack," the nurse should focus on this breakthrough.

Fantasy   Fantasy is a form of nonrational mental activity that enables the individual to escape temporarily the demands of the everyday world. Fantasies are not confined by the reality considerations of cause and effect and time and space. Fantasy normally characterizes the thinking of children before they are able to engage in consensually validated communication. Adults revert to fantasy during times of stress to obtain a symbolic satisfaction of wishes. For example, we can escape from financial difficulties temporarily by planning how to spend an imaginary fortune. This type of thinking is not rational, because it involves denying the actual economic situation. Fantasy may offer temporary relief from pressures, but people who spend too much time in fantasy may be unable to meet the requirements of reality.

Imagination does have a creative aspect, however. Fantasies have a richness and variety that is lacking in the everyday world. In fact, certain artists, such as Dali and Picasso, enrich their works of art through fantasy. Evidence also exists that insights into scientific discov-

ery do not come about as the result of step-by-step logical thinking. Rather, they are created through fantasy. Clients who are very ill may fantasize that when they recover many good things will happen to them. They may imagine that they will receive special recognition in their work, or that they will get along better with their families. These fantasies may help such clients deal with the deprivations caused by illness. However, they may also cause unrealistic expectations. Such clients may expect to be paid back for their suffering. They may cherish "suffering hero" fantasies. These fantasies provide some measure of compensatory gratification but interfere with problem solving.

Clients who are engaging in fantasy related to their illness need gradual help in assessing the responses others are likely to make and the achievements they themselves may realistically expect. Clients who fail to adjust to reality will be very disappointed when their grandiose expectations are not met. A helpful approach that will not devastate clients who need to hold onto some fantasy is to ask them to discuss their specific future plans. Examining the details of work and interpersonal adjustment may help a person to relinquish unrealistic expectations and make more realistic plans. For example, a woman who believes that a diagnosis of cancer will improve her marriage because her husband will appreciate her more fully must recognize that this is improbable. She needs to examine the real effects her illness will have on her husband. She must plan how to make specific improvements in their communication by anticipating problem areas. The nurse may also decrease this woman's need for fantasy by offering support for reality-based achievements, such as changing her own dressing. This enables her to receive gratification in a realistic way.

Rationalization   Rationalization is the substitution of acceptable reasons for the real reasons for our behavior. It is used to justify specific behavior or to deal with disappointment. For instance, a student fails an examination because he can't understand the material. However, this truth causes him an intolerable amount of self-doubt. He may resort to the rationalization that he did not prepare adequately or that the teacher did not clarify the material sufficiently. Many people use rationalization because they wish to prove to themselves or others that their actions are governed by reason and common sense—even though they may not fully understand the reasons for their own behavior. Such explanations may be essential to maintain personal integrity. They are not destructive as long as they do not prevent one from solving everyday problems.

Rationalization becomes more of a hindrance when it prevents us from making necessary changes in our behavior by interfering with our ability to examine that behavior. One sign of rationalization is an active search for reasons to justify our behavior or beliefs. Another is an inability to recognize inconsistencies in our beliefs. A third is being upset when our reasons are questioned, since such questioning threatens our defenses. The student who repeatedly claims that she failed in mathematics only because she didn't study may remain in a field for which she is unsuited. It would be more productive for her to recognize that she has little ability in mathematics. Then she might change to a more suitable career.

Clients may use rationalization to soften the blow of losses caused by illness. Work interrupted by illness may be given up prematurely if the client rationalizes that he or she wouldn't have been successful in that field anyway. Such unnecessary restrictions deprive us of possible achievements. Clients who cannot deal emotionally with illness may try to explain away their unwillingness to discuss their treatment by saying that they are too stupid to deal with medical matters. A client who cannot look at his incision may rationalize that he was "always bothered by illness." These rationalizations close off the possibility of developing new capacities to understand and deal with illness. Nurses must respect their clients' need to rationalize fears and insecurities they cannot face. However, nurses must hold open the possibility for change. Such clients must be helped to face the reality of their situation by being encouraged to explore ways in which they can change to deal with it more effectively. One way is to help them explore in detail past instances in which they did change to cope with a stressful situation. Believing that we have real strengths helps us to face areas of insecurity.

Reaction Formation   Reaction formation is a means of defense whereby an undesirable impulse is kept out of awareness by emphasizing its opposite. To protect ourselves from recognizing dangerous feelings, we develop conscious attitudes and behavior patterns that are just the opposite of those feelings. Hostility may be concealed behind a facade of love and kindness. The desire to be sexually promiscuous may be concealed behind a moralistic demeanor. People who use this defense are not conscious of their true feel-ings, because reaction formation reinforces repression.

People who crusade passionately against alcohol, pornography, or cruelty to animals may be dealing with an underlying wish to enjoy these things. Of course, this is not true of everyone who is devoted to a cause. Clues that reaction formation is occurring are an inappropriate intensity of feeling and the inability to consider alternative points of view. The person who is always unnaturally sweet and loving, and who cannot consider the possibility of being angry, is probably using this excess of feeling to counteract an unacceptable anger.

Reaction formation can be useful. It can help us maintain socially approved behavior and avoid aware-ness of desires that are not socially acceptable. But this defense, too, results in self-deception, because it is not under conscious control. Therefore, it may result in exaggerated or rigid behaviors that leave us un-equipped to deal with crisis. People who feel they can never express annoyance and discomfort may need to be "good" clients, who never question their care or make demands. Such clients may not be able to allow themselves to depend on others. They may not be able to acknowledge their needs and seek fulfillment. This rigid stance is a reaction formation against the uncon-scious wish to be completely dependent. It is destruc-tive because it masks the individual's needs. It also prevents the person from meeting a crisis with flexibili-ty, because many possible actions are blocked from awareness. People who use this particular defense may also be excessively harsh in dealing with other people's weaknesses. They may be unable or unwilling to help them because they think everyone should be able to solve their own problems.

Coping with reaction formation requires essentially the same approach as coping with repression. The nurse should respect and support the client's defenses while providing a secure relationship in which to ex-plore feelings and new behavioral alternatives. Nurses must also be aware that it is easy to be annoyed at clients who cannot face their true feelings. The rigid and excessive display of what seems to be an insincere emotion can be frustrating. It is important to remem-ber that these clients are not "lying" or pretending. They are unconsciously protecting themselves against having to recognize threatening feelings.

Displacement   Displacement is the discharging of pent-up feelings, generally hostility, on an object less dangerous than the object that aroused the feelings.

This defense is used when emotions are aroused in a situation where it would be dangerous to express them.

John has just failed an important examination. He believes his failure was the instructor's fault. He cannot express the full extent of his anger, because that would get him into worse trouble with the instructor. John goes quietly back to the dormitory. But when his roommate turns the stereo on too loud, John explodes. He doesn't fear retaliation from his roommate—they are peers and friends.

In some cases, anger aroused by another person may be turned inward on the self. When this happens, the individual will experience exaggerated self-accusations and guilt.

Clients may express inappropriate anger to the nurse when they are actually angry at someone or something else. The client may feel more secure with the nurse, who offers a safe target for displaced feelings. Displacement differs from projection in that people who use displacement are not distorting their feelings and attributing them to someone else. The feelings are clear, and the person acknowledges them. They are simply being directed at the wrong person. Therefore, it may be easier to help these clients acknowledge the real situation. This may be achieved by remaining calm and accepting during an angry outburst. After the outburst is over, the nurse should question the client: "You seem so angry. I wonder if you really are angry that your breakfast is cold or if there might be some other reason." Opening up the possibility for a discussion of anger may help these clients to sort out just who they are angry at and why.

Intellectualization   Intellectualization is the process of separating the emotion aroused by an event from ideas or opinions about the event because the emotion itself is too painful to acknowledge. The painful emotion is avoided by means of a rational explanation that divests the event of any personal significance. Failures are made less significant by telling oneself that the situation could have been worse. A husband may deal with his wife's death by saying objectively that sudden death is better than chronic illness. A girl who breaks her leg skiing seeks consolation by reminding herself that she could have broken her neck.

People who feel guilty about certain behaviors may relieve their guilt by verbalizing their good intentions for changing. Clients may use intellectualization to blunt the emotional impact of their problems. This may be difficult for the nurse to perceive, because such clients often seem to know a great deal about their condition. They may be able to discuss in great detail the metabolic processes in diabetes or the psychodynamics of anxiety. At the same time they cannot apply these concepts to their own situation in an emotional sense. Intellectualization resembles rationalization in that it provides a verbal means of dealing with anxiety. Its use closes off the possibility of accepting and working out problems. Clients often use intellectualization at the onset of a crisis, and the need for this defense may decrease in a supportive nurse–client relationship. The nurse can help the client relate emotionally to a problem by not forcing the expression of feeling. This will only frighten the client further. Asking these clients to explain how their knowledge relates to them personally may encourage them to accept and explore their emotional reactions.

SELYE'S STRESS-ADAPTATION THEORY

Another framework for understanding how people react to stress is Hans Selye's stress-adaptation theory (Selye 1956). Selye defines stress as the rate of wear and tear on the body. He disputes the idea that only serious disease or injury causes stress. Selye thinks that any emotion or activity causes some degree of stress. Stress can be produced by any factor that requires a response or change in the individual. Stressors can be physical, chemical, physiological, developmental, or emotional. Playing a game of tennis, going out in the rain without an umbrella, having an argument, or getting a promotion are all examples of stressful events. Life itself is basically stressful, since it involves a process of adaptation to continual change. Though the experience of adaptation is stressful, it is not necessarily harmful. Indeed, it can be exciting and rewarding under certain circumstances, and although we cannot avoid the stress of living we can learn to minimize its damaging effects.

Feelings of anxiety, fatigue, or illness are subjective aspects of stress. Though stress itself cannot be perceived, it can be appraised by the objectively measurable structural and chemical changes that it produces

Table 10–6	SELYE'S STRESS ADAPTATION SYNDROME		
Stage	**Function**	**Physical Manifestations**	**Psychological Manifestations**
Stage I: alarm reaction	Mobilization of the body's defensive forces	Marked loss of body weight Increase in hormone levels Enlargement of the adrenal cortex and lymph glands	Person is alerted to stress Level of anxiety increases Task-oriented and defense-oriented behavior Symptoms of maladjustment, such as anxiety and inefficient behavior, may appear
Stage II: stage of resistance	Optimal adaptation to stress	Weight returns to normal Lymph glands return to normal size Reduction in size of adrenal cortex Constant hormonal levels	Intensified use of coping mechanism Person tends to use habitual defenses rather than problem-solving behavior Psychosomatic symptoms may appear
Stage III: stage of exhaustion	Body resources are depleted and organism loses ability to resist stress	Weight loss Enlargement and depletion of adrenal glands Enlargement of lymph glands and dysfunction of lymphatic system Increase in hormone levels and subsequent hormonal depletion If excessive stress continues, person may die	Personality disorganization and a tendency toward exaggerated and inappropriate use of defense mechanisms Increased disorganization of thoughts and perceptions Person may lose contact with reality, and delusions and hallucinations may appear Further exposure to stress may result in complete psychological disintegration (involving violence or stupor)

in the body. These manifest themselves as the General Adaptation Syndrome (GAS) when stress affects the whole body, and as the Local Adaptation Syndrome (LAS) when only a limited part of the body is exposed to stress. The entire body, as well as its individual organs and tissues, responds to stress. Some of these responses are signs of the damage caused by stress. Other changes are produced by the adaptive reactions of the body or its mechanisms of defense against stress (see Table 10–6).

The General Adaptation Syndrome

The General Adaptation Syndrome (GAS) occurs in three stages: alarm, resistance, and exhaustion. An example of the GAS can be found in combat soldiers. These men are exposed to ever-present threats of death and mutilation. They also experience the severe psychological shock of witnessing the destructiveness

of war. Other psychological and interpersonal factors contribute to their overall stress load. One such factor is the reduction of personal freedom and gratification. Another is separation from loved ones. The experiences of combat soldiers will be used to illustrate the three stages of the GAS.

Alarm Reaction When the soldier first encounters the stress of war, he experiences the alarm reaction. In alarm the body undergoes biochemical reactions as the adaptive hormones are stimulated. These adaptive hormones fall into two basic groups. The anti-inflammatory hormones include the adrenocorticotrophic hormone, cortisone, and cortisol. The proinflammatory hormones include the somatotrophic hormones, aldosterone, and desoxycorticosterone. The biochemical reactions that occur during alarm result in an enlargement of the adrenal cortex and lymph glands and increases in hormonal levels. These changes lower the subject's overall resistance. For example, soldiers may show such behavioral changes as increasing irritability, disturbances of sleep, and recurrent nightmares. Soldiers are described as being hypersensitive to minor stimuli. For instance, they will leap up in fright at the sound of a branch cracking. This behavior generally indicates failure to maintain psychological integration.

Stage of Resistance   Many men are able to adjust to combat. As they do so, the next stage, resistance, occurs. In the stage of resistance the biological changes in hormonal levels, adrenal cortex, and lymph glands are reversed. These men can maintain their psychological integrity. They may become used to killing and may even take pride in it. They may be able to maintain a fatalistic attitude about their own and their comrades' survival. A soldier who has made this adjustment may be able to resign himself to fate and believe that his role has an important purpose, even though he cannot fully understand it. He may take comfort in hoping that the combat will not last long, or that he will soon be rotated out of the combat area to a less stressful role. The nature of this adaptation seems to depend on many psychological and social factors. These include the stability of the soldier's personality, the morale of the combat unit, the sense of security and control provided by the leadership, and the friendships the soldier forms with other soldiers, which provide emotional support.

Exhaustion   The third stage, exhaustion, occurs if stress continues over a prolonged period of time. It also occurs when multiple stressors are active simultaneously, or when the subject undergoes repeated or overwhelming stress. When too many life changes occur within a short time, there is not enough time for the body to accommodate and adjust. When this happens, adaptive energy is exhausted, and the body surrenders to stress. The adrenal glands again enlarge and then are depleted. The lymph glands enlarge, producing a subsequent dysfunction of the lymph system. There is an increase and then a decrease in hormonal levels.

The longer a soldier is in combat, the more vulnerable and anxious he is likely to feel. Prolonged combat lowers stress tolerance. It may produce increased anxiety, depression, tremulousness, and impairment of judgment and self-confidence. This decompensation results in disturbances in interpersonal relationships. The soldier may lose all sense of loyalty to his comrades. In some cases, the residual effects of combat exhaustion persist for a long time. Combat experience may continue to disturb a man after he has returned to civilian life. He may experience guilt about killing and have nightmares about his war experiences.

Exhaustion may be reversible if the total body is not affected, and if the individual is eventually able to eliminate the source of stress. However, if stress is unrelieved, or if the body's defenses are totally involved, the individual may not regain psychological stability.

The Local Adaptation Syndrome

Selye also described a Local Adaptation Syndrome (LAS), which he defined as the manifestation of stress in a limited part of the body. In the LAS, body tissues have been directly subjected to stress, as in the example of an infected wound. These injured tissues convey chemical alarm signals to the central nervous system and the endrocrine glands, especially the pituitary and adrenals, which produce adaptive hormones. As in the GAS, the effects of these hormones can be modified by such factors as diet, heredity, and emotional reactions to stress.

The LAS evolves in the same three stages as the GAS. The LAS differs from the GAS in that the LAS is a local response to stress, while GAS is generalized. The LAS and the GAS function together to combat the effects of all stress. Both involve a tripartite mechanism. The first part of this mechanism is the direct effect of the stressor on the body. The second part is the internal responses that stimulate defense against the effects of stress. The third part is the internal responses that inhibit defense and stimulate surrender to stress. Selye's theory has important implications for a holistic approach to behavior in its emphasis on the totality of the body's reaction to stress.

Intervention at Various Levels of Stress

Seyle's stress-adaptation theory also provides a general framework for interventions at various points in the reaction to stress. It corresponds to some extent to the levels of primary, secondary, and tertiary prevention in health care. The goal of primary prevention is to prevent a stressor from disrupting the state of wellness that is considered normal for a particular person. For example, a man who feels that he would be particularly vulnerable to the stress of combat could be encouraged to investigate alternative means of meeting his military obligations. If stress cannot be avoided, another goal of primary prevention is to lessen the degree of reaction. This may be done by reducing the possibility of encounter with the stressor, by reducing the strength of the stressor, or by strengthening the individual's immediate state of wellness. A soldier could request duties off the battlefield, or he could avoid putting himself into extremely dangerous situations whenever possible. If he could not avoid stress, he could strengthen his adaptive powers by forming strong loyalties to his commander and unit.

Secondary prevention focuses on interventions initiated after contact with stress. It is concerned with the early detection of stress reactions and the treatment of symptoms. Soldiers who display increased anxiety, sleep disturbances, and tremors should be removed from combat and treated in aid stations. It has been demonstrated that three or four days after such treatment many soldiers are emotionally ready to return to duty and seem to be able to adapt. Such early treatment can aid the process of resistance to stress and prevent the stage of exhaustion.

Tertiary prevention is intervention initiated after treatment. It focuses on readaptation to stress and maintenance of stability. Tertiary prevention is appropriate for those individuals who seem to be unable to resist stress, and who develop serious and prolonged symptoms such as high levels of anxiety and nightmares. Serious and prolonged readjustment problems among returning veterans may indicate a state of exhaustion when adaptive energies are depleted. Supportive treatment with a focus on adjustment to civilian life may prevent further personality decompensation.

Lazarus, another noted theorist on the subject of stress, adds to Selye's explanation the idea that individualistic interpretations of the meaning of stress to a person must always be considered when evaluating stress and coping experiences (Lazarus 1966).

THEORIES OF GROWTH AND DEVELOPMENT

The Relativistic Nature of Theories

In their adaptations to life, humans are characterized by a basic openness to the world. They differ in this respect from other mammals, whose world is firmly structured by their instinctual organization. Human drives are highly unspecialized. This makes possible a wide range of adjustments. The great variety of cultures throughout the world is evidence of this adaptability. However, this intrinsic openness to the world is limited to some extent by social order. This limitation is necessary because the inherent instability of the human organism requires a stable environment in which to structure conduct.

People adopt certain behavior patterns that relieve them of the need to make continual decisions about their behavior. The reinforcement of habitual behavior in interaction with others produces shared agreements about the nature of reality. These unspoken agreements become social rules, which are built up over time to control society. After a period of time, systems of shared agreements become institutionalized. That is, they possess a reality of their own and cannot readily be changed. Democracy and monogamy are examples of systems of shared agreements that have become institutionalized. Social agreements have an objective reality. Any great deviation from these agreements is a departure from reality.

Theories of growth and development can also be viewed as human creations that have become so accepted that they have a reality of their own. Viewing life as a series of stages, each of which involves certain developmental tasks, gives one's life order and meaning. People move through life like actors playing out the roles and expectations of each developmental phase. A person who deviates significantly from these role expectations is assigned an inferior status in the society. Thus, people institutionalize their conduct to make their behavior understandable and predictable to others and also to minimize their awareness of the basic precariousness of social reality.

Phases of the Human Life Cycle

The human life cycle can be divided into ten phases. These are infancy, early childhood, late childhood, the juvenile period, adolescence, postadolescence and the psychosocial moratorium, young adulthood, adulthood and the mid-life crisis, middle age, and old age. Each stage has specific tasks of development that lead to a restructuring of the individual's personality organization.

Infancy, early childhood, late childhood, and the juvenile period are thoroughly discussed in Chapter 19. Adolescence is the focus of Chapter 20, and old age is the concern of Chapter 22; those stages of the human life cycle are discussed in those chapters. Three phases of the human life cycle—postadolescence and the psychosocial moratorium, adulthood and the mid-life crisis, and middle age are the focus of the following discussion.

Postadolescence and the Psychosocial Moratorium (Twenty to Twenty-Eight Years)

In his discussion of identity formation, Erikson speaks of prolonged adolescence. He characterizes this stage as a second period of delay after adolescence. During this time we postpone the choice of a mate while experimenting with various role possibilities. This period is not merely a delay of adult commitments. It is a period permitted by the culture for adventures that coincide with social values, such as travel, the Peace Corps, involvement with political groups, or religious quests.

Part of our motivation during this period is to prolong the irresponsibility of youth. But frequently we undertake experiments in responsible, adult behavior. Two conflicting wishes are operating simultaneously. We want to build a secure future by making intelligent commitments, and we also want to explore without being confined to a permanent structure. We may see ourselves striking out in a new and creative way rather than following cultural rules for adulthood, or we may value a scholarly or nonmaterialistic life in contrast to society's competitive and materialistic values. This process may take as long as eight years to complete. On the surface it may seem to be a period of wasteful aimlessness. A person may have many different jobs during this time, move around constantly, and become involved in many relationships.

This period is crucial for some people. Even though they have consolidated their social roles, selected their life tasks, and disengaged from their parents during adolescence, they may not be completely integrated. The psychological purpose of the moratorium is to harmonize the component parts of the personality. Adolescence must be completely assimilated in order to achieve an adult functioning identity. Sheehy (1976) and others believe that such a process is necessary to fix the identity completely.

RESOLUTION Certain signs indicate that we are settling down. We begin to limit ourselves to meet goals of work or relationships. We begin to locate a peer group, sex role, and anticipated occupation or ideology. We recognize in ourselves the powers of self-reliance that we once admired in others who seemed

stronger. People who pass through a long psychosocial moratorium have the satisfaction of finding a place in society that is uniquely theirs. They may feel that their choice of life-style is the one true course in life.

People who fail to achieve such a degree of integration often feel that their identity was foreclosed too early. They may feel that they chose a career and mate in conformity with peer standards rather than with their own wishes. These people may always have uniform and shallow personalities.

During the period of prolonged adolescence, we shape an ideal version of life, but we also fear that our choices are irrevocable. We are strengthened by the illusion that we can do anything we want to do and can change ourselves and others through sheer power of will. This self-deception may be necessary to energize our first difficult commitments sufficiently.

INTIMACY VERSUS ISOLATION According to Erikson, people achieve intimacy with others only after developing the capacities associated with identity development. This intimacy involves true mutuality. In true mutuality we can merge ourselves in friendships or sexual relationships without fear of losing our sense of self. The ability to love results in a new and shared identity.

The counterpart of intimacy is isolation. Isolation manifests itself in withdrawal from relationships or in an active repudiation of people and ideas that seem foreign to the self. Isolated people may avoid close relationships or involve themselves in a series of highly stereotyped relationships that lack any sense of fusion.

Sheehy (1976) describes the "urge to merge" that occurs during the end of the psychosocial moratorium. Women have a more difficult time with identity formation than men. There is a general cultural expectation that they will marry and share in the prestige of the identity earned by their husbands. Some women may wish to marry in order to be as safe and secure as they were in their parents' home. These women may give birth to a child to prove their worth. Sheehy believes that many women are immature because early marriage has foreclosed their identities. However, the recent increased tolerance for a diversity of life-styles supports a variety of forms of commitment and intimacy. Living together or marriage without children are becoming viable situations in which women have an increasing variety of ways to demonstrate their worth.

Men may also marry for reasons of conformity or they may marry in order to have someone to depend on emotionally. They hope their wives will help them define and carry out their career ambitions. Whether the decision is made on the basis of genuine wishes for intimacy or is simply a matter of conforming to societal expectations largely depends on the degree of identity formation.

ADULT DEVELOPMENTAL TASKS   Daniel Levinson first proposed the theory that there is an underlying order to the course of adult life, and that each period involves specific tasks (discussed in Sheehy 1976). He thinks that developmental cycles in adulthood last about seven years. According to Levinson adults move from one period to the next only when they begin working at new developmental tasks and build a new structure for their lives. Each period must follow in sequence and is linked to a particular age. The appropriate age for each cycle varies within a very narrow range.

Adulthood and the Mid-life Crisis (Thirty to Forty-Two Years)

By adulthood we are assumed to have achieved maturity. We see ourselves as independent agents, free to choose intimates and implement decisions and able to love and influence others. Mature people can tolerate uncertainty, open themselves to new experience, and find common elements between themselves and people who are different from themselves. The late twenties are crucial for the development of these abilities.

CHANGE OF LIFE-STYLE   Sheehy's investigations have revealed that most people between the ages of twenty-nine and thirty-two want to change their life-style. They want to break out of old restrictions, change their occupations, or choose a new career. The single person considers marriage, and the childless couple considers children. Career women suddenly want to become housewives, and men want to return to graduate school. The work of this phase involves much turmoil as people change the life structure they have built during their twenties. It is only in the early thirties that a person really begins to settle down. Typically, men concentrate on the groundwork necessary to be successful in their field, and women concentrate on child rearing. Social life outside the family is reduced as the couple turn their attention to raising children.

BIRTH OF CHILDREN   The birth of a first child represents a crisis for the couple. Though it is usually a joyful experience and a manifestation of their common

bond, it involves adjustments in life-style and self-image. Social and recreational activities may be modified as the child makes demands on the couple's time and money. The wife may leave her job to care for the child, or the couple may move to larger living quarters. Changes in self-perception involve a transition from the early ideal of romantic love and marriage to a more practical sense of the marital relationship as the couple concentrates on the concrete tasks of establishing a family. Couples may view their marriage as more permanent and become less self-centered and more family centered. They may become interested in community and educational activities as they plan social and economic supports for child rearing.

Current social structures make adjustment to parenthood difficult. The isolated nuclear family system and the geographic mobility often linked with career advancement make it difficult to develop a close social network of family and friends. Intimates are frequently not available to serve as role models and help out during difficult periods.

PARTICULAR STRESSES ON WOMEN   Women may have problems with the role requirements of maternity. They may see motherhood as depriving them of opportunities to pursue their interests and social expectations. Cultural pressures on women to assume a maternal role are equal to pressures on men to work. A woman must usually assume this role to gain adult status, though cultural pressures in this respect fluctuate according to economic conditions. The current debate about women's participation in politics and work has eased these pressures in certain socioeconomic groups. So has the women's liberation movement, with its emphasis on restructuring traditional male and female roles. It is becoming more acceptable for parents to share equally in all parental functions. Thus the stress of parenting is more equally shared between husband and wife.

THE EFFECTS OF BIRTH ORDER ON CHILDREN   Additional children further alter the family relationship. Birth order research examines the influence of siblings on each other. It also examines parental attitudes toward male and female children in relation to birth order. These studies point out the effects of birth order on personality development. For instance, firstborns achieve more because their closer relationships with their parents have given them a greater need for approval and have internalized adult values. Lastborns are likely to be more sociable because they have had to gain the attention of a parent who may be less interested in them than in the firstborn child.

CHANGES BETWEEN AGES THIRTY-FIVE AND THIRTY-NINE   The years between thirty-five and thirty-nine are particularly important for careers because we feel the pressure of time as the age of forty approaches. The career person becomes less dependent on mentors, bosses, and colleagues. Couples may experience particular difficulties at this time, for a husband and wife do not necessarily develop emotionally and intellectually at the same rate and in the same ways. The husband may have experienced rapid economic and social change as he advances in his career. He may feel more competent and no longer need the emotional protection he once sought from his wife. He may urge her to change as well, go to school, or become more social. She may see these requests as threatening. She, too, wishes to expand at this age, but this may be difficult if she lacks the necessary confidence and skills to develop her abilities. If his wife cannot change, the husband may find another woman—possibly one connected with his career—who will validate his professional achievement in a way his wife cannot.

THE MID-LIFE CRISIS   At the age of forty we are impressed by the fact that we are at the midpoint of life. As we enter what may be the stage of greatest occupational and interpersonal fulfillment, we become vividly aware that death lies ahead. At forty we are no longer promising young people with potential. The degree of affirmation we have received professionally thus far is a good indicator of the amount of success that we will achieve, and current interpersonal commitments may represent the degree of intimacy we will attain.

During the years between thirty-nine and forty-two, people pass through a period of acute discomfort as they face the discrepancy between their youthful ambitions and their actual achievement. Until recently, developmental psychologists have generally ignored middle age. Now interest in this period is increasing. The mid-life crisis is important because it marks the passage between early maturity and middle age. The onset and duration of this crisis vary with the individual. Most women pass through it between thirty-five and forty and most men between forty and forty-five.

CHARACTERISTICS OF THE MID-LIFE CRISIS   The crisis is characterized by feelings of boredom, dissatisfaction with the way life has developed, and ambivalence and uncertainty about the future. During this time we re-

evaluate what we have done to date and assess our goals. We view with dismay the signs of aging—greying hair, wrinkled skin, and changes in eyesight. Women may anticipate the climacteric, which occurs in the late forties or early fifties.

At forty we must reconsider life in the light of the reality of aging and death. The optimism of earlier years that enabled us to shrug off disappointments gives way to depression. We recognize that our productive time is limited and fear that we cannot accomplish all we had hoped to accomplish before time runs out. Our teenage children suddenly seem intellectually and sexually mature and may challenge our sense of omnipotence. Parents—whom we looked to once for security and comfort—may now need taking care of. When a parent contracts a terminal illness or dies, we become next in line in the generational progression. Now we directly confront the threat of aging and death.

As we face early signs of physical deterioration and question social roles we used to take for granted, our personality changes. A woman may challenge traditional definitions of femininity and become more assertive. A man may become more introspective and sensitive to emotions. The sense of time passing us by produces a feeling of urgency about our last chances to accomplish a given goal. A woman may ask herself what she is giving up to maintain her marriage, or whether her concentration on a career is depriving her of happiness. She may wonder why she had three children or, if she is childless, ask herself if there is still time for childbearing. The sense of deadline that a woman experiences about the age of thirty-five is compounded by life events. The average mother sends her last child to school at this age. It is the time when the average married woman reenters the work force. If she is divorced, a woman is likely to remarry around this age.

Men also feel the pressure of time but generally not until the age of forty, and they may handle this crisis differently. Women tend to reevaluate their life as a whole, while men concentrate on their present goals. Many men accelerate their efforts to achieve success in their career. They are acutely aware of their employer's evaluations of them at this age. Most men have to adjust their goals downward. If they do succeed, they face pressure to outdo themselves in their next endeavor. Men may concentrate on making external changes. They may improve their appearance, marry a younger woman, or take up skiing or motorcycle racing in an attempt to retain their youth. However, a man must gradually give up the idealized self of the early twenties for a more realistically attainable self. He may have to relinquish early hopes of making important discoveries in his field and settle for the more modest goal of competence. Dreams of romance and sexual fulfillment may be replaced by the satisfactions of friendship and companionship.

Loss of youth and the faltering of physical powers produce a crisis that makes personality change possible. This struggle may cause depression, mood swings, and lowered self-esteem. Gradually, this emotional upheaval will lead to greater growth as the person develops a new sense of purpose. Without such a mid-life crisis, development may become restricted, and the vitality necessary for further developmental tasks may be lost.

Middle Age (Forty-Two to Sixty-Five or Seventy Years)

The person in the mid-life crisis is very different from the person who has restabilized around middle age. People in the mid-life crisis define their situation in relation to others. They relate their career plans to competition with younger people. They maintain their physical attractiveness in the face of what they see as a struggle to keep up with younger rivals. Their marriage partner or lover is crucial to their self-definition. These people feel they are at their peak in ability. But as we reach middle age, we look back on the mid-life crisis as only a stage in the ongoing life cycle. We cease to blame our marriage partner for our problems, and we relax our sense of competitiveness. A new freedom to be independent and follow our individual interests opens up. Sheehy defines this change as a movement from "us-ness" to "me-ness." We can now enjoy the prerogatives of middle age without making invidious comparisons with others, and we no longer fear aging and death.

GENERATIVITY VERSUS STAGNATION In Erikson's view, the developmental choice in middle age is between generativity and stagnation. Erikson defines generativity as a concern for establishing and guiding the next generation. We evaluate our productiveness and make inferences about what we can look forward to accomplishing. If we have been able to contribute something to society or care for dependents, we have resolved the issue of generativity in a positive way. If we refuse to assume the power and responsibility of middle age, we become stagnant. Erikson thinks that people who cannot expand their interests at this point

in life suffer a pervading sense of boredom and impoverishment. If the crisis is resolved constructively, we will have a greater capacity for responsible involvement and will shift our values away from physical attractiveness and strength to intellectual abilities. A corresponding shift from sexuality to platonic relationships may widen our circle of acquaintances in the community and vocational world. Our stature as an experienced person may provide contacts with people over a wide age range, and relationships may become more varied and differentiated.

THE PRODUCTIVITY OF MIDDLE AGE People who have done the work of self-confrontation and change in the early forties enter what may be the most productive period of their lives. Sheehy describes the period between forty-three and fifty as a time of restabilization and flowering. We come to terms with the fact that our life is finite and reconcile what is with what might have been. Children previously loved as extensions of ourselves are respected as individuals, and we are able to modify early illusions about our capacities. A well-developed sense of judgment makes more efficient and well-reasoned decisions possible.

In middle age interests left dormant during early struggles to establish a family and a career can be redeveloped. Previous hobbies or secondary interests can blossom into serious work. A teacher can retire and turn her hobby of weaving into a small business. A lawyer can concentrate on his interest in photography. Development of alternative abilities releases new energies.

Sheehy finds that men and women have different cues for changes in their status as they grow older. Men define themselves in terms of career position and health changes. Women define themselves in terms of family events, such as the marriage of children and the birth of grandchildren. A woman must find interests to replace housekeeping and child rearing or she will experience the depression of the "empty nest syndrome." Men face the problem of enforced retirement between the ages of sixty and sixty-five, when they may still be capable of productive work. Physical health becomes a concern as signs of chronic illness may begin to develop. However, the stereotype of mental, physical, and sexual decline in the middle years has now been challenged. Recent studies show that there is no significant decline in learning ability or sexual interests during this period, and increasing judgment compensates for decline in physical abilities (Bromley 1966, p. 249). The preoccupation with psychosomatic complaints that characterized many middle-aged people in the past is disappearing as other behavioral options become available. Marriage may offer more satisfaction as companionship develops between the couple who have left the stresses of child rearing behind.

THE EMPHASIS ON ONE'S OWN VALUES   Experience brings with it certain psychological benefits. Other people's opinions become less important as the middle-aged person becomes more preoccupied with inner life and philosophical and religious concerns. We may come to approve of ourselves ethically and morally in a way that is independent of the standards of others. The early habit of trying to please everyone, a particularly difficult problem for women, may be overcome. A woman may find she can tell the truth more often, instead of hiding her thoughts to protect other people's feelings.

We may understand, finally, that even if we have not achieved what we hoped for, we are good enough or successful enough. This feeling comes with self-respect. Outward manifestations of success, such as physical strength and material possessions, become less important. We appreciate everyday human experience more as we relinquish the search for glamour and power. The awareness of death may cause some people to value life in a deeper way.

CRITIQUE OF THE PARADIGM OF GROWTH AND DEVELOPMENT

This conception of the life cycle as a complex sequence of events from birth to death is based on the assumption that it is possible to describe such a sequence of events. Each stage of the cycle is accompanied by specific social roles. These roles are associated with appropriate norms of behavior and social expectations. In the mid-life crisis, for instance, one is expected to experience some emotional turmoil as one assesses the direction of one's life.

Each social role is appropriate to a particular age range, and people within one age range generally move through life together. Age norms are accepted social phenomena. Most husbands and wives are about the same age. Friendship groups and social organizations may have a restricted age range. Most promotions and retirements take place within certain age limits. Family and friends compare individuals within their

social group with respect to the individual's progress through the life span. This is particularly true in childhood, as parents compare their children's development with that of their friends' children. Normal development follows a standard path sequence that represents the typical progression through the life span. Various levels of achievement are thought to be possible at each stage. For example, development of social abilities during the juvenile period may range from the optimal level, at which social situations are undertaken with ease, to a merely adequate level, at which the child can manage social situations but is not particularly skillful in them. Development is said to follow a deviant path when it differs substantially from the standard. An example would be a school-age child who withdraws from all peer relationships.

The Standard Path of Development

The standard path of development varies somewhat from one person to another. This variation is due to differences in biological predispositions and environmental and social factors, all of which may constrain or encourage growth. Societal norms tolerate a wide range of developmental differences. However, behavior that falls outside this range is classified as abnormal or deviant. In today's achievement-oriented, competitive society, people who are markedly different are not readily accepted. American cultural values do not generally encourage individual solutions to problems; they exert a strong pressure to adjust to cultural patterns. Furthermore, certain areas in American culture fail to meet the individual's basic needs consistently, and this complicates the issue of adjustment. For example, in some cities it is difficult to establish an intimate social network because the social system is impersonal and mobile. Thus the individual's needs for intimacy may not be met. Even American developmental scales are structured in terms of achievement and continual progress, and people who adhere to these values receive the greatest reinforcement from the culture.

The Developmental Model of Behavior

The developmental model of behavior is based on the functionalistic-evolutionary model. The latter model assumes that in order to actualize oneself, one must unfold through a process of change. The developmental model of behavior originated in the biological model of development, and it is here that its weakness lies. There are crucial methodological differences between natural and cultural sciences. The natural sciences supplement observations of nature with hypotheses about their meaning. The cultural sciences cannot separate theory and observation in this way. The scientist of culture is not observing a neutral natural event but a preinterpreted world. The events in this world already have a particular meaning. They have this meaning because humans have preselected and preinterpreted the world by making a series of constructs about the meaning of everyday life.

We cannot deal with psychosocial development in the same way we deal with physical development. We can observe actual changes in height and weight. But we cannot make comparably precise observations of identity and intimacy, because those concepts are socially constructed. That is, they are formed by social processes that are determined by the social structure. Psychological theories only legitimate the identity-maintenance procedures that have been established in the society. This does not mean that such constructs are not useful: on the contrary, they are essential in structuring reality. But they must be used with caution—particularly where the placing of labels, such as "normal" or "abnormal," is concerned.

The Benefits of a Social Interaction Model

A social interaction model helps correct the faulty reasoning that characterizes absolute theories of development. It reveals theoretical structures as existing in constant revision determined by an ongoing process of interpretation. Concepts used in the cultural sciences should not be fixed and absolute. They should guide the observer's exploration, rather than precisely defining the characteristics of what is being investigated.

Using a fixed developmental model gives us a preconceived notion of what we are looking for. Rather than discovering reality, we rediscover our own preconceptions. This is harmless enough if we are merely theorizing. But using progress in developmental tasks as an absolute indicator of what is normal and abnormal distorts human experience. Such labeling of behavior becomes a means of social control and violates the rights of the individuals involved. Deviants from official definitions of reality may be given "therapy" to ensure that they do not trespass institutional definitions of reality. Another way of dealing with deviation is to negate it by denying its reality. This can be accomplished by giving deviants the inferior status of "immature" or "mentally ill" so that people do not take their actions seriously.

THE PROCESS OF DEVELOPING A DEVIANT IDENTITY

Development involves a sequence of recognized role behavior. Friends and family are continually judging the degree of developmental progress a person is making in life. Others judge the appropriateness of a person's behavior in relation to age norms. Developmental concepts enable us to compare adolescent identity development with the norm or to assess the preschooler's achievement of autonomy.

Deviance as Created by Society

Inappropriate behavior causes anxiety because it is meaningless and unpredictable. A man gesturing and talking to himself on the street goes beyond the usual social rules of propriety in public places. But, according to Howard Becker, deviance is not merely a failure to obey group rules (Becker 1973) or a disruption of the stability of society. In his view, the central fact of deviance is that it is *created* by society. A man who talks to himself in a public place is deviant because he is so labeled by people who are discomfited by his behavior. It is conceivable that in other settings his behavior would be tolerated.

Becker thinks that social groups create deviance, first, by making rules the breaking of which constitutes deviance, and second, by labeling as deviant people who break these rules. If society did not make such strict rules or socially segregate people who break them, deviance would not exist. "Deviants" do not exist naturally, and there is nothing inherently deviant in any human act. Deviance is an artificial category. This does not mean that there is no such thing as deviance, or that the deviant individual is merely an innocent victim of society. The individual generally chooses to engage in behavior that may be labeled deviant. But it does mean that society is actively involved in producing the phenomenon called deviance, and that we must look at these societal processes as well as at the deviant individual when we seek to deal with an instance of deviance.

From this point of view, deviance is not an aspect of the act the person commits. It is a consequence of rules applied by others to the so-called offender. The deviant is not a person who commits a certain act but a person who has been labeled deviant. A homosexual relationship, for instance, is not in itself deviant, according to this point of view. Society has made it deviant by deciding that such behavior is an infraction of rules and by categorizing as deviant a person who engages in homosexual behavior. More specifically, deviance is produced by a transaction that occurs between a particular social group and an individual who is seen by that group as a "rule breaker."

Classifying Behavior as Deviant   The classification of behavior as deviant depends on how people react to it. Just because a person has broken a rule does not mean that other people will consider the behavior deviant. In some social groups, homosexuality is not considered deviant, for instance. It may be seen as chic or adventurous, or as a political act.

People's responses to deviance vary over time. The same people may respond to deviant acts leniently at one time and strictly at another time. It has been noted, for instance, that police crackdowns on prostitution and pornography in urban areas intensify before mayoral elections. At other times, these infractions are more or less tolerated.

The degree to which an act will be treated as deviant also depends on who has committed the act and who feels harmed by it. Rules tend to be applied more strictly to some people than to others. It is well known that lower-class boys are much more likely to be convicted and sentenced for a crime than are boys from the middle and upper classes. The light jail sentences and pardons for high government officials involved in the Watergate affair also illustrate this inequality.

Some rules are enforced, not because of the act itself, but because of the consequences of the act. People who engage in premarital intercourse are not severely censured for doing so. However, if the girl becomes pregnant, she may be ostracized. Unmarried fathers usually escape social censure.

The Social Function of Deviance   Deviance is not simply behavior that disrupts the social stability. It may actually be an important factor in preserving that stability. Deviant people are placed outside the boundaries of society because they engage in certain behaviors. They illustrate the difference between the inside and the outside of the social group. In this way they dramatize the group norms and the punishment that can be expected to befall anyone who transgresses the rules. The definition of homosexuality as deviant behavior both reinforces the heterosexual norm and prevents people who might otherwise engage in homosexual behavior from doing so if they fear social censure.

The Process of Labeling Behavior Deviant
Only after behavior has caused repeated concern or interpersonal problems do others decide what, if anything, should be done about it. One achieves a deviant identity through a specifically delineated process of social definition. Suppose that a man continues in psychosocial moratorium well into his thirties. If his associates do not define his behavior in a negative way, the behavior will go unlabeled. If his intimates or the man himself defines his behavior as irresponsible or disturbed, it becomes a problem.

Redefinitions of Identity   Once an observer has defined a particular behavior as deviant, he or she must get other people—including the person who is being labeled—to agree. When this happens, the person's identity is redefined. The deviant is no longer normal but is suffering from a "fixation" or a "developmental lag." This redefinition of identity alters future interpersonal relationships by lowering the person's status and creating negative expectations of his or her behavior. Deviant people come to think of themselves in terms of a spoiled identity. This, in turn, may influence their present and future role behavior.

Class Differences in Development of Deviant Identity

What kinds of people formulate what kinds of problems? Upper-class people are likely to define deviant behavior in psychological terms and to seek psychiatric intervention. They tend to think that deviant behavior can and should be changed. If a person exhibits deviant behavior, psychologically sophisticated family members and friends may help that person define the problem and decide what to do about it. They help the potential client conquer initial fears and hesitations about therapy and offer specific guidance about where to seek help. Kadushin (1969) calls these helpers "Friends and Supporters of Psychotherapy." These friends of psychotherapy also tell the person what to expect from psychotherapy. They explain, for instance, that clients are expected to talk freely about what is on their minds and may relate their dreams. The deviant person's problems will also be defined in terms of the model to which the therapist adheres. For instance, a Freudian therapist might focus on the Oedipus complex. A Sullivanian therapist might focus on collaboration with peers. Kadushin found that as clients are initiated into a particular therapeutic model or style, they tend to increase the number of appropriate

KEY NURSING CONCEPTS

✔ The creation of a self begins at birth and ceases only at death.

✔ Through the process of socialization, individuals learn how to be human.

✔ Theories of life and growth are useful in understanding how human behavior changes throughout life. According to a holistic perspective, the complexities of behavior cannot be explained by any one theory alone.

✔ Four ways of organizing explanations of the life process include theories of growth and development, stress adaptation, basic human needs, and cognitive functions.

✔ Symbolic interactionists emphasize social definitions of behavior and reject any concept of development that depends on rigid standards of normalcy.

✔ A symbolic interactionist perspective views development as a progressive and directional process that involves the sequential acquisition of new abilities and is influenced by genetic, environmental, and important interpersonal relationships.

✔ Optimal emotional health is characterized by self-esteem, self knowledge, satisfying interpersonal relationships, environmental mastery, and stress management.

✔ Stress, changes, and threats to one's self-concept cause anxiety and place additional coping demands on the individual.

✔ Defense mechanisms may be used by anyone to cope with anxiety or stress, but a healthy person will more often use problem-solving methods.

✔ Defense mechanisms include repression, dissociation, suppression, identification, introjection, projection, denial, fantasy, rationalization, reaction formation, displacement, and intellectualization.

✔ Selye's stress-adaptation theory provides an explanation of the physiological reaction to stress.

✔ In the growth and development paradigm, the concept of life cycle refers to a complex sequence of events from birth to death, each stage of which is accompanied by specific roles, norms of behavior, and social expectations.

✔ The individual's behavior is formed by the way each developmental stage is completed.

✔ Satisfactory resolution of developmental phases is influenced by the events of earlier stages and has an important impact on the remainder of the life cycle.

✔ The development of a deviant identity and undergoing psychotherapy are social processes.

✔ Deviation from society's expectations for behavior at any point in the life cycle poses problems for the culture and for the individual who may be labeled abnormal by others.

problems and eliminate the inappropriate problems. For example, the client of an analytic therapist will bring in more dreams for analysis and gradually stop talking about physical symptoms.

One prepares a great deal for the role of client before one actually sees a therapist. The subsequent interaction between the therapist and client is a screening process in which the therapist decides who will be accepted for therapy and who will benefit. Not only is normal behavior socially defined, but the progress of

therapy for abnormal behaviors necessitates the adequate performance of a given role.

Lower-class people have not learned the social role of the psychotherapy client, which involves talking about feelings and engaging in free association. Therefore they are poorer candidates for psychotherapy than upper-class people. They are more likely to act like the typical medical client. That is, they will be compliant and passive, and seek relief of immediate symptoms.

References

Becker, H. S. *Outsiders.* New York: Free Press, 1973.

Bromley, D. B. *The Psychology of Human Aging.* New York: Penguin Books, 1966.

Dunn, H. *High Level Wellness.* Arlington, Va.: R. W. Beatty, 1961.

Illich, I. *Medical Nemesis.* New York: Pantheon Books, 1976.

Jung, C. *The Development of the Personality.* London: Routledge and Kegan Paul, 1954.

Kadushin, C. *Why People Go to Psychiatrists.* New York: Aldine Publishing, 1969.

Lazarus, R. S. *Psychological Stress and the Coping Process.* New York: McGraw-Hill, 1966.

Maslow, A. *Toward a Psychology of Being.* Princeton, N. J.: D. Van Nostrand, 1962.

Miller, J. B. *Toward a New Psychology of Women.* Boston: Beacon Press, 1976.

Murphy, L., and Moriarty, A. *Vulnerability, Coping and Growth.* New Haven: Yale University Press, 1976.

Peplau, H. *Interpersonal Relations in Nursing.* New York: G. P. Putnam, 1951.

Piaget, J. *The Origins of Intelligence in Children.* New York: International Universities Press, 1952.

————. *The Growth of Logical Thinking from Childhood to Adolescence.* New York: Basic Books, 1958.

Selye, H. *The Stress of Life.* New York: McGraw-Hill, 1956.

Sheehy, G. *Passages.* New York: E. P. Dutton, 1976.

Further Reading

Beauvoir, S. de. *All Said and Done.* New York: Warner Books, 1975.

Bernard, J. *The Future of Motherhood.* New York: Penguin Books, 1974.

Bettelheim, B. *The Uses of Enchantment.* New York: Alfred A. Knopf, 1976.

Chesler, P. *With Child . . . A Diary of Motherhood.* New York: Berkley Publishing, 1979.

Erikson, E. *Young Man Luther.* New York: W. W. Norton, 1958.

————. *Childhood and Society.* New York: W. W. Norton, 1963.

————. *Identity, Youth, and Crisis.* New York: W. W. Norton, 1968.

Fried, B. *The Middle-Age Crisis.* New York: Harper and Row, 1976.

Goble, F. *The Third Force.* New York: Pocket Books, 1970.

Hammer, S. *Daughters and Mothers—Mothers and Daughters.* New York: Signet Books, 1975.

Harris, J. *The Prime of Ms. America: The American Woman at 40.* New York: Signet Books, 1975.

Klein, M., and Riviere, J. *Love, Hate and Reparation.* New York: W. W. Norton, 1964.

Koestler, A. *The Act of Creation.* New York: Dell Publishing, 1964.

Land, G. *Grow or Die.* New York: Delta Books, 1974.

Levinson, D. *The Seasons of a Man's Life.* New York: Ballantine Books, 1978.

Lugo, J., and Hershey, G. *Human Development.* New York: Macmillan, 1974.

Mitchell, J. *Psychoanalysis and Feminism.* New York: Pantheon Books, 1975.

Newgarten, B., ed. *Middle Age and Aging.* Chicago: University of Chicago Press, 1968.

Pearce, J., and Newton, S. *The Conditions of Human Growth.* New York: Citadel Press, 1969.

Rich, A. *Of Women Born.* New York: W. W. Norton, 1976.

Scarf, M. *Unfinished Business.* New York: Ballantine Books, 1980.

Smelser, N., and Erikson, E. *Themes of Work and Love in Adulthood.* Cambridge, Mass.: Harvard University Press, 1980.

Sullivan, H. S. *The Interpersonal Theory of Psychiatry,* edited by M. L. Gawel and H. S. Perry. New York: W. W. Norton, 1953.

Sze, W. *The Human Life Cycle.* New York: Jason Aronson, 1974.

Valliant, G. E. *Adaptation to Life.* Boston: Little, Brown, 1977.

11

Life Turning Points: Crisis Theory, Assessment, and Intervention

CHAPTER OUTLINE

Crisis Defined

Stress and Crisis Development

   The Effect of Life Changes

   Using the Life Change Scale

The Emergence of Crisis Theory and Crisis Intervention

Crisis Intervention as a Therapeutic Strategy

The Crisis Sequence

Developmental Crises

   The Mid-life Crisis

   Retirement

Situational Crises

   Death and Loss

   Body Image Alterations

Victim Crises

   Family Violence

   Natural, Accidental, and Man-made Disasters

Suicide as a Coping Mechanism

   Self-destructive People

   Social Variables

   Demographic Variables

   Clinical Variables

   Suicidal Clues or Cries for Help

   Assessing Lethality

   Intervention with Suicidal Clients

   The Victims Left Behind

Crisis Intervention Modes

   Individual Crisis Counseling

   Crisis Groups

   Family Crisis Counseling

   Telephone Counseling

   Home Crisis Visits

Key Nursing Concepts

LEARNING OBJECTIVES

After reading this chapter, students should be able to

- Identify the role of stress in crisis development
- Help clients assess the effects of life changes
- Relate developmental and situational crises to strategies of crisis intervention
- Identify the social, demographic, and clinical variables that influence suicidal behavior
- Describe the process of lethality assessment
- Develop a plan for nursing intervention with suicidal clients
- Identify the major crisis intervention modes

CHAPTER 11

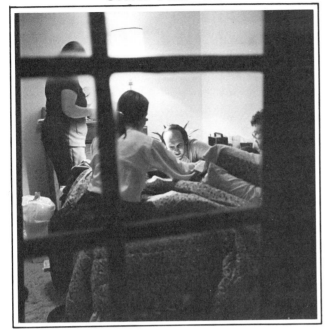

People in crisis experience a period of disorganization. Successful negotiation of life's passages turns life's obstacles into opportunities.

Early writers have described crises in Western culture since writing about Adam and Eve leaving the Garden of Eden. In finding ways to cope with this first crisis, Adam and Eve engaged in what must have been the first example of crisis intervention. We have since come to a better understanding of just what a crisis is, why people behave the way they do in crisis situations, and how to help people in crisis.

Nurses are in a unique position to function as crisis intervenors. Clients and families in crisis come to their attention in the multitude of health care settings in which nurses work. However, crisis intervention is not the specialty of any one professional group. Crisis intervenors come from the fields of nursing, medicine, psychology, social work, and theology. Police officers, teachers, school guidance counselors, rescue workers, bartenders, and barmaids, among others, are often on the spot in moments of crisis. Crisis intervention can be the business of all these persons and others.

CRISIS DEFINED

The word *crisis* stems from the Greek *krinein*, "to decide." In Chinese, two characters are used to write the word *crisis*—one is the character for *danger* and the

other the character for *opportunity*. A crisis is a situation in which customary problem-solving or decision-making methods are not adequate. Crisis situations are life turning points or junctures. Successful negotiation of a crisis leads either to a return to the precrisis state or to psychological growth and increased competence. Unsuccessful negotiation leaves the person undergoing a crisis feeling anxious, threatened, and ineffective. Persons may also handle a crisis event by disturbed coping patterns or disintegrative life patterns (see Chapters 14 and 16).

A crisis is self-limiting. It lasts a few days to a few weeks and will eventually run its course with or without intervention. However, the person who experiences a crisis alone is more vulnerable to unsuccessful negotiation than the person who works through a crisis with help. Working with a helping person increases the likelihood that a crisis will be resolved in a positive way.

Basically, there are two types of crises.

1. Internal or developmental crises are the anticipated crises of human maturation.

2. External or situational crises are stressful life events that may or may not be anticipated.

Table 11–1 defines and gives examples of each type. Selected crises are discussed later in this chapter. Victim crisis, a type of situational crisis, may lead to what DSM-III calls Post-traumatic Stress Disorder, and for that reason it is discussed separately.

STRESS AND CRISIS DEVELOPMENT

Stress is a situation that causes a person to experience strain or tension. People are stressed at many times in the normal course of living—when they move from one developmental level to another, when they lose someone or something of importance to them, when their car stalls at a busy intersection and the person

Table 11-1   THE TYPOLOGY OF CRISIS

Type	Definition	Examples
Developmental	Crisis that occurs in response to stresses common to all persons in periods of human maturation and transition	Birth, early childhood, preschool, puberty, adolescence, young adulthood, adulthood, late adulthood, old age
Situational	Crisis that occurs in response to stressful or traumatic external events	
Anticipated	Person experiencing crisis is involved to some extent through participation in event	Beginning nursery school, birth of sibling, divorce of parents, dating, promotion
Unanticipated	Unexpected and usually chance event that involved person has not predicted and is unprepared to meet	Death of significant person before old age, imprisonment, hospitalization for acute illness
Victim	Traumatic event involving physically aggressive and forced act by another person or by environment	War, rape, civil riot, murder, assault, incest

behind them honks furiously for them to move. Many corporations lose money because of lost or decreased employee productivity due to stress. The high number of heart attacks experienced on Monday (25 percent) in the face of a stressful week ahead have led many companies to offer stress-management programs for their employees. A stress situation becomes a crisis when people find they are unable to handle the distressing event.

The Effect of Life Changes

Most people are accustomed to thinking of untoward events as stressful, but they do not realize that desirable events such as job promotions, vacations, or outstanding personal achievements may also prove stressful. Life changes as stressful events were studied by Holmes and Rahe (1967) to learn the amount of social readjustment required to cope with them. These authors believe that the life events that require coping behavior tend to decrease a person's ability to handle illness or subsequent stress. Their research assigned ratings to forty-three different life changes, called *life change units* (LCUs). They asked subjects to indicate what life changes had occurred in the past year and then add up the points assigned to each identified life event. A low score indicated that the subject was not likely to have an adverse reaction. A "mild" score meant that there was a 30-percent chance that the impact of stress would be experienced through physical symptoms. Persons in the "moderate" category had a

50-percent chance of a change in health status, and a "high" score meant an 80-percent chance of major illness in the next two years. High LCU scores also correlated with an increased probability of accidental injury.

Marcia M, a twenty-two-year-old woman in group therapy, had recently been divorced from her husband (LCU 73) after attempting to achieve a marital reconciliation (LCU 45). Marcia's pregnancy (LCU 40) earlier in the year was uneventful, and the Ms' healthy son was born on June 2 (LCU 39). At six weeks of age, the child suddenly and unexpectedly died in his crib (LCU 63). The Ms began to argue frequently (LCU 35) before they made the decision to divorce. After the divorce, Marcia found herself short of funds (LCU 38) and went to work as a waitress in a pizza restaurant (LCU 36). She found it necessary to move to a smaller and less expensive apartment (LCU 20). In the short period of one year, Marcia accumulated an LCU score of 390 and was in the high-risk group.

During the course of group therapy, Marcia shared her desire to return to college and complete the junior and senior years of a medical technology program in which she had been enrolled before her marriage. In order to do so, she would have to make a number of changes—move to an apartment close to the college because she could not afford to own a car, change her working hours or job so that she could attend day classes, change her sleeping habits, change her recreational and social activities, and reduce her other expenses in order to pay school-related costs. The changes required would add almost 200 LCUs to her score.

In group, Marcia was able to consider this information and reevaluate her goals. She decided to delay her return to school until she could get on her feet financially. She chose not to make any other changes in her life for the present time.

In the early 1970s, other researchers correlated life stress events and mental health. In a study of 720 households in a metropolitan area, J. Meyers and his associates (1972) found a relationship between a high number of life changes and changes in the mental status of individuals. For example, an increase in the number of life changes preceded worsening of psychiatric symptoms, while a decrease in life changes brought improvement. The more stressful the life changes, the greater the likelihood of mental ill health. Meyers and his associates also found that entrance-related life events (those involving the addition of a new person into one's social sphere, perhaps through marriage or the birth of a child) produced less symptomatology than did exit-related life events (those associated with the loss of a valued individual or status).

Using the Life Change Scale

The Holmes and Rahe (1967) scale called *Schedule of Recent Experience* (SRE) is useful in a variety of ways. It is an assessment guide that helps people become aware of the stress they face in their lives. It is also useful in planning for the future. Clients can use it, much as Marcia did, to decide when it is advantageous or disadvantageous to engage in life change. It helps them make responsible decisions about the directions their lives will take. Nurses may find the SRE a valuable interviewing tool to guide the discussion of specific life changes and their circumstances with clients. Williams and Holmes (1978, p. 81) list the following ways in which clients can be helped to cope with life change using the SRE:

1. Orient clients to the life event items and the amount of change they require.
2. Have clients place the SRE where they can see it easily several times a day.
3. Help clients to recognize when a life change occurs.
4. Encourage clients to think about the meaning of the change and identify some of the feelings experienced.
5. Discuss with clients the different ways they might best adjust to the event.
6. Encourage them to take time in arriving at decisions.
7. If possible, encourage clients to anticipate life changes and plan for them well in advance.
8. Encourage clients to pace themselves. It can be done, even if they are in a hurry.
9. Encourage clients to look at the accomplishment of a task as a part of daily living and to avoid looking at such an achievement as a stopping point or a time for letting down.
10. Remember that the more changes clients experience the more likely they are to get sick. Of those people with over 300 LCUs for the previous year almost 80 percent get sick in the near future; of those with 150 to 299 LCUs about 50 percent get sick in the near future; of those with less than 150 LCUs only about 30 percent get sick in the near future. Thus the higher the LCU score the harder one should work to stay well.

THE EMERGENCE OF CRISIS THEORY AND CRISIS INTERVENTION

Two events in the 1940s can be said to have provided the starting point for contemporary crisis theory and intervention. One was the report by psychiatrist Erich Lindemann (see Lindemann 1944; Cobb and Lindemann 1943) on his observations of the crisis response many people had in their direct or indirect experience with the tragic Cocoanut Grove nightclub fire in Boston, in which hundreds of people lost their lives. Lindemann's observations and theoretical developments formed a landmark in understanding the behavior of people facing emergency situations and the grieving behavior of people whose relatives or friends died in the fire or its aftermath.

The other was the observation and treatment by military psychiatrists of battle-weary and emotionally upset military men. In most instances, men who received immediate help at the front lines were able to return to duty rather than being sent to inpatient psychiatric facilities. This immediate front-line treatment was therefore the preferred mode. Later studies and observations during the Korean War added to the knowledge of human behavior under stressful conditions.

James Tyhurst (1957) contributed further to the understanding of people's responses to natural disasters. He also studied transition states such as parenthood and retirement. Similar interests were held by Gerald Caplan (1965), who is best known for his work in preventive psychiatry and anticipatory guidance. Many of his methods were tested in the early days of the Peace Corps.

The report of the Joint Commission on Mental Illness and Health (1961) was an important development in crisis work. Its far-reaching mental health recommendations have been discussed in Chapters 1 and 28, among others. Conclusions of the Joint Commission specific to this chapter are:

• People in crisis did not receive immediate help but instead were put on lengthy waiting lists.

• When they did receive attention, it was often through lengthy and expensive psychotherapy.

• Extended and/or late psychotherapy is often not helpful to people in crisis.

• When people in crisis needed help, almost 50 percent sought out their clergyman, family physician, or other non-mental-health professional.

• Interested persons with minimal training could be helpful to people in trouble.

• A large group of interested persons in the community had been neglected as a resource for helping people in crisis.

Soon after publication of the Joint Commission report, large amounts of federal funding were made available for community-based mental health programs. One result was the establishment of suicide prevention and crisis services throughout the country. These were spearheaded by the efforts of mental health professionals on the West Coast. Crisis telephone counseling services, known popularly as *hot lines,* proliferated. So did the use of both paid and volunteer nonprofessional crisis workers. As community-based mental health programs became more firmly established and organized, many of them took on these crisis intervention functions.

Norris Hansell (1976) has developed a contemporary approach to people in crisis. Hansell's work with those in distress is based on findings of the theorists and researchers discussed earlier. In Hansell's social framework approach, the reestablishment of severed social attachments is necessary for successful crisis resolution. In this view, the emphasis is on social factors as the sources of problems. Others whose work has influenced modern-day crisis intervention are Abraham Maslow (1970) and Erik Erikson (1963). Their important developmental theories are discussed in Chapter 10.

CRISIS INTERVENTION AS A THERAPEUTIC STRATEGY

Crisis intervention as a therapeutic strategy is strongly humanistic. It views people as capable of personal growth and able to control their own lives. According to the humanistic orientation, effective planning for crisis resolution must be:

• Based on careful assessment

• Developed in active collaboration with the person in crisis and the significant others in that person's life

• Focused on immediate, concrete, contributing problems

• Based on an understanding of human dependence needs

• Appropriate to the crisis-ridden person's level of thinking, feeling, and behaving

• Consistent with the person's life-style and culture

• Time-limited, concrete, and realistic

• Mutually negotiated and renegotiated

• Organized to provide for follow-up

A plan with these components demonstrates respect for the crisis-ridden person's self, values, culture, and abilities. Table 11–2 compares the crisis model with other models of mental health delivery.

THE CRISIS SEQUENCE

Howard Parad and Harvey Resnik (1975) have identified a crisis sequence that involves three time periods—precrisis, crisis, and postcrisis.

An individual in the precrisis period is operating in a way to ensure that most of his or her needs get met. The person in crisis experiences a period of disorganization. This period is characterized by trial-and-error disequilibrium responses, in which the person attempts to reduce the feelings of discomfort. The resolution of the crisis or postcrisis period can result in either an increase or a decrease in the person's level of functioning or a return to the level of functioning evident in the precrisis period.

Table 11–2   COMPARISON OF CRISIS, PSYCHOTHERAPY, AND MEDICAL INSTITUTIONAL MODELS

Characteristic	Crisis Intervention Model	Psychotherapy Model	Medical Institutional Model
People served	Individuals and families in crisis or precrisis states	Those who wish to correct dysfunctional personality or behavior patterns	People with serious mental or emotional breakdowns
Service goals	Growth-promotion; personal and social integration	Working through of unconscious conflicts; reconstruction of behavior and personality patterns; personal and social growth	Control adjustment; recovery from acute disturbance
Service methods	Social and environmental manipulation; focus on feelings and problem solving; may use medication to promote goals; decision counseling	Introspection; catharsis; interpretation; free association; use of additional techniques depending on philosophy and training of therapist	Medication; behavior modification; electric shock; use of additional techniques depending on philosophy of institution
Activity of workers	Active/direct (depends on functional level of client)	Exploratory; nondirective; interpretive	Direct, noninvolved; or indirect
Length of service	Short—usually six or fewer sessions	Usually long-term	Short or long (depends on degree of disability and approach of psychiatrist); high repeat rate
Beliefs about people	Social—people are capable of growth and self-control	Individualistic or social (depends on philosophy of therapist)	Individualistic—social aspect secondary; institution and order often more important than people
Attitudes toward service	Flexible, any hour	Emphasis on wisdom of therapist and fifty-minute hour; flexibility varies with individual therapist	Scheduled; staff attitudes may become rigid and institutionalized

Source: Adapted from L. A. Hoff, *People in Crisis: Understanding and Helping* (Menlo Park, Calif.: Addison-Wesley Publishing Co., 1978), pp. 54–55.

The three periods of the crisis sequence are depicted in Figure 11–1. They are distinguishable in the following case example:

Mike was relatively free of emotional and physical stresses for most of his early adult life, and those that he did experience he was able to handle. At the time of his thirty-fifth birthday, Mike was offered the opportunity to purchase a deteriorating bar and restaurant on prime urban property near a large university. He went into debt to revamp the bar and restaurant into Dante's Disco, a discotheque Mike hoped would bring him financial success. After the first two years of its existence, it *became apparent that Dante's Disco would not return the financial investment that Mike had in it. Early one Sunday morning, Dante's Disco burned to the ground, a total loss.*

A year later, Mike was arrested and charged with arson for setting the fire. He had collected a quarter of a million dollars from the company that insured Dante's Disco, but the insurance company investigator considered the fire to be of suspicious origin, and had continued to investigate even after the claim was paid. The breakthrough in the case came when Mike's fifteen-year-old daughter provided the arson investigator with the evidence needed to arrest her father.

Mike was unable to handle this stressful event. His

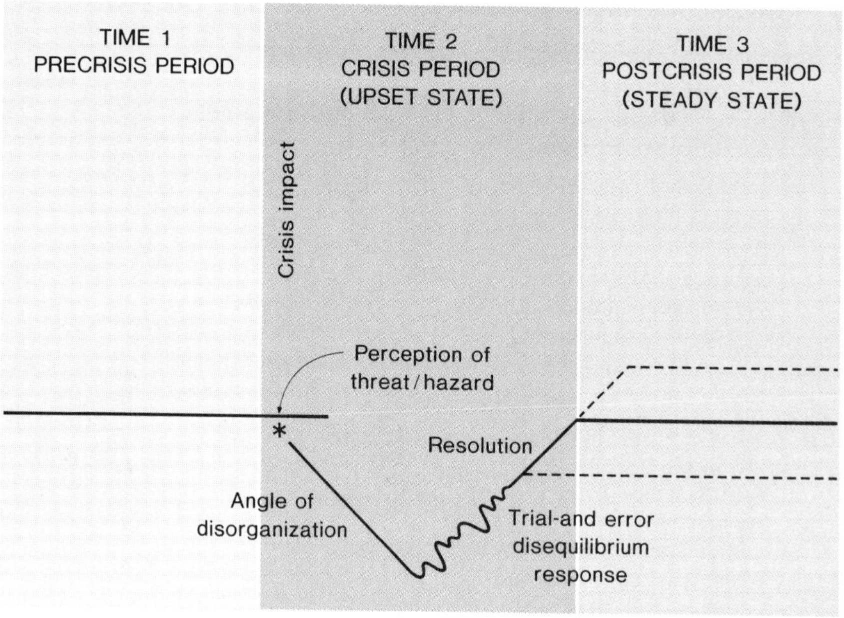

Figure 11-1

Crisis sequence diagram. The asterisk indicates the onset of a crisis period, which occurs directly after the crisis impact. An angle of disorganization develops during the crisis period and may vary from steep to gradual. This variance also occurs during the resolution (recovery or reorganization) phase. During time 3 (postcrisis period) the level of functioning may be about the same as during time 1 (precrisis period), or it may be higher or lower, depending on the nature of the stress, available resources, and whether the crisis resolution is adaptive or maladaptive. (From H. J. Parad and H. L. P. Resnick, "A Crisis Intervention Framework," in *Emergency Psychiatric Care*, edited by H. L. P. Resnick and H. L. Ruben. Bowie, Md.: Charles Press, 1975, p. 4.)

business prospects seemed to be ruined, and he faced a jail term if convicted. On top of it all he perceived his daughter's behavior as a betrayal. His current coping mechanisms were overtaxed, and he experienced a crisis state. Mike's lawyer obtained bail, and Mike was able to go home, but he became highly anxious and felt hopeless. He also began to experience severe migraine headaches. Three days later Mike shot himself and died in the ambulance on the way to the hospital.

DEVELOPMENTAL CRISES

The anticipated crises of postadolescence and adulthood are covered in Chapter 10. Chapters 19 and 20 address the crises of children and adolescents. Two adult-specific crises are considered below.

The Mid-life Crisis

An authenticity crisis occurs for some people between the ages of thirty-five and forty-five. Gail Sheehy (1976) calls this the *deadline decade*, for at this time people discover visible signs of their own aging and become somewhat preoccupied with the notion of their mortality. This is the period when they feel as if time is running out. Those with careers feel that it is now or never that they will accomplish unmet goals or move ahead. Women who have stayed at home to raise children find at this period that their children are leading socially active lives, embarking on academic or work careers of their own, and in some cases even contemplating marriage. Time, for these mothers, seems to drag. In the past, women were said to be experiencing the "empty nest syndrome"—depression because they no longer had children to nurture. Rubin (1981) found that the women she interviewed spoke of the departure of their children with a sense of relief combined with some sadness. In fact, it was the fathers, who had missed much of the children's development, who suffered more "empty nest" depression. Persons in mid-life need to assess the meaning of time and rebalance their notions of the future against the time they have left.

The mid-life stage is a time of reevaluation. People reexamine careers, marriages, children, and family life, considering pros and cons of each. Career changes and mate changes are not uncommon at this stage. The anxious and forlorn feelings experienced by a person in mid-life can presage adventuresome self-discovery and a reinvigorated passage into middle age. They are too painful for some people to handle, however.

Joshua handled the midstation of life by denial. Unable to see himself as growing older, he refused to permit himself to grieve for his "old" self so that he could accept a "new" self. Joshua played more tennis, ran more laps, and took a younger partner to bed. He eventually left his wife and two children to pick up the pieces of their lives and cope without him. A decade later Joshua had not yet moved through the mid-life passage. His wife and children were able to resolve the crisis of Joshua's departure by widening their boundaries. With supportive help from a crisis intervenor and a large network of interested friends and family, they mourned his loss and could move on.

According to Sheehy (1981) the key to successful negotiation of life's passages is willingness to take risks in order to turn life's obstacles into opportunities. Seven other helpful elements are:

- Timing
- Capacity for living
- Strong support systems
- Accumulated wisdom
- Sense of purpose
- Recognition of life's spiritual elements (not necessarily religion)
- True grit

Retirement

Work is central to human beings. People work not only for physical sustenance, but also for social reasons. Various writers have described the moral, economic,

and social status dimensions of work. Some say that work is a bond with the community, others that it is simply the best way to fill up a lot of time. Most agree that work responds to something basic and profound in human nature. Because it plays a pervasive and powerful role in the psychological, social, and economic aspects of people's lives, it can be called a basic or central institution. The example below speaks to some of the disruptive effects of early retirement from work.

"My God, what'll Lorraine do with Howard around all day? I'd go crazy if Alan retired early," said Eleanor. The talk of this upper-middle-income suburban community was Howard's retirement at age fifty from his job as an aviation engineer. Howard, the sole heir of his two aunts, came into a large sum of money when they died. Eleanor's reaction echoed that of many of her female friends and neighbors.

As it turned out, Howard and Lorraine discovered that their interests were not shared. While Howard had devoted most of his energy to success at his job, Lorraine had devoted hers to being the perfect homemaker. Their house was spotless, and Lorraine saw that it was kept that way. She baked, cooked, and grew and canned her own vegetables. With all three children away from home, the couple had little to say to each other and even less to do together.

Howard found he did not enjoy hobbies, sports, reading, or other leisure activities. As their unhappiness with each other escalated, Howard purchased a small vending machine business. He viewed this as a hobby, an interesting way to spend his time. But the business soon proved unsuccessful, and Howard and Lorraine were back where they started. This time, however, they enrolled in an adult education course on the pursuit of leisure at a local college. Through this they discovered an interest they could both enjoy. Howard's aunts had left him two old Victorian homes in a nearby small community, and both were completely furnished in antiques. It seemed natural to open a small antique store. Lorraine and Howard soon found they were able to value each other's skills and abilities in an enjoyable activity that was satisfying to both.

In our culture, a person may opt for *early* retirement, but most people find themselves faced with *forced* retirement. Some view retirement as a pleasurable experience. To others, it is a distressing, painful time of life, signaling old age and the approach of death. To all, it is a time of stress when people feel unwanted, unvalued, and unproductive.

A person's life-style influences how that person approaches retirement. For example, hobbies and interests that are primarily pleasure-related rather than work-related help persons look forward to retirement. A specifically planned retirement project, such as travel, a course of study, or learning to play a musical instrument, provides a positive reason for retirement. Another major influencing factor is the degree of comfort or ease with which a person can retire. Retirement is less stressful when health, income, and living environment are sufficient to make the person comfortable. Retirement is further discussed in Chapter 22.

SITUATIONAL CRISES

Death and Loss

Death and bereavement are universal and inevitable experiences. People are most familiar with grief as a response to the loss of a loved person through death or separation, but grieving follows the loss of anything, tangible or intangible, that is highly valued—a material possession, a position of status, a body part, a home, or a country, for example. An understanding of the reactions common to loss in general will help in understanding grief reactions to the death of a loved person.

Like most other universal and inevitable experiences, mourning has been treated historically as an accepted state of affairs. It is given little thought and is poorly understood. Mental health professionals originally were interested in grieving when it signaled disturbed coping. Scattered throughout the psychological and psychiatric literature are a number of references to grieving from a psychoanalytic point of view. These relate grief to depressive psychosis or agitated depression, or explore it as a psychopathological response in time of war. Few researchers were interested in the grieving process that is a necessary concomitant of daily living activities.

The well-known therapeutic efforts of Cobb and Lindemann (1943) with bereaved disaster victims and their families following Boston's Cocoanut Grove nightclub fire paved the way for more recent concerns about those who mourn. Shortly thereafter, Lindemann expanded his observations (1944) to include the bereaved in more common settings. His classic work identified acute grief as a definite syndrome with psychological or somatic manifestations. The syndrome may appear immediately, be delayed, be exaggerated, or apparently be absent. His work also identified distortions of the typical syndrome. These can be successfully transformed into a normal grief reaction and achieve resolution.

Experiences of Grieving Persons According to Lindemann (1944), there are five general classes of symptoms of normal grief. They are described in Table 11–3. Although a painful process, grieving is important. When a person attempts to handle these uncomfortable symptoms by avoiding encounters with others and increasing interpersonal distance or deliberately excluding from the thinking process all references to the deceased, a morbid grief reaction may result. Morbid grief reactions, as identified by Lindemann, are described in Table 11–4.

Stages of Successful Mourning George Engel (1964) built on Lindemann's work to identify a process of *grief work* necessary to successful grieving. Grief work, or the work of mourning, can be identified as emancipation from bondage to the deceased, readjustment to the environment in which the deceased is missing, and formation of new relationships. Successful grieving consists of three phases: shock and disbelief, developing awareness, and restitution or resolution.

SHOCK AND DISBELIEF   The first phase, shock and disbelief, can be characterized as the "Oh no!" stage. The need to deny the loss is paramount, and the resulting behavior may run the gamut from verbal denial to incapacitation. Each individual has a personal style of loss denial, determined partly by cultural factors and partly by previous experiences with loss and separation.

Behavior in the shock and disbelief phase reflects attempts by bereaved persons to protect themselves either against recognition of the event or against the painful feeling it evokes. While some deny the event or refuse to believe that it has occurred, others shut themselves off from the pain evoked by the stress and may move to comfort friends and relations in their grief. It is important for intervenors to be guided by the knowledge that the mental mechanism of denial in this phase serves a therapeutic purpose. It protects bereaved people from painful knowledge with which they may be unable to cope. Lengthy maintenance of denial in the face of reality, however, signals distress. Resolution of grief cannot be achieved until the bereaved successfully completes each stage of mourning. Continued

Table 11-3 SYMPTOMATOLOGY OF GRIEVING

Symptom Classification	Characteristics
1. Somatic distress	Occurs in waves lasting from twenty minutes to one hour
	Deep, sighing respirations most common when discussing grief
	Lack of strength
	Loss of appetite and sense of taste
	Tightness in throat
	Choking sensation accompanied by shortness of breath
2. Preoccupation with image of deceased	Similar to daydreaming
	May mistake others for deceased person
	May be oblivious to surroundings
	Slight sense of unreality
	Fear that he or she is becoming "insane"
3. Feelings of guilt	Accuses self of negligence
	Exaggerates existence and importance of negative thoughts, feelings, and actions toward deceased
	Views self as having failed deceased—"If I had only. . . ."
4. Feelings of hostility	Irritability, anger, and loss of warmth toward others
	May attempt to handle feelings of hostility in formalized and stiff manner of social interaction
5. Loss of patterns of conduct	Inability to initiate or maintain organized patterns of activity
	Restlessness, with aimless movements
	Loss of zest—tasks and activities are carried on as though with great effort
	Activities formerly carried on in company of deceased have lost their significance
	May become strongly dependent on whoever stimulates mourner to activity

Table 11-4 MORBID GRIEF REACTIONS

Symptom Classification	Characteristics
1. Delayed reaction	Most common and most dramatic morbid reaction
	Postponement may be brief or prolonged for years
	Usually occurs when bereaved is confronted with necessity of carrying out important tasks or maintaining morale of others
2. Distorted reactions	Excessive activity with no sense of loss
	Development of physical symptoms similar to those experienced by deceased just before death
	Medical illness of psychophysiological nature, developed close in time to loss of important person
	Continued and progressive social isolation with alteration in relationships with friends and relatives
	Extreme hostility against specific persons somehow connected with death event
	"Schizophreniclike" wooden and formal conduct, masking hostile feelings
	Lasting change in patterns of social interaction
	Activities detrimental to own social and economic existence
	Agitated depression

denial prevents the mourner from moving on. A therapeutic maneuver that may be helpful is expression of the nurse's own perceptions of the facts in the situation ("although the divorce has been finalized you're hoping your wife will change her mind"), while avoiding arguments based on logic.

DEVELOPING AWARENESS Reality begins to assert itself in the second phase. This may begin very soon after the bereavement or may take longer to develop. At this phase awareness of the loss becomes acute.

Crying is one of the most evident activities in this stage. Because tears are a vital and important part of the process of normal grieving, they should not be discouraged but rather allowed. Nurses should not be afraid to shed tears or to see them shed. On the other hand, they may encounter family members who do not cry as expected. These people may be unable to cry because they feel hostility or ambivalence toward the deceased. Bereaved people frequently feel anger about the dead person's "desertion." The anger may be displaced onto others or turned onto the self, taking the form of self-injury or self-destructive behavior. When the deceased has been terminally ill for a long time, family members may have already completed their grief work in a process called *premortem dying* (discussed below).

Refusal to cry may also be viewed as a protective mechanism that prevents the release of painful emotions. People who do not cry should therefore not be viewed as heartless and inhuman. Encouraging persons to cry or otherwise express emotion, when in fact they are unable to do so, may increase the guilt that is a component of most grief reactions.

When mourners are able to express their emotions, however, it is usually helpful to allow them to do so. In many instances health personnel move too quickly to suppress the expression of emotion, often with sedatives. While some medication may be useful initially, overmedication only delays and prolongs the grieving process. In giving medication to bereaved persons, it is important to consider whether it will facilitate or subvert the grieving process.

RESTITUTION During the first two phases of mourning, nurses are usually present to assist relatives in their bereavement. Nurses need to be good listeners who are willing to spend time hearing expressions of grief and reminiscences. This helps grieving persons to move toward the third phase of normal and successful mourning.

Restitution completes the work of mourning. It is assisted by the traditional religious mourning practices of the wake, the funeral, and the expression of condolences by friends. Institutionalization of the mourning experience in rituals helps to bring grief work to a close. Not only is the reality of death emphasized, but also the rituals allow supportive interpersonal interactions to occur. Today it is rare to see mourners display emotion publicly, retain keepsakes such as locks of hair, or employ lavish mourning equipment, such as the plumed hearses of the Victorian era. These ostentatious expressions of grief, however, provided more relief than the modern stiff upper lips and requests for no mourning and no flowers.

An exception to the convention of stoicism occurred when the entire nation exhibited its mourning following the death of President John F. Kennedy. People mourned in their living rooms in front of their television sets, responding to the funeral dirge, the beat of the drum, the riderless horse, and the draped hearse. The nation became actively involved in burying the dead.

Another public example of coping with grief was demonstrated by Robert Kennedy's family after his assassination. The three eldest children participated in the vigil over their father at the hospital and in every aspect of the funeral ritual, including bringing the coffin to New York City and the day of public mourning in Saint Patrick's Cathedral. They were joined at the funeral mass by all the younger children, down to Douglas, who was then fourteen months old. Some of the older children participated as acolytes in the service. The entire family made the train journey together to Washington, D.C., and Arlington National Cemetery. The adults rallied around the children in a variety of ways. When adult family members were unable to meet the needs of the children, other adults took over. The flexibility of family and friends in assuming necessary role functions ensured that nurturing and control needs were met. In discussing how Senator Kennedy's family handled these events, Gerald Caplan (1968) particularly notes the comfort and steadfast support the children received from their participation and its positive influence on the grieving process. He believes that the behavior of the Kennedy family can serve as a model to help others cope with the death of a parent or a significant person.

Early in the restitution period, the memory of the dead person is elevated to a degree of perfection. Negative or socially unacceptable facets of the deceased's personality or behavior may be overlooked. It may take many months for the mourner to be able to see the deceased as he or she actually was. For instance, shortly after the assassinations of John and Robert Kennedy a number of books and articles extolling their virtues were published. These publications generally overlooked the brothers' less positive or socially unacceptable behavior and personality characteristics. However, after the passage of time, publications concerning the Kennedys began to present their virtues and failings more accurately.

Mourning is frequently completed within the year following the death. However, when the mourner has not experienced all three phases, grieving cannot be considered completed, and some of the work of mourning must still be done. Unresolved grief can be the prelude to the disintegrative pattern known as Major Depression. For these reasons it is important to help bereaved persons resolve their grief. Not until the work of mourning is finished can the work of living continue.

Another helpful approach to the completion of successful grieving has been suggested by Caplan (1965). He advocates that bereaved persons be allowed "mourning leave" with pay, analogous to the accepted business practice of "sick leave." Freeing bereaved persons from the demands of their jobs for a time lets them devote their energies to grief work. Since the health care delivery system is one of the biggest businesses in the United States, its adoption of such a practice would constitute a significant precedent. It would be appropriate for the profession having the greatest interest in improving and preserving the health of the public to make this first positive movement in the direction of mental health for its own workers.

Premortem Dying   Premortem dying, a phenomenon described by Weisman and Hackett (1961), may occur in interactions between a dying client and his or her family. The dying person is less and less often allowed to participate in decisions regarding family or personal interests. When the terminally ill client asks questions about what is happening outside the hospital, family members frequently respond, "Don't you worry," and "Everything is being taken care of." This phenomenon is particularly common when dying is prolonged. While family members generally perceive their behavior as protecting the dying person from participating in stressful situations, the behavior indicates a change in the family system and may imply that they already think of the client as no longer part of the family.

When mourning begins long before the actual death, families may finish grieving before the client dies. Glaser and Strauss (1965) caution that family members may not be able to help a client during the last stages of dying if, with too much advance warning, they prepare themselves so well that they give up the client before death occurs. Ambivalence may be experienced by family members who complete their grief work before the client dies. They may feel resentful about the time and effort spent in visiting the dying client and the money spent on hospital care. They often find

themselves wishing they could go on with their own lives, interests, jobs, and friends. Such feelings of hostility often provoke feelings of guilt.

Family members begin to take on the roles previously held by a dying person and exclude the client from the family system. Should the client recover, it may be difficult if not impossible for him or her to reenter the family system.

Joan, a nurse, was the wife of a client with chronic glomerulonephritis. For five years she personally cared for her husband during long and frequent hospitalizations. Eventually, she began to assume the role of nurturer, provider, and decision-maker. After her husband underwent a successful kidney transplant and was able to resume his job, she found it impossible to give up or alter the roles she had taken on during his illness. He expected to take over the decision-making again and to have Joan resume the dependent role she had taken during their courtship and early marriage. She, however, had finished her grieving and had become, in many ways, a different person. They were unable to resolve their interpersonal difficulties and ultimately separated.

The Nurse's Need to Grieve   It is seldom recognized that those who care for the dying may also need to mourn the loss of a client and work through their grief. Nurses may need a respite from hospital units where death often occurs, such as the intensive care unit. Periodic assignments to units where clients have high recovery rates and where the nurse's emotional investment may not be so prolonged might provide an opportunity for the respite.

Nursing educators can help by including grief work in their curricula. Nursing students who learn about grief and acquire the skills necessary to resolve their own grief can then help others toward resolution. Nursing administrators need to request budgets for providing in-service programs to help nurses become grief facilitators. Clinical specialists in psychiatric nursing can also help individual nurses face grieving problems squarely and can serve as consultants to them in formulating a plan of care that allows for grief work.

Body Image Alterations

The body image is the individual's concept of the shape, size, and mass of his or her body and its parts. This image allows a person to evaluate the space the body occupies and to move about freely in the environment. It is the internalized picture a person has of the physical appearance of the body. Sensations arising inside the body and the attitudes and responses of others influence the individual's concept of his or her own body. In this way, body image is closely allied with self-concept or self-image.

Changes in the body image are threatening. Of necessity, people attempt to maintain the integrity of their own bodies. One five-year-old about to undergo a tonsillectomy had this to say: "Why do I have to have my tonsils out? I do not like myself not being myself, and that is what will happen if even my littlest tonsils is taken away from me."

The body image extends beyond the physical body. Objects of daily use that are intimately connected with the body surface, such as a cane, clothes, a tattoo, makeup, and jewelry, are incorporated into the body image. Objects connected with and symbolizing a profession, such as the policeman's gun or the nurse's cap, may be even more intensely incorporated into the body image, not only by the wearer but by the public as well.

All these factors form an inner mental diagram called the body image. This diagram is fluid and dynamic—it changes in response to the current sensory and psychic stimuli it receives.

Evaluating Body Image Alteration Certain consistent elements are important in evaluating the significance of the body image and its alteration.

First, body characteristics that people have from birth or acquire early in life seem to have less emotional significance for them than those that arise in adolescence or later. The boy born lacking a limb formulates an image of himself that accounts for the limb's absence. His healthy self-concept naturally excludes that limb from the "me." Children with crossed eyes, buck teeth, or disfiguring facial birthmarks often similarly incorporate these features into their body images. The school nurse or teacher who recommends correction of such a "defect" is often astounded by the resentment that greets this well-meant suggestion. Attempts to change a characteristic are unwelcome and resisted because they require changing the loved "me."

A second factor to consider in evaluating the significance of alterations in body image is that a defect, handicap, or change in body function that occurs abruptly is far more traumatic than one that develops gradually. For example, crippling arthritis that eventually impairs the use of an extremity is less disturbing

than traumatic amputation of an extremity during an auto accident. A person has time to adjust to the effects of arthritis on body function and body image, while the person whose extremity has been suddenly amputated is not allowed the healing effects of time. This person suddenly discovers the absence or loss of function of a loved part of self.

Third, the location of a disease or injury greatly affects the emotional response to it. Internal diseases are generally less distressing than external diseases that can be seen by the person and by others. For example, radical head and neck surgery, with its consequent disfigurement, is devastating to the body image and to the psyche, since the face is one of the primary means by which people communicate. Most people focus on the face in interacting with others. When that face is rendered unaesthetic, radical changes in body image are also necessary.

People generally experience a great threat when the genitals or breasts are involved in change. Breast surgery is of particular significance to many women, for breasts symbolize femininity and sexual attractiveness in Western culture. The mass media drive that point home in the idolization of women with large breasts. In men, such surgical procedures as circumcision and inguinal hernia repair pose a far more disturbing threat to the body image than major operations such as gastrectomy or cholecystectomy. Fears about sexuality and virility are reawakened and reinforced when illness or injury threatens genital areas. Those parts of the body are important to people's mental view of themselves as men or women.

When one is not capable of loving one's own body and oneself, the body image loses its boundaries. This phenomenon is called *depersonalization*, and it is not uncommon among clients whose functioning is disintegrative. For example, a client's image in a mirror may appear distorted to the client, as if seen in a hall of mirrors in an amusement park. A research study by Richard Spire (1966) investigated such body image changes by conducting photographic self-image confrontations. Spire took Polaroid photographs of chronically ill female psychiatric clients and then discussed with them their responses to the photos. He found that body image distortion noted in the literature about schizophrenia was consistent with the difficulties experienced by clients in identifying themselves or parts of their bodies in photographs. Many of the women in the study had difficulty in acknowledging that the photos were of themselves. They thought the photos were of mothers, sisters, brothers, husbands—

even Shirley Temple. Such body image distortions are not unusual. Many emotionally disturbed persons have "Alice in Wonderland" experiences in which they believe they are taller, shorter, thinner, or fatter than they actually are.

Phantom Experiences among Amputees   The phantom experience can be defined as the sensation of feeling a part of the body that is no longer there. The phantom limb phenomenon is the most well known. It is far more common than is generally believed. Phantom limb experiences increase markedly if amputation occurs after four years of age, and they are almost universal after age eight.

Phantom experiences occur in an attempt to redefine the lost part and to maintain the stability and integrity of the body image. In fact, some theorists view the phantom as an indication of a stable body schema. Too stable a body schema can prove problematic, however, when the individual recognizes that the phantom is unreal and that others do not share the perception of it. Problems also arise when the phantom is experienced as painful.

Although phantoms are considered universal, painful phantoms are relatively rare and are considered psychopathological. People experiencing them have described the pain as acute, burning, grinding, tearing, and crushing. The severity of the pain may account for the high incidence of addiction to narcotics and suicidal tendencies among persons with painful phantoms.

The nonpainful phantom eventually disappears, although there are recorded instances in which phantoms have persisted for as long as twenty years. Phantoms of the upper limb are generally stronger and last longer than phantoms of the lower limb. They often begin to disappear through a process known as *telescoping*—that is, the hand or the foot appears to be shrinking toward the stump. The final parts to disappear are usually the thumb, index finger, and big toe.

Helping Resolve the Body Image Crisis   Loss is the general theme in all body image alterations. In order to cope with the loss of a loved person, loved object, or loved body part, it is necessary to mourn. Nurses can help clients move through the three phases of mourning by applying the suggestions given earlier in this chapter. Clients may need to be helped to acknowledge the loss in order to move from the stage of shock and disbelief into developing awareness. Health professionals sometimes believe that ignoring or minimizing the loss is helpful to clients and their families.

This is not true. Those who fail to acknowledge the loss or minimize it hinder grief work.

Clients need a supportive person to help them move toward the resolution phase of mourning. It may be necessary to create opportunities for discussing the disability, its meaning to the client, the problem of compensating for the loss, and the reaction of persons with whom the client will come in contact. Attitudes of disapproval, repulsion, or rejection toward a person with a physical disfigurement or defect will hinder the person's social adaptation. Nurses can help family and friends to overcome such attitudes, if they experience them, by creating similar opportunities for them to discuss their fears and concerns.

Anticipatory Guidance in Body Image Crises   Anticipatory guidance aims to help people cope with a crisis by discussing the details of an impending stressful occurrence and solving problems before the event occurs. Anticipatory guidance is needed not only for clients but also for the significant persons in their lives, both family and friends. It is believed that anticipatory guidance lays the foundation for effective grief work. It consists of brief psychotherapeutic intervention to discuss the meaning of the body part to the client and significant others, their beliefs and feelings concerning previous losses they have experienced, and the beliefs they hold about the body image. Therapeutic preparation of a person who is to undergo amputation can help prevent the painful phantom. A discussion of the phantom phenomenon should be included as well as exploration of the client's fears and indication of how the client wishes to dispose of the body part to be amputated. Fantasies and superstitious beliefs about amputated parts of the body can increase a client's anxiety and discomfort.

Although anticipatory guidance is discussed here specifically in relation to body image alteration, it is an appropriate primary prevention strategy for coping with any traumatic event that can be anticipated.

VICTIM CRISES

Victim crises are those life situations in which persons experience physically aggressive and forced action by another person, a group of people, or the environment. Rape, incest, assault, murder, war, civil riots, kidnapping or the taking of hostages, and natural disasters such as floods, earthquakes, and hurricanes are

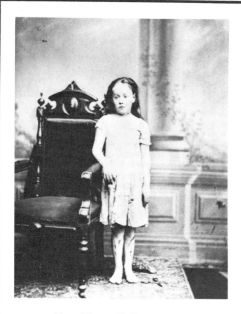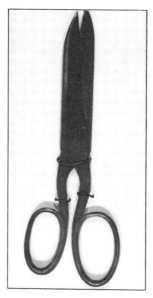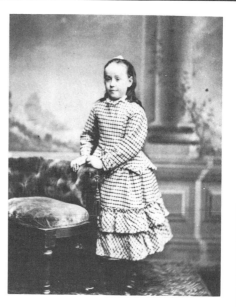

Mary Ellen, with the scissors used to abuse her, before and one year after the New York S.P.C.A. intervened.

examples of situations in which people are victimized. Increased interest by those involved in crisis work, criminology, and law has led to the proposal of the term *victimology* for the study of the victim. In these situations, the victim may be physically or emotionally injured or killed.

Family Violence

Family violence, although a centuries-old practice, gained public attention in the 1970s as a social problem of magnitude. Before that time, the beating of children, wives, and the elderly was often justified as a means of necessary discipline. Those who would intervene had no legal basis on which to do so. The problem is illustrated in the case below.

In 1874 a church worker in New York City was contacted by the neighbors of a local family. This family had a nine-year-old named Mary Ellen as an indentured servant in their household. Neighbors reported that the child was beaten daily, stabbed with scissors, and tied to a bed. When the church worker tried to intervene, she found that there was no legal way to rescue Mary Ellen from the people who were mistreating her. United States laws did not provide for the rescue of battered children. However, the church worker was persistent in her efforts, finally going to the Society for the Prevention of Cruelty to Animals (SPCA) for help. Using the rationale that Mary

Ellen was a member of the animal kingdom, the SPCA authorities were able to remove the child from the couple's home and bring them to trial, where the wife was sentenced to one year in prison. This led to the founding in 1875 of the New York Society for the Prevention of Cruelty to Children, the first such organization of its kind in the United States.

More recent public attention to family violence has been due mainly to the efforts of feminist organizations. For example, in 1976 the Ann Arbor, Michigan, chapter of the National Organization for Women (NOW) launched its Domestic Violence Project, offering a range of services to battered women: emergency housing, short-term peer counseling by volunteers, legal advice and referral, financial assistance, twenty-four-hour crisis phone coverage, and referral to appropriate social service and mental health agencies. Many other communities have established, or are in the process of establishing, similar services.

Stereotypes about battered women continue to exist, however. Three common stereotypes are: (1) Battered women are basically sadomasochistic. They need to be abused, and they enjoy it. (2) Battered women actually instigate assaults. If they would stop nagging and insulting their husbands, their husbands would stop beating them. (3) Battered women are "castrating females," domineering women who exploit their husbands. These stereotypes place blame on the victim and support the beating of women by men as part of the masculine mystique.

The Ann Arbor study by Bonnie Carlson (1977) indicates that alcohol was involved in 60 percent of the incidents that came to the researchers' attention, and drugs were involved in another 12 percent. Weapons were involved in 50 percent of the reported incidents, with 60 percent being household objects such as a shoe, a hockey stick, or a wooden cutting board; 25 percent of the weapons were guns, and 16 percent were knives.

Battered women tend not to leave their battering spouses. Many of them feel ill-prepared to meet the financial demands they would face if they lived on their own. Others are concerned that the abusing husband will cause them even greater harm if they leave. Some are intimidated by threats of further physical violence if they report the crime to the police.

In many instances police officers who answer domestic violence calls suggest that the couple "kiss and make up." They seldom do.

_____

Jim and Dorrie did not resolve their domestic problems when police arrived on the scene. Jim had been further angered by Dorrie's call to the local police precinct. After the two officers left, he barricaded Dorrie and the children in their home. The neighbors managed to alert the proper authorities before Jim could put a match to the gasoline he had poured around the house.

_____

The attention given by women's organizations to the problem of domestic violence has turned up a number of instances of husband beating. Although this is a less common occurrence, some husbands are subjected to significant physical abuse by their wives. Hospital emergency room personnel sometimes report that trade-offs occur within a family—one week the wife is treated, and the next week the husband.

Domestic violence may escalate to murder by either party—the battering spouse or the battered spouse who concludes that killing in self-defense is necessary. In one case, a 255-pound football defensive lineman was stabbed to death by his wife whom he had beaten regularly during their marriage. Once when she had called the police for assistance, the officers ended up talking football with her husband. More instances are becoming known of women who kill their mates because they have been battered once too often. A NOW report (1976) indicates that 33 percent of the murders

studied in one Michigan county were done by women who killed their battering spouses.

Although women are the primary victims of violence, children (see Chapter 19) and the elderly (see Chapter 22) may also be victimized. Figure 11–2 illustrates the wide-ranging potential effects that violence may have on a person. Nor is violence limited to the family setting. There are increasing reports of violence between persons who date or live together. Economic frustrations, tensions, and feelings of powerlessness are common wherever violence occurs, whether in the suburb, the inner city, the high school or college campus, or the psychiatric unit.

Violence has reached such alarming proportions that organizations have been developed to train health, education, and social welfare personnel in specific techniques and attitudes for therapeutic and safe management of aggressive, assaultive, and potentially acting-out individuals.

_____

Only recently Jim Z, a psychiatric nurse, was indicted for manslaughter. Fearful that a male client on an inpatient unit was about to hurt another client, Jim intervened by placing a stranglehold on his client in order to subdue him. However Jim's stranglehold was too powerful: it crushed the client's larynx, asphyxiating him. Jim lost not only his job but also his license to practice nursing.

_____

Had Jim known how to recognize the signs of escalating tension so that he could intervene earlier, or had he known noninjurious techniques of control, his client's death might have been avoided.

Appropriate crisis intervention for victims of family violence includes brief counseling plus the provision of alternative housing and child-care facilities. Couples in which one or both partners batter are likely to find family and marital counseling services useful. Self-help groups for persons interested in changing their battering patterns were originally established in England and have spread to North America. Self-help groups, in general, are quite successful and provide members with support and motivation.

Natural, Accidental, and Man-made Disasters

We have only recently begun to understand crisis intervention in disaster situations. Although federal aid for reconstruction of communities devastated by natural disasters has been available for many years, the provi-

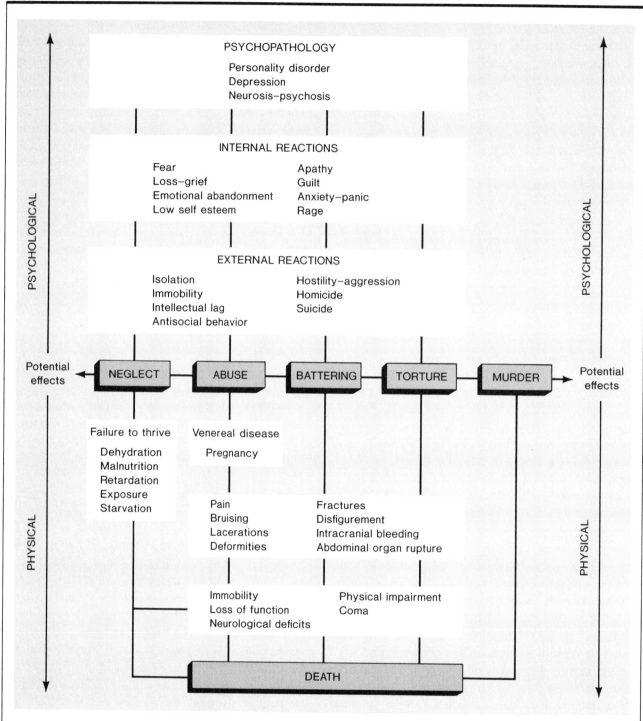

Figure 11–2

The continuum of violence. The diagram depicts the potential effects despite the variability in intent. (From M. Duggan, "Violence in the Family," in *Understanding the Family: Stress and Change in American Family Life,* edited by C. Getty and W. Humphreys. Norwalk, Conn.: Appleton-Century-Crofts, 1981, p. 258.)

sion of crisis intervention services through the National Institute of Mental Health (NIMH) was organized only as recently as 1972. Before then, a community in crisis depended on the voluntary help of social service and religious groups.

Nurses are often at the scene of natural disasters.

A number of nurses were in the Hyatt Regency Hotel—Kansas City, Missouri's newest hotel—in July 1981 when two skywalks in the four-story lobby collapsed, killing 111 and injuring 188 persons. These nurses, along with others who responded to calls for emergency personnel, assisted the injured and provided crisis intervention services. Some of the same nurses provided counseling services for people in the community, such as a fireman who was terrified to go on the next emergency call and 200 people from the community who attended a session to understand their responses and reactions. Some of the nurses themselves reported that since the disaster they have experienced shock, helplessness, nightmares, and difficulty in relaxing and concentrating.

The Dunlap article (1981) about the Kansas City disaster makes it clear that helpers on the scene may have many of the same responses to a disaster as its victims. These responses are delineated more specifically below.

Phases in Disaster Response   Three overlapping phases in response to disaster have been identified by James Tyhurst (1951, 1957). The first stage, *impact*, is stimulated by the catastrophe. The victims recognize what is happening to them and are concerned mainly with the present. During this acute phase the victim's major concern may be staying alive. According to Tyhurst, about 75 percent of the victims experience shock and confusion. Although they appear dazed, they also exhibit the physical signs of fear. Another group of people, up to 25 percent, are "together." They logically and rationally assess the situation and develop and implement a plan for dealing with the immediate problems the catastrophe brings. A third group, also up to 25 percent, may panic or become immobilized with fear. They may behave in hysterical ways, or they may be overlooked because they sit and silently stare into space.

In *recoil*, the second stage, the initial stress of the disaster has passed, and victims may no longer find their lives in immediate danger, although injuries and other discomforts come to their awareness. Emergency shelter, food, and clothing become available. Behavior of victims is usually dependent—they want to be taken care of. Weeping is common as survivors begin to realize all that has happened to them.

The full impact of the losses the victims have experienced comes in the third, or *post-trauma* period. Grief is a predominant response as persons mourn the losses in their lives. Disturbed and disintegrated responses may occur. DSM-III (1980) includes a syndrome called *Post-traumatic Stress Disorder*. Post-traumatic Stress Disorder occurs when the stressor (rape or assault, military combat, being taken hostage, floods, earthquakes, major car accidents, airplane crashes, bombing, torture, etc.) evokes significant distress. The syndrome appears to be more severe and to last longer when the stressor is man-made.

Many people essentially "relive" the experience in their dreams by having recurrent nightmares. Other sleep disturbances, including insomnia, often occur. Victims may feel a psychic numbing or emotional anesthesia in relationship to: other people; previously enjoyed activities; and feelings of intimacy, tenderness, and sexuality. They may have difficulty in concentrating and remembering. The survivors of trauma shared with others may also feel guilty about having survived, or about behavior they undertook in order to survive. When victims are exposed to situations or events that resemble or in some way symbolize the traumatic event, their symptoms may increase and they may feel even greater distress.

Post-traumatic Stress Disorder is known as the Acute subtype when symptoms begin within six months of the traumatic event and do not last longer than six months. In this instance the chances are good that the person can return to a precrisis level of functioning, particularly if the person's precrisis coping behaviors were effective. The Chronic subtype is diagnosed when a person's symptoms last for six months or more. The Delayed subtype exists when there is a period of latency (of six months of more) before the person first experiences the discomforts associated with this syndrome. Crisis counseling is helpful to persons who have experienced one of these disastrous events. Anticipatory counseling, such as that provided to the community by the Kansas City nurses after the Hyatt Regency disaster, is one form of primary prevention that can help circumvent the development of Post-traumatic Stress Disorder. The brief examples below illustrate the post-trauma experience.

Almost a year after the nuclear accident at the Three Mile Island nuclear plant near Harrisburg, Pennsylvania, sustained levels of distress and a high amount of demoralization have been identified among 100 residents living within 20 miles of the nuclear facility.

After the flooding caused in southern New York State by Hurricane Agnes in 1972, leukemia, lymphoma, and miscarriages were significantly higher than normal for more than a year after the June flood. The "wets" (persons who were flooded out) expressed resentment and hostility toward the "drys" (those who lived further from the river on higher land and were spared the effects of the flood).

Five years after the blizzard of 1977 that howled into Buffalo, New York, off Lake Erie, Buffalonians, who once took winter weather in their stride, still look fearfully out their windows checking weather conditions. Supermarket shelves are sold out as soon as local weathermen predict significant snow accumulations, and abseenteism rates in schools and businesses rise.

One year after fifty-two hostages were held captive in Iran for 444 days: four of their marriages have ended in divorce and others are coming apart; two ex-hostages have required extensive psychiatric care and more than a dozen others are receiving some psychiatric care; and there are a half a dozen cases of ulcers, weight loss, high blood pressure, skin rashes, migraine headaches, and intestinal and colon disturbances, as well as several cases of T-M syndrome (a stress disorder with constant grinding of the teeth or clenching of the jaws), nightmares, flashbacks, and insomnia.

One year after a Southern Airways DC–9 crashed in rain and hail near New Hope, Georgia, in 1977, one of the flight attendants was still overcome with guilt that she had survived and her passengers had died. It was two and a half years before she was able to go back to work as a flight attendant.

Crisis Management of Disaster Victims   Lee Ann Hoff (1978, p. 233) suggests that disaster victims need an opportunity to:

- Talk out the experience and express their feelings of fear, panic, loss and grief.
- Become fully aware and accepting of what has happened to them.
- Resume concrete activity and reconstruct their lives with the social, physical, and emotional resources available.

To assist victims though the crisis, the crisis worker should:

- Listen with concern and sympathy and ease the way for the victims to tell their tragic story, weep, express feelings of anger, loss, frustration, and despair.
- Help the victims of disaster accept in small doses the tragic reality of what has happened. This means staying with them during the initial stages of shock and denial. It also may mean accompanying them back to the scene of the tragedy and being available for support when they are faced with the full impact of their loss.
- Assist them to make contact with relatives, friends, and other resources needed to begin the process of social and physical reconstruction. This could mean making telephone calls to locate relatives, accompanying someone to apply for financial aid, giving information about social and mental health agencies for follow-up services.

People who are hysterical or panicked should be given attention to avoid the contagion of panic that sometimes occurs among large groups of people. It sometimes helps hysterical or panic-stricken persons to give them a small but structured task to focus their energies in a constructive direction. Nurses should remember, however, that assigning tasks beyond the person's capabilities at that time will add to the person's anxiety and feeling of helplessness.

Nurses will also find that in disaster situations they will be incorporating the concepts and intervention strategies related to death and loss described in detail earlier in this chapter.

SUICIDE AS A COPING MECHANISM

Suicide is destructive aggression turned inward. Although statistical reports indicate that suicide is the eleventh-largest cause of death in the United States and that 25,000 people are known to commit suicide per year, it is conservatively estimated that 250,000 people will *attempt* suicide each year. These estimates are really only guesses—no one knows for sure how many deaths labeled accidental are suicides. Some are called accidents because the determination is difficult to make, while others are so labeled for social or economic reasons—to avoid stigmatizing a family in a community or to collect on insurance policies that do not pay off when the cause of death is suicide.

Suicide is a behavior fraught with mystery. It has evoked some age-old tales and myths. Myths that con-

Table 11–5 SUICIDE MYTHS AND REALITIES	
Myth	**Reality**
A suicide threat is just a bid for attention and should not be taken seriously	All suicidal behavior should be taken seriously; a bid for attention may be a cry for help.
It is harmful for a person to talk about suicidal thoughts. The person's attention should be diverted when this occurs	Of prime importance in planning nursing care is an accurate assessment of the lethality of the person's suicide plan.
Only psychotic persons commit suicide.	The majority of successful suicides are committed by persons who are not psychotic.
People who talk about suicide won't do it.	Most people do talk about their suicide intention before making a suicide attempt.
A nice home, good job, or an intact family prevents suicide.	Complex sociocultural, physiological, or psychological stressors may all be related to suicide.
A failed suicide attempt should be treated as manipulative behavior.	Failed suicide attempts are more likely to be evidence of a person's ambivalence toward killing himself or herself.

tinue to surround it include those presented in Table 11–5.

Self-destructive People

Self-destructive people are those who harm themselves in any of a variety of ways, from nail biting, head banging, wrist cutting, cigarette smoking, drug and alcohol abuse, failing to take insulin or necessary medications, and reckless driving to the ultimate self-destruction, suicide. Four broad groups of self-destructive people are:

1. Those who actually do commit suicide
2. Those who threaten to commit suicide
3. Those who attempt suicide
4. Those who are chronically self-destructive in more indirect ways

There are a number of social, demographic, and clinical variables that affect suicidal behavior. They are outlined in the lists below.

Social Variables

Low suicidal rates are noted among the following:

- Developing communities and groups in which hope and optimism are high
- Cultures that are warm and nurturing, such as the Irish, Italians, and Norwegians
- Communities in which there is strong disapproval of suicide as an act, such as Italy, Spain, and Ireland, where the Catholic Church is highly influential

High suicidal rates are noted among the following:

- Societies in which social unrest, internal governmental problems, or pessimistic outlooks for the future predominate
- Cultures that are uncaring and cold and lack concern for people in trouble, such as skid rows and disorganized inner-city areas
- Societies, such as the United States, Japan, Russia, and Germany, that value independence and individual performance
- Social roles, occupations, and professions in which people exhibit high concern and nurturance toward others (physicians and police, for example)

Demographic Variables

Suicide rates are higher among the following:

- Single people and married people without children
- Men in general, although rates for white women have increased 49 percent and for black women have increased 80 percent in the past twenty years
- White people, although the rate for young, urban black persons between twenty and thirty-five years of age is twice that of white persons in the same age group

• Persons above the age of forty, although rates for adolescents are rising (persons over 65 account for 25 percent of the total number of reported suicides)

Clinical Variables

Suicide rates are higher among the following:

• People who have attempted suicide before

• People who have experienced the loss of an important person at some time in the past or the loss of both parents early in life, or the loss of or threat of loss of their spouse, job, money, or social position

• People who are depressed or recovering from depression or a disintegrative life pattern

• People with physical illness, particularly when the illness involves an alteration of body image or life-style

• People who abuse alcohol and drugs, thus decreasing their impulse control

Suicidal Clues or Cries for Help

People bent on suicide almost always give either verbal or nonverbal clues of their intent. Suicidologists and crisis workers who work with suicidal people believe that people bent on self-destruction actually make a powerful attempt to communicate to others their hurt and desperation; they are crying out for help.

Sometimes suicidal people state their intent directly. At other times, the message may be indirect or more subtle. A person may say: "I just can't take it anymore," "There's no reason to go on," "Sometimes I think I'd be better off dead," "I won't be seeing you anymore," "Take care of my dog and cat," "Too bad I won't get to see my little brother grow up," "Will you be sorry when I'm gone?" Sometimes their behavior provides the clue. They may give away prized possessions; make out or change a will; take out or add to an insurance policy; cancel all social engagements; be despondent or behave in unusual ways; be unable to sleep; feel hopeless; have trouble concentrating at school or on the job; or suddenly lose interest in friends, organizations, and activities.

Nurses and others who may have contact with potentially suicidal people must be alert to both clear and veiled communications about suicide. Once clues have been identified, the next step is to undertake an accurate lethality assessment.

Table 11–6 LETHALITY OF SUICIDE METHODS	
Low Lethality Methods	**High Lethality Methods**
Wrist cutting	Gun
House gas	Jumping
Nonprescription drugs (excluding aspirin and Tylenol)	Hanging
	Drowning
Tranquilizers	Carbon monoxide poisoning
	Barbiturates or other prescribed sleeping pills
	Aspirin and Tylenol (high doses)
	Car crash
	Exposure to extreme cold

Source: Adapted from L. A. Hoff, *People in Crisis: Understanding and Helping* (Menlo Park, Calif.: Addison-Wesley Publishing Co., 1978), p. 119.

Assessing Lethality

A *lethality assessment* is an attempt to predict the likelihood of suicide. An accurate lethality assessment is essential in formulating a plan for helping a suicidal person. It also gives the nurse cues about the client's possible need for hospitalization. Carrying out a lethality assessment requires direct communication between client and nurse concerning the client's intent. Lee Ann Hoff (1978, pp. 119–26) suggests that an adequate lethality assessment includes the following:

1. Suicide plan. Does the person have suicidal ideas? Is the person considering a highly lethal method, or one of low lethality? (The lethality of various suicide methods is categorized in Table 11–6.) Are the means for carrying out suicide available—that is, does the person have access to a gun, pills, ammunition? Has a specific plan been worked out?

2. History of suicide attempts. Has the person attempted suicide before? Is the method the same, or is it more or less lethal? What was the outcome of the previous suicide attempt? Was the person rescued accidentally? Has the person been hospitalized for attempting suicide in the past?

3. Resources and communication with significant others. What are the person's internal and external resources? Is the person alienated from others?

4. Age, sex, and race. (See the demographic variables identified earlier.)

5. Recent loss. (See the clinical variables identified earlier.)

6. Physical illness. (See the clinical variables identified earlier.)

7. Drinking and drug abuse. (See the clinical variables identified earlier.)

8. Isolation. Is the person physically alone or emotionally isolated? Are significant others rejecting? Do others fail to approve of the person's role performance?

9. Unexplained change in behavior. Change in behavior from careful to careless or impulsive may indicate suicide risk.

10. Depression. A significant number of suicide victims are depressed.

11. Social factors. A broken home, delinquency and truancy, family discord, unemployment, forced retirement, or a move to another residence may increase a person's risk of suicide.

12. Mental illness. If a person's hallucinations command him or her to commit suicide, the risk of suicide is increased. However, it is erroneous to believe that only mentally ill persons commit suicide. Persons with disintegrative life patterns should be assessed according to the other criteria.

Hoff indicates that a person who fits the first three criteria above is a high suicide risk regardless of other factors, although the others do increase the risk.

Assessment of suicidal risk is not easily accomplished. It is, however, the basis on which the nurse's response to the self-destructive person is formulated. An accurate lethality assessment can be used to determine whether to hospitalize a suicidal person and what alternatives the person has other than suicide. It serves as a guide for the intervenor.

An algorithm giving step-by-step instructions for gathering data about a depressed client who may be considering suicide is presented in Chapter 14.

Intervention with Suicidal Clients

Do people have the right to commit suicide, and can or should nurses intervene when people try to kill themselves? These questions of ethics are discussed in

Chapter 5. Nurses should know that, ethical concerns aside, they may be prosecuted under state laws, making it a crime to aid or abet a suicide, under any circumstance, even when a terminally ill person decides to end his or her life. Questions about a client's right to suicide and society's right to control suicide have not been answered. The nursing interventions discussed below are based on the traditional belief that mental health professionals should do everything possible to prevent suicide. Engaging in the process of ethical reflectiveness suggested in Chapter 5 will help nurses in their search for a personal position.

The first priority in intervening with suicidal clients is to protect them from themselves. The nurse may begin by telling the client of the nurse's concern about the client's welfare, of the nurse's interest in the client and the client's well-being, and of the nurse's intent to prevent the client's suicide. If the nurse is a hot-line counselor or is working with the client in the community, he or she may take steps to ask for immediate intervention by the police, a crisis team, or the client's own family or friends. In an inpatient setting, the nurse would take steps to remove dangerous objects, such as knives or other sharp implements, glass, matches, ropes or scarves, or other objects that could be used in a suicide attempt. However, it may be impossible to make an environment absolutely safe especially when a client is determined to commit suicide, as illustrated by the historical example that follows.

A San Quentin convict, sentenced in 1930 to be hanged, vowed that he would never be executed for his crime. The prison guards were especially careful to keep all objects that could be turned into tools for self-destruction out of the prisoner's reach. As the date of his execution drew nearer, he busied himself in his cell, seeming to play solitaire with a deck of cards. However, he knew something his guards didn't. The red spots on the heart and diamond cards contained the explosive ingredients nitrate and cellulose. He tore the red spots out of the cards and soaked them in water. Then he put them into a hollow iron leg from his bunk and sealed the ends, making a pipe bomb. The night before his execution, the prisoner committed suicide by placing the bomb on the hot oil heater in his cell, placing his head on top, and waiting for the explosion.

Once the environment has been made as safe as possible, the nurse should carefully observe the suicidal client. It used to be the practice to isolate suicidal clients. However, this measure appears to be for the convenience of staff rather than the benefit of the client, since isolation only furthers the client's loneliness and alienation. Careful observation is important until the suicidal crisis has passed. The mental health team determines when the immediate danger is over after a suicide attempt. The determination may be based on the client's happiness to be alive, failure to express further suicide plans, ability to explore the attempt and deal constructively with the stressors that preceded it, or ability to mobilize external resources (family, friends, community agencies, self-help groups, and so on).

It is important to recognize that suicidal risk increases for severely depressed clients as they begin to feel better and their depression lifts. Making a suicide plan and following through on it requires energy. For this reason, severely depressed people are at greater risk when their drive and energy begin to return. Nurses should recognize the need for careful observation at this stage as well. Some clients, previously ambivalent about committing suicide, may appear to be in better spirits because their ambivalence has dissipated and they have made a firm commitment to suicide. Nurses must be alert to this circumstance as well.

A long-term goal is to provide the suicidal client with continued supports both through a therapeutic relationship that gives the client the opportunity to explore the event and what precipitated it and through a support network or other interested persons such as family, friends, or community groups.

The Victims Left Behind

Last summer, a twenty-seven-year-old woman called her former boy friend and told him to look out of his window so that he could watch her die. He hung up on her. Only minutes later he heard a crash. She had driven her car into a tree in front of his apartment building. The impact killed her instantly.

A seventeen-year-old high school student killed himself in his home after holding his mother hostage for three hours and forcing her to type his suicide notes. The young man tied his mother to a chair and forced her to type four suicide notes. When she finished, he shot himself in the head.

There are thousands of "survivor victims" of suicide every year who are left behind to mourn, and often to feel guilty, ashamed, and angry. They need to be helped to mourn and express their feelings. The crisis intervention modes discussed below are useful for survivors as well as for persons who have attempted, or are thinking of attempting, suicide.

CRISIS INTERVENTION MODES

Earlier in this chapter, we identified the humanistic features of a good plan for crisis intervention. They should be kept in mind when using any of the following modes.

Individual Crisis Counseling

Crisis counseling is brief (five to six sessions) and issue-oriented. The counsellor makes an assessment and helps the client explore assessment issues. (See Chapters 7 and 8.) Hoff (1978) suggests that healthy crisis coping can be achieved when the nurse uses the following techniques:

- Listen actively and with concern
- Encourage the open expression of feelings
- Help the client gain an understanding of the crisis
- Help the client gradually accept reality
- Help the client explore new ways of coping with problems
- Link the client to a social network
- Engage in decision counseling or problem solving (see Chapter 7) with the client
- Reinforce newly learned coping devices
- Follow up the case after resolution of the crisis

Crisis Groups

The purpose of crisis groups is to resolve crises through the group process. Group members are individuals who are experiencing crisis. They usually meet for six sessions, although some groups have extended to ten. Chapters 9 and 18 present thorough discussions of group dynamics and group strategies.

Family Crisis Counseling

Family crisis counseling involves the entire family for approximately six sessions. It is the preferred mode for most children and adolescents in crisis. Chapter 21 discusses strategies of family counseling in general.

KEY NURSING CONCEPTS

✔ Everyday living brings desirable and undesirable changes that result in stresses and tensions with the potential for becoming crises.

✔ A crisis is a self-limiting situation in which usual problem-solving or decision-making methods are not adequate.

✔ A crisis offers the opportunity for renewal and growth.

✔ Working with a helping person increases the likelihood that a crisis will be resolved in a positive way.

✔ Nurses are often in key positions to help clients grow through the crisis experience.

✔ Crises may be classified into two types: internal or developmental (the anticipated crises of maturation), and external or situational (stressful life events that are usually not anticipated).

✔ The crisis episode may be understood as a sequence that involves three time periods— precrisis, crisis, and postcrisis.

✔ Crisis intervention as a therapeutic strategy is strongly humanistic in that it views people as capable of personal growth and able to control their own lives.

✔ Intervention strategies such as individual crisis counseling, crisis groups, family crisis counseling, telephone counseling, and home crisis visits are appropriate modes for dealing with either internal or external crisis.

✔ Suicide is a maladaptive response to crisis.

✔ Suicidal behavior is affected by a number of social, demographic, and clinical variables.

✔ A lethality assessment is the first step in helping self-destructive persons and is the basis on which the nurse's subsequent responses are formulated.

Telephone Counseling

Suicide prevention and crisis intervention centers rely heavily on telephone counseling by volunteers. Such "hot lines" have been successful because they give the person in crisis immediate help. They remove the necessity of long travel to an office to visit a counselor hours or days after the crisis has begun. Telephone counseling is also a cost-effective intervention.

Home Crisis Visits

Home visits are made when telephone counseling does not suffice, to obtain additional information by direct observation, or to reach a client who is unobtainable by telephone. Home visits are more common in circumstances where the crisis intervenors initiate contacts rather than waiting for clients to come to them— for example, when a telephone caller is assessed to be highly suicidal, or when a concerned neighbor, physician, clergyman, or the like informs the agency of potential clients in crisis.

References

Caplan, G. *Principles of Preventive Psychiatry*. New York: Basic Books, 1965.

———. "Lessons in Bravery." With V. Cadden. *McCall's* (September 1968): 85.

Carlson, B. E. "Battered Women and Their Assailants." *Social Work* 22 (1977): 455–460.

Cobb, S., and Lindemann, E. "Neuropsychiatric Observations after the Cocoanut Grove Fire." *Annals of Surgery* 117 (1943): 814.

Diagnostic and Statistical Manual of Mental Disorders. 3d ed. Washington, D.C.: American Psychiatric Association, 1980.

Duggan, M. "Violence in the Family." In *Understanding the Family: Stress and Change in American Family Life*, edited by C. Getty and W. Humphreys, pp. 253–271. Norwalk, Conn.: Appleton-Century-Crofts, 1981.

Dunlap, M. J. "Nurses Assist Injured at Hyatt Disaster." *The American Nurse* 13 (September 1981): 1.

Engel, G. L. "Grief and Grieving." *American Journal of Nursing* 64 (1964): 93–98.

Erikson, E. *Childhood and Society.* 2d ed. New York: W. W. Norton, 1963.

Glaser, B. G., and Strauss, A. L. *Awareness of Dying.* Chicago: Aldine, 1965.

Hansell, N. *The Person in Distress.* New York: Human Services Press, 1976.

Hoff, L. A. *People in Crisis: Understanding and Helping.* Menlo Park, Calif.: Addison-Wesley, 1978.

Holmes, T. H., and Rahe, R. H. "The Social Readjustment Rating Scale." *Journal of Psychosomatic Research* 11 (1967): 213.

Joint Commission on Mental Illness and Health. *Action for Mental Health.* New York: Basic Books, 1961.

Lindemann, E. "Symptomatology and Management of Acute Grief." *American Journal of Psychiatry* 101 (1944): 101-148.

Maslow, A. *Motivation and Personality.* 2d ed. New York: Harper and Row, 1970.

Meyers, J., et al. "Life Events and Mental Status." *Journal of Health and Social Behavior* 1 (December 1972): 398-406.

National Organization for Women. *Do It NOW* (bulletin), June 1976, pp. 3-8.

Parad, H. J., and Resnick, H. L. P. "A Crisis Intervention Framework." In *Emergency Psychiatric Care,* edited by H. L. P. Resnick and H. L. Ruben, pp. 3-7. Bowie, Md.: Charles Press, 1975.

Rubin, L. *Women of a Certain Age: The Midlife Search for Self.* New York: Harper and Row, 1981.

Sheehy, G. *Passages: Predictable Crises of Adult Life.* New York: E. P. Dutton, 1976.

————. *Pathfinders.* New York: William Morrow, 1981.

Spire, R. H. "An Experimental Study of the Use of Photographic Self-Image Confrontation as a Nursing Procedure in the Care of Chronically Ill Schizophrenic Female Patients." Master's thesis, State University of New York at Buffalo, 1966.

Tyhurst, J. S. "Individual Reactions to Community Disaster." *American Journal of Psychiatry* 107 (1951): 764-769.

————. "The Role of Transition States—Including Disasters—in Mental Illness." Paper read at the Symposium on Preventive and Social Psychiatry, Walter Reed Army Institute of Research and the National Research Council, Washington, D.C., April 15-17, 1957.

Weisman, A. D., and Hackett, T. P. "Predilection to Death: Death and Dying as a Psychiatric Problem." *Psychosomatic Medicine* 23 (1961): 232.

Williams, C. C., and Holmes, T. H. "Life Change, Human Adaptation, and Onset of Illness." In *Clinical Practice in Psychosocial Nursing: Assessment and Intervention,* edited by D. Longo and R. Williams, pp. 69-85. New York: Appleton-Century-Crofts, 1978.

Further Reading

Aguilera, D. C., and Messick, J. M. *Crisis Intervention: Theory and Methodology.* 3d ed. St. Louis: C. V. Mosby, 1978.

Bandman, E. L., and Bandman, B. "The Nurse's Role in Protecting the Patient's Right to Live or Die." *Advances in Nursing Science* 1 (April 1979): 21-35.

Engel, G. *Psychological Development in Health and Disease.* Philadelphia: W. B. Saunders, 1962.

Farberow, N. L., ed. *Suicide in Different Cultures.* Baltimore: University Park Press, 1975.

Gelles, R. J. "Abused Wives: Why Do They Stay?" *Journal of Marriage and the Family* 38 (1976): 659-668.

Golan, N. *Passing Through Transitions: A Guide for Practitioners.* New York: Free Press, 1981.

Kneisl, C. R. "Grieving: A Response to Loss." In *The Dying Patient: A Supportive Approach,* edited by R. E. Caughill, pp. 31-46. Boston: Little, Brown 1976.

McCloskey, J. C. "How to Make the Most of Body Image Theory in Nursing Practice." *Nursing 76* (May 1976): 68-72.

McGee, R. K. *Crisis Intervention in the Community.* Baltimore: University Park Press, 1974.

Perlin, S., ed. *A Handbook for the Study of Suicide.* New York: Oxford University Press, 1975.

Petit, M. "Battered Women: A (Nearly) Hidden Social Problem." In *Understanding the Family: Stress and Change in American Family Life,* edited by C. Getty and W. Humphreys, pp. 272-297. New York: Appleton-Century-Crofts, 1981.

Schneidman, E. S., ed. *Suicidology: Contemporary Developments.* New York: Grune and Stratton, 1976.

Spitzer, T. *Psychobattery.* Clifton, N.J.: Humana Press, 1980.

12

Human Sexuality

CHAPTER OUTLINE

Normal and Abnormal Sexuality
Physiological Sexuality
  The Female Genitals
  The Male Genitals
  Physiology of Sexual Responses
  Sexual Arousal and Intercourse
  Masturbation
  Arousal Techniques
  Coitus
  Anal Intercourse
Psychological Sexuality
  Gender Identity
  Theories of Gender Development
Sociological Sexuality
  Sex Roles
  Sex and Social Problems
Alternative Sexual Patterns
  Homosexuality
  Bisexuality
  Transsexualism and Transvestism
  Other Alternative Sexual Patterns

Sexual Problems and Their Treatment
  Impairments in Physiological Functioning
  Sexual Problems Associated with Other Coping
  Problems
  Therapeutic Counseling
Key Nursing Concepts

LEARNING OBJECTIVES

After reading this chapter, students should be able to

- Discuss normal physiological sexuality in females and males
- Define common terms used in sexual counseling and teaching
- Compare the advantages and disadvantages of a variety of coital positions
- Contrast concepts of gender identity, gender role, and sexual conduct
- Relate sexual acts considered to be social problems to the concept of consent
- Describe major alternative sexual patterns
- Comprehend the process of conducting a sexual assessment

CHAPTER 12

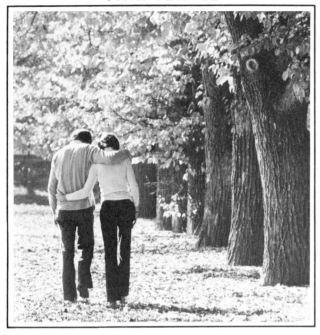

Human sexuality is more than a physiological act. It includes tenderness, warmth, and a sensitivity to the needs of another.

NORMAL AND ABNORMAL SEXUALITY

In the 1960s sex came out of the closet. Henry Miller and D. H. Lawrence—once circulated underground—are now required reading in college courses. Intercourse scenes in cinema—once hinted at by a train racing through a tunnel and blackout to next morning—are now almost compulsory in a commercially successful film. *Esquire's* suggestive pinup photos have been replaced by more explicit ones in *Playboy* and *Hustler*.

Yet human sexual interaction is still complex and mysterious, shrouded in myth and misunderstanding. Ironically, while human beings know an immense amount about distant phenomena—such as the movement of the galaxies—the nature of human sexuality is only partially mapped and rarely explored. Much of the new openness about sex is superficial, and while the language may be different, the anxieties and questions remain the same.

Health professionals have only recently recognized human sexuality as a subject for scientific analysis and therapeutic intervention. Appropriate or "normal" sexual interaction may be defined according to one of three perspectives. These are the physiological perspective, the psychological perspective, and the socio-

logical perspective. Each perspective has wrestled with the question of what constitutes "healthy" sexuality.

Professionals nowadays are far less judgmental about fixations and compulsions than Freud and his immediate successors were. They believe only that whatever the sexual activity is, it should be pleasurable and noninjurious to both partners. Thus the range of so-called normal sexual behavior has broadened enormously over the last five years. What society defines as normal sex depends partly on current definitions of sexuality itself as well as on the question of normal versus abnormal behaviors. Society once judged only reproductive sex to be normal. Now society also accepts relational sex and is moving toward sanctioning recreational sex.

In any society people learn how to express their sexuality through their culture. They learn norms, values, ideals, and ideology (see Chapter 26). They also learn to use a material technology that may include contraceptives, vibrators, and so forth. Normality, then, is a constantly changing concept. This concept is formed by the shifting interplay among discovery, invention, dissemination of information, and behavioral and attitudinal change. Yet the question "Am I normal?" reflects an anxiety about sexuality common to many clients. Some writers suggest that the greatest contribution a nurse can make is to reassure the client, "Yes, you are normal." A sensitive nurse must be prepared to counsel a woman who has never been able to enjoy sex, a man who is unable to achieve sexual gratification with his spouse, a couple feeling anxious, uncertain, and hopeless about their sex life after one of them has become handicapped, and so on. How do such problems affect the client's relationships, self-esteem, joy in living, and productivity in work?

Human sexuality is best understood through the holistic approach that characterizes other chapters in this text. A knowledge of physiological sexuality, psychological sexuality, sexual role behavior, and social contexts all contribute to an understanding of sexuality.

PHYSIOLOGICAL SEXUALITY

The study of physiological sexuality focuses on the nature of female and male sexual responses and on the structure of the sexual and reproductive organs.

The Female Genitals

The external female genitals (Figure 12–1) are collectively called the *vulva*. They consist of the mons veneris, labia majora, labia minora, clitoris, and the outer portion of the vagina. The *mons veneris* is the rounded, hair-covered, fatty cushion over the pubic bone. Nerve endings concentrated in the mons area can produce pleasurable sensations when stimulated by touch and pressure. One of the functions of the pubic hair, which is present from puberty onward, is to trap scent gland secretions that occur during sexual excitement. These secretions have a characteristically erotic, stimulating odor. Because of the conditioning of current American cultures—among others—many people find these odors offensive.

The *labia majora* are folds of fatty tissue on either side of the vaginal opening. They are also covered with pubic hair. In women who have never had children, the labia majora may meet in the middle. The *labia minora* are the small lips composed partially of erectile tissue that frame the sides of the vaginal opening. In some mature women, the labia minora protrude beyond the labia majora. They are pink or reddish and meet just below the mons to form a kind of hood for the clitoris.

The *clitoris* is apparently the only human organ that has the sole function of producing pleasure. It is located below the mons and above the urinary meatus and may be anywhere from less than .25 inch to over one inch long. It is composed of a shaft and a glans, the tip of which is like a small bump beneath the hood. The clitoris is often described as the primary female sexual organ in that orgasm depends physiologically on adequate clitoral stimulation. The clitoris has a nerve net three times as large as that of the penis in proportion to its size. During sexual stimulation the erectile tissue of the clitoris fills with blood, and the clitoris becomes stiff. During intercourse there is usually no direct stimulation of the clitoris by the penis. Instead, traction exerted on the labia as a result of the thrusting movements of the penis going into the vagina stimulates the clitoris sufficiently to produce orgasm.

The *vestibule* is the area that includes the vaginal opening and the urinary meatus. It is rich in nerve endings and blood vessels, making it highly sensitive to stimulation. The urinary *meatus* is the opening through which urine is released from the body after it passes from the bladder through the urethra. It lies between the clitoris and the vaginal opening. The *Bartholin's glands* are small, mucus-producing glands located in the groove between the hymen and the labia minora about one-third of the way up from the lower boundary of the orifice. These glands lubricate the vaginal entrance.

The *hymen* is a stretchable membrane across the lower portion of the vaginal entrance. An intact hymen has traditionally been regarded as a sign of virginity. In reality, the hymen can be stretched or torn in many ways that do not involve sexual activity. Some women

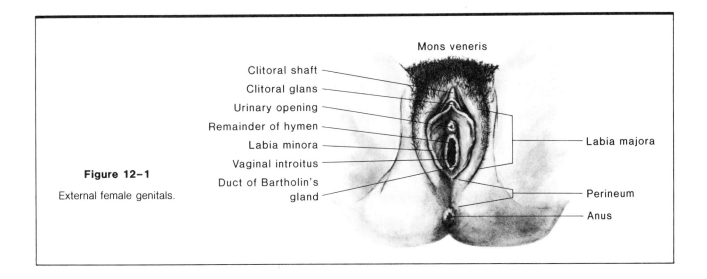

Figure 12–1

External female genitals.

Mons veneris

Clitoral shaft

Clitoral glans

Urinary opening

Remainder of hymen

Labia minora

Vaginal introitus

Duct of Bartholin's gland

Labia majora

Perineum

Anus

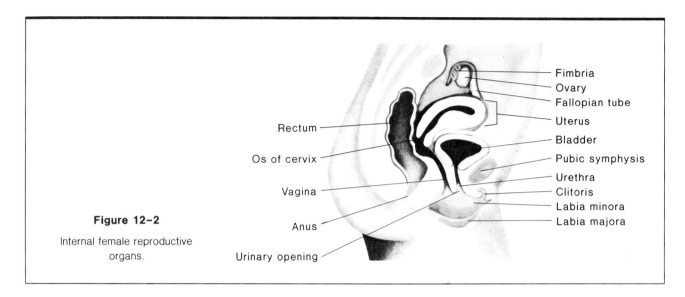

Rectum

Os of cervix

Vagina

Fimbria
Ovary
Fallopian tube
Uterus
Bladder
Pubic symphysis
Urethra
Clitoris
Labia minora
Labia majora

Figure 12–2

Internal female reproductive
organs.

Anus

Urinary opening

choose to stretch their vaginal opening before their first act of intercourse in order to avoid the pain that sometimes is experienced from the act of rupturing an unstretched hymen.

The *vagina* is positioned between the bladder and the rectum. Most of the time it is a potential rather than an actual space, since its walls are usually touching. In the unaroused state the vagina is three to five inches long. During sexual excitement it may lengthen as much as two inches, and it may dilate to a diameter of two inches. During childbirth the vagina may dilate to a diameter of five inches. The vagina is moist inside, the type and amount of moisture varying with the age of the woman and the phase of the menstrual cycle. Vaginal lubrication occurs in a biorhythmic cycle of approximately ninety minutes. In childhood and after menopause, when levels of circulating estrogen are low, the vaginal mucous membrane is thin, fragile, and less stretchable than it is during the childbearing years.

The *cervix* blocks the vagina at its upper end. The cervical *os* is the opening in the center of the cervix. It is about the size of a small drinking straw in the nonpregnant woman. Through the os sperm travel upward to the Fallopian tubes. The contents of the uterus are discharged through the os during menstrual flow, and the baby passes through it during childbirth, when it dilates to approximately ten centimenters. The *uterus,* also called the womb, is the organ in which the baby develops. In some women, it is a source of sexual pleasure as well.

It is through the *Fallopian tubes* that an ovum passes each month on its way to the uterus of the menstrual age woman. Each of these two tubes is four

or five inches long and about the thickness of a drinking straw. The *ovaries* are located one on each side of, and somewhat behind, the uterus. They have the dual function of producing the female sex hormones, estrogen and progesterone, and of producing the female ova. At birth each ovary contains forty thousand to four hundred thousand microscopic follicles. Each follicle consists of a ring of cells containing a premature ovum. The organs of the internal female reproductive tract are represented in a side view in Figure 12–2.

The Male Genitals

The external genitals of the normal adult male include the penis, scrotum, testes, epididymis, and parts of the vas deferens. The internal genitals include the vas deferens, seminal vesicles, ejaculatory ducts, and prostate. The male sexual organs fulfill two reproductive functions: the production of sperm and the depositing of viable sperm into the female reproductive tract. Figure 12–3 shows the external male genitals, while Figure 12–4 presents a side view of the internal organs.

The *penis* is the primary male sexual organ. It also serves as the passageway for urine. The skin of the penis is extremely loose, so that erection can occur, and it is hairless. The penis consists of the glans, shaft, and root. The shaft comprises three parallel tubes, two *corpora cavernosa,* which lie side by side, and beneath them the single *corpus spongiosum,* which is traversed by the urethra. The anterior end of the corpus spongiosum fits over the corpora cavernosa and is called the *glans.* Its rich supply of nerve endings makes the glans very sensitive to tactile stimulation. Most sensi-

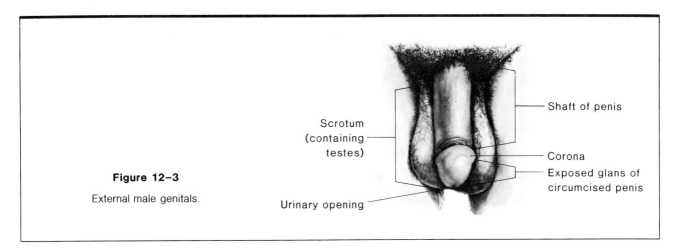

Figure 12–3

External male genitals.

Scrotum (containing testes)

Urinary opening

Shaft of penis

Corona

Exposed glans of circumcised penis

tive of all is the *frenulum,* which is the thin fold of skin on the lower surface of the glans where the glans connects to the *foreskin.* The *corona,* or ridge at the junction of the shaft of the penis and the glans, is also highly sensitive.

The penis is composed primarily of erectile tissue. When the corpora fill with blood, the penis becomes erect. The erective firmness is produced entirely by the blood trapped in the erectile tissues. There are a number of pathological conditions that interfere with the erective process. These include diabetes, alcoholism, and the routine use of certain drugs such as tranquilizers. In a rare condition known as *priapism,* erections become painful and prolonged. Priapism sometimes occurs with sickle cell disease and with leukemia.

Most theorists label as myth the idea that the larger his penis, the more effective a man is as a partner in intercourse. In general, a small flaccid penis will in-

crease proportionately more in size than a large flaccid penis. The normal range of flaccid penile length varies from 3 to 4 inches. The average is 3.75 inches. Erect, the male penis averages 6.25 inches.

The *testis,* or male gonad, is an oval gland measuring approximately 1.5 inches by 1 inch by .75 inch. There are two testes, each enclosed in the scrotal sac. The *scrotum* is the bag of skin that hangs between the thighs. It responds to temperature change by contracting when cold and expanding in response to warmth and sexual stimulation. The primary male hormone, *testosterone,* is manufactured within the testes, as are the male sex cells or *spermatozoa.* An adult human male usually produces several hundred million sperm per day. It takes an average of sixty to seventy-two days for sperm to become mature, and sperm are present in the testes in all stages of development.

Sperm pass through the epididymis, vas deferens, ejaculatory duct, and urethra before they are ejaculat-

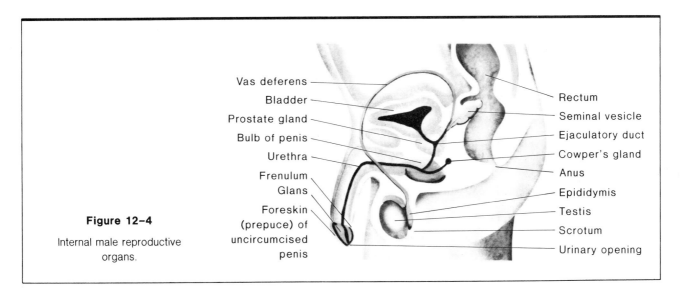

Figure 12–4

Internal male reproductive organs.

Vas deferens

Bladder

Prostate gland

Bulb of penis

Urethra

Frenulum

Glans

Foreskin (prepuce) of uncircumcised penis

Rectum

Seminal vesicle

Ejaculatory duct

Cowper's gland

Anus

Epididymis

Testis

Scrotum

Urinary opening

ed through the external opening. On the way secretions are added to the sperm by the seminal vesicles, the prostate gland, and the Cowper's glands. Contact with these secretions enhances the fertilizing capacity of the sperm and gives them maximum motility. Male semen is composed of sperm cells and fluids from these organs.

Physiology of Sexual Responses

A sexual response is a continuum of experience. This experience may ebb and flow in intensity. For descriptive purposes, however, arousal levels and certain behaviors have been labeled. This makes it possible to speak of stages or phases of the sexual response cycle. Since Masters and Johnson published their *Human Sexual Response* in 1966, their descriptive language has become the one most sexologists use. Masters and Johnson divide the continuum of sexual response into four phases. These are excitement, plateau, orgasm, and resolution. Variations among individuals are striking, yet some basic physiological responses are uniform. Table 12–1 gives a general description of the four phases of sexual response. Table 12–2 describes the physiology of the phases of female response. Table 12–3 describes the physiology of the phases of male response.

Orgasm in the Male   Orgasm and ejaculation are two separate events in the male, and one can occur without the other. Very few men are nonorgasmic, however. Masters and Johnson (1966, p. 215) have formulated a composite description of the male orgasm based on interviews of 417 men ranging in age from eighteen to eighty-nine years. As the plateau phase ends, a sensation of ejaculatory inevitability develops an instant prior to the accessory organ contractions that initiate the ejaculatory process. The man can no longer delay or control the process once this stage is reached, and ejaculation occurs within two or three seconds. At least two different contractile sensations are perceived during the ejaculatory phase. Two or three expulsive contractions of the penile urethra are followed by slow, almost tensionless final contractions.

A twenty-three-year-old sexually active male, offered the following description:

Before I have an orgasm I am usually concentrating on the woman I'm making love to and on my own erotic thoughts. About thirty seconds to a minute beforehand, I

Table 12–1	PHASES OF SEXUAL RESPONSE
Phase	**Response**
Excitement	Muscle tension increases (myotonia), particularly in striated muscles of arms and legs. May be some tensing in smooth muscles of abdomen late in phase. Heart rate and blood pressure increase moderately. Sex flush (more common in females) may appear late in phase. Nipple erection occurs (with greater reliability in females).
Plateau	Myotonia becomes quite pronounced throughout the body. Heart rate increases just before orgasm; blood pressure continues to elevate. Breathing becomes faster and deeper. Sex flush becomes more pronounced or may appear at this phase.
Orgasm	Involuntary muscle spasm occurs throughout body with reduction in voluntary muscle control. Blood pressure and heart rate reach highest levels. Hyperventilation and heart rate peak. Sex flush, if present, usually persists through orgasm. External rectal sphincter muscle contracts involuntarily.
Resolution	All signs of myotonia are absent usually within 5 minutes after orgasm. Heart rate, blood pressure, and breathing rate begin to return to normal. Nipple erection subsides slowly (more rapidly in females).

can feel the semen start to move in my body. It's a totally lovely sensation and then my body takes over completely and during ejaculation my mind is totally blank. It's a purely physical feeling centered in my groin and sometimes reaching down to my knees.

Orgasm in the Female   Female orgasm begins with a sensation of suspension or stoppage. This sensation lasts only an instant and is accompanied or followed immediately by a thrust of sensual awareness, clitorally oriented but radiating upward into the pelvis. Often there is a sense of bearing down. In the second stage a sensation of warmth pervades the pelvic area and spreads throughout the body. The third stage of

Table 12-2   PHYSIOLOGY OF FEMALE SEXUAL RESPONSE

Phase	Body Part	Response
Excitement	Vagina	Lubrication within ten to thirty seconds of effective stimulation. Barrel lengthens, inner two-thirds distends. Irregular expansive movements of walls late in phase; wall color changes to darker, purplish hue.
	Labia majora	Thin and flatten against perineum in nulliparous women; become markedly distended with blood in multiparous women.
	Labia minora	Expand markedly in diameter.
	Clitoris	Shaft increases in diameter through vasocongestion, elongates in some women (less rapidly than vaginal lubrication occurs; vaginal lubrication, not clitoral erection, is the "neurophysiological parallel" to male penile erection). Vasocongestion of glans varies from barely discernible to two-fold expansion of glans, depending on whether stimulation is direct or indirect and on individual variations in anatomy.
	Uterus	Pulled slowly up and back if initially in normal anterior position.
	Breasts	Nipple erection due to involuntary contracting of nipple muscle fibers. Vein patterns in breast extend and stand out. Actual breast size increases and areolae markedly engorge toward end of phase.
	Sex flush	In some women a rash appears between the breastbone and navel late in this phase or early in the plateau phase.
	Myotonia	Initial total-body responses include increasing restlessness, irritability, and rapidity of voluntary and involuntary movement. *Myotonia* [muscular rigidity] increases in long muscles of arms and legs; abdominal muscles involuntarily tense; involuntary contractile rate of muscles between ribs increases, increasing respiratory rate.
	Other	Heart rate and blood pressure increase.
Plateau	Vagina	Marked vasocongestion further reduces central opening of the outer third by at least one-third. Base of vasocongestion encompassing outer third of vagina and engorged labia minora is called the *orgasmic platform,* which "provides the anatomic foundation for the vagina's physiological expression of the orgasmic experience," and is regarded as a sign that plateau stage has been reached. Further increase in inner width and depth of vagina during this phase is negligible. Production of lubrication slows, especially if phase is prolonged.
	Labia majora	No further changes.
	Labia minora	Vivid color changes; nulliparous from pink to bright red; multiparous from bright red to deep wine. Orgasm invariably follows if stimulation continues once this "sex-skin" color change occurs.
	Clitoris	Retracts from normal position late in phase; withdraws; at least 50 percent overall reduction in length of total clitoral body by immediate preorgasmic period.
	Uterus	Full elevation is reached.
	Breasts	Markedly increased areolar engorgement. Unsuckled breast increases one-fifth to one-fourth over unstimulated size by end of phase; little or no increase in breast that has been suckled.
	Sex flush	Spreads over breasts in some women; may have widespread body distribution by late plateau stage on those affected.
	Myotonia	Overall increase. Involuntary facial contractions, grimaces, clutching movements; involuntary pelvic thrusts late in phase near orgasm.

Table continues on next page

		Table 12-2 continued	
Phase	**Body Part**	**Response**	
	Other	Hyperventilation develops late in phase. Further increase in heart rate and blood pressure	
Orgasm	Vagina	Strong, rhythmic contractions of orgasmic platform (three to fifteen), beginning at intervals of eight-tenths of a second and gradually diminishing in strength and duration; may be preceded by spastic contraction lasting two to four seconds. Inner vaginal area remains essentially expanded.	
	Labia	No changes.	
	Clitoris	Retracted and not observed.	
	Uterus	Contracts irregularly.	
	Breasts	No specific reaction.	
	Sex flush	Peaks.	
	Myotonia	Muscle spasms and involuntary contraction throughout the body. Loss of voluntary control.	
	Other	Hyperventilation, heart rate, and blood pressure peak. Urinary meatus will occasionally slightly dilate, returning to usual state before orgasmic platform contractions have ceased. Rectal sphincter sometimes rhythmically contracts involuntarily.	
Resolution	Vagina	Central opening of orgasmic platform rapidly increases in diameter by one-third. Cervix and upper walls of vagina descend toward vaginal floor in minimum of three to four minutes. Vaginal color returns to pre-excitement state, usually in about ten to fifteen minutes. Occasionally production of lubrication continues into resolution phase; suggests remaining or renewed sexual tension.	
	Labia majora	Rapidly back to pre-excitement levels if orgasm; slowly if only plateau levels were reached.	
	Labia minora	Sex-skin color returns to light pink within five to fifteen seconds after orgasm. Further color loss is rapid.	
	Clitoris	Returned to pre-excitement position within five to fifteen seconds after cessation of orgasmic-platform contractions. Vasocongestion of glans and shaft usually disappears five to ten minutes after orgasm, ten to thirty minutes in some women; may take several hours if plateau phase but no orgasm.	
	Uterus	Cervical os dilates early in phase; observable in nulliparous women.	
	Breasts	Rapid detumescence of areolae. Nonsuckled breasts lose size increase in about five to ten minutes. Superficial vein patterns may last longer.	
	Sex flush	Rapidly disappears from body sites in almost opposite sequence of appearance.	
	Myotonia	Obvious muscle tension usually disappears within five minutes of orgasm. Overall myotonia resolves less rapidly than superficial or deep vasocongestion.	
	Other	Heart rate and blood pressure return to normal. Hyperventilation ends early in stage. A sheen of perspiration appears over the bodies of some women.	

Source: J. S. De Lora and C. A. B. Warren, *Understanding Sexual Interaction* (Boston: Houghton Mifflin Co., 1977), pp. 43–46; developed from W. Masters and V. Johnson, *Human Sexual Response* (Boston: Little, Brown and Co., 1966).

Table 12-3   PHYSIOLOGY OF MALE SEXUAL RESPONSE

Phase	Body Part	Response
Excitement	Penis	First physiologic response to effective stimulation is erection, within three to eight seconds; erection may wax and wane throughout excitement phase.
	Scrotal sac	Decreases in internal diameter; outer skin tenses and thickens; dartos-layer muscle fibers contract. Localized vasocongestion.
	Testes	Elevate toward perineum; if phase is prolonged, may redescend and re-elevate several times. Spermatic cord shortens.
	Breasts	Nipple erection and tumescence develop in some men late in phase; remain throughout rest of sex cycle.
	Sex flush	Sometimes appears late in phase. Occurs or fails to occur with wide variation in same individual and between individuals.
	Myotonia	Observed late in phase. Similar to female pattern. Both voluntary muscle tension and some involuntary.
	Other	Heart rate, blood pressure, and respiration increase as sexual tension increases. Rectal sphincter contracts irregularly after direct stimulation.
Plateau	Penis	Increase in coronal area of glans due to increased vasocongestion. Glans deepens in color in some men.
	Scrotum	No further reactions.
	Testes	Continue to increase in size until about 50 percent larger than in unstimulated state. Further elevate until in pre-ejaculatory position against perineum.
	Sex flush	First appears late in plateau more frequently than in excitement phase. Indicates high levels of sexual tension.
	Myotonia	Voluntary and involuntary tensions increase. Pelvic thrusting becomes involuntary late in phase. Total body reactions of male and female quite similar.
	Other	Further increases in heart rate and blood pressure. Hyperventilation appears late in phase.
Orgasmic (Ejaculatory)	Penis	Ejaculatory contractions along entire length of penile urethra. Expulsive contractions start at intervals of eight-tenths of a second and after three or four reduce in frequency and expulsive force. Final contractions are several seconds apart.
	Scrotum	No specific reactions.
	Testes	No reactions observed.
	Myotonia	Loss of voluntary control. Involuntary contractions and spasms.
	Other	Heart rate, blood pressure, and hyperventilation peak. Degree of sexual tension is frequently indicated by physiological intensity and duration of hyperventilation. Involuntary contractions of rectal sphincter.
Resolution	Penis	Two stages: Rapid reduction in size to about 50 percent larger than in unstimulated state; less rapid if excitement or plateau stages have been intentionally prolonged. Slower disappearance of remaining tumescence, especially if sexual stimulation continues to take place.
	Scrotum	One of two patterns: Rapid decongestion, or decongestion occurring over one or two hours. Typically, but not true of everyone, individuals consistently follow one pattern or the other. In general, within the individual pattern, the more prior stimulation has occurred, the longer the resolution process.
	Testes	Rapid or slow resolution relative to scrotal pattern.
	Breasts	Loss of nipple erection if present; may occur slowly.

Table continues on next page

		Table 12–3 continued		
Phase	**Body Part**	**Response**		
	Sex flush	Disappears rapidly in reverse order of appearance.		
	Myotonia	As in female, rarely lasts more than five minutes, but not lost as rapidly as many of the signs of vasocongestion.		
	Other	Heart rate and blood pressure return to normal. Perspiration sometimes appears on soles of feet and palms of hands. Hyperventilation resolves during refractory period. Ejaculation cannot again occur until this refractory period has passed.		

Source: J. S. De Lora and C. A. B. Warren, *Understanding Sexual Interaction* (Boston: Houghton Mifflin Co., 1977), pp. 46–48; developed from W. Masters and V. Johnson, *Human Sexual Response* (Boston: Little, Brown and Co., 1966).

subjective awareness is the perception of involuntary contractions focused in the vagina, sometimes described as throbbing. Some women attain satisfaction and complete relaxation without the involuntary contractions.

THE VAGINAL-CLITORAL ORGASM CONTROVERSY In 1927 Sigmund Freud implied that vaginal orgasms were more mature than clitoral orgasms. This implication was introduced into marriage manuals and gynecology textbooks, where it was coupled with the further implication that women who did not have vaginal orgasms were frigid.

The findings of Masters and Johnson's physiological research (1966) made the issue of the vaginal versus the clitoral orgasm a debating point for scientists and clinicians in the field. Until then, therapists had accepted Freud's vaginal transfer theory, which holds that the woman who fails to transfer the seat of excitability from her clitoris to her vagina is immature. To be sure, the inability to have coital orgasm does signify an inhibition. But the clitoral and labial mechanisms must work together to produce an orgasm, and sexual counselors have begun to recognize the importance of clitoral stimulation in all healthy orgastic processes.

MULTIPLE ORGASMS Women are potentially multi-orgasmic. They have the potential for an additional orgasm at any point in the resolution phase, if effective stimulation is reapplied. Sometimes the clitoral glans will be extremely sensitive to touch immediately after an orgasm. In this case the woman will not welcome direct stimulation of the glans, although she may enjoy stimulation of other areas.

Sexual Arousal and Intercourse

Nurses who counsel clients on ways to enjoy their sexual interaction must understand the anatomy and physiology of the genitals and the way the human body reacts during arousal and orgasm. In considering the techniques that follow, nurses should bear in mind that sexual pleasure is closely related to feelings and social variables. Thus what is effective with one partner in one situation may not be effective with another. The type of relationship one has with one's sex partner is an important variable. Some people are most susceptible to sexual arousal when they have a very intimate relationship with their partner.

A thirty-year-old woman described her preference for sexual partners this way:

I don't have to be in love with a man to be sexually aroused by him, but I do have to know him quite well and like him a lot on other terms. I'm absolutely turned off by the idea of making it on a date with a stranger who expects it as part of the evening from any woman he's with. I really prefer someone who is much more discriminating, especially if he cares a lot for me personally.

Masturbation

Masturbation may refer to any kind of hand stimulation during sex play, such as mutual masturbation by two or more people exploring and manipulating one another's genitals. More commonly the term is used to mean self-stimulation (often to orgasm) using hands, sexual fantasies, vibrators, or other devices. Stores in the United States and elsewhere stock a variety of masturbatory aids, including artificial genitals and vibrators. For example, there are devices designed for use by women that have an artificial penis attached to a motor that moves the vibrator in a thrusting manner to simulate intercourse. Similar in concept are automatic masturbation machines designed for use by males. These machines have a sleeve that fits over the penis and provides a massaging action through alternating air suction and compression.

Ben-Wa balls have been used by Japanese women as a masturbatory aid for centuries. One of the two Ben-Wa balls is solid and is inserted deep in the vagina, touching the cervix. The second ball, which is filled with mercury, is placed in the vagina in contact with the first ball. The slightest body movement causes the mercury ball to jostle the solid ball, which stimulates the cervix, uterus, and vagina. With the Ben-Wa balls a woman could enjoy an afternoon of rocking in a hammock. In the American version of this ancient device, the balls are attached by a cord to an electronically operated vibrator.

Ordinary household items may also be drafted into use as masturbatory devices. "J.," the author of *The Sensuous Woman*, recommends female masturbation by holding the genitals against a washing machine while it is operating. However, most masturbatory aids are variations on artificial genitals. It is interesting to note that masturbation is still condemned by some religious leaders as a grave moral disorder. This attitude may be seen as a throwback to earlier times, when all sexual activity except marital procreative sex was condemned.

Female Masturbation   The most common technique for female masturbation is stimulation of the clitoral shaft, clitoral area, or mons veneris with the hand. Some women rub up and down along one side of the shaft, while others use a circular motion around the shaft and glans. Others rub from the shaft down across the glans and the urinary opening to the vaginal opening and minor lips and then back up to the shaft again. A few tug on the minor lips, which causes the loose skin covering the glans of the clitoris to slide back and forth. Occasionally women will not use direct or indirect clitoral stimulation but will move their fingers in and out of the vagina, stimulating the vaginal opening or jostling the uterus.

Male Masturbation   Men show less versatility than women in their masturbatory techniques. Most grip the penis, using an up and down movement to stimulate the glans and shaft. The degree of pressure, the speed of movement, and the extent of contact with the glans vary greatly with individual preference. Most men increase the speed of movements as they approach orgasm. At orgasm most slow their movements or stop altogether, because further stimulation is uncomfortable or painful. Other methods of male masturbation involve lightly touching or tugging at the skin around the frenulum or lightly flicking the penis with fingers or other objects. A few men use vibrators, which they rub along the shaft and glans or on the testicles or insert into the anus.

Sexual Fantasies and Masturbation   Many people fantasize during masturbation and intercourse. Although sexual fantasies are highly individualized, their content is often influenced by social taboos and myths. Some sexual fantasies are likely to involve a relatively impersonal encounter where one partner is powerful and aggressive in getting sex. For example:

My fantasy is that I spank this really beautiful woman on the butt—hard but not too hard, you know. And then I make violent love to her from behind, holding her down under me so she can't move. Sometimes I think about this story I read once about a man who was really strong and could lift and move a woman about, bringing parts of her body up to his mouth to kiss or bite.

In contrast, some fantasies either are highly romantic or involve a sexual situation in which a partner is forced to submit. For example:

My fantasy is usually the same. I am watching a woman being made love to forcibly by two men. One is licking her vagina and the other is penetrating her anus. When she has orgasm, the man inside her does too, and it's a combination of pleasure and pain.

The context of such sexual fantasies is apparently highly influenced by the cultural norms of acceptable behavior. Many couples use fantasies to relieve the monotony of a long-term sexual relationship. Clients need to be assured that a rich variety of sexual fantasy is normal and a readily available source of sexual stimulation.

Arousal Techniques

Sex play can focus on stimulating the erogenous zones, using the same techniques of arousal that are used in effective masturbation. Or it can focus on sensual arousal through mood-setting techniques. *Erogenous zones* are parts of the body that produce sexual arousal when stroked. The more typical erogenous zones are the genitals, breasts, lips, and thighs, but any area of the body may be an erogenous zone for a given individual.

Kissing   The lips and tongue are very commonly used in sex play. Kissing may simply consist of gently touching one's lips to the lips of another. With the use of teeth and tongue as well, kissing may assume many other forms. Sex partners may alternate tiny caresses with the tongue around the lips with deep thrusts of the tongue in and out of each other's mouths. Gentle and sometimes not so gentle biting of the partner's lips and tongue represent another variation. Kissing need not be confined to the partner's mouth. It may be used on any part of the body for erotic stimulation—eyelids, earlobes, breasts, genitals, navel, toes, and buttocks.

Breast Stimulation   Many men and women find that breast stimulation is one of the more arousing forms of sex play, and a few can reach orgasm by breast stimulation alone. Breast sensitivity varies from person to person. It is not related to the size of the breasts. Breasts may be stimulated with the hands or mouth. They may be massaged or kneaded, or the nipple may be sucked, flicked with the tongue, gently nibbled with the teeth, or pinched or tugged with the fingers. A man may stimulate a woman's breast by rubbing his penis or testicles over it.

Hand Stimulation of Female and Male Genitals   Many methods of stimulating the genitals can produce sexual arousal. Hand stimulation can be used to prepare for intercourse or to induce orgasm. The most effective method for manually stimulating a woman's genitals is with the flat of the hand on the vulva. The middle finger is inserted between the lips, and its tip moves in and out of the vagina while the ball of the palm presses hard just above the pubis. Gentle tugging on the penis or massaging the penis and testicles may

produce an erection in the male. Rolling the penis between the palms of both hands or applying pressure at the midpoint between the penis and the anus can also induce an erection. When the penis is erect, hand stimulation usually involves rubbing the shaft. The thumb and forefinger encircle the shaft just below the corona and the hand is moved up and down. Many men find direct rubbing of the unlubricated glans uncomfortable. The amount of pressure, speed of the movement, and timing can be varied by an empathic partner.

Oral Sex   Oral genital stimulation is called *cunnilingus* when performed on the woman and *fellatio* when performed on the male. It is highly stimulating and sexually exciting. In cunnilingus the focus is most often on the clitoral area, interspersed with a general exploration of the entire genital area with tongue and lips. Some women prefer having the tongue thrust in and out of the vaginal opening or having the minor lips sucked and licked. A woman may like slow or rapid motions, side-to-side, up-and-down, or circular. Some enjoy some other object, such as a finger, stimulating their anus during cunnilingus. For fellatio the techniques are varied. The most common is sucking on the glans of the penis and licking the glans and frenulum. Some variations including gentle nibbling along the shaft of the penis, sucking on the testicles, or placing the entire shaft or testicles or both in the mouth. Sucking motions can alternate with blowing ones, and the tongue can be flicked over the penis while it is being sucked.

Many men and women intensely enjoy oral sex. Some women find it the preferred method of reaching an orgasm. This preference should not be confused with immaturity or abnormality in the woman or homosexuality in the man. Both cunnilingus and fellatio are common forms of sex play in American culture despite some moral and legal sanctions against them.

Coitus

Coitus means coming together. Generally it refers to the penetration of the vagina by the penis. Many of the difficulties clients bring to a nurse–counselor may be alleviated by teaching them about variations in physical positions. Needless to say, no position is more "normal" than any other. Different positions are practiced more commonly in different societies. What follows is a brief discussion of positions commonly practiced by people in contemporary American society. Each couple can experiment to discover which position they prefer. Such choices are a highly individual matter.

Face-to-Face, Man Above   This is the most commonly accepted position in the United States. Like other face-to-face positions it allows the couple to kiss or engage in other stimulation. Its disadvantage is that the woman may be unable to move freely if the man rests much of his weight on her body. This position can be varied in several ways. The woman may place her legs together between the man's, allowing less vaginal penetration, or she may draw her knees up to facilitate deeper penetration. The man can prop himself up to keep his weight off her body and help her move more freely. He may also sit back on his heels and lift her buttocks onto his thighs, which makes manual clitoral stimulation possible.

Face-to-Face, Woman Above   In any variation of this position the woman has more freedom of movement than the man, and this position is more tiring for her. However, in this position most men have more ejaculatory control than in some of the other positions where the man must take a more active role.

Face-to-Face, Side-by-Side   This is probably the least tiring position for both partners. It permits them to move and touch each other freely and can be varied by the relative positions of their legs.

Rear Entry Position   The man can face the woman's back and enter her vagina from behind. This can be done with the woman resting on her knees and elbows while the man kneels behind her and holds her waist. Other variants are standing or sitting on the man's lap. Most of the rear entry positions, except the one in which the woman lies flat on her stomach, allow deep penetration. They also provide an opportunity for manual clitoral stimulation.

Other Positions   Most of the positions described above assume that the couple is making love in bed. However, some couples like to make love standing or sitting in a chair. These positions may be exciting and enliven a sexual relationship, but some people find them too strenuous.

Anal Intercourse

Anal intercourse means placing the penis in the anus of another person. It occurs occasionally among younger heterosexual couples and often in sexual relations between two men. Some men find anal intercourse more exciting than vaginal intercourse, both because it has a forbidden aspect and because the anal opening is smaller and tighter. Since the anus is not naturally lubricated as the stimulated vagina is, a lubricant such as surgical jelly is usually used to avoid pain. Bacteria found in the anus may be infectious to the vagina, so it is important to wash the penis after anal intercourse.

PSYCHOLOGICAL SEXUALITY

Freud's ideas on the stages of psychosexual identity tend to dominate the literature on psychosexuality. These ideas are presented in Chapter 2. The present section describes a few key concepts that are relevant to psychological and sociological sexuality.

Gender Identity

Gender identity is that psychological state in which a person comes to believe "I am female" or "I am male." It is the first stage in gender development. In contemporary society, the biological "male" or "female" are not necessarily seen as coterminous with the social psychological categories "masculine" and "feminine."

The term *gender role* refers to learning and performing the socially accepted characteristics and behaviors for a given sex. However, contemporary psychological theory tends not to link specific psychological characteristics—such as active or passive—with either sex. Rather, it holds that psychological characteristics are distributed according to culture and temperament.

A distinction is generally made between gender identity and *sexual object choice*. A homosexual male may have a male gender identity yet choose other men as sexual objects. A male with a female gender identity is termed a transsexual, not a homosexual.

Although core gender identity is fixed in early childhood, social interaction throughout the life span modifies and expands it. Gender identity in a mature person may be elaborated in statements such as "I am a somewhat masculine female." The recent prominence of people such as Dr. Renee Richards and author Jan Morris has brought to the public attention situations in which an individual is born with one biological gender yet develops a gender identity of the opposite sex.

Theories of Gender Development

Biological Imperative How do gender identity and gender roles develop? One contemporary theory rests on the notion that for the most part anatomy is destiny, and that because men and women are biologically different, they have innate characteristics and styles of interacting. According to this position, the fetus has a biological mechanism that directs it to become male or female.

Cognitive Switch Another theory argues that children are born more or less neutral, but that one of the central developmental tasks of childhood is to label oneself male or female. According to this theory a *cognitive switch* occurs at age three or four. After this point the process of acquiring gender identity is irreversible.

Social Learning and Labeling The third theory is the one subscribed to in this text. This theory focuses on social learning. It holds that gender identity and roles are continuously constructed and maintained throughout the life span. The stability of one's gender identity depends on biological differences. But it also depends on the fact that *everyday situations continuously provide expectations, demands, and feedback for one or another conception of oneself.* Figure 12–5 is a developmental conceptualization of the complex set of factors that influence the development of gender identities, gender roles, and sexual conduct.

SOCIOLOGICAL SEXUALITY

A society's economic system, changes in its religious values, the world of politics, and social class distinctions all may seem unrelated to human sexuality. However, it has been argued that one of the keys to understanding sexual interaction in the United States today lies in understanding the transition from an agrarian to an industrial society. In an agrarian society, children are an economic asset. However, in an industrial economy, children tend to consume more than they produce. The lessening of the economic need for children at the onset of the Industrial Revolution released sexuality from its solely procreative function. At the same time, however, it downgraded women's roles in society without allowing for any role changes. Women still had to be wives and mothers, but those functions ceased to be considered very valuable to society as a whole.

Sex Roles

A challenge to the male sexual domination of females and the traditional structure of both male and female sex roles has arisen in recent years especially in relation to the feminist social movement. The issues identified as relevant vary with the ideological nature of various groups. The more conservative organizations, such as NOW, are concerned with matters of discrimination and equality. They seek passage of the Equal Rights Amendment, for example, and enforcement of civil rights in cases of sex discrimination. The more radical organizations are attempting to restructure the female sex role. They see this role as one of dependence on men—a dependence maintained by the woman's childbearing and child-rearing responsibilities. They seek to restructure society dramatically by advocating test tube babies, voluntary sterilization, and homosexuality.

Sex and Social Problems

In American culture most sexual norms reflect a central concept of *consent*. Even when individuals are violating laws, such as the laws against prostitution, the social sanctions focus on the issue of consent. The following categories of sexual behavior violate the concept of consent in our society.

- Sex acts with partners who are legally unable to consent
- Sex acts accompanied by force or violence
- Invasion of other people's privacy without their knowledge
- Public nudity or display of genitals

Sex Acts with Partners Unable to Consent All sexual relations between adults and children are viewed as criminal in the United States. These acts are legally considered to be sex without consent because presumably minors do not have sufficient knowledge of the consequences of their acts to consent meaningfully. The medical or diagnostic term for an adult who gains sexual satisfaction from engaging in sexual activities with immature children is *pedophile*. When force is used on the child, the act is called *rape*. When no force is used, it is called *child molesting*. In many states the penalty for the offending adult is life imprisonment, and in a few it is death.

Some sex offenses against children involve only touching and fondling. Most child molesters are men unable or unwilling to seek gratification with other

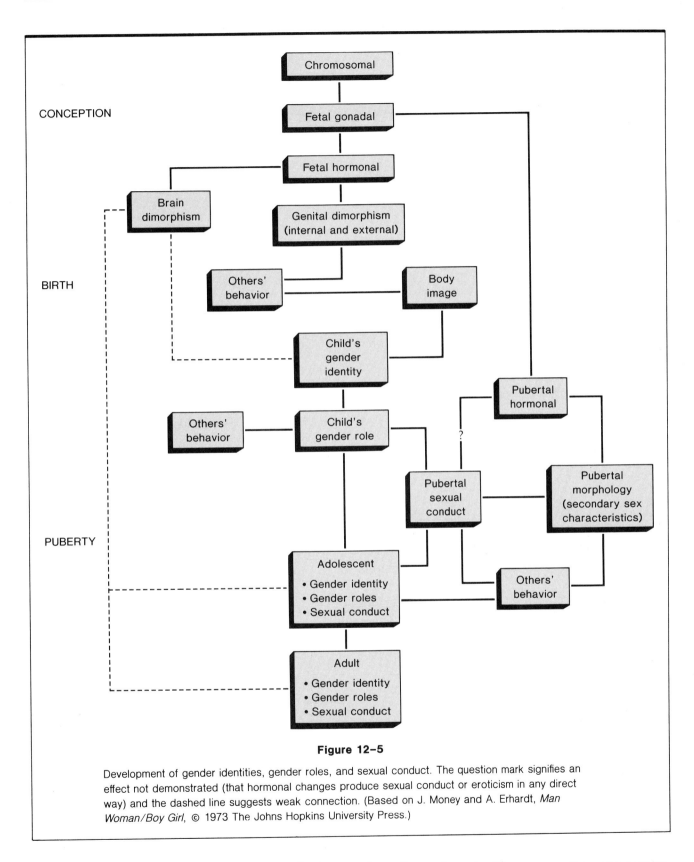

Figure 12–5

Development of gender identities, gender roles, and sexual conduct. The question mark signifies an effect not demonstrated (that hormonal changes produce sexual conduct or eroticism in any direct way) and the dashed line suggests weak connection. (Based on J. Money and A. Erhardt, *Man Woman/Boy Girl*, © 1973 The Johns Hopkins University Press.)

adults. Often the nurse may be asked to counsel a family about the effects of the actual molesting or of the reporting process on the child involved. The parents must decide whether they wish to expose their child to the police and courts. These reservations are counterbalanced by the fact that many pedophiles have a long history of child molesting for which they have never been arrested or convicted.

Sex relations with animals, called *bestiality* or *zoophilia,* and sex with a corpse, called *necrophilia,* also occur without the consent of the object, of course. As many as 17 percent of male adolescents brought up on farms have had sexual contact to orgasm with animals. A few large cities have prostitutes who cater to these preferences.

INCEST   Incest is defined as the occurrence of sexual relations between blood relatives. A broader definition includes sex between two persons related to one another by some form of kinship tie. Social taboos against incest have roots in psychological as well as sociological factors. While accurate figures of the incidence of incest are difficult to obtain because of the shame associated with it, most authorities believe that contemporary social, cultural, physiological, and psychological variables have all contributed to a breakdown in the incest taboo. For example, incestuous behavior has been associated with alcoholism, overcrowding, and rural isolation. Major mental illnesses and intellectual deficiencies are also associated with cases of incest. Father-daughter incest is reported to be more common than mother-son or sibling incest. Incest is usually considered as a form of child abuse or in extreme cases, rape.

Counseling focuses first on the disclosure of incestuous behavior and then on family therapy designed to develop internal restraints and more acceptable means of gratifying needs (see Chapter 21). Of particular long-term significance is counseling of the victim who has kept the matter secret because of fears of punishment, repercussions, abandonment, or rejection. Often disclosure causes a crisis for the entire family and must be dealt with as such (see Chapter 11). The sexual victimization of children is a growing social concern. Nurses are often in crucial positions to identify and assist children who are the targets of such abuse (see Chapter 19).

Sex Acts Accompanied by Force or Violence

Violent sex constitutes a continuum that runs from *sadomasochism* to forcible *rape. Sexual sadism* is obtaining sexual pleasure from pain inflicted on another person. *Sexual masochism* is obtaining sexual pleasure from having pain inflicted on oneself. The two terms are often linked because it is believed that people who are stimulated by one activity will be stimulated by the other. The word "sadism" is derived from the name of the Marquis de Sade, who wrote extensively of his cruel erotic fantasies and exploits. The term "masochism"

is derived from the name of an Austrian novelist, Leopold von Sacher-Masoch, whose greatest sexual pleasure came from being mistreated by the women in his life.

While some sadomasochism involves violence with a real lack of consent, at least 3 percent of the women and 10 percent of the men Kinsey and his associates studied reported that they experienced definite and frequent erotic responses to sadomasochistic stories (Kinsey 1953, pp. 676–678). In actual practice, most deliberate infliction of pain occurs in foreplay by biting, spanking, scratching, and pinching. Actual bondage and discipline—being tied and whipped—is relatively rare. However, some couples use sado-masochistic games as part of their lovemaking. These games involve devices such as leather clothing, whips, and chains.

RAPE   The legal definition of rape varies from state to state. According to most definitions, however, rape is sexual intercourse without the consent of the other person. *Statutory rape* is the seduction of a minor. It is distinguished legally from *forcible rape,* in which the victim is over eighteen. Rape is usually committed by men against women, although reports of rape committed against men by women as well as other men are increasing.

Rape has increased over the last decade, but the actual extent of the increase is unknown, since many cases of rape go unreported. It is said that over thirty years a Los Angeles woman has one chance in ten of being raped. Rapes go unreported for many reasons. One reason is that there are ambiguities in the legal and social definitions of forcible rape. Some women fear that the courts will say they did not resist hard enough and therefore were not legally raped. Another reason is that many women fear the publicity and the stigma associated with being a rape victim. They therefore may decide not to report the experience. Some women do not want to be subjected to a rigorous and sometimes brutal cross-examination by the personnel in the police or district attorney's office, most of whom are men.

Because these fears are so common, many nurses have become involved in rape victim counseling. Nurses realize that the fear of such consequences is difficult to face alone. Rape counseling offers rape victims a sympathetic hearing and advice on how to proceed with legal action. Of particular value are the following:

- Explaining procedures and services to the victim
- Negotiating the victim's request
- Accurately recording data

Rape prevention counseling generally emphasizes three strategies.

1. Women should avoid isolated areas. Women who are alone should also avoid being helpful to strangers.
2. A woman who is attacked should resist from the very beginning. Screaming, running away, or fighting back may induce a would-be rapist to look for a more cooperative and easily intimidated victim.
3. If the assailant has a knife or gun, however, the woman who resists risks being injured or killed. In such cases it is sometimes wiser to submit.

The physical consequences of rape include injury, pregnancy, and venereal disease. The emotional consequences include the trauma associated not only with the experience itself but also with the humiliation of the legal procedures. Nursing interventions can offer rape victims information and psychological support.

Voyeurism   A *voyeur* or Peeping Tom is someone who obtains sexual gratification from looking at other people's bodies, sex organs, or sex acts without their knowledge or consent. Unlike people who merely enjoy looking at naked bodies, voyeurs obtain all their sexual satisfaction from the act of peeping and the masturbation that usually accompanies it. Peeping usually fulfills a sense of sexual adventure and participation, a heightened sense of power. Voyeurs are rarely dangerous, though a few are peeper-burglars or peeper-rapists. Nevertheless, people are frightened to find themselves the object of a peeper's attention, and rightly resent the invasion of their privacy.

Exhibitionism   An *exhibitionist* is a person who exposes his or her sexual organs to the opposite sex in situations where the exposure is socially defined as inappropriate, for the exhibitionist's own sexual arousal and gratification. In nearly all instances, exhibitionists expose themselves to strangers. Exposure is commonly an expression of anger and hostility resorted to primarily by men. It represents the desire to shock women. This desire often occurs among men who are suffering from transitory stress or sexual deprivation. The shock that the woman shows is what excites the exhibition-

ist. Exhibitionists are generally quiet, submissive people who do not want to hurt anyone.

Prostitution   *Prostitution* is the sale of sexual services, most commonly by women to men although male prostitution is not uncommon. People go to prostitutes for a variety of reasons. They may want sex without negotiation or sex without responsibility. They may be seeking eroticism and variety. They may even be looking for company. A few people go to prostitutes because they have physical or mental handicaps that prevent them from seeking out conventional partners.

Prostitution is both fostered and suppressed by contemporary societies. It is illegal in most jurisdictions, even those where it flourishes most openly. Since there is a great deal of money to be made from a prostitute's earnings, however, there is little pressure for prostitution to be decriminalized.

The prostitution of women represents a difficult issue for the women's movement. It cannot approve of prostitution, since prostitution is a commercial use of a woman's body most of the profits of which go to men. In addition, the fact that prostitution exists is an indictment of the economic status of minority and poor women, a status that recruits them into criminal lifestyles. Yet to argue for the continuation of laws against prostitution limits the control women have over their own bodies.

One source of original thinking on the issue of prostitution has been *COYOTE*, the new prostitute's union organized in California. This union is dedicated to self-help, consciousness raising, political change, and social protection. The strength of a prostitute's union is in its moral appeal as the representative of an exploited underclass. Its future will depend on its ability to find allies in the women's movement, law reform groups, and other sectors of society committed to opposing the oppression of minorities.

Pornography   *Pornography* is the other area where sex and money meet. Pornography is the sale of sexual depictions or live sexual displays. The struggle between those who defend the current statutes on pornography and those who oppose them has mostly been fought out in the courts. The legal struggle over control of erotic materials has centered on the question of what impact these materials have on society or on a particular industry. The conservative position has been that nearly any noncondemnatory public discussion of sexuality is likely to lead to sexual activity.

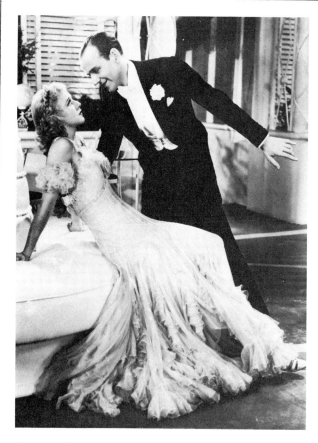 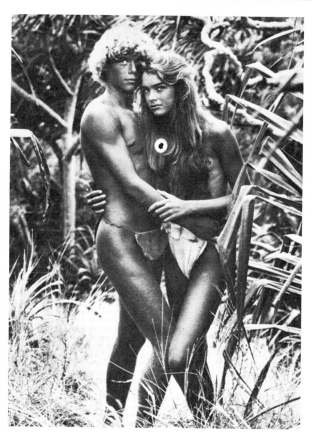

The romantic image of heterosexuality suggested by Fred Astaire and Ginger Rogers in 1934 (left) contrasts with the natural and more explicit media sex image of Brooke Shields and Christopher Atkins in 1979 (right).

Those who take this position believe that people have powerful and dangerous sex urges, which automatically express themselves when they are presented with erotic stimuli. They believe that obscenity can immediately and irretrievably corrupt the viewer. In fact, there is no evidence to support this belief. Most people use pornography simply as a sexual ritual that relieves the tedium of normal social life.

American social norms prescribe that sexual interaction should take place in private. People who do not wish to observe it should not be obliged to do so. In fact, however, a certain amount of sexual contact does occur in public places. People kiss and touch in parks, in movie theaters, and on beaches. It is difficult to specify exactly what distinguishes a romantic encounter from a sexual one. Although the topic of public sex is an interesting one for psychosocial analysis, little research has been done in this area. An exception is Humphreys's *Tearoom Trade: Impersonal Sex in Public Places* (1975). This book describes the sexual interaction between homosexual males in public restrooms.

ALTERNATIVE SEXUAL PATTERNS

In the United States the ideal norms for sexual behavior specify partners of the opposite sex. Homosexuals, bisexuals, and transsexuals violate this norm, since they engage in sexual relations with people of the same sex. *Homosexual* behavior means engaging in sexual relations specifically with others of the same sex. *Bisexual* behavior means engaging in sexual relations with people of both sexes. *Transsexuals* can be distinguished from homosexuals and bisexuals by their unique gender identity. Transsexuals consider themselves to be people who have the bodies of the wrong sex. Transsexualism may also represent a deviation from the heterosexual norm, since some transsexuals have sexual relations with partners of the same biological sex.

Until fairly recently most people in the United States assumed that there were only three sexual categories—homosexuality, heterosexuality, and bisexuality—and that everyone fell into one or another of the three. The typical stereotyped assumption was that only heterosexuals were normal. Homosexuals and bisexuals were perverted objects of pity or scorn, in need of psychiatric attention and perhaps of institutionalization. Modern sex research has demolished this assumption. Kinsey and other sex researchers use a seven-point scale to rate people on a continuum. One extreme on this scale represents exclusive heterosexuality and the other exclusive homosexuality. According to the continuum idea, however, homosexuals are defined as people who engage only in physical homosexual acts. It is probably more accurate to recognize that there is not just one kind of homosexuality. There are many different ways to organize a homosexual preference into a commitment and an ongoing lifestyle.

Homosexuality

As Sickness   In recent decades the religious conception of homosexuality as "evil" has been partially replaced by the medical conception of it as "sick." Until the 1970s homosexuality was on the American Psychiatric Association's diagnostic list of categories of mental illness. It was revised and limited to Ego-dystonic Homosexuality only after a great deal of conflict among psychiatric professionals. Though Ego-syntonic Homosexuality is no longer officially an illness, psychiatrists still tend to search for a cause and cure. The medical view of homosexuality is based on the implicit assumption that people are born with a tendency to be heterosexual. It is probably more accurate to say that human sexual behavior varies widely and that it depends more on learning and social experiences than on inborn tendencies. For this reason, the causes of homosexuality are best sought in a general theory that explains how all sexual preferences are acquired.

Male Homosexuality   Some men who have experienced homosexual fantasies label themselves as "gay." Others who have experienced these fantasies do not. The sexual options open to active homosexual males are fellatio, anal intercourse, oral-anal contact, hand stimulation, friction or rubbing the penis against the partner's body, the use of vibrators and dildos for anal stimulation, and insertion of the fingers into the anus.

In order for a homosexual to join the gay community, he must "come out." The gay subculture can be extremely important to a homosexual, because it provides places to meet lovers—such as gay bars. However, the public gay culture is often limited in its emotional diversity. Homosexuals who have not "come out" are referred to as "closet queens."

Many people believe that a male homosexual may be easily recognized because he is effeminate. Some homosexuals do indulge in extravagant mannerisms or appear in "drag" (women's clothes). However, many homosexuals are indistinguishable from other men. In sum, homosexuality is as varied as heterosexuality in its cultural, social, and sexual aspects.

Lesbianism   Like male homosexuality, lesbianism can be defined as a form of sexual behavior, an emotional preference, a part of one's identity, or a social role. As a form of sexual behavior, lesbianism can include masturbation, cunnilingus, rubbing the genitals against the partner's body, and use of vibrators and dildos on the internal or external genitals. Very little is known about the psychological and social characteristics of lesbians. Many lesbians are married women with children and are secretive about their lesbian affairs.

Lesbians may play mutual lovemaking and social roles with each other. A *butch* plays the masculine role, and a *femme* plays the feminine role. In some instances—in prison, for example—partners play either a butch or a femme role exclusively. In other lesbian relationships neither partner plays a specifically masculine or feminine role. The sexual and social roles can vary with the lesbian setting.

Many lesbians do not belong to any lesbian community or group. However, several types of lesbian communities are emerging. These include the lesbian bar community, the overt lesbian feminist activist community, lesbian affiliations with the gay male community, and lesbian familial organizations in single households and communes.

Bisexuality

In contemporary society more and more people are claiming a bisexual identity. It is possible that this trend is influenced by the mass media and by such public role models as bisexuals Joan Baez, David Bowie, Lily Tomlin, Kate Millett, and Billie Jean King. The most notable aspect of bisexuality is its increasing institutionalization as an alternative life-style and identity.

Transsexualism and Transvestism

Transsexuals are members of a sexual minority who find themselves profoundly uncomfortable with their gender. Their sense of gender, the psychosocial com-

Table 12-4 UROLOGICAL TIMETABLE FOR TRANSSEXUAL MANAGEMENT	
Male to Female	**Female to Male**
Live as a female for up to 5 years	Live as male for up to 5 years
Female hormone Rx 1 + years (testicular atrophy; adequate breast enlargement in minority)	Male hormone Rx 2 + years (testosterone enlarges clitoris, beard, etc.)
Breast augmentation surgery at least 6 months prior to vaginoplasty	Lower abdominal penile tube graft
Vaginoplasty	Stage I. Insert prosthesis
(Preliminary orchiectomy if adequate atrophy)	Six months later release upper end tube graft and glans penis phalloplasty
Penectomy, partial perineal dissection and perineotomy	Stage II. Combined with
Skin grafts and penoscrotal inversion and clitoroidallabial construction	Mastectomies Salpingo-oophorectomies Hysterectomy
Follow-up:	Stage III. Insert inflatable F. Brantley Scott type of prosthesis
IVP's	Follow-up:
Vaginograms	Urethral calibration
Hormone therapy	Hormone therapy
Prostatic-vaginal exams	Psychological and behavioral rehabilitation
Psychosocial and behavioral rehabilitation	

This chart first appeared in the *Humanist*, March/April 1978 and is reprinted by permission.

Table 12-5 SEXUAL VARIANTS	
Variant	**Definition**
Coprophilia	Sexual pleasure with the desire to defecate on a partner or be defecated on.
Coprophagia	Sexual pleasure associated with eating feces.
Urolangia	Sexual pleasure associated with the desire to urinate on a partner or be urinated on.
Coprolalia	Obtaining sexual pleasure from using obscene language.

logical, endocrinological, and preoperative management as well as for psychological and psychiatric screening. The complex and involved process is presented in Table 12–4.

Transvestites are men who dress in women's clothes. In most instances the cross-dressing is *fetishist*—that is, it is associated with erotic arousal. Specific articles of clothing most conventionally converted into fetishes include bras, women's panties, negligees, garters, stockings, shoes, and gloves.

Other Alternative Sexual Patterns

Libertarian groups and the media have begun to call people who engage in certain forms of sexual conduct "sexual minorities." This shift in rhetoric has both political and scientific consequences. To describe people as members of a minority group or as engaging in an alternative sexual style rather than as pathological and perverted is to record a major change in cultural emphasis. Table 12–5 presents additional sexual patterns found more rarely than those discussed in detail above.

ponent of masculinity or femininity, does not match their anatomy. Most transsexuals do not identify with the homosexual community, because transsexuals consider themselves to be heterosexual. Transsexuals also resent being labeled as transvestites, because unlike the transvestite, they see cross-dressing as appropriate to their true sex, while for the transvestite it is a fetish.

Many transsexuals fervently wish to change their physical sex. In recent years an increasing number of people have sought surgical sex change operations. The schedule for such procedures must allow for socio-

SEXUAL PROBLEMS AND THEIR TREATMENT

Sex therapy per se is a relative newcomer to the nurse's intervention repertoire. It is distinguished from other therapies by the fact that it focuses on sexual activity itself, rather than relying on insight and personality change. Sex therapy programs are springing up around the United States. Many are patterned after

Table 12–6   INTERVENTIONS FOR SEXUAL DIFFICULTIES

Sexual Difficulty	Guidelines for Therapeutic Intervention	Sexual Difficulty	Guidelines for Therapeutic Intervention
Premature ejaculation The man tends to ejaculate before the woman has an orgasm	Reestablish a climate of comfort and acceptance for sexual interaction Encourage client to masturbate and enjoy touch and body stimulation in general The man or woman is instructed to stimulate the erect penis until the premonitory sensations of impending orgasm are felt. Then penile stimulation is abruptly stopped. This process is repeated in order to train the threshhold of excitability to be more tolerant of the stimuli. Sometimes the woman uses the squeeze technique, in which at the point of orgasm she squeezes the head of the penis with thumb and first two fingers for 3 to 4 seconds. This stops the urge to ejaculate The couple is also instructed in ways to reduce the tactile component of friction in the vagina by limiting the frequency of thrusts or the extent of movement within the vagina	**Primary orgasmic dysfunction** The woman has never had an orgasm by any method Situational orgasmic dysfunction The woman is able to have orgasms under certain conditions and at certain times but not others. For example, she may be able to masturbate to orgasm but not achieve orgasm during intercourse	The couple is advised to assume a nondemand position for female stimulation The woman is to place her hand lightly on her partner's to indicate her preference for contact The emphasis is not on achieving orgasm but on learning erotic preferences The couple is instructed to use the lateral side-by-side position, which enables both partners to move freely with emphasis on slow, exploratory thrusting The goal is to develop an ability to enjoy pelvic play with the penis inside the vagina
Primary impotence The man has never been able to maintain an erection sufficient to accomplish sexual intercourse	Intercourse is avoided, and nongenital caressing exercises begin with man and woman alternating as the initiator of a session of caressing, thus sharing responsibility for sexual interaction	**Functional vaginismus** An involuntary tightening or spasm occurs in the outer third of the vagina that can be so severe as to make intercourse impossible	The initial step is physical demonstration of her involuntary vaginal spasm to the woman by inserting an examining finger into her vagina Then Hegar dilators in graduated sizes are inserted by the man into the woman's vagina. At first she manually controls his insertion of the smallest dilator. Later he can insert larger dilators following her verbal instructions
Secondary impotence The man currently cannot maintain or get an erection but has had a history of success. Occasional impotence that most men experience is not considered secondary impotence	Next genital stimulation is added to provide the couple with positive sexual experiences without intercourse When intercourse is attempted, the woman is instructed to assume the superior position and insert the man's penis into her vagina When setbacks occur, the couple is advised to rely on sexual techniques that do not involve intercourse		After larger dilators are successfully inserted, she is instructed to retain the dilator for several hours each night. Most involuntary spasms can be relieved in three to five days with the daily use of dilators In addition to physical relief from spastic constriction, therapy is directed toward alleviating the fear that led to the onset of symptoms

Source: Compiled from W. Masters and V. Johnson, *Human Sexual Inadequacy* (Boston: Little, Brown and Co., 1970), pp. 30–56.

the therapy offered by William Masters and Virginia Johnson at the Reproductive Biology Research Foundation in St. Louis. Most of these programs accept only married couples for treatment, and the concept of a marital problem is basic to the therapy. Both partners are involved in a relationship in which there is sexual distress, and both must participate in the therapy program. Treatment is short term and behaviorally oriented. Since most forms of sexual inadequacy involve ignorance and performance anxiety, the couples are specifically prohibited from any sexual play other than that prescribed by the therapists. Beginning exercises focus on heightened sensory awareness. Couples learn how to communicate nonverbally in a mutually satisfying way. At the same time they learn that sexual foreplay is as important as intercourse and orgasm. Genital stimulation is eventually added to general body stimulation. The couples are then instructed to try various positions for intercourse, one at a time, without necessarily completing the union. The overall approach is intended to diminish fears of performance and to facilitate communication. The Masters and Johnson techniques described below have contributed numerous strategies to the repertoire of sexual counselors. However, many therapists find them too mechanical and feel that they overemphasize physical interventions.

Impairments in Physiological Functioning

Impairments in physiological sexual functioning might well have been discussed in Chapter 17 under the heading of psychophysiological disorders, since these problems usually have psychological and social components. Although generalists in psychiatric nursing may not be engaged in specialized sexual counseling, they may encounter the problems listed in Table 12–6 among clients who are having difficulty coping with their lives.

Sexual Problems Associated with Other Coping Problems

Many arguments have been advanced about the relationship between sex and other coping problems. It appears most accurate to assume that sexual function or dysfunction is simply one facet of behavior. It may or may not be affected by the presence of physical illness or other coping problems. In general most sexual problems associated with illnesses can be classified in four general groups:

Table 12–7	SEX AND MEDICAL–SURGICAL PROBLEMS
Medical–Surgical Procedure/Condition	**Associated Sexual Difficulties**
Sterilization without hormonal therapy	Loss of potency and low sperm counts
Prostatectomy	Retrograde ejaculation and loss of urethral phase of orgasm
Perineal prostatectomy	Impotency and loss of urinary control
Ostomies	Disorders of potency
Bilateral oophorectomy	Loss of libido

1. Disinterest in or lack of desire for sexual activity
2. Physical incapacity for or discomfort during sexual activity
3. Fear of precipitating or aggravating a physical illness through sexual activity
4. Use of illness as an excuse to avoid feared or undesired sexual activity

Tables 12–7 and 12–8 summarize information about these and other sexual and coping problems. Sexuality and aging is discussed in detail in Chapter 22.

Therapeutic Counseling

The commonest questions asked of a nurse engaged in psychological sex counseling are the following:

- Do you think it is normal to wait until marriage?
- Is it normal to want to have sexual relations with one person when you're already having them with another person?
- Is abortion wrong?
- How do I know I'm in love?
- Should we break up our marriage when we're no longer in love?
- How young is too young?

Guidelines for counseling are based on the following questions:

- Does the behavior in question enhance the self-esteem of those involved?

Table 12–8	SEX AND OTHER COPING PROBLEMS		
Condition	**Commonly Occurring Sex-related Problem**	**Condition**	**Commonly Occurring Sex-related Problem**
Mental retardation	Limitation to sexual behaviors such as individual and mutual masturbation Risk of being sexually exploited by others	Aging	Menopausal women may experience lack of vaginal lubrication, less frequent and less intense orgasm, and less sexual desire Men may not wish to ejaculate as often, may experience difficulty maintaining erections, and may find that their erections are less firm
Organic brain syndromes	Occasional bizarre hypersexuality Loss of social control with retreat toward more primitive sex behaviors at inappropriate times or circumstances Decreased interest in sexual activity due to related depression	Taking medications	Antihypertensives, psychotropics, antidepressants, antispasmodics, sedatives, tranquilizers, and narcotics may all impair clients' ability to perform sexually
Affective disorders	Decreased libido and potency associated with depression Increased incidence of promiscuity during manic episodes Increased sexual preoccupation during manic episodes Sexual delusions	Use of alcohol	Alcoholism is associated with impotence and the man's ability to achieve an erection. Women may experience a decline in ability to experience an orgasm or to become aroused
Disintegrative coping patterns	Sex often associated with unusual patterns and variations	General stress from job or living situation	May experience performance anxiety about engaging in sexual activity that includes sweating, nausea, palpitations, and hyperventilation
Disturbed coping patterns	Sexual inhibitions		
Disruptive coping patterns	Sexual indifference with hysterical life-styles Sexual offenses associated with compulsions; promiscuity	Lack of affection	May result in sexual disinterest

- Is it entirely voluntary?
- Does it offer pleasure and gratification?
- Does it prevent unwanted pregnancy?
- Does it prevent the spreading of disease?

It is remarkable how health professionals neglect sexual assessment. Physicians rarely ask clients about their sexual health. They seldom discuss menstruation, the use of contraceptives, libido gratification, or emo-

tional well-being. The well-informed nurse can play a crucial role both in sex education and in helping clients integrate their sexuality with their total personhood. But talking about sex can be an extremely delicate business. Sometimes it is embarrassing for both client and nurse. Neither may have a vocabulary that is comfortable and facilitates communication for both. Table 12–9 summarizes a format for conducting an effective sexual assessment interview.

In order to confirm that the nurse has heard and

Table 12–9   SUGGESTED FORMAT FOR ASSESSMENT INTERVIEW

Interview Step	Rationale	Interview Step	Rationale
1. Open the discussion of sexual matters subtly with an open-ended question. "People with your illness or stresses often experience other difficulties, sometimes with sexual functioning."	This gentle opening lets the client know that other people have difficulties, too. It gives the client permission to talk with the nurse about sexual matters without labeling these matters as problems.	4. Ask about the severity and duration of the dysfunction. "Is it always difficult to control your ejaculation?" "Tell me when you first noticed this."	These questions are directed at identifying the specific problem.
2. Follow up with another open-ended question about the client's current status. "Has your illness or stresses made any difference in what it's like for you to be a wife or husband (lover, boy friend, girl friend, sexual partner)?"	The phrasing of this question enables the client to acknowledge a problem without admitting a shortcoming.	5. Ask about the effects on the client's sexual partner. "Has this affected your relationship with your partner?"	This question is directed toward exploring the interactional aspects of the identified problem.
3. If the client speaks of having a dysfunction, ask about its effect. "How does this affect you?" or "How do you feel about it?"	This indicates that the nurse is willing to explore sexual matters more completely.	6. Ask what the client has already done to alleviate the situation. "Have you made any adjustments in your sexual activity?"	This question yields data that will help the nurse to formulate an intervention plan.
		7. Ask the client if and how he or she would like the situation changed. "How would you like to change the situation to make it more satisfying?"	This question conveys the negotiated nature of the therapeutic relationship, in which the client's own goals play an important part.

Source: Adapted from M. P. Whitley and D. Willingham, "Adding a Sexual Assessment to the Health Interview," *Journal of Psychiatric Nursing and Mental Health Services,* Vol. 16, No. 4, April 1978, pp. 17–27.

understood the data, it is wise to summarize what the client has said. The nurse should pay particular attention to paraphrasing street language or slang expressions that the client may have used. This is a good way to make sure that the nurse understands what the client is talking about.

To assess a client's sexual status accurately and sensitively, the nurse must feel comfortable with the subject of sex. Nurses who have unresolved sexual conflicts often avoid dealing with issues of sexuality or let their own sexual problems interfere with the assessment. A self-review to gain insight into our own sexual attitudes might cover the following points:

• "What does my own sex mean to me?" "How does it feel to have the body I have?" "Would I prefer to be the opposite sex?" Such questions will help

nurses focus on and recognize their own personal values when clients discuss their concerns about gender identity.

• "Am I content with the style in which I live out my gender role?" "Can I accept expressions of gender roles that are different from my own?" Questions like these clarify the nurse's expectations and assumptions regarding "normal" gender role behavior.

• "Am I satisfied with the mode of sexual activity I have chosen?" Both celibates and sexually active people need to accept their own life-styles in order to relate comfortably to other alternatives.

• "How do I feel about sexual behavior that differs from mine?" The nurse's attitudes on this subject can cause problems, especially when a client's behavior provokes a negative reaction from the nurse.

KEY NURSING CONCEPTS

✔ Human sexuality is best understood through a holistic approach that takes into account physiological, psychological, and sociological perspectives.

✔ Sexual normality is a changing concept defined by society's norms, values, ideals, and ideology. The central concept of consent is reflected in sexual norms in American culture.

✔ In any society, people learn how to express their sexuality through their culture.

✔ Sexual pleasure is closely related to feelings as well as to social variables.

✔ Human sexuality is a critical component of self-actualization and self-expression.

✔ Sexual dysfunctions trouble many clients.

✔ Theoretical explanations of gender development include the ideas of biological imperative, cognitive switch, and social learning and labeling.

✔ The social learning and labeling theory is consistent with humanistic psychiatric nursing practice and holds that gender identity and roles are continuously contructed and maintained throughout the life span.

✔ In contemporary society, there is a growing trend toward accepting alternative sexual styles rather than necessarily labeling them as pathological and perverted.

✔ Nurses need up-to-date knowledge about human sexual functioning.

✔ The treatment of sexual problems is short term and behaviorally oriented. It is intended to diminish fears of performance and to facilitate communication.

✔ The well-informed nurse can play a crucial role both in sex education and in helping clients integrate their sexuality with their total personhood.

✔ Nurses need to be aware of their own personal attitudes toward sex in order to respond helpfully to clients.

References

Humphreys, L. *Tearoom Trade: Impersonal Sex in Public Places.* 2d ed. Chicago: Aldine Publishing, 1975.

De Lora, J. S., and Warren, C. A. B. *Understanding Sexual Interaction.* Boston: Houghton Mifflin, 1977.

Kaplan, H., and Sadoch, B. J. *Modern Synopsis of Comprehensive Textbook of Psychiatry.* III. Baltimore, Md.: Williams and Wilkins, 1981.

Kinsey, A.C., et al. *Sexual Behavior in the Human Female.* Philadelphia: W. B. Saunders, 1953.

Masters, W., and Johnson, V. *Human Sexual Response.* Boston: Little, Brown, 1966.

———. *Human Sexual Inadequacy.* Boston: Little, Brown, 1970.

Whitley, M. P., and Willingham, D. "Adding a Sexual Assessment to the Health Interview." *Journal of Psychiatric Nursing and Mental Health Services* (April 1978): 17–27.

Winer, J. H., and Bloomberg, S. D. "Transsexual Surgery." *The Humanist* (March–April 1978): 27–28.

Further Reading

Belliveau, F., and Richter, L. *Understanding Human Sexual Inadequacy.* New York: Bantam Books, 1970.

Berkman, A. H. "Sexuality: A Human Condition." *Journal of Rehabilitation* (January–February 1975): 13–15.

Brandt, R. S. T., and Tisza, V. "The Sexually Misused Child." *American Journal of Orthopsychiatry* 47 (1977): 80–90.

Browning D. H., and Boatman, B. "Incest: Children at Risk." *American Journal of Psychiatry* 134 (1977): 69–72.

Brownmiller, S. *Against Our Will: Men, Women and Rape.* Simon and Schuster, 1975.

Bullough, B. "Sex Counselors." *The Humanist* (March–April 1978): 32–34.

Burgess, A. W., and Holmstrom, L. L. "Crisis and Counseling Requests of Rape Victims." *Nursing Research* 23 (1974): 196–202.

Canfield, E. "Am I Normal?" *The Humanist* (March–April 1978): 10–12.

Christensen, E. W.; Norton, J. L.; Salisch, M.; and Gull, S. "An Effective Sexual Awareness Program for Counselors." *Counselor Education and Supervision* (March 1977): 153–157.

Coleman, T. F. "Sex and the Law." *The Humanist* (March–April 1978): 38–41.

Cuthbert, B. L. "Sex Knowledge of a Class of Student Nurses." *Nursing Research* 10 (1961): 145–150.

Dearth, P., and Cassell, C. "Comparing Attitudes of Male and Female University Students Before and After a Semester Course on Human Sexuality." *Journal of School Health* 46 (1976): 593–598.

Elder, M. S. "The Unmet Challenge . . . Nursing Counseling on Sexuality." *Nursing Outlook* 18 (1970): 38–40.

Elder, R. G. "Orientation of Senior Nursing Students toward Access to Contraceptives." *Nursing Research* 25 (1976): 338–345.

Gagnon, J. H. *Human Sexualities.* Glenview, Ill.: Scott, Foresman, 1977.

Glass, D., and Padrone, F. J. "Sexual Adjustment in the Handicapped." *Journal of Rehabilitation* (January–March 1978): 43–47.

Halstead, L. S.; Halstead, M. M.; Salhoot, J. T.; Spock, D. D.; and Sparks, R. W., Jr. "A Hospital-based Program in Human Sexuality." *Archives of Physical Medical Rehabilitation* 58 (1977): 409–412.

Hartman, W. E., and Lithian, M. A. "The Center for Marital and Sexual Studies." *The Humanist* (March–April 1978): 26.

Hoch, A. "Sex Therapy and Marital Counseling for the Disabled." *Archives of Physical Medical Rehabilitation* 58 (1977): 413–415.

Jacobson, L. "Illness and Human Sexuality." *Nursing Outlook* (January 1974): 50–53.

Johnson, W. "Sex Education and the Nurse." *Nursing Outlook* (November 1970): 26–29.

Lief, H., and Payne, T. "Sexuality Knowledge and Attitudes." *American Journal of Nursing* 75 (1975): 2026–2029.

Lobsenz, N. M. *Sex After Sixty-five.* New York: Public Affairs Committee, 1975.

Paradowski, W. "Socialization Patterns and Sexual Problems of the Institutionally Chronically Ill and Physically Disabled." *Archives of Physical Medical Rehabilitation* 58 (1977): 53–59.

Payne, T. "Sexuality of Nurses: Correlation of Knowledge, Attitudes and Behavior." *Nursing Research* 25 (1976): 286–293.

Pease, R. A. "Female Professional Students and Sexuality in the Aging Male." *Gerontologist* (April 1974): 153–157.

Silverman, D. "Sharing the Crisis of Rape: Counseling the Mates and Families of Victims." *American Journal of Orthopsychiatry* 48 (1978): 166–173.

Smith, R. W. "Research and Homosexuality." *The Humanist* (March–April 1978): 20–22.

Stoeler, R. J. *Sex and Gender: On the Development of Masculinity and Femininity.* New York: Science House, 1968.

Warren, C. A. B. *Identity and Community in the Gay World.* New York: John Wiley, 1974.

Weinstein, S. A., and Borok, K. "The Permissiveness of Nurses' Sexual Attitudes: Testing a Stereotype." *Journal of Sex Research* 14 (1978): 54–58.

Withersty, D. "Sexual Attitudes of Hospital Personnel: A Model for Continuing Education." *American Journal of Psychiatry* 133 (1976): 573–575.

13

Parenting

by Pamela Burton

CHAPTER OUTLINE

The Process of Parenting
    Parenting and Psychiatric Nursing Practice
    The Difficulties Inherent in the Parenting Role
    Bonding and Attachment: Beginning of the Interactive Process
    Mothering and Fathering
Different Structures of Parenting
    Single Parents
    Adoptive, Foster, and Stepparents
    Communal Parents
    Working Parents
Parents and Children under Stress
    Poverty and Racism
    Sexism
    Adolescent Parents
    Battering Parents

Counseling Parents
    Prenatal Assessment of Parenting Skills
    Working with Parents Postnatally
    Parent–Child Fit
    Intervention Strategies
Key Nursing Concepts

LEARNING OBJECTIVES

After reading this chapter students should be able to
- Explain the relevance of parenting as an area for study by health care professionals
- Discuss key characteristics of different structures of parenting
- Identify stress factors for parents and children
- Identify and discuss counseling and assessment strategies for working with parents
- Recognize key bonding and attachment elements

CHAPTER 13

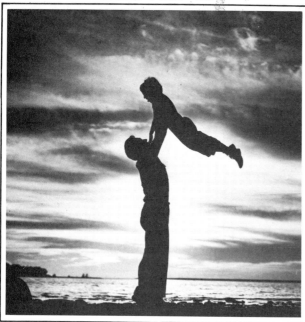

Psychiatric nurses work with healthy parents, recognizing that no other single factor affects the psychological development of children more dramatically than parenting.

THE PROCESS OF PARENTING

Parenting and Psychiatric Nursing Practice

Probably no other single factor affects our psychological development, either positively or negatively, as much as the parenting we receive. Yet this area has been virtually ignored by medical and nursing schools and mental health workers, unless it is related to a child's current psychopathology. Thus we are approaching the problems of parenting only after dysfunctional parenting has produced an emotionally disturbed child. One of the broad goals of nursing is optimum wellness (see Chapter 10) for the client and prevention of disorder whenever possible. Optimum wellness, unlike the absence of disease, is a dynamic and positive concept. One of the major nursing interventions in achieving the goal of optimum wellness for a client is an assessment that forms the basis for primary prevention. In working with parents and prospective parents, the psychiatric nurse is in an excellent position to promote optimum wellness among both parents and children by using assessment approaches geared to primary prevention.

Nursing is also committed to meeting the needs of the health care consumer. The popularity of how-to-parent books, the current interest in parent effective-

ness training, and the eagerness with which most parents seek advice or reassurance about their parenting skills, all tell us, directly and indirectly, that parents want help with the difficult task of parenting.

Most nursing school curricula include enough growth and development to enable the graduate to answer questions about children knowledgeably. The same programs rarely include parenting as a separate and important area of study. The parent–child relationship is a highly interactive process. We can't claim to understand children without trying to understand parents. This chapter presents an overview of the parenting role and the parent–child interactive process from the parental perspective. It explores ways in which the nurse can help meet the needs of both parent and child.

The Difficulties Inherent in the Parenting Role

Decline of the Traditional Family American society expects all parents to be "good" parents. At the same time, it offers them very little support or instruction. It is almost as if the new parent is expected to know instinctively how to parent successfully.

However, parenting involves a complex set of skills and knowledge. These skills do not emerge fully developed with the birth of the first child. Where does the new parent learn how to parent?

Traditionally, parenting skills were taught by families. As children, future parents learned from their parents and extended family what parents did, how they behaved, what the parent role included and did not include. Usually there were younger siblings available to practice on, so the mechanics of infant care were no mystery. Later, when the child in turn became a parent, the extended family was still available to provide parental role models, advice, and support. It also validated the importance, difficulty, and joys of the parenting role.

In today's highly mobile society, the support and instruction of the traditional extended family are available to very few new parents. Few schools offer education in parenting. Where do new parents turn for the support, advice, and validation they need—usually desperately?

Support for Parents   If there are two parents, and the relationship between them is satisfactory, they can provide some support and validation for each other. If parenting friends are available, peer support can furnish the comfort of shared experiences. However, friends can rarely give authoritative advice on the process of optimal parenting.

In the absence of available parenting classes or knowledgeable family or friends, the new parents may turn to books for advice. Unfortunately, the advice in parenting books is often contradictory and dogmatic.

One of the most widespread parenting models is furnished by the mass media. However, the media model is also one of the most unrealistic. Media parents are usually joyful, serene, effortless mothers and fathers. They always delight in their children. Their greatest concerns are getting the grass stains out of Susie's jeans or deciding which disposable diaper to use. If one accepts the media parent for a role model, one is bound to feel angry, guilty, and inadequate.

Parents also seek advice from health care professionals. On hospital wards, in psychiatric outpatient settings, at parties, in clinics, or in casual conversation, nurses are often asked for information on child rearing and parenting. The nurse who is knowledgeable about parenting will have many opportunities to use this knowledge professionally.

Bonding and Attachment: Beginning of the Interactive Process

The psychology of pregnancy and expectant parenthood includes fantasies, expectations, and unconscious processes that can affect postnatal parent–child interaction. However, the interaction itself begins with bonding and attachment. Bonding and attachment are the interactive processes by which the infant and parent commit themselves to each other. They are opposite sides of the same coin. *Attachment* is the infant's tie to the parent, *bonding* the parent's tie to the infant. Though they are both part of the same interactive process, bonding and attachment vary with the psychological development of parent (usually the mother) and infant.

Attachment   The process by which human infants become attached to their mothers has been carefully studied by researchers, notably Bowlby (1958, 1969). Bowlby described five basic, biologically determined

modalities by which infants attach to their mothers. These are smiling at the mother, sucking, clinging, following, and crying.

Bonding   Klaus and Kennell (1976) have examined the parental side of the attachment process, describing the development of bonding from parent to infant. The importance of bonding is enormous. The human infant, who goes through a relatively long dependency period, must rely on the parents for physical and psychological survival. Psychologically, the parent–infant bond is the basis for all the infant's subsequent attachments. The quality of this attachment will directly affect the quality of all future attachments.

Klaus and Kennell's description of the bonding process is based on the belief that a sensitive period exists during the first minutes and hours of life. To insure optimal bonding, it is necessary for one or both parents to have close contact with the neonate during this time. This has obvious implications for routine hospital labor and delivery practices.

Components of the Bonding Process   According to Klaus and Kennell (1976), the sensitive period is one of the seven critical components of the bonding process.

1. A sensitive period exists during which close contact with the neonate is necessary.
2. Parents exhibit species-specific responses to the infant when making contact.
3. Parents will become optimally attached to only one infant at a time.
4. Infant response to the parent, such as body or eye movements, is necessary for bonding.
5. Being present at the birth increases one's attachment to an infant.
6. Some adults find it hard to bond to one person while mourning the loss or possible loss of the same or a different person.
7. Some early events, such as anxiety about a baby with a temporary disorder, can have long-lasting effects on bonding.

When one looks at the critical components of the bonding process and the attachment behaviors by which the infant attaches to the parents, the interactive nature of this process is obvious. Nurses who are knowledgeable about the bonding–attachment process can often facilitate it.

Mrs. C had just delivered her second child. Mr. C had been present throughout labor and delivery. The nurse asked Mr. and Mrs. C if they would like some time with the baby. Mrs. C was pleased but surprised. She wondered if the baby didn't need to be cleaned and weighed. The nurse replied that there were some routine procedures to be done, but that they could be postponed for a bit if the parents wanted to be with the new baby for a while. The parents spent thirty minutes with their new infant, getting to know him before he was taken to the newborn nursery. Later, both parents commented that they felt much closer to this newborn than they had to their older son. "It seems like he belonged to us and us to him right away," Mrs. C commented.

Hospital procedures that interfere with early parent–infant contact need to be reevaluated. The practice of separating mother and infant immediately after birth and limiting the amount of time the family is allowed with the newborn interferes with the bonding and attachment process. With a goal of primary prevention in mind, nurses should be promoting, not interfering with, the bonding and attachment process between infant and parents.

Mothering and Fathering

Recent events, notably the women's liberation movement, have resulted in a reevaluation of traditional masculine and feminine concepts of role. Men and women are critically examining their values and assumptions about masculinity and femininity. These values and assumptions have a great deal of influence on the parenting role.

In American society, the father is traditionally expected to fill the instrumental parental role. He provides for the family financially, makes and implements the important decisions, and is the authority figure for the children. In this traditional model of parenting, the mother fills the complementary expressive role. She provides the nurturance, being consistently available to the children, and her role is essentially subordinate to that of her husband.

Currently, many parents are reevaluating traditional roles. These parents are finding that they are more effective and comfortable when they share the instrumental and expressive roles on the basis of inclination and capability rather than of gender. Fathers are getting in touch with their own nurturing qualities. In turn, this allows more liberalization and flexibility in the mothering role.

In a very real sense, shared roles can introduce liberalization and flexibility into both mothering and fathering. The mother has more freedom to stay in touch with other aspects of her life. The father has more freedom to become involved in child care. Current legal issues about father's rights reflect this new freedom.

Dan and Janet D, a young couple with a six-month-old infant, were becoming increasingly resentful of and alienated from each other. During a routine visit to the pediatrician, Mrs. D confided to the nurse-practitioner that she missed the job she had held before the birth of the baby and felt stifled by being in the apartment so much. With encouragement from the nurse, she added that she felt her marriage was in trouble. She resented the baby because she felt he was breaking up her marriage. The nurse offered support and referred Mrs. D to a mental health clinic where she and her husband could be seen together. In the course of conjoint counseling by the psychiatric nurse, Mr. D said he resented being the sole breadwinner for the family and was jealous of the time his wife had at home with the baby. With the nurse-counselor's help, the Ds were able to work out a different parenting pattern that met their individual needs. Mrs. D found a part-time job that provided the outside stimulus she missed and took some of the financial pressure off Mr. D. Mr. D was able to cut down his work hours, giving him more time and energy to be with his family. Mrs. D was delighted to share the child-rearing responsibilities with her husband, and the Ds now felt able to share their concerns and feelings with each other.

Parenting behaviors are derived from a complex combination of many factors. These include the mothering care received by the parent, the marital relationship, prenatal fantasies and events, cultural practices, current relationships to the family of origin, the parent's knowledge of child development, and the parent's financial and emotional stability and general ego functioning. Many of these factors are givens that the parents cannot manipulate. However, parents are now recognizing that the expressive and instrumental parenting roles are not inalterably sex linked. Rather, they represent one area where parents can tailor the parenting role to fit their individual needs while still meeting the needs of their children.

DIFFERENT STRUCTURES OF PARENTING

Single Parents

The single parent role can be created by divorce, separation, desertion, death, or unwed parenthood. Each of these situations, and the individual's response to the situation, can create unique stresses. However, some factors are common to all forms of single parenthood.

First of all, with the exception of an occasional tv situation comedy that stresses the "amusing" aspects of single parenthood, role models and validation of the single parent role are difficult to find. In spite of social evidence, American society perceives the parenting role as one shared by two married parent-partners who are the biological mother and father of their children. In addition, American society in general still disapproves deeply of the single parent, with the possible exception of the widow or widower. AFDC (Aid to Families with Dependent Children) payments reflect this disapproval. The community will not allow the single parent family to starve, but it will not subsidize them above the poverty level.

Inadequate income is one major stress most single parents face. With shared parenthood, one parent can assume daily child care while the other parent is employed outside the home. If both parents work, they can usually afford adequate child care outside the home. The single parent's options are more limited. Single parents can either remain home with the child or children and try to make do on AFDC or work outside the home and spend a large portion of their wages on child care. Divorced and separated single parents may have court-enforced child support payments, and widowed parents may have Social Security benefits. These sources of income help relieve the stress but rarely confer financial independence.

Ms. G had not planned to have a baby, but when she became pregnant, she chose not to have an abortion or relinquish the baby. A year after his birth, she was delighted with her son and was enjoying motherhood, but she was bitter about the difficulty of making ends meet. She felt it was important for her to stay home and provide her son with good mothering, but she was discouraged by trying to live on AFDC payments. She returned to her job as a telephone installer, but found that after paying the excellent but expensive day care

center she had found for her son, she had very little more money than when she stayed home. She expressed her anxiety about the situation to a children's psychiatric nurse who was on the staff of the day care center as a consultant and counselor. The nurse offered Ms. G the option of meeting with her for an hour a week to explore her situation and her feelings. Ms. G eagerly accepted. During the course of the next six months, the nurse-counselor did not produce any easy solutions to the stresses of single parenthood, but she did offer Ms. G a chance to explore and verbalize her feelings about her son and about herself as a woman and a mother. The nurse also offered Ms. G information on child development and management techniques. During their final session, Ms. G told the nurse, "Well, you haven't helped me solve my money problems, but I feel a lot less uptight. I know myself better and understand my kid better. I'm clear now about some things—like my wanting to work for a lot of reasons other than money."

The nurse in this case study was unable to solve the client's financial problem, and she did not provide long-term, insight-oriented psychotherapy. But she did offer Ms. G the following things:

- An opportunity to share and explore her feelings with an understanding and supportive adult
- Information on child development to help her understand and meet her child's needs
- Validation of the difficulties of the single parent role and positive feedback for the concerned, caring mothering she was giving her son
- Information and help with child management that wasn't available to Ms. G from a close extended family
- An opportunity to share her parenting experience—especially important since Ms. G had no spouse or close significant others

Ms. G's financial dilemma highlights what is currently a critical problem in this country—the lack of reasonably priced, readily available, high-quality child care services for families where the parents work, from either choice or necessity. Many two-parent families also need child care, but for the single parent family with limited resources, the need is often desperate.

Another stress on the single parent family is the lack of support and sharing a partner provides. Single parents must be both mother and father; they don't have the option of sharing the instrumental and supportive parental functions. Those who succeed must redefine and rework the parenting role again if they remarry.

Mike was divorced a year after the birth of his son, Allan, and assumed custody of the baby. He found single parenthood rewarding but emotionally and physically exhausting. Mike had great difficulty setting any limits on his now three-year-old son, and Allan's behavior and insecurity showed it. When Mike remarried, he was delighted that his wife was easily able to establish and enforce limits for Allan. However, he found himself frequently interfering and undermining her attempts. After discussing this openly with his wife, Mike realized that he was reluctant to relinquish the sole control to which he had become accustomed. The parents were able to work this out by assuming the parental tasks to which each was most suited, thus meeting Allan's needs and their own.

The single parent also lacks the companionship of an intimate who can share the parenting experience. A two-parent family, when the parents are also good friends, can share the fun, disappointments, joys, and sorrows of parenting. The single parent can sometimes share with a friend or extended family. But in a highly mobile society the best chances for this kind of sharing are with a spouse.

The parent who does not have custody of the child also faces difficulties. Often this parent would like to remain in the child's life as something more than a visiting Santa Claus figure, but this is difficult when the parent does not see the child every day. At present, divorced fathers seem particularly vulnerable to this kind of missing out.

The Ls had been divorced for a year, and their three children lived with Mrs. L. Mr. L had visiting privileges on Sundays. Because the strain between them was so disruptive, he did not want to stay around Mrs. L when he visited the children. He was living in a small, furnished room, so on Sundays he took the children out to a place they selected. This was usually a movie, amusement park, or some other setting that gave him little chance to interact with them on more than a superficial level. Mr. L thought he was losing all real contact with his children and felt powerless to do anything to change the situation.

Parenting is demanding and challenging even under ideal circumstances. Single parents lack the emotional support and regular companionship of a spouse. They have no one to help with routine child care and housework and to share the responsibility of parenthood with. Finally, they seldom enjoy the financial security of the two-parent family.

Children in single parent families lack a close male or female role model.

They are usually deprived of a second adult who could offer them affection, set limits, and provide additional emotional support.

Adoptive, Foster, and Stepparents

Adoptive, foster, and stepparents have one thing in common. They are parenting a child who is not biologically theirs and who has had parenting experiences they didn't control. An exception would be adoptive parents who assume care of an infant immediately after birth or hospital discharge. However, not many adoptive parents do this.

Adoptive Parents Adoptive parents, once the adoption is final, enjoy the same rights and responsibilities as biological parents. When the adopted child is an infant, adoptive parenthood has essentially the same structure as biological parenthood—minus the pregnancy and birth experiences. How the loss of these experiences is resolved depends largely on the adoptive parents. Adoption procedures are usually cumbersome enough to allow the prospective parents more than the biological nine months to prepare psychologically for parenthood. However, a nurse who surveyed 167 parents found that adoptive parents—particularly those who adopted their first or second child—had greater needs for information and reassurance than biological parents (Walker 1981). Awareness of the needs of adoptive parents can help nurses formulate interventions on a primary level.

Nowadays most adopted children are not infants. The availability of abortion and effective birth control, and some change, especially among young people, in social attitudes toward single parenthood, have reduced the number of infants available for adoption. Adoption of an older child requires difficult adjustments on both sides, even when both sides desire the adoption. The adoptive parents are dealing with psychological needs and emotional fallout from the child's previous relationships with a parent or parent substitute.

Seven-year-old Katie had been adopted by Mr. and Mrs. S shortly after her sixth birthday. Until she was two years old, Katie had lived with her mother. She was then removed by court order because her mother was suspected of abusing her. During the next four years Katie was in three different foster homes, as well as the group home where children awaiting foster placement lived.

Six months after Katie's adoption, Mrs. S arranged for her to see a child psychiatric nurse-therapist. She was concerned about Katie's tantrums, nightmares, and excessive fears. The nurse suggested that Mr. and Mrs. S participate in conjoint counseling with another nurse. They were reluctant initially, and in the first several sessions they focused exclusively on Katie's problems and how to manage them. As rapport and trust were established between the nurse and the parents, they were able to use the sessions to explore their own feelings, hopes, and frustrations. They talked about their inability to have their own child, the unavailability of adoptable infants, the various parenting experiences Katie had had, and the difficulties they were having with Katie. After a year of conjoint counseling and individual therapy for Katie, Katie's problem behavior was markedly decreased. The individual members expressed a sense of integration as a family. As Mrs. S put it, "We really belong together now."

The nurse did four things in her work with Mr. and Mrs. S.

1. She offered them support and validated the difficulty of adoptive parenting.
2. She gave them information on child rearing and psychological development, especially as these related to Katie's life history.
3. She facilitated their efforts to explore and understand themselves.
4. She helped them explore ways to meet their own and Katie's needs.

Foster Parents   The role of the foster parent is not as clearly defined as that of the adoptive parent. Foster parenting is a paid job, yet it has neither the advantages of regular employment nor those of traditional parenthood. Foster parents are paid by social work agencies to parent other people's children, but they are not paid much. It is a twenty-four-hour-a-day, seven-day-a-week job without sick leave, overtime, or vacations. While biological parents receive no wages for parenting, they have parental rights. Foster parents

usually do not have the option of adopting the child, and the agency has the right to remove the child at any time. In short, the foster parenting role demands the commitment of traditional parenting in a situation structured to weaken this commitment. Ideally, foster parents would be child care experts, paid well by society to parent children in need of first-class parenting. The distance between this ideal and the current reality reflects the low status of parenting in American society.

Stepparents   Stepparents are usually created by the inclusion of another adult into a single parent family, either with or without a legal marriage. The stepparent faces the task of working out a parenting role with a child who has been influenced by a previous parent of the same sex, and whose ideas about mothering or fathering have been at least partly determined by the behavior of that parent. The child will compare the stepparent with the previous parent. Whether the previous child–parent relationship was good or bad, the stepparent (like the adoptive parent of an older child) will have to deal with emotional fallout from that relationship.

Children who have had one parent all to themselves may view the addition of a stepparent as an unwarranted intrusion. The emotional demands of establishing an intimate adult relationship while simultaneously working out a new parenting role can be very difficult.

After several months of dating, Jack and Mary decided to live together. Because she and her two children were already established in a house they liked, Jack moved in with them. Mary's daughters, two and three and one-half, seemed to adjust quickly to the situation, calling Jack "Daddy" and wanting a lot of attention from him. Jack, however, quickly began to feel overwhelmed by the demands of two young children on top of his relationship with Mary. He said he felt unable to meet the needs of the children, Mary, and himself. He had had a satisfactory relationship with the children as their mother's friend, but he felt unable to fill both the father and mate roles successfully. After six months he moved out, though he continued to visit.

Communal Parents

Communal parenting is a move away from isolated nuclear family life. It offers many of the advantages of a large extended family. These include readily available companionship of both adults and children; commitment to mutual goals; and shared talents, capabilities, and duties.

Communal organization, including the philosophy and practice of child rearing, varies with the structure, membership, and general purpose of the commune. In the United States today, it varies from the highly structured and cohesive organization of Synanon to the loose organization of The Family in Taos, New Mexico, which shares all the commune's children in common without making any distinctions about biological parenthood. Still other urban and rural groups share chores, child care, and expenses while maintaining distinctly separate nuclear family constellations within the communal structure.

Communal life generally offers children the opportunity to have their needs met by, and to learn from, a variety of adults and peers. It also includes them as valuable, contributing members of the group. Communal life offers parents an alternative to isolated nuclear family life. It reduces many of the problems and stresses inherent in contemporary nuclear family living.

Communal child rearing does have one disadvantage. There are no long-term longitudinal research results that suggest its long-range effects on the child. Multiple caretaking, multiple role models, the increased importance of peer relationships as a socializing force, and other aspects of communal life may or may not expose the child to risks. Many parents who have opted for a communal life-style think these possible risks are negligible compared to what they perceive as the certain disadvantages of isolated nuclear family life. However, the success of communal versus traditional child-rearing practices cannot be objectively assessed until the results of further evaluative research become available.

Working Parents

Working parents are so common today that they are included in this section on "different" structures of parenting only because they are different from the traditional family, which allotted home and child care to the mother and work outside the home to the father. The combination of economic pressures and the trend toward the maximum use of individual potential espoused by the women's liberation movement have caused many women to seek jobs who might otherwise have opted for the traditional homemaker role. For single parents, outside employment is often the only

alternative to the marginal existence provided by programs such as AFDC.

The extent and type of parental role changes that occur when both parents work varies with the individual family. Some parents attempt to divide household and child care responsibilities evenly while both hold full-time jobs. In other families one or both parents work part-time, and the parents share home duties. In still other families husband and wife may reverse traditional roles, with the wife employed outside the home and the husband assuming the homemaker's responsibilities. Finally, the wife may be employed full-time outside the home and still assume full responsibility for home and child care. The single largest problem faced by working parents, regardless of their specific parenting style, is the lack of high-quality, affordable, accessible child care facilities.

Bob and Chris are both employed full-time, and both would like to remain so. They enjoy both the work they do and the occasional luxuries that two incomes provide. Unable to find a child care center they liked and could afford, and having no extended family in the area, they have employed a series of sitters for their twenty-three-month-old daughter. Most of these sitters have not remained more than three or four months. Lately, they have become concerned about their daughter's increasing fearfulness, crying, and nightmares. Currently they are trying to decide which of them will relinquish outside employment to provide stable care for her. Neither wants to work part-time, for this would mean losing all job benefits and seniority. Since neither of them wants to quit, yet both agree that one or the other must do so, they're unsure how to decide which of them will assume full-time child care. Chris says, "We'll probably end up flipping a coin."

The rigidity of the traditional American work structure—forty hours per week, nine to five, fifty weeks per year—is a major obstacle to the successful combination of parenting and employment. Current employment schedules are designed to suit the traditional family structure. They are ludicrously unsuited to the family in which both parents work. Current demands for paid maternity and paternity leave and the laudable (though still extremely rare) provision of child care facilities at the place of employment are moves in the right direction. But as yet these benefits are not widely enough demanded or provided to help out more than a few fortunate families.

PARENTS AND CHILDREN UNDER STRESS

Poverty and Racism

Although the United States owns almost half the world's wealth, a significant number of American children are not receiving the minimum necessary food, shelter, and emotional care. Poverty and racism are basic social conditions that encourage the development of disturbed coping patterns. In American society, poverty and racism are linked in many ways, both subtle and obvious.

Lowered self-esteem and a (usually realistic) lack of faith in and commitment to the future is the legacy passed on to the child by the impoverished parent. This perpetuates the vicious circle of poverty. Society's response to the major mental health problems of both poverty and racism has failed to meet the needs of many segments of the population. Programs such as food stamps, unemployment compensation, Social Security, and Federal Aid to Dependent Children attempt (not always successfully) to meet the physiological needs of impoverished ethnic groups. But they do not repair the psychological damage inflicted by the covert social message that some people are more equal than others.

The Joint Commission on Mental Health of Children has studied poverty and racism. Their Committee on Children of Minority Groups stated unequivocally that racism is the "number one public health problem facing America today, presenting a clear danger to the mental health of all parents and children" (Joint Commission on Mental Health of Children 1969, p. 216). The committee went on to identify poverty and the education system as factors that compound the problem of racism.

The Vicious Circle of Poverty   The high rate of poverty within minority groups provides another significant environmental stress. Poverty places minority children at extremely high risk physically and psychologically. Growing up in a racist society impairs the minority child's self-image and fosters a sense of alienation and isolation. An educational system based on white middle-class mores, cultural ideals, knowledge, and achievement contributes little to a sense of worth or opportunity in the minority child. In addition, ghetto schools are notoriously poor and understaffed and

have larger classes than other schools. These factors lead to a high rate of educational retardation and dropouts, which, together with racist attitudes that influence employment practices, leads to high rates of youth unemployment or underemployment. This in turn reinforces the young person's feelings of alienation, isolation, and worthlessness. The vicious circle of poverty and racism closes, trapping the individual inside (Joint Commission on Mental Health of Children 1969, p. 244).

The following case study describes a family that did receive the psychiatric intervention necessary to mitigate the psychological effects of poverty and racism. Unfortunately, there are not enough mental health resources to solve the problem in this way, on the tertiary level of prevention, for more than a fraction of the population.

Tamecah was an eight-year-old black child who was referred to the child guidance center for evaluation because of her poor academic performance and severe behavioral problems. The evaluation team ruled out learning disabilities and recommended individual therapy, for they had diagnosed Tamecah's difficulties as being emotional in origin. During the course of play therapy with a psychiatric nurse, Tamecah revealed her extremely low self-esteem and fears of destruction. Tamecah repeatedly played out situations in which one small, "bad" girl was at the mercy of hordes of wild animals, large malevolent people, or fatal accidents the child could not prevent.

The therapist thought Tamecah's low self-esteem and insecurity were a result of her home situation. The father had deserted the family when Tamecah was six months old, leaving her mother to raise her and her four older siblings on assistance from social services. The mother often expressed to her children her own sense of helplessness and hopelessness by saying things like "It doesn't matter how hard you try. We're black and we're poor, so we're nothing."

The therapist felt that it was crucial for Tamecah that her mother also receive psychiatric help so that the home environment would be altered. Financially this was feasible, since state Medicaid covered the cost of therapy for all family members. Tamecah's mother began seeing another therapist at the clinic.

After two years of therapy, Tamecah's self-esteem had increased, her anxiety and fears had decreased, and she was doing well in school. Her therapist judged that a great deal of Tamecah's improvement was due to her mother's continued involvement in therapy and the resulting change in the home environment. At this time the therapist and Tamecah's mother and her therapist were considering family therapy including Tamecah, her mother, and the two siblings who were still living at home.

Factors Associated with Poverty   Examining poverty specifically, the Joint Commission (1969) identified eight major factors strongly associated with poverty. These were

1. Little education
2. The poverty environment
3. Chronic unemployment
4. Life-styles that are a product of impoverishment
5. Low income
6. Poor physical and mental health
7. Large families
8. Broken families

These factors all interact, forming the intergenerational poverty cycle.

Intervention in the Problems of Poverty and Racism   The Joint Commission's recommendations (1969, pp. 213–14) included

- Free high-quality education for all children
- Radical and immediate improvement of the poverty environment
- Vocational training, job opportunities, and wages for the unemployed and underemployed
- Provision of a decent standard of living administered in ways that foster dignity
- Free, high-quality physical and mental health and social services available to all
- Full and equal opportunity to help plan and develop these services given to parents and youth of all ethnic and socioeconomic backgrounds

The solution to the major problems of poverty and racism is both simple and extremely complex. Poverty, racism, and the conditions that create them must be eradicated. This sounds overwhelming. How can the individual have any impact on the alleviation of problems this large? What can we, as nurses and mental health care professionals, do about poverty and racism?

On a personal level, we can

- Be willing to analyze our feelings about people of different races and classes
- Be aware of, and knowledgeable about, the problems of poverty and racism
- Use this awareness and knowledge in our professional practice when we formulate assessments, interventions, and evaluations of our interventions
- Use our professional role to educate others about the existence and significance of the problems
- Support legislation designed to alleviate poverty and racism
- Support public educational programs in ethnic history and family life

As a professional group, we can

- Collect data about poverty and racism that can be used on local, state, and federal levels to formulate interventions
- Support nursing research on poverty and racism
- Be politically active; lobby for legislation designed to alleviate the problems
- Use the media, including professional journals, to educate ourselves and the general public about the crippling effects of poverty and racism
- Develop and implement courses dealing with poverty and racism that will meet the continuing education requirements for nurses
- Include the study of these major public health problems in the basic curriculum of nursing education
- Lobby for and help implement changes in basic education in public schools that are necessary for the eradication of racism, such as the development of nonracist textbooks

Nurses who are committed to the eradication of poverty and racism will find ways to contribute personally. The basic requirement is involvement. As individuals, as nurses, as mental health professionals, we can contribute to the fight against poverty and racism.

Sexism

The effects of sexism are not as obviously detrimental as the effects of poverty and racism, but this does not justify dismissing the problem. Like racism and poverty, sexism is a barrier to the full development of the individual. People must be allowed to develop on the basis of capability, talent, and inclination rather than on the basis of ethnicity, income, or sex.

The women's liberation movement has provided the impetus for a reappraisal of traditional stereotypes of masculinity and femininity. It has shown how these stereotypes create artificial and unnecessary barriers to growth and choice. The practice of sexual stereotyping does not always operate to the benefit of men, as many male nursing students and nurses—men in a traditionally "feminine" occupation—can attest. Sexism is a problem for both men and women, just as racism is a problem shared by all. As with ethnicity, the deleterious effects are more obvious in the subordinate group, but it doesn't follow that there are no adverse effects on the dominant group.

The following case study illustrates one family's failure to understand a basic tenet of liberation from sexual stereotypes. Liberation means informed and conscious freedom of choice. The deliberate choice of a traditionally feminine role by a girl, or of a masculine one by a boy, is as valid and acceptable as rejection of those roles. Traditional roles are not detrimental in themselves. Being forced to choose traditional roles is detrimental.

Tom and Elizabeth consider themselves enlightened parents. They are well aware of the adverse effects of sexism. Throughout her life, they have consistently given their twelve-year-old daughter, Megan, trucks, tool sets, and chemistry labs rather than dolls, cooking sets, and other toys considered traditionally feminine. Lately, Megan has been reading books about nurses, and has said she wants to become a nurse. Her parents have responded by advising Megan to go into medicine if she wants to enter health care. They assure her that it is totally acceptable for a young woman to enter this traditionally masculine field. Though Megan insists that she would prefer nursing to medicine, her parents continue to urge her to select medicine.

When sexist attitudes and practices are eradicated, men, women, and children of both sexes will be liberated from arbitrary, predetermined options. This does not mean that unisex will, or should, prevail. It simply means that each individual will have maximum freedom of choice within the cultural framework.

Adolescent Parents

Adolescent parents face special, often overwhelming, stresses. Adolescence is a stage of great turmoil and change. During this period the individual gradually, and with difficulty, moves from childhood to adulthood. The psychological work involved in this transition is enormous. (See Chapter 20.)

While the adolescents are still in the process of establishing self-identity, adolescent parents suddenly become responsible for a totally dependent infant. Adolescent psychosocial tasks require most of the individual's time and energy. But so does infant care. The adolescent parent is in a bind. Either the parent's own developmental needs or those of the infant will be shortchanged. After infancy, the needs of child and adolescent parent will continue to clash until the parent's developmental needs are resolved.

Pregnancy and parenthood frequently separate the adolescent from peers. This separation is particularly significant in adolescence, because one's primary values at this time are those of the peer group. The peer group is one of the major tools adolescents use to build their own identity. Isolation from the peer group deprives the adolescent parent of this important tool.

Jill and Allan had married at sixteen, as soon as Jill realized she was pregnant. Alan worked and went to night school, so Jill was alone most of the time with their three-month-old son. She urged her high school friends to stop by, for she was lonely and felt out of place with the older mothers in the neighborhood. Her friends talked about what was happening at school and at home—the usual chatter Jill had been a part of until a year ago. Though she felt divided from her friends' life, Jill longed to belong to it again. She felt guilty for not being happy and satisfied with the baby and her new life. At the same time she resented the baby, whose presence excluded her from the life-style she'd enjoyed before her pregnancy.

Feeling very depressed one day, Jill went to a neighborhood drop-in clinic and asked to talk to someone. The staff psychiatric nurse interviewed Jill and suggested she come in once a week to talk. The nurse assessed Jill psychiatrically as basically healthy with good ego strength, but with an adjustment reaction of adolescence precipitated by the crisis of parenthood. The nurse structured the sessions to provide support for Jill, rather than focusing on intrapsychic processes. Eight months later, Jill commented, "We don't seem to do much, and I sure didn't think I needed a shrink, but I feel so much better every time I leave, it must be doing something.''

Adolescent parenthood is usually unplanned parenthood. Unplanned parenthood for the unwed at any age offers three alternatives—adoption, marriage (possibly unwanted), or single parenthood. Each of these alternatives entails problems and stresses not usually associated with parenting. For the adolescent parent, there is usually the further complication of financial dependence. Career choice may well be severely restricted. If an adolescent girl does get pregnant on purpose, she may do so in an attempt to meet her own needs (often for intimacy or companionship). These needs will probably not be met by pregnancy or parenthood.

Gwen had been in twenty foster homes in the course of her fifteen years. She was sexually active at fourteen and used no birth control. When she became pregnant shortly after her fifteenth birthday, Gwen began to plan all the things she and the baby could do together. Abortion or adoption were presented as options by the maternity clinic nurse. Gwen rejected both immediately. She told the nurse that the baby would be one thing that would always be hers. She said they would have a lot of fun playing together.

Alerted by this unrealistic attitude, the maternity nurse referred Gwen to the psychiatric nurse, who functioned as a staff consultant and counselor for patients one day a week at the clinic. The psychiatric nurse saw Gwen weekly throughout her pregnancy, focusing on Gwen's psychological developmental needs. Gwen had little interest in exploring or questioning her motivations about her pregnancy and her decision to keep the baby. However, the nurse did help Gwen to see how her stated desire of ''having something all mine'' related to her deprived childhood and to her expectations that her baby would meet needs that hadn't been met in the past. After the baby was born, Gwen continued to see the nurse once a week. They continued to focus on Gwen, but the nurse also talked to Gwen about the baby's psychological needs and how she could meet them.

Like Gwen, many adolescent parents have unrealistic expectations of parenthood. Admittedly, so do many adult parents. But the additional stresses of unmet adolescent developmental needs, financial dependence, peer group exclusion, and societal disapproval combine to place the adolescent parent at extremely high risk for unsuccessful parenting.

Battering Parents

Child abuse is an emotionally laden issue. It's not a comfortable topic to deal with, and so, unfortunately, health care professionals often avoid it or ignore it. This attitude usually conveys to the battering parents the message that child abuse is too horrible even to discuss, and that no normal parent is capable of it.

On the contrary, every parent is potentially abusive at times. Most parents manage to vent their pain and frustration in other ways, but some do not. It is a common misconception that abusive parents are usually members of an ethnic minority, or poor, or both. Racism and poverty certainly contribute to the situational stresses involved in parenting. But child abuse is not limited to any particular segment of the population.

What is child abuse? What is the difference between maltreatment and punishment? A national nursing journal recently addressed these questions, and provided the following guidelines for use by nurses when assessing the possibility of child neglect or abuse (Nursing 79 and Leaman 1979).

Child neglect includes physical neglect, or failure to provide adequate food, shelter, medical care, and so on, and emotional neglect or failure to nurture the child's sense of self. Child abuse includes

- *Physical abuse,* which consists of one or more episodes of inappropriate disciplining.
- *Battering* (battered child syndrome), which includes serious injury that is both severe and repetitive and is usually found in a child under four years.
- *Sexual abuse* which ranges from fondling or exposing the genitals to rape.
- *Emotional abuse,* which is continued and inappropriate debasement of the child's feelings and can be more subtle and difficult to assess than physical abuse or neglect and more difficult to mobilize intervention for, but no less crippling to the child.

When assessing the possibility of neglect or abuse, the nurse needs to be aware of cultural norms and differences. For example, a parent who is a member of the Jehovah Witnesses Church may not consider it neglect to refuse a medically necessary blood transfusion for a child, and disciplining that seems inappropriate to one cultural group may be the norm in another. However, they may be perceived as neglectful or inappropriate by the larger society. For further discussion of the sociocultural context of psychiatric nursing, see Chapter 26.

The Child Abuse Pattern The Department of Health, Education, and Welfare, in a publication dealing with the problem of child abuse (Helfer 1975, p. 15), has identified a combination of events that often lead to physical abuse when they occur in a certain sequence at a certain time:

1. The presence of potential within the family, which includes

   a. Parents reared in a physically or emotionally traumatic manner

   b. Parents who are isolated and distrustful

   c. Parents who give each other little help

   d. Parents who have a poor self-image

   e. Parents who have unrealistic expectations of children

2. The presence of a special child who

   a. Is seen as different

   b. Really is different

   c. Is both different and seen as different

3. The presence of a crisis or crises that are

   a. Physical (no food, money, heat, lights)

   b. Personal (death, separation)

   c. Both physical and personal

Mr. and Mrs. B and their five-year-old daughter, Samantha, came to the psychiatric clinic on a court order. They had been referred to protective services by the school nurse after Samantha had come to school several times with unexplained bruises and burns. ("Protective services" refers to the division of the local department of social services that deals specifically with families in which child abuse is suspected.) The parents told the psychiatric nurse that Samantha was the one who needed to see a mental health worker. They said she had always been different from her four brothers and sisters. When asked to clarify, Mrs. B said that Samantha had been "whiny and a crybaby" since she was an infant. She said they didn't have any problems with the other children. She added that she couldn't stand Samantha's "whining" and punished her to stop it.

Further questions elicited the information that Mr. B had been unemployed for several months, and the family was in severe financial stress. Asked for his assessment of Samantha, Mr. B replied, "Raising the kids is her job, not mine." Both parents were suspicious of the clinic staff and very resentful about what they termed interference. The intake recommendation was for

individual psychotherapy for each parent and Samantha, with possible couple or family therapy later. Initially, the parents insisted that only Samantha be seen but were told it was agency policy not to treat the child in an abuse situation unless the parents were also in treatment. They reluctantly agreed to therapy for themselves. Working with Mrs. B, the nurse planned to maintain a nonjudgmental and sympathetic attitude to establish a therapeutic alliance. She also planned to help Mrs. B to resolve her own unmet dependency needs.

While it frequently is one child who is identified as "different" and is therefore the target of parental abuse, the nurse assessing the family should carefully consider siblings as potential, if not yet actual, victims. As a nurse and two physicians found when studying sexual abuse, both victims and their siblings are at high risk of repeated abuse (Tillelli, Turek, and Jaffee 1980). Child abuse, like poverty and racism, is a vicious circle. Abused children frequently become abusive parents. Knowing this enables the nurse to maintain an empathic attitude when dealing with battering parents, and empathy is crucial when working with these parents. Low self-esteem and guilt are part of the syndrome that creates the problem. The health professional who blames the battering parent will only compound the problem by intensifying these feelings and making the parent more resistant to intervention.

While making a home visit, the public health nurse noted a large bruise on two-year-old Carrie's face. When questioned, Ms. T explained that Carrie had fallen a few days before, angrily adding, "I suppose you think I hit her." The nurse responded, "You sound pretty mad that I might think you hit Carrie, but it's not an unusual way for a parent to respond to a lot of pressure." The nurse's matter-of-fact attitude allowed the mother to confide that she never had hit Carrie but had frequent impulses to do so, and was really afraid she would seriously injure her child if she ever "let go." The nurse helped Carrie's mother verbalize and explore her feelings, maintaining a sympathetic and nonjudgmental manner. After the nurse reassured her that it was not for "crazy people," the mother accepted a referral to a mutual support group for parents run by a psychiatric nurse and psychiatric social worker through protective services. The group was structured to offer mutual support through sharing feelings, fears, and experiences. It also offered information on child rearing. The group leaders helped the parents recognize what feelings or events precipitated abuse or potential abuse incidents. Then, as a group, they explored alternative ways to deal with the feelings and events. During the second meeting she attended, Ms. T told the group, "I'm so grateful I found this group. I felt like such a bad person and a bad mother for wanting to hit Carrie when she was bugging me. Now I feel like there's some hope for me."

Most abusive parents can be helped. Essentially, they need to learn a new pattern of parenting. Exactly how this is accomplished will vary with the parents and the available resources. Intervention strategies include personal therapy for the parent, support groups, group therapy, parenting classes, and the development of a support system. Family therapy is viewed by many mental health professionals as the most effective single intervention in working with battering families. Chapter 21 outlines the process of family therapy. In working with abusive parents, the first requirement is to establish a therapeutic alliance. Unfortunately, the parent and health worker in an abuse case often perceive each other as enemies.

Establishing a Therapeutic Alliance To establish a therapeutic alliance with the abusive parent, mental health nurses must do the following things:

- They must be in touch with their own feelings about child abuse and abusive parents.
- They must recognize that battering parents have many of the same needs as their children—primarily severe and unmet dependency needs.
- They must be able to accept the parent as a worthwhile person.

Abusive parents may have unrealistic perceptions of both the child and the child's relationship to them. Frequently they perceive their children as being much more capable and self-controlled than they really are. They may interpret crying as the infant telling them that they are bad parents. They see it as a sign that the infant doesn't love them rather than as an expression of the helpless and dependent infant's needs.

Nine-month-old Kenny was admitted to the hospital for evaluation and treatment of multiple small burns. The admitting physician, suspecting child abuse, reported the case to protective services. The pediatric nurse who was caring for Kenny talked to the mother, commenting on her obvious anger and dismay when she learned of the referral. The mother told the nurse, "It wasn't my fault.

He wouldn't leave me alone. I kept telling him if he didn't stop crying, I'd have to punish him, and he kept disobeying me."

Working with battering parents is a challenging and difficult task, but well worth the effort. As health professionals, psychiatric nurses should be aware of and informed about the problem of child abuse. Specifically, nurses can

- Refer to local protective services all cases of confirmed or suspected child abuse
- Be alert for potentially abusive parents (such as those who experienced childhood deprivation and are now under stress) and attempt primary prevention
- Talk about the problem of battering parents and child abuse; use opportunities in professional and private life to share information about it
- Be aware of their own feelings about child abuse and battering parents
- Be honest and empathic when dealing with abusive parents

COUNSELING PARENTS

Prenatal Assessment of Parenting Skills

Like other nursing interventions, counseling parents begins with assessment. Ideally, the assessment of the potential parents begins before pregnancy. Adult and child psychiatric nurses; public health nurses; maternity, family planning, and pediatric nurses; and nurse-practitioners are frequently in a position to do significant primary prevention when working with prospective and expectant parents.

Interview Guide In working with prospective parents, the psychiatric nurse can assess many factors significant to successful parenting. The following guide presents some relevant areas and sample interview questions.

FANTASIES ABOUT THE CHILD. Be alert for rigid fantasies that may cause problems if the infant does not meet them. Parents who fantasize nothing except a beautiful, quiet, cuddly girl may feel surprised, upset, and cheated if they have an active, noisy boy who frequently kicks when held. The nurse might ask:

- Do you want a boy or a girl?
- What if it's (the opposite gender to the one the parents want)?
- What do you think the baby will be like?
- Would you like a quiet baby or an active one?

FEELINGS ABOUT AND EXPERIENCE WITH PARENTING.
How the prospective parents were parented themselves and their feelings about the parenting they received affect how they will parent their own child. They will be more successful in the parenting role if they have resolved their feelings about their own parents. The nurse might ask:

- How was your mother (father) as a parent?
- How was it for you as a child?
- What things did you enjoy doing with your parents when you were a child?
- How do you want to be like or different from your parents?
- How are things now between you and your parents?

AVAILABLE SUPPORT SYSTEM. Given the stresses inherent in the new parent role, support outside the immediate nuclear family is important for the parents' mental health. The nurse might ask:

- What do you do when you're happy or sad and want to share it with someone?
- Do you have friends or family in the area?
- Do you see them as often as you'd like to?
- Are they interested in the new baby?
- Have you thought of any ways you (you and your mate) will be able to have time alone (together) after the baby's born?

MATES' RELATIONSHIP If the parents' relationship is a close and sharing one, they can give each other support, companionship, and validation. If both parents are present at the interview, their relationship can be assessed indirectly by observing their interaction and by asking:

- How are things between the two of you?
- How do you feel about the baby?
- Do you have as much time together as you'd like?

- If you're worried or upset, do you share it with anyone?
- What kind of things do you enjoy doing together?
- What kind of things does each of you like to do alone? How is that for your partner?
- What is important to you both?

KNOWLEDGE OF GROWTH AND DEVELOPMENT. A basic working knowledge of physical and psychological growth and development and infant care increases the chances for successful parenting. The nurse should avoid creating an examination atmosphere by quizzing the parents on developmental milestones. It is better to ask indirect questions. If necessary, the nurse can recommend books on growth and development, classes, a resource person, or another source of information that will match the parents' cognitive style. The nurse might ask:

- Did you have younger brothers and sisters?
- Did you help care for them or other babies?
- Do you think it will be easy or hard for you to care for the baby?
- What would you like to provide for your baby? What do you think babies really need?

ECONOMIC AND SOCIAL STABILITY. Economic and social stability reduce the stress experienced by the new parents. Their economic and social situation may be appraised to some extent without asking direct questions by observing living conditions, dress, and speech. The nurse might also ask:

- Have you been married (living together) long?
- How long have you lived in this area? In your present house or apartment?
- Do you enjoy your work? Does your mate (wife; husband) enjoy (hers; his)?
- Will the expense of a child be difficult for you?

Specific Interventions The specific interventions will depend on the assessment made from the information obtained in the interview. The nurse may focus on helping the parents be aware of their fantasies about the baby and parenting. Nurse and parents can mutually assess their fantasies for their realistic and unrealistic aspects and explore alternatives to fantasized ideals. Or the nurse may teach parents about the psychological aspects of pregnancy, birth, parenting, and infant development. A single mother without friends or family may need support and help to determine what her needs are and how she can meet them.

Ellen had been seen regularly at the family planning clinic for two years. On this visit, she told the maternity nurse-practitioner that she and her husband had decided to have a baby and requested removal of her IUD. During the procedure, the nurse asked if Ellen wanted a boy or girl and what she thought the baby would be like. Alerted by the rigid and unrealistic fantasies Ellen voiced about her prospective baby, the nurse made time to talk with her further. During this conversation, Ellen confided that her own mother had left her when she was very young, adding that she wondered if she could be a good mother herself. The nurse suggested that she wait awhile before getting pregnant, adding that counseling before pregnancy might make both pregnancy and parenthood easier. Ellen was receptive, so the nurse made several referrals to places where Ellen could obtain counseling at a reasonable cost. The nurse also discussed alternative birth control methods with Ellen. After several months of counseling, during which the psychiatric nurse-counselor helped Ellen gain insight into her feelings about her mother, the parenting she had received, and her own ambivalence about motherhood, Ellen decided again to become pregnant. When her baby was born, she enjoyed mothering him and did so successfully.

Working with Parents Postnatally

What New Parents Need   New parents have two major postnatal needs. The first is the need for factual information. The second is the need for support and reassurance.

The enduring popularity of such classics as Benjamin Spock's *Baby and Child Care* (1976) and the many current books on how to be a successful parent reflect the new parents' need for factual information. The current bewildering choice of life and parenting styles, and the frequent lack of role models formerly provided by the extended family, intensify these parents' needs for information and support. Psychiatric nurses are uniquely suited to meet these needs, for they can offer both counseling and child care information and skills.

Nurses must be aware of their own feelings when they work with parents. It is easy to lay all a child's problems at the parents' doorstep. This is simplistic. It is also therapeutically counterproductive and can reinforce the parents' feelings of helplessness. It is essen-

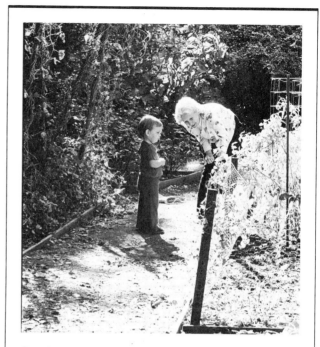

Grandparents, when they are interested and available, can provide an important source of support to parents.

tial to assess the strengths, as well as the weaknesses, of an individual's parenting ability. Within limitations imposed by factors beyond their control, most parents do their best to raise physically and psychologically healthy children. The nurse should give the parents positive reinforcement for the things they have done right, rather than focusing exclusively on their deficiencies.

Postnatal Assessment   Specific things to assess postnatally include

1. Parental expectations of the infant
   a. Are they realistic in terms of normal growth and development?
   b. Are the parents basically happy and pleased with the baby?
2. Competence of primary caregiver in meeting infant's needs
   a. How competent is this parent at meeting the infant's psychosocial needs—holding, talking to the infant, providing or reducing stimulation at appropriate times?
   b. What is this parent's attitude toward meeting the infant's needs? Does the primary caregiver seem to enjoy the care-giving tasks? Both what

is done and the style in which it is done should be assessed.

3. Support system for parents

    a. If it is a two-parent family, what kind of support are the parents able to furnish one another?

    b. If it is a single parent family, does the parent have someone to share the parenting experience with?

    c. Is there support available outside the nuclear family?

        (1) Are there friends or family in the area?

        (2) Are they willing and able to furnish support?

    d. Do the parents have interests outside the home to meet their needs for adult companionship?

        (1) Is the primary caregiver isolated in the home with the infant most of the time?

        (2) If it is a two-parent family, are the parents able to have time alone?

4. Temperamental match between infant and primary caregiver

    a. Is the primary caregiver sensitive to the baby's needs?

    b. Does this parent derive satisfaction from the baby and from parenting?

Once the nurse is familiar with the general categories and rationale of infant–parent assessment, this postnatal assessment can usually be done in one visit. Ideally, it should take place in the home. Psychiatric wards and well baby clinics are other obvious settings for this type of assessment.

When Mr. G brought Jennifer in for a routine checkup, the child psychiatric nurse associated with the pediatrician noted that he seemed depressed. While Jennifer was with the physician, the nurse interviewed Mr. G. After talking about Jennifer's needs and how Mr. G, as the primary caregiver, was meeting them, the nurse asked about their friends and family. Mr. G replied that he and Mrs. G had family in another state and didn't have many friends "now." The nurse pursued this lead. Mr. G explained that he and his wife had had a small circle of friends before Mrs. G became pregnant. This group, with the exception of the Gs, were philosophically opposed to having children and had tried to dissuade the Gs from opting for parenthood. The Gs resented their friends' disapproval and had gradually dropped out of the group. The nurse had previously assessed the infant–

caregiver interaction between Jennifer and Mr. G as a positive and mutually satisfying one. It was now apparent that the Gs had no satisfactory support system. With Mr. G, the nurse explored ways they could make peer contacts and establish other supports.

The following excerpt from a novel by Norma Klein illustrates the feelings of a mother whose actual child does not match her prenatal fantasies. Prenatal counseling could have helped her to identify and explore alternatives to her fantasy infant before her child was born. Postnatal psychiatric nursing intervention could help her deal with her distress and establish a positive relationship with her infant.

At one, after I've gobbled up a huge lunch, they wheel in a small basket. "Here he is!" the nurse says cheerfully, handing something to me.

He! It really is a he! I sit there dumbfounded, looking down at the wool-wrapped creature in my arms. It can't be! I was going to have a girl. It was all planned. It can't be a boy, it just can't. I can't even move, I feel so distressed, as though they had handed me a two-headed child. How can it be a boy? Explain that to me, please. Okay, I'll explain it. There are two sexes. When a woman becomes pregnant, she has roughly, a fifty-fifty chance to have a boy all along. Why am I so shocked, so horrified? Where is all this much vaunted common sense that I always attribute to myself?

No one would believe this, but I have never once, in all these nine months, seriously considered for even one minute that I would not have a girl. Not once. How is that possible? I'm not that kind of a person. I'm never taken by surprise, I always foresee all possibilities.

But I wanted a girl! I don't want a boy. Oh, no! A boy! How can this have happened? The whole point of this was to have a girl, a little girl like Elizabeth, not someone to raise grossly in my own image, but that was there, sure it was, someone who would be like me, whom I could joke with, have fun with.

A boy? What will I do with a boy? Boys like baseball cards and motorcycles and . . . Jesus, where do I get these stereotypes? Usually I fight them tooth and nail, but deep down I do believe boys, little boys anyway, can't be as much fun as girls. They mature slower, they have more emotional problems, they aren't as verbal. . . . It's true! It's all true! I can cite thousands of examples.

Anyway, that's not the point, I wanted a girl. Most people if you ask them what you want say, "Oh anything . . . as long as it's healthy." I never said that. Are there any witnesses? I never said it, not once. I always said I want a girl. Wasn't anyone listening? It was already a boy, right when I was saying that, it was growing a tiny penis, it was all over right then, only I didn't know.

There ought to be a way to set this right. There must be dozens of women right here, right in this hospital who wanted boys and got girls, whose husbands wanted boys. Maybe a little switch? No one will know. Why not? We won't tell anyone. The nurses won't notice if the armbands are switched.

So why didn't I adopt a child? Wouldn't that have been easier? Then I could have specified the sex. No, I wanted my own. I really did. I wanted the experience of childbirth, and I wanted my own child. I knew my peculiarities. I knew I might not be the mother type, and I felt if it were my own child, that would make a difference. I still feel that. I don't really want to trade him. *

Parent–Child Fit

How much of a child's personality, character, and temperament is innate and present at birth is yet to be determined. But it is now generally accepted that individual differences do exist. The question of heredity versus environment is by no means resolved. Many scientists believe that the child is neither the exclusive product of the genetic program nor of the environment. Rather, the child is the product of the interaction between the two. These scientists are usually referred to as *interactionists*.

The *tabula rasa* theory of child development conceives of children as blank slates written on by environment. This theory has been effectively disputed by research such as that conducted by Chess, Thomas, and Birch (1959). Such studies have demonstrated that infants have individual patterns of responses and temperament. So have parents. Consideration of the parent's needs, capabilities, and temperament, as well as those of the infant offers a basis for assessing parent–child fit, a major component of parent–infant interaction.

Parents' comments have long reflected the basic concept of parent–child fit.

- "He was such a good baby, so easy to take care of."
- "It's really great how that little kid knows what she wants. She has a mind of her own."

These are comments about infants whose temperaments are very different. But in each case the parent–child fit is positive. Had it been negative, the same infants could have elicited these parental comments:

*Reprinted by permission of Joan Daves and by G. P. Putnam's Sons from *Give Me One Good Reason* by Norma Klein. Copyright © 1973 by Norma Klein.

- "He doesn't respond to me enough. He's always so quiet."
- "It drives me crazy. She never does what I want her to."

Parent–child fit is an interactive process that tends to reinforce itself, as Figure 13–1 illustrates. Figure 13–2 illustrates the effect of parent–child fit on one aspect of infant behavior (alertness) and the subsequent effect of this one behavior on the parent–child interactive process. These diagrams illustrate the fact that both the infant and the parent contribute to and mutually reinforce their temperamental interaction. As Rexford, Sander, and Shapiro (1976, pp. xvi–xvii) state: "The infant and the caretaking milieu are the constitutents of an open, interactive and regulative system, each component member participating in exchanges which mutually influence and regulate the behavior of the other."

There is no single right or wrong, better or worse temperament for infant or parent. The important factor is how their temperaments fit together. Like the other subjects of postnatal assessment, parent–child fit is ideally assessed in the home during the course of the family's daily routine. Table 13–1 presents the basic areas to be assessed. In a two-parent family where one parent is the primary caregiver, the other parent may be assessed in those areas in which he or she is involved with the infant. Support given to the primary caregiver by the second parent may also be evaluated, since a supportive partner will make it easier for the caretaking parent to meet the infant's psychological needs.

Making a postpartum visit to a single mother and her one-week-old son, the nursing student observed mother and infant during waking, changing, and feeding. The mother responded to the baby's cries by going over to the crib and talking to the baby as she changed him. "You little devil, it seems like you never sleep more than a few minutes at a time. Your poor mom will be run ragged by the time you're six months old." While these words could have been interpreted as angry, the mother's amused and happy tone of voice implied otherwise. The nurse noted that the mother handled the baby in a gentle, competent way. While feeding the baby, the mother held him closely and securely, frequently smiling and making eye contact with him. When the nurse asked specifically about the baby's activity level, the mother commented that he seemed much more active and harder to quiet than a younger sister she had cared for when she was in high school. The nurse then asked

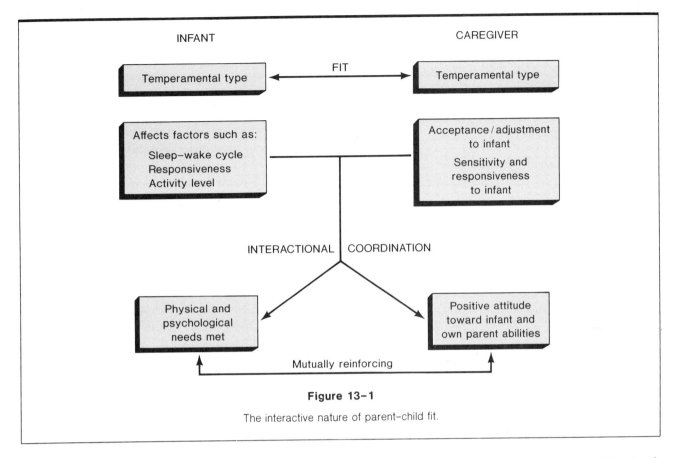

Figure 13-1

The interactive nature of parent–child fit.

how this was for the mother. She replied that she enjoyed it—the baby was much more company than a lot of "good, quiet" babies she knew. She added that she felt that her son really needed her and seemed to like her. The nurse assessed the mother as competent in caregiving activities and the mother–child fit as a positive one.

The parent–child fit can change with the child's developmental stage. A parent who competently and happily meets an infant's dependency needs may have difficulty meeting the same child's needs for separation and autonomy a year later. If the parent has unresolved conflicts left over from childhood, these can be reawakened when a child enters the developmental stage where the parental conflicts originated.

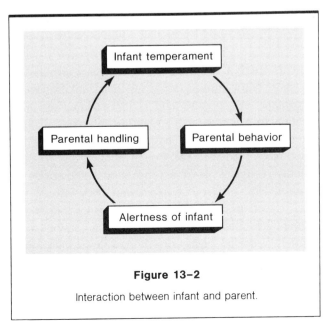

Figure 13-2

Interaction between infant and parent.

Table 13-1   ASSESSMENT OF TEMPERAMENTAL FIT BETWEEN INFANT AND PARENT

Child	Events	Parent
Reaction to delay	Feeding	Response to infant's reactions
Reaction to separation	Changing	
	Sleeping	Is parent empathic / flexible in meeting infant's needs?
Tense or relaxed	Waking	
Responsiveness	Playing	
		Does parent seem comfortable?

Ms. S had come to the child guidance center for an intake interview with her six-year-old son, Tai, who had been referred by the family pediatrician for psychiatric evaluation and intervention. While her son was with the psychiatrist, Ms. S was interviewed by the psychiatric nurse. She had brought her four-month-old baby, Arron, with her rather than leave him with a sitter.

The nurse noticed that Arron's hands were painted red. When questioned, the mother replied that she was trying to keep him from sucking his thumb by painting bad-tasting fluid on his hands. She added that he was "old enough to stop thumb sucking." The nurse explained Arron's need for oral gratification and exploration with his mouth as well as his hands. Ms. S agreed to stop using the paint.

Seeing Ms. S and Arron in the lobby a month later waiting for Tai to finish his play therapy session, the nurse noticed immediately that Arron's hands were bundled in mittens. Ms. S told the nurse she had tried, but she just "couldn't stand his sucking on his hands," so she had begun keeping them in mittens. The nurse responded sympathetically, reflecting that it was very hard for Ms. S to watch Arron suck his thumb. Ms. S agreed. She added that she would be glad when Arron could use a cup because she didn't like having him drink out of a bottle. She said she had already started trying to wean him. The nurse assessed Ms. S as being uncomfortable with Arron's infant dependency. She suspected that Ms. S was subconsciously dealing with conflicts generated in her own infancy. Recognizing the unfeasibility of working on an intrapsychic level with Ms. S, because Ms. S was extremely resistant to any therapy for herself, the nurse set up an appointment with her to discuss Arron's current needs and to describe how they would change. When she was given reassurance and specific information about the duration of the infancy stage, Ms. S was able to allow Arron to gratify his oral needs. Seeing mother and child a year later, the nurse was struck by how supportive Ms. S was of Arron's toddler needs for independence, exploration, and autonomy, and how comfortable she seemed to be with them.

Intervention Strategies

Assessment of parenting skills and parent–child fit forms the basis for therapeutic intervention. The specific intervention will depend on the assessed needs. It can range from simple presentation of information about growth and development to psychotherapy for help with intrapsychic disturbances that are affecting parenting ability.

The following section describes some interventions not previously considered in the chapter.

Parenting Classes   Ideally, these would begin in junior high. They would furnish prospective future parents with theoretical material about parenting and normal growth and development. In addition, clinical work could provide experiential learning by requiring actual child care.

Prenatal Classes   Most prenatal classes focus exclusively on pregnancy, labor, and delivery. While these subjects certainly need to be covered, this approach betrays an "and then they got married and lived happily ever after" mentality. Prenatal classes could also be used to teach parents about infancy, temperamental differences, and parental and infant needs. A teaching team composed of a nurse-midwife or maternity nurse-practitioner and a child psychiatric nurse could meet this need.

New Parent Groups   This is a pressing need for new parents. The chance to get together with other adults who are also experiencing new parenthood to exchange ideas, feelings, questions, frustrations, fears, and joys would go a long way toward alleviating the sense of isolation most new parents feel. Ideally, a nurse or other professional trained in child development would be part of the group. Parents often form groups like this spontaneously in playground or park settings. The OB unit, maternity care clinic, obstetrician's or pediatrician's office, and well baby clinic are obvious places to generate such groups.

Health Care Curriculum   Health care professionals, particularly nurses and physicians, are frequently in contact with parents and children. They are in a position to assess (and if necessary intervene in) parent–child interaction. In addition, parents frequently ask them for advice. Yet though nursing and medical schools require at least a fundamental knowledge of childhood growth and development, they virtually ignore parenting. Since the parent makes up half of any parent–child interaction, this interaction cannot be accurately assessed unless one knows something about parenting. Nursing and medical schools should include a basic working knowledge of parenting in the curriculum.

KEY NURSING CONCEPTS

✔ Due to the decline in the traditional extended families, parents frequently have little support or instruction in parenting skills. The nurse is frequently in a key position for counseling prospective, expectant, and actual parents on parent-child problems.

✔ Contemporary structures of parenting that have unique stresses include single parents; adoptive, foster, and stepparents; and working parents.

✔ The psychiatric nurse needs a basic working knowledge of the parenting process and appropriate counseling techniques.

✔ Because of the inherent stresses of parenthood, every parent is potentially abusive at times.

✔ New parents need factual information, support, and reassurance.

✔ Parent-child fit is an interactive process that tends to reinforce itself, although it can change with the child's developmental stage.

✔ Assessment of parent skills and parent-child fit forms the basis for the nurse's therapeutic interventions.

✔ Parenting intervention strategies include parenting classes, prenatal classes, new parent groups, and health care curricula.

References

Bowlby, J. "The Nature of a Child's Tie to His Mother." *International Journal of Psychoanalysis* 39 (1958): 350–373.

———. *Attachment*. Attachment and Loss Series, vol. 1. New York: Basic Books, 1969.

Chess, S.; Thomas, A.; and Birch, H. "Characteristics of the Individual Child's Responses to the Environment." *American Journal of Orthopsychiatry* 29 (1959): 791–802.

Helfer, R. *Child Abuse and Neglect: The Diagnostic Process and Treatment Programs*. DHEW Publication no. 75-69. Washington, D.C.: Government Printing Office, 1975.

Joint Commission on Mental Health of Children. *Crisis in Child Mental Health: Challenge for the 1970's*. New York: Harper and Row, 1969.

Klaus, M., and Kennell, J. *Maternal-Infant Bonding*. St. Louis: C. V. Mosby, 1976.

Klein, N. *Give Me One Good Reason*. New York: G. P. Putnam's Sons, 1973.

Nursing 79 in consultation with Leaman, K. "Recognizing and Helping the Abused Child." *Nursing 79* 9 (February 1979): 65–67.

Rexford, E.; Sander, L.; and Shapiro, T., Eds. *Infant Psychiatry*. Monographs of the *Journal of the American Academy of Child Psychiatry* (no. 2), New Haven: Yale University Press, 1976.

Spock, B. *Baby and Child Care*. Rev. ed. New York: E. P. Dutton, 1976.

Tillelli, J. A.; Turek, D.; and Jaffee, A. C. "Sexual Abuse of Children—Clinical Findings and Implications for Management." *New England Journal of Medicine* 302 (February 1980): 319–323.

Walker, L. "Identifying Parents in Need: An Approach to Adoptive Parenting." *American Journal of Maternal Child Nursing* 6 (March–April 1981): 118–123.

Further Reading

Bowlby, J. *Separation*. Attachment and Loss Series, vol. 2. New York: Basic Books, 1973.

Brazelton, T. *Toddlers and Parents*. New York: Delta Publishing, 1974.

Carr, J. "Communicating with the Child-abusing Family." *Topics in Clinical Nursing/Communication* 1 (October 1979): 41–48.

Norris, G., and Miller, J. *The Working Mother's Complete Handbook*. New York: E. P. Dutton, 1979.

Scharer, K. "Nursing Intervention with Abusive and Neglectful Families within the Community." *American Journal of Maternal Child Nursing* 8 (Summer 1979): 85–94.

Senn, M. J. E. "Hospitalism: A Follow Up Report." *Psychoanalytic Study of the Child* 2 (1946): 113–117.

Wilk, J. "Assessing Single Parent Needs." *Journal of Psychiatric Nursing* 17 (June 1979): 21–22.

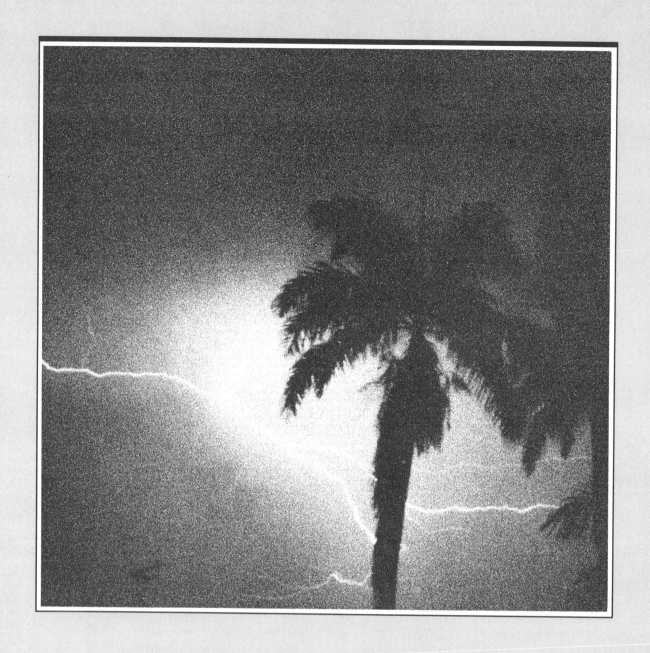

PART FOUR

Human Distress
and Dysfunction

IN PART FOUR WE EXAMINE *the application of the psychiatric
nursing process to clients whose distress and dysfunction in
personal, social, and occupational aspects of their lives place
them at the illness end of the health–illness continuum. The clients
discussed here are those generally diagnosed as having mental disorders
by the interdisciplinary psychiatric team. Here, we detail the content
usually associated with psychopathology in most psychiatric nursing texts.
All the chapters are fully updated to correspond with the terminology and
diagnostic criteria published in the American Psychiatric Association's third
edition of the* Diagnostic and Statistical Manual *(DSM-III) and the ninth
edition of the* International Classification of Diseases *(ICD-9). In Chapter
14 we cover non-psychotic clinical syndromes traditionally called
"neuroses." From a nursing perspective, in Chapter 15, we address the
life-style problems of clients' with Personality and Substance Abuse
Disorders. We offer an analysis of clients with psychotic conditions in
Chapter 16, emphasizing the nurse's role in promoting their self-care and
self-determination. Finally, in Chapter 17, we bring together conditions that
exist on the border between the biological and psychosocial models by
focusing on Psychophysiological Disorders, Organic Mental Disorders and
Developmental Disorders, historically termed "Mental Retardation." Our
emphasis in all these chapters is on nursing assessment, diagnosis, and
intervention strategies applied flexibly and creatively to this challenging
array of individual client problems.*

14

Disturbed Coping Patterns: Nonpsychotic Clinical Syndromes

CHAPTER OUTLINE

The Contours of Disturbances
The Need for a Holistic View
A Humanistic Interactionist Approach
  Control
  Balance
  Stress
  Anxiety
  Coping Strategies
  Inability to Cope Using Everyday Strategies
Therapeutic Intervention
  Specific Patterns Requiring Intervention
  Anxiety Disorders
  Dissociative Disorders
  Somatoform Disorders
Affective Disorders
Key Nursing Concepts

LEARNING OBJECTIVES

After reading this chapter, students should be able to

- Compare historical nosologies with contemporary ones
- Assess clients with disturbed coping patterns and plan interventions for anxiety, dissociative, somatoform, and affective disorder patterns
- Discuss the dynamics of the concepts of control, balance, stress, and anxiety in relation to the major disturbed coping patterns identified above

CHAPTER 14

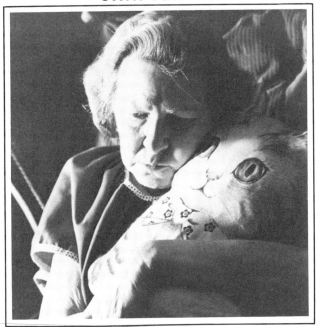

People for whom everyday coping strategies no longer ward off stress and anxiety feel troubled and unhappy and experience increased pain and distress.

Psychiatric *nosologies* are the ways in which emotional problems have been classified by psychiatric professionals who seek to understand them. These nosologies may be highly complex, including genera, species, types, and entities. Or they may be as simple as a single holistic concept of mental illness. The following list is an example of a complex nosology. It is Immanuel Kant's classification of weaknesses and diseases of the "soul" (quoted in Menninger 1963, p. 441) dating from the Enlightenment (1600–1700).

1. Weaknesses of the soul in regard to its cognitive faculties
   a. Partial weaknesses
      (1) Stumpfsinn: lack of wit
      (2) Dummheit: lack of judgment
      (3) Einfalt: lack of comprehension
      (4) Zerstreuung: lack of attention
      (5) Thorheit: sacrificing valuable things for worthless ones
      (6) Narrheit: foolishness that is insulting to others
   b. Total weaknesses
      Blodsinnigkeit: idiocy, for instance, cretinism
2. Sicknesses of the soul
   a. Grillenkrankheit (whimsical disease)

   (1) Hypochondrie: excessive preoccupation with one's body, with exaggerated mirth, wittiness, joyous laughter, moodiness . . . originates in a childish, anxious fear of the thought of death"
   (2) Raptus: sudden change of mood. . . . manifestations can be suicide
   (3) Melancholia: "a delusion of misery, created by the gloomy person"
   b. Mania or "the disturbed disposition" (das gestorte Gemut)
      (1) Amentia (Unsinnigkeit): "the impossibility of bringing one's representations into sufficient coherence for enabling [personal growth] experience"
      (2) Dementia (Wahnsinn): systematic delusions, for instance, of persecution
      (3) Insania (Wahnwitz): unsystematized delusions
      (4) Vesania (Aberwitz): delusion of a man who "pretends to comprehend the incomprehensible," for instance, the squaring of the circle or perpetual motion

The current official psychiatric nomenclature published in 1980 by the American Psychiatric Association appears in Appendix B. It identifies some conditions that are neither organic disorders, personality disorders, nor psychotic conditions, yet are associated with functional disability or the experience of distress. These mental disorders, termed "psychoneuroses" in recent history, are the focus of this chapter. They occur without tangible cause or structural changes in the brain or nervous system.

THE CONTOURS OF DISTURBANCES

People can go awry in a variety of ways more bewildering than the neat categories of any nosology would lead us to believe. To illustrate this principle, consider the following example (adapted from Kovel 1976, pp. 3–9):

David M was forty-three years old. He had lived all his life in the great decaying city for which he worked as a police inspector. His uncle and father had both been lawyers, and although he was never able to achieve his ambition of going to law school as they had done, David took comfort in being able to check up on other people's lives.

David had been relatively content with his work until the last two years or so. Then things began to go to pieces. Some of his associates in the police force had been caught taking bribes. Others had been beaten up by adolescent gangs. David's best friend had been in a car accident, and now he was confined to a wheelchair. Demoralization and worry replaced the sense of pride that David once had taken in his work. Then one day, during an interrogation, a suspect cursed him and knocked him down. Although he felt no anger—only fear—it was necessary to press charges. But his assailant got off with a suspended sentence, and David's fear continued to increase. Furthermore, it began to take a new form. He became obsessed with worry about an old wound.

Fifteen years before, David had lain on the verge of death. He had suffered a cerebral aneurysm—a weakness in the wall of his cerebral artery—which bled. The aneurysm was ligated, and a neurosurgeon reinforced it with a metal clip. The doctor had said there was no need to worry—the clip could not give way and the vessel could not open up. Yet David M could never quite shake the fear that it might. He had been too close to death, and he had always been fussy about his health. Now, under the pressure of stress, the fear became a preoccupation.

He withdrew from his weekly bowling league. His sex life suffered too, although he was quick to attribute this to aging. Despite his doctor's reassurances, he couldn't dismiss the idea that the suspect's blow might have loosened the clip in his head. He took a leave of absence from his job. He talked about leaving the city, but he had no clear goals. His behavior was deteriorating completely when he brought his fear to a therapist.

There is more to David's story, of course. A therapist can never confidently say, "Now I know enough, now I understand this client." Still, no matter how little we know of our troubled clients, we are constantly forming hypotheses about what we do know.

It is important to take some of David M's story as he presents it. His fear does have a lot to do with the danger of the decaying city, his thoughts of approaching death, and the attack by the suspect. Yet, as is usually the case with disturbed people who come to the attention of psychiatric nurses, there is more to it than that. Why wasn't Mr. M angry at his assailant? Why is his sex life suffering? Why do his eyes dart about as the logic of his explanations breaks down? His class, race, and occupation have given form and structure to his identity. His work as a police inspector in particular has given him a sense of being somebody—a proof of his life's value. If that is taken away, he is primed for trouble.

THE NEED FOR A HOLISTIC VIEW

In order to understand David M even partially, it is necessary to take a holistic view. No matter how circumscribed a disturbed pattern may seem, it is always part of the client's total reality. Yet the holistic approach makes matters far more complicated for psychiatric nurses. It would be simpler to select from the client's total experience some single factor that would explain the problem—some infantile trauma, fixated libido, schizophrenogenic mothering, or destructive conditioning. Not only would the task of understanding David M be much simpler, but the strategies for restoring his well-being would be equally clear-cut. To paraphrase psychiatrist Joel Kovel (1976), what is missing is an appreciation of the richness of human reality. A survey of the landscape of disturbed coping patterns reveals two common features:

1. A loss of inner freedom to make choices
2. Domination by hateful and frightening aspects of experiences

---

A HUMANISTIC INTERACTIONIST APPROACH

In thinking about disturbed coping patterns it is best to adopt a viewpoint that emphasizes processes and change. People have certain physical, chemical, and psychological resources with which they interact with the other people and situations in their environment. From time to time most people's coping patterns break down. The breakdown may be no more than a slight impairment to smooth adaptive control and organization. Or it may be as serious as the regressions, disorganizations, and failures of ego function that lead to hospitalization. Understanding the continuum of disturbed coping patterns permits some useful distinctions to guide helpful nursing interventions.

This book takes a humanistic interactionist perspective somewhat broader than is customary in psychiatric theory. It does so by using five major concepts to explain the dynamics of commonly recognized disturbed coping patterns. These five concepts are control, balance, stress, anxiety, and coping defenses.

Control

The word *ego* has many meanings. In psychology it means that part of the personality that experiences, perceives, reflects, suffers, decides, and controls behavior. In Freudian psychiatry it means a group of psychological parts or functions that control and direct human instinctual drives. Ego gives personality its firmness and its boundaries. Without ego functions, people become helpless manikins buffeted by the powerful forces of their instincts. Ego is equated with personality or character structure. In fact, the nature of the ego has been a subject of much speculation and research. Most theorists agree that the concept of ego refers to the processes that are used in the self-regulation of human behavior (see Chapter 10). These processes, called ego functions, are:

- Perception
- Control of voluntary movement
- Management of memory
- Production of adaptive delay between perception and action
- Decisions between "fight" and "flight"
- Selection of needs to be gratified
- Judgment and evaluation of internal and external conditions
- Problem solving
- Learning
- Reality testing

The ego regulates the self, maintains the balance between drives and values, and preserves the integrity of personal identity. Like a periscope it constantly scans the environment for possibilities, necessities, threats, and opportunities. At the same time, it remains in constant contact with the urges of somatic functioning.

Drives and moral values are constantly being reconciled, often without any strain or tension. However, some circumstances can distress ego processes to the threshold of extinction. Because it has the capacity to perceive anxiety, the ego serves a signal function. In order to perform its adaptive function of discrimination, it must also perceive and test reality. In short, the ego or *self-system* is a controlling agency that recognizes messages, receives input, stores memories, discriminates among perceptions, integrates life experiences, and guards the adaptive balance between the person and social world.

Balance

The "Health–Illness" Continuum   In process-oriented theory, a disturbed coping pattern is a troubling, uncomfortable state of existence. It is troubling to the afflicted person, or the afflicted person's companions, or both. The total disturbance is the focus of clinical attention. People with disturbed patterns frequently become psychiatric clients. In these people a shift in balance has occurred that lowers the effective quality of living.

Everyone undergoes constant shifts in balance. Usually the balance is easily restored. But certain events can upset the balance of social functioning beyond the point where it can be righted immediately. When this happens, a crisis occurs, and special restorative maneuvers are instituted. All these considerations—the circumstances, the person's perception of the circumstances, and reactions to that perception—make up the clinical picture that we encounter in psychiatric clients. Disturbed coping patterns, then, are associated with an imbalance—a disequilibrium between a person and the social world. Most nurses accept the idea that there is such a mutual process of adaptation between person and social world. Yet we often take refuge in oversimplification by relying on intrapsychic explanations of neurosis. The concept of balance enables us to incorporate this interactive adaptation and maladaptation into our assessment and interventions with disturbed clients.

Homeostasis   The principle that all organisms react to changing conditions in such a manner as to maintain a relatively constant internal environment or a *steady state* was introduced into physiology from chemistry. The combination of processes that maintain an organism's steady state is called *homeostasis*.

The concept of homeostasis may be extended beyond the regulation of the body. It then accounts for the conservative and defensive reaction patterns that influence the mobilizations of energy to maintain personal harmony. However, some critics believe that the concept of homeostasis fails to account for more complex forms of behavior. These include creativity, the search for novelty and uniqueness, and continued maturation and growth. Life cannot be satisfying without stability, yet the completely stable life seems less than human.

The concept of a *vital balance* combines both the conserving and the exploring capabilities of human beings. Its disruption is described by clients who exclaim, "I feel like I'm going to pieces!" or "I'm falling apart!" By using expressions like "upset" or "unbalanced" or "going to pieces," the client implies an awareness of a natural equilibrium and of a stress that threatens that equilibrium.

Stress

While there is no generally agreed-on definition of stress, Axis IV of DSM-III offers some general parameters for assessing the severity of stress (see Chapter 8). Some theorists define mild stresses as those whose effects last from seconds to hours. A mild stress might be caused by missing a train or burning the dinner. Moderate stresses are those whose effects last from hours to days. Moderate stress might be caused by overwork, an unwelcome guest, or a marital quarrel. Severe stresses are those whose effects last over weeks, months, or even years. Severe stresses might be caused by the death of a loved one, poverty, or a degenerative illness. In general, however, it is useful to apply the word *stress* or *stressor* to the source or the producer, not to the effects. The internal state that the stress usually produces is one of tension, anxiety, or strain.

Conflict as a Stressor   The concept of conflict is useful in identifying the stresses that help cause disturbed coping patterns. *Conflict* is a state in which opposing desires, feelings, or goals coexist. Conflict often explains such observable behaviors as hesitation, vacillation, blocking, and fatigue. Conflict is frequently seen in the behavior of psychotic clients, who may have difficulty making even the simplest decisions.

The following conflicts are the most likely to cause anxiety:

- Conflicts that involve social relations with significant people
- Conflicts that involve ethical standards
- Conflicts that involve meeting unconscious needs
- Conflicts that involve the problems of everyday family living

A conflict proceeds according to the following four steps:

1. The person holds two goals simultaneously.
2. The person moves in relation to both of the goals, using
   a. Approach–avoidance movements, or
   b. Avoidance–avoidance movements.
3. The person shows hesitation, vacillation, blocking, or fatigue.
4. Resolution occurs either temporarily or permanently.

Conflict with Approach–Avoidance Movements   When a person holds two incompatible goals at the same time, the goals usually constitute an either–or situation. If the person chooses one goal, the other goal will be rejected or abolished automatically. This situation is called a double approach–avoidance conflict. Here is an example:

Mrs. R holds two goals. She wants to talk with the nurse about her fears of her scheduled surgery. At the same time, she wants not to be perceived as weak or "a bother." Mrs. R makes a movement in relation to her first goal—talking to the nurse—by ringing the bell. When the nurse enters the room, Mrs. R asks some superficial question about her supper. In this way she avoids discussing her real concerns. When the nurse offers an opening to talk further, Mrs. R avoids the conversation she needs by saying she wants to rest. An hour later, she rings the bell again with an apologetic but vague question about her scheduled operation.
Vacillation describes Mrs. R's behavior.

Principles that Explain Vacillation   In order to understand how vacillation comes to be the manifest behavior, and what is going on during a conflict situation like the one described above, it is necessary to understand four key principles.

1. As you near a desirable goal, the approach tendency is strengthened.

2. As you near an undesirable goal, the avoidance tendency is strengthened.

3. The strength of the avoidance tendency always increases more rapidly with nearness to the goal than does the strength of the approach tendency. That is, the avoidance gradient is steeper than the approach gradient.

4. The strength of both tendencies varies with the strength of the need basic to the tendencies. That is, an increased need can strengthen both tendencies and intensify the conflict, while a decreased need can weaken both tendencies and lessen the conflict.

Avoidance–Avoidance Conflict   In avoidance–avoidance conflict, a person is faced with two undesirable goals at the same time. The person will attempt to avoid the nearer of these two goals, but with the retreat from the nearer goal, the tendency to avoid the second goal will increase. Unless the tendency to avoid one of the goals overpowers the tendency to avoid the other, or unless there is a third way out of the conflict the person will feel trapped by the conflict.

Robert P, the thirty-five-year-old son of well-to-do parents, was strongly attracted to "the good life." He wanted to live in a creative, esthetic environment, read good books, attend the opera, drink quality wine. Simultaneously he both wanted to avoid working to earn the money for the life-style he desired and rejected the idea of depending on his parents to support him. His life-style became one of waiting to find a resolution to his conflict. He neither worked nor accepted "handouts" from his family, but his preferred life-style became one that he talked about rather than lived.

Conflict and Anxiety   Conflict is a compelling experience. It increases tension and provides energy, and thus it is a crucial factor in behavior. When we cannot use the energy to resolve the conflict, we are often left with a stalemate. Or we may make a maladaptive response to allay the anxiety associated with the conflict. A client in this situation may show hesitation, blocking, vacillation, tension, and withdrawal.

Anxiety

Anxiety is the internal feeling caused by conflicts and frustrations (see also Chapter 10). It is usually experienced as unexplained discomfort. It is frequently coupled with guilt, doubts, fears, and obsessions. Anxiety is a potent force, for the energy it provides can be converted into destructive or constructive action. When it is used destructively, anxiety can immobilize a person with problems. When it is used constructively, anxiety can stimulate the action necessary to alter the stressful situation, fill a painful need, arrange a compromise, and so forth. It is easier to use anxiety constructively when a client understands its source.

People could not live without anxiety. It arises from many sources—dangers of the outer world and inner feelings. However, past a certain point anxiety can become a problem in its own right. When this happens, it is a signal that the forces behind the anxiety are calling for attention.

Degrees of Anxiety   THE ANXIETY CONTINUUM Many theorists conceptualize anxiety in the continuum presented in Figure 14–1. Mild to moderate anxiety can be functionally effective in that it helps us focus our attention and generates energy and motivation. Thus anxiety is an aspect of problem solving in that it alerts us to the need to concentrate our resources. However, severe anxiety and panic narrow our attention to a crippling degree. Under these conditions alertness is greatly reduced, and learning does not usually take place.

OBSERVABLE BEHAVIOR AT EACH STAGE ON THE CONTINUUM   In *mild anxiety* (+) the perceptual field—that is, sensory reception—is broad. We may be more alert than usual and better able to observe what is going on in ourselves and in our environment. We can see connections between events and explain them to others.

In *moderate anxiety* (++) the perceptual field is narrowed, but we may be more alert and better able to

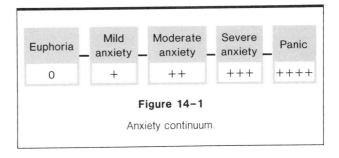

Figure 14–1

Anxiety continuum.

concentrate on one specific thing. We engage in selective inattention by shutting out what is irrelevant to the task or issue at hand. We can still perceive and understand connections between events.

In *severe anxiety* (+++) what we perceive is greatly reduced. We focus on a small detail or scattered details of the experience and cannot perceive the connections between these scattered details and the experience as a whole.

In *panic* (++++) a detail that previously served as a focal point is distorted and enlarged, or the perceptual field is completely disrupted. Most of what we attempt to communicate is unintelligible to the listener. A panic state could be described as the disintegration of personality organization and control into innumerable bits. A person experiences this disintegration as the most intense terror.

Selective Inattention and Dissociation Selective inattention and dissociation are both closely related to anxiety. *Selective inattention,* a filtering out of stimuli, occurs in moderate and severe anxiety. We may notice what we had not particularly attended to previously. If the noticed event is a disturbing one that could be ignored before, we may experience some discomfort in noticing it.

When we experience severe anxiety, we tend to *dissociate* anxious feelings from ourselves—to deny their existence in awareness. This dissociation protects the self from a threatening awareness of uncomfortable feelings resulting from stress and thus prevents possible panic. Dissociation actually helps us not to notice what is going on.

Cues to Anxiety Mild anxiety underlies such observable irritations as restlessness, sleeplessness, hostility, belittling, misunderstandings, and the like. It also underlies such persistent behavior as curiosity, repetitive questioning, constant attention seeking, and approval or reassurance seeking.

Anxiety Distinguished from Fear Although most psychiatric nursing literature distinguishes anxiety from fear, it is probably important to note that all emotions are complex. We experience them in many mixtures and degrees. However, the usual theoretical distinction is that fear occurs in response to a real danger or threat, whereas anxiety occurs in response to situations that are not actually dangerous. Sometimes anxiety occurs with no specific stimulus.

Most people have a pretty good idea of what an extreme fear response is like. It is important to appreciate the intensity of this emotion. Fear is sometimes so intense that it severely impairs, or even totally blocks, functioning. Few situational stresses compare with war in their potential for arousing incapacitating fear. The collection of behaviors and manifestations fear excites was called shell shock in World War I. In subsequent wars, it was called war neurosis, combat fatigue, combat exhaustion, and Post-traumatic Stress Disorder. If war is truly a situational stress, however, the manifestations should diminish when the person is removed from the field of combat. Unfortunately this does not always happen, leading some people to the speculation that perhaps war is more than a situational stress.

Anxiety is an uncanny, unpleasant feeling that something is not right. It is usually stimulated by a threat to some value that we hold essential to our existence as personalities. In some instances the threat is obvious; in others, it is obscure. The values threatened are unique to each person. To one person, power and prestige are essential; to another, freedom; to a third, the love of others. Whatever the value, we see it as necessary, and when it is threatened we experience anxiety.

Data that Indicate Fear Usually the experience of fear is inferred from three kinds of data:

1. Reports of subjective experiences, including apprehension, fright, tension, inability to concentrate, going to pieces, the wish to flee, and physical sensations, such as a pounding heart or a sinking feeling in the pit of the stomach

2. Behavorial manifestations, including flight, disorganization of speech, motor incoordination, impairment of performance, and sometimes immobilization

3. Measurable physiological responses that represent activation of the sympathetic nervous system, including restlessness, frequent urination, increased blood pressure, rapid rate and changed quality of respirations, increased perspiration, and change in pupil size

Mild and moderate anxiety usually speed up physiological operations, whereas severe anxiety slows them down and can even paralyze them. Prolonged panic can result in a complete paralysis of functioning, culmi-

Table 14-1 AUTONOMIC NERVOUS SYSTEM RESPONSES		
Organ	Sympathetic Response	Parasympathetic Response
Adrenal medulla	Secretes epinephrine and norepinephrine	None
Heart	Rate increases Force of contraction increases	Rate decreases

Blood vessels,
  To skeletal muscles,
  heart, brain
	Dilate; blood flow increases	Constrict; blood flow decreases

To viscera (stomach, intestines, colon)	Constrict, blood flow decreases	Dilate; blood flow increases
Lungs	Air passages dilate	Air passages constrict
Stomach	Inhibits secretion of acid and pepsin	Secretes acid and pepsin
Salivary glands	Secretion is inhibited	Secrete saliva
Liver	Releases sugar	None
Colon	Action is Inhibited	Tone increases
Rectum	Action is Inhibited	Releases feces
Genitals	Ejaculate (males) Blood vessels constrict (females)	Firm erection (males) Blood vessel dilation (females)
Pupils of eyes	Dilate	Constrict
Sweat glands and palms of hands	Secrete sweat	None

nating in death. This observation illustrates the relationship between the mind and the body. Anxiety is a multidimensional phenomenon in that the total person is involved in *every* aspect of it. Our perception of the threat, our interpretation of it, the way in which our past and present and our estimates of the future influence how we cope, our own interpersonal and cultural milieu—are all involved in anxiety. Consequently, most clinicians acknowledge that while both sympathetic and parasympathetic effects are observed among the bodily changes in anxious persons, the specific patterns of physical manifestation are determined by the balance of involuntary functions characteristic of each specific client. (See Table 14–1 and Figure 14–2.)

Sources of Anxiety   People experience anxiety in many different kinds of situations and interpersonal relationships. The stimulus varies with the individual. However, the general causes of anxiety have been classified into two major kinds of threats.

1. Threats to biological integrity: actual or impending interference with basic human needs such as the need for food, drink, or warmth

2. Threats to the security of the self:

   a. Unmet expectations important to self-integrity

   b. Unmet needs for status and prestige

   c. Anticipated disapproval by significant others

   d. Inability to gain or reinforce self-respect or to gain recognition from others

   e. Guilt, or discrepancies between self-view and actual behavior

Operational Definition of Anxiety   To deal effectively with clients who are anxious, nurses must understand the operational definition of anxiety. Manaser and Werner (1964, p. 127) summarize it as follows:

• Expectations or needs are present.

• Expectations or needs are not met.

• Unexpected discomfort (anxiety) is felt.

• Anxiety is controlled and power is restored through some automatic behavior (e.g., anger, withdrawal, somatization) that has been effective in restoring control in the past.

• The relief behavior is rationalized or justified rather than being explained or understood.

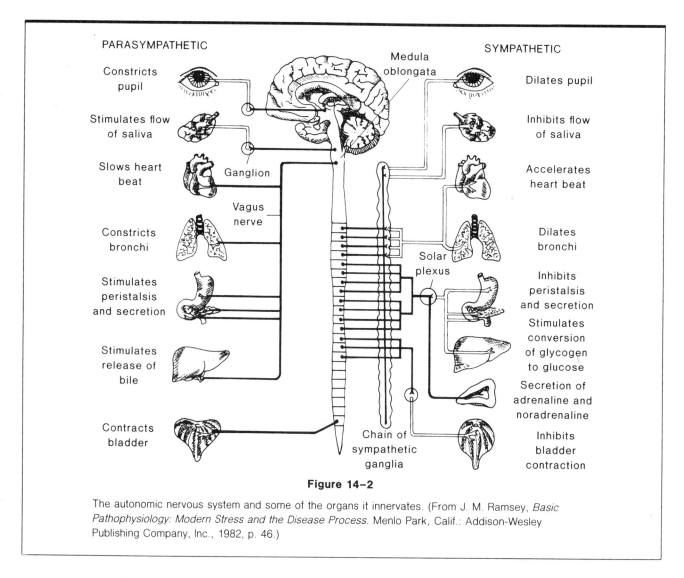

PARASYMPATHETIC

Constricts
pupil

Stimulates flow
of saliva

Slows heart
beat   Ganglion

                        Vagus
                        nerve

Constricts
bronchi

Stimulates
peristalsis
and secretion

Stimulates
release of
bile

Contracts
bladder

Medula
oblongata

SYMPATHETIC

Dilates pupil

Inhibits flow
of saliva

Accelerates
heart beat

Dilates
bronchi

Solar
plexus

Inhibits
peristalsis
and secretion

Stimulates
conversion
of glycogen
to glucose

Secretion of
adrenaline and
noradrenaline

Chain of
sympathetic
ganglia

Inhibits
bladder
contraction

Figure 14–2

The autonomic nervous system and some of the organs it innervates. (From J. M. Ramsey, *Basic Pathophysiology: Modern Stress and the Disease Process*. Menlo Park, Calif.: Addison-Wesley Publishing Company, Inc., 1982, p. 46.)

Coping Strategies

Stress is part of modern life. However, the devices people choose to cope with stress depend on many factors. Among them are the external circumstances, the suddenness and intensity of the stress, the resources available to the person, and the person's predisposition to one or another coping pattern. Certain coping patterns are established in the course of one's development. One man who is late for an appointment because he gets caught in a traffic jam may react with a furious outburst of anger. Another may begin to daydream and forget where he is going. A third may use the time to solve some problem. Everyone develops strategies to cope with stress.*

*Special acknowledgment is made to Joel Kovel (1976) for his ideas on everyday coping strategies.

Turning to a Comforting Person   No doubt the earliest coping strategy is the familiar method of turning to a mothering figure for soothing and protecting. To get love is to be reassured that one is lovable. Love from supportive others may take the form of physical touching, rocking, patting, or verbal reassurances of various kinds ("Don't be afraid, I'll stay with you"). This category also includes the function of eating in times of stress and for general support. Alcohol, nicotine, and other chemicals are often used to enhance well-being in the face of stress. Many theorists view these alternatives as substitutes for the dependent comfort of being a baby in the care of a mothering parent.

Relying on Self-Discipline   While some people under stress tend to turn to the comfort of friendly company, food, or alcohol—all of which are reminiscent of childhood dependency—others rely on self-discipline. Self-control ranks high in the value system of many cultures and subcultures. This coping style involves pride in the ability to laugh off problems, endure frustrations, and discount anxiety. Keep a stiff upper lip, bite the bullet, and get over it—are all admonitions that people address to themselves when self-discipline is their patterned response to stress. These people are unlikely to want the company of supportive others and may even push them away. They are often unresponsive when others seek comfort from them, for they see such dependency as weak.

Intense Expression of Feeling   Crying, swearing, and laughing all tend to relieve tension. Swearing loses its usefulness as an escape valve if it becomes a habit. This is less likely to be true of crying and of laughing. Crying and laughing tend to release energy and exert a soothing effect on a person who is experiencing tension.

Avoidance and Withdrawal   While some people find it hard to sleep when they are under tension, others react to worries, bad news, or an argument with somnolence. Still others respond with a form of waking sleep like apathy or emotional withdrawal, which accomplishes the same thing.

Talking It Out   Many people relieve tension by talking it out. Talking implies establishing and maintaining a contact of sorts with another human being. In addition, it enables new ideas to emerge and new perspectives to be entertained. Obviously, this device is the medium of most therapeutic intervention.

Privately Thinking It Through   Some people believe that the unexamined life is not worth living. When faced with a problem that causes them anxiety, they become introspective about it. The rationalizations that emerge serve as effective tension relievers.

Working It Off   Acting to relieve tension may range from pointless activity such as finger tapping, floor pacing, and door slamming to activities purposely designed to alter the tension-producing circumstances. In addition, some tense individuals feel a lot of aggressive energy. Physical exertion in the form of demanding sports, like soccer or tennis, or manual labor, like washing walls or scrubbing the floor, uses this energy constructively.

Using Symbolic Substitutes   Stress may be relieved by ascribing symbolic values to acts or objects. These acts or objects may or may not have other meanings. There are symbolic devices for the management of tensions in religious conventions like meditation, confession, prayer, or sacrifice. For some people, the automobile has a symbolic significance; for others, it is an annual income or their physical appearance. The list is almost endless, but the principle is always the same. Some people attach a meaning beyond the obvious one to objects, experiences, and people. Through their involvement with these meanings, they find a means to reduce their tensions.

Somatizing   Many organs have an expression and communication function. This is sometimes known as *somatizing* or *organ language*. Some organs communicate their messages only to their owner. For example, the heart may communicate by means of palpitation. Other organs communicate publicly, for example, in blushing or stuttering. Urination and defecation, increased sweating, and altered sexual activity are other familiar examples of organ language.

Inability to Cope Using Everyday Strategies

The coping strategies described above are considered normal. They are simply ways of getting along. In some people, however, what passes for a normal adjustment is actually a very tenuous one with few outlets for controlled aggression, few sublimations, few love objects, few opportunities for satisfaction and growth. These people find it more and more difficult to cope with additional stress. Ultimately the external stress that the person is trying unsuccessfully to ward off is matched by a mounting internal stress. The person suffers both from increased anxiety and from the strain on overworked stabilizers.

People in this situation feel troubled. They may define their situation in one way, while family members define it in another, and psychiatric professionals making an assessment define it in still a third way. These judgments place the person somewhere on a health–illness continuum that ranges from happy, healthy, contented, and constructive at one end to disintegrating at the other.

Disturbed Coping Patterns   Threatened disorganization occurs when anxiety evoked by stressors exceeds the powers of the person's habitual coping devices. The person then resorts to coping patterns that are usually associated with diminished satisfactions and increased pain and distress. These coping patterns may consist of manifestations of the anxiety as it is directly felt and expressed. Or they may consist of efforts to control the anxiety by means of defenses such as conversion, dissociation, displacement, phobia formation, or repetitive thoughts and acts. These feelings or manifestations of anxiety usually have three characteristics. They are repetitive, unchanging in character, and representative of some behavior that was gratifying at an earlier stage of development. Sometimes the particular coping pattern affords a clue to the fundamental problem. More often it is best understood in terms of the function it serves.

Distinctions between "Neurotic" and "Psychotic" Patterns

For many years psychiatrists emphasized a supposed distinction between neuroses and psychoses. Now, however, most psychiatrists agree that there is little evidence to support this distinction. The distinction is often a function of the characteristics of the person making it. The classifications currently in use have omitted the old diagnostic class of "neuroses" based on the recognition that no consensus exists in contemporary psychiatry about the definition of "neurosis." In DSM-III the neurotic disorders are included in Affective, Anxiety, Somatoform, Dissociative, and Psychosexual Disorder categories. (Psychosexual Disorders are covered in Chapter 12.)

Some theorists still distinguish between neuroses and psychoses. One group believes that psychoses are major reactions and neuroses minor ones. Another group views neuroses and psychoses as successive stages on a continuum of the same mental process.

Distinctions between Healthy and Disturbed Patterns

To define a pattern of behavior as disturbed, we must first define mental health. The concept of mental health should not be confused with adjustment to societal norms. Everyone has values—including the ability to love; to act with inner freedom; and to be steadfast, affirmative, and affirming—that may be affected by disturbed coping patterns. However, it is probably an error to confuse virtue with health. In DSM-III a *mental disorder* is conceptualized as a behavioral or psychological pattern that occurs in an individual and is associated with either a painful symptom (distress) or inpairment in important areas of functioning (disability). In addition, the disturbance does not

merely reflect conflict between an individual and society.

In our therapeutic role we must try to answer three questions:

1. How do we recognize genuinely disturbed coping patterns?
2. How are these patterns constructed?
3. What constitutes therapeutic intervention appropriate to each pattern?

Recognizing Disturbed Coping Patterns Disturbed coping patterns can be recognized by the way the person manages anxiety. Although stress and anxiety are universal conditions of life, some people follow a distinctive course in developing a disturbed rather than functional coping style.

• The person is faced with a conflict so serious or anxiety laden that the usual problem-solving steps will not lead to a solution. These steps yield only a vague or inaccurate notion of the nature of the problem and offer no plan of constructive action.
• The person retreats from the conflict by attempting to block it out and avoid future situations that tend to reactivate it.
• Because most conflicts are not totally avoidable, the anxiety tends to recur regularly, but the person is not aware of its cause.
• The person mobilizes one or several defense mechanisms to control or manage the pervasive anxiety.

Properties of Disturbed Coping Patterns Disturbed coping strategies take several forms. However, they all have certain properties in common.

They are characterized by a loss of the ability to make choices. The outer world may permit a range of choice, but some subjective obstacle blocks the way. A student finds that he cannot finish his term paper, no matter how much opportunity he gives himself. A woman leaves her husband for another man, only to find that the man she thought she wanted now fails to excite her. A man desperately in need of a job won't answer an ad in the paper because something tells him he will be rejected. A teenager can't leave the house until she checks the lock four or five times. A young, attractive newlywed who wants a more exciting sex life is chronically tired or ill when her husband tries to make love to her.

Disturbed coping patterns are characterized by the presence of conflict. More specifically, the internal conflict is locked in a struggle that is outside conscious control. The battle rages simultaneously on two fronts—between the person and the external world and within the person's own self. This complex interplay of inner and outer events explains why several different therapeutic intervention strategies can be used to alleviate a given disturbed coping pattern.

Disturbed coping patterns are characterized by repetition and a feeling of blindness. The coping strategy is repeatedly attempted—even though it has failed before—in an effort to restore harmony and balance. Most disturbed or neurotic behavior is rigid and inappropriate as well as repetitive. Although it provides some benefits in warding off anxiety, in the long run it is ineffective. Everyday coping strategies offer an immense repertoire of defenses to maintain control and balance in the face of stress. A disturbed pattern, however, is a state of sustained imbalance. Sometimes the stress gets too strong—for example, when a child enters adolescence or a woman faces the role changes associated with new motherhood. Sometimes the defenses get too weak—for example, a person becomes physically ill or intoxicated. Sometimes both things happen at once—especially following a loss, such as a hysterectomy or a facial disfigurement. In all three cases the inner system of control goes haywire and cannot handle the external social context and all its sources of stress. Then the person feels unable to see new solutions and lapses into old patterns.

Disturbed patterns are characterized by alienation, because disturbed patterns fail to hold and leave people with a sense of being split. They feel estranged from their own bodies, feelings, thoughts, moods, and fears, as well as from other people. Disturbed coping patterns are thus said to be *ego dystonic*—that is, they distress the person. Yet although these people are genuinely troubled by their coping patterns, they cannot alter their behavior for fear of what they sense as unidentified, impending dangers. They are captives both of their own anxiety and fear and of the behaviors they use to control them.

People can use coping patterns for *secondary gain*, that is, they seek sympathy, psychological support, financial aid, and special treatment by virtue of being labeled ill. Secondary gain must be distinguished from *primary gain*. Primary gain refers to the function of the symptom itself. For example, a person who develops a conversion disorder paralysis may derive primary gain

from symbolic punishment for unconscious misdeeds.

In summary, the properties associated with disturbed coping patterns are:

- Loss of ability to make choices
- Presence of conflict
- Repetition, rigidity, and ineffectiveness of "solution"
- Alienation and feeling of being troubled and distressed
- Secondary gain

How Disturbed Patterns Are Constructed   Social forces play an enabling role in the construction of disturbed coping patterns. However, most clinicians believe that they are the unfinished madness of childhood carried forward. Prolonged dependency, intense self-centeredness, unbounded yearnings, and unique patterns of thought are peculiarities that children and people with disturbed coping patterns share.

In normal, favorable development the child's fears and conflicts are blotted out by continual reaffirmation of parental regard. Fears are put to rest by parental benevolence, and wants are neither aggravated nor ignored. Thus there is no reinforcement of childhood fears by the social environment. The child's capacity to love is nurtured, and the child is subjected day by day to civilizing influences.

However, some children experience repeated stress or *trauma*, a noxious state of any duration in which they feel overwhelmed, flooded with stimuli beyond their capacity to master and control. Physical injury can cause trauma. So can prolonged separation from caring parents. Ordinarily children have considerable resources for dealing with potentially traumatic situations. However, some situations overwhelm even the stoutest everyday coping strategies. When this happens, less effective patterns are called into action to defend the child against stress and anxiety. Because they worked to control anxiety, these patterns reappear later in life in an almost automatic way. At this point they have become disturbed coping patterns.

THERAPEUTIC INTERVENTION

So far, this chapter has described the nature of disturbed coping patterns and how they are experienced. The next section will consider the need for intervention. How is this need to be assessed? More specifically, how can one tell when things have gone too far? And what can be done about it?

The following discussion is based on the humanistic-interactionist idea that the external situation and the inner state of mind must both be considered when planning intervention—not separately, but rather as they interact with one another. It might help to consider a spectrum at one end of which are problems caused mainly by external factors and at the other end of which are problems caused mainly by internal factors. The following case study is an example of a mixture of both.

Ellen N thought she was "going crazy" and indeed gave a fair impression of being right. At nineteen she had begun sleeping with her boy friend and was terrified of her parents' judgment. Some years later she found herself sleepless, agitated, and wildly anxious. She had left her parents to marry someone with whom she had little in common. For a time she coped with the separation from her mother by adopting her mother's ways and protected herself from guilt with a self-effacement that other people found excessive. Then her mother died. Ellen became depressed. She felt she was a faithless daughter, even though she had nursed her mother through a long decline, and she lost interest in life. Instead of rallying after a few months of mourning, Ellen kept sliding downhill to the point of functional incapacity. She suffered major interferences with sleeping, eating, and bowel function, and she began to entertain bizarre ideas about her body and to consider suicide. In addition, her husband and children considered their family life to be chronically miserable. They said sexual incompatibility, hatred, and lack of communication had alienated them from Ellen for years.

Where and with what goals does a therapist begin in this example? In general, to the extent that a client's subjective world is rich, flexible, and open to experience, we should choose objective interventions. Ellen and her parents could have gone to a family counselor and talked out their differing moral views early in her story. Ellen and her husband could have sought sexual counseling when their relationship began to deteriorate. A nurse might have provided therapeutic support to assist Ellen through the steps of the grieving process when her mother died.

On the other hand, to the extent that a client's subjective world is deadened, twisted, empty, or closed, the client will not be helped by objective intervention. In this case, therapeutic attention should focus on the client's subjective world. An example of such a client might be a striving young businessman who achieves outwardly in order to avoid inner guilt, anxiety, and depression. The outer, material rewards of success only increase his inner sense of hollowness or guilt, and this, in turn, spurs him on to further outer achievement. The end is a perfect life—job, family, possessions, pleasures all in place—that feels like a cage to the client. In this case, the therapist might focus on the intrapsychic processes of the client. Assessing the nature of the client's problem and planning creative and versatile interventions is a challenging task. The following descriptions of disturbed coping patterns are designed to provide the foundation on which to build unique approaches.

Specific Patterns Requiring Intervention

The clinical picture of most disturbed coping patterns is often a mixed one—that is, most patterns combine several elements of each labeled type. However, certain major types are identified as syndromes in the nosology of the American Psychiatric Association. These are Anxiety Disorders, Dissociative Disorders, Somatoform Disorders, and Affective Disorders. The following section examines each of these syndromes and some related intervention approaches in depth.

Anxiety Disorders

In this group of disturbed patterns, anxiety is either the predominant disturbance or a secondary disturbance, which is confronted if the primary symptom is taken away. Panic and Generalized Anxiety Disorders are examples of the first case and Phobic and Obsessive-compulsive Disorders are examples of the second.

Generalized Anxiety Disorders   In Generalized Anxiety Disorder, the anxiety is not displaced or automatically controlled by some repetitive thought or act. Instead, it remains diffuse, free-floating, and painful. Some of the many subjective experiences described by persons suffering from generalized anxiety are found in Table 14–2.

Panic Disorder   In addition to a chronic state of tension and anxiety accompanied by the experiences listed above, people with this coping pattern may be subject to acute, terrifying, paniclike attacks lasting

Table 14-2 SYMPTOMS OF GENERALIZED ANXIETY DISORDER		
Physiological	**Emotional**	**Intellectual**
Increased heart rate	Irritability	Forgetfulness
Elevated blood pressure	Angry outbursts	Preoccupation
Tightness of chest	Feeling of worthlessness	Rumination
Difficulty in breathing	Depression	Mathematical and grammatical errors
Sweaty palms	Suspiciousness	Errors in judging distance
Trembling, tics, or twitching	Jealousy	Blocking
Tightness of neck or back muscles	Restlessness	Diminished fantasy life
Headache	Anxiousness	Lack of concentration
Urinary frequency	Withdrawal	Lack of attention to details
Diarrhea	Diminished initiative	Past- rather than present- or future-orientation
Nausea and/or vomiting	Tendency to cry	Lack of awareness of external stimuli
Sleep disturbance	Sobbing without tears	Reduced creativity
Anorexia	Reduced personal involvement with others	Diminished productivity
Sneezing	Tendency to blame others	Reduced interest
Constant state of fatigue	Excessive criticism of self and others	
Accident proneness	Self-deprecation	
Susceptibility to minor illness	Lack of interest	
Slumped posture		

from a few moments to an hour. The person usually experiences palpitations, rapid pulse, nausea, diarrhea, dyspnea, and a feeling of choking or suffocation. The pupils are dilated, and the face is flushed. The person may feel dizzy or faint and often has a sense of impending death. Restlessness is acute, and the person may make pleading, apprehensive appeals for help. In its most developed state panic creates a symptom constellation totally mimicking severe cardiac disease. This symptom complex is seen most frequently in young adults and is called *cardiac neurosis*.

Symptoms involved in cardiac neurosis are: palpitations, tachycardia, chest pain, dyspnea, easy fatigability, dizziness, sweating, irritability, faintness, and a feeling of impending doom.

L was a thirty-two-year-old, married, male social worker who was employed as a case worker at a child welfare agency. He sought psychiatric help on the advice of his family physician. L reported an eighteen-month history of anxiety attacks, increasing in intensity and frequency, about which he had become quite frightened. The attacks seemed to occur mostly when he was alone,

often in his car or in a large store. He felt palpitations, tightness in the chest, shortness of breath, and dizziness. He would hyperventilate and was intensely fearful of collapsing in the street and dying. He had previously been to a cardiologist and had been given EKGs, stress tests, a complete workup. All results were negative. An especially serious development was that L found he was staying in his apartment, since attacks did not seem to occur there. This presented difficulties at his job and frightened both him and his wife.

L was almost totally preoccupied with his symptoms. The knowledge that he had no organic disease and reassurances that he was in no physical danger had little beneficial effect. After much patient, gentle probing, however, L said that his wife had been pressuring him to buy a house and that he was extremely frightened of the responsibility he felt such a move would place on him. It turned out that this had been a conflict in his parents' relationship as well, with his mother having been the frightened one. L identified strongly with her feelings, which had been more direct in preventing his parents from moving. In L's case some normal physiological sensations had most likely gradually been elaborated into a full-blown "cardiac neurosis," based on an especially stressful situation that had deep personal significance.

Both the acute attack of cardiac neurosis and the more lasting anxiety pattern require therapeutic intervention.

Intervention Strategies Most clinicians believe that clients who cope with stress through anxiety disorders can grow and change with therapeutic intervention. Usually this optimistic prognosis is related to the absence of highly systematized and established defense mechanisms. Several guidelines are useful in providing effective intervention for such clients.

First, the nurse should take direct measures to reduce intense anxiety. During an acute panic attack, perception is narrowed and disrupted to such a degree that the client cannot engage in problem solving. The panic must be dealt with first. The sample nursing care plan in Table 14–3 puts this principle into practice. The goal of the plan is to reduce the client's immediate anxiety to more moderate and manageable levels, since learning cannot occur in stage four anxiety (panic).

A nurse can frequently detect subtle indications of mounting anxiety and intervene to prevent a severe attack. Some clients are adept at covering up their anxiety, but they usually transmit something to the sensitive observer. Often the nurse's own feelings of increased tension are a useful cue that the source of anxiety is in the client. Anxiety may make people excessively demanding. The nurse's response to the demands must take into account the consequences for the course of the client's anxiety. In some cases it may be reassuring to set limits and deny the request. In other cases such a response may place further stress on the client.

Second, the nurse must know how to treat clients who suffer from prolonged anxiety patterns. Here the intervention strategies are intended to help clients use their anxiety to learn about themselves and their coping strategies. This requires that the client endure the anxiety while searching out its causes. The client must then develop more effective and satisfying coping strategies to replace the old ones. To help clients learn to cope more effectively with anxiety, the nurse must first detect the anxiety, and second make thoughtful observations and responses that facilitate learning. The operational definition of anxiety presented earlier in this chapter provides a framework for the care plan for an anxious client presented in Table 14–4.

The nurse who is working through this step-by-step intervention approach must avoid getting bogged down in the client's usual justification of his or her automatic coping pattern. Usually clients try to give plausible explanations for their ineffective anger, withdrawal, or somatization. However, they do not explain the relief in terms of the factors that caused the anxiety. The temporary feelings of relief afforded by the

Table 14–3 NURSING CARE PLAN FOR CLIENT IN PANIC

Step of Plan	Rationale
Assessment of Need	
Client is pacing and wringing her hands in a pointless, agitated manner. Tearfully she begs for help, says she is falling apart, can't concentrate, feels like she's going crazy.	
She is experiencing palpitations, chest pain, a feeling of choking, and trembling.	
Nursing Intervention Strategy	
1. Stay physically with client.	Often being left alone further aggravates person in panic.
2. Maintain calm, serene manner.	Anxiety is easily communicated from staff to client.
3. Use short, simple sentences and firm, authoritative voice.	Convey sense of ability to provide external controls.
4. Encourage client to move to a smaller physical environment, such as her room, to minimize the stimuli.	Client is already overwhelmed by stimuli.
5. Sometimes it is useful to focus client's diffuse energy on some physically tiring task such as moving furniture or scrubbing the floor.	Physical exercise can sometimes drain off high levels of anxiety.
6. It may be wise to recommend that antianxiety medication be ordered for client.	Certain somatic interventions are highly specific and effective in relieving panic.

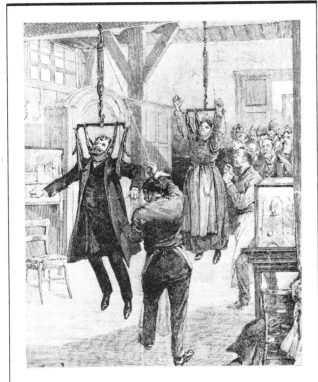

The Suspensory Treatment for Nervous Ataxia used at Salpêtrière Hospital, Paris.

automatic coping pattern do not last long, because the needs or expectations that originally caused it still exist. They may even become more intense. Only when these clients understand what their unmet needs are, what they did instead of fulfilling these needs, and what they felt then, can they begin to alter their disturbed coping patterns.

At this point, clients have two alternatives. They can reduce or change their hopes and expectations. Or they can try new tactics or resources to get their needs met. The nurse should discuss these options with the client and negotiate a contract to work on one or both goals. (See Chapter 7.) Realizing either option often involves problem solving. Nurse and client must find ways to alter structural features of the client's environment to reduce or meet the need.

Mrs. K, a working wife and mother, played out a superwoman role by bearing 75 percent of the family responsibilities, only to find that her husband, from whom she expected appreciation and admiration, resented her and her accomplishments. Her unmet needs for his approval and love created automatic coping patterns of anger or depression, and he withdrew even further from her demands. Strategies for Mrs. K might include

Table 14–4   NURSING CARE PLAN FOR ANXIOUS CLIENT

Step of Plan	Nursing Intervention
1. Observe client for increased psychomotor activity, anger or withdrawal, excessive demands, and tearfulness.	Verbalizations intended to help client recognize and name his experience as anxiety.
	"Are you feeling uncomfortable?" "Are you anxious or nervous now?"
	When client says "Yes," he is ready for Step 2.
2. Connect feeling of anxiety with relief behavior. Client acknowledges, describes, and names feelings of nervousness or anxiety.	Ask client what he does to feel more comfortable when he feels anxious.
	When client understands that when he feels anxious he gets angry, withdraws, or somatizes, he is ready for Step 3.
3. Investigate situation that immediately preceded feeling of anxiety.	Encourage client to recall and describe what he was experiencing immediately before he got anxious (including thoughts, actions, and other feelings).

4. Help client observe, describe, and analyze connections between what led to his anxiety and what happened after he felt anxious. Only through seeing all parts of this experience can client understand why he became anxious.

5. Formulate causes of anxiety. Help client state causes of the anxiety. Then help him observe and recall similar instances in his experiences of anxiety. Through such extensive discussions, client will eventually be able to recognize and perhaps alter his pattern of handling anxiety.

Source: H. Peplau, "Interpersonal Techniques: The Crux of Nursing." Copyright © 1962, American Journal of Nursing Company. Adapted with permission from the *American Journal of Nursing*, June, Vol. 62 No. 6.

redistributing the workload more equitably, so that she no longer feels that she deserves any special appreciation, or helping her gain support and admiration from friends and relatives who find it easier to give than her husband does. Of course, Mrs. K could also seek and find another partner more responsive to her feelings and better able to meet her needs.

Phobic Disorders

A *Phobic Disorder* is an intense, irrational fear response to an external object, activity, or situation. Like all the disturbed patterns discussed in this chapter, a Phobic Disorder is a response to experienced anxiety. Unlike a Generalized Anxiety Disorder, however, where the anxiety is free-floating, a phobia is characterized by persistent fear of specific places or things. The major dynamic mechanisms of Phobic Disorders are thought to be *displacement* of the original anxiety from its real source and *symbolization* of the stressor in the focus of the phobia. The hallmark of phobias is that they are irrational and persist even though the person recognizes that they are irrational. The unconscious operations involved in phobias help the person control anxiety by providing a specific object to attach it to. The phobic person can then control the intensity of the anxiety by avoiding the object to which the anxiety has become attached.

TYPES OF PHOBIAS   The Phobic Disorders are divided into three main types.

1. Agoraphobia—fear of being alone or in public places
2. Social Phobia—fear of situations that may be humiliating or embarrassing
3. Simple Phobia—residual fears not either of the above

There are many subtypes of Simple Phobias. Their names derive from their Greek origins. The commonest ones include *claustrophobia* (fear of closed places), *acrophobia* (fear of heights), *mysophobia* (fear of germs), and *zoophobia* (fear of animals). Although these Simple Phobias are most common among the general population, Agoraphobia is the most common among people seeking treatment.

LIFE-STYLE CONSEQUENCES OF PHOBIC DISORDERS   A phobic person who is forced to confront the feared object may become extremely afraid or even panic. The mere possibility of contact may cause sweating, faintness, nausea, and other symptoms of anxiety. The most obvious and debilitating consequence of phobic

reaction as a coping strategy is the incredible restrictions it imposes. People who hold several phobias concurrently, as is often the case, may become walled off and isolated from many normal activities. A housewife who is afraid of crowds and vehicles becomes gradually less able to carry out her responsibilities of grocery shopping, car pooling, and so forth. The multimillionaire Howard Hughes died a wasted recluse because he had grown so afraid of germs that he refused to leave his hotel room or wear clothing. Such people often consciously recognize the irrationality of their fears but cannot help experiencing them intensely.

INTERVENTION STRATEGIES   Most clinicians agree that phobic coping patterns are highly resistant to most insight-oriented therapies. These therapies require that clients confront and at least temporarily experience some of their originating anxiety. It is not surprising that they are ineffective with phobic clients, since the phobic's style is basically one of *avoidance*. In recent years, however, some relatively dramatic symptomatic improvements have been made using techniques derived from behaviorist learning theory (see Chapter 2). The most commonly used interventions are desensitization and reciprocal inhibition.

- In desensitization, the client is exposed serially to a predetermined list of anxiety-provoking situations graded in a hierarchy from the least to the most frightening. Through techniques of progressive relaxation, the person becomes desensitized to each stimulus in the scale and then moves up to the next most frightening stimulus. Eventually the stimulus that originally provoked the most anxiety no longer elicits the same painful response. For example, a client who is irrationally afraid of ordinary earthworms might first talk about earthworms until the topic no longer evokes the same anxiety. Then he might be shown pictures of earthworms until he masters that level of closeness—and so on, increasing contact until he can actually hold a live earthworm in his hand.

- In reciprocal inhibition, the anxiety-provoking stimulus is paired with another stimulus that is associated with an opposite feeling strong enough to suppress the anxiety. Through the use of tranquilizing medications, hypnosis, meditation, yoga, or biofeedback training, clients are taught how to induce in themselves both psychological and physical calm (see Chapter 25). Once they have mastered these techniques, they are taught to use them when faced with the anxiety-provoking hierarchy of stimuli.

RATIONALE FOR NURSING INTERVENTION   In seeking intervention strategies for people who cope by developing phobias, the nurse must consider three things. First, an assessment must be made to determine the degree of impairment caused by the phobia. Many people manage to lead successful productive lives by binding their anxiety up in an object that can be avoided without unduly restricting their quality of life. Second, forcing clients to come into contact with the feared object or the basic source of their anxiety can create in them an intense, disorganizing flood of panic. The nurse who chooses this mode of intervention must be prepared to deal with the panic. Third, using behavioral conditioning techniques to rid the client of a phobia merely eliminates the symptom without removing the original stressor or conflict. If a client gives up a phobic reaction without learning a more effective coping strategy, one can usually expect some alternative and equally troublesome disturbed pattern to emerge.

Obsessive-compulsive Disorders

Phobic people fear that someone or something will harm them. Obsessive-compulsive people usually fear that they will harm someone or something. In other respects these two patterns are similar. Both rely heavily on avoidance. Both are best understood in terms of control. Individuals who develop them are characterized by high needs to control themselves, others, and their environment.

DEFINITION   An *obsession* is a recurring thought that cannot be dismissed from consciousness. These thoughts are sometimes trivial or ridiculous, often morbid or fearful, and always distressing and anxiety provoking. An example of a strange but trivial obsession is that of a young adolescent man who was unable to get the rhyme "Snips and snails and puppydog tails" out of his mind. An example of a much more ominous obsession is that of a woman who could not stop thinking that she must kill her children to prevent a worldwide race war.

A *compulsion*, on the other hand, is an uncontrollable, persistent urge to perform certain acts or behaviors to relieve an otherwise unbearable tension. There are two kinds of compulsive acts—those that give expression to the primary impulses, and those that are attempts to undo or control these impulses. The first kind is rare. Most compulsive acts are attempts to control or modify obsessions, either because the people fear the consequences or are afraid that they will not be able to control the primary impulse. Typical com-

pulsive acts are endless handwashing, checking and rechecking doors to see if they have been locked, and elaborate dressing and undressing rituals. Such defensive compulsive acts are used to contain, neutralize, or ward off the anxiety related to the primary impulse. In the case of the young man who could not dismiss the rhyme from his mind, compulsions that involved ritualistic washing of his genitals emerged to ward off the anxiety generated by his apparently silly obsession. The woman obsessed with thoughts about killing her children engaged in symbolic rituals of touching religious objects in order to repel evil influences through magical interventions by the saints. Compulsive acts like counting and elaborately checking routine duties are frequently associated with the fear of failing or making a mistake, or with the need to be perfect.

COMMONALITIES OF OBSESSIONS AND COMPULSIONS   Obsessions and compulsions have certain features in common.

- An idea or an impulse insistently, persistently, and impellingly intrudes itself into the person's awareness.
- A feeling of anxious dread accompanies the primary manifestation and often leads the person to take countermeasures against the forbidden thought or impulse.
- Both the obsession and the compulsion are egoalien—that is, foreign to one's self-perception.
- No matter how compelling the obsession or compulsion is, the person has enough insight to recognize it as irrational and experience it as a significant source of distress.
- Many of the personality traits associated with obsession and compulsion are highly valued in American culture. Success in many professions and occupations demands cautiousness, deliberateness, and rationality. These traits are usually associated with the tendency toward being obsessive or compulsive. It is when these personality traits are carried to an extreme, or when the balance between control and impulse expression leads to paralysis, that they become a liability.

PSYCHODYNAMICS OF OBSESSIVE-COMPULSIVE DISORDERS

- *Isolation* is an ego defense mechanism that protects a person from experiencing anxiety by separating feelings and impulses from ideas and pushing them out of consciousness. When isolation is completely successful, both the feelings and the ideas are repressed. When isolation is less complete, the person is aware of the impulse without realizing its significance. For example, a man might experience violent sexual impulses toward casual acquaintances without knowing why.

- Obsessive-compulsive people are under a constant threat that an impulse may escape the primary defense of isolation and break free. Secondary defense may emerge to quiet the anxiety that this threat arouses in the individual. *Undoing* is a compulsive act that is performed in an attempt to prevent or undo what the person irrationally anticipates as the consequences of the frightening impulse. In the example given above, the man might need to wash his hands to undo his sexual obsessions.

- *Reaction formation* is the formation of character traits that are exactly the opposite of the underlying impulses. The man in the example might appear unduly preoccupied with cleanliness when his impulses are actually to commit vile and "dirty" acts.

- *Magical thinking* is a regression to a phase of development when one believed that merely thinking about an event could make it happen. Inherent in magical thinking, then, is the idea of omnipotence of thought. Therefore an impulse to commit vile acts is equated by the person with actually doing them.

SOCIOCULTURAL DYNAMICS IN OBSESSIVE-COMPULSIVE PATTERNS   Nurses who understand only the intrapersonal mental dynamics of disturbed coping patterns will not fully understand their clients. It is important to take into account the function obsessive-compulsive acts serve in the context of interpersonal relationships. In some cases, the client becomes so involved with obsessions and compulsions that these behaviors substitute for relating to other people. In other cases, the obsessions and compulsions are used in negotiating interaction and social roles. It is not unusual for people to establish a reciprocal pattern of interaction based on obsessions.

Mr. O constantly complains that his wife does not keep the house clean enough. Actually he is using reciprocity to express his own wish to be untidy. He need never feel guilty, because he can blame the mess on his wife. In this rather convoluted way, Mr. O avoids some of the anxiety he would experience if he allowed himself to create some of the mess. His wife's messiness also enables him to spend time cleaning up the house, thus further undoing his own impulses. Finally, the housecleaning gives both Mr. and Mrs. O a focus for some level of interaction and communication—albeit a low one. As it turns out, this kind of wife is the perfect complementary foil for a man with such a compulsive coping style. Mr. O would probably have difficulty establishing a safe relationship with someone as controlling and compulsive as himself. He can regard Mrs. O's sloppiness as somehow inferior because she obviously has difficulty managing. In this way he enhances his own shaky self-esteem. If Mr. O had nothing to complain about, he might well develop more severe problems, because he would be denied meaningful behavior patterns, and because his wife might demand a more mature relationship with him.

As this example suggests, nurses who plan intervention strategies for obsessive-compulsive clients should first assess the impact on the whole family system of intervening in one member's coping style (see Chapter 21).

INTERVENTION STRATEGIES   Unless nurses are involved only in private practice, they will sooner or later encounter an obsessive-compulsive client whose problem is severe enough to require hospitalization. Even with long-term, intensive psychotherapy, however, most clinicians agree that these clients have certain character traits that make them poor candidates for growth and change. These traits include:

- A dominant pattern of rigidity in thinking and behavior
- Immature and dependent relationships with people
- A poor ability to tolerate anxiety and depression
- A limited ability to express emotion
- An inability to be insightful and introspective

The nurse should assess the client for these characteristics and should also try to place the client's behavior in its social context. The third clue to the probable outcome of psychotherapy is how chronic and fixed the symptom pattern has become. In general, the more chronic and fixed it is, the less likely it is to be changed through psychotherapy—or any other intervention approach, for that matter.

If both the client and the nurse attempt to substitute more mature and satisfying coping patterns for obsessions and compulsions, the nursing strategies should include:

• Coping with the compulsive behavior. Compulsive rituals are employed to undo and control anxiety. Therefore any interference with them must be carefully weighed and timed to match the client's progress in psychotherapy. In some cases, psychiatric professionals do attempt to modify the client's behavior prematurely, but only when this behavior seems to threaten the client's life or health. For example, clients with washing compulsions may completely remove the skin from their hands, and nurses have successfully intervened by suggesting surgical gloves. However, it is not usually fruitful to hurry an obsessive client. These people often have a strong tendency toward negativism, which may cause them to become more firmly entrenched in their defenses should modifications be introduced prematurely. Nurses should attempt to develop an affirming, dependable relationship with clients before suggesting that they change their behavior patterns. The nurse must balance the value of intervening in behavior that protects clients from mental anguish against the need to prevent physical deterioration caused by the behavior.

• Dealing with the client's communication problems. It is frustrating to try to communicate with people who cope by developing an obsessive-compulsive disorder. If we use the customary techniques of paraphrasing and reflecting, these clients will say that we have failed to get the details right. They will then go on to correct, qualify, and clarify what we've said. Curiously, this pedantic striving for accuracy produces greater vagueness and confusion. It's as if parallel conversations are going on. Clients hear only themselves repeating and correcting insignificant details and completely lose the overall meaning of the message. Consider the following example:

CLIENT: *Well, you won't have to make any more arrangements for my wife to come down here next month and talk.*

NURSE: *The arrangements are settled now?*

CLIENT: *We made the reservations, but the airlines put us on the wait list. That travel agent never knows what he's doing anyway. I got another ticket for her on a different airline, United Flight #744 that leaves there at 6:47 P.M.*

and arrives here at 9:22 P.M., but she may not even be able to get off work on time.

NURSE: *Are you disappointed that she might not be able to come?*

CLIENT: *Well, if I had just booked the excursion in advance instead of leaving it up to that damn travel agent, she would have been here by 8:00 P.M. on the eighteenth. (He continues to go over the various flights, arrivals, and departures.)*

• Working with the client's dependency conflict. Most psychoanalytic therapists believe that obsessive-compulsive clients are fixated or regressed to the level of infantile dependence. And, in fact, nurses who are working with such clients usually encounter the dependence–independence conflict in one form or another. These clients ask everyone for advice and then ignore it. They avoid any involvement with a therapist for fear of becoming obligated. Their general behavior pattern pushes people away while they complain of loneliness. Nurses who expect these clients to learn how their behavior interferes with their needs to be cared for must recognize that such a complete alteration in style requires enormous growth, change, and awareness. Few clients are capable of making such a change.

• Discovering the source of the original anxiety that the client used obsessive-compulsive behavior to avoid. Most of these strategies are techniques of long-term insight therapy designed first to identify the source of anxiety, then to confront it, and finally to develop alternative modes of coping with it. This is a lengthy process even with an ideal client. Furthermore, it must usually be supported by the client's family and friends. Communication techniques used in this process are discussed in Chapter 6.

Dissociative Disorders

Dissociative coping patterns are somewhat uncommon and often bizarre defensive reactions to stress. There are five types of dissociative reactions: Sleepwalking Disorder, Psychogenic Amnesia, Psychogenic Fugue, Multiple Personality, and Depersonalization Disorder. Dissociative reactions are complex and are usually difficult to distinguish from one another. They share one common characteristic. In any dissociative reaction a cluster of recent, related mental events is beyond the client's power of recall but can return spontaneously to conscious awareness. Depersonalization Disorder is included because in it the client's feeling of personal reality, an important component of identity, is lost. The most common forms of dissociative reactions are described below. None is attributable to an Organic Mental Disorder.

Forms

SLEEPWALKING DISORDER   In sleepwalking a person exhibits an altered state of conscious awareness of the surroundings resembling sleep. Such people often have vivid recollections of emotionally traumatic events that they have consciously forgotten. In DSM-III, although Sleepwalking Disorder has the essential features of a Dissociative Disorder, it is classified among disorders first evident in childhood.

PSYCHOGENIC AMNESIA   Sufferers from Psychogenic Amnesia suddenly become aware that they have a total loss of memory for events that occurred during a period of time that may range from a few hours to a whole lifetime. In localized amnesia, the most common form, a person loses the memory only for specific and related past times, usually surrounding a disturbing event.

PSYCHOGENIC FUGUE   In Psychogenic Fugue a person wanders, usually far from home and for days at a time. During this period clients completely forget their past life and associations, but, unlike people with amnesia, are unaware of having forgotten anything. When they return to their former consciousness, they are amnesic for the period covered by the fugue. Fugue clients are generally seclusive and quiet, and as a consequence their behavior rarely attracts attention.

MULTIPLE PERSONALITY   Clients with Multiple Personality are dominated by two or more distinct personalities, each of which determines the nature of their behavior and attitudes while it is uppermost in consciousness. The transition from one personality to another is often sudden and dramatic. There are many popular stories about people with multiple personalities. Two of the best known are *Sybil* and *The Three Faces of Eve*. However, this portrayal is more classic and colorful than that commonly occurring among clients today.

DEPERSONALIZATION DISORDER   The essential feature here is one or more episodes of alteration in the perception or experience of the self so that the usual sense of personal reality is temporarily lost or changed with subsequent social or occupational impairment. All the associated feelings are ego-dystonic.

Intervention Strategies   In choosing intervention strategies for clients with Dissociative Disorders, the nurse must decide whether to alleviate the problematic symptom or reintegrate the anxiety-producing conflict. Some clinicians emphasize the disruptions in day-to-day functioning occasioned by Dissociative Disorders. These include unexplained disappearances, absences from work, unreliability, and unpredictability. The dread associated with them justifies intervention strategies designed to change the disruptive behavior pattern. Others believe that it may simply create new problems to remove the so-called symptoms without considering how they help the client control internal anxiety and maintain some balance in external social life. Nurses should keep in mind that although clients may complain about the difficulties associated with their symptoms, the symptoms often form the basis of relationships with other significant people in their lives. These clients' roles in social groups are likewise built around their coping styles. If we remove these coping styles, we must offer clients more effective and satisfying ways to handle anxiety and to be supported in their social network. Such a learning task usually requires long-term psychotherapy. On the other hand, we can alleviate symptoms using strategies of behavior modification discussed in Chapter 2. Specific guidelines for dealing with a client with a Dissociative Disorder are given in the care plan in Table 14–5.

Somatoform Disorders

Historical Considerations   Conversion Disorders, previously termed hysterical conversion reactions, were among the earliest disturbed coping patterns described by Sigmund Freud. They were often associated with the repressive sexual conventions and passive-dependent women's role of the Victorian period. One of Freud's most famous patients was Anna O., a woman whom he worked with in the 1880s in association with Josef Breuer. Anna O. was an intelligent, strong-minded woman of twenty-one. After her father's illness and death, she had developed a set of symptoms including paralysis of the limbs, contractures, anesthesias, visual disturbances, disturbances of speech, anorexia, and a nervous cough. Anna had been very close to and fond of her father. She had nursed him on his deathbed. Using hypnosis as a primary tool, Breuer made the connection between inhibited sexuality and the production of symptoms such as Anna's that have no organic basis. Breuer and Freud described their clinical experience in the treatment of hysteria in an 1895 volume

Table 14–5	NURSING CARE PLAN FOR CLIENT WITH DISSOCIATIVE DISORDERS		
Therapeutic Action	**Rationale**	**Therapeutic Action**	**Rationale**
1. Physical Assessment A meticulous assessment should be made of the client's physical condition to rule out organic causes for the dissociative disorder, such as brain tumor (see Chapter 8). The nurses' observations of the descriptive character, duration, frequency, and context of the Dissociative Disorder contain crucial firsthand data.	Many of the behaviors exhibited by a client with a Dissociative Disorder resemble organic conditions, including postconcussional amnesia and temporal lobe epilepsy. Tables 14–6 and 14–7 summarize the central differentiating points. Physical examinations and assessments will not be continued as part of the long-term intervention program because they reinforce the symptom and provide secondary gain. Therefore the completeness and accuracy of the decision to rule out organic causes are of the utmost importance.	3. Family Counseling Inclusion of the family members in the therapeutic relationship may be indicated to help them learn new ways to deal with the client. 4. Environmental Manipulation It may be necessary to assist the client in problem solving with the goal of minimizing other stressful aspects of the environment.	Considerable secondary gain is often associated with dissociative behavior. The client can use the illness to escape responsibilities and get special treatment. Families may need support in learning to avoid reinforcing dissociative behavior by acting as the source of secondary gain. In learning to confront and become desensitized to the underlying conflict, the client will experience some anxiety and discomfort. This anxiety must be kept within manageable limits. Therefore, more obvious and alterable sources of stress and anxiety should be minimized during the therapy period.
2. Psychosocial Assessment The fundamental source of the anxiety should be identified as early as possible. Strategies include those effective for recovering unconscious content, such as free association or dream description. At times more active strategies are used. These may include projective psychometric tests (Rorschach, Thematic Apperception Test) and hypnosis or I.V. Pentothal.		5. Supportive Insight Therapy Clients in whom the dissociative phenomena arise primarily against a background of intrapsychic or subjective conflict may benefit from longer-term therapy aimed at surfacing and integrating traumatic experiences and learning new modes of coping with future anxiety.	Repression is the basic ego defense mechanism in Dissociative Disorders. The behaviors are mechanisms for protecting the client from the emotional pain of experiences or conflicts that are repressed. The behaviors are reactivated by current situations that arouse emotional pain—such as the anniversary of a loss, a major role transition, or the accumulation of multiple, diffuse anxiety.

Table 14-6 DIFFERENTIATION OF POSTCONCUSSIONAL AMNESIA AND PSYCHOGENIC AMNESIA	
Properties of Postconcussional Amnesia	**Properties of Psychogenic Amnesia**
1. History of a head injury	1. No history of head injury
2. Retrograde amnesia does not extend beyond a week into the past	2. Retrograde amnesia extends indefinitely into the past
3. Amnesia disappears slowly and memory is not completely restored for events that occurred during the amnesic period	3. Client can recover suddenly with total restoration of memory

Table 14-7 DIFFERENTIATION OF TEMPORAL LOBE EPILEPSY AND DISSOCIATIVE TRANCES	
Properties of Temporal Lobe Epilepsy	**Properties of Dissociative Trances**
1. Presence of positive electroencephalographic evidence of temporal lobe dysfunction	1. No such evidence
2. Usually does not occur in conjunction with other patterns	2. Often occurs with other behavior (stigmata, sleepwalking)

entitled *Studies in Hysteria* (1966). This succinct book outlined a "theory of hysteria" that placed early repressed traumatic sexual experiences, such as seductions, at the root of hysterical symptoms. Later Freud was to modify this hypothesis by abandoning the notion of actual physical seduction and placing a new emphasis on the inner fantasy life of the child.

Current Definition   The essential features of Somatoform Disorders are physical symptoms suggesting physical disorders for which there is no positive evidence of organic or physiological causes. Somatoform Disorders include four major clinical pictures:

1. *Somatization Disorder.* Clients have sought medical attention for recurrent and multiple somatic complaints of several years duration but there is no evidence of physical disorder. This problem usually begins before the age of 30 and has a chronic course often accompanied by anxiety and depressed mood. Clients believe they have been sickly for a good part of their lives and report lengthy lists of symptoms including blindness, paralysis, convulsions, nausea, and painful menstruation.

2. *Conversion Disorder,* previously termed Hysterical Neurosis, Conversion Type. Clients report loss or alteration of physical function that suggests a physical disorder but in fact is related to the expression of a psychological conflict.

3. *Psychogenic Pain Disorder.* Clients complain of pain in the absence of physiological findings and the presence of possible psychological factors.

4. *Hypochondriasis.* Clients are preoccupied with the fear or belief that they have a serious disease, which on physical evaluation is not present. The unrealistic fear or belief persists despite medical reassurance and causes impairment in social or occupational functioning.

The Symbolism of Conversion Disorder Symptoms   The point of view advocated in this book leads us to search beyond repressed infantile sexuality for the meaning of Conversion Disorder. Some communication theorists believe that manifestations are really nonverbal body language intended to communicate a message to significant others. Sometimes the message is as general as "pay attention to me" or "take care of me." At other times the particular form that the conversion of anxiety takes actually symbolizes the nature of the specific underlying conflict. For example, a woman who wants to strike her children may develop a paralysis of her arm. A girl who feels guilty about reading erotic books may become blind. Both realize the primary gain of protection from their anxiety-provoking impulses, and both get secondary gains of attention and sympathy as well. These patterns are most likely to occur among clients who do not have more aggressive alternatives.

Other Behavioral Characteristics   Clients who deal with anxiety by converting it into physical symptoms usually show no other psychological symptoms, such as disturbed thoughts or depressed moods. However, they are often said to exhibit subtler behavior patterns. Characteristics that have come to be associated with conversion disorder clients are self-dramatization, exhibitionism, narcissism, emotionalism, seductiveness, dependency, manipulativeness, childishness, and suggestibility. It is interesting to note, however, that these characteristics have usually been attributed to female clients by male psychiatrists.

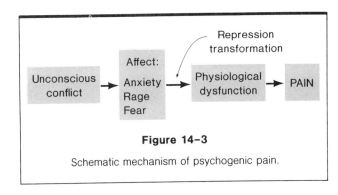

Figure 14–3

Schematic mechanism of psychogenic pain.

Pain* Pain is associated with a great many disease processes (see Chapter 24), including many of the organ-specific somatoform disorders. Pain can be an adaptive or a maladaptive response. It often indicates real danger to the organism, but sometimes it interferes with functioning.

Consciousness, attention, perception, and cognition are all necessary for the experience of pain. Modern theories of pain perception postulate that humans have a control system over pain that operates as a "gate." Pain stimuli can be "allowed in" to or "shut out" from the cerebral cortex, depending essentially on the meaning the person attaches to the stimulus. This underscores the importance of meaning, symbol, and affect in the experience of pain sensation.

MECHANISM The basic schematic mechanism for so-called psychogenic pain is depicted in Figure 14–3. In psychoanalytic concepts, the unconscious conflicts are a result of traumatic or frustrating childhood experiences that are reawakened in adult life by an analogous stress or frustration. Usually this theory postulates that the person cannot express the affect that is aroused because of feelings of guilt, fear of loss of love, fear of retribution, etc. The affect is therefore repressed and transformed into physiological correlates.

CLINICAL SYNDROMES Some of the clinical syndromes in which Psychogenic Pain may be the predominant complaint are conversion disorders, workers' compensation injuries, and masochistic personality styles. In Conversion Disorders, pain symbolizes an unacceptable wish, perhaps sexual or aggressive, aroused by a frustrating life situation, and the punishment for having such a wish. In workers' compensation cases, the client may unconsciously use pain, and the monetary com-

pensation received for the suffering, to strike back against employers or others by whom the client feels unfairly treated. Some individuals seem to need to suffer in order to achieve any sort of gratification without guilt. They seem to assume they are otherwise unworthy of any pleasure. Often their entire lives are conducted according to a self-destructive pattern of expecting punishment and eliciting it from the environment.

Ms. G was a twenty-six-year-old separated female working as a truant officer in a suburban school system. One day, in the course of tracking down a particularly truant child, she became embroiled in an argument with the child's father. The argument escalated to the point where Ms. G threatened to recommend the child for suspension, if the father did not take more responsibility in ensuring the child's school attendance. At this point, the father struck her in the face with his fist and knocked her to the ground.

Ms. G sustained a fracture of the mandible and in addition became severely depressed over the following two weeks. She complained of agitation, irritability, inability to sleep, and fits of uncontrollable crying, which she related to her unremitting pain. These symptoms continued unabated for six weeks. Although the jaw's healing progressed well, she refused to return to work, saying it was physically impossible to do so. She applied for workers' compensation insurance. Eventually, four months after the incident, she was referred for psychiatric evaluation.

The therapist noted that Ms. G's clinical depression was significant and was struck by the intensity of her antagonistic feelings. She focused rage and hatred on the assailant, although he had become contrite about the incident. Ms. G spoke as if the incident had occurred the previous day and maintained this intensity during six months of treatment. She also persisted in contending that she was incapable of any work. She viewed the Compensation Board's requests for justification with bitter contempt. Ms. G's past history had been problem-free.

After a year's psychotherapy, Ms. G finally developed

*This section appeared in a chapter entitled "Life Enhancement for Clients with Medicopsychiatric Conditions," authored by A. E. Skodol in the first edition of *Psychiatric Nursing* by H. S. Wilson and C. R. Kneisl, (Menlo Park, Calif.: Addison-Wesley, 1980).

a sense of trust in the therapist and revealed that, as a child, she had been subjected to severe beatings by an alcoholic father. It developed that all the client's repressed and suppressed feelings about this period in her life were being focused on her present assault. The assailant, the school, the Workers' Compensation Board all embodied, in her frame of reference, the abusiveness of her father. With this special meaning attached to the assault, it bore a heightened significance that immobilized her far more than the physical injury. The nurse working at this level enabled Ms. G to become less depressed and go back to work, although not in her former position.

RECOGNITION AND INTERVENTION   In most clients suffering pain that may be psychologically influenced or generated, there is evidence of a stressful life situation that the client cannot handle because of particular past experiences or present states. The inability to cope is often intimately tied to the particular, special, and individual meaning the client attaches to the situation, which may make it seem more complex than it superficially appears. Thus, some clues to Psychogenic Pain are:

• Life stress
• A complaint that is excessive for the observable injury
• Pain that is nonanatomical in distribution
• A demanding personality
• A history of repeated extensive medical-surgical procedures without relief

Effective intervention involves:

• Recognizing and understanding the life problem or adjustment the client is facing
• Recognizing and understanding the client's self-perception as helpless to cope
• Helping the client learn more effective ways of adapting

These steps may be accomplished by insight-oriented or supportive psychotherapy, behavior modification, hypnosis, acupuncture, or any of several other psychological, as well as some physical, therapies. None can claim superior effectiveness, and new approaches and techniques are indicated when traditional ones prove inadequate.

Differentiating Somatoform Disorders from Physical Illness   The earliest manifestations of central nervous system disease—such as the temporary weakness of an arm or disturbed vision in one eye, heralding the onset of multiple sclerosis—may be confused with Somatoform Disorders. However, if nurses observe the client carefully, using the information contained in Table 14-8, they can avoid confusing the two.

Differentiating Somatoform Disorders from Factitious Disorders   Factitious means not genuine or natural. In the DSM-III this category of disorders includes conditions in which a client has physical or psychological symptoms that are actually produced by the client under conscious, voluntary control. Clients who have Factitious Disorders may produce a symptom like hematuria (blood in their urine) by taking anticoagulants or a self-induced dislocation of the shoulder for no other reason than to assume a patient role. The distinction between Factitious and Somatoform Disorders is based on the determination that the physical symptoms present are under voluntary control in Factitious Disorders and not under voluntary control in Somatoform Disorders. Both conditions must be thoughtfully assessed for the possible presence of a true, primary physical disorder (see Chapter 8).

Intervention Strategies   Once organic problems and Factitious Disorders have been ruled out and a client's behavior is confirmed as representing an example of a Somatoform Disorder, the following guidelines may be used to plan an intervention strategy.

• *Be aware of personal responses to the client.* Many nurses find people who employ physical symptoms irritating to deal with. Often these people are self-centered, self-indulgent, and manipulative. In a hospital setting, they often create scenes that bring them the attention they need without regard for the needs of either fellow clients or staff. In short, nurses frequently find it difficult to be kind, understanding, and nonjudgmental with these clients. Nurses who cannot cope with their own reactions to these clients cannot work with them effectively. It may help to remember that these clients do not intentionally produce their symptoms, nor do they appreciate the effects of their behavior on other people. Nurses who appreciate the whole story can sometimes feel a bit more empathy for a client's basically pathetic coping style.

Table 14-8 PROPERTIES OF CENTRAL NERVOUS SYSTEM DISEASE AND SOMATOFORM DISORDERS	
Central Nervous System Disease	**Somatoform Disorder**
Presence of emerging positive neurological signs	Absence of positive neurological signs
No history of disturbances of interpersonal relationships, such as a recent death, related to onset of symptoms	History of disturbance in interpersonal relationships associated with onset of symptoms
Authentic concern about the symptoms	Indications that symptoms may be useful in manipulating others for secondary gain
	Presence of one or more of the following other major deviations from characteristic neurological conditions:
	• No incontinence during seizures
	• Absence of true clonus and Babinski reactions
	• Forearm in hemiplegia is extended instead of flexed as in organic hemiplegia
	• Leg is dragged instead of swung in circumduction
	• No wasting of paralyzed extremities
	• Sensory disturbances are usually of functional incapacity and do not follow the anatomic distribution of the nerve

• *Try to avoid reinforcing the client's symptoms.* A well-known psychiatric axiom that applies to clients in this general category is "ignore the symptoms but never the client." To concentrate on the physical symptom by trying to get a "paralyzed" client to walk or a "blind" client to see again is to give the symptom more importance than it merits, thus increasing the secondary gain associated with it. Ultimately this merely makes it harder for the client to relinquish the symptom.

• *Assess the symbolic meaning of the client's symptom.* Interpersonally oriented psychiatric theorists intervene with clients who employ physical symptoms based on the symptom's meaning. They propose that people who cope with anxiety by converting it into hystrionic physical symptoms have difficulty communicating verbally. What these people do articulate often contains many gaps. It is usually necessary to help these clients tone down their characteristic extravagances and to express respectful skepticism regarding their oversimplifications and overdramatizations in order to plan effective interventions. The nonverbal communicative function of the symptom itself should also be considered. The common symptoms of blindness, deafness, pain, numbness, itching, swelling, vomiting, paralysis, and so forth may be communicating something as general as "take care of me," "pay attention to me," or "I

want out of these responsibilities." Specific symptoms may also be associated with more exact meanings. The "blind" person may be saying, "I don't want to see something, because not having to see it allows me to escape my feelings about it." After assessing the meaning behind the client's communication patterns, the nurse can plan intervention strategies that enhance the client's functional verbal communication and self-esteem to the point where the clients feels ready to face problems. A hypothetical nursing care plan for a client who develops somatoform symptoms is given in Table 14–9.

Affective Disorders

Depression, grieving, sadness, and "blue spells" are all feeling states or moods that weigh heavily on the person who experiences them. Affective Disorder is the name given to a disturbed personal pattern in which the client feels extreme sadness, withdraws socially, often feels guilty, and expresses self-deprecatory thoughts or experiences an elevated expansive mood with hyperactivity, pressure of speech, inflated self-esteem, decreased need for sleep, and involvement in activities that have a high potential for painful consequences. These mood disturbances may occur in a number of patterns of severity and duration alone or together (see Appendix B). The former is usually

Table 14-9 NURSING CARE PLAN FOR CLIENT WITH SOMATOFORM DISORDER	
Client Problem	**Intervention**
Client is moody, demanding, self-centered, and complaining. This creates strong feelings of resentment and anger in both staff members and fellow patients, who all avoid her.	1. Have client participate in communication and feelings group with goal of giving feedback about effect of her behavior on others. 2. Staff need to set limits with client and stick to them. 3. Staff members need to discuss their feelings in supervisory session and find problem-solving strategies that will enable some of them to relate helpfully to the client. (Assigning one or two constant staff may be compared with assigning multiple caretakers to determine which is preferable.)

Client relies on physical symptoms to manage anxiety and communicate needs.	1. Make systematic behavior observations to assist the team in ruling out physical reasons for symptoms.
	2. Subsequently avoid focusing on physical symptoms to decrease secondary gain.
	3. Establish therapeutic relationship in which
	  a. Nurse works to enhance client's self-esteem.
	  b. Nurse helps client to use verbal communication to get needs met.
	  c. Nurse attempts to explore the source of the client's anxiety, if long-term therapy is feasible.

termed a Major Depressive Episode or Disorder and the latter, a Manic Episode or Disorder. Common features of Depressive Disorders are a loss of ambition, boredom, and numerous physical complaints. The latter include fatigue, loss of appetite (anorexia), sleep disturbances (including both excessive sleeping and insomnia), and loss of libido. Although Depressive Disorders come in several forms (see Table 14–10), clinicians tend to agree that they share certain typical features. These are:

- An alteration in feeling toward sadness, loneliness, and apathy
- Vegetative physical changes
- Alteration in activity level toward either retardation or agitation
- Lowered self-esteem associated with self-reproaches and blame
- History (usually recent) of an experienced loss

Dynamics of Depressive Disorders   Depressive Disorders usually originate with an experience of loss. The loss may be anything valued that the client once

had or wanted and now cannot have. People who sustain this kind of loss feel as if they had lost part of themselves. They feel angry and helpless at first. Then they feel guilt, leading to lowered self-esteem. This combination of feelings is especially likely when the depressed person has had ambivalent feelings about the lost person or object.

Some people are particularly vulnerable to depression. These people are convinced that the security and status of being loved depend on their meeting requirements set for them by significant others. People who are prone to depression feel that if they fail to meet others' requirements, they will disrupt their relationships and render themselves worthless and helpless. They feel that they alone are responsible for these disruptions. Somehow they have developed the feeling that they are completely unlovable. Depression originates when people suffer a loss—of love, of status, of self-esteem. They then direct their actions toward reducing their losses. People who depend on depressive coping patterns are those who have experienced so many losses that their sense of security is highly conditional. They only feel secure as long as they have direct signs from important people around them that

---

Table 14-10   DIFFERENTIATION OF MAJOR DEPRESSIVE EPISODE, BIPOLAR DISORDER, AND DYSTHYMIC DISORDER

Criteria	Major Depressive Episode	Bipolar Disorder	Dysthymic Disorder
Intensity	Depressive symptoms prominent	Depressive symptoms prominent	Depressive symptoms are mild
Ego impairment	May have psychotic features	May have psychotic features	No psychotic features
Pattern	No history of manic episode	Has had manic episode	Alternating depressed and hypomanic periods over two-year period

---

Table 14-11   FACTORS RELATED TO THE DEVELOPMENT OF DEPRESSION

Biological	Psychological	Cognitive	Sociocultural
Possible genetic influence Hormonal influence (drop in estrogen and progesterone) Biochemical activities of monamine oxidase (MAO) and catecholamines (high levels)	Dependency Low self-esteem Powerlessness Ambivalence Guilt	Narrow, negative perpective called "cognitive triad": view of self, world, and the future Conclusions drawn on inadequate or contradictory evidence Overgeneralizations from one instance Focus on a single detail rather than on the whole Distortion of long-range consequences, hence bad judgment	Social situations that contribute to feelings of powerlessness and low self-esteem: 1. Status of minority groups 2. Status of women in male-oriented professional and business culture 3. Role loss such as loss of parent role in empty nest phase 4. Being the object of cultural stereotypes (e.g., blacks, aged, Jews)

they are approved and loved. Women have been particularly susceptible to depression (see Chapter 5).

Classical Clinical Picture of Depression In severely depressed people the muscles of the face droop, giving them a glum, dispirited appearance. Sometimes the eyeballs are sunken due to weight loss. These clients assume a slumped position when seated, and when they walk their gait is slow and dragging. The voice is flat and colorless. These clients cry a lot, and sleep problems are common. They are uninterested in personal hygiene and appear dirty and disheveled. The physical changes associated with depression are caused by retardations in the various systems. For example, retardation in the gastrointestinal tract leads to belching, constipation, and appetite loss.

Depressed clients typically engage in harsh self-criticism. They harp on their supposed worthlessness. They may openly cry as they talk about their problems. Depending on their relationship with the nurse, they may exhibit a passive, clinging, beseeching dependency. Above all, it is lowered self-esteem that constitutes the hallmark of this disorder. From time to time everyone suffers from lowered self-esteem, but most people have ways of restoring their emotional equilibrium. This is not true of people who rely on depressive reactions as a coping strategy. These people have few inner resources to combat threats to their self-esteem and become extremely despondent.

Table 14-11 presents a comparative summary of theoretical notions about depression from biological, psychological, cognitive, and sociocultural perspectives that nurses can use to develop an integrated understanding of a depressed client.

Assessment and Intervention Strategies

The prototype for depression is found in basic grief reactions. *Grief* is a process that accompanies all loss. It follows a pattern of physical and psychological distress over the loss, and it is resolved when clients find some way of replacing the loss and restructuring their lives. The steps a nurse takes in helping a client reach this resolution are discussed in Chapter 11.

In a Depressive Disorder the grieving process is short-circuited. When a person does not successfully complete this process, there is an exaggerated reaction to the loss in which the grief is heightened and distorted.

A DEPRESSION ALGORITHM Nurses functioning in a wide variety of settings, including schools, clinics, industry, emergency rooms, and so forth, may encounter clients experiencing Depressive Disorders and considering suicide. An algorithm such as the one provided in the following chart offers a set of step-by-step instructions for collecting data about a depressed client. Essentially the depression algorithm includes a review of all the possible symptoms and characteristics of the various types of depression. It then guides the nurse through an assessment of suicide potential. If the risk is significant the nurse may recommend hospitalization; if not, the severity of the identified depression symptoms becomes a major factor in deciding on the client's disposition. Nursing intervention for depressed clients is then geared toward helping them to meet their needs for safety, hygiene, rest, activity, nurition, elimination, self-esteem, and affiliation.

SAFETY Severely depressed clients are liable to die. They may die of starvation or—more commonly—from suicide. A complete discussion of the nurse's role in assessing the probability of suicide and of strategies for crisis intervention is presented in Chapter 11. Severely depressed clients may also become so racked with self-doubt and sadness that they become immobilized and stuporous. If left to their own resources, these clients may well die of starvation or infection, because they do not mobilize their energy to protect their physical safety. Therefore the nurse may need to intervene on their behalf. In caring for these people, nurses must not assume that they will respond to a fire alarm, avoid falling down, or even take care not to cut themselves while shaving. The nurse may have to plan actions that will substitute temporarily for the client's own protective devices.

HYGIENE A filthy, unkempt body not only risks invasion by pathogens and infection, but it also perpetuates the client's low self-esteem. It may be necessary for the nurse to groom depressed clients who are unable to do it for themselves.

REST AND ACTIVITY Fatigue and sleeping disturbances reinforce depression. Any measures that the nurse can take to help the client get adequate rest are important. Sometimes encouraging clients to take part in some kind of activity will help them rest. The best form of activity for depressed people is often work at their usual occupation. Working frequently enhances their self-esteem and distracts them from morbid ruminations. Often helping clients develop new activities and goals can redirect their attention from the past to the future.

NUTRITION AND ELIMINATION The depressed client is subject to malnutrition and serious changes in normal bowel activity. There are several ways to minimize problems in these areas. One is to encourage some physical activity. Another is to modify the client's food intake. A third is to monitor the client's output for evidence of serious and prolonged constipation.

Increasing a depressed client's physical activity is not an easy task, since these clients would prefer to sleep away the day in a darkened room. But a consistent, firm approach may be effective in getting them to do something useful. In addition to strengthening their self-esteem and providing distraction, physical activity relieves gastrointestinal tract retardation and helps these clients develop an appetite.

Gastric motility can be influenced by the quantity of food ingested at a given time. If smaller portions are provided more frequently, there is less to empty from the stomach, and the miserable feeling of bloatedness can be alleviated. Foods that are high in fiber are also indicated.

Constipation is a chronic problem among depressed clients. While appropriate food and physical activities are preferable to the use of enemas and laxatives, one or both of the latter may be indicated. In an inpatient setting, it may be the nurse's responsibility to convey this need to the prescribing physician.

SELF-ESTEEM AND AFFILIATION The nurse deals with the whole client by meeting biological needs and psychosocial needs. Psychosocial needs of depressed people require that the nurse plan interventions directed toward meeting the client's needs for self-esteem and affiliation. The following guidelines may be used to fashion the nursing care plan for a depressed client:

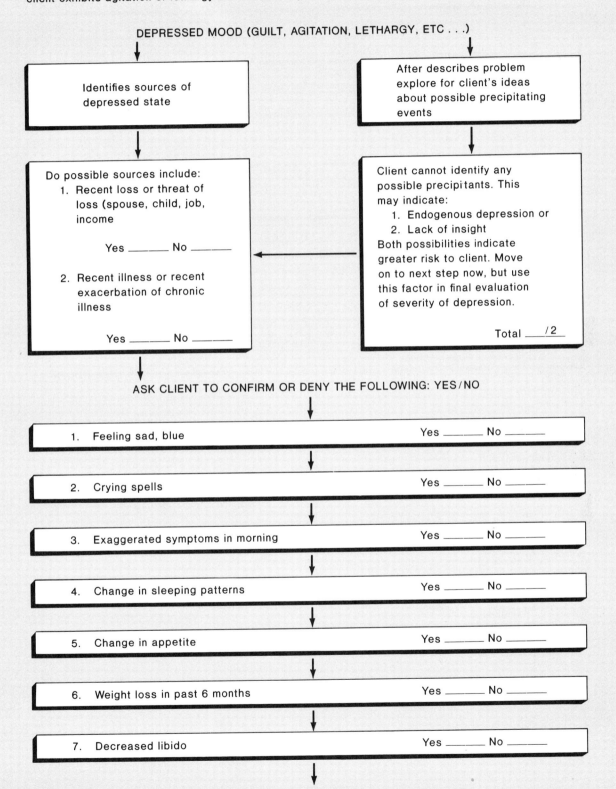

ALGORITHM FOR DEPRESSION

For use when client indicates problem related to depressed mood, feelings of guilt or shame, or when client exhibits agitation or lethargy not immediately attributable to organic cause.

DEPRESSED MOOD (GUILT, AGITATION, LETHARGY, ETC . . .)

Identifies sources of depressed state

After describes problem explore for client's ideas about possible precipitating events

Do possible sources include:
1. Recent loss or threat of loss (spouse, child, job, income

   Yes _____ No _____

2. Recent illness or recent exacerbation of chronic illness

   Yes _____ No _____

Client cannot identify any possible precipitants. This may indicate:
1. Endogenous depression or
2. Lack of insight
Both possibilities indicate greater risk to client. Move on to next step now, but use this factor in final evaluation of severity of depression.

Total ___/2___

ASK CLIENT TO CONFIRM OR DENY THE FOLLOWING: YES/NO

1. Feeling sad, blue   Yes _____ No _____

2. Crying spells   Yes _____ No _____

3. Exaggerated symptoms in morning   Yes _____ No _____

4. Change in sleeping patterns   Yes _____ No _____

5. Change in appetite   Yes _____ No _____

6. Weight loss in past 6 months   Yes _____ No _____

7. Decreased libido   Yes _____ No _____

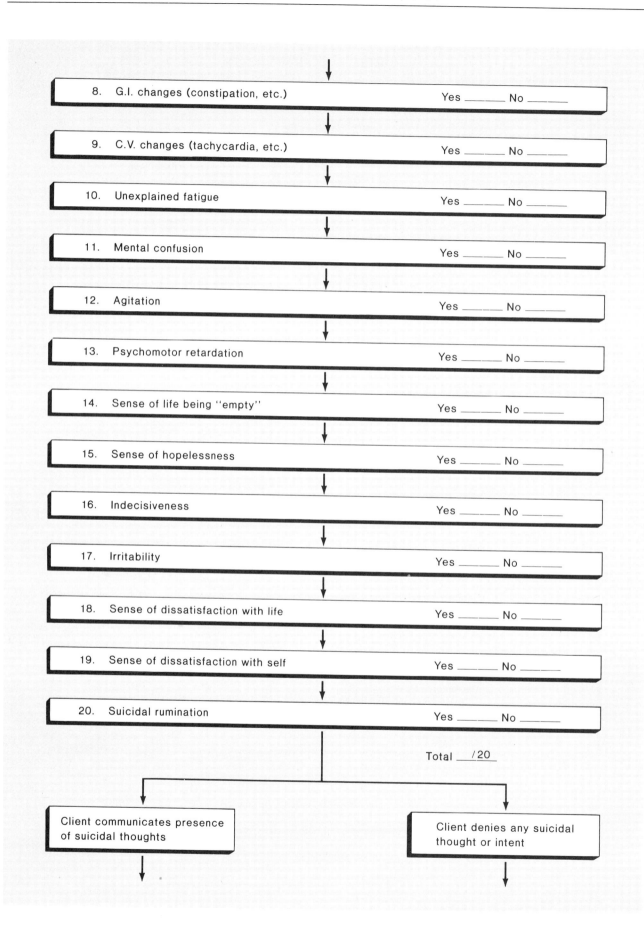

8. G.I. changes (constipation, etc.)   Yes _____ No _____

9. C.V. changes (tachycardia, etc.)   Yes _____ No _____

10. Unexplained fatigue   Yes _____ No _____

11. Mental confusion   Yes _____ No _____

12. Agitation   Yes _____ No _____

13. Psychomotor retardation   Yes _____ No _____

14. Sense of life being "empty"   Yes _____ No _____

15. Sense of hopelessness   Yes _____ No _____

16. Indecisiveness   Yes _____ No _____

17. Irritability   Yes _____ No _____

18. Sense of dissatisfaction with life   Yes _____ No _____

19. Sense of dissatisfaction with self   Yes _____ No _____

20. Suicidal rumination   Yes _____ No _____

Total ___/20

Client communicates presence of suicidal thoughts

Client denies any suicidal thought or intent

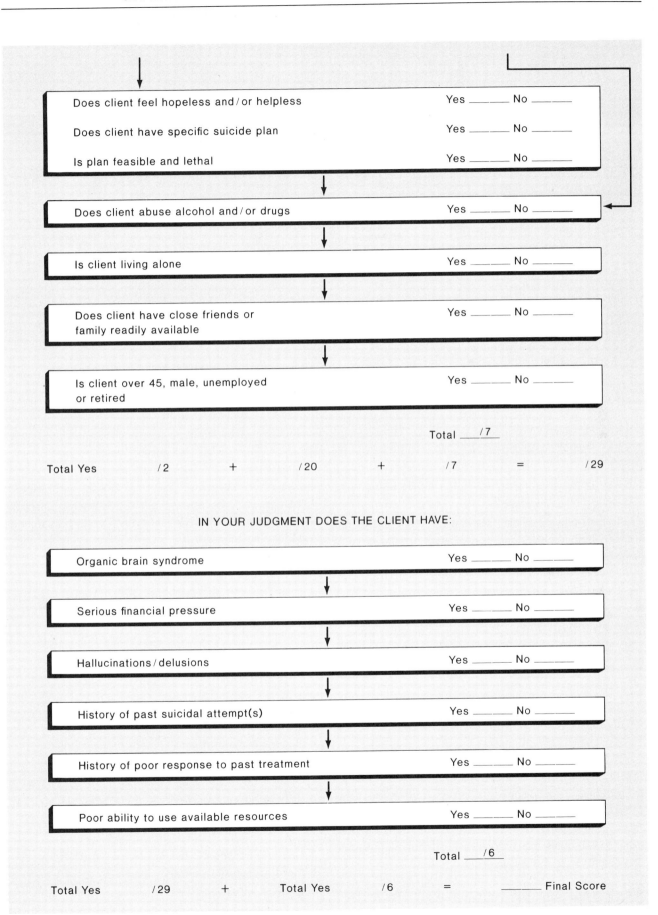

Does client feel hopeless and/or helpless   Yes _____ No _____

Does client have specific suicide plan   Yes _____ No _____

Is plan feasible and lethal   Yes _____ No _____

Does client abuse alcohol and/or drugs   Yes _____ No _____

Is client living alone   Yes _____ No _____

Does client have close friends or
family readily available   Yes _____ No _____

Is client over 45, male, unemployed
or retired   Yes _____ No _____

Total ___/7

Total Yes   /2   +   /20   +   /7   =   /29

IN YOUR JUDGMENT DOES THE CLIENT HAVE:

Organic brain syndrome   Yes _____ No _____

Serious financial pressure   Yes _____ No _____

Hallucinations/delusions   Yes _____ No _____

History of past suicidal attempt(s)   Yes _____ No _____

History of poor response to past treatment   Yes _____ No _____

Poor ability to use available resources   Yes _____ No _____

Total ___/6

Total Yes   /29   +   Total Yes   /6   =   _____ Final Score

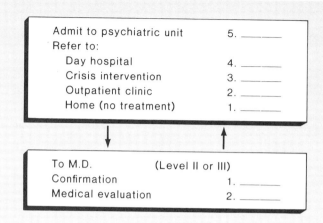

ALGORITHM SCORING

Add the number of "Yes" responses in each subsection to provide a final score. Scoring has been included in the algorithm's construction from the outset in order to facilitate future analysis of data. Correlations of disposition decisions, and possibly other outcome measures, with these subtotal and total scores can be completed.

Reprinted with permission from Journal of Psychiatric Treatment and Evaluation, Marcia Orsolits and Murray Morphy, "A Depression Algorithm for Psychiatric Emergencies," Vol. 4, pp. 137–145, April 1982, Pergamon Press, Ltd.

- Make therapeutic use of self in the form of empathic presence and listening.

- Establish a nurse–client relationship that conveys respect, both verbally and nonverbally, for the dignity of the client. This may be done by keeping promises, following agreements about time structure, and avoiding false reassurances.

- Provide an organized, well-planned schedule to help the client fend off the decline to a vegetative state.

- Build new communication patterns in which the depressed client can learn to express negative feelings openly instead of turning them inward.

- Observe precautions against suicide as discussed in Chapter 11.

The nurse has two primary goals in caring for depressed clients. One is to help these clients to change or redefine some oppressive external situation that evokes feelings of powerlessness. The other is to help them learn more optimistic and effective coping strategies. These goals apply to all the disturbed patterns examined in the preceding pages.

Assessment and Intervention with Manic Behavior   In some instances depression is but one phase of an Affective Disorder. Clients with Bipolar Disorder and the less severe Cyclothymic Disorder have numerous periods of mania or hypomania as well. During the depressive periods the client exhibits:

- Insomnia or hypersomnia
- Low energy and chronic fatigue
- Feelings of inadequacy
- Decreased effectiveness and productivity
- Decreased attention and concentration ability
- Loss of interest in or enjoyment of sex
- Restricted involvement in pleasurable activities
- A slowed-down feeling
- A pessimistic attitude
- Tearfulness or crying

During hypomanic periods, there is an elevated, expansive or irritable mood and some of the following:

- Decreased need for sleep
- More energy than usual
- Inflated self-esteem
- Increased productivity

- Sharpened thinking
- Extreme gregariousness
- Hypersexuality
- Involvement in activities without concern for the consequences
- Physical restlessness
- Unusual talkativeness
- Exaggeration of past achievements
- Inappropriate laughing, joking, and punning

Some clients experience manic episodes without experiencing depression. Nursing intervention with clients who have nonpsychotic disturbances of affect in the form of mania is guided by the following principles:

- Decrease environmental stimulation. Hyperactivity among manic clients can become life threatening. Therefore the nurse should decrease environmental stimuli for these clients by keeping the noise level down, the lighting low, and the surroundings as simple and calm as possible. The nurse should also remove hazardous objects and substances.
- Provide adequate hygiene, nutrition, and rest. Not unlike depressed clients, manic clients may need help from the nurse in meeting their basic human needs. High-calorie foods and drink are recommended. A place to take short but frequent naps may encourage the client to get adequate rest. The client may need reminders to wash or bathe.
- Provide activities that decrease energy and tension. Such activities may include vigorous housekeeping chores, jogging, and exercise.
- Monitor medication. Most manic clients are treated with lithium carbonate (see Chapter 23). Nursing intervention includes assessing the effects of the medication and identifying the side and toxic effects.

However, the major emphasis of nursing intervention should be directed toward teaching clients on lithium therapy about their treatment. The nurse should discuss the fact that the medication must be taken regularly and perhaps for life. Clients should be taught to recognize the symptoms of lithium toxicity and to notify their physician immediately if any symptoms appear. Such symptoms include:

- A feeling of sluggishness
- Lethargy
- A fine tremor or muscle twitching
- Ataxia
- Slurred speech
- Anorexia
- Nausea and vomiting
- Diarrhea

If untreated these early toxic symptoms can progress to semiconsciousness and coma. Seizures can also occur in association with electrolyte changes. Thus the client must be aware of any other conditions that alter electrolyte balance like vomiting, diarrhea, or excessive perspiration. Side effects of lithium include:

- Fine tremor of the hands
- Abdominal cramps
- Nausea, vomiting, and diarrhea
- Thirst and polyuria
- Fatigue
- Weight gain

A client on lithium therapy is often committed to a lifelong regimen of drug therapy. The nurse can provide crucial health education about the implications of this treatment program.

KEY NURSING CONCEPTS

- ✔ Disturbed coping patterns are characterized by loss of freedom to make choices, presence of conflict, repetition despite ineffectiveness, feelings of distress or pain, and the potential for secondary gain.
- ✔ Disturbed patterns have been known as psychoneuroses in traditional psychiatric terminology.
- ✔ The dynamics of disturbed coping patterns may be explained by an understanding of the concepts of control, balance, homeostasis, stress, and anxiety.

Key Nursing Concepts continued

✔ Anxiety is the uncomfortable internal feeling that results from conflict and frustration.

✔ General causes of anxiety may be classified into threats to biological integrity and threats to the security of self.

✔ The choice of coping strategy often depends on external circumstances, the suddenness and and intensity of the stress, the resources available to the person, and a predisposition to a certain coping pattern.

✔ No sharp boundaries separate disturbed coping patterns from the general conduct of life.

✔ The humanistic interactionist perspective purports that the interaction of the external situation and the inner state of mind must both be considered when planning intervention.

✔ Commonly recognized disturbed coping patterns include anxiety, dissociative, somatoform, and affective disorder patterns.

✔ The clinical picture of most disturbed coping patterns is a mixture of several elements from each labeled type.

References

Breuer, J., and Freud, S. *Studies in Hysteria.* New York: Avon Books, 1966.

Kovel, J. *A Complete Guide to Therapy.* New York: Pantheon Books, 1976.

Manaser, J. C., and Werner, A. M. *Instruments for the Study of Nurse–Patient Interaction.* New York: Macmillan, 1964.

Peplau, H. E. "A Working Definition of Anxiety." In *Some Clinical Approaches to Psychiatric Nursing,* edited by S. F. Burd and M. A. Marshall. New York: Macmillan, 1963.

McConnell, J. *Understanding Human Behavior.* New York: Holt, Rinehart and Winston, 1974.

Menninger, K. *The Vital Balance.* New York: Viking Press, 1963.

Orsolits, M., and Morphy, M. "A Depression Algorithm for Psychiatric Emergencies." *Journal of Psychiatric Treatment and Evaluation* 4 (April 1982): 137–145. New York: Pergamon Press.

Further Reading

Angefal, A. *Neuroses and Treatment: A Holistic Theory.* New York: John Wiley, 1965.

Akiskal, H., and McKinney, W. "Overview of Recent Research in Depression." *Archives of General Psychiatry* 32 (1975): 285.

Burd, S. F., and Marshall, M. A., eds. *Some Clinical Approaches to Psychiatric Nursing.* New York: Macmillan, 1963.

Crumb, F. W. "Behavioral Pattern of a Depressed Person." *Perspectives in Psychiatric Care* 64 (1964): 40.

Davenport, Y., et al. "Couples Group Therapy as an Adjunct to Lithium Maintenance of the Manic Patient." *American Journal of Orthopsychiatry* 47 (1977): 495–502.

Deutsch, H. *Neuroses and Character Types.* New York: International Universities Press, 1965.

Drage, E. "Recall of Panic Episodes." *American Journal of Nursing* 68 (1968): 1254–1257.

Fenichel, O. *The Psychoanalytic Theory of Neuroses.* New York: W. W. Norton, 1945.

Garber, K. D. "Depression Following an Acute Schizophrenic Episode." In *Current Perspectives in Psychiatric Nursing: Issues and Trends,* vol. 2, edited by C. R. Kneisl and H. S. Wilson, pp. 94–103. St. Louis: C. V. Mosby, 1978.

Lagina, S. "A Computer Program to Diagnose Anxiety Level." *Nursing Research* 20 (1971): 491.

Lazare, A. "The Difference Between Sadness and Depression." *Medical Insight* 2 (1970): 23–31.

May, R. *The Meaning of Anxiety.* New York: Ronald Press, 1950.

Peplau, H. E. *Interpersonal Relations in Nursing.* New York: G. P. Putnam, 1952.

Ruesch, J. *Disturbed Communication.* New York: W. W. Norton, 1957.

Swanson, A. "Communicating with Depressed Persons." *Perspectives in Psychiatric Care* 13 (1975): 63–67.

White, C. L. "Nurse Counseling with a Depressed Patient." *American Journal of Nursing* 78 (1978): 436–439.

15

Disruptive Life-styles: Personality Disorders and Substance Abuse Disorders

CHAPTER OUTLINE

The Concept of Life-style
Types of Disruptive Life-styles
Development of Disruptive Life-styles
    Styles of Defense and General Life-styles
    Interaction of Factors in Style Preference
Impulsive Life-styles
    Development of Impulsive Life-styles
    Common Features
    Nursing Intervention
Addicted Life-styles
    Alcohol Addiction
    Drug Dependence
Compulsive Life-styles
    Rigidity
    Style of Paying Attention
    General Mode of Activity
    The Subjective Quality of Trying
    The Consequences for Quality of Life
    Nursing Intervention

Dependent Life-styles
    Characteristics
    Nursing Intervention
Eccentric Life-styles
    Characteristics of a Paranoid Personality
    Characteristics of Schizoid and Schizotypal Personalities
Key Nursing Concepts

LEARNING OBJECTIVES

After reading this chapter, students should be able to
- Compare and contrast characteristics of disturbed coping patterns and disruptive life-styles
- Explain the concept of life-style
- Analyze impulsive, addicted, compulsive, dependent, and eccentric life-styles
- Plan nursing intervention for the disruptive life-styles presented

CHAPTER 15

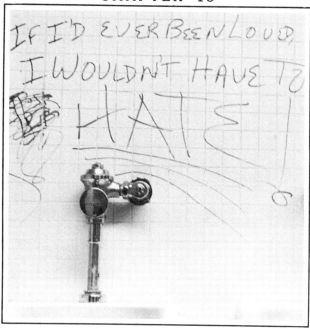

> People with disruptive life-styles are storm centers in their social relations and sometimes thrive on the trouble they create. Underlying their behavior and attitudes may be feelings they seldom express.

Disturbed personal patterns, traditionally called neuroses, characterize *troubled* people. In response to inner or outer stress, these people fall back on some relatively ineffective coping mechanism. In so doing they sacrifice some of the quality of their lives. In addition, they usually experience distressing feelings of alienation and emotional pain.

Disruptive life-styles are those categories of behavior conventionally called personality disorders, character disorders, and personality trait disturbances. People with disruptive life-styles are often the *troublesome* members of society. Unlike "neurotics," they are relatively free of emotional pain. Their interpersonal life-style is therefore called *ego syntonic,* that is, not at odds with their sense of self. These people are storm centers in their social relations, but they seem to thrive on the turmoil they create. They are often indifferent to the trouble their behavior causes others.

THE CONCEPT OF LIFE-STYLE

A life-style is an enduring pattern of perceiving and functioning. It includes ways of thinking and perceiving, ways of experiencing emotion, modes of subjective experience that are generally consistent patterns over broad areas of living. People whose life-styles are characteristically disruptive are often among society's marginal members. Their clash with the dominant social and cultural environment brings them into contact with agencies of public assistance such as police departments, correctional systems, mental hospitals, and child placement facilities. Disruptive life-styles are both social problems and maladaptive coping styles.

TYPES OF DISRUPTIVE LIFE-STYLES

Before the publication of DSM-III, the psychiatric literature offered no consistent, clear-cut definitions of the major disruptive life-styles. DSM-III's accepted definitions are presented briefly in Table 15–1.

Although each of the disruptive life-styles has certain unique characteristics, they also have many properties in common.

- They are primarily defensive modes of living.
- They make it extremely difficult for the person to adjust to social relationships.
- They are usually related to some form of arrested behavior development or to the overdevelopment of a particular pattern or trait.
- Problems are expressed through general behavior, rather than through the development of any particular symptoms in response to stress.
- The behavior that expresses these problems is troubling to others. It usually does not cause guilt, anxiety, or depression in the person who engages in it.
- Disruptive life-styles become deeply ingrained and are very difficult to modify or change.
- People with disruptive life-styles usually come into conflict with others, either in their immediate families or in society at large.
- Most of the behavior is governed by infantile, pleasure-oriented forces, with inadequate control in the form of moral sensitivity (superego) or problem-solving and reality-testing skills (ego functions).

Table 15-1 CHARACTERISTICS ASSOCIATED WITH MAJOR TYPES OF DISRUPTIVE LIFE-STYLES (PERSONALITY DISORDERS)	
Type	**Characteristics**
Histrionic life-style	Behavior that is overly dramatic, reactive, and intense. Engages in attention-seeking, self-dramatization, and irrational outbursts of emotion. Perceived by others as shallow, self-indulgent, vain, demanding, dependent, inconsiderate. Prone to manipulative threats and gestures.
Narcissistic life-style	Grandiose sense of self-importance. Preoccupied with fantasies of unlimited success, power, beauty, brilliance, etc. Need for attention and admiration. Indifference or marked feelings of rage, inferiority, or humiliation in response to criticism. In relations with others expects special favors, takes advantage of others, shifts between overidealizing others to disregard of them. Lacks ability for empathy.
Antisocial life-style	Behavior that causes conflicts with society such as thefts, vandalism, fighting, delinquency, truancy, and other crimes. Inability to sustain consistent work, lack of ability to function as a responsible parent, failure to exhibit lawful behavior. Unable to maintain enduring attachment to sexual partner. Lack of respect or loyalty, irritability and aggressiveness, conning others for personal gain, failure to plan ahead, tendency not to feel guilt or learn from experience and to blame others.
Borderline life-style	Impulsive and unpredictable in areas of life that are self-damaging, a pattern of unstable but intense interpersonal relationships, inappropriate displays of temper, mood instability, uncertainty about identity, intolerance of being alone, physically self-damaging, chronic feelings of boredom or emptiness.
Compulsive life-style	Overconscientious, overmeticulous, perfectionistic. Excessive concern for conformity. Rigid adherence to strict standards. Prone to self-doubt, unhappiness, and worry. Restricted ability to express warm and tender emotions, preoccupation with trivial details, rules, schedules, and lists.
Avoidant life-style	Hypersensitivity to rejection and interpretation of innocuous events as ridicule. Unwillingness to become involved with others unless given a guarantee of uncritical acceptance. Social withdrawal in interpersonal and work roles. Desire for affection and acceptance. Low self-esteem and overly dismayed by personal shortcomings.
Dependent life-style	Passively allows others to assume responsibility for major areas of life. Subordinates own needs to those on whom client depends to avoid possibility of having to rely on self. Lacks self-confidence.
Passive-aggressive life-style	Resistance to demands for adequate functioning through indirect methods such as procrastination, dawdling, stubborness, intentional inefficiency, and forgetfulness.
Paranoid life-style	Pervasive, unwarranted suspiciousness and mistrust evidenced by jealousy, envy, and guardedness. Hypersensitivity, usually feels mistreated and misjudged. Restricted feelings evidenced by lack of sense of humor; absence of sentimental, tender feelings; and pride in being cold and unemotional.
Schizoid life-style	Emotional coldness and aloofness. Indifference to praise or criticism from others. No desire for social involvement. Tendency to be reserved and seclusive.
Schizotypal life-style	Presence of various oddities of thought, perception, speech, and behavior, such as ideas of reference, bizarre fantasies, and preoccupations. Suspiciousness and hypersensitivity to real or imagined criticism. Social isolation.
Addicted life-style (Not identified in DSM-III as Personality Disorder but meets criteria for life-style.)	Continued use of alcohol and drugs to impairment of health, relationships, and economic security. Uneasy and dissatisfied with life. Selfish, domineering, and self-destructive.

- The ability to develop meaningful relationships with others and to communicate effectively is seriously impaired.

- The person rarely recognizes or acknowledges that any problem exists. Most of these people come to the attention of the nurse through an agency such as a public health department, a general hospital, or a detention home.

DEVELOPMENT OF DISRUPTIVE LIFE-STYLES

Styles of Defense and General Life-styles

Our style of functioning and thinking shapes our defensive operations. Our style of defense may be dictated by our general life-style, which in turn is dictated by constitutional, maturational, and experiential factors. Consider the following clinical example:

Steven, a compulsive man of thirty-two, was sober, technically minded, and active. However, he usually showed a conspicuous lack of enthusiasm or excitement in circumstances that seemed to warrant them. On one occasion, as he talked about an important promotion that he was almost certain to get, his sober expression was momentarily interrupted by a smile. After a moment more of talking, during which he maintained his soberness with difficulty, he began to speak of this promotion and then broke into a grin. Almost immediately, however, he regained his worried expression. "Of course," he said, "I don't know if I'm going to get it." This was said in a tone that suggested that the promotion was almost certain to fall through. After ticking off all the things that could go wrong, he seemed to become himself again.

Steven experienced a feeling or idea that made him visibly uncomfortable. A defensive process was immediately set into operation, and he regained his comfort. For Steven, expressions of slight optimism were associated with childish and unrealistic, premature hopes. One part of Steven didn't believe that the mere expression of enthusiasm would magically diminish his chance of success—but another part of him thought it might. Enthusiasm, according to Steven, could lead one to believe in a fool's paradise and thus to reckless behavior.

When he feels in danger of recklessly overestimating his position, this careful man takes precautions. He did not decide to become a careful man, he simply is one. The defensive process may therefore be regarded as a special case of the operation of a general style of functioning.

The following factors shape the style of functioning:

- Original psychological equipment, capacities, or tendencies

- Demands, opportunities, and forms of early external reality

- Later, generally stable modes of functioning

Most theorists acknowledge that innate endowments and their products—for example, thinking and language—influence a preference for a way of functioning. However, social forces also influence and reinforce development of a particular life-style.

Interaction of Factors in Style Preference

The interaction of the factors enumerated above in explaining life-styles is apparent in the following example:

Let us imagine that we observe an Indian, whose culture is unfamiliar, performing a strange dance with great intensity. As we watch, we may notice that the Indian belongs to an agricultural community, and that there is a drought. We consider the possibility that the dance is a prayer dance designed to bring rain and an expression of apprehension as well. Nearby, however, is a non-Indian farmer who also suffers from the drought, but who does not join in the dancing. It does not occur to him to perform these gestures. Instead, he goes home and worries. The Indian dances not only because there is a drought, but also because he is who he is. His dancing follows from certain attitudes and ways of thinking that are likely to be long standing and relatively stable.

Much the same sort of thing can be said of people who engage in disruptive life-styles. Compulsive persons, for instance, are interested in doubts, worries, and rituals. They perform their rituals not only because of their innate drives and conflicts but also because they are people with relatively stable ways of thinking, cognition, attitudes, and ways of feeling and responding to their environment. It is only when we understand the style and general tendency of the individual's mind and interest that we can reconstruct the subjective meaning of a thought or behavior for that person.

This chapter examines in some depth five of the commonest disruptive life-styles: impulsive, addicted, compulsive, dependent, and eccentric. The discussion follows the ideas expounded by David Shapiro (1965) modified to correspond with DSM-III categories of Personality Disorders.

IMPULSIVE LIFE-STYLES

People who have impulsive life-styles repeatedly come into conflict with society. These people are typically incapable of significant loyalty to individuals, groups, or social values. They are often selfish, callous, irresponsible, impulsive, and unlikely to feel guilt or to learn from experience or responsibility. In addition they usually have many of the following characteristics:

- Inability to postpone gratification
- Superficial charm and good intelligence
- Absence of delusions and other signs of irrational thinking
- Unreliability
- Untruthfulness and insincerity
- Lack of remorse, shame, guilt, or anxiety except under external stress
- Inadequate motivation
- Poor judgment and failure to learn by experience
- Egocentricity and incapacity for love
- General poverty in other major affective reactions
- Specific loss of insight
- Inability to form close, lasting relationships with friends or family
- Impersonal, trivial, and poorly integrated sex life
- Failure to follow any life plan
- Inability to tolerate frustration

Development of Impulsive Life-styles

Impulsive life-styles are generally associated with people who have been poorly or inadequately socialized. The individual often grew up in a chaotic home environment. Some theorists specifically connect maternal

Table 15–2   EARLY LIFE EXPERIENCES ASSOCIATED WITH DEVELOPMENT OF AN IMPULSIVE LIFE-STYLE

Experience	Rationale
Parental rejection or neglect that negates or limits development of emotional bonds.	This is often associated with the development of unsocialized aggressive behavior.
Separation or divorce in a marriage fraught with discord or similar antisocial life-styles.	Parental problems correlate highly with development of problems in the children.
The absence of adequate discipline or the presence of leniency in both parents.	This represents an extension of socialization deficients.
EEG findings show an excess of bilateral rhythmical slow-wave activity.	This finding is associated with lower baseline anxiety level and difficulty with impulse control.

deprivation in early life and development of an impulsive life-style. This somewhat deterministic idea is surrounded by controversy, but there is evidence that relates affectionless life-styles to an early lack of close emotional ties. A number of other early life experiences have been associated with adoption of an impulsive life-style. These are summarized, along with the dynamics of their rationales, in Table 15–2.

The predominant characteristics of a person living out an impulsive life-style are portrayed in the following clinical example:

S was an attractive, charming man of thirty-nine. He invariably impressed others as being intelligent and witty. In fact, his forte was superficial cocktail party conversations, in which he was both entertaining and attractive. Only the few people with whom he developed some slight intimacy knew how unreliable, untruthful, and insincere he was. He often demonstrated a lack of anxiety or concern that was inappropriate to the situation. The most frustrating aspect of his behavior was its unpredictability. His charming facade might predominate for weeks at a time. When he did lie or cheat, he was skillful at projecting the blame on others or justifying his behavior through some rationalization. He was well known for being able to avoid the consequences of his acts. He was a highly narcissistic person whose interests were centered on satisfying his own needs. He was unable to sustain any lastingly meaningful relationships and failed to follow any life plan unless some well-meaning individual provided it for him. Ultimately much of his behavior was self-defeating in that it was contrary to his own self-interest. His background involved desertion by his mother at the age of eight, physically violent family battles, and setting off to make his own way in the world by age sixteen.

Were we to examine this man's life for additional cues, we might find these typical adult problems:

- Frequent job changes
- Lengthy periods of unemployment
- Financial dependency, including total or partial support by relatives, social agencies, or institutions
- An arrest record
- Marriages characterized by verbal and physical fighting, separations, and divorces
- Desertion and nonsupport of spouses and children
- Alcohol and drug abuse
- Sexual promiscuity
- Vagrancy
- Belligerency
- Military records of desertions and absences without leave
- Social isolation, with no true friends but many casual acquaintances

Common Features

The DSM-III has grouped Histrionic, Narcissistic, Antisocial, and Borderline Personality Disorders together on the basis that individuals who are so diagnosed often appear dramatic, emotional, erratic, and impulsive. Impulsive life-styles also have certain additional features in common.

Distinctive Features of Subjective Experience   In any impulsive life-style, normal feelings of deliberateness and intention are impaired. This impairment is manifested to the individual as an irresistible impulse. The whim is paramount in the person's mental life.

It is worth mentioning that not all impulsive action is vivid and dramatic, but the subjective experience of

giving in to external temptation is the same for both passive and active impulsive people. They feel carried along by moment-to-moment events and execute significant actions without a clear and complete sense of motivation, decision, or sustained wish. When asked why they behaved as they did, they may say:

- "I just felt like it."
- "I didn't want to do it, but somehow I just did."
- "I didn't really want to do it, but I just gave in."
- "I was just carried along by the events."

All these explanations reflect an abrupt, transient and partial experience of deciding in which the sense of active intention is impaired.

Distinctive Features of Action and Motivation   In an impulsive life-style, actions reflect a deficiency in the mental processes that translate incipient motives into actions. The short-circuiting of these processes results in rapid, abrupt action without planning. Because their behavior has no anchor in stable aims, the whims of impulsive people tend to shift erratically. They experience an urge instead of a rich, sustained intention, and they take more interest in their own satisfaction than in objects, experiences, or other people.

ABSENCE OF JUDGMENT   Poor judgment and a conspicuous lack of long-range planning are characteristic of an impulsive life-style. The judgment of impulsive people is often arbitrary or reckless. They rush into unlikely business deals or ill-advised marriages, because the deal looks good or the person they met last night is their love of a lifetime. They believe they can "carry it off," though anyone else would recognize that the prospects are dim.

The active, searching, critical process known as *judgment*—a process that the compulsive person carries out in the manner of a dutiful prayer and at great length, and that the normal person carries out relatively smoothly—is abbreviated or eliminated in the impulsive person. These people remain partially or totally oblivious to drawbacks and complications that would give another person pause, and therefore have no stabilizing force against their tendency to speedy action.

MORALITY AND CONSCIENCE   Moral values, such as justice, truth, or personal integrity, are ideals. Their development depends on a capacity for self-critical examination. In most impulsive people moral values are comparatively underdeveloped and uninfluential, and conscience is perfunctory. These people do not reject morality on principle; they are simply uninterested. This holds true even though they may be well aware of morality as a fact to be dealt with or deferred to when it is practical to do so. From a moral standpoint, these people are cynical. From a practical standpoint they are expedient.

INSINCERITY AND LYING   Insincerity and lying are also characteristic of an impulsive life-style. Obviously they are somehow related to the lack of moral values just discussed. Impulsive people may merely lack any sense of responsibility to be truthful. However, even more obvious is the impulsive individual's ability to lie so easily and glibly. Their lies are not always deliberate, the product of serious reflection. Sometimes they tell lies "off the top of their heads"—leading them to contradict themselves. Ultimately they are motivated by some practical gain or advantage. They are immersed in opportunities to "operate" to win favor or disarm or impress someone. It seems reasonable, then, to suppose that a good deal of the antisocial impulsive behavior of so-called psychopaths or sociopaths is not simply the consequence of deficient moral values or defective conscience. Rather, it results from a combination of egocentricity; a general lack of direction; an absence of other than selfish, superficial values; and quick, involuntary modes of action.

The Impulsive World View   Impulsive people see the world as a discontinuous, inconstant composite of opportunities, temptations, frustrations, sensuous experiences, and fragmented impressions. They do not search beyond the immediately relevant present, because their interests and emotional involvements are limited to immediate gains and satisfactions.

Nursing Intervention

Intervention for people whose impulsive life-style is disruptive enough to warrant change is aimed at helping them control their behavior. This end is accomplished by maintaining a firm but accepting attitude toward clients, while imposing external limits on their actions. Often such a therapeutic plan is undertaken in a total inpatient milieu. Nurses are most likely to encounter these clients in a correctional institution or general hospital.

Essential Properties of the Nurse   The nurse who works with clients who have impulsive life-styles needs to be

- Patient
- Able to control personal resentment
- Intuitive
- Insightful
- Warm without being seductive
- Firm without being punitive
- Able to accept the client's feelings without identifying with the modes of behavior
- Able to use authority rationally and judiciously for the client's benefit
- Able to give unconditionally
- Able to accept the client's idiom and behavior without adopting them
- Able to persevere kindly but tenaciously when faced with manipulation of limits
- Able to tolerate verbal abuse from the client when enforcing limits

All of these qualities are used in intervention that is designed primarily as an educational experience. This form of intervention is not intended to resolve unconscious conflicts. Rather, it is meant to further the maturational process. Any effective intervention is likely to be long-term, because the client's fundamental behavior is based on some interference with or distortion of the normal process of personality growth.

Common Sources of Frustration   Nurses who set out to change the behavior of impulsive clients must be prepared to cope with some special problems. One is the client's immature behavior. Because these clients are relatively insensitive to anxiety, they are usually unaware of the immaturity of their responses. Another problem is their idiosyncratic or poor communication skills. They find it difficult to talk to others about how they feel. They may also be unwilling to acknowledge other people's feelings. Rather than use the customary adult modes of dealing with feelings, they tend to exhibit explosive, erratic, and inappropriate reactions. The nurse must provide consistent feedback about the behavior to increase the client's awareness of it. Modeling appropriate expression of feelings can be effective in coping with the second major source of frustration.

Goals of Intervention   Impulsive people often have unusual ability and demonstrate superior intelligence. They succeed brilliantly for a while in their studies and human relations. But sooner or later, inevitably and repeatedly, they fail, losing their jobs, alienating their friends, perhaps abandoning their families. It is usually difficult to account for these failures. They deprive impulsive people of what they claim are their chief objectives and can bring sorrow, hardship, and even disaster to those who know them.

If a client is firmly wedded to the impulsive life-style and feels no ambivalence or anxiety about its consequences, goal-centered therapy focused on changing behavior will probably fail. However, not all of these clients are committed to their life-style. Some exhibit some of the behaviors and characteristics discussed in the preceding pages, but not all. These people sometimes become internally motivated to change by a life crisis. Or friends or spouses may convince them to modify their patterns. When this happens, a plan of therapy focused on redefining and maturing the client's personality beyond its present state of development can work.

The general goals of this treatment in the context of a one-to-one, long-term relationship are to:

- Provide a model of mature behavior
- Develop a positive relationship
- Mobilize some anxiety in the client while encouraging the client to persist in the therapeutic relationship
- Convey concern and interest in the client
- Use problem-solving techniques to help the client make environmental changes, such as stable living arrangements and work plans
- Encourage the client to inhibit acting-out behaviors and rely more on verbal communication, thereby enhancing both self-control and self-esteem
- Help the client who has developed a more positive and realistic self-concept to continue the process of personal growth, which has usually been arrested in the preadolescent and adolescent years
- Anticipate and deal with depression in clients who gradually develop enough insight to realize and accept the responsibility for behavior that has injured others

The potential for achieving these goals with impulsive clients varies greatly from one client to another. Among the factors that influence the likelihood of successful change are

- The severity of the client's emotional deprivation
- The rigidity of the client's personality structure
- The client's ego strengths

- The client's superego development and potential for moral sensibility
- The client's motivation to change
- The nurse's skill and commitment
- Social support systems in the client's family or milieu that favor the desired changes

Education and maturation for these people require a willingness to engage in the self-examination they have so skillfully avoided. However, the reward for engaging in the process is liberation from the fundamental fears and low self-esteem carefully hidden beneath layers of defenses.

ADDICTED LIFE-STYLES

Addiction to alcohol and drugs is a complex social problem. It has physiological, psychological, and sociological dimensions—all of which are poorly understood by health professionals. Some professionals view addiction as an illness. Others prefer to consider it from a social or legal point of view. In the case of alcoholism, developmental theorists propose that there are psychological components caused by early experiences in family relationships. Some geneticists believe that there is a genetic susceptibility to alcohol addiction. Social scientists attribute it partly to high levels of stress in modern life and partly to social customs concerning drinking. The DSM-III categorizes it as a clinical syndrome, but in our view nurses most often encounter it as an enduring, maladaptive life-style. A genuinely holistic assessment of addiction takes organic, personality, and social factors into account.

Alcohol Addiction

Alcohol is a mind- and mood-altering substance classified as a central nervous system depressant. Its consumption at low levels may have no apparent effect on the drinker. At moderate levels it may produce euphoria. At high levels it acts as a sedative. Excessive use of alcohol usually occurs in one of two ways: *substance abuse* and *substance dependence*.

Abuse is distinguished from recreational or medical use by three criteria.

1. A pattern of use including intoxication during the day, inability to cut down or stop, need for daily intake in order to function, blackouts, and so forth.

	Table 15-3 BASIC FACTS ABOUT ALCOHOL AND ALCOHOLISM		
Definition	**Illnesses Associated with Long-term Use of Alcohol**	**Physiological Action**	**Public Health Issues**
An intoxicating beverage is one that produces a blood level concentration of alcohol of 0.15 percent or more. This concentration is the legal test for inebriation in many states	Alcoholic hepatitis Chronic gastritis Anemia Wernicke-Korsakoff syndrome (amnesia, confabulation, disorientation, peripheral neuropathic clouding of consciousness, and sometimes coma) Peripheral neuropathy Beriberi Pellagra Laennec's cirrhosis Alcoholic cerebellar degeneration	Absorbed in small intestine 2 to 10 percent excreted through lungs, kidneys, and skin Remainder broken down in liver Acts as CNS depressant Stimulating qualities felt as result of release of inhibition In large doses acts as a severe depressant of respiratory centers Simple intoxication does not last longer than 12 hours and is usually followed by a hangover	An estimated 9 million Americans suffer from alcoholism They are associated with an annual toll of 25,000 traffic fatalities, 15,000 homicides and suicides, and 20,000 deaths Alcoholism affects 40 million spouses and children Alcoholism accounts for half the 5 million arrests each year Alcoholism costs this country $20 to $25 billion in medical expenses, lost wages, and reduced productivity

2. Impairment of social or occupational functioning evidenced by failure to meet important business obligations, inappropriate displays of impulsive behavior or aggressive feelings, absenteeism from work, legal difficulties incurred because of incidents during the intoxicated state.

3. Duration of at least one month according to the most current psychiatric nomenclature. Isolated instances of problematic use are diagnosed as a specific Organic Brain Syndrome associated with the use of some substance such as alcohol.

Dependence is a severe form of Substance Use Disorder evidenced by the development of *tolerance* or *withdrawal*. Tolerance means that increased amounts of the substance are required to achieve the desired effect or that there is a diminished effect with regular use of the same amount. In withdrawal, a specific syndrome of symptoms develops when the person abruptly stops drinking. Alcohol withdrawal symptoms are:

• Tremors

• Excessive perspiration

• Nausea

• Vomiting

• Anorexia

• Restlessness

• Hallucinations

• Convulsions

• Delirium tremens

In popular usage the term *alcoholic* is reserved for those whose continued or excessive drinking results in impairment of personal health, disruption of family and social relationships, and loss of economic security. Some basic facts about alcohol are summarized in Table 15-3.

Some people drink because of social pressure. Others drink because they have strong emotional conflicts that remain unsolved. One of the first effects of alcohol is to depress the inhibitory centers of areas in the frontal lobes of the brain. This reduces self-criticism and judgment and produces a comfortable feeling of sureness and self-confidence. Under the influence of alcohol, a person can express emotions that normally are suppressed—for example, deep resentment and hostility. In doing so, the person experiences some relief. When the person is sober again, however, tension is usually increased by the feelings of guilt and the fear of retaliation that follow the expression of hostility. So the person drinks again to release the tension. The effect of alcohol is two-fold. It blurs the sharp edges of reality, and it makes the individual feel more competent to deal with reality. For people who tolerate anxiety poorly, alcohol can be a quick and effective solace.

Personality Traits of Alcoholics Most psychiatric literature concludes that no specific personality type is predisposed to alcoholism. However, we can make some generalizations about the personality structure of alcoholics. These include

• Difficulties in interpersonal relationships

• General uneasiness and dissatisfaction with life

• Tendency to excess in work, sex, and recreation

• Low tolerance for frustration

• Extreme dependence coupled with resentment of authority

• Flagrant selfishness

• Insistent demands for immediate satisfaction of needs

• Tendency to be domineering

• Tendency to self-destructive acts, including suicidal tendencies

As with most exclusively psychological theories, it is difficult to determine whether these characteristics are typical of the potential alcoholic or are the result of drinking.

Labeling the Alcoholic Differentiating normal drinking from an alcoholic life-style depends, like all psychiatric labeling, on both intrapsychic and social factors. If interference in social and occupational functioning is a criterion, a business executive with an efficient secretary to do much of his work and a lot of flexibility in how he chooses to accomplish it may be able to avoid the label of alcoholic, even though he consumes three double martinis at lunch *every* day and drinks steadily all evening. Different cultures also influence the manner in which labels are distributed. (See Chapter 26.) In France, where the quantity of wine drunk regularly exceeds the limits set in most other cultures, a man who drinks wine with breakfast would rarely define himself as having a drinking problem. Labeling may also depend on the amount a person consumes. People who are intoxicated as seldom as four times a year or as often as twice a week may be classified as alcoholic.

Nursing Intervention Health professionals must view alcoholic life-styles holistically if they wish to generate effective approaches to treat them. Alcohol Dependence is more than an addiction, a toxic state, a disease, a bad habit, a criminal offense, or a mental illness. It is also a social problem with effects on the client's body, behavior, and interpersonal relationships.

The nurse usually encounters alcoholics first when they are acutely ill from the toxic effects of the drug and require hospitalization. See Figure 15–1. The symptoms during this acute phase may include

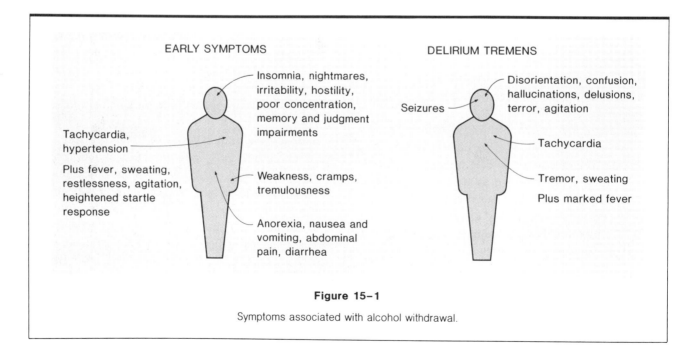

Figure 15–1

Symptoms associated with alcohol withdrawal.

- Nausea and vomiting
- Perspiration and weakness
- Severe tremors, especially of hands and face
- Myoclonic jerking of arms, legs, head, and neck, which may increase to the severity of generalized convulsions
- Dilated pupils
- Insomnia
- Loss of appetite, or even inability to tolerate food
- Dehydration
- Slurred, often rambling and incoherent speech
- Motor activity ranging from wild restlessness to a state of stupor
- Emotional symptoms including anxiety, depression, irritability, hypersensitivity to light and sound, impaired memory, disorientation, inappropriate behavior, visual and auditory hallucinations, and impaired insight and judgment
- Tendency to develop intercurrent respiratory infections, which may develop into pneumonia
- Apparent poor hygiene and poor nutrition
- If alcoholism is prolonged, nutritional and vitamin deficiencies, liver cirrhosis, chronic brain damage, and mental deterioration

OVERVIEW The nurse may play a key role both in identifying alcoholics and referral and in coordinating a

system of treatment that includes the following services:

- Crisis intervention or acute emergency care
- Detoxification
- Medical or psychiatric inpatient follow-up
- Halfway houses to bridge the transition to some stable social situation
- Aftercare

Intervention for an alcoholic life-style can occur on a medical, behavioral, social, or psychological level. The nurse must recognize that the client may have problems in all four areas. When this happens, a broad-based treatment program is necessary. Whether these clients say they drink to relieve loneliness, reduce tension, be sociable, combat boredom, unwind, make themselves feel good, or drown their sorrows, the basic issue is always the same. Why do clients continue to drink when to do so ruins their lives on every level—physical, emotional, social, and economic? The nurse should encourage dialogue, listen carefully, help the clients bear their painful feelings, and convey an attitude of acceptance and optimism. In this way the nurse can support the alcoholic toward the achievement of negotiated treatment goals.

TREATMENT IN ACUTE PHASE Initial treatment for the acute phase of alcoholism is often referred to as "dry-

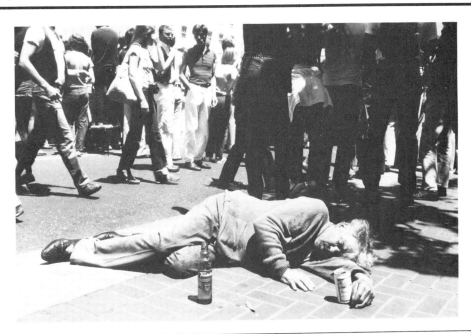

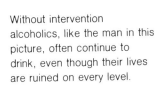
Without intervention alcoholics, like the man in this picture, often continue to drink, even though their lives are ruined on every level.

ing out" or detoxification. Support measures directed toward relieving the symptoms include

- Some type of sedation or tranquilizers
- Medication to relieve symptoms of nausea and insomnia
- Adequate diet
- Replacement of fluids
- Vitamin therapy
- Antibiotics if infections are present

Acute phase treatment usually occurs in a well-controlled environment such as a hospital.

FOLLOW-UP TREATMENT   Like the other people discussed in this chapter, alcoholics rarely consider themselves in need of prolonged psychological treatment. They tell themselves and others that this binge will be the last. Some of their biggest difficulties stem from their inability to face their own problems and fears, their skillful rationalizations, their ability to hide and minimize their problem drinking, their characteristic ambivalence, and the critically rebellious attitude they develop toward hospitalization. Their minimization of their difficulties and rationalizations of their behavior often help them avoid follow-up treatment. Consider the following clinical example:

Mr. C, a man in his early sixties, was admitted to the medical floor of a community hospital by his family. After a period of prolonged drinking, he was in poor physical condition. At first he was concerned about himself and eager to be helped. He seemed ashamed and embarrassed about his drinking problem. As he improved physically, he became congenial and eager to become involved in his life and work again. As soon as he began to feel physically well, he began demanding to go home—saying that he had only come in for a routine checkup and now that it was complete, he was ready to deal with his life again. Any suggestion that he come to grips with his underlying problem evoked first evasiveness and then criticism and hostility toward the health care professionals. Mr. C signed himself out of the hospital. Within two months he was back into his cyclical drinking pattern.

For long-term treatment, goals to prevent a script like Mr. C's include the following:

- Alcoholics must give up alcohol for the rest of their lives. No treatment can restore their control so that they can drink moderately.
- Generally alcoholics need to restructure their everyday living patterns to develop a satisfactory life without alcohol.
- The therapeutic relationship should focus on increasing the alcoholic's self-confidence, feelings of self-worth, and attempts to become more independent.

In short, the long-range general goal for the alcoholic is social recovery. These people must regain the ability to live as accepted members of society with every function restored except the ability to drink. Most therapists agree that the conditions listed in Table 15–4 contribute to the probability that such a long-range goal can be achieved.

ALCOHOLICS ANONYMOUS   A number of the conditions listed in Table 15–4 are provided by Alcoholics Anonymous. This organization of ex-alcoholics will go to great lengths to assist alcoholics who are willing to ask for help. They will come any hour of the day or night, nurse alcoholics through hangovers, even take them to their own homes. Membership in Alcoholics Anonymous is voluntary, and there are no fees associated with any of its services.

Prevention Measures   Most health professionals are beginning to view prevention of alcoholic life-styles as a community responsibility. A number of strategies have been proposed as primary prevention measures. They include the following:

- Training people to tolerate increased stress and to learn improved coping patterns
- Preparing people in advance for difficult or painful events
- Reducing irritating or frustrating environmental stress
- Reducing social isolation
- Attempting to alter alcoholic beverages chemically to lessen their addictive qualities
- Instituting measures to regulate their sale and distribution
- Promoting educational programs in schools on the use and abuse of alcohol
- Finding substitute tension-reducing strategies

Table 15-4 THERAPEUTIC CONDITIONS FOR ALCOHOLIC RECOVERY	
Therapeutic Condition	**Rationale**
Group therapy	Most alcoholics find the self-examination and introspection of individual psychotherapy intolerable and find support, understanding, and influence to change their behavior from other former alcoholics.
Family involved in long-range treatment plan	With more research it becomes apparent that alcoholism does not involve just one individual. It has its roots in the family of origin and its source of maintenance in the current family constellation.
Nurses with special knowledge of problems of alcoholism could follow up with clients providing continuity and consistency	Some of the failure in treatment of alcoholics has occurred because clients get lost between referrals or drop out of treatment in the episodes between binges.
Therapist available at critical times	The alcoholic has difficulty tolerating delays in help or disinterested attitudes in the therapist. These people usually require immediate support to avoid drinking.

Drug Dependence

Life-styles are either supported and reinforced by other aspects of a culture or they are discouraged and denied. A glance into the average American medicine cabinet or an assessment of advertising on television or in the popular press reveals that contemporary American culture contributes both directly and indirectly to drug dependence. While the chemical characteristics of drugs determine their effects on the individual, cultural norms dictate the circumstances under which various drugs are used and the consequences of using them. People in most societies need to avoid or minimize pain, fatigue, and anxiety. They also sometimes need to feel euphoria. They use drugs for both purposes.

Alcohol, tobacco, and coffee are commonly used. These substances qualify as drugs, and all three have become important adjuncts to daily life in most of the civilized world. The following discussion, however, examines drug dependence that has become a *disruptive life-style.*

Definitions   Many people are confused about the precise meanings of the terms *drug use, drug abuse,* and *drug addiction* or *dependence.* Table 15–5 clarifies the meanings of these terms.

Psychological Theories on Causes   Theorists explain the development of a drug-dependent life-style in different ways. Most theories may be classified as psychological, sociological, or physiological. We will begin by considering the psychological theories.

In the psychoanalytic literature people with drug-dependent life-styles are said to be regressed and fixated at pregenital, oral levels of psychosexual development. In some of the literature the pattern of drug taking is related to parental inconsistency, self-centeredness, and inner dishonesty. The following personality traits are often associated with disruptive drug use:

- Dominant and critical behavior with underlying self-doubts and passivity
- Tendency to describe own parents as self-reliant and efficient but not emotionally warm
- Personal insecurity
- Problems with sexual identification
- Rebellious attitudes toward authority
- Tendency to use defense mechanisms that are primarily escapist
- Inability to form close and lasting affection ties
- Absence of a strong and efficient superego
- Marked narcissistic trends

There is no real agreement about whether certain personality traits are sufficient to account for drug dependence, yet those who become dependent on drugs to relieve anxiety or suppress conflict do so at least partially because of their particular personality structure.

Sociological Theories on Causes   Many social scientists view the drug-dependent life-style as a product of a particular social context and as a reflection of a particular social role. In other words, the patterns of

	Table 15–5 DEFINITIONS OF TERMS COMMONLY USED IN DISCUSSING DRUG USE	
Term	**Definition**	**Example**
Drug use	Ingesting in any manner a chemical that has an effect on the body	Taking an aspirin for headache
Drug abuse	A state of chronic intoxication detrimental to the individual and produced by repeated consumption of a drug. Characterized by	Street use of heroin
	1. Overpowering need or desire to take the drug despite legal, social, or medical problems	
	2. Willingness to obtain the drug by any means, including illegal ones	
	3. Tendency to increase the dose	
	4. Physical dependence on effects of drug	
Drug dependence	Dependence on a drug such that	Regular and increasing use of sedatives and hypnotics like valium
	1. The body requires it to continue functioning.	
	2. The body develops a tolerance for it, so the person must increase the dose.	
	3. The body develops physical withdrawal symptoms if the drug is stopped.	
	4. The person feels that it is impossible to get along without the drug.	

behavior and attitudes characteristic of this life-style are learned by many members of a particular culture. In the early fifties, many writers argued that socioeconomically deprived cultures were those most likely to produce drug addicts. However, the steady increase in the number of addicts from privileged and middle-class homes suggests that this may not be true. Drugs are used to relieve anxiety, and much anxiety is the product of an economically and socially deprived environment. But it is not only the ghetto resident who turns to drugs to block out life's harsh realities.

SOCIAL CONTEXT: A BROADER VIEW Life's harsh realities come in many forms. There is the sense of hopelessness and defeat that comes of living in an urban slum. There is the adolescent's feeling of impotence and alienation. There is the social vacuum of unloving families, where meaningful attachments are dissolved or dissolving. All of these social conditions and contexts help create and sustain drug addiction. In addition, however, people who become addicts tend to live in environments where access to drugs and initiation into their use are widespread. Deviant subcultures encourage their members to adopt a drug-dependent life-style. The sociologist Howard Becker (1963) studied

the process by which a person becomes a marijuana user. His study emphasized the role the subculture plays in teaching people to disengage from conventional social controls. It also teaches them the definitions of experience and the techniques that insure that they will enjoy using the drug. Many people who use marijuana today do not make a full transition to a drug-dependent life-style. Another sociologist, Alfred Lindesmith (1965), observes that people recognize that they are addicted at the moment when the appearance of withdrawal symptoms makes voluntary abstinence impossible. At this point they are ready to be assimilated into a genuine drug-dependent life-style, for they must begin planning how to assure their future supply. They must learn the sources, devices, and customs by means of which their problems can be solved.

ELIMINATING MYTHS ABOUT DRUG DEPENDENCE There is no evidence to support a number of common myths about drug dependence. The following list of statements is intended to correct these myths.

• Drug dependence and addiction are not exclusively problems of residents of inner city ghettos.

		Table 15–6 ADDICTIVE DOSES OF SEDATIVE-HYPNOTICS	
Generic Name	**Trade Name**	**Dependence-producing Dose (Mg per Day)**	**Number of Days Necessary to Produce Dependence**
Chlordiazepoxide	Librium	300–600	60–180
Diazepam	Valium	80–120	42
Chloral hydrate	Noctec	2,000–3,000	
Meprobamate	Equanil Miltown		
Glutethimide	Doriden	200–3,000	
Sodium secobarbital	Seconal	800–2,200	35–37
Sodium pentobarbital	Nembutal	800–2,200	35–37
Methaqualone	Sopor Quaalude	2,100–3,000	21–28

Source: Reprinted with permission of STASH, Inc. from the *Journal of Psychedelic Drugs*, Volume 3(2):81, Spring, 1971. Copyright © 1971.

- The major shift in drug use patterns has been a trend away from heroin and back to alcohol, except that now alcohol is being used in combination with barbiturates and other sedative-hypnotics.

- The drug user now tends to use a combination of drugs rather than a single one.

- It is unclear whether the use and abuse of hallucinogens such as LSD have really leveled off, or whether the user of these drugs is more knowledgeable and sophisticated than before and so less likely to be seen in psychiatric, medical, or legal settings.

- While heavy drug abuse is incompatible with a normal life-style, millions of Americans use marijuana on a regular basis.

- The punitive approach used to provide social control over drug traffic has done little to solve the problems associated with the drug-dependent life-style.

- Beyond the early states of addiction there is little euphoria and much misery associated with most addictive drugs.

- Internal psychodynamics and social and familial experiences both seem to differentiate an adolescent or young adult who adopts a drug-dependent life-style from one who does not.

- Less is known about the personality deviance associated with adult drug addicts than with adolescents.

- Evidence shows that crime and narcotics use do exist side-by-side, but that neither opiates nor marijuana leads to crimes of violence. Arrests for nonviolent theft predominate among addicts.

- While most addicts to opiates began by smoking marijuana, there are no data to suggest that the use of marijuana actually leads to the use of opiates or other addicting drugs.

Biochemical Theories on Causes   Many researchers are dissatisfied with the inconclusiveness of psychological and sociological theories of drug dependence. These researchers focus their attention on biochemical factors that might be related to drug use. Certainly many addictive drugs do produce actual physical dependence. This fact does not explain how or why people begin to use drugs, but it does explain why they may continue to use them. A post-addictive syndrome among heroin addicts includes anxiety, depression, and craving experienced under stress even after prolonged abstinence. Even though the exact mechanisms have not been identified, most proponents of biochemical theories account for readdiction in terms of the effects of the opiate molecules on the central nervous system. Studies of addictive doses and length of regular use of common sedatives and hypnotics have also yielded findings that are important to nurses who advise, educate, and counsel clients. Some of these data are presented in Table 15–6.

Specific Drugs Commonly Abused In order to assess a client who is abusing drugs, it is important to collect the following data:

• What drug is being used?
• How much is being used on a daily basis?
• How frequently is it used?
• How long has the client been using it?
• What combination of drugs is being used?

The nurse must evaluate the category of drug in use and its effects in order to plan effective immediate and long-term intervention. Some clients are ashamed of their drug habits and believe that the nurse would be shocked by them. Yet, questions about substance use patterns are part of every good psychiatric history (Chapter 8). Experienced clinicians suggest that questions directed particularly to *street users* of alcohol and other drugs are more likely to elicit the truth if the nurse begins with an overstatement then allows the clients to offer the correct information.

NURSE: *Are you drinking about a gallon a day now?*
CLIENT: *No, not that much. More like a quart and a half.*
NURSE: *What do you have, a two hundred dollar a day habit?*
CLIENT: *No, only about half that.*

The major categories of drugs are sedative-hypnotics; narcotics; marijuana; central nervous system stimulants; hallucinogens; cocaine; and inhalants—glue, gasoline, and solvents. The slang names of these drugs, their routes of administration, the usual desired effects, the observable effects, the untoward and long-term effects, the symptoms of overdose, and the methods of immediate first aid or intervention are all presented in Table 20–8. Here we will touch briefly on several of the seven categories.

SEDATIVE-HYPNOTICS Used therapeutically for insomnia, barbiturates have many of the same effects and pose many of the same dangers as alcohol. However, it would be difficult to consume a fatal dose of alcohol at one sitting. Barbiturates, on the other hand, are frequently used to commit suicide. Many barbiturates have a synergistic action with other drugs, narrowing the margin between maximum and lethal doses. Overdoses of these drugs are often medical emergencies

that require hospitalization. All the drugs in this group have a potential for physical and psychological dependence. All produce tolerance leading to progressively higher dosages.

CENTRAL NERVOUS SYSTEM STIMULANTS This group of drugs includes caffeine, nicotine, cocaine, and amphetamines. Nicotine is unique in that it acts both as a stimulant and as a depressant. Interestingly, it is a highly toxic drug. Sixty milligrams make up a lethal dose. Nicotine has also been related to lung cancer, coronary artery disease, and emphysema. Amphetamines have effects similar to those of ephedrine: constriction of peripheral blood vessels, stimulation of heart, increased blood pressure, relaxation of bronchial and intestinal muscles, and a decrease in appetite. These drugs are used as mood elevators and appetite depressants. They are also used to combat drowsiness. As tolerance to these drugs develops, the sense of well-being is increasingly blurred by apprehension, and emotional lability—particularly characterized by hostile impulsiveness—increases. Withdrawal from amphetamines usually causes depression and somnolence.

COCAINE Cocaine acts as a topical anesthetic. Among users in the drug culture it is usually sniffed or snorted rather than injected intravenously. If taken in sufficient quantity, it induces euphoric excitement and hallucinatory experiences. Despite its comparatively high cost in the street market, its use is increasing. As with amphetamines and other stimulants, users experience depression when they stop using it. Heavy use of this stimulant can cause a particular kind of drug-induced psychosis called *cocaine bugs,* in which sufferers feel that bugs are crawling under their skin.

HALLUCINOGENIC DRUGS Hallucinogenic drugs—LSD, mescaline, psilocybin, and THC—are not physically addictive, but they can produce psychological dependence and tolerance. Some of these drugs, such as LSD, are synthetic. Others, such as mescaline and psilocybin, are contained in certain cactuses and mushrooms, which are important in the spiritual rites of certain Indian cultures in the United States and Mexico. The most characteristic effect of these drugs is a kaleidoscopic visual hallucination of vivid colors and forms. Moods and perceptions may also vary dramatically. The major problems usually associated with use of these drugs are bad trips and flashbacks.

Bad trips are acute anxiety and panic reactions that occur among users of psychedelic drugs who are not prepared for the physical and psychological sensations associated with use of the drug.

The following guidelines are useful in caring for clients experiencing a bad trip:

- Place them in a quiet room, either with a trusted friend or with a professional who can "talk them down."
- Quietly reassure them that what they are experiencing is drug related and will go away shortly, and that they won't suffer any permanent damage.
- Counter distortions of reality by careful reality orientation.
- Be careful not to threaten or upset these clients, because they feel extremely vulnerable. Any slightly hostile comment can set off an extreme panic reaction.

Persons using hallucinogens may experience flashbacks. Flashbacks may be either visual distortions (intense colors, trails, geometric forms in objects) or emotional flashbacks, in which the person relives an intense emotional experience that occurred during a previous drug experience. Both kinds of flashback are more likely to occur when the person is undergoing stress or is falling asleep. These are times when ego functions are somewhat disturbed, making the person susceptible to invasion by feelings.

INHALANTS   Young people are increasingly using inhalants—glue, gasoline, and solvents—to attain a state similar to alcohol intoxication. The media have published widespread information about the potentially dire consequences of this practice. However, there is only a limited amount of valid and reliable research on its effects.

Nursing Intervention   There are three steps in developing an effective intervention plan with a drug-dependent person. The first is to assess the person's drug use pattern. The second is to offer support during detoxification or withdrawal. The third is long-term rehabilitation. Key considerations relevant to each of these steps are presented in Table 15–7.

Many addicts seem to need to create a pattern of failure in their lives. They often do this by setting unrealistic goals. This perpetuates their low self-esteem and sense of failure. The will to fail makes these clients extremely difficult to deal with, and nurses who attempt to intervene in their life-style are often frustrated.

COMPULSIVE LIFE-STYLES

People who have a compulsive life-style demonstrate an excessive conformity and conscientiousness. They are excessively meticulous and perfectionistic. Among the features generally associated with compulsive life-styles are rigidity, the distortion of the experience of autonomy, and the loss of consensual reality. Extremely maladaptive forms of this life-style involve elaborate and at times health-threatening compulsive rituals covered in Chapter 16.

Rigidity

The term *rigidity* has several meanings. It can refer to a stiff body posture, a stilted social manner, or a tendency to persist in a course of action that has become irrelevant—even absurd. Most of all, however, rigidity refers to a dogmatic or opinionated way of thinking. Consider the following casual conversation between a father and his son. They are discussing an upcoming holiday visit.

FATHER: *I know your wife doesn't like me to stay long, so I'm only coming from December 20 to January 6. I couldn't get a flight any earlier that would connect with the limo to my house.*

SON: *Well, Dad, based on past visits, I think seventeen days is probably too long without everyone getting a bit on each other's nerves. Let me help you arrange an earlier flight back.*

FATHER: *Well, my friend is the travel agent for American and does all the sports bookings, and I could have got one on January 4, but it gets here too late for the limo.*

SON: *I'd be happy to pay for the taxi home. Let's change the reservation to December 30. I know there's space available then.*

FATHER: *I'd only be there for nine days then, and it wouldn't be worth the money for that short a time.*

SON: *Nine good days are probably worth more than a seventeen-day visit that wears thin by its end, though.*

FATHER: *That flight wouldn't get back until after the last limo has left, and there's no other way to get to my house from the airport except by taxi.*

In this conversation, the father doesn't exactly disagree with his son. He simply does not pay attention. Furthermore, his inattention has a special quality. It is,

	Table 15–7 NURSING INTERVENTION WITH DRUG-DEPENDENT CLIENTS	
Step	**Key Considerations**

1. Assessment of the drug use pattern.	1. Find out what drug or drugs are being used.
	 2. For each drug, note
	   a. The quantity on a daily basis
	   b. The frequency of use
	   c. How long drugs have been used
	 3. Collect data to establish whether alcohol is being used in combination with other sedative-hypnotics.
	 4. Remember that more accurate information may be obtained by interviewing the client's parents or friends, or by a physical exam and blood and urine lab tests, than by questioning the client directly.

2. Support during detoxification or withdrawal	1. Gradual withdrawal or detoxification is essential for persons addicted to barbiturates, nonbarbiturate hypnotics, and tranquilizers. Abrupt withdrawal can be fatal. 2. Detoxification takes from two to three weeks and should take place in a structured inpatient setting. 3. Phenothiazines may be used as an adjunct to treatment. 4. The nurse should attend to accompanying physical problems, such as abcesses at the injection site, hepatitis, malnutrition, and respiratory and gastrointestinal disease. 5. It may be necessary to give verbal reassurance and reality orientation to reduce feelings of panic during withdrawal. It is essential to stay with a person who is on a bad trip until the effects of the drug wear off. 6. Fatigue and depression lasting for several weeks accompany withdrawal from stimulants.
3. Rehabilitation	1. Long-range treatment is based on helping the person learn better mechanisms for coping with stress and problems. 2. In programs such as methadone treatment, the nurse may need to learn to administer methadone and supervise such medical procedures as the proper collecting and processing of urine samples. 3. Selection of clients for a long-term rehabilitation program should be based on a thorough evaluation of the individual. Not all drug users are hardcore junkies. Rehabilitation programs exist for drug experimenters and social users as well as established addicts.

for example, quite different from the wandering attention of a tired person. It has a principled quality (Shapiro 1965). This inattention to new information or points of view is what we are referring to when we speak of rigidity.

Style of Paying Attention

Compulsive people cannot seem to receive a casual or immediate impression. Instead they always seem to concentrate on insignificant details. In general, the compulsive person will have some sharply defined in-

terest, stick to it, get the facts about it, but usually miss those aspects of it that give it its flavor or impact.

William was visiting Europe for the first time in his fifty years. Every day he sent home lengthy postcards from each new city or town. The cards were filled with technical details ranging from the price of gasoline to the time he woke up, ate each meal, or retired. Nowhere among those many cards and letters was a single comment about how any of his experiences made him feel.

Most people can concentrate or entertain impressions equally well. The compulsive person lacks this mobility of attention and flexible cognitive mode. That is why, in conversation, these people exhibit selective inattention to any new idea or external influence. Perhaps this is also why they often seem insensitive to the emotional tone of social situations.

General Mode of Activity

To understand a particular life-style, we must understand three things. The first is the individual's way of thinking. The second is the unique modes of action associated with that life-style. The third is the affective experience associated with it. Each of these three things may influence the person's overall functioning to varying degrees. In the hystrionic life-style, for instance, affective experience or feelings virtually dominate the person's functioning. In the compulsive life-style, feelings have very little influence; activity predominates. The activity is conspicuous both for its sheer quantity and for its intensity. These people may be enormously productive, especially in work that requires routine and attention to technical detail. Equally often they devote themselves to minor or irrelevant details. For example, a young man may spend weeks carefully collecting, preparing, and transcribing on index cards detailed information on all the colleges he might attend so that someday he can choose the "best." In the meantime, his high school grades plunge below minimum qualification for even the most ordinary of colleges.

The Subjective Quality of Trying

The compulsive life-style has another, equally distinctive, quality. This is the sense of deliberate trying that is almost a continuous experience for compulsive people. They can even bring tense deliberateness to activities that most people enjoy—Christmas shopping, taking family photos, or scheduling holidays to have the most fun. As one client put it, "I always try hard to schedule my social life to be as spontaneous as possible." Sometimes compulsive people are also characterized as "driven." This term is apt, since their activity actually seems pressed or motivated by something beyond their own interest. They do not seem enthusiastic about the activities that they pursue with such intensity. Instead, they act and feel as though they were being pressed by some necessity that they are at pains to satisfy.

Peter J set himself a deadline in early fall for ordering his family's Christmas gifts. His family found this deadline something of an annoyance to deal with. Yet Peter persisted in his attempts to get commitments from everyone about what they wanted. As often as not, his early purchases would be mislaid by the time Christmas finally arrived, and he would rush out to do last-minute shopping anyway.

Peter J not only suffers under the pressure of his deadlines, he also sets them. He constantly functions like his own overseer—issuing commands, directives, reminders, warnings, and admonitions about what should be done. People like Peter J are also keenly aware of society's and other people's expectations; of the threat of possible criticism; of the weight and direction of authority; of rules, regulations, and conventions; and of a great assemblage of moral or quasi-moral principles. These people feel and function like hardworking automatons, pressing themselves to fulfill unending duties, responsibilities, and tasks that are, in their view, not chosen but simply there.

The Consequences for Quality of Life

Obviously these people's lives are severely restricted by their compulsive style of functioning. Sometimes their restriction of feeling is mistaken for overcontrol. This is misleading, for these people do not deliberately curb their whims, playfulness, and spontaneity. Their whole orientation prevents them from feeling really comfortable with any activity done simply for pleasure. Often even vacations become exhausting tours meticulously planned to cover every possible sight and event available in as short a time as possible.

Decision-making   It comes as no surprise that people who are cut off from their own wants and feelings, driven by a sense of pressure, and guided by what they perceive as moral direction, shrink from making decisions. Free choice for them is extremely disagreeable. Usually they attempt to reach a solution by calling on some rule or external requirement. In short, they seek some means other than their own resources to make the decision at hand. They choose the cheapest movie—not the one they would enjoy—or the most logical community to live in. When they cannot reach a decision by formula or rule, they stew and struggle to find the "right" solution and go on stewing long after they have worn out the facts and exhausted any possibility of gaining new understanding from them.

The Loss of Consensual Reality   Sometimes the compulsive's worries border on the delusional. People in this position may believe that they have been contaminated by some unlikely and integrated chain of events, or are developing symptoms of some unnamed disease, though doctors assure them that they are in perfect health. They experience dogma and doubt simultaneously, because they have no real convictions of their own. These people's narrow interest in technical indicators prevents them from seeing things in their real proportions, recognizing the rich shading or substance of the world.

Nursing Intervention

People with compulsive life-styles are usually poor candidates for growth and change because their ego functions are often too weak to handle the anxiety that would be released if the behavior patterns were removed. However, a few guidelines can be advanced for nurses working with these clients.

- Study how the coping mechanisms of compulsions operate.
- Work to help the client feel safer in relationships and in making some decisions.
- Avoid attacking or interfering with coping mechanisms unless prepared to work with the anxiety that results from such interference.
- Introduce new, potentially threatening experiences to the client carefully to minimize anxiety.
- Provide an environment that relieves the client from as much anxiety-provoking decision making as possible.
- Set consistent, firm limits about rituals that seriously interfere with the client's welfare.

The guidelines reflect the principle that compulsive life-styles are adopted by people to avoid the anxiety that is often related to decision-making. In most instances it is futile to work toward developing insight about these behavior patterns. Clients know only that they behave this way because it makes them feel better. Attacking any of the compulsive defense mechanisms will cause the client intense anxiety. A nurse

who chooses to make such an attack must therefore be prepared to stay with the client and work with the anxiety that surfaces.

DEPENDENT LIFE-STYLES

Characteristics

Avoidant, Dependent, and Passive-aggressive Personality Disorders are grouped together and characterized in DSM-III as having the common characteristic of fearfulness. The avoidant personality is hypersensitive to potential rejection yet experiences a strong need for affection and acceptance. Dependent personalities passively allow others to assume responsibility for major areas of their lives because of a similarly low self-esteem and lack of self-confidence. Passive-aggressive personalities also appear dependent and lack self-confidence, but their most consistent characteristic is resistance to demands for occupational and social performance expressed indirectly through such maneuvers as procrastination, dawdling, stubborness, inefficiency, and forgetfulness. These behaviors persist even under circumstances in which more assertive and effective patterns are possible.

Nursing Intervention

There is a widespread tendency for nurses to avoid involvement with dependent clients out of fear or dislike for their clinging demands. It is crucial that the nurse break the cycle of avoidance leading to increased anxiety in the dependent client, leading to increased demands for help and attention, leading to further avoidance. Guidelines for effective intervention with clients who present with dependent life-styles include the following:

- Anticipating clients' needs before they demand attention
- Setting realistic limits about what can and cannot be done for clients
- Helping clients manage anxiety that occurs when others do not spontaneously meet their needs
- Teaching clients to express their ideas and feelings assertively

• Supporting clients who are gradually making more of their own decisions

The above guides for nursing intervention rest on the premise that dependent people usually lack confidence in the willingness of others to help as well as in their own ability to be self-sufficient. Consequently they have a pattern of dependent clinging, fearing that if others are permitted any distance, they will be abandoned.

ECCENTRIC LIFE-STYLES

Eccentric life-styles impair normal functioning more severely than the other patterns discussed in this chapter. In its most extreme form the eccentric life-style can plunge the person into a complete alternative reality.

Paranoid, Schizoid, and Schizotypal Personality Disorders are grouped together in DSM-III and considered to be examples of odd or eccentric life-styles.

Characteristics of a Paranoid Personality

Suspicious Thinking The word *suspicious* is usually used to describe someone with certain ideas, preoccupations, or unwarranted apprehensions such as a continual expectation of being followed. But suspiciousness is also a way of thinking.

Rigidity Suspicious thinking is remarkably and impressively rigid. Suspicious people look at the world with certain fixed and preoccupying expectations and search for confirmation of them. They pay no attention to rational arguments. Anyone who tries to persuade a suspicious person will not only fail, but will probably become an object of suspicion. Suspicious people do not ignore a new bit of information; they examine it quite carefully. But they examine it with an extraordinary prejudice, dismissing what is not relevant to their suspicions and seizing on anything that confirms them. Suspicious people are not simply people who are apprehensive and imagine things. They are in actual fact keen and penetrating observers. They not only imagine, they also *search* with an intensity of attention and an acuteness that may easily surpass the normal person's capacity. For example, a client who was afraid that she would be hypnotized

became extremely upset when she noticed one book on the subject among the hundreds in the hospital library. This cognitive mode—characterized by active, intense, searching action—enables suspicious people to impose their own conclusions virtually anywhere. Thus they can be at the same time right in their perception and wrong in their judgment. Among the manifestations of suspiciousness are:

• Expectations of trickery or harm

• Guardedness or secretiveness

• Jealousy

• Doubt of others' loyalty

• Overconcern with hidden motives and special meanings

Hypersensitivity and Alertness Paranoid people avoid surprise by anticipating it. They are ready for any unexpected event and are immediately aware of it when it happens. They must then scrutinize it and bring it into their scheme of things. A police car that arrives at an intersection is noticed, carefully observed for details, and then integrated into a system of beliefs the person has about being followed by the authorities. There is also a tendency to be easily slighted, to make mountains out of mole-hills, and to find it very difficult to relax.

Distortions of Reality Paranoid people construct a subjective world in which facts, accurately enough perceived in themselves, are endowed with a special interpretive significance. Thus the subject matter of their interest has to do with hidden motives, underlying purposes, special meanings, and the like. They do not necessarily disagree with the normal person about the existence of any given fact—only about its significance. Therefore, even severely paranoid people can recognize various essential facts well enough to achieve a limited adjustment to the normal social world. At the same time, however, they continue to interpret substantial portions of this world autistically. For example, a paranoid woman may recognize the necessity of paying her income taxes but may regard their collection as part of some government action directed toward her personally.

Use of Projection Projection is an ego defense mechanism in which paranoid people attribute to external figures the motivations, drives, or other feelings

Table 15–8 COMPARISON OF COMPULSIVE AND PARANOID STYLES

Factor	Paranoid	Compulsive
Mode of attention	Extremely acute, intense, and narrowly focused; fixed on its own idea, searching only confirmation; biased	Acute, intense, and narrowly focused; fixed on what is relevant to its own idea and interest
	Characterization: suspicious	Characterization: rigid
Object of attention	The clue	Technical detail
Response to the novel or unexpected	Sharply attentive but not to apparent content ("mere appearance"); searches out confirming clue to "real" meaning; the unexpected regarded as threatening	Refuses attention; the unexpected regarded as distraction from its own fixed line of thought
Experience of reality	World constructed of clues to hidden meaning; apparent, substantial reality disdained; extreme manifestation is projective delusion	World constructed of technical indicators; loss of sense of conviction and sense of substantial truth; extreme manifestation is logical absurdity

Source: Table I, adapted from *Neurotic Styles*, by David Shapiro, p. 105, copyright © 1965 by Basic Books, Inc., New York. Reprinted by permission of the publisher.

that are present in, but intolerable to, themselves (see Chapter 10). Some psychiatric theorists contend that paranoid people use projection to attribute to others the evil intentions that they themselves feel. In this way the idea that they may be harmed really reflects their own wish to harm others.

In certain respects the paranoid life-style resembles the compulsive life-style. The two styles are compared in Table 15–8. The paranoid life-style may be regarded as a more primitive form of the compulsive style. A paranoid life-style is differentiated from a Paranoid Disorder or Paranoid Type of Schizophrenia in DSM-III in that there are no persistent psychotic symptoms, such as delusions and hallucinations, in the paranoid life-style. However, the latter two diagnoses may be superimposed on a paranoid personality.

The Process of Exclusion The process begins with persistent strains between the person and family and friends. The person earns the reputation of being "difficult." The troublesome behavior is interpreted at first as a variation of normal behavior. People say, "He's just ornery," or "There's something odd about her."

At some point in the chain of interactions, the definition changes. The person is no longer seen as a normal variant. Now he or she is "unreliable," "untrustworthy," "someone you wouldn't want to get involved

with." Relationships with others become patronizing, evasive, spurious. These interactions have three effects. They stop the flow of information to the person, create a discrepancy between expressed thoughts and feeling among those with whom the person interacts, and make the image of the others ambiguous for the person.

The next step is usually some form of crisis that formalizes the informal exclusion. Often this takes the form of a job promotion or demotion. During this phase, gross misstatements, termed *pretexts,* become justifiable ways of getting the person to cooperate—for example, to submit to a psychiatric exam. This aspect of the process of exclusion has been termed a "betrayal funnel" through which the client may be admitted to the mental hospital (Goffman 1953).

The next step is the growth of *ideas of reference.* The idea that paranoid people are simply imagining conspiracies against them is somewhat oversimplified. Many paranoid people recognize that their behavior is causing them to be isolated by others, or that they are being excluded and manipulated. But since channels of communication are closed to them, they have no means of getting feedback on the consequences of their behavior. Yet feedback is essential for correcting their interpretations of social relationships. The need for communication and the sense of identity that comes with it go far to explain the preference of paranoid people for formal, legalistic, written communications and the care with which many of them preserve records of their contacts with others.

The last step is the reinforcement of their interpretations or ideas of reference. These people's needs and dispositions and their self-imposed isolation are significant factors in perpetuating their interpretations. However, there is an important social context through which these interpretations are reinforced.

Paranoia can become a way of life for some people, because it provides them with an identity not otherwise attainable. Their overriding tendency to contest issues that other people dismiss as unimportant becomes a central theme in their lives. However, paranoid people may also fulfill certain marginal functions in society. One is the scapegoat function, through which they strengthen other people's feelings of consensus and homogeneity. Another is the mouthpiece function, through which they articulate the dissatisfactions of those who fear to criticize their leaders openly. As long as labeled deviants serve society, it is more likely to interact with such deviants in ways that perpetuate their behavior. The exclusion pattern described above is one such example.

Nursing Intervention   Nursing intervention with people who have paranoid life-styles is often made difficult by their lack of insight, rigidity of thought, and lack of tender, kind feelings. As with most labeled psychiatric conditions, however, it is helpful to consider the interpersonal context of persons labeled "paranoid." The interactionist approach focuses on a process of exclusion that arises in a paranoid person's relationships with others. Thus while it is true that paranoid people react differently to their social environment, it is also true that others react differently to them. Nursing intervention with these people would benefit from an understanding of paranoid styles as the product of interactive relationships in which communication has been disrupted by exclusion, and mutually perceived trust is lacking.

GUIDELINES FOR INTERVENTION   Nursing interventions for persons with paranoid life-styles should take into account the idea that reciprocal relationships produced the informal and formal exclusion of these persons. Interventions should therefore

- Reestablish attenuated communication and feedback with the client
- Diminish the social isolation that reinforces the client's idea that something is wrong

- Keep verbal and nonverbal messages clear and consistent
- Avoid engaging in pretexts, trickery, and deception to enlist the client's cooperation
- Offer a basis for establishing consensual validation of reality without belittling the client's experience of it (for example, it is preferable to state, "I don't interpret things in that way, but I understand from what you've said that you do," than to assert, "You're wrong, it's not that way at all").

The fundamental principle in working effectively with these clients is to convey to them that you do not perceive reality in the same way they do but are willing to listen, learn, and offer feedback about their experiences and concerns. Other guidelines in working with suspicious clients include:

- To foster trust, follow through on commitments made to the client.
- To help minimize anxiety, plan several brief contacts with the client rather than one prolonged contact.
- Provide environmental supports that may decrease fear, such as a night light.
- Respect the client's privacy and preferences as much as is reasonable.
- To avoid misinterpretation and enhance trust, be as honest and open with the client as possible.

Characteristics of Schizoid and Schizotypal Personalities

The essential feature of a schizoid personality is a defect in the capacity to form warm, tender relationships. These people tend to feel indifferent to the praise, criticisms, and feelings of others. They usually prefer to be loners and have few if any close friends. They appear reserved, withdrawn, and seclusive and pursue solitary interests that keep them away from the occupational or social mainstream. Others perceive them as aloof, cold, vague about goals, indecisive, detached, and generally "not with it" or "in a fog." Unlike people with avoidant personalities, who choose social isolation out of fear of rejection by others, these people have no apparant desire for social relatedness. While some authorities believe that schizoid personalities may deteriorate into schizophrenia, no eccentricities of speech, behavior, or thought are present in the schizoid personality except for the incapacity to form relationships with others.

People with schizotypal personalities are also characterized by social isolation, but they experience social anxiety or hypersensitivity to real or imagined criticism; suspiciousness; magical thinking; ideas of reference; recurrent illusions; and vague, circumstantial, and metaphorical speech patterns.

Nursing Intervention Nursing intervention with persons whose major difficulty is in the area of establishing relationships is particularly difficult and frustrating. Such clients rarely respond quickly to sincere attempts at establishing rapport. In a classic article on intervening with withdrawn clients in an inpatient setting, Tudor (1952) emphasized three areas:

- Attending to the clients' basic daily needs for nutrition, elimination, activity, hygiene, and so on
- Attempting to establish some basis for therapeutic interpersonal communication (see Chapter 6)
- Enhancing the client's social interaction with others through structured group or family situations (see Chapters 18 and 21)

All the approaches mentioned are based on the assumption that even though withdrawn people may seem indifferent to others, their apparant lack of concern is probably a defensive posture that interferes with the quality of their lives. Nursing interventions for clients with extreme oddities of thought, speech, perception, and behavior are covered in Chapter 16.

KEY NURSING CONCEPTS

✔ A life-style is a mode of functioning that includes ways of thinking and perceiving, ways of experiencing emotion, and modes of subjective experience that are generally consistent patterns over broad areas of living.

✔ Disruptive life-styles are those categories of behavior engaged in by society's troublesome members.

✔ Disruptive life-styles have been called personality or character disorders in psychiatric terminology.

✔ Disruptive life-styles are best understood as a social problem rather than a psychiatric illness.

✔ Examples of disruptive life-styles include those that are impulsive, addicted, compulsive, dependent, and eccentric.

✔ Nursing intervention in disruptive life-styles is based on the understanding that the life-style allows the client to avoid anxiety.

✔ The impulsive life-style is generally associated with people who have been poorly or inadequately socialized; nursing intervention for these people is aimed at helping them establish inner controls over their behavior.

✔ Explanation and intervention for the alcoholic and drug-dependent life-styles may occur on medical, behavioral, social, or psychological levels.

✔ The compulsive life-style is characterized by rigidity, distortion of the experience of autonomy, and loss of consensual reality.

✔ An interactionist view of eccentric life-styles focuses on the process of exclusion that arises in relationships with others.

✔ The fundamental principle in working with clients with eccentric life-styles is to convey the idea that the nurse does not perceive reality the same way as the client but is willing to listen, learn, and offer feedback about his or her experiences and concerns.

References

Becker, H. *Outsiders*. N.Y.: Free Press, 1963.

Goffman, E. *Stigma*. Englewood Cliffs, N.J.: Prentice-Hall, 1953.

Lindesmith, A. *Opiate Addiction*. Bloomington: Indiana University Press, 1965.

Shapiro, D. *Neurotic Styles*. New York: Basic Books, 1965.

Tudor, G. "A Sociopsychiatric Nursing Approach to Intervention in a Problem of Mutual Withdrawl on a Mental Hospital Ward." *Psychiatry* 15 (1952): 193. Reprinted in *Perspectives in Psychiatric Care* 8 (1970): 11.

Further Reading

Aichorn, A. *Wayward Youth*. New York: Viking Press, 1935.

Cahalan, D., et al. *American Drinking Practices: A National Survey of Drinking Behavior and Attitudes*. New Brunswick, N.J.: Rutgers Center for Alcohol Studies, 1969.

Chein, I., et al. *The Road to H: Narcotics, Delinquency and Social Policy*. New York, Basic Books, 1964.

Cleckley, H. *The Mask of Sanity*. St. Louis: C. V. Mosby, 1964.

Densen-Gerber, J. *We Mainline Dreams: The Odyssey House Story*. New York: Doubleday, 1973.

Didion, J. *Play It as It Lays*. New York: Bantam Books, 1970.

Estes, N. "Counseling the Wife of an Alcoholic Spouse." *American Journal of Nursing* 74 (1974): 1251–1255.

Estes, N., and Heinemann, M. E. *Alcoholism. Development, Consequences, and Intervention*, 2d ed. St. Louis, Mo.: C. V. Mosby, 1982.

Estes, N.; Smith-DiJulio, K.; and Heinemann, M. E. *Nursing Diagnosis of the Alcoholic Person*. St. Louis: C. V. Mosby, 1980.

Foreman, N. J., and Zorwekh, J. "Drug Crisis Intervention." *American Journal of Nursing* 71 (1971): 1736–1739.

Grinspoon, L. *Marijuana Reconsidered*. Cambridge: Harvard University Press, 1971.

Livingston, J. *Compulsive Gamblers: Observations on Action and Abstinence*. New York: Harper and Row, 1974.

Matza, D. *Delinquency and Drift*. New York: John Wiley, 1964.

Melville, H. *The Confidence Man*. New York: New American Library, 1964.

Morgan, A., and Moreno, J. "Attitudes toward Addiction," *American Journal of Nursing* 73 (1973): 497–501.

Piaget, J. *The Moral Judgment of the Child*. Glencoe, Ill.: Free Press, 1932.

Reich, W. *Character Analysis*. New York: Orgone Institute Press, 1949.

Disintegrative Life Patterns: Psychotic Conditions

by Patricia R. Underwood

CHAPTER OUTLINE

Behavior Associated with Disintegrative Life Patterns

    Disintegration of Perception

    Disintegration of Thought

    Disintegration of Affect

    Disintegration of Motivation

Defining Disintegrative Behavior

    Personal Definition

    Social Definition

    Legal Definition

    Statistical Definition

    Medical Definition

Examples of Disintegrative Behavior

The Study and Treatment of Psychotic Conditions: 1950 to 1970

    Institutionalization

    Psychoactive Drugs

    Community Mental Health

Contemporary Study and Treatment of Psychotic Conditions: 1970 to Present

    Descriptions of Psychotic Conditions

    Past History Associated with Psychotic Conditions

    Explanations of Psychotic Conditions

    Treatment of Psychotic Conditions

Contemporary Nursing Approaches

    Factors that Influence Care Planning

    Nursing Strategies

    The Nursing Care Plan

Key Nursing Concepts

LEARNING OBJECTIVES

After reading this chapter, students should be able to

- Compare and contrast the characteristics of disintegration of perception, thought, affect, and motivation
- Distinguish between medical, personal, social, legal, and statistical definitions of disintegrative behavior
- Identify key elements in the classification and treatment of psychotic conditions
- Recognize factors that influence the planning of care for clients with psychotic conditions

CHAPTER 16

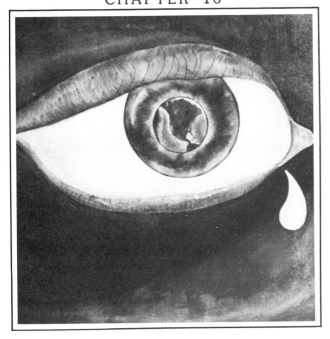

People with disintegrative life patterns often experience frightening disturbances of perception, thought, affect, motivation, and behavior.

People with disintegrative life patterns may be called eccentric, strange, gifted, talented, bizarre, or crazy. If they come to the attention of the mental health system, they will probably be called *psychotic*. The etiology of psychosis is unknown. Therefore the cause of the disorder cannot be treated specifically, and the outcome of the available treatment cannot be readily predicted. Nonetheless, many people who enter the mental health care system are, and will probably continue to be, labeled psychotic.

It is virtually impossible to study behavior completely without using diagnostic categories, because the literature on human behavior is often catalogued by diagnostic category. In the latest official nomenclature of psychiatric conditions, DSM-III, psychotic conditions in adults are limited to Schizophrenic Disorders, Paranoid Disorders, and Psychotic Disorders Not Elsewhere Classified, which includes Schizophreniform Disorder, Brief Reactive Psychosis, Schizoaffective Disorders, and Atypical Psychosis. Other conditions, such as Bipolar Affective Disorder (Manic-Depression), may be classified as having psychotic features but are no longer under the psychotic classification (see Chapter 15). Delusions, hallucinations, and grossly bizarre behavior are considered evidence of a psychotic condition. Regardless of the finer points of the present nomenclature, in general practice the majority of psychotic conditions will be identified as Schizophrenic Disorders or

the Manic phase of the Bipolar Affective Disorder. Furthermore, in the case of acute and severe disturbances the official psychiatric diagnosis rarely alters a client's actual nursing care. The nurse deals with persecutory delusions the same way with the person diagnosed as having a Schizophrenic Disorder as with a person diagnosed as having Bipolar Affective Disorder. The focus of nursing care is the person with symptoms of psychotic proportion rather than the schizophrenic or manic disorder. When the nurse has learned to care for the person in a manic or schizophrenic episode she will be prepared to care for most clients with psychotic conditions regardless of the name or cause. This chapter describes the behavior associated with psychotic conditions, reviews the history of the condition, and discusses contemporary explanations, treatments, and nursing care. It is intended to provide the reader with the best possible understanding of one of the least understood human conditions.

BEHAVIOR ASSOCIATED WITH DISINTEGRATIVE LIFE PATTERNS

Disintegrative life patterns are characterized by disturbances in verbal and motor behavior that reflect disintegration of perception, thought, affect, and motivation. These categories of disintegration are rarely observed in a pure form. Most disintegrative behavior overlaps all four categories. For clarity of presentation, however, disintegration of perception, thought, affect, and motivation will be dealt with separately.

Disintegration of Perception

Perception is the response of sensory receptors to external stimuli. More broadly, perception is not only a response to a stimulus but the knowing of the object, image, or thought. Perception includes both cognitive and emotional knowing of the perceived object.

Perception is one of the most studied and least understood functions of human behavior. There is agree-

		Table 16–1 DISINTEGRATION OF PERCEPTIONS
Type of Disintegration	**Sense**	**Example**
Illusions	Visual	Chairs or tables or other inanimate objects are seen as sinister beasts.
	Auditory	The ticking of a clock is heard as a constant countdown to disaster.
	Tactile	Human flesh feels like the cold, damp skin of a toad.
	Gustatory	Water is tasted as if it were blood.
	Olfactory	Cooking meat has the smell of burning hair.
Hallucinations	Visual	Family members long dead, or God, or the devil appear. A man sees his own death or witnesses some dreadful act being performed as if on a movie screen.
	Auditory	A woman hears the voice of God or a world-famous person (J. Edgar Hoover, Ronald Reagan) repeating her thoughts or talking about some dreadful, perverted act that she is supposed to have performed.
	Tactile	A man feels the hand of God on his shoulder. His body feels to his touch like wood or plaster.
	Olfactory	The environment is heavy with the smell of death. A woman smells an offensive body odor coming from herself or others.
	Gustatory	A man tastes mother's milk in his mouth. He tastes burnt food even when he does not eat.
	Kinesthetic (somatic distortions)	The individual has strange body sensations that may or may not be part of the delusional system. A man feels as if rats or worms are crawling through his brain. A woman feels as if her heart has stopped and turned to concrete. The individual may not recognize ordinary body sensations, such as hunger or the need to urinate or defecate.

ment, however, that within a wide range of sensory functions certain perceptions can be out of the ordinary, different, or altered. Disintegration of perception may include one or more of the auditory, visual, tactile, olfactory, or gustatory sensory processes.

Disintegration may be mild and transitory. Almost everyone has experienced waking in the night and perceiving a familiar object as an unfamiliar object (e. g., a chair as a beast). This is a mild and transitory experience, and we easily regain a reality orientation. The chair is a chair. In this chapter, *reality* means that which can be consensually validated by others. That is, most would describe the same object as a chair. Disintegration of perception is not uncommon. When perception is constantly disintegrating, however, the resulting behavior may be identified as strange or even bizarre.

The most common disintegrations of perception are illusions and hallucinations (see Table 16–1). *Illusions*

are misperceptions and misinterpretations of externally real stimuli. Visual and auditory illusions are much more common than tactile, olfactory, and gustatory illusions. Misperceiving the chair is an example of an illusion. *Hallucinations* are perceptions of objects, images, sensations that have no counterparts in reality. Visual and auditory hallucinations are the most common in psychiatric conditions. Tactile, olfactory, and gustatory hallucinations are most often related to organic disorders. In psychiatric conditions, tactile, olfactory, gustatory, and kinesthetic hallucinations may be mixed with illusions and delusional systems. The following case study is an example of an hallucination.

Cathy, a twenty-three-year-old Greek exchange student, was brought to the hospital by her roommate. Cathy has exceptional grades and is evaluated by her teachers and her peers as extremely bright. She is tearful but cooperative. However, she is so preoccupied that she has difficulty participating in the interview. On the unit, she does not initiate any interaction and pays only minimal attention to the activities of daily living. She often sits with her head tilted as if listening and may suddenly go to her room as if she has seen or heard something very frightening. The nurse sits with Cathy and says, "You seem to be frightened." Cathy is tearful and says, "Yes, I keep hearing myself called a whore and a pervert and a whole chorus of people accusing me of awful things. My body is being pulled apart. I can feel hands pulling my spinal cord, and when I walk my feet begin to rot. Sometimes I believe I am in Hell."

Disintegration of Thought

Thought represents reason, intellect, and judgment. The term *cognition* is often used interchangeably with the term *thought*. Cognition means the mental process of obtaining knowledge. At one time or another, almost everyone has experienced the inability to think clearly. In times of fear, stress, or anxiety thought may not come or may not make sense. Judgment may not be reality oriented. The most common disintegrations are in the form, content, and flow of thought.

Form of thought is usually described as realistic, rational, and logical. However, it can change to unrealistic, irrational, and illogical to become dereistic or autistic. In *dereistic* thought, thinking is disconnected from reality. In *autistic* thought, thinking is focused on internal processes. Common disintegrations of thought form are *symbolic associations* and *concrete associations*.

Content of thought, except in special situations such as dreams, is controlled by the individual and is reality oriented. Delusions reflect inability to control the content of thought or to maintain a reality orientation. A *delusion* is a false set of ideas that seem real to the individual. It is not an accurate reflection of cultural or social ideas or beliefs, and it cannot be corrected by logic, reason, or argument. Delusions are defined by the content of thought involved. Some common delusions are: delusions of being controlled, delusions of grandeur, delusions of persecution, delusions of reference, bizarre delusions, and somatic delusions.

Flow of thought is the rate at which thoughts are expressed. Thoughts usually occur and are expressed in a regular, even way. The inability to regulate and pace thoughts results in *flight of ideas, retardation,* and *blocking.*

The various disintegrations of thought are described in Table 16–2.

Disintegration of Affect

Affect is emotion. It consists of both internal feelings and the external demonstration of feelings. Common affects are happiness, sadness, fear, anger, disgust, and surprise. Affect is expressed verbally and nonverbally, in tone of voice, facial expression, and body movement. It may be directed toward persons, ideas, or thoughts. Disintegration of affect is recognized in change in intensity of affect, inappropriate affect, or labile affect (see Table 16–3).

All cultures have rules about the appropriate expression of affect. These rules also influence the accurate interpretation of affective behavior. Disintegration of affect is often judged by an individual's own cultural interpretation of what affect and how much is appropriate in a given situation.

Disintegration of Motivation

Motivation is what prompts an individual to action. Like perception, it is widely studied and poorly understood. It is generally viewed as an internal force, such as a drive, a need, or an instinct. Different theories of human behavior explain the exact nature of that force in different ways. In disintegration of motivation the individual cannot, for whatever reason, recognize or control motivation. Disintegration of motivation is recognized in regression, withdrawal, impulsive behavior, hyperactivity, and ambivalence (see Table 16–4).

DEFINING DISINTEGRATIVE BEHAVIOR

Behavior that results from the disintegration of perception, thought, affect, and motivation can be defined personally, socially, legally, statistically, and medically.

Personal Definition

A personal definition is a subjective definition. People are "normal" if they believe they are "normal." They suffer "psychoses" only if they believe they suffer them. Personal definitions of sanity have rarely been accepted by health professionals, the courts, or the public. Even today, people who are identified as psychiatrically ill are rarely evaluated on the basis of their

Table 16-2   DISINTEGRATION OF THOUGHT

Characteristic Affected	Disintegration	Example
Form of thought	*Symbolic associations* Symbols such as words that should have common meanings take on specific meanings known only to the individual.	Mona, a sixteen-year-old girl, continually runs out of cigarettes. She insists on giving them to everyone—other patients, staff, and visitors. She smokes very little herself and agrees she does not have a "real habit," but she becomes distressed, agitated, and tearful if she does not have a pack of cigarettes stuffed in the top of her blouse. She eventually tells her primary therapist that the cigarettes have always represented her heart and her love for her fellow man because she has always carried them over her heartbeat. She says that she sometimes feels drained and empty of emotion, but by giving away her cigarettes, she believes she makes herself symbolically at one with all, and as a result, all are at one with her. She has universal love and is filled again. Cigarettes are a symbol of love and giving to Mona, not just something to smoke.
	Concrete associations The ability to make abstract associations and to generalize ideas is lost.	Proverb: People who live in glass houses shouldn't throw stones. Abstract association: You should not criticize others without expecting criticism yourself. Concrete association: If you throw rocks at a glass house, you will break it. George was continually putting all kinds of objects in the toilet and had to be accompanied to the bathroom to protect the plumbing. On one such occasion the nurse said to George, "Please let me have the book, George, and please don't put anything else in the toilet." George entered the cubicle and urinated on the floor. He did not put *anything* else in the toilet.
	Blocking The expression of a thought is stopped in midstream, and in a few seconds a new, unrelated thought is expressed.	Jane and the nurse are in Jane's room talking about an outing in the park. Jane says, "Parks are really lovely this time of year. The grass is all green and the flowers are starting to bloom. It's nice to take off your shoes and walk in the grass. I hope we take blankets and lots and lots . . . The walls of this room are a dreadful color. Do you suppose they will ever paint them anything but this dreadful yellow? I swear I will never be able to see this color without thinking about this room."

Table continues on next page

own opinions of their conditions. The negating of personal opinion, particularly in chronic conditions, has prompted state and federal legislation to ensure clients' increased participation in identifying their mental condition by requiring informed consent and setting forth the client's rights (see Chapter 5).

Individuals have also banded together to protect their right to define themselves. These individuals believe that they may have problems, but that they are "sick," "insane," or "psychotic" only because the psychiatric establishment has so defined them. California has one such group called Network Against Psychiatric Assault (NAPA). In the psychiatric establishment, several prominent persons have taken a similar stand, notably the physician Thomas Szasz. His books (1961, 1976, 1977) proclaim his belief that most so-called psychiatric illnesses are not illnesses at all. Like Szasz, R. D. Laing contends that schizophrenia is not a dis-

Table 16-2 continued		
Characteristic Affected	**Disintegration**	**Example**
Content of thought	*Delusions of grandeur* Individuals place themselves in a special relationship to the world. They may believe themselves to be prominent people, living or dead, or to be related to such people, or to be influential in important affairs.	John, a forty-seven-year-old man, raised in an orphanage with no known relatives, joined the Army during the Korean War. He received a medical discharge for psychiatric problems. At present he believes himself to be the illegitimate son of Albert Einstein. John believes that through telepathy he invented all the spacecraft for all American space flights and settled the Vietnam War. John's delusion is expansive, and he continually incorporates scientific and military advances into the system. On the whole he is a pleasant, friendly man until his delusional system is challenged. Disagreements usually end in a fight, an arrest, and a brief hospital stay.
	Delusions of persecution Individuals believe themselves to be harassed, in danger, under investigation, or at the mercy of some powerful force. They may be driven to drastic acts by these delusions.	Jane, a forty-five-year-old, unemployed schoolteacher, has always been an isolative person with few friends and few interests. When busing was begun to enforce integration, Jane believed that the school district and her fellow teachers had plotted to give her the most difficult students. Jane eventually incorporated childhood friends, relatives, and even the governor of the state into her delusional system. She resigned her position and moved several times. Jane was hospitalized when she tried to burn down her house. Jane was discharged in three months with no change in her system except that she was no longer driven to act on her delusional thoughts.
	Delusions of reference Individuals believe that certain events, situations, or interactions are directly related to themselves.	Jim, a thirty-five-year-old man, is watching the street from the hospital window. Two people get off a city bus and walk down the street. Jim tells the nurse, "Did you see them? They are from the Symbionese Liberation Army, and now they know I'm here."
	Somatic delusions Individuals believe that their bodies are changing or responding in some unusual way. They may be unaware of ordinary sensations such as hunger or thirst.	Lynn, a twenty-nine-year-old woman, has lost forty pounds in the last two months. She had not eaten in three days when she was admitted to the hospital. She believes that as punishment for a secret crime God has closed up her bowels, and that if she eats she will not be able to swallow.

Table continues on next page

ease (Laing 1967). However, Laing does believe that specially trained individuals, psychiatrists and lay-people alike, are the most appropriate persons to deal with the process labeled schizophrenia. He believes that the condition will respond to "treatment" as he has identified it. Neither Laing nor Szasz contends that behavior labeled psychosis does not exist. They simply contend that this behavior is not a disease. While both Laing and Szasz have wide followings, their views are by no means universally accepted. However, both theorists raise issues and offer insights that deserve serious consideration. Other commentators, such as

Characteristic Affected	Disintegration	Example
	Delusions of being controlled Individuals believe that their feelings, impulses, thoughts, or actions are not their own but are imposed from some external source.	David, a twenty-year-old man, tells the nurse during the admission interview that he is being controlled by his father and that he can speak only when his father puts words in his mouth.
	Bizarre delusions The content of the delusion is so absurd that there is no possible way it could be based in fact.	Mark, a thirty-five-year-old man, is referred to psychiatry from the dentistry department, where he reported that while he was in Vietnam a military dentist replaced the fillings in his teeth with transistors. Since then he has been the radio receiving and sending unit for all communications between the United States and China. He believes that since relations between the two countries are better, he can replace the fillings without jeopardizing the safety of the United States.
Flow of thought	**Flight of ideas** Thoughts come so fast and bring so many associations that no single thought can be clearly expressed. Ideas occur in a rapid and endless variety of ways, connected only by a single, slim thread.	Mary approaches the nurse before dinner and says, "I hope we have chicken tonight. (Angrily) Chicken is exactly what my husband was. He called the police to bring me here. (Calmly) The cops wore blue. Have you ever noticed how blue the sky is? (Happily) I'm sky-high on life and love and pursuit of happiness. Just like the constitution, not like this institution. (Angrily) This institution locks me up against the constitution. (Happily) I have rights, but right here is just fine with me."
	Retardation Thoughts come very slowly and are difficult to express. There may be such a dearth of thought that communications are monosyllabic. There may even be mutism.	Ann explains that her thoughts are like a record being played at a slow speed.

Table 16-2 continued

Scheff (1970) and Goffman (1961), hold similar positions.

Social Definition

Social definitions are based on the behavior the family, tribe, or community will accept. As long as we live within the norms and standards of our social group, we are accepted as normal. Unfortunately, or perhaps fortunately, not all social groups have the same norms and standards (see Chapter 26). Furthermore, standards change, as the recent experience of American society demonstrates. In the sixties, "hippies" were seen as abnormal by most of the "straight" establishment. They were so labeled because their behavior did not meet social norms, and people who lived by those norms rarely understood it. By the seventies, however, the hippies' behavior had become somewhat

Table 16–3 DISINTEGRATION OF AFFECT	
Disintegration	**Example**
Change in intensity of affect—recognized in over- or underresponse to stimuli	
Overresponse	A man responds to the death of a minor public official whom he never knew by mourning so intensely that he is unable to work.
Blunted affect	A woman recounts her recent vicious mugging with mild sadness and regret.
Lack of affect	When told that his brother has died in an accident, a man neither shows nor feels grief, shock, or relief.
Inappropriate affect—response to an event, situation, or interaction is out of sync with the stimulus	A man recalls his wife's death with good humor and laughter. A woman becomes enraged when asked if she has eaten yet.
Labile affect—abrupt, rapid, and repeated changes in affect for no apparent reason	Linda is watching television and laughing. She suddenly slips from the chair to the floor. Before the nurse can reach her she is up and walking down the hall cursing in a loud tone of voice.

institutionalized; "Doing your own thing" had become acceptable.

Social definitions of normal and abnormal change as society and culture change. However, people with disintegrative life patterns are often viewed as abnormal—or more precisely, unacceptable—because their behavior is not in keeping with social norms.

Legal Definition

People are defined as legally insane if they do not know what they are doing, or if they know what they are doing but do not know that it's wrong. To be legally sane, they must be able to accept responsibility for their behavior and understand legal action being taken against them. A related but somewhat different legal approach defines who should be committed to mental institutions. In California, only homicidal, suicidal, and gravely disabled persons may be involuntarily hospitalized. In the past, laws were less specific, and many persons, especially those identified as having chronic disintegrative life patterns, were committed to state mental institutions, often for life. Legal definitions are a reflection of public attitudes. As the public becomes more knowledgeable about and tolerant of disintegrative behavior, laws will change accordingly (see Chapter 27).

Statistical Definition

Statistical definitions are based on the mathematical model of average. This model requires that one determine mathematically what is average and to what degree deviance will be accepted before it can be labeled nonaverage. It is frequently used to explain the human condition. We have average IQs, average heights and weights, average years of education, average-sized families. People who demonstrate psychiatric chronicity are rarely viewed as average. Any person who deviates from the average may be defined as abnormal.

Medical Definition

Medical definitions are based on subjective and objective signs of illness that physicians agree indicate mental illness (see Chapter 2). Medical definitions are *diagnoses*. In the medical model, psychopathology was introduced to denote the study of the etiology, symptomatology, and process of mental disorders in the same way that pathophysiology denoted the study of the etiology, symptomatology, and process of physical disorders. However, in contemporary thinking it is generally accepted that while psychopathology may be a disorder of the mind (psyche), it does not follow disease principles in the same way as disorders of the body (soma) do.

The most widely accepted classification system is the medical system developed by the World Health Organization. This system is interpreted for American use by the American Psychiatric Association in the Diagnostic and Statistical Manual of Mental Disorders (DSM-III). While this classification is widely disputed, it is also widely used, and it influences the way in which certain behaviors are understood. Although medicine may be the discipline most often identified with medical diag-

Table 16-4 DISINTEGRATION OF MOTIVATION	
Disintegration	**Example**
Regression—the return to earlier and less sophisticated adaptive behavior. Regression may be to early childhood or even to infantile adaptive patterns.	Jane is a twenty-six-year-old woman whose mother died three months ago. Shortly after the funeral, Jane felt frightened to be alone in her apartment and returned to her father's home. She seemed to get great comfort and satisfaction out of being in her old bedroom. She began to bring out her dolls and childhood toys. She maintained contact with her friends but spent most of her time at home caring for her father. She refused to return to work when her leave of absence was up. About a month after her mother's death, she began to carry around a favorite doll and a blanket from childhood. She was no longer doing housework but was still cooking meals for her father. She began to spend more and more time in bed with her doll and blanket. Eventually, she would not get out of bed at all. She sucked her thumb and talked to her father in a childish way. Two months after her mother's death, Jane was admitted to the hospital, mute and sucking her thumb.
Withdrawal—retreat from life. Withdrawal may be a total break with reality. In this case the individual is no longer in touch with the real world. Withdrawal may also be an emotional (affective) break with the real world. In this case the individual is reality oriented but is unable to show affective responses to external stimuli.	Greg is a twenty-three-year-old graduate student at a local university. He did well in undergraduate work and was admitted to a competitive graduate program. Shortly after his admission, he met and began living with a girl in the same program. Greg has been going to school full-time and working part-time for the last two years. Several months ago, he told his girl friend that he had feelings of overwhelming despair and fear and was afraid he couldn't complete the graduate program. At her insistence, he sought help at the student health service. He visited with a counselor once a week for two months. His girl friend believed everything was going well until she came home unexpectedly and found him sitting, staring at the blank tv screen. He confessed he had dropped out of school, had quit his part-time job, and was no longer talking to anyone but her and his therapist. Greg continued to stay in the apartment. He assumed the responsibility for cleaning and cooking. He eventually quit seeing his therapist. Then he began staying up all night and sleeping most of the day. He no longer carried on conversations with his girl friend, cooked, cleaned, or watched tv. He sat for hours staring into space. He finally told his girl friend that he understood the cosmic order of everything, and that it was his duty to sit forever. This so frightened her that she contacted his parents. They brought him to the emergency room.
Impulsive behavior—behavior that appears unpredictable and unmotivated by observable events. The individual is unable to exert socially expected controls and may be verbally or physically destructive, aggressive, or violent.	Billy is a twenty-one-year-old man. He answers in monotones or not at all. He interacts only minimally. Billy spends most of his day listening to the radio with the radio very loud and very close to his ear. Suddenly he jumps up and throws the radio across the room, barely missing another client.
	Joyce is a quiet sixteen-year-old girl. She does not interact with others. She is sitting at the dining room table eating lunch. Suddenly she gets up and starts clearing both her own and all the other clients' dishes. She is unable to stop and moves from table to table, clearing all the dishes despite attempts of clients and staff alike to prevent her. Just as suddenly she stops. She returns to her seat at the dining room table and sits staring into space.
Hyperactivity—an increase in the rate of activity. It may include emotional lability and flight of ideas.	Elizabeth is a forty-seven-year-old, married woman. She was brought to the hospital by her husband of twenty-five years. Elizabeth has been hospitalized four times in the last year. She has not slept much in the last few nights. She talks incessantly and paces back and forth in the hallway. She interrupts anyone to talk about her previous hospitalizations. She cannot sit down to eat. She is

Table continues on next page

Table 16–4 continued	

Disintegration	Example
	labile and fluctuates from being extremely happy to being extremely sad. She can become angry at the slightest interruption in her behavior. She refuses medication because she says she feels ''too good to need meds.'' After several attempts, the nurse gets Elizabeth to take a cup of water and her pills. Elizabeth is holding them and laughing and chatting with the nurse. In a teasing voice, Elizabeth says, ''Oh, no you don't. I told you, no pills.'' The nurse responds, ''But you need the medication.'' Elizabeth says angrily, ''Like hell I do,'' and she throws the water in the cup at the nurse. Other clients laugh and so does Elizabeth. Elizabeth says, ''We'll get along fine as long as you don't try to give me those pills. I really like you, dearie, I really do. Come on and I'll help you find a towel and dry you off. I'm really sorry I did that, but you shouldn't have tried to give me the pills.''
Ambivalence—the coexistence of positive and negative feelings about objects, events, situations, or interactions. These feelings produce the desire to do two opposite things at once. The resulting indecision is observable in exaggerated inaction and constant action.

Exaggerated inaction—in extreme compliance (automatic obedience, robot responses) the individual will not act at all unless told what to do and often how to do it.

In negativistic behavior, the individual refuses to participate. The refusal may be verbal or nonverbal or both. As ambivalent feelings intensify, the individual attempts to avoid these feelings by refusing to stop, or to change, or to start action. | Gary is a nineteen-year-old high school graduate brought to the hospital by his parents. His parents report that he refuses to leave his room to eat or to get a job. They seem frustrated by his behavior and are unable to deal with it any longer. On the unit, Gary will do nothing unless he is told. He will stay in bed all day if he is not assisted verbally and often physically to get up. He must be told step-by-step what to do to maintain minimal functioning. He will eat only if he is told to put the bite in his mouth, to chew, and to swallow. Several weeks after admission, Gary is demonstrating less extreme compliance but has become very negativistic. He refuses to get up in the morning, and he must be physically assisted with day-to-day care. He refuses to eat but finally agrees and then refuses to stop eating. He refuses to go to occupational therapy but once there refuses to leave when the activity is over. When Gary watches tv, it sometimes takes him ten minutes to find the appropriate chair. He sits down, gets up, and sits down again. When he is finally settled, he will not move from the chair. At times, his refusal is so adamant that he sleeps in the chair through the night, and only in the morning is he able to leave it. |
| Constant action (mannerisms, ritualistic acts, stereotyped behavior) that appears meaningless to the observer, often accompanied by repetitive speech, autism, and regression. | John is a forty-five-year-old man who immigrated to this country at the age of twenty-five after completing his degree in business administration in Mexico. He also studied flamenco dancing and still dances regularly. He was unable to find work commensurate with his education. He has been a night janitor at a large bank for the last seventeen years. He has few friends and considers dancing his only interest. He was admitted to the hospital when he was found dancing in the bank lobby after his night shift. John is mute upon admission and moves his hands over his body in a continuous, ritualistic, exaggerated dance motion. The movement continues wherever he is. He is unable to eat, sleep, or use the bathroom because he cannot stop his ritualistic dance movement. John will stop if his hands and arms are restrained, but as soon as the restraints are removed, the ritualistic movements begin again. |

nosis, these diagnoses are also accepted by nursing, social work, psychology, and other fields designated to deliver mental health services (see Chapter 8).

EXAMPLES OF DISINTEGRATIVE BEHAVIOR

Behavior may be defined in any of the ways described above. The medical definition of behavior is a diagnosis. Diagnoses often override personal, social, legal, and statistical definitions. A wide range of socially unacceptable behavior is diagnosed as mentally ill, for example, Substance Abuse Disorder, Voyeurism, Schizophrenia, and Mania. Psychiatric professionals, mainly psychiatrists, judge individuals legally sane or insane and in some cases recommend confinement to mental institutions. Clinicians collect data that are used to determine average mental health. The people described below would probably be labeled psychotic no matter what other definitions were used.

Sharon, a thirty-one-year-old woman, is brought to the hospital by her parents. Her eyes are shut tight. She is dressed in an adult-sized, one-piece pajama suit of the kind most often seen on small children. She dropped out of high school at age sixteen and has been home with her mother ever since. She has been withdrawn and noncommunicative for ten years. Recently she has refused to eat anything but Fig Newtons and Coke. She will eat only if her parents aren't in the house. She has not had a bath or washed her hair in eighteen months. Neither she nor her parents have ever sought psychiatric assistance before.

Eleanor is a thirty-three-year-old woman married to a telephone company executive. They have no children and live in an expensive high-rise apartment. Eleanor is brought to the hospital by her husband and a private detective he hired to find her. A month ago, Eleanor began to spend enormous amounts of money. Her husband was unaware of this until the bills began to come in. She bought several fur coats and several sets of china and refurnished two rooms in the apartment. Her husband went on a business trip a week ago. While he was gone, Eleanor used her credit cards and her checking account to book a trip around the world on an international airline. She took with her a young college student she picked up in a bar at the airline terminal. The private detective found her in Tahiti three days ago. She is being brought to the hospital, even though she claims she has done nothing to deserve hospitalization.

John, a twenty-four-year-old man, came to the outpatient department because he thinks his wife and new baby are in danger. He has a premonition that they will die, and that he will somehow be involved. These thoughts started when his wife was eight months pregnant. They became so intrusive that he lost his job because he could not concentrate. His daughter is now eighteen months old, and he has not worked since she was born. The family is presently living with friends, and his wife works two days a week as a librarian. His wife has threatened to leave him if he does not get assistance.

George is a thirty-five-year-old executive in a large corporation. He has worked for this firm for the past eight years. He is married and the father of three. He and his wife are considered pillars of the community. George is hardworking and dedicated to his family. He got a long-sought promotion several months ago. He and his wife were able to buy a larger house and move the family to a better neighborhood. Shortly after that, George began to worry about finances. His worries seemed unfounded, since his promotion brought with it a considerable raise. However, no amount of reassurance would help. He continued to worry and became so preoccupied with money that he sold his car and began taking the bus to work. He lost his appetite, and his weight went down twenty pounds in one month. He is not sleeping well either. He has not been to work for two weeks and refuses to talk with his boss. He no longer bathes or shaves. His wife brings him to the family doctor for a checkup.

Mary, a thirty-one-year-old, attractive, well-dressed, divorced woman, comes to the medical clinic complaining of a vaginal discharge and odor of two years' duration. Mary has previously been to eight private physicians and six clinics. The doctor finds neither discharge nor odor. Mary has moved six times in the last year because the "smell" in her apartment has become so bad. She is a retail clerk, and she has changed jobs four times. When asked why, she says that wherever she worked, her coworkers avoided her because of the smell. She is presently unemployed. Mary is now living in a transient hotel in the least desirable section of town. She moves nightly from one room to another. She has used up most of her savings but believes that she must have the odor stopped before she can look for work again.

Jim is a twenty-nine-year-old father of four. He teaches high school science and lives with his family in a quiet suburb. He is brought to the emergency room by his wife and the pastor of his church. Six months ago, Jim believed that he had received a calling from God to preach and began plans to enter a seminary. His wife and pastor both supported Jim's plans. Jim became increasingly withdrawn and spent most of his time in prayer. He began to question the scientific principles he

Table 16–5 MAJOR CHANGES IN HOSPITALIZATION AND TREATMENT BY DIAGNOSTIC CATEGORY, 1950–1970			
	1950	**1960**	**1970**
Schizophrenia			
Hospitalization	Long-term custodial care, several years to a lifetime	Long-term custodial care and some treatment, months to years	Short-term, active treatment; long-term very limited
Treatment	1. Electroconvulsive therapy 2. Insulin coma 3. Limited psychotherapy (one-to-one)	1. Phenothiazines introduced in 1954 2. Electroconvulsive therapy 3. Resocialization activities (one-to-one and groups) 4. Supportive psychotherapy (one-to-one and groups)	1. Many major tranquilizers 2. Supportive psychotherapy; (one-to one, group, and family) 3. Socialization activities 4. Vocational rehabilitation
Manic-depression			
Mania			
Hospitalization	Long-term custodial care, several months to several years; repeat admissions	Fewer hospitalizations; short-term, several months; fewer repeat admissions	Short-term, if at all, several days to several weeks; fewer repeat admissions
Treatment	1. Electroconvulsive therapy 2. Limited psychotherapy (one-to-one)	1. Phenothiazines 2. Electroconvulsive therapy 3. Supportive psychotherapy (one-to-one, group)	1. Lithium 2. Many major tranquilizers 3. Supportive psychotherapy (one-to-one, group, and family)
Depression			
Hospitalization	Long-term custodial care, several months to several years	Fewer hospitalizations; short-term, several months; fewer repeat admissions	Short-term, if at all, several weeks to a few months; fewer repeat admissions
Treatment	1. Electroconvulsive therapy 2. Limited psychotherapy (one-to-one)	1. Tricyclics introduced in 1957 2. Electroconvulsive therapy 3. Supportive psychotherapy (one-to-one and group)	1. Tricyclics and monamine oxidase (MAO) inhibitors 2. Electroconvulsive therapy 3. Supportive therapy (one-to-one, group, and family)

taught in school and was generally irritable and labile. At his wife's insistence, he saw his family doctor, who reported that he was in good health but under stress because of his decision to follow God's calling. Jim continued to pray and meditate, and his wife and family accepted his devotion. At the regular Sunday night church service, Jim entered the church in a white sheet and began to proclaim that he was Christ, the Son of God. He was verbally and physically abusive to the pastor. With the help of the police, Jim's wife and his pastor brought him to the emergency room.

This introduction has described and defined disintegration of behavior. Since medical diagnoses are the most widely accepted definitions of this behavior, this chap-

ter will use psychiatric diagnoses of psychoses to study psychiatric chronicity.

THE STUDY AND TREATMENT OF PSYCHOTIC CONDITIONS: 1950 TO 1970

Through the late 1940s people who were labeled psychotic were little better off than their counterparts 100 years before (see Chapter 1). However, this situation was about to change.

The 1950s were a whirlwind of activity in mental health (see Table 16–5). The domination of American psychiatry by the psychoanalytic school was changing.

Emphasis was shifting from the study of neuroses to the study of psychoses. More and more psychological theories were broadened to include environmental processes. Social science introduced family and group dynamics along with other social and cultural variables. Communication and cybernetic theories were being explored. Biological research flourished, and there were new insights into the genetic and biochemical origins of psychosis. Treatment began to include psychosocial, as well as somatic, therapy. However, the major change in the treatment of psychoses occurred when the consequences of institutionalization were identified and psychoactive drugs were discovered. This led to the development of community psychiatry, which introduced a new era in the study and treatment of psychoses.

Institutionalization

Since insane asylums were first established in the 1700s, most psychiatric clients have been confined to mental institutions. And until the 1950s, long-term hospitalization was the rule, not the exception. Psychoses, by definition, were chronic illnesses. This chronicity necessitated large custodial institutions designed to deal with people who could neither make decisions nor care for themselves. Active treatment was available to only a few psychotic clients. Most received custodial care.

The effects of prolonged confinement to an institution had been hinted at down through the ages. But not until the mid-fifties did professionals in the United States begin to suspect that the treatment might be worse than the disease. Then several things happened. Erving Goffman (1961) published his observation of social deterioration in state hospitals. Prompted by the results of changes in custodial care in Europe, Greenblatt, York, and Brown (1955) began to restructure three eastern hospitals to create therapeutic rather than custodial care settings. Other major treatment centers followed suit, initiating the open-door policy, the therapeutic community, a new focus on staff–client relationships, and family involvement. Surprisingly, the clients were not as chronic as they had appeared to be.

Mentally ill adults were subject to at least two types of chronicity: chronicity attributable to the actual disease process or to the process of care and treatment. The latter is an iatrogenic disorder known as *institutionalization* and is a two-part phenomenon of process and effect. The process of institutionalization is the

care and treatment that produces the disorder, and the effect of institutionalization is the individual behavior that results from the process. Institutionalization occurs when routine, structure, and control are used to create a care-giving environment that systemically dehumanizes people by denying their self-care and self-determination (process). This produces a chronic condition in which a person's ability for self-care and self-determination in living day-to-day is so markedly impaired that often life outside institutional care is not possible (effect).

Originally, researchers believed that only long-term confinement produced institutionalization. They assumed that if hospital stays could be prevented or shortened, institutionalization would eventually disappear. This is not the case, however; institutionalization is caused by the process of care and treatment, not by its duration or setting.

Psychoactive Drugs

Until the early 1950s no drug had been identified as psychotic-specific. Most attempts at chemical control of psychotic processes had failed. Chlorpromazine was introduced as a psychotic-specific agent in 1954 (see Chapter 23). Early reports were no less than miraculous. Clients became calmer, and their thought processes improved. Clients labeled schizophrenic or manic and identified as chronic and untreatable responded to the new drug. Discharge rates soared, but so did readmission rates. Many clients were social cripples. Even with the psychological process under control, clients were unable to live in the community. Psychoactive drugs might stop the psychological processes in psychoses, but they could not offer social rehabilitation.

Mary was admitted to a state hospital in 1925 at the age of fifteen. She was withdrawn, heard voices, and believed she was controlled by the Devil. Mary stayed in the hospital until the early 1950s. She received both insulin coma and electroconvulsive treatment, but her condition did not improve much. She was a quiet, good client and worked daily in the hospital laundry.

In 1955, when Mary was forty-five, she was one of the first clients to be given Thorazine. She responded well and was judged ready for discharge in the late fifties. The hospital found Mary an apartment and a job in a laundry similar to the one she had held in the hospital for twenty years. She was discharged with the assistance of hospital personnel.

However, the world had changed so much between 1925 and 1958 that Mary was a stranger in a strange land. She had not traveled outside the hospital in thirty years. She did not know the public transportation system and had no idea there were so many cars. She had not cooked a meal for herself in all her time in the hospital. She had few personal belongings and no personal clothing. Though she had ironed state clothing all day, she had never cared for her own clothes. Mary could not care for herself despite the remission of the psychotic process. She pleaded to be readmitted to the hospital and signed herself back in as a voluntary client. This was somewhat irregular, but it was clear that, while Mary was no longer actively psychotic, she was unable to live outside the hospital.

There were many Marys in state hospitals in those days. Even if these clients were judged asymptomatic, many could not function outside the sheltered environment. This had long been attributed to the illness itself. In reality, it was often a side effect of having been labeled psychotic for so long. As phenothiazines began to be widely used and the major symptoms of psychosis began to be controlled, the effect of institutionalization became increasingly apparent. The psychiatric establishment believed it had found the long-sought "cure" for at least some of the clients labeled psychotic, but for many the cure was too late. They were chronic clients because of institutionalization, and drugs could not treat that.

Community Mental Health

The long-sought "cure" for psychoses in the form of psychoactive drugs, the discovery of the effects of institutionalization, and pressure by public organizations on federal and state legislators worked together to initiate community psychiatry. (For complete details, see Chapter 28.) Emphasis now began to be placed on preventing hospitalization or on providing only short-term hospitalization when this was absolutely essential. Clients were to maintain their place in the home and the community by being treated there. These were the new goals, but there were few new tools available to attain them.

Most communities were not ready to receive or provide services for a large group of chronic psychiatric clients. Furthermore, while the public and the professionals were ready to change the location of care, many were not ready to change the approach. Institutionalization had been more than putting a person in the place of treatment. It had been a process of eliminating self-care and self-determination. Deinstitutionalization through community care had to be more than removing a person from the place of treatment. It had to be the process of assuring self-care and self-determination. Community mental health needed to be redesigned to give psychotic or chronically ill people services in their own community without relinquishing the right to self-care or self-determination and without fear of involuntary long-term confinement. Many communities have not and will not be able to provide the essentials for such service.

CONTEMPORARY STUDY AND TREATMENT OF PSYCHOTIC CONDITIONS: 1970 TO PRESENT

In the last decade, there has been a shift in emphasis in both the explanation and the treatment of the psychotic conditions (see Table 16–5). The study of the psychotic conditions has moved away from psychological explanations. Breakthroughs in technology have allowed increasingly sophisticated research into the genetic and biochemical aspects of the conditions. There is an ever-growing body of evidence that the vast majority of persons diagnosed as psychotic have some biological malfunction that plays a primary role in the illness. The primary method of treatment is drug therapy. Psychosocial interventions focus on rehabilitation and social adjustment and are seen more and more as an adjunct to drug therapy rather than a replacement or substitute. The site of treatment is the community. Inpatient services have decreased and the length of hospitalization sharply reduced. However, because of the severity of the conditions, most psychotic individuals will continue to need some form of inpatient care at some point in their lives.

The Department of Health and Human Services estimated that 3 million Americans suffer an episode of severe mental illness every year. Of this 3 million, 2.4 will become moderately to severely disabled and 1.7 million will become chronically ill. The vast majority of the chronically ill are psychotic and over half of them continue to be cared for in inpatient or residential care facilities. Only about 170,000 chronically ill individuals actually live with their families; 120,000 are on the streets without a permanent residence; 110,000 are in community hospitals; 400,000 are in board and care homes; 150,000 are in state hospitals; and 700,000 are in nursing homes (Department of Health and Human Services, 1981, p. 2–1). This pattern is likely to continue until definitions, causes, and cures can be identified.

Descriptions of Psychotic Conditions

The more that psychotic conditions are studied and the more attempts that are made to refine descriptions, the clearer it becomes that the behaviors associated with the conditions are more alike than different. From observation alone it is difficult to determine if a person ought to be called Manic, Schizophrenic, or Schizoaffective. Depressive episodes of the Bipolar Affective Disorder are usually easier to recognize, but, if the depression is of psychotic proportions, it may be mistaken for a Schizophrenic, Schizoaffective, or Paranoid Disorder. The similarity of behavior leads to speculation about the nature of the psychotic conditions. Are they really separate and distinct disorders? Or are they a continuum of the same disorder? This speculation has led Belmaker and Van Praag (1980, p. 4) to state: "We have in front of us a fruit called psychosis, and we don't know whether it is a citrus that will divide itself into separate sections or an apple that we must divide along arbitrary lines."

John P. Docherty and his colleagues (1978) first began to develop the concept of the stages of schizophrenic decompensation. However, they now suggest these stages of decompensation and recovery can be applied to all psychotic episodes and are not limited to Schizophrenia. Docherty identified the following stages:

Equilibrium People in this stage, are in control, well-adapted to their environment, with minimal anxiety, and a positive sense of the future. They are capable of meeting current situational demands.

Overextended People in this stage are beginning to feel overwhelmed. They are irritable, anxious, and distractible. Their work performance declines, and they feel pressured and have difficulty maintaining control of their lives.

Restricted Consciousness In this stage, there is social withdrawal. People are apathetic and listless and feel hopeless, dissatisfied, and lonely. Their range of thought is limited, and obsessional and phobic symptoms may appear.

Disinhibition This stage resembles hypomania. Impulse control is lowered. There may be rage attacks, unre-stricted spending, sexual promiscuity, uncharacteristic risk-taking, and elevated mood as previously repressed material begins to surface.

Psychotic Disorganization In this stage, there are three substages.

1. Destructuring of the external world. The person begins to demonstrate increased disturbance in perception, thought, affect, and motivation. Perceptual and cognitive disorganization increase particularly. Ideas of reference are common.

2. Destructuring of the self. The person loses a sense of self, and severe anxiety, panic, and horror set in. Hallucinatory experiences begin. Behavior may change from minute to minute as the person searches for self-identity.

3. Total fragmentation. The person in this substate experiences complete loss of self and control.

The stages above are the stages of psychotic decompensation and may be used to describe Schizophrenic, Bipolar, or any other condition of psychotic proportion. However, the most popular way of describing psychotic conditions is still to separate them by classification. The next section discusses descriptions of Schizophrenic and Bipolar Affective Disorders separately.

Labels can be based exclusively on the behavior exhibited. When known organic conditions, such as Pellagra, are ruled out, a person can be diagnosed Schizophrenic or Manic-depressive on the basis of his or her current behavior. This kind of diagnosis depends very little on early history.

Schizophrenia   Bleuler's (1950) four A's are still used to identify Schizophrenia. In order to be classified as schizophrenic, the individual must demonstrate *autism, ambivalence, inappropriate affect,* and *loose associations.* Another theory differentiates between first-rank and second-rank symptoms. First-rank symptoms are

- Hearing your own thoughts spoken out loud
- Auditory hallucinations that discuss your own behavior
- Somatic hallucinations
- The feeling of having your thoughts controlled
- The feeling of having your thoughts spread to others
- Delusions that focus on being controlled

Second-rank symptoms are

• Other hallucinations
• Perplexity
• Depression and/or euphoric disorders of affect
• Emotional blunting

Freedman, Kaplan, and Sadock (1981) identify the key symptoms of Schizophrenia as loose associations and bizarre behavior. Obviously, any and perhaps all of these symptoms might be present in one form or another in many conditions. All sources on diagnoses warn that recognizing Schizophrenia from symptoms alone is difficult. When it is possible at all, an accurate diagnosis depends on extensive clinical experience.

Bipolar Affective Disorder   Kraepelin's original delineation of manic-depressive behavior is still widely accepted. He identified flight of ideas, exalted mood, and pressure of activity in mania and sadness, or anxious moodiness and sluggishness of thought and action in depression. The key factor, however, is a history of previous depressive or manic episodes. In contemporary thinking, manic symptoms are

• Unstable mood
• Pressured speech
• Increased motor activity
• Delusions of grandeur

These symptoms could easily be confused with those of Schizophrenia or any number of other conditions. Depressive symptoms are the reverse of manic symptoms. They are

• Depressive mood
• Difficulty in thinking,
• Psychomotor retardation
• Delusions of persecution, somatic in nature

Again, these symptoms can easily be confused with those of other conditions. To complicate the issue further, both mania and depression are categorized on the basis of severity and intensity. Mania may be identified as hypomania or hypermania. Depression may be identified as mild, moderate, or severe. Key symptoms in mania are said to be excessive spending and excessive sexual encounters, and in depression, vegetative signs such as weight loss.

Past History Associated with Psychotic Conditions

Past history provides more information that can be used in making a diagnosis. This source identifies other family members with psychiatric conditions, describes the client's early growth and development, and provides insight into life adjustment before the onset of the disturbed behavior. Information from social and family history (see Chapter 8) helps the diagnostician distinguish between the major disorders and between subtypes within the major disorders. A diagnostician who knows the client's past history will understand the client better, have more options for treatment, and be able to predict its outcome to some extent.

Schizophrenia   Clinical observations support two distinct pathways to Schizophrenia. Some people show a slow and insidious deterioration, while others show a sudden, severe onset. In 1939, Langfield developed the concepts of *process* and *reactive* schizophrenia to depict these two pathways. The determination was based on both observable behavior and social and family history. The concepts of process and reactive schizophrenia were later refined by Kantor and Herron (1966).

The process schizophrenic is the potentially chronic client. There is some speculation that process schizophrenia may be an organic disorder. Process schizophrenics are poorly adjusted, marginally functioning individuals. Family and social history usually reveal that they have had difficulty in the family and have always been dominated by the caretaking parent. They have had few, if any, friends and were never very successful in school. Their social skills are often severely limited. They may present a picture of early asocial behavior and may even have been labeled juvenile delinquents. It is difficult to pinpoint the precipitating factor, and it appears that families usually seek help only after many years of unsuccessful attempts to cope with the disintegrative behavior.

Reactive schizophrenics have a more hopeful prognosis. Their condition seems to be related to social and psychological stresses rather than to an organic process. Reactive schizophrenics are average to well-adjusted individuals with no history of abnormally difficult family or peer relationships. They have been successful in school and work and have not usually appeared to have any serious problems. Their social skills are average or above. The precipitating factor is clear—a breakup with a fiancee, a death in the family—and the onset is acute and disruptive.

Some investigators and clinicians believe that only process schizophrenia should be called Schizophrenia, and that reactive schizophrenia should be called *Schizophreniform Disorder*. Schizophreniform Disorder may look like, but is not, true Schizophrenia. It is neither long-term nor persistently disintegrative. The person will probably recover fully and have no residual impairment. In true Schizophrenia, the course is long-term and persistently disintegrative.

The labels process schizophrenia (true Schizophrenia) and reactive schizophrenia (Schizophreniform) can be used to determine treatment. Both conditions may improve with drugs, or electroconvulsive therapy, or both. However, reactive schizophrenia will not require management or therapy after the episode is past and the symptoms have subsided. Process schizophrenia, on the other hand, may require lifelong management with drug therapy and repeated hospitalizations. In reactive schizophrenia, treatment must be rapid, and every attempt must be made to prevent institutionalization and the chronicity that may result. In process schizophrenia, complete recovery may not be possible, and chronicity is most often the result of the condition.

The DSM-III incorporates some of these concepts. It makes duration of illness a critical factor in Schizophrenia, which allows nonschizophrenic psychotic conditions to be identified more easily. Table 16–6 shows the criteria for a Schizophrenic Disorder and a Schizophreniform Disorder (APA, 1980).

Bipolar Affective Disorder   Manic depression has always been considered less debilitating than Schizophrenia and since it is difficult to determine from behavior alone what psychotic condition is present, clinicians have focused on past history to distinguish a Manic or Depressive Episode with psychotic features from a Schizophrenic Episode. The DSM-III identifies the behavioral criteria for a Manic Episode of a Bipolar Affective Disorder (see Table 16–7 APA, 1980), but there is more confidence in such a diagnosis if the following are part of the past history:

- The individual in question had a rather normal development and good premorbid adjustment.
- The person has exhibited earlier hyperactive behavior and/or an early and critical loss of a significant other and/or a family of high expectations.
- The person belongs to certain nationalities and ethnic groups, such as Scandinavians and Jews (Belmaker and Van Praag 1980, p. 10).

- Other family members have had Bipolar Affective Disorders. (Schizophrenia in the family is less likely.)
- The person has had previous mild mood disturbances.

However, it is possible to have a diagnosis with none, all, or some of the above. The diagnosis of Manic Episode of Bipolar Affective Disorder can best be supported when the illness is established as episodic, or the manic individual improves on lithium and deteriorates without it.

A Case Study   The following case study presents both the behavior and past history of a young woman with a psychotic condition.

Jane H appears to be in her early twenties. She is 5 feet 5 inches tall and weighs 125 pounds. Jane is labile, irritable, and negativistic. Her speech is often pressured and shows flight of ideas. She refuses most prescribed activities and prefers to remain in the dayroom playing records. She rarely lets a record finish, usually changing it halfway through. She laughs and jokes with other clients and is often loud. At times she says she is a spy hiding from the CIA. She is unable to finish a meal and often walks in the hall eating her dessert. She goes to bed late, if at all, and gets up early. She is disheveled, and she wears extremely heavy makeup—fire engine red lipstick and emerald green eye shadow. She has long hair and puts it up and down several times a day. She says "likes the patients, hates the staff" and is disruptive in community living meetings and group therapy. She is seductive with male staff and clients.

Precipitating Events

Jane is a twenty-one-year-old college student who works part-time as a waitress. She lives at home with her divorced mother and three younger siblings. Jane's mother brought her to the emergency room on Monday night. Jane had returned from a skiing weekend with her boy friend on Sunday afternoon. She seemed fine until about 9:00 P.M., when she began laughing and crying and refused to go to bed. She stayed up all night and was extremely agitated in the morning. She called her mother a "bitch" and refused to go to school or work. When her mother returned home at 6:00 P.M. Monday, Jane was sobbing uncontrollably and begged for help. Her mother took her to the emergency room. When Jane met with the intake therapist alone, she reported that she had had sexual intercourse with her boy friend for the first time. As a result, she said, her body was contaminated and rotting, and she was filled with sin.

Schizophrenic Disorder	Schizophreniform Disorder

A. At least one of the following during a phase of the illness:
 	
1. Bizarre delusions (content is patently absurd and has no possible basis in fact), such as delusions of being controlled, thought broadcasting, thought insertion, or thought withdrawal
 	
2. Somatic, grandiose, religious, nihilistic, or other delusions without persecutory or jealousy content
 	
3. Delusions with persecutory or jealousy content if accompanied by hallucinations of any type
 	
4. Auditory hallucinations in which either a voice keeps up a running commentary on the individual's behavior or thoughts, or two or more voices converse with each other
 	
5. Auditory hallucinations on several occasions with content of more than one or two words, having no apparent relation to depression or elation
 	
6. Incoherence, marked loosening of associations, markedly illogical thinking, or marked poverty of content of speech if associated with at least one of the following:
  a. Blunted, flat, or inappropriate affect
  b. Delusions or hallucinations
  c. Catatonic or other grossly disorganized behavior
	A. Meets all the criteria for Schizophrenia except for duration
	
	B. The illness (including prodromal, active, and residual phases) lasts more than two weeks but less than six months

B. Deterioration from a previous level of functioning in such areas as work, social relations, and self-care.

C. Duration: Continuous signs of the illness for at least six months at some time during the person's life, with some signs of the illness at present. The six-month period must include an active phase during which there were symptoms from A, with or without a prodromal or residual phase, as defined below.

Prodromal phase: A clear deterioration in functioning before the active phase of the illness not due to a disturbance in mood or to a Substance Use Disorder and involving at least two of the symptoms noted below.

Residual phase: Persistence, following the active phase of the illness, of at least two of the symptoms noted below, not due to a disturbance in mood or to a Substance Use Disorder.

Prodromal or Residual Symptoms:

1. Social isolation or withdrawal

2. Marked impairment in role functioning as wage-earner, student, or homemaker

3. Markedly peculiar behavior (e.g., collecting garbage, talking to self in public, or hoarding food)

4. Marked impairment in personal hygiene and grooming

5. Blunted, flat, or inappropriate affect

6. Digressive, vague, overelaborate, circumstantial, or metaphorical speech

7. Odd or bizarre ideation, or magical thinking, e.g., superstitiousness, clairvoyance, telepathy, "sixth sense," "others can feel my feelings," overvalued ideas, ideas of reference

8. Unusual perceptual experiences, e.g., recurrent illusions, sensing the presence of a force or person not actually present

D. The full depressive or manic syndrome (criteria A and B of Major Depressive or Manic Episode), if present, developed after any psychotic symptoms, or was brief in duration relative to the duration of the psychotic symptoms in A.

E. Onset of prodromal or active phase of the illness before age 45.

F. Not due to any Organic Mental Disorder or Mental Retardation.

Table 16–7   DSM III DIAGNOSTIC CRITERIA FOR MANIC EPISODE OF BIPOLAR AFFECTIVE DISORDER

Manic Episode	Manic Episode
A. One or more distinct periods with a predominantly elevated, expansive, or irritable mood. The elevated or irritable mood must be a prominent part of the illness and relatively persistent, although it may alternate or intermingle with depressive mood. B. Duration of at least one week (or any duration if hospitalization is necessary), during which, for most of the time, at least three of the following symptoms have persisted (four if the mood is only irritable) and have been present to a significant degree: 1. Increase in activity (either socially, at work, or sexually) or physical restlessness 2. More talkative than usual or pressure to keep talking 3. Flight of ideas or subjective experience that thoughts are racing 4. Inflated self-esteem (grandiosity, which may be delusional) 5. Decreased need for sleep 6. Distractibility, i.e., attention is too easily drawn to unimportant or irrelevant external stimuli 7. Excessive involvement in activities that have a high potential for painful consequences, which is not recognized, e.g., buying sprees, sexual indiscretions, foolish business investments, reckless driving C. Neither of the following dominates the clinical picture when an affective syndrome is absent (i.e., symptoms in criteria A and B above): 1. Preoccupation with a mood-incongruent delusion or hallucination (see definition below) 2. Bizarre behavior D. Not superimposed on either Schizophrenia, Schizophreniform Disorder, or Paranoid Disorder. E. Not due to any Organic Mental Disorder, such as Substance Intoxication. (Note: A hypomanic episode is a pathological disturbance similar to, but not as severe as, a Manic Episode.) Fifth-digit code numbers and criteria for subclassification of manic episode	6— In Remission. This fifth-digit category should be used when in the past the individual met the full criteria for a Manic Episode but now is essentially free of manic symptoms or has some signs of the disorder but does not meet the full criteria. The differentiation of this diagnosis from no mental disorder requires consideration of the period of time since the last episode, the number of previous episodes, and the need for continued evaluation or prophylactic treatment. 4— With Psychotic Features. This fifth-digit category should be used when there apparently is gross impairment in reality testing, as when there are delusions or hallucinations or grossly bizarre behavior. When possible, specify whether the psychotic features are mood-incongruent. (The non-ICD-9-CM fifth-digit 7 may be used instead to indicate that the psychotic features are mood-incongruent; otherwise, mood-congruence may be assumed). Mood-congruent Psychotic Features: Delusions or hallucinations whose content is entirely consistent with the themes of inflated worth, power, knowledge, identity, or special relationship to a deity or famous person; flight of ideas without apparent awareness by the individual that the speech is not understandable. Mood-incongruent Psychotic Features: Either (a) Delusions or hallucinations whose content does not involve themes of either inflated worth, power, knowledge, identity, or special relationship to a deity or famous person. Included are such symptoms as persecutory delusions, thought insertion, and delusions of being controlled, whose content has no apparent relationship to any of the themes noted above. or (b) Any of the following catatonic symptoms: stupor, mutism, negativism, posturing. 2- Without Psychotic Features. Meets the criteria for Manic Episode, but no psychotic features are present. 0- Unspecified.

Recent Social and Family History—Informants: Mrs. H and Jane

Jane is the oldest of four children. She has a seventeen-year-old brother, a fifteen-year-old sister, and a twelve-year-old sister. Her parents were divorced when Jane

was thirteen. Her mother went to work at the time, and Jane assumed much responsibility for the care of her younger siblings. Both Jane and Mrs. H are bitter toward Mr. H, Jane because she believes his leaving increased her responsibilities, and Mrs. H because he left for another woman. The younger children have seen their father regularly, but Jane refused to visit with him or even speak to him until six months ago. At that time she said she "just wanted to know what he was like." Jane has always had several girl friends but no close ones. She has not had a boy friend until recently. She has been seeing her present boy friend for about six months. She is planning to be a laboratory technician and is enrolled in a community college. Both she and Mrs. H report that generally she has been doing well in school, at work, and at home.

Early Social and Family History—Informants: Mrs. H and Jane

Jane was born in 1961, while her father was stationed in Vietnam. Her mother was alone in San Francisco. The mother's family was in Oklahoma. Mrs. H reports the birth as normal but says she was very frightened during and after the birth. Mrs. H was only eighteen and had been married less than six months when her husband was sent to Vietnam. They had just been transferred to San Francisco, and Mrs. H could not afford to go back home. Jane was reported to be a colicky baby, and Mrs. H was often fearful when caring for her. Jane's eating problems did not subside until she was 1½ years old and her father returned home. Mrs. H readily admits that she believed Jane to be a difficult baby and "a lot of work" for her. She was glad when her husband returned. He seemed to be less frustrated by the child than she was.

Mrs. H reports that she and her husband had a second honeymoon on his return, and although they did some things as a family, she preferred to be with him alone. Jane was often cared for by the teenage girl next door.

When Jane was 2½, her father was transferred to Tokyo, and she and her mother remained in San Francisco. Her mother took a sales job to start a savings account to buy a house. Jane was cared for by an older woman. She was not toilet trained until she was over three years old. Her father returned about that time, and her mother quit her job and became pregnant again immediately. Her brother, Joseph, was born shortly after Jane's fourth birthday. Under pressure from Mrs. H, Mr. H did not reenlist but took a civilian job in San Francisco. They bought a house and, Mrs. H reports, "became a real family." Jane and her mother both report that Jane was very attached to her father and extremely jealous of his attention to the new baby. Jane began wetting her bed again after Joseph was born and was severely punished by her mother. Mrs. H reports that Joseph was an excellent baby, unlike Jane, and at last she enjoyed being a mother. She has told Jane that continually ever since Jane was old enough to remember. Jane's first sister, Mary, was born when Jane was six and had just started school. Jill was born when Jane was seven.

Mrs. H reports that when Jane started school she was a model child and a good student. She presented no further problem until her parents divorced when she was thirteen. At that time Jane ran away from home several times and had a few encounters with the juvenile authorities. However, by the time she was fourteen she had returned to her previous style and was a help to her mother and the younger children. Mrs. H believes that part of this change was due to Jane's having joined a church. Jane has been active in that church ever since and still attends.

Mrs. H reports no mental illness on either side of the family. Jane had the usual childhood diseases but is in good health.

Using both behavior and social and family history, the nurse can often recognize the person who demonstrates a disintegrative life pattern. From the history the nurse will also learn something about life events before the disintegration. However, the cause of the condition will still be unclear. The next section explores the possible causes of psychoses.

Explanations of Psychotic Conditions

The cause of psychotic conditions is unknown. In fact, there is probably no single cause. However, there is increasing evidence that psychotic disorders are actual diseases with a biological bases. Nonetheless, theory and research support the idea that social and psychological factors also influence the development of a psychotic condition.

Biological Factors   Biological theories and research in psychoses are at once the simplest and the most complicated. They are simple in that psychoses are thought to be caused by organic malfunction. Therefore, the process and outcome of the condition depend on isolating and correcting the malfunction. They are complicated because the human organism is complicated and not well understood.

Psychoses were originally believed to be caused by brain lesions. The discovery that metabolic, nutritional, and endocrinologic malfunctions could also produce aberrant behavior broadened the biological perspective to include the total organism. Today genetic and biochemical research are the major areas of interest.

GENETIC STUDIES   Genetic research originally attempted to answer the question, Are psychoses inherited, or are they environmentally produced? If consistent genetic links could be found, it would support the contention that the conditions are not only biological but also inheritable. Genetic factors are explored primarily through twin studies, and family studies.

Twin studies date from Franz Kallmann's (1953) work in the 1930s. Original studies focused on Schizophrenia but later work included manic-depressive conditions as well. Twin studies identify how often the twin of an identified client is also psychotic and compare the prevalence of this psychosis to that in the population as a whole. Reports on concordance (similar traits in twins) vary widely and depend greatly on the caliber of the research design. However, concordance is three to six times greater for monozygotic than for dizygotic twins. Concordance is the same for dizygotic twins as for nontwin siblings. Manic-depression studies are fewer than schizophrenic studies, but they also show a higher concordance in monozygotic (50 to 90 percent) than in dizygotic twins (16 to 38 percent).

Family studies also seek to determine genetic links. Again, research design has a substantial effect on findings. Findings suggest that

- Biological families of adoptives who develop chronic Schizophrenia have higher rates of Schizophrenia than biological families of adoptives who do not develop Schizophrenia.

- When biological parents diagnosed as schizophrenic give children up for adoption, higher rates of pathological conditions are found in those children than in children adopted from nonschizophrenic parents.

- Birth risks for children of schizophrenic parents are higher than for the general population.

Since low birth weight and deafness at birth may predispose individuals to Schizophrenia, this suggests a familial, although not a genetic, link.

Few family studies have been done on Bipolar Affective Disorders, but there are two major findings:

1. Prevalence seems to be greater in families with bipolar cases than in families with unipolar cases

2. Schizophrenia in one twin and Manic-depression in the other rarely occurs in monozygotic twins.

Although genetics is not the only factor to be considered when reviewing families, genetic research leaves little doubt that heredity plays some part in both Schizophrenia and manic-depression. Close relatives of persons with either disorder are at greater risk than

the general population. Research has not yet been able to determine how these conditions are transmitted, or even what it is that is transmitted. In time, investigators believe that genetic research will be able to answer these questions.

BIOCHEMICAL STUDIES Drugs were known to be effective in treating psychotic conditions even before the brain chemistry involved was understood. At present, many neuropharmacologic mechanisms are proposed to explain the effectiveness of drugs. For instance, it is known that the *dopaminergic system* is involved in Schizophrenic Disorders and that *dopaminergic blockage* is crucial in decreasing psychotic symptoms. It is also known that the antidepressants are a satisfactory treatment for most depressed persons, that lithium is a satisfactory treatment for most manic persons, and that the neuroleptics, drugs that alter thinking, are satisfactory treatment for most schizophrenics. What appears to be most baffling at this time is why lithium may work in some schizophrenic persons and neuroleptics in some manic persons. Certainly our inability to make totally accurate diagnoses plays a part, but perhaps the psychotic conditions have biological commonalities yet to be discovered.

Current understanding of brain chemistry has developed slowly. While the intricate process of neurotransmission is not completely understood today, there is general agreement that acetylcholine, catecholamines, norepinephrine, dihydroxyphenylalanine (dopamine), indoleamine, and serotonin are among the various amino acids that somehow are affected in psychotic conditions. The work has progressed so well in recent years that it has been suggested that scientists are on the threshold of a major breakthrough in the understanding of brain chemistry and psychotic conditions. (See Chapter 23 for a discussion of psychotropic drugs.)

Psychological Factors: Personality Theory

Psychological theories and research in psychoses have traditionally focused on individuals who were already labeled psychotic. Personality theory has developed out of this approach. It is concerned with the development, motivation, and behavior of the psychotic individual. Theory and research have two major focuses. The first is to develop the personality theory through case study. The second is to test the effect of psychotherapy. Research is predominantly clinical. Psychotic individuals are studied by case study methods to develop an understanding of the interactions among psychological factors that have produced the observable condition. When these are identified, normal personality development is described by omitting possible psychopathological factors. Personality theory tends to offer understandings of normal as well as neurotic or psychotic conditions. Personality theories are perhaps as much a reflection of the theorists' own philosophies of life as anything they study. The effects of treatment are studied by comparing various psychotherapies with each other and with other forms of treatment. If the outcome is positive, it reinforces the personality theory on which the psychotherapy was based.

Psychological personality theory offers an explanation for the cause and outcome of psychoses. It also prescribes treatment within a psychodynamic formulation. This formulation combines all the available information about the client into a statement that

- Shows how events, interactions, and situations interrelate to produce the present behavior
- Predicts the outcome of the psychosis on the basis of events, interactions, and situations
- Prescribes treatment

Psychodynamic formulations attempt to relate past experience to present behavior to show how and why the individual is motivated toward the psychotic process. The exact nature of the formulation depends on the theorist. Personality theories vary in their emphasis on internal conflicts, external conflicts, cultural and social factors, families, mothers, fathers, and any number of other persons and situations encountered in the individual's development over time from infancy to maturity and finally old age.

TYPICAL DEVELOPMENTAL PICTURE FOR SCHIZOPHRENIA The schizophrenic process is believed to start very early in life, usually during the first year. Theorists agree that the relationship between the child and the caretaking parent is in some way inadequate and impaired. The result is that the child has difficulty relating to other people. The child may also distort events, situations, and interactions. Freud assumed that the development of the ego was impaired. He believed that this impairment resulted in a weak ego. The ego psychologists are more specific in identifying the impairment of certain ego functions, for example, reality testing. Erik Erikson, using an approach based on ego psychology, states that the caretaking parent and child do not develop mutual trust, and therefore the child's ability to trust self and eventually others is impaired (Erikson 1968). Sullivan (1960) proposes that

the caretaking parent is filled with anxiety, which spills over into the parent–child relationship. In this case the child has a poor personification of self. Self-esteem is low, and the self-system may be permanently impaired. Sullivan explains that the caretaking parent's anxiety may or may not be directly related to the child.

All theories, with the exception of classical Freudian theory, hold that even though these children get a poor start early in life, they have the opportunity at later stages of life to strengthen their egos, increase their trust, and repair their self-system. Most often, however, this opportunity goes unused, and they continue to have difficulty throughout their lives. There is some general agreement that the increased responsibility of adulthood precipitates the schizophrenic episode. The difference between process and reactive schizophrenia is explained in terms of degree, rather than kind, of impairment. Symptoms and outcome also depend on the degree of impairment.

TYPICAL DEVELOPMENTAL PICTURE FOR A BIPOLAR AFFECTIVE DISORDER The Bipolar Affective Disorder, like Schizophrenia, is believed to begin early in life, but it is usually traced to the second or third year. At this point the ego is more stable and stronger than it is during the first year. Trust has been established, and the self-system has developed from early positive personifications. The child is less dependent and more mobile, and verbal communication has begun.

Freud and Erikson and the ego psychologists trace the onset of manic-depression to loss of mother's or mother surrogate's love. This could occur if the mother is ill or absent, if her attention is directed elsewhere (for example, to a new baby), or if the child feels her disapproval harshly, as in toilet training. Sullivan considers the influence of both parents. He assumes that some situation (for example, the parents' money worries) creates anxiety in the parents and thus in the child. As a result the child grows anxious, self-doubt develops, and the child's self-system is impaired. Children who develop Bipolar Affective Disorder may have difficulty with the stages, phases, or tasks of the second and third years. Like children who develop Schizophrenia, they may have many opportunities to repair the damage later, but most often they fail to do so. In Bipolar Affective Disorder the individual usually weathers the stresses of adolescence but enters adulthood with vague fears and doubts about failure and rejection. Symptoms emerge when these people experience an event, situation, or interaction that they interpret as a loss, failure, or rejection. Manic symptoms are a desperate attempt to ward off depression and to deny the loss. Depression is seen as the response to loss. (See Chapter 11 for an in-depth discussion of loss.)

DYNAMIC FORMULATION OF SCHIZOPHRENIA The history and symptoms presented by the client Jane, in the case study earlier in this chapter, may be interpreted as either a Bipolar or a Schizophrenic Disorder. If Schizophrenia is selected, the original stress would occur in the first year of life as a result of the strain between mother and child. By history, Jane was a colicky child. Her mother was fearful and frightened and felt lost and lonely. She felt that Jane was a burden to her. As a result, Jane's early ego development, early development of trust, early development of self-system, or all three were impaired. This is further supported by the fact that Jane continued to have difficulty until she started school. She is then reported to have been a model child. The behavior identified as "good" could actually be withdrawn and compliant behavior, the result of Jane's inability to relate to others, or of her fear of rejection, or both. At age thirteen, when her father left, she became disruptive and rebellious. The father's leaving coincides with the onset of adolescence and the introduction into adult responsibilities. The present episode seems to be precipitated by intercourse, which is also indicative of adult responsibility. When faced with adult responsibilities, especially those involved in developing an intimate relationship with another person, Jane panicked, her defenses shattered, and she developed schizophrenic symptoms. If Jane is labeled schizophrenic, she would be expected to have a weak ego, lack trust, and have low self-esteem.

DYNAMIC FORMULATION FOR A BIPOLAR AFFECTIVE DISORDER On the other hand, if Jane suffers a Bipolar Disorder, her conflict would originate in the second or third year of life. It would begin when her father returned home and Jane lost part of her mother's attention. This period also coincides with toilet training, when there may be conflict between mother and child. Later the history reports that Jane developed a great attachment to her father. After the birth of her brother, Jane clearly came second with both of her parents. Jane's behavior as a model child could be interpreted as her attempt to prevent disapproval and, therefore, loss of love from parents and other adults. However, at thirteen, when she lost her father despite her behavior, she lashed out at all authority. Her symptoms seem to have been precipitated by intercourse with

her boyfriend. Intercourse could have precipitated a sense of loss—that is, she actually lost her virginity, and she may have symbolically felt that she was losing part of herself. Her symptoms developed as a result of this sense of loss.

Jane's case was specifically selected to illustrate how confusing the distinction between a Bipolar Affective Disorder and a Schizophrenic Disorder can be. There is no question that Jane is psychotically disturbed, but how should she be diagnosed? Psychodynamic formulations are an attempt to clarify the nature and the process of the specific psychotic condition and to develop appropriate approaches to treatment. However, as this example illustrates, psychodynamic formulations do not always provide definitive answers. Both Bipolar Affective and Schizophrenic Disorders have any number of other dynamic formulations.

Psychological Factors: Behavior Theory
General psychology has tended to study specific conditions in normal people—for example, cognition, perception, affection, and decision making—in order to understand the behavior of the population at large. The knowledge so developed has had little bearing on the understanding and treatment of psychoses. The exception is behavior theory.

Behavior theory has grown out of laboratory research into conditioning (see Chapter 2). It is one of the few research-derived theories used in clinical practice. This theory assumes that maladaptive behavior is learned through conditioning and can be corrected through conditioning. The maladaptive behavior—not personality, character structure, or underlying conflict—is seen as the primary problem. Like personality theory, behavior theory formulates the problem, but it does so in terms of maladaptive responses rather than of psychodynamics. It then devises a plan to eradicate the maladaptation, or to teach new behavior, through conditioning. One technique for implementing behavior theory is behavior modification.

Both personality theory and behavior theory state that psychotic conditions originate in childhood. This makes it difficult to validate the theories through research, because research on origin would require the experimental manipulation of children and families. Personality theories have tended to obtain validation through the case study method. Behavior theories have tended to obtain validation through laboratory study. Both personality theory and behavior theory depend on retrospective studies for validation of maladaption. If the treatment was effective, the proposed etiology must have been correct. Treatment and outcome will be discussed later in this chapter.

Social Factors   Social theories focus on the individual's relationships to society. While these theories have studied the influence of social attitude and social stress on the psychotic process, their major contribution to the understanding of psychoses has come through the study of family interactions and transactions. Biological theories have studied families as genetic links. Psychological theories have studied the influence of family in personality development. But social theories have actually placed the origin of psychotic behavior in the family transactions.

The study of the family as a social system is concerned with three things. The first is the relationship between the family and the individual. The second is the family structure and function and family interrelationships. The third is the relationship between the family and the external systems. The study of the family as a social system offers several approaches to understanding psychoses, especially Schizophrenia. It is less useful in understanding Affective Disorders. Notable contributors to the understanding of the schizophrenic family system are Gregory Bateson and his associates (1956) and R. D. Laing (1967) (see Chapter 21).

BATESON'S DOUBLE-BIND COMMUNICATION   Bateson identified the double-bind phenomenon. This is the old "damned if you do, and damned if you don't" situation. The mother gives the child a double-bind message, which is really two messages at once. She tells the child, "Come here and give mother a kiss to show her that you love her." But as the child approaches, mother pulls back, extends her arms, almost blocking the child's approach, and offers a very small part of her cheek. Mother has asked for a kiss to show love, but at the same time her behavior (pulling back with her body and pushing away with her arms) tells the child that she does not want either child or kiss. The father and other family members do not interrupt the process. They appear to be as helpless to deal with the mother as the child is. In rage, helplessness, and frustration, the child withdraws into the psychotic process.

LAING'S SCHIZOPHRENOGENIC FAMILY   R. D. Laing focuses almost exclusively on social factors in psychoses, especially as they arise and are played out in the schizophrenic family. Laing believes schizophrenia to be the response of the individual to an impossible situation. The impossible situation is the continual social

and cultural pressure on the individual to be like everyone else in the society and therefore "normal." This pressure precipitates personal fragmentation, confusion, and loss in some individuals. These individuals realize that there is a split between their inner and outer worlds. They are further fragmented and confused as the inner world leaks into the outer and vice versa. Terrified, they use every process at their disposal—withdrawal, projection, and denial—to cope with the societal pressure and the resulting psychotic process.

Laing does not actually offer an approach to treatment, since he believes that for people to enter an inner world from their outer world and return to the outer world is a normal, natural process. Rather, he offers the person guidance through the inner world. He believes that people must be allowed to go deeper and deeper into their inner world and then be guided back in a kind of existential rebirth that provides them with a new self.

Treatment of Psychotic Conditions

What is and is not treatment for the psychotic, especially the schizophrenic, client is a hotly debated issue. Since neither etiology nor outcome is completely understood, treatment can hardly be called "illness-specific." Because the natural course of the psychoses varies, it is difficult to predict future outcome. Freedman, Kaplan, and Sadock (1981) list five possible outcomes for Schizophrenia:

1. Full recovery
2. Full remission with one or two future episodes
3. Social remission with the need for supervision and protection, or social remission with self-support
4. Stable chronicity
5. Terminal deterioration

Since DSM-III ties Schizophrenia to duration of illness, recovery rates are likely to decrease. There may be an increase in chronic cases of Bipolar Disorder now that it will be more difficult to rediagnose those persons as schizophrenic.

When psychotic people enter the health care delivery system, they will probably be prescribed some form of treatment, most likely drug therapy with or without psychosocial interventions. In the majority of cases drugs relieve symptoms, though how they do this is not yet completely understood. As a better understanding of the brain chemistry of psychotic conditions has developed, there has been increasingly less reluctance to use medication and, in most cases, they have replaced other somatic approaches. Electroconvulsive therapy is still available in some locations but is less frequently used than in the past. These treatments are discussed in depth in Chapter 23.

All the major psychosocial therapies have been used to treat psychoses with limited reported success. Psychotherapy does not cure the condition, but it can improve social functioning.

Contemporary research emphasizes the specific effects of various treatments on psychoses. There is good evidence that some psychotics can improve with somatic therapies, psychotherapies, or a combination of both. There is less evidence to indicate when and with whom a given treatment will be effective. Nor is it always known which treatment will lead to the most effective long-term outcome for a given person. The question is no longer, Can the psychotic respond to treatment? Rather, it is, What person should have which treatment, and what will the long-term outcome be?

Effects of Somatic Therapies Somatic therapies—especially the use of neuroleptic drugs—are by far the most effective in interrupting the psychotic process. Psychoactive drugs are also effective in promoting long-term social functioning. The National Institute of Mental Health reports that in chronic Schizophrenia, relapse rates after one year are only 10 percent when injectable medication is used and 35 percent when oral medication is used. They rise to 65 percent when a placebo is used (Segal 1975, p. 335). Research indicates that 70 to 80 percent of the clients with Bipolar Affective Disorders respond to lithium (Segal 1975, p. 336). Clinical studies, as well as empirical observation, show that psychoactive drugs decrease disintegration in perception, thought, affect, and motivation for the majority of clients labeled schizophrenic. Tricyclics and monoamine oxidase (MAO) inhibitors can alleviate depression. Lithium can adjust a manic mood. A common cause for readmission in psychoses is discontinuation of drug therapy by the client. However, psychoactive drugs have been widely used only since 1955. The effects of lifetime ingestion are only now beginning to be studied. Long-term drug therapy may turn out to have disadvantages similar to those of long-term hospitalization.

The major criticism of the positive findings for drug therapy is the lack of stable populations and controlled research designs. Readmission rates represent only those people who discontinue medication and are readmitted. There is no way to know how many people discontinue medication but never come to the attention of the health care system. Regardless of the ambiguity of clinical research, however, empirical observation supports the effectiveness of psychoactive drugs for the majority of acutely disturbed, psychotic individuals, whether the condition is Schizophrenia, Mania, or Depression.

Effects of Psychosocial Therapies Every conceivable type of psychosocial therapy has been attempted with the various psychotic conditions. Research into the effects and outcome of these therapies is on the whole less well controlled than research on the somatic therapies. Some studies report "miraculous" recoveries. But for every study that validates the effect of a specific treatment, there is another study that invalidates it. The vague definition of psychoses, the mobility of the subject group, and the lack of strict criteria for applying psychosocial therapies make many findings questionable and replication often impossible. Somatic and psychosocial therapies used together seem more effective than either used separately. Here, too, however, the results are inconclusive.

In clinical practice psychotherapy is being used as an adjunct to drug therapy rather than as a primary therapy. Very few practitioners continue to believe that therapy can "cure" psychotic conditions. However, some forms of psychotherapy, particularly family work, may assist psychotic individuals to cope with the condition and with living in the community. Since many such people do not have families or do not have interested families, researchers and clinicians have begun to look into other support systems for the psychotic person. The whole area of social networks and networking has begun to be investigated. It is too early to assume this may provide a new treatment approach but it is clear that social supports and social networks are important to the community survival of psychotic individuals (Hammer 1980; Pattison and Pattison 1981).

Generalizations about the Effects of Therapy from Research Findings The following generalizations may be made about the effects of therapy when the body of research is taken as a whole.

• Most acutely disturbed people, regardless of how they are labeled, respond to medication with a decrease in symptoms even if no other therapy is offered. Most people identified as schizophrenics function more easily if they are maintained on drugs. People identified as manic-depressives who respond to lithium are less likely to have further episodes if they are maintained on lithium. While the long-term consequences of drug maintenance are not yet known, short-term results support the use of drugs to interrupt the psychotic process.

- Acutely disturbed people, regardless of how they are labeled, are generally hospitalized. Most therapists believe that the acutely disturbed are not amenable to psychotherapy. Reports by Sullivan, Rosen, Laing, and others on the use of psychotherapy with extremely disturbed clients are the exceptions rather than the rule. Even when clients have been in therapy for years, they are usually hospitalized in acute exacerbation. Hospitalization and medication are the most common approaches to the control of acute symptoms. When medication is unacceptable, hospitalization is still ordered, and hydrotherapy, seclusion, and restraints provide time-limited external controls in acute periods.

- People who suffer from Bipolar Affective Disorder rarely seek or remain in any form of psychotherapy when the episode is past. These people seem to manage life fairly well except during acute episodes. Insight therapy has little value for most of them. Supportive or relationship therapy may help them understand the process of a specific condition and the treatment associated with it. Whether or not these people participate in any psychotherapy, it is extremely important that they be seen periodically by a physician or by a clinic to evaluate medication intake. People suffering from Bipolar Affective Disorder will probably reenter the health care system in an acute episode when they stop medication.

- Insight therapy is less than effective with people diagnosed as schizophrenic. There are various explanations for this. According to many ego psychologists, the schizophrenic's ego is too weak to withstand the pressures of insight therapy. On a more pragmatic basis, the schizophrenic will rarely accept the rigorous requirements of insight therapy and will either drop out of the therapy or escape into a psychotic episode if pressures become too great. Intensive insight therapy has sometimes been successful (Sullivan 1960; Laing 1967). In these cases the therapy was undertaken in a long-term residential treatment center where the individual client re-

ceived supervision, support, and protection during the process.

- People diagnosed as schizophrenic seem better able to tolerate the low stress level of supportive therapy. However, it may be necessary to continue this approach for some years. Many individuals maintain regular contact with therapists for ten to fifteen years and more. The goal of the therapy is not to cure but to provide support to the client in day-to-day living. Chronic schizophrenics often have little or no family involvement, and long-term supportive therapy can to some extent replace absent support systems.

- Family work can provide an opportunity to clear up communication, develop an atmosphere of change within the family, and help family members recognize that the client's problem is a family problem. This reassures the client that he or she is not the only one responsible for change. If the family is not committed to treatment, family work will teach family members about the process of the client's condition and help both the family and the client cope with the client's disturbing behavior. Unfortunately, not all psychotic clients have families, or families who are willing to work with their problems.

CONTEMPORARY NURSING APPROACHES

Psychiatric nurses use problem solving, interpersonal relations, and knowledge of human behavior to help psychotic clients cope with the problems of living from day to day. Most often they are the only professional people who interact with clients on this day-to-day basis. This section discusses nursing interventions with psychotic clients in inpatient, day care, and crisis units. In these settings, the nurse is the person who spends the most time and has the most opportunity to interact with the clients. Therapeutic nursing interventions grow out of nurses' experiences living day to day with the clients. Unlike most other health professionals, nurses are there when clients get up and when they go to bed. Nurses interact with clients around the tasks of living—eating, sleeping, getting to appointments, using leisure time, etc. No other mental health professional has such an opportunity to affect the client's life. The nursing care presented here was developed from day-to-day experience with clients.

Factors that Influence Care Planning

The care planning and implementation process can be influenced by factors other than the nurse's knowledge and skill. In working with psychotic clients, these factors are

- The nurse's attitude toward and role with the client
- The way in which the client enters the health care system
- Services contracted for between the client and the facility

The Nurse's Attitude and Role with Clients Labeled Psychotic

The art of nursing is the implementation of the science of nursing in a humane and caring way. The most brilliant approach to care is useless if it is implemented in a cold, uncaring way. Being therapeutic is rarely, if ever, a justification for being harsh or unkind to clients.

CLIENTS ARE ALWAYS PEOPLE FIRST   Clients labeled psychotic have the same experiences in life as other people. They are not innately good or evil, although by society's norms their behavior may sometimes be defined as bad. They are neither mentally retarded nor stupid. Intellectual capacity differs from person to person for these clients as it does for everyone else. Psychosis does not render these people incapable of all self-care or self-determination, nor does it deprive them of their individuality. Psychosis does not make them second-class citizens or subhuman. They are still entitled to respect and courtesy, even in their most bizarre moments. Because their perceptions and thoughts are distorted, clients may be dangerous to themselves or others, but the danger they actually pose is often determined by how they are approached. Even the most passive people will protect themselves if they believe they are being attacked. While nurses must be cautious, they must learn to view the client as a person first and as a "psychotic process" second, if at all.

CLIENTS WANT TO COMMUNICATE   Clients' fears may prevent them from communicating in a way that is easily understood. They are not attempting to confuse or baffle the nurse; they are reflecting their own confusion. They will continue to attempt to communicate until they are understood. Clients labeled psychotic appear to be unpredictable. However, only rarely is behavior truly random. Psychotic clients may not re-

spond to common cues in a common way, but with patience the nurse can determine how they do respond and can predict their behavior. Very few people are "psychotic" twenty-four hours a day, seven days a week. The nurse may assume that because certain clients can think logically at some times, they are not really "sick"—just obstinate or uncooperative. This is rarely the case. People do not choose to be "psychotic," and they cannot choose to be "not psychotic." They can, however, be assisted to maintain contact with reality.

PUNISHMENT IS NOT THE ANSWER   Punishment may produce compliance with the punisher, but that is not a true change in behavior. Helping clients control their behavior through limit setting can be done in a caring way. Child psychologists say that discipline, fairly and equitably administered, is a sign of concern from the parent to the child. The nurse can set limits in a fair and equitable way, and this can be a sign of concern to the client. Punitive attitudes or actual punishment for psychotic behavior will not help the client cope.

CLIENTS AND NURSES HAVE RIGHTS   Regardless of behavior, the client is a human being, not a thing. Manifestations of disintegrative behavior do not give the nurse the right to negate, ridicule, lie to, or abuse the client—even in the name of therapy. Clients retain their full rights as human beings no matter how bizarre their behavior. They may have momentarily lost the capacity to exercise their rights, but they do not lose those rights. Nurses sometimes violate the client's rights in the course of treatment. When this happens, they must recognize that they *have* violated the client's rights.

The nurse also has rights as a human being. The nurse must not be expected to tolerate physical abuse from clients. No matter how bizarre, clients can—and must be expected to—abstain from physically abusing staff and other clients. Nurses must believe in their own rights and the clients rights to physical safety, for this is the first step in developing the skill to deal with potentially explosive behavior. Nurses who have taken this step are less likely to abuse the client physically or provoke the client into physically abusing them.

CLIENTS MAKE VALID OBSERVATIONS   If institution food is bad, as is often the case, and the client says so, then the food is bad because it is bad, and not because the client is psychotic. Hospitals are regimented, and they do deprive clients of certain freedoms. Clients who complain of these restrictions are making valid observations that should not be attributed to the client's psychiatric condition. Clients will also make valid observations about the staff and their behavior. Like anyone else, they can be assisted to discuss their observations directly with the person involved. Clients of different cultural backgrounds may respond in different ways to being hospitalized. Cultural attitudes, too, are valid and should not be confused with pathology.

Note that clients can and do confuse valid observations with distorted perceptions and thoughts. When this happens, the confusion, not the observation, must be the focus of nursing interventions.

EMPATHY IS ESSENTIAL   Empathy is the single most essential quality in the delivery of nursing care. Clients labeled psychotic are often unattractive, difficult, ungrateful, and hostile to the nurse. Without empathy the nurse can develop a callous attitude in response to these clients' behavior. This only further complicates the nurse–client relationship. Nurses who believe that they know what is "best" for the client and ignore the client's input run the risk of losing their empathic approach. When this happens, the nurse–client relationship will probably disintegrate into a power struggle. When nurses insist on having power and control over the client, they cease to be nurses and become keepers. Maintaining one's empathy with clients and recognizing their human rights are the best ways to avoid becoming a keeper.

ON BEING A NURSE RATHER THAN A KEEPER   Psychotic people have been considered less than human for so long that it may be extremely difficult for the nurse to develop and maintain empathy with a psychotic client. Many nurses, as well as other health care workers, believe that a nurse who does not have control over the client is ineffective, or worse, a bad nurse. Nurses who maintain an empathic attitude, recognize and protect client rights, and encourage clients to participate in their own care may be considered weak, unskilled, inexperienced, or all three. These nurses may be viewed as unable to control clients, rather than as following a thought-out, conscious approach to nursing care. Many health professionals still believe that all psychotics are chronically ill and incapable of exercising self-care or self-determination unless their behavior is controlled, primarily by nursing staff. These coworkers believe that clients who are not controlled can do untold damage to themselves and others. Since psychotics cannot control their own behavior, in this view, nurses must force them to behave in an "acceptable" way. In fact, the role of nurses is to exercise control over clients

and force them to behave appropriately. This attitude advocating control and enforced conformity does not give way easily to an empathic approach that includes client participation.

Inexperienced nurses may find themselves becoming keepers in order to maintain their position with the health care staff. While mental health care has come a long way since the early insane asylums were established, the attitudes of society in general and health care workers specifically about "psychotically disturbed" persons have not changed that much. Despite overwhelming evidence to the contrary, individuals diagnosed as psychotic can still be redefined as incapable human beings by virtue of that diagnosis. Nurses who oppose these attitudes are likely to need support and fortitude to withstand the drift from nurse to keeper. However, the hope for better understanding, and therefore better care, of psychotic clients depends largely on the nurse's ability to withstand these pressures and to maintain an empathic, human, caring approach to these clients, despite the clients' bizarre behavior and criticisms from other staff members.

The Client's Entry into the Health Care System

Why did the individual client, or other people in the client's name, seek assistance? Did the identified client come voluntarily to the hospital, day care, or crisis service seeking assistance? Or did someone else (family, police) bring the client because they believed him or her to be disturbed? If the client did not actually initiate the attempt to get assistance but was forced by others, the nurse can expect him or her to be angry, uncooperative, and resistant to interventions. This kind of behavior is sometimes a function of the client's delusional system. Some clients believe they will actually be harmed. On the other hand, people who do not believe that there is anything wrong with them or that they need assistance will naturally be angry and uncooperative. These people will probably not agree to treatment unless they are forced. They will probably then be admitted to a hospital as involuntary clients if they are believed to be dangerous to themselves or others. Most people labeled psychotic do not voluntarily seek assistance. This fact has implications for planning their care.

The Contract for Service between the Agency and the Client

People labeled psychotic are offered services in a wide variety of settings. Since the cause, treatment, and outcome of psychoses are often vague, facilities may develop a wide range of service

Table 16–8   CONTEMPORARY SERVICES AVAILABLE FOR CLIENTS LABELED PSYCHOTIC

Type of Facility	Length of Stay	Primary Service	Goal
Inpatient			
Crisis service	Short-term, seven days to two weeks	1. Evaluation 2. Rapid interruption of the psychotic process 3. Referral	Rapid return to community living situation
Hospital	Moderate stay, two weeks to two months	1. Evaluation 2. Interruption of the psychotic process 3. Beginning treatment 4. Referral	To establish treatment of choice, i.e., medication or medication and psychotherapy
Hospital or residential treatment	Long stay, indefinite	1. Evaluation 2. Treatment 3. Social rehabilitation if needed	Recovery and/or social rehabilitation
Three-quarter or halfway house	Depends on client and program but usually one to six months	1. Rehabilitation 2. Socialization	1. Social recovery 2. Vocational rehabilitation
Board and care home	Indefinite, six months to a lifetime	1. Socialization 2. Supervision	1. Social recovery with protection 2. Stabilization of chronicity
Outpatient			
Emergency service	Short-term, one to six visits	1. Evaluation 2. Referral for further treatment	1. Time limited treatment 2. Referral
Outpatient clinic	Indefinite	1. Evaluation 2. Psychotherapy 3. Medication follow-up	1. To coordinate treatment 2. To maintain at present level of functioning
Private practitioner	Indefinite	1. Evaluation 2. Psychotherapy 3. Medication follow-up	1. To coordinate treatment 2. To maintain at present level of functioning
Day care	Indefinite	1. Socialization activity 2. Supportive therapy	1. To maintain social recovery 2. To stabilize chronicity

programs (see Table 16–8). Each program may be based on a specific method of treatment, and nursing care will be planned to augment that method. For example, acutely disturbed people are usually treated in a residential or inpatient center. However, they are treated differently in different settings. A short-term crisis service seeks to evaluate the person's condition, intervene rapidly in the psychotic process, and return the person immediately to the community. Further

treatment takes place in community day care centers, community service programs, or outpatient clinics. The person's actual hospital stay is short, and the nursing care is planned to alleviate the acute condition.

At the other end of the continuum is the long-term residential treatment center, often based on a specific model or philosophy of treatment. Kingsley Hall in England, Soteria House in California, and Chestnut Lodge in Maryland are examples of such facilities. In long-term facilities, clients are offered evaluation, treatment, and rehabilitation. Depending on the facility, the psychosis may be interrupted with medication, or the client may be allowed, with staff assistance, to live out the natural course of the condition. The most common service falls somewhere between crisis and long-term care and provides evaluation, interruption of the psychosis, and beginning treatment.

Few psychotic people are able to function independently on discharge from an inpatient facility. Board and care homes, halfway houses, and day care centers offer them the chance to adjust gradually to life outside the institution. These facilities provide social rehabilitation primarily. They increase the person's ability to function independently, rather than treating the psychotic condition.

Depending on the program offered the client, the nurse may plan care primarily for the acute phase, the treatment phase, the rehabilitation phase, or some combination of the three. It is important that both nurse and client understand the limits and scope of the program, so that the goals of care can be developed realistically. For example, social rehabilitation would not be an appropriate goal for most short-term crisis settings.

Nursing Strategies

A nursing strategy includes the procedure and process of a nursing act. A strategy is a plan for reaching a specific goal. Any number of nursing strategies are effective with clients labeled psychotic. New strategies need not be developed for each client who exhibits behavior common to the psychoses. The same strategies are used over and over with different clients who have different problems. Nursing care is individualized by the way in which the strategies are implemented. This section discusses strategies that may be used to intervene in disintegration of perception, thought, affect, and motivation.

Interventions in Disintegration of Perception

Disintegration of perception may take the form of illusions, hallucinations, or less dramatically, of distorted reality. Nurses should not attempt to convince clients that their perceptions are wrong. However, they should not validate the client's distorted perceptions. Nurses work with clients to validate reality, to reassure them when their perceptions are frightening, and to protect them from external danger that may result from their distorted perception (see Table 16–9).

Table 16–9   SUGGESTIONS FOR INTERVENING IN DISINTEGRATION OF PERCEPTION

Observation	Rationale
Don't argue about hallucinations.	These clients truly believe that their distorted perceptions are real. If you question them or argue with them, they must try to convince you that what they believe is real. They know that what you believe is not real.
Point out your reality, but don't try to rob clients of theirs.	Clients have a distorted reality because your reality is more frightening than theirs. You must not validate or enter the client's reality, but neither can you expect that the client will enter, and accept without question, your reality.
Offer the client gentle reassurance.	Even though the client's reality is less frightening than yours, it is often cruel and painful. Recognize the client's fear, pain, and despair, and be gentle in bringing him or her back to reality.
Don't touch clients without telling them first.	These clients may not know where they begin and end, and if you touch them without telling them, you may break into their space. They may lash out to protect themselves.
If you are frightened by the client or the client's distorted perceptions, ask someone to help you.	The client is probably more frightened than you are. However, these clients are also more sensitive to strong affect and so will sense your fear. Because their perceptions are distorted, they may not know where the fear is coming from and may become still more upset and frightened. Frightened clients must be approached with calm firmness, and this takes time to learn. The important thing is to help the client cope, not to prove that you are not afraid.

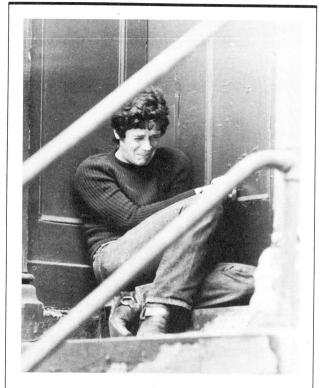

Disintegrations of perception in the form of hallucinations may be frightening and confusing to the client.

VALIDATING REALITY

Jane is sitting alone in the dayroom with her head slightly tilted as if listening. She is gazing into space. Lunch has arrived, and the nurse approaches Jane to tell her.

NURSE: *Jane, Jane. (Jane does not acknowledge the nurse's presence.)*

NURSE: *Jane, you are listening to the voices again. But only you can hear them. Jane, listen to me, not to the voices. (Jane looks at the nurse.)*

NURSE: *Jane, lunch is here. I'll take your hand. (Nurse takes Jane's hand and Jane stands up.)*

NURSE: *Jane, I am going to be your nurse today. (Jane looks puzzled.)*

NURSE: *Jane, I know the voices seem real to you, but I do not hear them. You are in the hospital. It's Tuesday noon and time for lunch.*

JANE: *I guess I lost track of time.*

NURSE: *The voices are bothering you again?*

JANE: *Yes. I'm really not very hungry.*

NURSE: *I'll walk with you to the dining room and sit with you there. You can try to eat a little something.*

The nurse recognized by Jane's behavior that she was probably hearing voices. The nurse was patient and waited until she got Jane's attention. She did not argue about the voices but recognized that Jane was confused. The nurse validated reality by stating who she was and where the client was. The nurse recognized that Jane might not be aware of her hunger. The nurse did not argue with Jane but was firm and took Jane in to lunch. Recognizing that Jane might be ambivalent and indecisive, the nurse did not ask questions or offer alternatives.

REASSURANCE WHEN PERCEPTIONS ARE FRIGHTENING

Margaret is the thirty-five-year-old mother of a five-year-old child. She is divorced. Margaret reports having had a psychoticlike episode at seventeen with what she believed was a full recovery. At the birth of her child she had a mild depressive episode. After her divorce she began to feel depressed and then increasingly sure that God was talking to her. On a day-to-day basis Margaret functioned very well, and until recently she was able to ignore God's voice. However, as soon as she began to date again, Margaret heard God call her a whore and condemn her to death. Lately she has not only heard God but seen him. He looks like the Devil, and Margaret is afraid that God is changing to the Devil because of her behavior. When her visual and auditory hallucinations become extremely severe, Margaret freezes and panics.

Margaret is sitting in the dayroom. She stands up quickly and begins to cry and shake. Two nurses recognize that Margaret is going into a panic. They approach and take her quickly to the quiet room. She is wrapped in a blanket, and one nurse sits and holds her.

NURSE: *Margaret, I am here. Listen to me. I know you are frightened. I'll help you. You will not be hurt. Listen to me, Margaret. (The nurse continues to hold Margaret and talk with her, attempting to interrupt the voices and to reassure her.)*

Several weeks later as Margaret is getting ready to be discharged, she tells the nursing staff how effective this intervention was.

MARGARET: *I believed you were there with me, helping me fight those frightening feelings.*

When their clients' perceptions are especially frightening, nurses must recognize this and acknowledge the client's fear. At the same time they should reassure these clients that they will stay with them and help them with their fears. By working with these clients to maintain contact with reality, the nurse helps them decrease their focus on fearful perceptions and thus decreases their fear.

PROTECTING THE CLIENT FROM EXTERNAL DANGER

Gail, a nineteen-year-old girl, is admitted from her community mental health center. She has been a client in the day care program there since she was sixteen. At that time she refused to go to school because "a man might rape me." She has had no medication and has been treated with group therapy and special education classes. Her fears of rape have become so great that she regularly calls the police, the ambulance, and the sheriff's office to rescue her. Her parents and the community mental health center can no longer cope with her behavior. She actively hallucinates and believes that all men will rape her and all women will betray her. There is an early history of child abuse and perhaps incest in her family. Gail demonstrates negativism and answers in monosyllables. She is animated only when "The People" attack her.

GAIL *(walking down the hall)*: I told you to bug off. Now stop it. *(She swings with her right hand and barely misses the wall.)* I can't take this any more from you. *(She turns and swings. She grazes the wall, ripping the skin off her knuckles.)*

NURSE *(approaches Gail but stands at a distance)*: Gail, Gail.

GAIL *(looks at the nurse)*: Yes?

NURSE: Gail, there is no one here. I can see you believe that "The People" are after you again, but there is no one here.

GAIL: I know, but I'm going to get them. *(She walks briskly down the hall.)*

The nurse asks two other staff members to join her and approaches Gail.

NURSE: Gail, I can see you feel really pressured by "The People," and you may hurt yourself. Look at your hand. Mary, Barbara, and I are going to walk with you to the quiet room, give you some medication, and bandage your hand.

Gail and the nurses go to the quiet room. Gail changes to pajamas, has her hand bandaged, and takes medication.

NURSE: We are going to leave you. We are going to wrap you tight in a blanket, and you can rest for a while. We will talk with you every few minutes.

Gail relaxes in the bed wrapped in her blanket. She is safe for now.

Everyone experiences inaccurate perceptions now and again. However, when perceptions are so distorted that they make day-to-day living impossible, or terrorize or endanger the person who has them, that person needs assistance.

Interventions in Disintegration of Thought

Verbal communication is a valued skill in contemporary culture. People are often judged on their ability to make themselves understood. Clients often demonstrate disintegrative thought in verbal behavior. Because these clients speak English, we may think we understand them. In reality, understanding "psychotic language" is often extremely difficult. Nurses must be willing to admit when they don't understand, to recognize when they do understand, and to keep trying (see Table 16–10).

ADMITTING LACK OF UNDERSTANDING

Charlene is a twenty-five-year-old woman who carries a plastic bag full of baby clothes with her all the time. She has had the bag since she was admitted and refuses to let go of it. Charlene will take a bath five to ten times a day if she is not redirected. At present she is only allowed to bathe in the morning, in the afternoon, and before bed. She always has her bag with her. Over time the contents have become damp and foul smelling. A nurse who does not understand (but does not know it) initiates the following interaction:

NURSE: Charlene, holding that bag is ridiculous. Let me have it while you bathe.

CHARLENE: No, no. *(She pulls on the bag, sits on the bathroom floor, and holds the bag, her clothing, her towel, and all her other bathroom paraphernalia to her chest.)* Let me be, you bitch.

NURSE: Have it your own way. No bag, no bath tonight!

After a struggle Charlene leaves the bathroom. She refuses to go to bed and is up pacing most of the night. The next morning a nurse who does not understand (but knows it) initiates the following intervention:

NURSE: Charlene, I don't understand what the bag means, but I know it is very important. Everything in there is damp, and it is really getting ruined. Let's you and I take everything out and put it in the washer and dryer. You can bathe and you and the bag will be ready at the same time.

CHARLENE: No, no *(holding the bag tightly)*. Leave me be, stupid.

NURSE: I can wait while you think about it.

Table 16–10   SUGGESTIONS FOR INTERVENING IN DISINTEGRATION OF THOUGHT

Observation	Rationale	Observation	Rationale
If you don't understand, say so.	Clients will often talk with you in what appears to be English, and you may find yourself responding as if you understood. If you suspect that you actually do not understand, encourage these clients to keep trying, but let them know that you do not understand what they are saying. Communication is less difficult if both you and the client are clear about what you do and do not understand.	Listen very carefully.	Keep listening to the client very carefully. When you think you understand, share what you understand with the client. If it is not accurate, the client will keep telling you until you get it.
Recognize the feeling, if not the content, of the communication.	Feelings may be much more apparent than the actual content of the communication. Be aware of what clients are telling you about feeling with their verbal and nonverbal communications. You may recognize the feeling before the content, and that will help you to understand the content.	Don't argue or agree with delusions.	Delusions are very real to the client, no matter how farfetched they sound to you. If you try to argue or reason with clients about their delusions, they will feel compelled to convince you that they are right. This only solidifies the delusional system. Since a delusional system is not real, don't agree with the client. Let these clients know you think it seems real to them but not to you.
Help the client regulate the verbal production so you can understand.	If clients are communicating many ideas rapidly, ask them to slow down and try to take one idea at a time.	Really understanding disintegrative communications takes a long time and lots of patience.	Confused, disoriented, distorted, or disintegrative thought is extremely difficult to understand. Don't rush. Take your time. Eventually you will learn something about "psychotic" language and be better able to help the person to cope.

CHARLENE: *Wait until you rot.*

NURSE: *I have some things to do while you think. Come with me. (Charlene stays with the nurse.)*

(Some time later . . .)

NURSE: *Well, Charlene, it's time for your bath. Let's get your bag cleaned too.*

CHARLENE: *Well, okay, But you have got to stay with it.*

NURSE: *Okay, Charlene, you bathe, and then we will do your bag together.*

Charlene left the hospital six weeks later. She never did tell the nurse what the bag meant, but she left without it.

The bag had a special meaning for the client, and the nurse accepted this, even though she did not under-

stand. At this point the client was not amenable to logic, and attempts to take the bag would have provoked an outburst. As the client's thoughts cleared, the bag lost its symbolic meaning, and she was able to give it up.

Clients with delusional systems may be difficult to understand and to work with.

Gloria is a fifty-year-old woman who was referred for hospital treatment by her family physician. She had been seeing an outpatient therapist and had developed an active delusional system around that therapist. She would have her sister and daughter drive her around looking for the therapist's house. She would go and sit in his office or call him continually. Gloria is preoccupied and labile. The nurse approaches her.

NURSE: *We are going out for coffee. Will you join us?*

GLORIA: *Okay. You are wearing a cross around your neck. You are religious. Well, you will understand me. Only religious people do understand, don't you know? Dr. G [her outpatient therapist] wants me to marry him. I have prayed about this, because it would be a mixed marriage—color and religion. I am black, he is white. I am Christian, he is Jewish. But God has spoken to me and to Dr. G. We will be married. He will call today and tell me.*

NURSE: *I know these thoughts are real to you. I don't fully understand, but they are not real to me.*

GLORIA: *You wear a cross but you are not one of God's children!*

NURSE: *Gloria, let's walk over to the cafeteria and talk about your weekend plans.*

GLORIA: *I will see Dr. G then.*

NURSE: *I know that is real to you but not to me. Let's not talk about it any more now, Gloria.*

GLORIA: *You will see. I know Dr.—*

NURSE (interrupting): *Gloria, what time will your sister be here to pick you up?*

The nurse may not understand the delusional system. But when the nurse has validated that it is a delusional system and has listened once, he or she redirects the client to something else. Talking about the system or subjecting the client to a logical explanation only reinforces the system. Occasionally the nurse may have to interrupt the client to stop the discussion of the delusional system.

RECOGNIZING WHAT IS UNDERSTOOD

Tom, a twenty-one-year-old man, meets the nurse as she comes on duty every day. He always asks, "Who are you? A policeman? No, an FBI man?" The nurse explains every day that she is a nurse. After several weeks the nurse realizes that Tom has never identified her as a woman in a common female role. He has always said "policeman," "FBI-man," "hatchetman," "man to do me in." He appears to be using the word man to mean human. He doesn't see the nurse as male, but neither does he see her as female. At the next opportunity, she uses this understanding.

TOM: *Who are you? A Man for All Seasons?*

NURSE: *Tom, I am not a man. I am a woman. You are a man.*

TOM: *You are a woman?*

NURSE: *Yes, Tom, I am a woman. You are a man.*

TOM: *Well!*

NURSE: *Okay?*

TOM: *Yeah, that's really okay I guess. I am a man, and you are a woman.*

Tom never again asked who the nurse was.

What is obvious to the nurse may be less obvious to the client. Tom had been asking all along to be reassured that he was a man. The nurse did that by identifying herself as a woman and telling him he was a man.

Joe is a seventeen-year-old boy with no address who was picked up by the police. He confessed to several bizarre crimes and was admitted to the hospital. He believes he is being poisoned by the medication.

JOE: *Hey man, I need a cane. These pills are killing me and making me weak. I can hardly stand up. I can hardly walk. My whole body is in bad shape because of this here pill. Get me a cane, somebody!*

The nurse tries to figure out what Joe is saying. She thinks, "A cane helps you walk. A cane is support."

NURSE: *Joe, we will help you. You need support right now and it's okay to lean on us. We know your body feels in bad shape. We will support you while your body gets better.*

JOE: *You will, huh? My body does need help. I need help.*

When we believe we have some idea of what these clients are saying, we can tell them. If we have interpreted their communication accurately, they will let us know. If we have not, little harm is done, because if encouraged they will continue to communicate until someone understands them.

CONTINUING TO TRY

Nancy, a twenty-seven-year-old woman, is married to a college professor. She has three daughters, four years, two years, and six months old. After the birth of her last baby she seemed listless. The child was fretful, and Nancy began staying up all night to watch her. After a couple of months Nancy seemed to readjust. But last month she suddenly refused to talk to her husband and finally threatened to divorce him. Since that time she has *been staying up night and day and has had only a few hours of sleep in the last two or three weeks. Her husband admitted her a few days ago because she is manic. Nancy is always moving and talking. On admission she is labile and demands a female therapist.*

NANCY *(to the nurse): Listen, you, I have the message. I have talked with Steinem and Helene Deutsch. She's dead, you know, but I have talked to her anyway. And I know a wedding band means three but now we are four. Me, Charles, Lisa, Janice, and Tam. Tam was the mistake. Tam is really my mother. I am the child.*

NURSE: *Nancy, I'm not understanding you. I don't know what you are saying. Let's walk and you try and tell me again.*

NANCY: *You bet your sweet life. Life. What a drag. Drag queen. That's what my husband is.*

NURSE *(gently): Nancy, stop. Let's just walk. Be quiet for a while. I know you are trying to tell me something, but I can't understand.*

NANCY: *Try, my little chickadee. Try again. Try. That's what I need is a try to die.*

NURSE *(recognizing that Nancy is frightened, says gently): Nancy, let's keep walking and let's not talk so much. Take my hand. We will communicate this way.*

When we do not understand, we must say so. But we must also demonstrate that we want to understand and are willing to keep trying. If we can't understand the content, we may understand the feelings—and those feelings should be recognized.

Interventions in Disintegration of Affect   Disturbance of affect is painful for clients but often more painful for nurses. Modern American culture tends to deny emotion and does not encourage the expression of negative or intense feelings. Cultural rules call for polite conversation. In dealing with disintegration of affect, nurses are acting in opposition to cultural norms. They accept negative and intense feelings and do not require polite conversation. Nurses must recognize affect and accept it as a reflection of how the client feels. They must also attempt to help the client regulate affect (see Table 16–11).

RECOGNIZING AND ACCEPTING AFFECT

John is an attractive young medical student who attempted suicide when he failed an exam. His mood is labile. He cries or is extremely angry. He is feeling very guilty about his failure, both on the exam and at suicide.

He is embarrassed about being in a "nuthouse" and concerned about not being able to "control" his emotions. John is on his bed crying. The nurse approaches.

NURSE: *John?*

JOHN *(in an angry voice): What do you want? You can't help. Nobody can help. I just messed up. I hate myself. I hate you.*

NURSE: *John, you seem to be in pain. I'll stay with you for a while.*

JOHN *(sarcastically): Yeah, you bet I'm in pain. Why don't you get the hell out of here and leave me alone. (He turns his face to the wall.)*

NURSE: *I'll come back later.*

The nurse recognizes John's pain and anger. She does not push him by staying. By saying she will be back, the nurse gives the message of acceptance. Later she approaches John again.

NURSE: *How is it going?*

JOHN *(head down): I'm sorry I yelled at you. I don't hate you. Please forgive me.*

NURSE: *I forgive you. I don't like to be yelled at, but I'll try to understand. I still like you, John.*

John is not actually angry at the nurse, but he does take his anger out on her. The nurse recognizes this and accepts John by not retaliating in anger or increasing his guilt by refusing to forgive him.

John is eating lunch. Suddenly he puts his hands to his face and begins to sob. The nurse quickly approaches.

NURSE *(taking John by the hand): Come with me, John. (John follows and tries to stop crying.)*

NURSE: *John, I know it hurts. It's okay to cry. Crying sometimes helps. I know you're embarrassed, so let's go into your room and shut the door.*

The nurse knows John is embarrassed about crying in front of others. She has encouraged him in group to talk about his feelings and to discuss crying with other clients. However, when he begins to sob in the dining room, the nurse recognizes that he needs both to cry and to have privacy in which to do it.

	Table 16-11	SUGGESTIONS FOR INTERVENING IN DISINTEGRATION OF AFFECT	
Observation	**Rationale**	**Observation**	**Rationale**
If you are angry with these clients, tell them in a matter-of-fact way. Avoid making them feel guilty or depriving them of care.	Nurses get angry at clients, sometimes with good reason. Being a nurse does not put you above common, ordinary emotion. You do have a responsibility to know when you are angry and to let the client know what made you angry. By recognizing your own anger and dealing with it in an open way, you can better recognize your clients' anger and help them deal with it. You are also less likely to punish the client because you are angry.	Don't encourage the client to express feelings if you are not comfortable with the feelings, don't have time to listen, or are not interested.	When you cannot give your full attention to clients, it is better to ask them to wait to talk with you. Clients often have low self-esteem and believe themselves to be unworthy. Thus they may interpret your lack of attention, for whatever reason, as a rejection.
Learn to accept the client's anger calmly. The client is rarely angry at the nurse personally.	These clients may take their anger out on you even when they are not angry at you. The nurse is a safe, dependable person to these clients, and they may feel they can be angry with you without fearing loss of self-esteem or retaliation. Sometimes clients are just so upset that they lash out at the first person they run into.	Don't encourage clients to express feelings unless you have a purpose in mind.	Catharsis may be good, but if you are having clients express feelings because it will "help them," it is best to understand clearly why it will help. Expression of feelings is not always therapeutic.
Clients are influenced by social norms and so may be embarrassed by their own display of emotion. Be alert to the client's feelings about showing feelings.	American society has tended to frown on the display of emotion. Although social attitudes are becoming more open, not all clients feel free to express their feelings. If the client is unwilling to cry in front of others, help him or her to find a place to cry in privacy. You can use group therapy, family therapy, and community living meetings to discuss the display of emotions and help these clients be more comfortable not only with their emotions, but with the display of them.	Learn to distinguish ruminations from the expression of feelings.	Going over and over the same thing is not necessarily good. It will not always help the client to cope. When you recognize that a client is ruminating, don't dismiss the feeling, but don't encourage the person to talk more about it. The more the client talks, the more overwhelming the issue may seem. Redirect these clients into an activity that will help them to refocus their attention.
		Emotions can be painful even to the extremely bizarre individual.	No matter how out of contact or out of control clients may seem, they may still be painfully aware of their emotions. Even with clients who seem to have suffered a complete break with reality, be compassionate.

REGULATING AFFECT

Ursula is a fifty-year-old widow. Her husband died three years ago, and she has become increasingly depressed. She blames herself for his death and wishes she had died. She believes she should be punished and often scratches her arms until they bleed. She ruminates and cries constantly. Crying has not helped Ursula resolve her feelings.

URSULA *(crying): Nurse, nurse, help me. I feel so bad. My husband is dead. It's my fault. He was such a good man and I treated him so poorly. I never deserved him. I've got what I deserve now.*

NURSE: *Ursula, you know you get upset when you talk about this. Let's do something to get your mind off of your troubles.*

URSULA: *But you don't understand. I hurt so bad.*

NURSE: *You've said you hurt, Ursula, but going over and over it doesn't help. Come on, let's play Scrabble. (The nurse finds two other clients and they start a game.)*

Ursula will become increasingly upset if she is encouraged to talk. If the nurse asks Ursula to talk about her concerns or offers her consolation, Ursula will begin to feel more and more guilty about her husband's death and punish herself more for what she thinks she did. If the nurse matter-of-factly accepts what Ursula is saying and joins her in an activity, the nurse can change the focus of attention, and Ursula will be able to stop punishing herself for a while.

After three weeks in the hospital on tricyclics, Ursula is generally improved and her feelings are less intense. She needs little assistance during the day, but at bedtime she asks for medication and a sleeping pill and then sits up and cries.

As bedtime approaches Ursula has less and less to occupy her mind and her time, and she remembers over and over how her husband died and finds more and more fault with her behavior toward him. If the nurse responds to Ursula's tears with sympathy or consolations, Ursula only feels worse. She does not believe she is entitled to any understanding. Ursula can better regulate her emotions if she has a schedule and firm, kind direction from the nurse.

URSULA: *Nurse, I'm ready for my pill.*

NURSE: *Ursula, it's only ten o'clock. Taking your pills at ten o'clock doesn't seem helpful, because then you stay up till midnight crying.*

URSULA: *Oh nurse, I can't help it. I feel so bad at night.*

NURSE: *Let's try something different tonight. Your roommate is usually in bed by ten-thirty. You go take a warm bath at ten-thirty. Let me know when you are finished. You go to bed and I'll bring your pills and stay with you a while.*

Later, when Ursula has taken her bath, the nurse comes in with her pills.

NURSE: *Okay, I'll just sit here. (Ursula starts crying.)*

NURSE *(in a firm but gentle voice): Ursula, no crying. Think of something pleasant, breathe deeply, and concentrate on sleep. (Ursula tries, and the nurse stays almost an hour until she is asleep.)*

The nurse is firm with Ursula in telling her to stop crying. The nurse knows that Ursula will become increasingly upset if she begins to cry and think about her husband.

The next night the nurse has Ursula do the same thing but tells her she will only stay a half an hour. In a week's time the nurse does not have to stay with Ursula at all. Ursula continues to improve on medication, and the nurse helps her maintain her improvement by helping her to deal with her feelings more effectively. The week before discharge the nurse approaches Ursula.

NURSE: *Ursula, you will be going home next week, and I won't be there to give you your pills. Let's figure out a way for you to handle this by yourself. Before you take your bath, I will show you how to take your medication by yourself. Then when you have had your bath, you can pour your own medication before you go to bed.*

URSULA: *Oh, do you think I am ready?*

NURSE: *Yes, Ursula, I really do.*

Ursula learns to take her own medication and does so every night until she is discharged. She does not have a problem sleeping.

The nurse recognizes Ursula's increasing ability to regulate her emotions. She supports Ursula by encouraging her to take more and more reponsibility for herself.

Interventions in Disintegration of Motivation

Disintegration in perception, thought, or affect may re-

Table 16–12	SUGGESTIONS FOR INTERVENING IN DISINTEGRATION OF MOTIVATION		
Observation	Rationale	Observation	Rationale
Be alert to understanding what clients tell you in whatever way they can. Take time to observe.	Behavior is rarely random. Many behaviors that look meaningless have autistic meaning for the client. When you have learned enough about the client, some of this autistic behavior may have meaning for you, too.	Use physical force only as a last resort to protect the client and others, not to make clients do what you want them to do.	Occasionally it is necessary to use physical force. However, force should never be used as punishment, or to make the patient comply so the nurse can save face. The use of physical force is serious in any setting. In a therapeutic setting it must be viewed as an extreme measure.
Don't talk past clients or talk about them in their presence.	When clients are regressed, withdrawn, or out of contact, they can still see and hear. Talking past clients or talking about them makes them feel less than human.	Help clients regulate their behavior to meet their needs, not yours.	Clients do not always behave in a socially acceptable way. As long as the behavior is not harming anyone, concentrate on helping the client cope, rather than on encouraging "acceptable" behavior.
Clients may not be able to stop their behavior just because you have asked them to. If the behavior is not harmful to themselves or others, go away and try again later.	Clients who have disintegrated motivations rarely refuse to follow directions because they are stubborn or obstinate. Ask these clients once or twice and then give them some space. They may be able to comply after you leave. If your request is not absolutely essential to the client's welfare, let it be. Approach the subject again later. The client may be able to comply in a few minutes, in a few days, or maybe never.	Never try to restrain even the smallest client alone.	If the client is sufficiently out of control to need physical restraint, you probably can't do it alone. Call for help. If you try it alone and are hurt, the client will have the added burden of guilt.
Avoid using physical force by avoiding power struggles.	One person cannot make another person do what he or she absolutely does not want to do—except by using physical force. When you approach clients about something that you believe they might resist doing, ask yourself if you are willing to use physical force to get what you want. If you are not, don't push these clients to the point where they have to lash out to make their position clear.	The client rarely wants to hurt you.	Even though clients may hurt themselves, each other, or staff, they rarely intend to do so. Usually they are only trying to escape their own thoughts, perceptions, or affects, or are lashing out in response to their delusions and hallucinations. Anyone who tries to stop them may accidentally be hurt.

sult in disintegration of motivation and vice versa. Disintegration of motivation produces a wide variety of behavior that is difficult to understand. Nurses must try to understand what is motivating the client, but even when they cannot understand, they must try to help the client to handle the behavior that results from disintegration of motivation. This includes *ambivalence, withdrawal, impulsive behavior,* and *hyperactivity* (see Table 16–12).

REGULATING AMBIVALENCE

George is a twenty-five-year-old man. He has to be assisted onto the unit, for he stops at the door and seems unable to walk in. The nurse must gently push him into his room.

NURSE: *George, put your things on that bed.*

GEORGE: *Is that a good bed? What about the other bed?*

NURSE: *George, this is your bed. Please sit down. I will be right back.*

When the nurse returns, George is moving his suitcase from one bed to the other.

NURSE: *George, that is your bed. Please leave the suitcase there.*

GEORGE (*as he moves the suitcase*): *Okay.*

The nurse recognizes that George is so ambivalent that even when he appears to agree, he continues to be undecided. Since there are no private rooms, the nurse moves the vacant bed into the hallway, so that George can accept one bed. The nurse decides against helping George to unpack for the time being.

Later that day George is prescribed psychoactive drugs. Since the nurse recognizes that George is extremely ambivalent, she does not attempt to take medication to George in the dayroom but has him join her in the medication room.

NURSE: *George, these are pills that Dr. M ordered for you. Hold out your hand. I will put them in your hand, and you put them in your mouth.*

George looks at the pills, puts them in his mouth, and spits them out into his hand. He does this several times.

NURSE: *I know it is hard for you to decide, so follow my instructions. Put the pills in your mouth. (Holds a cup of water to his lips.) Drink, George. Okay, swallow the pills. Open your mouth.*

The nurse sees George drink water, but when he opens his mouth the pills are still on his tongue.

NURSE: *Spit them out in the sink, George. Pills are too hard to take. I will put your medication in juice for you so you can drink it.*

George watches the nurse mix the elixir in juice. She holds the cup and George drinks. George is not actually refusing medications. He is extremely ambivalent and is unable to decide what to do.

The nurse recognizes when George is ambivalent and in clear, simple, declarative statements makes the decision for him. If the nurse had asked George questions, she would have increased his ambivalence and his discomfort.

REGULATING WITHDRAWN BEHAVIOR

Peg is a thirty-one-year-old woman who sits in the dayroom all day listening to records. This afternoon she sits and sways her body in time with the music. She gets up from her chair and sits on the floor. She puts her head on her knees. Then she sits up and lies back on the floor. The nurse approaches. Peg is lying still and staring out into space. The nurse recognizes that Peg has withdrawn into her own world, and is out of contact with reality. Peg may be having auditory or visual hallucinations, or both.

NURSE: *Peg, Peg? (Peg does not respond.)*

NURSE: *Peg, I am going to touch you. (She takes Peg's hand.) Peg, listen to me. (She pulls Peg into a sitting position.) Peg, Peg, look at me. (Peg starts to cry and goes limp. The nurse holds her.) Come on, Peg. Get up. Let's walk. I know it is frightening and sad. (The nurse gets Peg to her feet.) Come on, Peg. Look at me. Walk with me. I am here and I am touching you. You are real. (Peg walks, but she is still crying.) Peg. Hey, Peg. Where are you, Peg?*

PEG: *I am in the hospital.*

NURSE: *What day is it?*

PEG: *Tuesday.*

NURSE: *That's right. What time is it, Peg?*

PEG: *I don't know. Afternoon, I guess.*

NURSE: *That's right. It's about two o'clock. Keep talking with me. Don't go back.*

PEG: *What do I talk about?*

NURSE: *Do you go to the movies?*

PEG: *Yes.*

NURSE: *What did you see last?*

The nurse recognizes that Peg is withdrawing and tries to help her maintain contact with reality. Peg's own world is frightening and attractive at the same time. The nurse helps Peg maintain a reality orientation by focusing on reality.

REGULATING IMPULSIVE AND VIOLENT BEHAVIOR

Jim has been pacing all day. He is unable to sit down. The nurse has been walking with him in the hallway at intervals. She recognizes that Jim is frightened by voices and is also delusional. He believes that he is the victim of a CIA plot. The nurse approaches Jim.

NURSE: *Hi, Jim. Are you still pretty upset?*

JIM: *Damn right. Everyone here is out to get me. I don't know which of you is a CIA agent, but I will find out.*

NURSE: *That sounds very frightening.*

JIM: *No, I just have to be careful. Can't let down my guard. I think I know who it is. It's Harry [the evening nurse]. He sneaks in and looks at me after I go to bed.*

NURSE: *Jim, you seem more upset. Let's go sit down in the dayroom. We won't talk, just sit.*

JIM: *No, if it's not Harry, maybe it's George [another client]. Where is George, anyway? (Jim is speaking now in a very suspicious voice.)*

NURSE: *He is at school.*

JIM: *Sure, CIA school. I'll get him.*

NURSE: *I'll see you in a while, Jim.*

No matter how impulsive the behavior looks to the nurse, it has meaning to the client, who may be responding to voices or visions or to a thought or affect. Usually these clients are out of contact with reality, or at least their reality is distorted. The nurse approaches such clients cautiously. If they are potentially explosive and violent, the nurse may need other staff assistance.

The nurse recognizes, from working with Jim all day, that he is becoming increasingly agitated and is losing control. She believes that if he were quiet for a while, he might be in better control. Talking with him seems to activate his delusional system. She asks two staff members to join her and approaches Jim.

NURSE: *Jim, you are extremely upset. You are having difficulty with the voices and with your fears. You need to be quiet and rest for a while.*

JIM: *It's you! Don't come near me. (He backs up to the wall.)*

NURSE: *Jim, we will not hurt you, but you must go to the quiet room. It is safer and less frightening there.*

JIM: *Not me. I'm safe here. I've got to get George before he gets me.*

NURSE: *Jim, come on and walk with us to the quiet room. We don't want to hurt you. You need to be safe, and we understand.*

JIM: *Don't touch me.*

NURSE: *Okay. (She moves back and puts her hands behind her back.) We won't touch you, but you walk with us. It is safe in the quiet room. You can put on your pajamas and lie down, and we will lock the door.*

JIM: *Don't touch me. (He is walking slightly ahead of the nursing staff.)*

NURSE: *Jim, I have to walk in front of you to unlock the door.*

JIM: *(stopping): Okay, you go ahead.*

The nurse unlocks the door and Jim enters. He changes his clothes and puts on his pajamas.

NURSE: *I'll take your clothes.*

JIM: *No, don't touch them.*

NURSE: *Okay, you pick them up and we will lock them in the bathroom.*

Jim takes his clothes to the bathroom and puts them in a corner. He covers them with paper towels. Then he comes back and lies down on his bed.

NURSE: *Jim, we will lock the door. We will look in every fifteen minutes. We will tell you before we open the door.*

JIM: *Okay. Just don't let George or Harry get in.*

NURSE: *We won't. We'll be back in fifteen minutes.*

The nurse recognizes that Jim is extremely frightened and in poor contact with reality. Therefore she works slowly with him to assure him that he will be safe. She also allows him to control the seclusion procedure. She believes that he wants to feel safe and that he will feel safe in a locked room. The locked room will help decrease his frightening feelings of losing control. However, if she insists on controlling the situation and does not respect his needs, she will provoke an explosive episode. As long as clients have control, they should be allowed to use it. The important thing is to get Jim into a quiet, safe room—not to have the nurse demonstrate her power over him. There must always be sufficient physical force available to call on should the client lose control, but it should not be employed unless that actually happens.

Later that evening Jim observes Harry and George talking together. He stands up and starts to yell.

JIM: *You're plotting to get me. I'm going to get you first. I am innocent.*

The nursing staff recognize that Jim is out of control and may hurt himself or others. Four staff members approach him from either side in a quiet, calm manner.

NURSE: *Jim, we are taking you out of the dayroom and into seclusion.*

JIM: *They're going to kill me. You are going to kill me. (He begins to struggle. The staff walk him down the hall.)*

NURSE: *Jim, there are more of us than you. We will not let you go. We will not let you hurt anyone.*

JIM: *It's not me, it's them.*

NURSE: *Okay, Jim. Just hang on. Walk with us to the seclusion room. (Jim struggles, but he is walked to the seclusion room.)*

NURSE: *We are going to help you change your clothes. (Two staff members hold Jim and two others change his clothes.)*

NURSE: *Lie down on the bed, Jim. (The staff wrap him securely in blankets.)*

JIM: *Don't let them get me.*

NURSE: *We won't. You'll be safe in here.*

When the nurse recognizes that the client needs physical assistance to control himself, she makes sure that there is enough. The staff members are firm but gentle, and Jim is constantly reassured.

Coping with violent and explosive behaviors in a psychiatric service is similar to providing a cardiac arrest code in a medical service. It happens sporadically but all staff must be prepared to assist when it does. The best way to deal with violent behavior is by preventing it. Staff can prevent it by knowing the clients well and by working with the clients to understand how the behavior occurs.

David is a twenty-eight-year-old male. Six months after enlisting at age eighteen, he was discharged from the service for explosive behavior. David has been hospitalized almost continually since then, but he had been in the community for almost a year. During that time, he married, but he and his new wife lived with his parents. He was admitted after breaking up his parents' home. Since his admission, he had had several violent episodes. The nurse in reviewing David's chart realizes that the episode always occurred on Thursday, always occurred in the bathroom and that David always had difficulty sleeping the night before. The nurse recognizes a pattern and attempts to work it out with David.

NURSE: *David, I've been looking back over the last few weeks and it seems to me that you usually have an outbreak on Thursday. Today is Tuesday. Maybe if we can find out what's happening we can help you avoid another.*

DAVID: *Well I have to do so much work Wednesday night that I'm tired on Thursday but nobody lets me rest.*

NURSE: *You are working Wednesday night?*

DAVID: *Sure, that's why I'm here. I was a medic in Nam and they knew the docs couldn't handle the load so they readmitted me.*

NURSE: *David, I'm afraid I don't understand all this. Tell me some more.*

DAVID: *Well, you know about Wednesday.*

NURSE: *No.*

DAVID: *Wednesday is when all the cheaters are out— when all the wives and husbands run around on each other. Then they catch each other and blow their brains out and I have to patch 'em up. They start coming in Wednesday night about midnight and I operate in the bathroom until 6 or 7 A.M. Then I'm real tired and I get real irritable and you all want me to get up and eat and act normal after I've operated all night, and what I really need is sleep and rest.*

NURSE: *We didn't know about Wednesday, David. What can we do to help you? I'll talk with the team if you tell me.*

DAVID: *Well, you could get the doctors to at least assist me and the nurses could let me rest on Thursday.*

The nurse reported her work to the team. A plan was developed: (1) to adjust David's medications, (2) to have his primary therapist work with him around his delusional system, and (3) to plan nursing care with David for several rest times on Wednesday and Thursday. David remained in the hospital for three more months but never had another violent episode. In reviewing his chart, that was the longest time in all his hospitalization that he had not been violent.

REGULATING HYPERACTIVITY

Mary, a thirty-five-year-old woman, is extremely hyperactive. She has not slept for two nights when she is admitted. She moves continually, talking and laughing. She is intrusive and upsets the other clients. She is too active to eat or drink. At lunch time the nurse approaches Mary.

NURSE: *It's time to eat.*

MARY: *Not me. I've got too much to do.*

NURSE: *I know you can't sit down, and that's okay. But you need some food. I'll bring a tray to the dayroom.*

MARY: *If you like.*

Mary continues to rearrange the books and magazines as she flips through them. The nurse leaves the tray where Mary can get to it. She sits apart from both Mary and the tray. The nurse does not want to interact with Mary and stimulate her further. Mary is able to eat a little. That night Mary has all her belongings out on her bed, folding and counting them at 11:00 P.M. Her roommate is unable to sleep.

NURSE: *Mary, you are keeping Joan awake.*

MARY: *That's tough. I've got things to do.*

NURSE: *Okay, but let's do them in the dayroom.*

MARY *(looking at her belongings)*: *Where will I put it all?*

NURSE: *Everybody is in bed, so you can use the pool table.*

Mary and the nurse take her belongings out to the pool table. Mary continues her activity until 3:00 A.M. The nurse checks on her at intervals.

The nurse recognizes that Mary cannot stop her activity. She could not stop to eat and could not stop to sleep. The nurse recognizes her need to have external stimuli decreased. Mary is so labile that if the nurse had secluded her, she would probably have been more agitated. Since all the clients were in the dining room and later asleep, the dayroom provided a quiet area. The nurse removed herself to decrease the stimuli still further, but she continued to observe Mary. Mary eventually calmed down enough to sleep for a few hours.

The Nursing Care Plan

The nursing care plan must focus on the goals and expected outcomes of care (see Chapter 4). Goals are general. They involve the client's total experience with nursing care and staff. A long-term goal might be to return the client to the previous level of functioning. A short-term goal might be to decrease the client's acute symptoms. Expected outcomes are specific. They are directly related to the identified problem. The identified problem might be: Mr. Jones is afraid he is being poisoned and refuses to eat any food. The expected outcome might be: Mr. Jones will take enough food and fluid to prevent malnutrition and dehydration. Nursing interventions are all those things the nurse does to bring about the expected outcome. The nursing care plan will be illustrated by presenting a case study. The study includes the client's admission history, the client's progress and unit behavior, the nursing care plans, and the goals of care.

Davis, Joe
ADMISSION HISTORY

Identification

Joe Davis is a twenty-year-old, male Catholic of middle-class background. He is presently unemployed. On admission he states, "I'm paranoid, and I need help. I want to better myself."

History of Present Illness

During junior high and high school, JD created problems in school (breaking windows and creating disturbances during assemblies). He also had frequent encounters with the law (stealing cars, going joyriding, speeding). All this irritated and upset his family. During JD's senior year in high school, his mother, age forty-eight, collapsed and died suddenly of unknown causes. The family was stunned and according to JD blamed him for "driving her to an early grave." Two weeks later, JD's father turned him out of the house to the care of the Juvenile Authorities. JD was placed with his widowed maternal aunt, Mrs. Jones, and lived with her and her fifteen-year-old daughter.

JD was profoundly upset by his mother's death and reports being withdrawn and isolative. He refused to have anything to do with his friends or relatives. He continued in school but was expelled for asocial behavior. He could not graduate with his class, and this upset him. His aunt took him to her internist, who reported that JD was a very, very troubled person and needed counseling. JD refused. JD reports being depressed, but he was able to get a part-time job and went to night school to complete his work for his high school diploma. He felt "good" after that but became depressed again when his girl friend broke up with him.

While Mrs. Jones and her daughter were on a Christmas trip, JD stole her credit cards and car. He put 5,000 miles on the car. When Mrs. Jones returned, she found JD hyperactive, with rapid speech and grandiose ideas about money. Mrs. Jones kicked him out of her house. A few days later he was found unconscious and taken to the county hospital emergency room for an apparent overdose of barbiturates and alcohol. JD denied any suicide attempt and claimed he had simply passed out by mixing drugs and alcohol. He returned to Mrs. Jones's home.

JD was soon agitated again. He had rapid speech and was described as extremely restless. He was physically abusive. He was arrested when he broke out a window and was taken again to the county hospital emergency room. He was admitted to the psychiatric unit on a fourteen-day legal hold and was then transferred to the state hospital. This was approximately one year after his mother's death.

JD reports that he was hospitalized for two months and that his diagnosis was "either bipolar affective disorder or schizophrenia." JD reports that he was treated with Thorazine. During his hospitalization, he reports that he went AWOL and stole two cars before he was apprehended. The state hospital listed his diagnosis as "adjustment reaction of adolescence" and reports that he was discharged to his aunt with no medications or follow-up plans.

Following discharge, JD stole a car. He was subsequently sent to the state medical center for the criminally insane for ninety days' incarceration and observation. At the facility JD claims to have met a man whom he had identified several years earlier as a neighbor who was sexually molesting children. JD feels guilty that he had any part in this man's confinement. He was also very frightened because, he says, "the guy said that he would kill me when he got out." JD presently believes that there is a contract out on him.

JD was released to a rehabilitation center on parole from a three-year suspended sentence. His aunt reports that he seemed to be "normal" after release, but JD says, "I was getting more and more paranoid about that joker in jail."

JD functioned well for several months. Then he saw his old girl friend. They had intercourse, and he asked her to marry him. She refused. He dates a dramatic increase in his paranoia from this point on. He began sleeping less and had a feeling of severe "pressure in my head." On Father's Day, JD went to his parents' home and had a terrible fight with his father. His father told him, "I regret the day you were born." JD's aunt reports that he was hyperactive, tense, agitated, and in a panic about losing his job. He was telling people wild stories about famous people he knew who were going to do wonderful things for him. He used ever-increasing amounts of marijuana to try to relax. Finally he turned himself in to the county hospital for treatment. He was transferred to the state hospital but signed out Against Medical Advice three days later. Four days after that, on his twentieth birthday, he returned to the county hospital and asked to be admitted.

JD was retained on a fourteen-day legal hold. He was believed to have a drug-induced psychosis. Laboratory reports were negative, and when he failed to clear in a few days, he was diagnosed as manic-depressive, manic type. While awaiting transfer to this hospital for treatment, JD received Haldol, Mellaril, Navane, Thorazine, and Vistaril at various times in an attempt to control his agitation. None was particularly effective, and he was placed in restraints each night.

Past History

Developmental and Social: Pregnancy, delivery, and early childhood were all unremarkable. Immediate family members do not recall JD being "hyperactive" as a youngster. They say he was simply full of energy like a normal, active boy. In grade school, junior high, and high school, JD maintained average to below average grades with secondary to poor study habits. He was able to obtain B grades without trouble when he applied himself. Family members rate him as "above average" in intelligence. He had a fair number of casual and close friends throughout his school years and was popular with

boys and girls alike. His aunt's daughter recalls that he was "always hyperactive" from the age of ten. She says she felt tense when she was around him. She also recalls that he was often labile and pouted and sulked.

Family History: JD is the third of five children. His father is a quality control supervisor at a factory where he has worked for twenty years. He currently earns around $16,000 per year. He is a chronic alcoholic who drinks daily. When drunk, he unmercifully beats his sons. JD believes that his father has never liked him. He hates his father for having beaten him as a child, for his alcoholism, and for the way he mistreated JD's mother. JD loved his mother deeply and felt very close to her. She regarded him as her favorite and gave him special privileges. JD's father made all the family decisions and controlled all the money. JD reports that his mother would have divorced his father if she had not been a devout Catholic and devoted to her five children. According to her sister, JD's mother always "dreaded sex" with his father.

JD feels close to all his sibs but says that they were jealous of him because he was his mother's favorite, and his sister confirms this. The sister says the children were not particularly close to one another. The two youngest children live with their father at home. The twenty-three-year-old lives with her boy friend. The twenty-four-year-old brother has a history of paranoid schizophrenia with a three-year hospitalization at the VA hospital. He was recently rehospitalized after failing to take his antipsychotic drugs. JD's aunt says that her brother-in-law is an "alcoholic." JD's sister says that the father is "schizophrenic." There is no other family history of serious mental or physical disease.

Medical History: Child: Not remarkable. Adult: Five instances between age thirteen and the present of blows to the head resulting in lacerations. Client lost consciousness in three of these episodes. Three involved minor automobile accidents, one a bicycle accident, and one a blow to the head with a hoe. Client denies residue from any of these.

Allergies: None. Dystonic reactions to antipsychotic drugs.

Tobacco: One pack per day since age thirteen.

Alcohol: Gets drunk once a month.

Street Drug Use: Marijuana: from age eleven to the present with frequent use over last few months. Barbiturates (Seconal): four pills per day in an on-and-off pattern from age thirteen to help the client get to sleep at night. He claims no use since January 1976 overdose episode resulting in ER visit. PCP: ten episodes of use since age sixteen. Mescaline: one time at age eighteen. Cocaine: claims intravenous use one time, one month before admission. Amphetamines: four episodes of use of three or four "double tablets" since age eighteen, with last episode two months before admission. Client's aunt notes that she and others have suspected drug use as the etiology of his emotional problems in the past but have no firm evidence other than his abnormal behavior.

Mental Status Examination

Young white male unable to sit in chair during periods of extreme volatility. Good eye contact with hypervigilance. Walks with a limp at times, favoring his left foot and leg. He forgets his impairment when he is distracted.

Speech is rapid, with slight to moderate pressure and occasional episodes of blocking. Speech is coherent and well organized but with some suggestion of flight of ideas.

Mood is moderately anxious, and he is tearful when talking about his mother's death. He reports he has been "depressed for years." Denies suicidal intention or ideation.

Thought: Content is marked by intense paranoid delusions that a prison inmate plans to kill him and/or his loved ones. He is somewhat grandiose. He displays ideas of reference and somatic delusions that his body is dying or decaying in various ways. The client knows that he is "anxious and paranoid" and feels that his "head is about to explode," but insists that this is so because of the pressure of living under a death threat.

Intellectual Functioning: He has a good fund of knowledge and seems to be of at least average intelligence. His judgment is impaired by his delusional system. The ability to abstract is impaired. Proverbs: "Rolling stone gathers no moss." JD: "Live fast, die young."

Diagnostic Formulation

JD appears to be a severely disturbed young man with a long history of social maladaptations. He is the third of five children born into what is reported to be a disrupted household. His mother was a long-suffering, devout Catholic who hated her alcoholic husband. JD, by all reports, was her favorite child. He apparently enjoyed a particularly close relationship with her. He was physically abused by his father, as were his two brothers. While JD has been hyperactive and asocial since early childhood, the sudden death of his mother seems to have precipitated the onset of his psychotic behavior. After his mother's death, he was faced with a rapid succession of stresses:

1. His father turned him over to the juvenile authorities.
2. He was then sent to live with his widowed aunt.
3. His behavior caused him to be expelled from school, and he was unable to graduate with his class.
4. He took a part-time job and went to night school.
5. His first girl friend rejected him.

The realization that he was facing adulthood culminated

in an acute psychotic break and hospitalization. JD was hospitalized over a year at the state hospital and state facility for the criminally insane. Despite what he reports as intense delusions, he maintained himself for six months in the community before the present episode. Even though he was diagnosed as bipolar affective disorder, his present intense paranoid delusional system, his poor judgment, and his kinesthetic hallucinations support a diagnosis of schizophrenia. However, although laboratory tests are reported to be negative, his drug and accident history may have influenced his present behavior. This is doubtful, however, in the light of his brother's similar paranoid condition.

DSM-III Multiaxial Diagnosis

Axis I   799.90 Diagnosis deferred
Axis II   301.70 Antisocial Personality Disorder
Axis III Physical Condition or Disorder—none at this time
Axis IV Psychosocial Stressors: Rejection by girlfriend and father seemed to exacerbate the psychosis. Severity—moderate
Axis V   Highest Level of Adaptive Functioning Past Year: 4—Fair

Treatment Plan

1. Physical: Rule out organic condition resulting from drugs or accidents.
2. Psychiatric: Evaluate for drug and psychosocial therapies
3. Nursing: Encourage participation in the milieu. Evaluate actual day-to-day function.

On admission, Joe is hyperactive, pacing, and agitated. He chain smokes. He stops staff and clients and tells them that he is here for help, or that he is here to avoid being murdered. He interrupts activities he is not a part of. He opens doors and inspects every room. If nursing staff members interrupt his behavior, he becomes verbally abusive. He says he wants medication, but he will not take Thorazine, Mellaril, Haldol, or Stelazine. He has had all these and says they "are not effective." He complains about a wide variety of somatic ailments, such as toothache, a broken foot, and an upset stomach.

While Joe denies having any problems, nursing staff who have observed him closely recognize that he is preoccupied with his delusions and extremely frightened. He seems unable to screen stimuli and becomes increasingly hyperactive and out of contact with reality when interacting in the milieu, i.e., at meals and at meetings. His resulting intrusive behavior is disturbing to other clients. Joe is labile and volatile. His extreme fear is expressed in hostility and verbal abuse. His behavior agitates others, and they may unintentionally provoke him to physical abuse.

The nurses also observe that Joe responds to firm but gentle reassurance. He is able to maintain reality orientation in a quiet, low stimulus environment. Joe's labile and volatile condition requires close observation and rapid intervention to protect him and other clients. The goal of care is to assist Joe through this acute phase. *The nursing staff will help Joe decrease stimuli and maintain reality orientation.*

Joe's Schedule

7:30 A.M.	Wake up
8:00 A.M.	Breakfast
8:30 A.M.	Morning cleanup
9:00 to 9:45 A.M.	Free time
9:45 A.M.	Group therapy
10:30 to 11:30 A.M.	Rest time
11:30 to 12 noon	Free time
12:00 to 1:00 P.M.	Lunch
1:00 to 3:00 P.M.	Occupational therapy
3:00 to 4:00 P.M.	Rest time
4:00 to 5:00 P.M.	Individual therapy
5:00 to 6:00 P.M.	Free time
6:00 to 7:00 P.M.	Dinner
7:00 to 9:00 P.M.	Informal unit activity
9:00 P.M. until bedtime	Free time

Joe has been hospitalized for two months. His acute episode is under control. He is no longer actively psychotic, but he is unable to function above a minimal level. He is less hyperactive, but he still cannot structure his time or meet day-to-day problems of living consistently without assistance. He is enrolled in the Vocational Rehabilitation Workshop but is unable to attend full-time. He needs to have time to himself. He is afraid that he will be forced to leave the hospital before he is ready. In fact the hospital has nothing further to offer Joe that is not more appropriately obtained in the community. Joe's family is unwilling to assume any responsibility for him and requests that he be sent to a state hospital if he cannot be discharged to his own care.

The treatment team meets with Joe to decide whether he will be discharged to a state hospital or to a halfway house. Joe does not want to go to a state hospital. He must increase his ability to function on a day-to-day basis to be eligible for placement in a halfway house. Joe and the nursing staff plan his care around assessing his ability to care for himself and helping him to take independent action. Joe will be discharged on medication, and a teaching plan is prepared for him.

Even though Joe has been included in the planning of his care and discharge, he is still angry at leaving and feels he is being rejected by the staff. Joe has usually managed to become so disruptive in his other hospitalizations that he has been discharged ahead of schedule and so has made his fear of being thrown out of the hospital come true. The nursing staff are aware of this past behavior. They will plan care and set goals to prevent it from happening again. The goal of care is to assist Joe to accomplish discharge and placement smoothly.

Joe's Activities

Monday
10:30 to 11:00 A.M.	Community living meeting
4:15 to 5:45 P.M.	Bowling

Tuesday
9:45 to 10:45 A.M.	Basic living skills
11:00 to 12 noon	Yoga
4:15 to 4:45 P.M.	Music appreciation

Thursday
9:30 to 10:00 A.M.	Community living meeting
10:15 to 11:15 A.M.	Movement group
1:00 to 3:00 P.M.	Outing

Friday
10:30 to 11:30 A.M.	Poetry group

Teaching Care Plan—Medication Teaching*

Goals

Joe will demonstrate an understanding of the possible side effects of, or adverse reactions to, Prolixin Decanoate (fluphenazine decanoate injectable).

Objectives

Joe will demonstrate an understanding of the possible side effects of, or adverse reactions to, Prolixin Decanoate by

1. Explaining them to his primary care nurse
2. Explaining them to his support system in the presence of the primary care nurse
3. Performing satisfactorily on a written test prepared and administered by the primary care nurse
4. Reporting any side effects or adverse reactions to his primary care nurse while he is an inpatient

Methodology

1. Administer pretest to Joe.
2. Present information from the fact sheet, and review it with Joe periodically.
3. In teaching, use language appropriate to Joe's age and education.

*Developed by Alex Anagnos, R.N., M.S.

NURSING CARE PLAN

Problem	Expected Outcome	Nursing Orders
1. Joe is hyperactive, intrusive, ambivalent, negativistic, fearful, and agitated. He has a short attention span and is actively delusional. As a result, he is unable to structure his time.	Joe will participate with staff in planning a schedule and will make every effort to follow his schedule (see copy attached).	1. Go over schedule with Joe each morning. 2. Verbally remind him of the time of each activity scheduled. 3. Joe is to attend all scheduled activities. He may leave if he is unable to tolerate them. 4. Assist Joe in structuring free time with short activities that require energy, e.g., pool, Ping-Pong, punching bag. 5. Allow Joe to use his room to decrease stimuli. He may use typewriter in his room. 6. Awaken Joe from his scheduled morning and afternoon rest times. Encourage him to get up but *do not force him.* 7. Make brief contacts with him every twenty minutes until he is able to leave his room.
2. He needs to dominate interactions with others. In so doing, he alienates them.	Joe will interact with staff and other clients for short periods of time without alienating them.	1. When Joe becomes loud, intrusive, and fragmented, redirect him into activities such as pool or Ping-Pong with staff, or have him use his room to decrease stimuli. 2. Provide Joe with adequate space in which to be active. If he is intrusive with other clients, intervene to prevent altercations. 3. Make brief (about ten-minute), frequent contacts with Joe throughout the day. Focus on concrete issues such as what he has done or plans to do that day. Reassure him that this is a safe place, and that he will not be hurt here.
3. He may not be able to maintain control in the unit milieu.	Joe will regain control when stimulation is decreased.	1. If Joe is extremely agitated, intrusive, or hyperactive, seclude him for brief periods to decrease stimuli. 2. Approach Joe in a calm, firm manner. Allow him time to walk to seclusion and to change his clothes. If he is cooperative, do not physically assist him. Do not raise your voice. Use simple, concrete statements. 3. If Joe is not responsive to verbal direction, physically assist him to seclusion. 4. Check him every fifteen minutes. He is usually considerably less agitated in about one hour.
4. Joe has no problems taking in adequate food or fluids. However, his hyperactivity, intrusiveness, and poor impulse control may increase with the stimulation of the dining room.	Joe will maintain adequate food and fluid intake.	1. Observe and document any difficulty with food or fluid. 2. If he becomes hyperactive or intrusive in the dining room, sit with him and quietly refocus his attention on eating. 3. If his behavior is excessively hyperactive or intrusive, allow him to eat in the dayroom. 4. If Joe refuses to eat, don't argue. Offer him frequent, small meals to support adequate nutrition, e.g., milk, toast, fruit.

Continues on next page

NURSING CARE PLAN continued

Problem	Expected Outcome	Nursing Orders
5. Joe has no problem with elimination at present. He is on dioctyl sodium sulfosuccinate (DSS) to facilitate regularity and avoid constipation that can be a side effect of psychoactive drugs.	Joe will maintain his normal elimination pattern of one bowel movement every day or every other day.	1. Each evening ask Joe if he has had a bowel movement and record. 2. Encourage adequate fluid and roughage intake daily.
6. During hyperactive periods, Joe is disorganized about hygiene. (He is presently growing a moustache.)	Joe will maintain hygiene with minimal assistance from staff.	1. Document any difficulty with hygiene. 2. Remind Joe to shower with antiseptic soap for body rash daily. 3. Remind Joe to brush his teeth every morning and evening. His teeth are in very poor condition. 4. Joe will do his laundry on Saturday. He will ask for staff assistance as needed. 5. Remind Joe to take care of his personal space every morning. He usually needs help with making his bed.
7. During hyperactive periods Joe is careless with smoking materials.	Joe will smoke only in designated areas.	1. Joe knows it is against fire regulations for him to smoke in his room. Have him go to the dayroom. Take the ashtray out of his room. 2. To conserve his cigarettes, Joe leaves them in the nursing station. When he asks for a new pack, help him look for the old one first.

Source: Developed in collaboration with Cecile Miranda. R.N., M.S.

NURSING CARE PLAN

Problem	Expected Outcome	Nursing Orders
1. In preparation for discharge to halfway house, Joe will need to be responsible for maintaining adequate food intake. When under increased stress, Joe refuses to go to dining room to eat.	Joe will maintain adequate food and fluid intake. He will eat all meals in dining room.	1. Observe and document any difficulties with food and fluid intake. 2. To assure consistency, follow this plan before all meals: a. In matter-of-fact voice remind Joe (only twice) that it's time for meal. b. If Joe does not go to dining room at appropriate time, he may not go later. Suggest he fix something for himself on unit. c. Joe may leave dining room and return to unit alone.
2. Elimination. Joe has one bowel movement every day or every other day, facilitated by DSS.	Joe will have bowel movement every day or every other day.	1. Observe and document any changes in elimination pattern. 2. Each evening ask Joe if he had a bowel movement and record. 3. Encourage fluids and roughage intake PRN.

Continues on next page

Problem	Expected Outcome	Nursing Orders
3. In preparation for discharge Joe needs to assume full responsibility for hygiene tasks. During increased stress he becomes disorganized about these tasks.	1. Joe will take a shower with antiseptic soap every day. 2. Joe will brush teeth each morning and evening. 3. Joe will make bed and straighten room every day. 4. Joe will do laundry PRN.	1. Document changes from self-care behavior. 2. Remind Joe of these activities once only, then document.
4. Joe smokes in room.	Joe will smoke in appropriate areas on unit.	1. Remove matches and ashtray from bedside. 2. Redirect Joe to appropriate areas to smoke.
5. Joe usually gets six to eight hours of sound sleep each night. He sometimes retires as early as 7:30 P.M.	Joe will continue to get six to eight hours of sound sleep each night. He will not retire before 9:00 P.M.	1. Document any changes from pattern of six to eight hours of sleep each night. 2. Encourage Joe to remain up until 9:00 P.M. Do not force him but remind him of his discharge goal.
6. During periods of increased stress, Joe withdraws to room. To prevent overuse of this pattern, Joe needs to minimize use of his room. In order for Joe to be discharged to halfway house, he will need to be occupied at least eight hours a day without rest period.	Joe will withdraw to his room only for half hour after lunch and half hour in late afternoon.	1. Allow Joe to sleep for agreed-on amount of time. 2. If Joe chooses to sleep longer or at other times, remind him of purpose of limiting rest periods. 3. Do not force Joe to alter his rest periods if longer. Just document them. 4. Offer alternative of pool game, walk, or TV to change focus of activity.
7. Joe has difficulty tolerating group activities for long periods. In preparation for discharge he needs to increase his participation for longer periods. Joe's delusional system concerns a former acquaintance of his attempting to kill Joe. When outside hospital he becomes increasingly fearful. He needs to work on this to increase his tolerance for being outside hospital.	Joe will maintain adequate activity for his age and size. He will slowly increase his tolerance for structured group activities.	1. Joe is to attend group therapy on Tuesday and Wednesday for full forty-five minutes. 2. Joe is to attend work program each afternoon. Document length of time he is able to stay (Monday through Friday). 3. Go over day's activities (see schedule attached), and encourage Joe to attend them. 4. Joe is to take evening walks with staff and other clients. 5. Encourage Joe to structure free time around pool, Ping-Pong, writing letters, or listening to music.
8. Joe can only tolerate brief interactions with staff and other clients. He needs to dominate interactions. In preparation for discharge, Joe needs structured time to express his concerns.	Joe will interact with staff and other clients at least for ten minutes without agitation.	1. Set up two ten-minute periods each morning and afternoon for Joe to express his concerns to his nurse for shift. Keep these periods flexible to allow Joe control, and do not force them. 2. Use positive feedback when Joe initiates longer periods of conversation.

Continues on next page

451

NURSING CARE PLAN continued		
Problem	**Expected Outcome**	**Nursing Orders**
9. Joe is demonstrating evidence of poor impulse control and acting-out behavior. This is interpreted as a sign of his difficulty with termination. Joe historically terminates program by provoking staff to anger and/or fear so that they reject him.	Joe will be able to control his impulses and demonstrate appropriate behavior throughout his termination phase with the aid of staff support and PRN medication.	1. Assess frequently for signs of agitation (i.e., motor restlessness, verbal abuse, swearing, combativeness, etc.) 2. Attempt supportive verbal interaction. 3. Give PRN medication if support is not effective within fifteen minutes.

Source: Care plan developed by Ellen Drevers, R.N., M.S.

4. *Hold a discussion (including question-and-answer session) between Joe and the primary care nurse and between Joe and his support system.*
5. *Administer posttest to Joe.*
6. *Review test results and misconceptions with Joe.*

Fact Sheet

Side effects of, and adverse reactions to, injectable fluphenazine include the following:

1. *It may impair the physical and mental abilities required to drive your car or operate heavy machinery.*
2. *It may increase the effects of alcoholic beverages.*
3. *It may cause you to be more drowsy than usual. You may feel tired and sluggish.*
4. *It may cause what are known as extrapyramidal symptoms. These may include tremors (trembling) in your hands, stiffness in your arms and legs (they may feel rigid and tight), and stiffness in your neck. Your tongue may feel swollen or otherwise "funny." Your legs may feel "jumpy," as if you can't sit still.*
5. *It may cause impotence (inability to achieve an erection) or diminish your sexual drives.*
6. *It may make you oversensitive to the sun. You may sunburn easily, and your eyes may hurt in normal sunlight. Sunglasses will help, and you should always apply sunscreen (which can be purchased at any drugstore without a prescription) before going out in the sun.*

These are the commonest side effects of fluphenazine. You may also notice that your appetite is poor, that you have too much or too little saliva, that you perspire more than usual, or that you have to urinate more frequently than usual. You may become constipated. You may also have occasional headaches.

You may experience any or all of these things, or you may experience none of them. If you do experience any of these things, please consult your nurse while you are in the hospital. Once you leave the hospital, talk with your doctor if you are experiencing something that you feel might be related to the fluphenazine.

Evaluation

1. *Joe will accomplish objectives 1 through 4.*
2. *The primary care nurse will evaluate effectiveness of plan and tool via pre- and posttesting.*

Joe is able to function at an increasingly higher level, and three months after admission he is discharged to a halfway house for young men. He is seeing a therapist in the outpatient department and will continue in the vocational rehabilitation program. Joe had begun a disintegrative life pattern and will probably continue to need assistance periodically in order to maintain life in the community. However, active nursing care during the acute phase of the condition and realistic discharge planning prevented Joe from becoming socially nonfunctional. Without them he would have been relegated to custodial care.

KEY NURSING CONCEPTS

✔ Persons whose life patterns contain disintegration of perception, thought, affect, and motivation usually are labeled psychotic by mental health workers.

✔ Disintegrated perception may include altered auditory, visual, tactile, olfactory, gustatory, or kinesthetic senses.

✔ Disintegrated thought involves disturbances in the flow and content of reason, intellect, and judgment.

✔ Disintegration of affect or feeling tone is recognized as a change in intensity or appropriacy.

✔ Disintegration of motivation is manifested in regression, withdrawal, ambivalence, impulsivity, and hyperactivity.

✔ Disintegrative life patterns may be defined medically, socially, legally, personally, and statistically; research supports the assumption that social, psychological, and especially biological factors influence the development of a psychotic condition.

✔ Psychiatric nurses use problem solving, interpersonal relations, knowledge of human behavior, and somatic and psychosocial therapies to assist pychotic clients to cope with problems of living.

✔ Nurses are in a key role to interact with clients around tasks of living since most psychotic conditions are more alike than different in the nursing problems they present.

✔ Factors that influence care planning with clients labeled psychotic include the nurse's attitude and role, the way the client entered the health care system, and the contract for services between the agency and the client.

✔ Goal-oriented nursing strategies are used to intervene in disintegration of perception, thought, affect, and motivation.

References

American Psychiatric Association. *Diagnostic and Statistical Manual of Mental Disorders.* Washington, D.C.: American Psychiatric Association, 1980.

Bateson, G.; Jackson, D. D.; Haley, J.; and Weakland, J. "Toward a Theory of Schizophrenia." *Behavioral Science* 1 (1956): 251–264.

Belmaker, R. H., and Van Praag, H. M. *"Manic: An Evolving Concept."* New York: Spectrum Publications, 1980.

Bleuler, D. *Dementia Praecox or the Group of Schizophrenias.* Translated by J. Zinkin. New York: International Universities Press, 1950.

Bowers, M. B. "Biochemical Processes in Schizophrenia: Update." *Schizophrenia Bulletin* 6 (1980): 139–148.

Department of Health and Human Services. *Toward a National Plan for the Chronically Mentally Ill.* DHHS Publication No. (ADM) 81–1077, 1981.

Docherty, J. P.; Van Kammen, D. P.; and Rayner, J. *"Toward a Definition of Psychotic Decompensation."* Unpublished monograph. 1978.

Docherty, J. P.; Marder, S. R.; Siris, S. G.; and Van Kammen, D. P. "Stages of Onset of Schizophrenic Psychosis." *American Journal of Psychiatry* 135 (1978): 420–426.

Erikson, E. H. *Identity: Youth and Crisis.* New York: W. W. Norton, 1968.

Freedman, A. M.; Kaplan, H. I.; and Sadock, B. *Modern Synopsis of Comprehensive Textbook of Psychiatry/III*, 3d ed. Baltimore: Williams and Wilkins, 1981.

Freud, S. *Three Case Histories.* New York: Macmillan Collier Books, 1970.

Fromm-Reichman, F. *Principles of Intensive Psychotherapy.* Chicago: University of Chicago Press, 1950.

Goffman, E. *Asylums.* New York: Doubleday, 1961.

Greenblatt, M.; York, R. H.; and Brown, E. L. *From Custodial to Therapeutic Patient Care in Mental Hospitals.* New York: Russell Sage Foundation, 1955.

Hammer, M. "Social Supports, Social Networks, and Schizophrenia." *Schizophrenia Bulletin* 7 (1980): 45–58.

Hersen, M. "Token Economies in Institutional Settings: Historical, Political Deprivation, Ethical and Generalization

Issues." *Journal of Nervous and Mental Diseases* 162 (1979): 206-211.

Kallmann, F. *Heredity in Health and Mental Disorders*. New York: W. W. Norton, 1953.

Kantor, R. E., and Herron, W. G. *Reactive and Process Schizophrenia*. Palo Alto, Calif.: Science and Behavior Books, 1966.

Kline, D. "Psychosocial Treatment of Schizophrenia or Psychosocial Help for People with Schizophrenia." *Schizophrenia Bulletin* 6 (1980): 122-130.

Kolb, L. *Modern Clinical Psychiatry*. Philadelphia: W. B. Saunders, 1977.

Laing, R. D. *The Politics of Experience*. New York: Pantheon Books, 1967.

Langfield, G. *The Schizophrenic States*. London: Oxford University Press, 1939.

Mosher, L. R., and Meltzer, H. Y. "Psychosocial Treatment: Individual, Group, Family and Community Support Approaches." *Schizophrenia Bulletin* 6 (1980): 10-21.

Pattison, M. E., and Pattison, M. L. "Analysis of a Schizophrenic Psychosocial Network." *Schizophrenia Bulletin* 7 (1981): 135-144.

Paul, G. L., and Lentz, R. J. *"Psychosocial Treatment of Chronic Mental Patients: Milieu vs. Social Learning Program*. Cambridge, Mass.: Harvard University Press, 1977.

Rosen, J. N. *Direct Analysis*. New York: Grune and Stratton, 1953.

Rothman, T. *Changing Patterns in Psychiatric Care*. New York: Crown Publishers, 1970.

Scheff, T. "Schizophrenia as Ideology." *Schizophrenia Bulletin*, fall 1970, 15-19.

Segal, J. *Research in the Service of Mental Health*. Report of the Research Task Force of the National Institute of Mental Health. Washington, D.C.: National Institute of Mental Health, 1975.

Sheldon, W. H. *Atlas of Men*. New York: Harper and Row, 1954.

Sullivan, H. S. *The Collected Works of Harry Stack Sullivan*, vols. 1 and 2. New York: W. W. Norton, 1960.

Szasz, T. *The Myth of Mental Illness*. New York: Harper and Row, 1961.

Further Reading

Alexander, F. *The History of Psychiatry*. New York: Harper and Row, 1966.

Arieti, S. *Interpretation of Schizophrenia*. New York: Basic Books, 1974.

Bachrach, L. *Deinstitutionalization: An Analytical Review and Sociological Perspective*. Series D., no. 4. Washington, D.C.: National Institute of Mental Health, 1976.

Bellock, L., and Loeb, L. *The Schizophrenic Syndrome*. New York: Grune and Stratton, 1969.

Brenner, C. *An Elementary Textbook of Psychoanalysis*. Garden City, N.Y.: Doubleday Anchor Books, 1974.

Cancro, R., ed. *The Schizophrenic Reaction: A Critique of the Concept of Hospital Treatment and Current Research*. New York: Brunner/Mazel, 1970.

————. *Annual Review of the Schizophrenic Syndrome 1974-75*. New York: Brunner/Mazel, 1976.

Englehardt, D., and Rosen, B. "Implications of Drug Treatment for the Social Rehabilitation of Schizophrenic Patients." *Schizophrenia Bulletin* 2 (1976): 454-464.

Freides, D. "A New Diagnostic Scheme for the Disorders of Behavior, Emotions and Learning Based on Organism-Environment Interaction." *Schizophrenia Bulletin* 2 (1976): 218-248.

Glassner, B.; Haldipur, C. V.; and Dessauersmith, J. "Role Loss and Working-class Manic Depression." *Journal of Nervous and Mental Diseases* 167 (1979): 530-541.

Gottesman, I., and Shields, J. "A Critical Review of Recent Adoptive, Twin and Family Studies of Schizophrenia: Behavioral Genetics Perspectives." *Schizophrenia Bulletin* 2 (1976): 360-400.

Keith, S.; Gunderson, J.; Reifman, A.; Buchsbaum, S.; and Mosher, L. "Special Report/Schizophrenia 1976." *Schizophrenia Bulletin* 2 (1976): 509-565.

Kolle, L. "Schizophrenia: The Potentials and Limitations of Public Care." *Journal: National Association of Private Psychiatric Hospitals* 10 (1979): 54-59.

Leff, J. "Developments in Family Treatment of Schizophrenia." *Psychiatric Quarterly* 51 (1979): 216-232.

Lidz, T. *The Origin and Treatment of Schizophrenic Disorders*. New York: Basic Books, 1973.

Ludwig, A. M. *Treating the Treatment Failures*. New York: Grune and Stratton, 1971.

MacVane, J. R.; Lange, J. D.; Brown, W. A.; and Zayat, M. "Psychological Functioning of Bipolar Manic-depressives in Remission." *Archives of General Psychiatry* 35 (1978): 1351-1354.

Mosher, L. R., and Keith, S. J. "Research on the Psychosocial Treatment of Schizophrenia: A Summary Report." *American Journal of Psychiatry* 136 (1979): 623-631.

Mullahy, P. *Psychoanalysis and Interpersonal Psychiatry*. New York: Science House, 1970.

Nathan, P. "DSM-II and Schizophrenia: Diagnostic Delight or Nosological Nightmare?" *Journal of Clinical Psychology* 35 (1979): 477-479.

Ozarin, L.; Redick, R.; and Taube, C. "A Quarter of a Century of Psychiatric Care, 1950–1974, a Statistical Review." *Hospital and Community Psychiatry* 27 (1976): 515–518.

Ramshorn, M. "The Major Thrust in American Psychiatry: Past, Present and Future." *Perspectives in Psychiatric Care,* July–August 1971, pp. 144–155.

Reifman, A., and Wyatt, R. J. "Lithium: A Brake in the Rising Cost of Mental Illness." *Archives of General Psychiatry* 37 (1980): 385–388.

Strauss, J. S.; Bowers, M.; Downey, T. W.; Flick, S.; Jackson, S.; and Levine, I. *"The Psychotherapy of Schizophrenia.* New York: Plenum, 1980.

Szasz, T. *Schizophrenia, the Sacred Symbol of Psychiatry.* New York: Harper and Row, 1976.

————. *Psychiatric Slavery.* New York: Harper and Row, 1977.

Wilson, H.S. *Deinstitutionalized Residential Care for the Severely Mentally Disordered: The Soteria House Approach.* New York: Grune and Stratton, 1982.

17

Medicopsychiatric Conditions

by Andrew E. Skodol

CHAPTER OUTLINE

Psychophysiological Disorders
    History
    Recent Theory
    Classification
    Syndromes
    Intervention
Mental Retardation
    Intelligence
    Definitions of Retardation
    Causes of Retardation
    Problems Encountered by the Retarded
    Intervention
Organic Brain Syndromes
    Myths and Reality about Organic Causes of
    Psychiatric Symptoms
    Assessment
    Classification
    Syndromes
    Intervention
Key Nursing Concepts

LEARNING OBJECTIVES

After reading this chapter, students should be able to

- Identify and discuss the etiology, characteristics, and treatments associated with the Psychophysiological Disorders, Developmental Disorders, and Organic Brain Syndromes presented in the text
- Explore psychiatric nursing interventions designed to help clients with these syndromes function at an optimal level
- Relate psychological to physiological forces and reactions in the syndromes presented
- Analyze ethical issues involved in the care and treatment of the developmentally disabled

CHAPTER 17

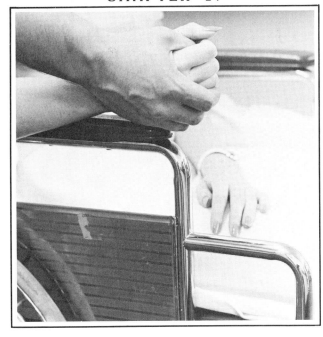

> *The clients in the categories presented in this chapter offer a unique opportunity to the psychiatric nurse who seeks to focus on the essential psychological and emotional aspects of these physical expressions of disorder.*

This chapter has a broad clinical scope, covering diverse syndromes associated with Psychophysiological Disorders (e.g. Psychological Factors Affecting Physical Condition), Organic Brain Syndromes, and Mental Retardation. There are unifying principles that justify clustering this material together in a book presenting a humanistic approach to psychiatric nursing practice.

First, of course, the material represents the areas of psychiatric interest in which the general medical community is most involved. One immediate implication of this is that clients with these problems may have their psychological needs ignored while concern is directed to their medical treatments. Thus the nurse, whether psychiatric or medical, needs to be well versed in both the physical and the psychological ramifications of these syndromes in order to offer appropriately balanced help to afflicted individuals. The intimate relationship between psychological and physiological forces and reactions in the various conditions to be described here emphasizes the criticism made earlier of the mind–body duality. By appreciating and understanding the complex interwoven pattern of emotional and physical elements in medicopsychiatric conditions, the nurse can fully comprehend the essential unity of human life and its disorders. This indicates the need for revised approaches to the ill person.

A second principle that groups these conditions together is that, to differing degrees, Psychophysiologi-

cal Disorders, Organic Brain Syndromes, and Mental Retardation are often treated as the "stepchildren" of psychiatry: not really wanted but accepted almost out of obligation. These clients traditionally are not considered desirable to treat and therefore are not eagerly sought on psychiatric wards or in outpatient practices. This bias results from several factors.

For the most part, these clients suffer from chronic and/or largely irreversible illnesses. The very nature of the conditions—that is, their natural course or history—makes them so, and few definitive or even very helpful treatments have been found using traditional approaches. This contrasts sharply with the effective psychiatric treatments available for Affective Disorders and even cases diagnosed in traditional terms as Schizophrenia.

Clients in the categories presented here are traditionally not highly verbal, insightful, or imaginative. They therefore do not appeal to the typical psychotherapist, who seeks such qualities in clients. The lack of verbal and imagery skills may result from organic deficits, psychological makeup, or both, but it definitely puts such clients at a disadvantage in traditional medical-psychiatric settings.

Lastly, no mystique surrounds clients with medico-psychiatric disorders. No one has ever argued that it might be desirable, for social, aesthetic, or existential reasons, to have some intellectual impairment, or to be experiencing the destruction of one's brain or other organ, or to be in chronic pain. In contrast, the more nebulous schizophrenic syndrome at times is portrayed in the literature as an alternative life-style, and as such it has fascinated social scientists and laypeople struggling with issues of conformity and socialization as part of human existence.

Thus, although traditional psychiatry necessarily recognizes and treats individuals with Psychophysiological Disorders, Organic Brain Syndromes, and Mental Retardation, the profession has a rather tenuous hold on these areas. The need for a renewed, fresh, and vigorous approach to enhancing the lives of individuals with these conditions will become apparent in this chapter, as we review what is known and much that needs to be explored about the relationship between psychological processes and organic illness. Each section presents the basic descriptive medical-psychiatric material that nurses need in order to become familiar with and be able to recognize the syndromes. The psychological phenomena related to each are discussed, and known treatments, inadequate as they may be, are covered. Some novel roles are suggested for the psychiatric nurse, to help these clients function maximally, given their unusual and distinctive frames of reference about themselves and the world.

PSYCHOPHYSIOLOGICAL DISORDERS

Clients who come to the attention of health care professionals because of physical complaints frequently have their psychological needs neglected, although those needs may be contributing to or even the primary motives in symptom development or the decision to seek help. Regardless of the quality of medical diagnosis and treatment for such clients, ignoring the psychological components of the illness can be disastrous. These problems can easily undermine medically adequate or appropriate treatment. Psychiatry has recognized the significance of psychological processes in the psychophysiological disorders, but effective use of this information has yet to be made.

Psychotherapy is recommended as an adjunct to medical treatment in the management of most disorders classified as psychophysiological. But, by using the standards of traditional insight-oriented treatment, the psychiatric community has sabotaged the chances for successful treatment of many of these clients. Typically, clients with Psychophysiological Disorders are not considered "good" psychotherapy candidates for several reasons:

- They are believed to be rather lacking in insight, since they express conflict through somatic complaints rather than verbalization.
- In psychoanalytic terminology, they are said to suffer from a large number of pregenital conflicts—that is, conflicts over unresolved dependency and aggressive wishes. This makes them difficult to relate to interpersonally.
- These clients focus steadfastly on their somatic complaints, apparently indicating that alternative defense

mechanisms are unavailable to or inadequate for them.
- They are rarely highly motivated to heighten their self-awareness, which is the goal of many forms of psychotherapy.
- Even when they are somewhat motivated, they are believed to be either unable or unwilling to delay gratification and thus are impatient with the slow process of growth usually required in psychotherapeutic work.

The humanistic symbolic interactionist approach offers the psychiatric nurse an innovative yet rational departure from traditional psychotherapeutic approaches to clients suffering from Psychophysiological Disorders. By focusing on the communication aspect of psychiatric symptoms and disabilities, the nurse zeros in on the essential features of the psychology behind these physical expressions of disorder. The client undoubtedly is making a profound statement about self-image, needs, aspirations, frustrations, prospects for the future, etc. Regardless of which theoretical framework is followed, the clinician who hopes to have an impact on the client's pattern of illness must be able to hear, understand, and respond to such statements. Successful treatment necessitates discovering the meaning the client attaches to or expresses through the symptom pattern. Then, through genuine interaction in the client's frame of reference, clinician and client may develop more effective, less personally destructive ways of making statements or solving problems.

History

The history of psychophysiological medicine is essentially a chronicle of humanity's struggle on philosophical and psychological levels with the so-called mind–body problem. Trying to understand the relationship between these concepts and debating the relative dominance of one over the other have preoccupied those interested in the healing arts since prehistory. It is only recently, in the twentieth century, that attempts to view the mind–body relationship holistically have flourished. Even so, the dichotomous view persisted in the area of the Psychophysiological Disorders until very recently. The anachronistic term *psychosomatic disorder* was in the official nomenclature until 1968.

Freud (1953) initially observed the intimate interrelationship of the emotions and physical responses in the conversion reactions. Karl Abraham (1927) and Sandor Ferenczi (1926) both proposed ways in which emotional expression was translated into tissue or organ responses. The later history of Psychophysiological Disorders, from a theoretical point of view, was characterized by a debate between the specific and the general hypotheses of emotional impact on certain disease processes.

The Specific Hypothesis   Franz Alexander (1950) was the father of the so-called specific hypothesis. His theoretical formulations on psychophysiological problems posited that a specific kind of stress, arousing specific conflicts for an individual, resulted in damaging effects on particular organs or organ systems. This implied that there was a rough one-to-one correlation between personality types with their prototypic conflict areas and specific Psychophysiological Disorders. For example, peptic ulcer occurred in passive-dependent individuals who were experiencing some frustration of their dependence wishes or needs. The pathophysiological process was mediated anatomically by the autonomic nervous system. An up-to-date version of this concept is the popular theory of Friedman and Rosenman (1959) describing the Type A personality—the aggressive, hard-driving individual—who has a high incidence of coronary artery disease and myocardial infarction.

The General Theory   In contrast, the general theory proposes that stress sufficient to cause anxiety acts in a general way to arouse the individual's psychological and physiological defenses (the fight or flight response of the autonomic nervous system). This view has been elaborated by Selye (1950) and others (see Chapter 10). If these defenses are inadequate coping mechanisms, one potential result is the transformation of the stress into an alteration in somatic functioning. According to this theory, any organ may show the resulting pathological changes. The one that actually does is determined more by physiological and genetic factors than by the nature of the psychological conflict or the client's personality style.

The Holistic Approach   One extremely important effect of the holistic approach to Psychophysiological Disorders has been an increased appreciation that the relationship between stress and disease state is not unidirectional. A final somatic expression of a problem in living is a result of a complex confluence of factors—genetic, environmental, physiological, psychological—

that impinge on one another in multidirectional ways. This is a more sophisticated view of the interactions of emotions and physical responses. Whether or not the nurse believes in the psychological determinism of a particular symptom constellation, the importance of the meaning a client attaches to life's stresses cannot be denied. The stresses include relationships to loved ones, success or failure in school or job, economic status, and aging, and these become the focus for psychologically oriented intervention.

Recent Theory

In recent psychiatric theory, a model has been developed for understanding the Psychophysiological Disorders. It consists of a system of multiple inputs relating in complex interactions, giving feedback to one another, and being transformed—through as yet undetermined coding mechanisms—from systems of perception, cognition, and feeling into physiological systems that themselves give feedback to the inputs and influence their occurrence (see Figure 17–1). The most thoroughly described and studied illnesses can be shown to operate in just this manner. The inputs undoubtedly involve social phenomena, such as noxious environmental stimuli and disruptions in life patterns. These have been outlined in studies such as the Midtown Manhattan Project and elaborated by many investigators (see Srole et al. 1962). In the more purely psychological sphere, intrapsychic conflict, interpersonal difficulties, and learned maladaptive responses all may contribute. In many of the diseases, genetic factors both provide a predisposition and influence many of the other environmental and psychological inputs.

There seems no doubt that meaning and symbol function in humans as the mediating mechanism between emotion and physiology, although the nature of this process is largely undefined. However, the practical implication of this notion for the psychiatric nurse is that the fulcrum for change lies in the realm of meaning and symbol. Clients and nurses must use these universal human phenomena effectively in order to achieve results.

Classification

Psychophysiological Disorders are now classified under the broad DSM-III diagnosis, Psychological Factors Affecting Physical Condition. The physical disorder or syndrome adversely affected by the psychological factors is noted on Axis III of the multiaxial evaluation

Figure 17-1

Model of current theory of Psychophysiological Disorders.

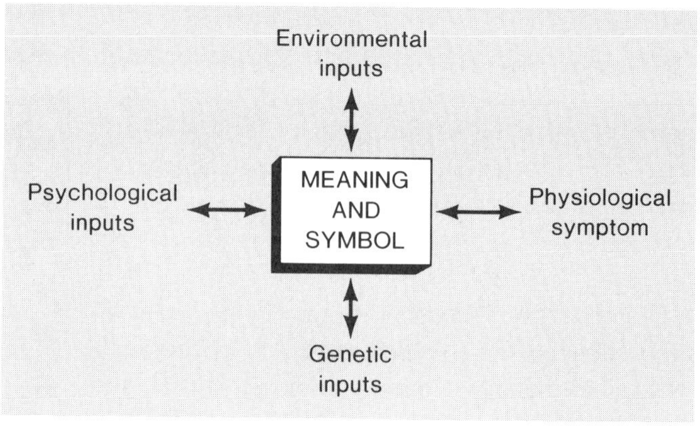

system (see Appendix B). This change in nomenclature parallels the shift away from simple, unicausational ideas about illness etiology implied by the anachronistic term *psychosomatic illness*. The new terminology is more consistent with the "systems" approach to the relationship between psychological and physical factors for patients who have illnesses with mixed organic and emotional components.

In fact, the revised DSM-III classification of these problems allows for the consideration of the role of psychological factors in the initiation, exacerbation, or maintenance of any physical illness. Therefore, even disorders not traditionally viewed as psychosomatic or psychophysiologic can be evaluated according to the model proposed above. The revised classification is expected to encourage greater collaboration between mental health professionals and other, strictly medical, professionals in the treatment of ill persons.

The following sections review the characteristics of syndromes traditionally considered Psychophysiological Disorders. Discussions of assessment and interventions with clients who have other medical illnesses or physical complaints without any documentable physical disorder appear in Chapters 8 and 14.

Syndromes

Ulcer Peptic ulcer, especially duodenal ulcer, has been one of the most thoroughly studied psychophysiological illnesses. Ulcer is the classic example of a disorder in which physical and psychological factors interact by means of feedback loops—that is, physical processes (in this instance, gastric hypersecretion) contribute to psychological processes that influence or determine the stressful circumstances under which the

client suffers pathophysiological changes. Frustration and stress in later life increase gastric secretion, which in turn leads to an increased risk of peptic ulcer formation.

The following case study illustrates this point.*

Ulcers

A 42-year-old trial lawyer, married and the mother of two children, is referred for consultation by her gastroenterologist following her third hospitalization for duodenal ulcer disease. Her ulcer disease was first diagnosed four years ago, but an upper gastrointestinal (GI) series at that time showed evidence both of an active ulcer and of scarring secondary to previously healed ulcers. The gastroenterologist has requested the consultation for help in considering the possibility of surgery, prompted by the seriousness of the bleeding episode that precipitated the patient's last admission and by the fact that she seems to "ignore pain." His referral note indicates that he sees no clear connection between the bleeding episodes and the patient's highly stressful occupation.

The patient appears exactly on time for her appointment; she is neatly and conservatively dressed. She presents an organized, coherent account of her medical problem and denies any past or immediate family history of significant mental disorder. She appears genuinely worried by her recent hospitalization, frightened by the prospect of surgery, and doubtful that speaking to a psychiatrist will produce any meaningful help. As she points out, "Ulcers are supposed to be related to stress, and that just isn't true with me." She then produces a detailed, written outline of her professional life over the past five years side by side with a chronology of her ulcer attacks. Indeed, there seems to be no temporal

---

*From R. L. Spitzer et al. *DSM-III Casebook*. American Psychiatric Association, Washington, D.C., 1981, pp. 23-24.

relationship between her attacks and several dramatic and highly taxing court cases in which she has appeared.

During the second evaluation session, the patient discusses her background. She is the oldest of four children and the clear favorite of her father, also an attorney. He had, and communicated, a strong expectation that she would become a lawyer and that she would succeed in this field. The patient experiences herself as having fulfilled this expectation admirably, and displays a rare smile while describing several of her more dramatic courtroom triumphs. There is no evidence that she herself experiences these difficult cases as stressful; in fact, she seems to enjoy them.

She married a law-school classmate, who is also quite successful and who works noncompetitively in an unrelated legal field. Their marriage seems sound. As she begins to talk about her two sons, aged eight and four, the patient becomes noticeably more tense, and appears much more concerned and upset than usual while describing minor crises they have experienced with friends or in school. With great surprise, she discovers that the chronology of these crises corresponds clearly to five of her seven ulcer attacks, including all of those that resulted in hospitalization. She admits that despite being upset by her sons' problems, she finds it difficult to share her concerns about parenting with her husband or friends. At the end of the session she comments: "You'd have made a good lawyer. I'm glad I'm not arguing against you." She herself suggests that some further sessions may be in order.

Discussion of Ulcers

In the past, certain disorders, such as duodenal ulcer, were assumed to be caused by emotional factors and were classified as Psychophysiologic Disorders. In DSM-III the corresponding category is called Psychological Factors Affecting Physical Condition, but it is to be used only in cases in which a relationship between psychologically meaningful environmental stimuli and the initiation or exacerbation of a physical disorder can be demonstrated. This case attests to the fact that it is often difficult to demonstrate the role of psychological factors and that the precise nature of the psychologically meaningful stimuli frequently is not obvious.

The dramatic demonstration of the relationship between her children's minor crises and the exacerbations of this woman's ulcer justify the Axis I diagnosis of Psychological Factors Affecting Physical Condition. The presence of the duodenal ulcer is noted on Axis III.

DSM-III Diagnosis:

Axis I: 316.00 Psychological Factors Affecting Physical Condition (p. 303)
Axis III: Duodenal ulcer

MECHANISMS Gastric functioning becomes intimately tied to dependence needs in humans through the feeding process from earliest infancy. The baby's mouth and digestive system are its early means of relating to the external world and its principal sources of gratification and frustration. Through complex learning processes, humans associate feeding and being taken care of and nurtured in a general sense. The mouth, through biting and chewing, also becomes the first mechanism through which the human infant can express anger and disappointment at being frustrated. It is well known that gastric secretion increases when infants and children are emotionally involved in either a positive or a negative sense.

The formation of a peptic ulcer is depicted schematically in Figure 17–2. While the mechanism has a logical consistency, this depiction accounts only for vulnerability to peptic ulcer. A great deal remains unknown, particularly about the varying degrees of stress presented by life events and the mediating variables of other personality attributes, defenses, and coping patterns.

Bowel Disorders   A classic example of a lower bowel disorder with psychophysiological characteristics is ulcerative colitis. In this disease of the large intestine, a psychologically traumatic event can precipitate severe inflammatory changes in the mucosa of the intestinal wall, leading to ulceration and bleeding. This disorder tends to be chronic, with remissions and relapses. It seldom disappears, exhibiting the same lasting characteristics as the personality constellation associated with it.

ASSOCIATED PERSONALITY   Clients with ulcerative colitis typically display the following personality characteristics:

• Neatness
• Orderliness
• Punctuality
• Indecisiveness
• Emotional guardedness
• Humorlessness
• Conscientiousness
• Obstinateness
• Conformity
• Overintellectuality
• Moral rigidity
• Worry

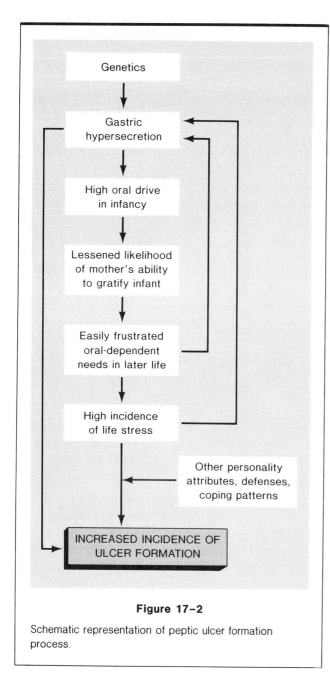

Figure 17–2

Schematic representation of peptic ulcer formation process.

Cardiovascular Disorders The cardiovascular system is a sensitive indicator of emotional arousal, whether fear, anger, or pleasurable excitement. High levels of stress are suspected to have deleterious effects on the heart and vascular system, especially if chronic or repeated. Experience, learning, and symbolic meaning, along with the accompanying affects, can influence the heart rate, heart rhythm, blood pressure, etc. These cardiovascular changes can in turn create emotions, mostly unpleasant, that affect perception and ideation by means of a feedback loop.

PREDISPOSING FACTORS A number of factors have been identified as associated with high risk of generalized heart disease. They include genetic, physiological, social, and psychological elements:

- Family history of heart disease
- Diet high in saturated fats, cholesterol
- High level of blood cholesterol, triglycerides, sugar, uric acid
- Hypertension, diabetes, hypothyroidism, renal disease, gout
- Low level of physical activity
- Heavy smoking and eating
- High-pressured life-style (Type A personality)

The highly competitive, driving Type A personality (see Friedman 1969) is the classic constellation of personality characteristics associated with coronary disease, angina pectoris, and myocardial infarction. Adverse conditions in the client's environment, either social or economic, can also create the stress that leads to cardiac dysfunction.

MECHANISMS Essential hypertension, cardiac arrhythmias, and so-called cardiac neurosis are three syndromes of cardiovascular functioning with major psychological inputs. The classical hypothesis in hypertension has been that people have conflict between their dependent and aggressive inclinations. This causes chronic repression of all displays of anger or resentment. The repressed emotions are eventually transformed into disorders of blood pressure regulation. Although this specific hypothesis has been difficult to prove, experiments have shown that fear, anger, frustration, and guilt all cause rises in diastolic blood pressure in vulnerable individuals. Likewise, anxiety, hostility, depression, interpersonal conflict, and disruptive life events have all been shown capable of precipitating arrhythmias such as sinus tachycardia,

This personality style is commonly known as *compulsive.* According to psychoanalytic theory, it develops in early childhood, usually from a relationship with a controlling, domineering mother who makes the child feel overwhelmed, helpless, and rejected. Such a pattern of rearing often leads the individual, once adult, to feel that relationships to important others are always threatened, highly dependent on his or her performance in meeting the demands or expectations of others, and constantly colored by impending disapproval, especially by authority figures. The client feels helpless to cope and unable or forbidden to express the emotions associated with this frustration.

paroxysmal atrial tachycardia, and both atrial and ventricular ectopic beats.

Asthma   Asthma has been among the most widely studied psychophysiological illnesses of the respiratory system. Because breathing is essential to life itself, much speculation has been made about the emotional and symbolic significance that can become attached to the processes of air exchange. Asthma is a disease characterized by labored breathing and wheezing resulting from spasm, secretion, and swelling in the bronchial tree.

There are allergic, immunological, and emotional inputs to asthmatic attacks. The emotional components may lead directly to alterations in bronchus size. They may also affect the allergic and immunological systems through hypothalamic nuclei in the central nervous system.

The typical asthmatic client has heightened dependence needs resulting from an induced exaggerated fear of loss of the mother at an early stage of infancy. These clients are therefore sensitive to separations or threats of separation, real or imagined, from people to whom they are attached and feel they need. The asthmatic attack is interpreted as a "repressed cry for a lost mother." It is unclear, due to the absence of controlled studies, whether the dependency, need for love, etc., are etiologic in asthmatic clients or consequent to the disease itself. Asthmatic persons may be extremely frightened by the attacks, particularly in childhood. This may make them feel more helpless and vulnerable, so that they adopt a clinging style of relating. The emotional and the physical aspects of the illness seem to interrelate in a complex system of feedback loops.

Arthritis   Rheumatoid arthritis has long been identified as an illness that is strongly influenced by emotional life. Written records over 1,500 years old attest to this. Basically it is a progressive inflammatory disease primarily of the joints, with unknown causes. Family prevalence studies indicate a genetic predisposition to the particular immunological abnormalities present in the disease.

MECHANISM   Psychological stresses are postulated to act as precipitants to attacks and exacerbations. The mechanism of transformation from idea or affect into tissue alteration appears, from research, to be by hormonal and autonomic nervous system pathways. Specifically, growth hormone, sex hormones, thyroid hormone, and adrenal corticosteroids all change in states of emotional arousal, and all are involved in the pro-

duction of connective tissue, especially collagen. The hypothalamus and the limbic system also mediate. Heredity and stress may operate in inverse proportion, according to a study by Rimon (1969). In that research, arthritic clients without genetic predisposition developed the illness under severe stress, and others with a heavy genetic loading developed it despite little evidence of life conflict.

ASSOCIATED PERSONALITY   Rheumatoid arthritic individuals appear to have difficulties with control, especially of hostility. Most clients appear to be overcontrolled, highly responsible, sensitive to criticism, and self-sacrificing. The diagnosis cannot be based on personality type, however, because there are many exceptions to the rule. Physical findings, deformities, subcutaneous nodules, and blood studies remain the criteria for identification.

Allergy   Allergic illnesses, particularly those involving the skin, have been shown to have psychological elements in etiology or course. The skin, with its critical sensory functions, becomes symbolically identified with the ego, or the part of an individual's psychological makeup that mediates between the outside world and internal states. Itching (pruritis), excessive sweating (hyperhidrosis), urticaria, and atopic dermatitis are all conditions commonly classified as psychophysiologic.

MECHANISMS   A variety of stressful or emotional states are associated with exacerbations of allergic skin disorders. Attempts have been made to correlate the following specific ones with individual disorders:

- Generalized pruritis: aggression
- Genital and anal pruritis: sexuality (heterosexual and homosexual)
- Hyperhidrosis: anxiety
- Urticaria: anger
- Atopic dermatitis: longing for love

In truth, these affective states and conflicts are ubiquitous to normal, neurotic, and other psychophysiological states. Nurses should therefore be cautious about accepting pathogenic mechanisms and explanations.

The location of the lesions has, historically, had symbolic significance. Thus, conflict over an extramarital affair has been associated with dermatitis in the wedding ring area. Head and face locations have been classically associated with conflict over affective display. Affliction of the hands is associated with practical or professional conflicts. A genital distribution is associated with concerns that are sexual in nature.

Eating Disorders   There is considerable psychiatric research on disorders of eating behavior. In general eating disturbances can be divided between *obesity,* or overeating with excessive fat accumulation, and *Anorexia Nervosa,* severe weight loss due to self-imposed dietary restriction to the point of malnourishment and even death by starvation. These conditions can be present in the same individual and sometimes are related to one another consciously or unconsciously (also see Chapter 20).

OBESITY   Hunger and satiety are under the control of the hypothalamus, which turns eating behavior on or off in response to the concentration of one or more substances in the blood. The mechanism is illustrated in Figure 17–3. Whether carbohydrate, fat, or protein is the triggering nutrient has been a matter of debate. How the hypothalamus is programmed to respond is influenced by a wide range of factors, including:

• Socioeconomic status
• Genetic determinants
• Developmental considerations
• Physical activity
• Brain damage
• Emotional factors

The net result is a wide range of specific eating patterns and a consequent wide variation in human body weights. Obesity, for example, is far more prevalent in members of lower socioeconomic classes, including children.

Body build among normal persons is an inherited trait. The so-called ectomorph, a thin, angular body type, is associated with a low incidence of obesity. In addition, studies have indicated that the number of fat tissue cells a person has is established in the first few months of life and remains fairly stable for the individual's entire life. Although increased physical activity generally causes increased eating, body weight remains stable, because more calories are being expended. With physical inactivity, however, the amount of food intake rarely decreases sufficiently, and weight does tend to go up. In humans, brain damage is an infrequent cause of obesity.

Many people, obese and normal, tend to overeat when they are emotionally distressed. Obese individuals, however, seem particularly susceptible to frustrations in love relationships. People with weight problems show poor self-control when it comes to eating behavior and a high response level to a variety of social cues, rather than physiological stimuli, to eat. These people frequently have body image disturbances that either help cause or result from their overeating patterns. Many obese individuals have a low self-concept and act out self-critical, self-punitive rituals with overeating, commonly in "binges."

A disorder characterized by binge eating, *Bulimia,* is commonly encountered in adolescent and young adult women. Individuals with Bulimia rapidly consume large quantities of high-calorie food, such as ice cream, cake, or candy, over a limited time, such as a couple of hours. These eating binges are commonly followed by severe self-deprecation that leads to self-induced vomiting. In between binges, the client may diet or use cathartics and/or diuretics to try to lose weight. Bulimic episodes may occur as part of Anorexia Nervosa, but not all individuals with Bulimia have the distur-

Figure 17–3

Schematic diagram of hypothalamic control of hunger.

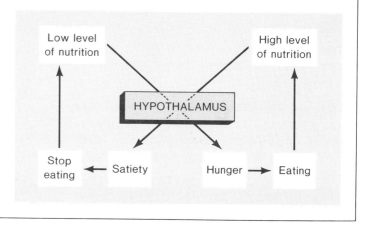

bances of body image characteristic of Anorexia Nervosa, and, although weight may fluctuate, clients with bulimia rarely become as emaciated as anorexic clients.

B, a twenty-five-year-old, female nurse came to the mental health center because of binge eating. She complained that although she was very concerned with her weight and very invested in her physical image, she regularly went on gluttonous eating binges for one to two days. These would leave her nauseated, exhausted, and disgusted with herself. Her inability to control the behavior voluntarily was making her depressed.

In the course of her therapy, it became apparent that although B consciously wanted certain improvements to occur in her job and social life, and in her appearance, she had subtle ways of sabotaging any movement in that direction. Binge eating destroyed any attempts she made to control her weight and thus feel positive about her body image.

Movement in a self-interested direction had become attached in B's mind to repudiation of her depressed mother, with whom she felt very close. Individual successes, she felt, were antagonistic toward her mother, since they might lead to her own greater independence. Although she wished such independence for herself, she also feared losing her mother's support, which she needed. Thus she developed ways of undermining her own efforts.

Psychotherapeutic work with B involved discovering these meanings, bringing her concerns to the surface for discussion, and attempting to resolve issues of fear of separation and dependency needs. When this material was directly discussed, B had less need for indirect expression of conflict, and the binge-eating behavior subsided.

ANOREXIA NERVOSA   Anorexia Nervosa is a condition characterized by severe emaciation due to an intense fear of becoming obese and a disturbance in body image such that the individual feels fat even when grotesquely thin. It must be distinguished from weight loss seen in a number of psychiatric disturbances, including:

- Psychotic disorders
- Depression
- Geriatric states
- Psychogenic malnutrition

In psychotic disorders, agitation, apathy, or delusions about poisoning and the like may be responsible for the reduction in eating, whereas in depression the general unhappiness results in loss of appetite. A host of adjustment and adaptive problems may lead the elderly to give up good dietary practices. There are four other major types of undereating clients with strong psychogenic components:

1. Obese adolescents with counterphobic behavior
2. Histrionic individuals with repressed and displaced sexual conflicts leading to difficulty in swallowing
3. Obsessional individuals with self-punitive behavior leading to starvation
4. Adolescent females with pregnancy fears

Fasting, which has a deep cultural history of ritualistic and symbolic significance, has also become interwoven into the symbolism of neurotic life-styles. In particular, the self-gratification and pleasure attached to eating becomes negatively perceived by certain people. It comes to represent selfishness and evil. Controlling the natural drive to eat then becomes a symbolic struggle of the will against the body's baser needs or desires. In addition, starvation can represent a repudiation of sexuality or can function as a punishment for real or imagined transgressions. In its severest state—starvation to near death—this behavior can be interpreted as a denial of self or the right to exist.

Cases have been reported in the literature of individuals, particularly adolescent and young adult females, whose body weight fell below fifty pounds, although more typically the weight may be in the range of sixty to eighty pounds. Often a major life change, such as the first sexual encounter or moving away from home, precipitates the onset of the syndrome. Some clients merely take in less food, while others eat but immediately self-induce vomiting. Typically, the client's resolve falters after a time, and binge eating occurs. This invariably is followed by guilt and further dietary restriction or vomiting.

The following physical signs and symptoms are associated with Anorexia Nervosa:

- Weight loss
- Amenorrhea
- Hyperactivity
- Constipation
- Hypotension

- Bradycardia
- Hypothermia
- Hyperkeratosis of skin
- Secondary sexual organ atrophy
- Leukopenia
- Anemia
- Hypoglycemia
- Hypercholesterolemia
- Hypoproteinemia
- Reduced basal metabolic rate
- Reduced gonadotropins
- Normal thyroid function
- Normal adrenal cortical function

Anorexia Nervosa is a life-threatening emergency. Up to 15 percent of cases die of malnutrition and another fraction are prone to suicide.

Headache   The experience of headache resulting from emotional tension is common enough to be familiar to most readers. Tension headache and other kinds of headache resulting from vascular changes, such as migraine, comprise the group of headaches not related to intracranial lesions, diseases, or either systemic or local infections.

Structural or disease-related headaches arise from:

- Systemic infections
- Primary or metastatic tumors
- Hematomas
- Abscesses
- Cranial infections
- Cranial nerve inflammations
- Eye, ear, nose, sinus, or tooth diseases

MECHANISMS   The mechanism of vascular headache seems to involve the release of various vasoactive substances in the brain, such as serotonin, catecholamines, histamine, bradykinin, and prostaglandins. This frequently occurs with stress. In genetically susceptible individuals, the substances cause vasodilation and inflammation of the arterial walls. There are generally prodromal symptoms of migraine attacks. These range from mood changes and gastrointestinal upset to gross neurological findings in the visual and contralateral sensorimotor systems. A number of upsets in physiological functioning can actually be migraine equiva-

lents. These include nausea and vomiting, diarrhea, tachycardia, cyclical edema, vertigo, periodic fever, pain, depression, confusion, and insomnia. Another mechanism of tension-induced headache is muscular contraction in the neck, shoulders, face, or scalp. These are steady, persistent headaches with no warning signs and commonly feel like a "band wrapped around the head."

Endocrine Disorders   A large number of disorders of endocrine functioning are intertwined with psychological factors. Studying the endocrine system has particular significance for psychiatry, because there is a close relationship between the emotions and a variety of neurohumoral processes. In physical medicine, the feedback loop has long been accepted as the model for the functioning of the endocrine organs.

MECHANISM   Extensive research on the endocrine feedback system has developed a sophisticated model that includes three kinds of feedback loops. The levels of circulating hormones released by endocrine glands, such as the thyroid or sex glands, are controlled by long feedback loops sending information to the cerebral cortex and limbic system, short feedback loops of pituitary hormones affecting the hypothalamus, and very short loops of releasing hormones from the hypothalamus determining their own production and control. Studies on the relationship of emotions to endocrine function have shown that:

- Various neurotransmitters have effects on hormone releasing factors.
- Psychoactive drugs whose action is mediated by neurotransmitters also affect the release of releasing factors.
- Stress stimulates the autonomic nervous system, which can stimulate the adrenal medulla to produce epinephrine or the pancreas to secrete insulin.
- Corticosteroid production of the adrenal cortex increases greatly during acute psychotic episodes of schizophrenic clients.
- Steroid levels also increase in agitated or anxious depressive people.

It seems fair to conclude that the emotional centers of the brain—that is, the cortex and limbic systems—are intimately tied to the endocrine organs, through the axis of the hypothalamus and the anterior pituitary, and use their secreted substances as communication

---

Table 17-1 NORMAL DEVELOPMENTAL ALTERATIONS IN ENDOCRINE FUNCTION

Development	Physical Evidence	Psychological Aspects
Puberty	Age, growth spurt, changes in fat and muscle proportions and distribution, changes in genitals, changes in secondary sex characteristics, menarche	Changes in popularity, prestige, self-confidence; increase in moodiness, hostility, depression, interpersonal difficulties
Menstruation	Menstrual bleeding cycles, cramps, backaches, headaches, alterations in estrogen-progesterone ratio	Irritability, mood swings, tension, depression
Postpartum	Pregnancy and delivery, vast prior increases in progesterone and estrogen levels during pregnancy fall to normal within ten days, changes in fluid and electrolyte balance, increased prolactin secretion	Emotional lability, body image changes, self-esteem issues, anxiety about adequacy as mother, sensitivity to father's responses to mother and baby
Menopause	Cessation or irregularity of menses, hot flashes, low levels of estrogen secretion	Anxiety, depression, irritability, decreased sexual interest, end of reproductive era, increased physical illness, loss of youth, issues of children being grown, parents dead or infirm, husband changing

messengers. It is not surprising, then, to find expressions of emotional arousal through endocrine changes and major effects on emotional states from endocrine diseases. These are both, in fact, common.

ALTERATIONS IN ENDOCRINOLOGICAL FUNCTION The major normal, developmental changes in the endocrine system are set forth in Table 17-1, while pathological, disease-induced changes are summarized in Table 17-2. Adequate preparation of a person for developmental changes by offering accurate information about likely physical and emotional alterations can help prevent severe psychiatric disturbances around these periods. Reliable support and open channels of communication are necessary. New coping strategies can be successful, if their ingenuity, timing, and presentation are appropriate.

Adrenal dysfunction characteristically produces prominent mental as well as distinctive physical symptoms. Thyroid disorders commonly are accompanied by cognitive or emotional changes. Stress has been implicated, though inconclusively, in the precipitation of thyrotoxic crises. Stress may influence the course of diabetes, either by promoting exacerbations directly or by causing the client to neglect a usually rigid medical regimen and thus indirectly worsen the disease. So many mental symptoms are associated with hypoglycemia that many clients are classified and treated as "classic neurotics."

Intervention

Because traditional biomedical approaches to illness focus predominantly on disease as it affects the body, the client as a person is often neglected in treatment plans. Even psychological approaches have focused on what is wrong with the individual's defense mechanisms or psychic makeup in a reductionistic, medical model way. Treatment based on contemporary, holistic theories of disease combines both humanistic and scientific approaches. Derangements of the body are accompanied by difficulties at the symbolic level as the individual attempts to cope with a changing reality. Even when disease can be observed at a cellular or organ level, illness and clienthood remain issues at the personal level.

Stress is the common denominator in the role psychological factors play in the initiation, exacerbation, or maintenance of Psychophysiologic Disorders. Degrees of stress are ubiquitous in human experience. Some stress appears actually to lead human beings to more productive, fulfilling, and successful functioning. On a biological level, the "fight or flight" response of the human body, mediated by the release of adrenaline, can enable the individual to adapt to a stressful event. Too much stress, however, appears to overwhelm people and increase their vulnerability to a wide range of bodily and emotional disorders.

Table 17–2	DISEASE-INDUCED ALTERATIONS IN ENDOCRINE FUNCTION		
Disease	**Physical Symptoms**	**Mental Symptoms**	**Diagnostic Test**
Cushing's syndrome (adrenal cortex hyperfunction)	Truncal obesity, moon facies, abdominal striae, hirsutism, amenorrhea, hypertension, osteoporosis, weakness	Impotence, decreased libido, anxiety, increased emotional lability, apathy, insomnia, memory deficits, confusion, disorientation	Increased 17-hydroxy-corticosteroids
Addison's disease (adrenal insufficiency)	Weakness, fatigue, anorexia, weight loss, nausea and vomiting, pigmentation of skin, hypotension	Depression, irritability, psychomotor retardation, apathy, memory defect, hallucinations	Decreased urine steroids, decreased sodium chlorides, bicarbonates, increased potassium
Hyperthyroidism	Staring, exophthalmos, goiter, moist warm skin, weight loss, increased appetite, weakness, tremor, tachycardia, heat intolerance	Anxiety, tension, irritability, hyperexcitability, emotional lability, depression, psychosis, or delirium	Increased PBI, increased T_3, T_4, increased radioactive iodine uptake
Hypothyroidism	Dull expression, puffy eyelids, swollen tongue, hoarse voice, rough dry skin, cold intolerance	Psychomotor retardation, decreased initiative, slow comprehension, drowsiness, decreased recent memory, delirium, stupor, depression or psychosis	Decreased PBI, decreased thyroid symptoms, increased cholesterol, hypochromic anemia
Diabetes mellitus	Polydipsia, polyuria, polyphagia, weight loss, blurred vision, fatigue, impotence, fainting, paresthesia	Stupor, coma, fatigue, impotence	Increased fasting blood sugar (FBS), increased two-hour postprandial (PP), abnormal glucose tolerance test
Hypoglycemia	Tremor, light-headedness, sweating, hunger, nausea, pallor, tachycardia, hypertension	Anxiety, fugue, unusual behavior, confusion, apathy, psychomotor agitation or retardation, depression, delusions, hallucinations, convulsions, coma	Abnormal glucose tolerance test

There are many sources of life stress. Conjugal relationships, parenting, occupational pursuits, finances, legal problems, developmental phases, and a host of other life experiences and situations may lead to severe stress. Individuals seem to vary widely in their capacity to deal with and master stress. In training people to cope with stress, the nurse may play an increasingly important role in a variety of settings, including the hospital, the workplace, and the community.

Since stress often seems to lead to Psychophysiological Disorders, reducing or overcoming stress naturally plays an important part in their treatment. Minimizing the effects of a potentially stressful life event, such as a change in job, depends on the ability to anticipate and thus prepare for or take steps to avoid certain stressful aspects of the event. How an individual handles stress also depends on the person's adaptive capabilities. Being flexible—that is, able to change some aspect of a usual way of behaving—can often turn a potential stressor into a positive life experience.

Approaches to mastering stress involve teaching the individual to mobilize both internal and external resources. This approach emphasizes teaching people to

- Develop new capabilities that will enable them to change the environment or their relationship to it
- Find ways of reducing threat
- Obtain alternative sources of satisfaction to replace those that are frustrated or lost

- Minimize the physiological and psychological arousal that often accompanies stress

Some of these tasks are cognitive in that stress usually results from stressed people's perception of a gap between their abilities to handle a situation and the demands placed on them by the situation. Reducing people's perception of what is expected or demanded is often very helpful in alleviating stress. Certain other tasks may involve increased or more effective use of social supports. Therefore, enhancing people's ability to call on and use individuals in their social network or developing a better network when the current system is not adequate may relieve stress. Finally, exercises in relaxation, meditation, and related activities can actually reduce physiological arousal levels so that morbidity from stress is reduced (see Chapter 25). In a more relaxed state, individuals can use their cognitive and intrapsychic coping processes more effectively.

When a specific problem or conflict appears to make an individual particularly susceptible to a Psychophysiological Disorder, attention must be directed toward some special concerns with each of the disorders discussed.

Ulcer An important feature of the frustration of dependence needs that may lead to ulcer formation is that in adult life the frustration may be real, remembered, or symbolic. The meaning attached to life events and the perceived ability to deal with them are of prime significance. Especially relevant is the fact that the individual caught in the maladaptive pattern has no confidence in his or her ability to cope with the circumstances and achieve a successful outcome.

Traditionally, psychological treatment involves partial gratification of the client's dependence needs without eliminating the possibility that the client can develop greater independence. Clients need new ways to satisfy their needs effectively and perhaps to decrease their sense of need. Thus far, no treatment has proved curative.

Bowel Disorders Effective treatment of clients with psychophysiological bowel disorders must also be allied to an understanding psychological approach. This is made especially difficult, however, by the fact that such clients are often exceedingly unrevealing about themselves. They may expect the practitioner to be omniscient and omnipotent—to know their needs and meet them without further information or requests.

Cardiovascular Disorders The treatments for physically documentable cardiac symptoms involve antihypertensive medications or beta-adrenergic blocking drugs. Almost always the client needs supportive therapy to handle fears associated with the potential failure of this essential organ system. Therapy should also lead the client toward more effective ways of dealing with conflicts and feelings of vulnerability, while shedding maladaptive coping mechanisms. Benzodiazepine antianxiety agents are also widely prescribed (see Chapter 23).

Arthritis Arthritic clients usually require work around issues of separation, insincerity, autonomy, and felt dependency needs. Psychotherapy is recommended to identify potential stressful life situations, such as a separation or loss, that may provoke anger. Therapy can also provide a stable, dependable interpersonal relationship for vulnerable people.

Allergy The pathogenesis of allergic reactions involves a relative balance between biological/constitutional and psychological factors. In many cases, psychotherapy, particularly family therapy, psychotropic medications, hypnosis, behavioral conditioning, and biofeedback training can all be of benefit.

Eating Disorders Traditional psychotherapy has not had impressive results with overeating clients unless their behavior was stress-related and the therapy led to less stressful, more gratifying adaptations to living. Behavior modification intervention has given more encouraging results. Key elements in the behavior modification approach to overeating are:

- Clients keep precise, complete, detailed records of the time, amount, and circumstances of eating.
- Discriminative stimuli to eating are controlled by limiting the time, place, and circumstances of eating.
- Delay techniques are introduced into the eating process.
- Such delays or other controls of eating are reinforced by other valued objects or gestures.

No specific therapy has a roundly acclaimed success rate for anorexia nervosa. As is usual in medical psychiatry, a range of treatment is employed, with successes and failures somewhat randomly distributed. At least one third of the clients who survive continue to suffer chronically from severe eating disorders.

Headache   Some persons with severe, recurring headaches require an extensive neurological examination to rule out organic disease (see Chapter 8). But in cases where anxiety, stress, or depression seems prominent, psychotherapy may reverse the emotional maladaptations.

Endocrinopathies   Psychiatry's role in the endocrinopathies includes diagnosis and management of the Organic Brain Syndromes, treatment of the major psychotic presentations, and counseling, therapy, and support of individuals whose lives are high in stress or whose personalities are likely to lead them to overresponse or maladaptive response to normal life cycles. Through therapy, individuals with endocrine disorders or with a propensity to develop them could conceivably become less vulnerable to unfavorable circumstances. Both the psychiatric and the medical-surgical nurse will have occasion to deal with these challenging problems, particularly in hospital settings.

MENTAL RETARDATION

The syndrome of Mental Retardation encompasses a vast array of disorders that are uncomfortably considered to fall in the domain of psychiatry. This uneasy assignment of responsibility resulted primarily from the frustrating nature of clinical work in retardation, which suffered both from a dearth of realistic and potentially successful treatment approaches and from the seemingly endless number of socioeconomic problems that need to be solved before substantial steps toward prevention can be taken. However, several recent scientific developments in the areas of detection and primary prevention are encouraging.

Intelligence

Intelligence represents the capacity to relate to problems of living in ways that generate solutions, show adaptive potential, reflect conceptual organization, and demonstrate augmentation through learning. Intelligence in humans obviously is a product of both biological and sociocultural factors. Attempts to distinguish the relative contributions of "nature" versus "nurture" in order to establish the primacy of either are usually unsuccessful. Traditionally, intelligence has been reflected in test scores such as the Stanford-Binet Intelligence Quotient (IQ), but considerable research has

demonstrated that such scores are valid mainly for estimating school success. They do not necessarily reflect an individual's true problem-solving ability in any broad sense. In addition, extraneous factors, such as anxiety, reduced attention span, low expectation level, race, and culture, alter scores on standard tests (see Chapter 8).

Piaget's Theory of Development   Modern conceptions of intelligence stress the quality of the thinking process as a measure of the degree of development, rather than of any specific performance. Jean Piaget (1953), a Swiss developmental psychologist, postulated that a constant interplay between the child and the environment develops, over time, the following specific conceptualizing stages:

1. Sensorimotor stage (birth to eighteen months)
2. Preoperational stage
   a. Preconceptual (eighteen months to four years)
   b. Intuitive (four to seven years)
3. Stage of concrete operations (seven to eleven years)
4. Stage of abstract operations (over eleven years)

Each stage exists potentially in the human brain. Given a biologically normal brain and sufficient appropriate opportunity to assimilate or accommodate to the external environment, the child passes through all the stages and achieves fully functional intellectual capacities (see also Chapters 10 and 19).

Abnormal Development   In general, a retarded person has difficulty learning. The more complex the learning task, the more evident the retarded person's limitations. Processes of cognition in which deficits or inabilities may account for difficulties in learning include:

- Arousal of attention
- Direction of attention
- Maintenance of attention
- Sensation
- Perception
- Inhibition of already learned responses
- Abstraction
- Generalization

In the broad sense, retardation may result from disordered brain functioning, either secondary to structural or metabolic disease or from a failure to develop physiological maturity due to genetic abnormality, disease, or profound lack of stimulation.

Definitions of Retardation

The definition of retardation offered by the American Association of Mental Deficiency (1961) is: "Mental retardation refers to sub-average general intellectual functioning which originates in the developmental period and is associated with impairment of adaptive behavior." The American Psychiatric Association's official categorization of mental retardation levels, as presented in DSM-III, is given in Table 17–3. By these criteria, it is estimated that 1 percent of the population in the United States is retarded. Since the DSM-III definition of Mental Retardation includes not only subaverage intellectual functioning but also deficits or impairments in adaptive behavior, borderline intellectual functioning (IQ 71–84) is now considered a V code (see Chapter 8) rather than a mental disorder. Not all individuals in this IQ range have significant functional impairment.

Causes of Retardation

The causes of retardation are generally grouped according to the time of influence of the offending factor—that is, prenatal, perinatal, postnatal, and sociocultural causes. These are outlined in the following sections.

Prenatal Causes The prenatal causes of Mental Retardation fall within the following general classifications:

- Inherited defects in metabolism
- Chromosomal abnormalities
- Developmental anomalies
- Maternal infections during pregnancy
- Maternal systemic diseases

INHERITED DEFECTS IN METABOLISM A wide variety of metabolic defects that can cause severe Mental Retardation can be inherited by the offspring of normal carrier parents. Generally, the pattern of inheritance is autosomal recessive, which means that any offspring, male or female, of two unaffected parents who carry the recessive gene has a one-in-four chance of being affected. Some defects, particularly those affecting fat metabolism, are found only in Jewish persons. The ba-

Table 17–3 CATEGORIES OF MENTAL RETARDATION	
Category	**IQ Level**
Profound	Below 20
Severe	20–34
Moderate	35–49
Mild	50–70

sic defect is almost universally an enzymatic one. The afflicted child is unable to synthesize a particular essential enzyme, so that a key metabolic operation cannot be carried out. This causes multiple deleterious effects, including profound Mental Retardation. The enzyme defects discovered thus far involve all the major metabolic pathways—protein, carbohydrate, and fat—as well as calcium, bilirubin, copper, and uric acid. Table 17–4 summarizes features of several widely studied metabolic disorders. The degree of Mental Retardation associated with these illnesses is usually quite severe. Many are fatal at an early age.

Biochemical research has led from identification of the enzyme involved to specific treatment approaches that in some cases can have dramatic effects. The treatments involve mainly dietary manipulations. Thanks to the development of early detection screening tests, treatments can prevent brain damage that would otherwise be inevitable. The schematic diagram in Figure 17–4 describes the essence of treatment in an illness such as the aminoaciduria, phenylketonuria.

CHROMOSOMAL ABNORMALITIES When the process of cell division in the early stages of the zygote following fertilization does not divide the genetic material from the egg or the sperm evenly or normally, such chromosomal abnormalities can lead to syndromes associated with Mental Retardation. One of the most common of these is Down's syndrome, also known as mongolism. The most frequent cause of Down's syndrome is a nondisjunction of chromosomal material, leading to an extra (third) chromosome 21. This pattern is known as trisomy 21, and affected individuals have a total of forty-seven chromosomes rather than the usual forty-six. The extra genetic material is known to cause several enzymatic defects, although it is presently unknown which ones are responsible for the various features of the syndrome. Down's syndrome occurs in about 1 in 700 births in the United States. The risk rises as the mother's age increases over thirty. Characteristic physical features associated with Down's syn-

	Table 17–4	METABOLIC DISORDERS ASSOCIATED WITH MENTAL RETARDATION		
Nutrient Affected	Example	Essential Defect	Clinical Features	Treatment
Amino acid (protein)	Phenylketonuria	Decreased phenylalanine hydroxylase	Blond hair, blue eyes, small size, light complexion, coarse features, small head, hyperactivity, autism	Decrease dietary phenylalanine
	Maple syrup urine disease	Decreased amino acid decarboxylase	Onset at one week of age, decerebrate rigidity, seizures, respiratory difficulties, hypoglycemia	Decrease dietary amino acids
Lipid (fat)	Tay-Sachs disease	Decreased hexoaminodase A	Onset at four to eight months of age, hypotonus, apathy, spasticity, primitive reflexes, cherry spot retina, convulsions	None
	Gaucher's disease	Decreased glucocere-brosidase	Onset (1) in infancy or (2) before ten years, hepatosplenomegaly, abdominal and cranial enlargement, hypotonia, opisthotonus	None
Carbohydrate (starch)	Galactosemia	Decreased galactose-1-phosphate uridyltransferase	Onset one week after birth, jaundice, vomiting, diarrhea, failure to thrive, hepatomegaly, cataracts	Decrease dietary galactose
	Glycogen storage disease	Absent glycogen metabolism	Onset in neonatal period, hepatomegaly, failure to thrive, acidosis, hypoglycemic convulsions	Symptomatic
Miscellaneous	Idiopathic hypercalcemia	Hypersensitivity to vitamin D	Irritability, elfin facies, short stature, hypotonia, hypertension, strabismus, nephrocalcinosis	Cortisone
	Wilson's disease	Decreased copper ceruloplasmin	Onset in juvenile or adult, cirrhosis, pseudobulbar palsy, wing-flapping, Kayser-Fleisher ring	Penicillamine, dimercaprol
	Hurler's syndrome	Increased dermatan sulfate or increased heparan sulfate	Bone and skull malformations, hepatosplenomegaly, dwarfism, hypertelorism	None

drome involve the *eyes, facies, skull, tongue,* and hands. Retardation is universally significant. As children, individuals with the syndrome are frequently easy to manage at home because they have rather pleasant dispositions. Once adolescence is reached, however, a variety of emotional difficulties and behavioral disturbances may provoke institutionalization.

H was a sixteen-year-old mongoloid male who was brought to the mental health center by his mother. He was the only child of divorced parents, and had lived with his mother. His father was not actively involved in family life, save for alimony and child support payments. The mother was devoted and extremely close to her son. She

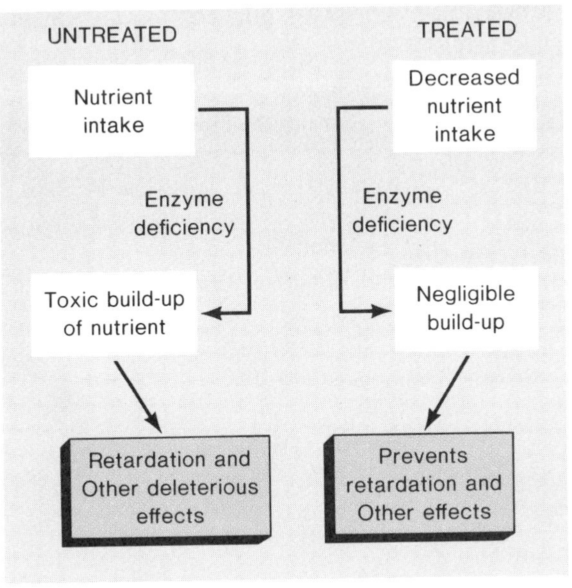

Figure 17–4

Treatment approach in metabolic disorders.

had gone to great lengths to keep him at home, had worked intimately with the Bureau of Child Welfare to obtain special schooling, and had resisted all suggestions that H might someday need to be institutionalized.

At about age fourteen, H had reached his present size of about five feet six inches and 160 pounds. Although he had been very friendly and docile to this point, he began to become somewhat more ornery and subject to outbursts of anger. These episodes occurred with increasing frequency at his school, until his mother elected to take him out and keep him at home. During the eight months before the psychiatric consultation, H had reacted to his confinement by destroying furniture and striking out at his mother, who was now his only human contact. His mother had been punched several times, until her fear of her son's anger and her own anger and resentment at him brought her to the point where she felt she could no longer care for him.

Intervention consisted of working with the mother about her guilt at having to give up the care of her son and her fear of loneliness. She had never really dealt with the dissolution of her marriage or with the responsibility she felt for H's condition. In addition to positive mother–son attachments, her devotion was being determined by unresolved problems in her own personality.

DEVELOPMENTAL ANOMALIES A number of conditions involving central nervous system damage at critical periods in development are felt to be due to endogenous (inherited) rather than exogenous causes. Some of these genetic determinants are autosomal dominants, with variable expressivity and penetrance, passed on with rare incidence in families where the afflicted person remains fertile (such persons are often sterile from the moment of sexual maturity). Sometimes the degree of retardation associated with these conditions is only slight. Distinctive characteristics and neuropathological findings of several of the classic syndromes of this variety are listed in Table 17–5.

Conditions thought to be genetic but with either recessive or unknown patterns of inheritance are presented in Table 17–6. These are not truly familial illnesses and may be affected by a variety of influences.

MATERNAL INFECTIONS DURING PREGNANCY Syphilis, rubella, toxoplasmosis, and cytomegalic inclusion disease are all infections that may cause neurological damage to the fetus and result in Mental Retardation when contracted by a pregnant woman. Rubella (German measles) is probably the most widely recognized and most common infection causing retardation today. Affliction during the first trimester of pregnancy is associated with a 10- to 15-percent chance of damage to the offspring. Rubella in the first month of pregnancy damages the fetus 50 percent of the time. The abnormalities associated with prenatal maternal rubella are:

• Mental Retardation

• Congenital heart disease

• Microcephaly

• Cataracts

• Deafness

• Microphthalmia

Part of good prenatal care is a routine check for German measles when a woman becomes pregnant.

MATERNAL SYSTEMIC DISEASES Poor health of a pregnant mother and poor prenatal care carry with them a high incidence of Mental Retardation in the offspring. Toxemia of pregnancy, malnutrition, poorly controlled diabetes, and injudicious use of drugs are all systemic conditions that may damage the fetus's central nervous system before birth.

Perinatal Causes In the perinatal period, the nearly full-term fetus or newborn infant runs considerable risk of central nervous system damage and mental retardation. The final stages of gestation and the birth

Table 17–5   DEVELOPMENTAL MENTAL RETARDATION SYNDROMES DUE TO AUTOSOMAL DOMINANT INHERITANCE

Disease	Clinical Characteristics	Neuropathological Findings
Tuberous sclerosis	Red or brown skin lesions; tumors of heart, kidney, liver, retina, leading to organ failure; epilepsy	Multiple glial tissue nodules in cerebral cortex and cerebellum leading to hydrocephalus
Neurofibromatosis (von Reckling-hausen's disease)	Brown patches along nerve distributions in skin (café au lait spots); epilepsy	Tumors of central nervous system, optic and acoustic nerves
Sturge-Weber disease	Facial nevus in distribution of trigeminal nerve; hemiparesis; convulsions	Intracranial angiomata
Hippel-Lindau disease	Cerebellar signs	Angiomata of cerebellum and retina
Marfan's syndrome	Tall, long extremities, spiderlike fingers and toes, lens dislocations, cardiac anomalies	None

Table 17–6   MENTAL RETARDATION SYNDROMES DUE TO RECESSIVE OR UNKNOWN PATTERNS OF INHERITANCE

Type	Clinical Characteristics	Neuropathological Findings
Anencephaly	Lethal	Absence of cranial vaults and at least both cerebral hemispheres, if not most of central nervous system
Hydranencephaly	Normal at birth; at several weeks or months spasticity, convulsions, rigidity, and hydrocephalus	Intact meninges and cranium, filled with fluid; absent cerebral cortex
Porencephaly	Hemiplegia; quadriplegia	Cysts in hemispheres communicating with ventricles or subarachnoid space
Microcephaly	Small head, birdlike face, sensorimotor disturbances, blindness, deafness, convulsions possible	Small brain, cortical atrophy, maldeveloped cerebral convolutions
Hydrocephalus	Large head after second or third month, tense fontanel, vomiting, papilledema, other central nervous system signs	Increased cerebrospinal fluid, large ventricles, ductal or foraminal atresia, other defects in central nervous system

process present a variety of dangers threatening normal intellectual development.

Failure to complete a full gestational term results in an infant of low birth weight who is susceptible to intellectual, sensorimotor, and emotional disorders. Problems are roughly inversely proportional to the degree of prematurity and the consequent birth weight. Prematurity is known to be increased by poor prenatal care. The following factors increase the risk of prematurity:

- Obstetrical complications
- Toxemia of pregnancy
- Multiple births
- Maternal malnutrition
- Maternal heavy smoking
- Maternal urinary tract infections

Improved obstetrical techniques and sophisticated practitioners of perinatology have increased the survival rate of premature infants and, paradoxically, the incidence of Mental Retardation from this cause.

Another group of infants susceptible to central nervous system damage are term births that are of low birth weight and are said to suffer from intrauterine growth retardation.

The birth process itself may cause significant intracranial damage. Usually, one of two pathological processes is involved:

1. Cerebral trauma leading to hemorrhage, which is associated with
    a. Cephalopelvic disproportion
    b. Breech presentation
    c. High forceps deliveries
    d. Prolonged, difficult labor
2. Cerebral anoxia causing direct tissue destruction, which is associated with
    a. Caesarian section
    b. Any obstetrical complication
    c. Tracheal obstructions in infant
    d. Analgesia or anesthesia used for delivery

A final group of perinatal pathological processes that cause Mental Retardation do so secondary to the deposit of unconjugated (indirect) bilirubin in the central nervous system. This phenomenon, known as *kernicterus*, results from conditions that cause neonatal jaundice, including:

- Low enzymatic activity in the premature infant
- Rh factor incompatibility
- Neonatal sepsis
- Drugs

Postnatal Causes   A wide variety of conditions and factors potentially present in the postnatal period can be associated with significant Mental Retardation. These can be categorized as:

- Infections
- Other exogenous noxious or toxic factors
- Diseases
- Nutrition

INFECTIONS   Severe infections of the meninges by bacteria or viruses can lead to Mental Retardation. Among the bacterial causes, pneumococcal infections are par-

ticularly severe on the central nervous system and have a high incidence of brain damage, while meningococcal infections are the most benign. An unfortunate result of advances in antibiotic therapy is that, while more children survive such serious infections, many of these suffer sufficient damage to cause Mental Retardation.

OTHER EXOGENOUS TOXIC FACTORS   Head trauma and poisoning, primarily lead poisoning from paint ingestion, are leading postnatal causes of retardation. Fortunately, if recognized early, lead poisoning is treatable and the serious results can be avoided.

DISEASES   Several diseases without known etiology affect infants in the postnatal period and are associated with high incidence of retardation. These include epilepsy, hypsarrhythmia or myoclonic seizures of infancy, nonspecific febrile illnesses, cerebral palsy, and Heller's disease. This last is a controversial syndrome of progressive mental deterioration in certain children after the third or fourth year. It is a poorly understood syndrome probably associated with a wide variety of undetected central nervous system insults that do not show their effects until this period.

NUTRITION   Postnatal nutrition can also affect the incidence of Mental Retardation. This subject is properly covered by pediatrics texts.

Sociocultural Factors   Statistics show that a disproportionate segment of the mentally retarded population comes from the groups that are most disadvantaged socioeconomically. To a greater degree than others, the underprivileged are subjected to a host of problems that can contribute to future intellectual deficiencies. In general these can be divided into three major areas:

1. Medical problems
2. Emotional/social problems
3. Environmental problems

Many of the strictly medical conditions that were described in preceding sections, which lead to Mental Retardation, arise at a higher incidence among the poor because of deficiencies in medical care. These problem areas include poor prenatal care, poor well-baby follow-up, poor nutritional status of mother and child, and increased incidence of lead poisoning and other traumatic or toxic brain insults. Factors of an emotional nature that may inhibit the development of full cog-

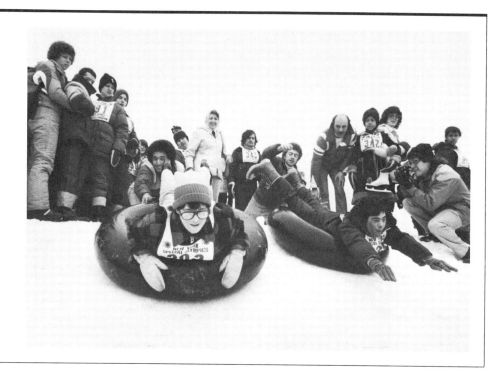

This snow-tubing event, held during the 1980 Fifth Annual New York State Winter Special Olympics, provides athletic and recreational opportunities for mentally retarded persons.

nitive capacities may also be seen with greater frequency among the poor. Such factors as lowered family cohesion, unstable object relatedness, poor limit setting on behavior, damaged sense of self, hopelessness, and tendency to act out, all have ramifications that can eventually interrupt the many processes that must operate smoothly for a child to develop full cognitive potential. Lastly, purely environmental deficits, such as reduced sensory or verbal stimulation, inadequate structure (limits, guidance, direction, and support), and insufficient nurturing are more frequent among poor people, whose needs are necessarily met on a subsistence level. These deficits undoubtedly influence the mental development of the children adversely. The implications of these observations for social policy change are obvious.

Problems Encountered by the Retarded

In addition to suffering intellectual limitation, the retarded individual is susceptible to a variety of personality and emotional problems. There is considerable debate about frequencies and relative risks of frank maladaptive development of personality to the point of clear-cut psychiatric pathology.

Emotional Vulnerability Short of demonstrable psychiatric illness, the retarded child does seem to run the risk of high vulnerability to emotional instability because of both constitutional deficiencies and inter-

personal inputs from family, and peers. Irritability, hypersensitivity to environmental stimuli, tendency to motoric hyperactivity, restlessness, short attention span, poor impulse control, and tendency to act out are all behavioral manifestations that can be problematic for the retarded child and that may stem from the central nervous system disturbance that causes the intellectual difficulties. Beyond these problems, the retarded person may have difficulty forming and maintaining meaningful human relationships because of reduced cognitive capacities. The effects of this deficiency can be devastating emotionally in early mothering interactions, general socialization, peer group formation, and so on throughout development toward emotional maturity.

In order to develop to the limits of their potential, retarded individuals need an environment geared to be supportive of their functional personality patterns and character traits. The environment must reinforce the child's independence and autonomy, impulse control, appropriate super ego restraints, and interest in others. Under optimal conditions, the natural family is the ideal setting, especially during the formative first five years of life.

Two immediate dangers to the smooth development of personality within the family system may arise on discovery of the retarded child's deficits. The first is rejection of the child by the parents, based on their own anxiety, fear, anger, insecurity, guilt, or threats to self-esteem. The second is overprotection, either to compensate for feelings of rejection or out of a heightened sense of compassion. In the former case, the child is unlikely to receive adequate mothering, love and nurturance and will surely fail to develop optimally. In the latter situation the child is unable to develop independent resources and becomes hopelessly and helplessly bound to caretakers.

Psychopathology   Studies on overt psychopathology of retarded persons indicate high frequencies of the diagnoses of Adjustment Disorders, Depressive Disorders, Organic Brain Syndromes, and certain psychotic disorders. This is not surprising in light of the emotional characteristics described in the preceding section. A personality profile typical of the pathological retarded person is:

- Autistic
- Repetitious
- Inflexible
- Passive
- Immature
- Deficient in ego function

In the realm of the ego functions, investigators have noted low stimulus barrier, poor drive regulation, and superficial object relations.

Intervention

Medical/Psychiatric Roles   Assessment and intervention are the roles generally adopted by the medical/psychiatric profession in the area of Mental Retardation. Perhaps a disproportionate share of resources has been spent on diagnosis and what would be tertia-

ry prevention—that is, treating the behavioral and emotional disorders in retarded individuals. While these remain necessary areas of professional activity, they have dominated the attention of the helping professions at the expense of secondary prevention (that is, early detection and reversal of treatable causes of retardation and enhancing the retarded child's potential development), and primary prevention (that is, eliminating the causes of retardation).

Diagnostic Evaluation   Diagnostic evaluation is primarily a medical role, although the observant nurse may provide significant data for the process. A detailed history, covering the family incidence of hereditary disorders and a careful recounting of the mother's pregnancy, labor, and delivery, is prerequisite to any thorough assessment of retardation. The client is then given a complete physical exam, with special attention to neurological signs because of their substantial association with retardation, augmented by routine and special laboratory procedures, including chromosomal karyotyping where indicated. A complete workup includes specialized speech and hearing tests, a psychiatric examination, and psychological testing with particular attention to measures of intellectual functioning. Though no intelligence tests currently in use are above criticism, there are some available for testing infants, including the Gesell, Cattell, and Bayley tests. Several can be used for older children, including the Stanford-Binet, Wechsler, and Peabody vocabulary test. The Peabody purports to avoid undue emphasis on purely language-based deficits. The Bender-Gestalt test is frequently used to test for brain damage (see Figure 17–5).

Plan of Care   Effective care for the retarded individual depends on formulating flexible treatment geared to changing problem areas during the client's

Figure 17–5

Examples of figures to be copied on Bender-Gestalt test. Subjects are asked to copy the figures on a single sheet of paper and then to draw them from memory. The clinician looks for distortion of the figures in terms of incompleteness, rotation, oversimplification, perseveration (giving more than is present in the stimulus), and looks at the use of space on the page. The recall drawings also test for memory deficits. (From L. Bender, *A Visual-Motor Gestalt Test and Its Clinical Use*, Research Monograph no. 3. New York: American Orthopsychiatric Association, 1938.)

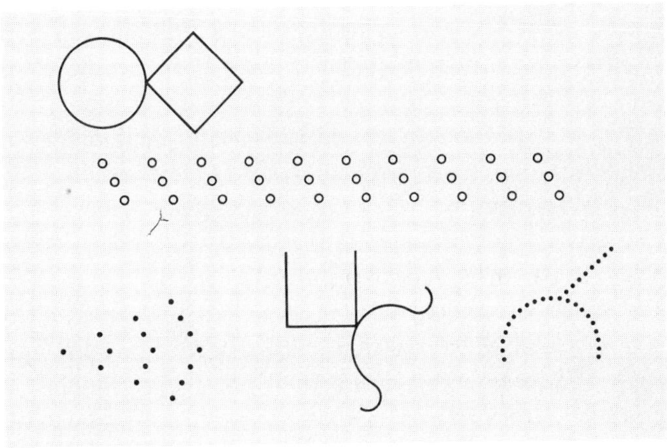

life cycle. Ideally, a single treatment team would follow a retarded child from birth through adulthood, thereby maximizing the client's potential for development. Retardation is a developmental disability and requires special patience on the part of health care personnel to avoid levels of frustration that will be detrimental to the client. Although retardation is by definition an intellectual deficit, client needs exist in all aspects of life, and the treatment approach must be holistic.

It must be expected that the life of the retarded individual will be characterized by crises, for both client and family. At these times, extra resources need to be made available and extra effort expended. Common crises include:

• Discovery of the retardation
• School failure
• Peer group rejection
• Birth of siblings
• Puberty
• Placement in a foster home, institution, etc.
• Vocational failure

In childhood, attention must be focused on habit training, gross motor development, socialization, and language skills. Specialized resources may be required. Learning to get dressed and eat independently will promote the child's future feelings of self-reliance and autonomy. Once school age is reached, learning appropriate behavior and controls, dealing with feelings of inadequacy in relation to peers, and achieving the maximum level of scholastic success are major areas of work. Problems can be anticipated, and each member of the health team should be alert for signs of difficulty.

Adolescence presents new tasks. Certainly, puberty can be a difficult period. Socially, relationships with others can present trouble for the mentally retarded. Sexually, some retarded individuals show little interest and have few problems, while others have normal drives and may encounter difficulty because of poor judgment. There can be considerable acting out and delinquency due to inadequate controls, impressionability, and a need to belong (to an adolescent group, for instance).

Care is aimed at enabling the retarded person to enter adulthood having developed as much independence as possible. Intervention and support are necessary to promote independent living and vocational capacities. Again, referral may be necessary to special-ized agencies, such as sheltered workshops and residential settings for vocational rehabilitation or training in activities of daily living appropriate for adults.

Nursing Roles   Treating the disturbed retarded child psychotherapeutically can be an arduous task, due to the difficulties in communication, particularly verbally. Simplicity, patience, and support are hallmarks of a successful approach. Very concrete, reality-oriented, and pleasure-oriented experiences can be therapeutic. Some have suggested group therapy as a potentially reinforcing experience, especially for retarded adolescents.

Psychiatric nurses undertaking the long-term therapy of a retarded person must create an accepting and affectionate atmosphere. Nurses must be willing to try to meet considerable dependency needs. Developing a sense of value or self-worth in the individual is essential, to counteract the forces that induce feelings of rejection and worthlessness. Behavior modification can be used when behavioral difficulties predominate. Family intervention, if not family therapy in a formal sense, is recommended virtually from the birth of the retarded person. Counseling parents can be an appropriate and useful role for the psychiatric nurse.

If the diagnosis of retardation is made at birth, the obstetrical nurse may be in a position to help the parents deal with the shock and sense of loss, thus preventing problems on the parents' parts, which compound the infant's difficulties. The nurse who accepts the caring role for a defective child can provide a valuable role model for ambivalent parents. An ambivalent mother should not be pushed into caring for the child but rather should be supported. The father should be encouraged to lend support as well.

Parents of retarded infants may encounter considerable emotional distress as a result of their stress. The treatment team must be aware of this possibility, be alert for signs of developing problems, and be prepared to intervene. Typical defenses encountered in parents include denial, projection, and blaming. Parental nonacceptance of the reality of the child's disability can have disastrous medical, psychological, and developmental consequences. Recognizing the intense disappointment the parents must feel and their wish for a magical solution, and empathizing with these feelings, may promote mature acceptance of the reality without undue stress. Guilt over the child's retardation may provoke parents to blaming behavior, and the nurse who can work with the family about these feelings is likely to do great service. At other times in the child's

---

NURSING CARE PLAN FOR A SEVERELY RETARDED THIRTEEN-YEAR-OLD CHILD

Michael is thirteen years old and weighs fifteen pounds. Only his wizzened face and long thin feet suggest his chronological age, for he cannot talk, crawl, feed himself, or use the toilet. He can and does smile and coo and clutch his favorite toy moose. He sucks the foods he likes (Jello, applesauce, crushed doughnuts, etc.) and spits out the foods he doesn't like (cottage cheese, etc.). Most of the time he is cared for in a progressive institution, but he is brought home for two weeks each summer and on school holidays. His loving parents and two adopted sisters (nine and ten years old) share in his arduous care needs. The plan developed collaboratively between Michael's family and the nurse is outlined below.

Goal	Intervention
1. *Nutrition* Michael must eat sufficiently nutritious and caloric foods to maintain or increase his present weight	1. Take the time required to allow him to suck in as much food as he can tolerate (usually 45 minutes per meal) 2. Have frequent, small feedings 3. Use high-calorie milk shakes and protein supplements as snacks and drinks 4. Use jaw control techniques when giving liquids in cups 5. Talk to him and praise him for eating his meals well
2. *Safety* Due to his extreme fraility Michael cannot be exposed to colds, coughs, and other contagious illnesses or health hazzards	1. Use face masks if there is a possibility of infection 2. Inquire about the presence of contagious illnesses before employing babysitters or "mother's helpers"
3. *Warmth* Because of Michael's lack of body fat, he must be kept warm	1. Even on a 70° day many layers of clothing are needed 2. Avoid temperature extremes like air conditioning
4. *Social interaction* Michael must feel loved and cared for Michael needs to modify some of his messiest behavior	1. Greet and talk to Michael in a warm friendly way 2. Touch him when interacting and feel free to say "I love you" 3. When he spits food, bangs his head, pulls his tongue, or is purposely messy firmly restrain him for a moment and say "No, rude!" with a serious facial expression

Source: Special acknowledgment for validating this care plan is made to Hillary Wilson (age 12) who serves as a "mother's helper" for Michael when he is with his family.

---

development, if the child's social network becomes unstable, family intervention may again be indicated (see Chapter 21).

Countertransference feelings, or negative feelings by the treating person toward the retarded child or the family, can be devastating. Given the difficulty of the problem, the limited knowledge about retardation, and the few opportunities for "cure," the nurse may feel frustration and anger. In addition, both the retarded person and the distraught and overtaxed family can, at times, be very demanding. The health care worker necessarily has a high level of investment in the retarded person and can become overinvolved, losing a necessary sense of perspective. The nurse may become angry at the family's deficiencies or problems or may join with the family in a sense of despair. The key to adaptive responses in nurse, client, and family is the maintenance of a reasonable degree of hopefulness by reinforcement of the retarded person's inherent value.

Institutionalization   Institutionalization remains a part of the treatment approach to the retarded individual. It may be needed to handle severe medical problems, such as seizures or physical handicaps, or when behavior is such that the retarded person cannot fit comfortably in the family or the general community. If parents are unable to overcome their own emotional difficulties surrounding the retarded child, the child may also receive better care or have a better chance for maximum development in a specialized institutional setting.

Conditions in institutions vary widely, but the enlightened philosophies that have developed in recent years provide the impetus for major institutional revamping. In general, there are indications of movement away from large, hospitallike, custodial institutions and toward smaller homelike cottage clusters, adequately staffed, and provided with classrooms, workshops, and recreational areas. Even after institutionalization, contact with the family is recommended and promoted. Vocational rehabilitation, physical rehabilitation, and special education are now considered necessary, integral parts of any comprehensive care plan for retarded persons, in or out of the institutional setting.

Early Recognition   Beyond treating the already retarded or disturbed child, much needs to be done at the levels of early recognition and special help for children with slow or deficient development. Phenylketonuria, galactosemia, and hypothyroidism are three conditions in which early detection can prevent irreversible damage. In deafness, blindness, poor motor coordination, hyperactivity, and aphasia, if intensive treatment efforts are brought to bear, future deficiencies may be minimized. Public health nurses may be in a particularly advantageous position to detect such problems in the community. Appropriate emotional counseling and support for children and their parents in cases of retardation detected early can head off many psychological difficulties. This may be an area for development of special expertise by the nursing profession, particularly the psychiatric nurse. To counsel effectively, nurses need to know the characteristics of retarded persons at various developmental stages. These are presented in Table 17–7.

Primary Prevention   The principal need in the area of Mental Retardation falls under primary prevention. Increasing efforts must be made throughout society to eliminate the host of factors responsible for this problem. Within the strict medical model, improvements in prenatal care, obstetrical practices, and pediatric care are indicated. Such changes are connected to social issues in that improved care must be extended into the poor communities where retardation occurs most frequently. Thus changes are a responsibility of voters and legislators as well. Genetic counseling has a definite role in prevention. General public education about retardation is also a mixed medical–societal responsibility. The community health nurse with an interest in psychiatry can aid in the prevention of Mental Retardation by disseminating information about the importance of regular prenatal checkups, the special relevance of certain diseases during pregnancy to the incidence of birth defects, and the significance of hereditary patterns.

Over and above the medical model, future efforts at the prevention of retardation require an improvement in the living standard for disadvantaged populations. This socioeconomic responsibility falls to all citizens, but any movement to achieve it may rely for some time to come on the health care community for its leadership and rationale.

ORGANIC BRAIN SYNDROMES

The Organic Brain Syndrome (OBS) is a confusing area to many psychiatric and medical professionals alike, and it is often neglected in training and treatment, sometimes with disastrous consequences. Clients suffering from OBS can often be misperceived as having some sophisticated psychiatric impairment that is causing a behavior change. Lacking proper treatment, they may die. (Conversely, a client with a treatable psychiatric disorder may be written off as having an irreversible progressive organic deterioration of the mental capacities.)

Relatively little attention has been paid to psychological approaches to clients suffering from Organic Mental Syndromes. While the field of geriatrics is growing in psychiatry, in many facilities treatments are mainly addressed to elderly clients who are mostly functional. Those who are more severely impaired cognitively are screened out of many programs by design (see Chapter 22).

Table 17-7   CHARACTERISTIC BEHAVIOR BY LEVEL OF RETARDATION AND DEVELOPMENTAL STAGE

Developmental Stage	Profoundly Retarded	Severely Retarded	Moderately Retarded	Mildly Retarded
Stage 1: Maturation and development (birth to five years)	Sensorimotor capabilities virtually absent, needs total nursing care	Minimal speech, motor abilities poor, little communication, little self-help training possible	Can communicate, has little social awareness, trainable in self-help, needs supervision	May be normal in communication and social skills, minimal sensorimotor deficiency
Stage 2: Training and education (six to twenty years)	Slight motor development reached, limited training in self-help possible	May communicate, can be trained in hygienic habits	Can learn social and occupational skills, academic level no higher than second grade, may move freely in limited areas	Academic skills to sixth grade level possible, social awareness may be fostered
Stage 3: Social and vocational adequacy (twenty-one years and over)	May develop rudimentary speech pattern, self-care capabilities do not preclude nursing care	Can aid in self-care but only under total supervision, can protect self in structured, monitored environment	Can do unskilled work in sheltered workshop, needs supervision for most stressful circumstances	Minimum self-support possible with social and vocational skills, stress requires support

Source: Adapted from U.S. Department of Health, Education, and Welfare, *Mental Retardation Activities* (Washington, D.C.: Government Printing Office, 1963), p. 2.

Organic Brain Syndromes are by no means phenomena of old age alone. Certain major physical conditions that lead to OBS occur with increased frequency among the elderly population, but the syndromes can complicate illnesses in all age groups.

Myths and Reality about Organic Causes of Psychiatric Symptoms

The relationship of organic variables to disturbances of behavior or emotion is exceedingly complex. Some commonly held but false beliefs about organic influences are:

- Organic factors are clearly secondary to environmental (social, learning, psychodynamic) influences in importance and relevance to psychiatric disorders.
- Conditions with a major organic contribution are largely intractable and therefore are outside the domain of psychiatry.
- Neurological causes of psychiatric disorders are rare.

- There are simple physical or laboratory criteria for establishing the presence or absence of neurological illness.
- Standard deficits are produced in mental status by all organic influences, so that the clinical features of an OBS are readily and easily defined.

Contrary to these myths, it is *crucial* to recognize organic influences on an individual's disturbed behavior or affective life, since a large number of psychiatric conditions with a predominant and detectable organic etiology are almost totally reversible. In fact, far from being rare, neurological illness accounts for up to 30 percent of all first admissions to psychiatric hospitals in the United States. Yet recognition is difficult because of the many ways in which organic factors can disrupt brain functioning and the myriad causes of OBS. The physical/neurological examination and the standard tests, including the electroencephalogram and computerized tomography scan (CT scan), may reflect wide variability even in the presence of real central nervous system disease. Likewise, the mental status examination of clients afflicted with OBS yields far from homogeneous results and can make detection a sophisticated, frustrating, yet essential enterprise (see Chapter 8).

The Organic–Functional Distinction   The distinction between organic and so-called functional disorders in psychiatry is more appropriately viewed as a continuum rather than a dichotomy. A functional disorder is usually considered to be an alteration in behavior or affective life that results from processes of learning that modify the brain through normal physiological mechanisms. In contrast, such a modification is viewed as organic if some change has occurred in the structure of the brain that tends to impair physiological functioning and consequently lessen the impact of learning processes, past, present, and future. Such a structural alteration can result from a destructive or discharging (seizure activity) lesion or a general biochemical change that impairs the normal transmission of nerve impulses through the brain's circuitry.

Holistic Views   The major thesis of this book is that the normal and deviant adaptations of human beings need to be seen in terms of systems incorporating all inputs and interconnections relevant to the individual's life situation. Holistic concepts of psychiatric disorder frequently lead to the conclusion that a host of factors may act in concert to determine the occurrence of a particular behavior or emotion. Such an approach must incorporate the role of physical illness, especially cerebral disorders, as potential etiological factors in cognitive and affective dysfunction.

In general, organic illness affects psychological functioning in one of two ways:

1. The Organic Mental Syndrome directly modifies brain functioning by either diffuse or localized damage to the cerebral structure or by metabolic derangement.

2. The individual may resort to maladaptive coping patterns in order to deal with the stress of illness. These patterns commonly present recognizable reactions, such as psychosis or neurosis, although they may be observed in less clearly definable but equally self-defeating patterns of behavior, such as denial of illness, noncompliance with medical treatment, and regressive dependence on loved ones or caretakers.

How a particular person responds to OBS depends on such factors as personality type, interpersonal relationships, past experiences, and the current environmental situation.

Problems from both sources are the domain of psychiatric professionals, because both cause alterations in the client's symbolic system. Alterations of the first kind involve damage to the substrate of symbolic processes, while the latter reactive patterns change the meanings attached to events in an attempt to cope with the realities and distress of illness itself.

Assessment

The assessment of organicity is a task relevant to psychological testing (see Chapter 8). Changes in cognitive functioning—alterations in the information processing systems of the brain—are usually interpreted as indicating organicity. Areas of impairment that identify organicity include:

- Attention span
- Concentration
- Language skills
- Memory
- Orientation
- Thinking
  a. Learning
  b. Abstraction
  c. Reasoning
  d. Concept formation

People with Organic Brain Syndromes usually manifest some degree of organicity as part of the clinical picture, but changes in behavior and emotion brought about by cerebral pathology are by no means limited to those commonly described as organicity.

M was a ninety-five-year-old female admitted to the hospital to await nursing home placement. Her seventy-two-year-old daughter, who had been caring for her, had herself been hospitalized for surgery. M was a pleasant member of the ward community, smiling and greeting clients and staff congenially. She did cause ward management problems, however, in that she could not remember the location of her room, the bathrooms, the dayrooms, etc. Although she greeted all personnel, she rarely knew anyone by name and frequently acted as if she were meeting ward personnel for the first time. She *insisted that she was in a hospital in Connecticut for a checkup, and she described her favorite activity as walking to the central staircase and looking down over the balcony into the lobby of the hospital to view its Renaissance art works. In fact she was in the most spartan of city hospital settings, with grey tile walls, locked doors, and barred windows. She also talked about the flowers outside, when it was the dead of winter. One day she said that she had grown up on an estate in Fairfield, Connecticut, while the next she told how she had been one of eight children living in a Lower East Side walk-up apartment. She could not count backwards from twenty to zero and, in fact, had to be reminded of the task. She thought that the proverb "People who live in glass houses shouldn't throw stones" referred to the fragility of glass walls and that apples and oranges were too dissimilar to have anything at all in common.*

M exhibited short-term memory loss, disorientation to place and time, confabulation (fabrication to fill memory gaps) in response to deficits, reduced attention span and concentration ability, and concrete thinking. Her assessment indicated organicity due to primary degenerative changes in her brain (Alzheimer's Disease).

The flavor of her Organic Brain Syndrome, however, suggested that M was finding it difficult to adjust to her lost life and was attempting to cope by conjuring up pleasant (real or imaginary) past memories to fill the void. Whether they were real or imaginary was less significant than their proper interpretation—as compensations for a present reality that was extremely disturbing to M. Her strengths may have been her vivid imagination and her sense of optimism. It seemed unnecessary for the ward staff to confront M with her fictions, since they did not interfere with her care or the well-being of other clients. Staff members did, however, push for M to be placed in a congenial nursing home atmosphere, and they stressed orienting experiences for M while she was hospitalized.

Classification

The classification of Organic Mental Syndromes, historically, has been riddled with ambiguities, which underscores how poorly such disorders have been understood by the medical/psychiatric community. The standard nomenclature of the American Psychiatric Association's Diagnostic and Statistical Manual (DSM–II [Committee on Nomenclature 1968]) defined OBS as a mental condition that can result only from *diffuse* impairment of brain tissue function. It divided such impairments into acute conditions—temporary and therefore reversible—and chronic conditions—permanent

and irreversible. Lastly, DSM–II attached labels distinguishing purported causative agents: degenerative, inflammatory, toxic, metabolic, traumatic, vascular, or neoplastic.

Several major problems existed in this schema of classification. First, it eliminated from consideration changes in mental or behavioral functioning that might result from a focal neurological disease. Secondly, the confusion that could result from the idiosyncratic use of the terms *acute* and *chronic* could be destructive to client care. Many fatal processes evolve suddenly, while many curable ones take months to develop. Potentially reversible causes of OBS are:

1. Vascular disorders
   a. Hemorrhage
   b. Hypertension
   c. Systemic lupus erythematosus
2. Infectious disorders
   a. Meningoencephalitis
   b. Brain abscess
   c. Tertiary syphilis
3. Traumatic disorders
   a. Hematoma
   b. Communicating hydrocephalus
4. Metabolic disorders
   a. Hepatic failure
   b. Renal failure
   c. Chronic obstructive pulmonary disease
   d. Electrolyte imbalance
   e. Inappropriate antidiuretic hormone
   f. Wilson's disease
5. Poisons
   a. Barbiturates
   b. Heavy metals
6. Endocrine disorders
   a. Thyroid disease
   b. Parathyroid disease
   c. Cushing's disease
   d. Addison's disease
   e. Hypoglycemia
7. Deficiency states
   a. Pernicious anemia
   b. Wernicke-Korsakoff's syndrome

Thus, the time course should not be equated with the prognosis. In addition, the reversibility of any pathological process is a relative, not an absolute, phenomenon.

The classification of Organic Brain Syndromes presented by Z. L. Lipowski (1975) stressed that brain impairment may be a global cognitive disruption or a disturbance limited to a portion of normal physiological functioning. Lipowski's classification had three main divisions:

1. Characterized by global cognitive impairment
   a. Delirium
   b. Subacute amnestic–confusional state
   c. Dementia
2. Characterized by selective psychological deficit or abnormality
   a. Amnestic syndrome
   b. Hallucinosis
   c. Personality and behavioral disorders
   d. Other limited cognitive or psychomotor disorders
3. Characterized by symptomatic functional impairment
   a. Schizophreniform syndrome
   b. Paranoid syndrome
   c. Depressive syndrome
   d. Manic syndrome

In general, focal lesions of the brain, often unclassified in standard terminology, receive appropriate attention here under the deficits of circumscribed nature. The course of onset is also distinguished, in this classification, from the prognosis.

The reclassification of mental disorders in the DSM-III incorporates much of the Lipowski classification schema into the sections on Organic Mental Disorders. Section 1 of the Organic Mental Disorders includes Organic Brain Syndromes whose etiology is associated with the aging process or a drug. The first group, called Dementias Arising in the Senium or Presenium, includes Primary Degenerative Dementia and Multi-infarct Dementia. The Substance-induced Organic Mental Disorders include diagnoses for all the types of brain syndromes encountered with various substances of abuse. There are separate classes of substances that include Alcohol, Barbiturates, Opioids, Cocaine, Amphetamines, Phencyclidine (PCP), Hallucinogens, Cannabis, Tobacco, and Caffeine. The syndromes themselves may be either Delerium, Dementia, Amnestic Syndrome, Delusional Syndrome, Hallucinosis, Affective Syndrome, Personality Syndrome, Intoxication, or Withdrawal, depending on the predominant clinical manifestations. These Substance-induced Organic Mental Disorders apply only when there is evidence of the direct effects of the drugs on the central nervous system.

Among the syndromes whose etiology is neither senility nor a drug-induced state, the classifications continue to distinguish qualitative types of deficits with the cause listed as a separate diagnosis from the International Classification for Diseases (ICD–9) on Axis III of the multiaxial evaluation system. This section of the DSM–III is:

293.00 Delirium
294.10 Dementia
294.00 Amnestic Syndrome
293.81 Organic Delusional Syndrome
293.82 Hallucinosis
293.83 Organic Affective Syndrome
310.10 Organic Personality Syndrome
294.80 Other or Mixed Organic Brain Syndrome

The reclassification efforts reflect the general dissatisfaction and inaccuracy of the former method in addition to a positive orientation toward classification according to type of deficit.

Table 17–8 summarizes the differences between the two global syndromes Delirium and Dementia. Among the syndromes with more circumscribed impairment, Amnestic Syndrome applies to losses of memory, due to organic factors, when other cognitive processes are relatively intact. Organic pathology tends to impair recent memory more than long-term memory. Confabulation may characterize a client who is attempting to deny or cover up a memory deficiency. Thiamine deficiency associated with alcoholism (formerly called Korsakoff's syndrome) is an example of a cause of an organic Amnestic Syndrome. Delusional Syndromes, Hallucinosis, and Affective Syndromes are, as their names imply, characterized predominantly by delusions, hallucinations, and manic or depressive symptoms, respectively. In these syndromes, *all* cognitive capacities may be spared and the organic etiology missed if a clinician was looking for the hallmark signs of traditional "organicity." In Personality Syndrome, there is emotional lability, impaired impulse control, apathy, suspiciousness, and other signs of personality change that can be traced to an organic cause. Differ-

	Table 17-8 CLINICAL FEATURES OF GLOBAL ORGANIC BRAIN SYNDROMES	
Feature	**Delirium**	**Dementia**
Onset	Acute	Either acute or insidious
Level of consciousness	Clouding with either hyperactivity or somnolence	No clouding
Cognitive impairment	Fluctuating, worse at night	Severe, recent memory impaired first
Disorientation	Present	Absent
Electroencephalogram pattern	Slowing	Unreliable, may be normal
Special characteristics	Disturbance of sleep pattern, hallucinations, delusions, incoherence	Impaired abstract thinking and judgment, evidence of cerebral cortical dysfunction, personality change
Prognosis	Depends on cause	Depends on cause

ent disease processes, often those that affect focal areas of the brain, tend to result in these heterogeneous brain syndromes. Figure 17-6 depicts the areas of brain damage that are related to various behavior changes and psychiatric symptoms.

Syndromes

This section briefly describes significant aspects of several classic illnesses encountered in medicine that can cause Organic Brain Syndromes. More elaborate discussions may be found in the further reading recommended at the end of the chapter.

Acute Intermittent Porphyria   Disorders involving the substance porphyrin, which is involved in cellular metabolism throughout the body, are commonly misdiagnosed because of their unusual and varied clinical presentations. This relatively rare disease may affect several members of the same family. Classically, females are more affected than males. Attacks, characterized by abdominal pain, are induced by ingestion of certain kinds of drugs, including barbiturates, alcohol, and sulfa drugs. Hypertension, photosensitive skin, peripheral neuropathy, and muscle wasting are physical signs. A wide variety of behaviors mimicking neurotic and psychotic states may occur with an attack. The urine turns maroon when exposed to sunlight. Treatment consists of chlorpromazine (Thorazine) for abdominal pain and prophylactic avoidance of precipitating drugs.

C was a nineteen-year-old woman with a history of behavior problems throughout her adolescence. Both mother and father complained that she kept bad company and had a very lax attitude toward school. They feared she was rather heavily into the drug and alcohol scene in their community. Attempts at setting limits were met with a variety of temper tantrums and manipulations.

Shortly after one such confrontation, C complained of feeling weak, with pain in her stomach and numbness in her fingers and toes. At first her parents were unconcerned, as it was typical of C to "invent" some symptoms of illness in order to evoke guilt in her parents and get them to soften their stance. The symptoms progressed, however, and after several days C seemed beside herself with pain. At the emergency room, the intern requested psychiatric consultation on hearing the story. At first the psychiatrist suspected hysterical conversion symptoms. Finally the client was able to confide to the psychiatrist that she feared she was bleeding following her last episode of intercourse, because her urine was dark red. The client was admitted to the medical service, where the urine was actually found to contain porphyrins, and the diagnosis of acute intermittent porphyria was made.

Addison's Disease   Adrenal cortical insufficiency may cause organic mental changes that are largely affective (anxiety or depression) or that are more frankly psychotic. Physical symptoms of Addison's disease in-

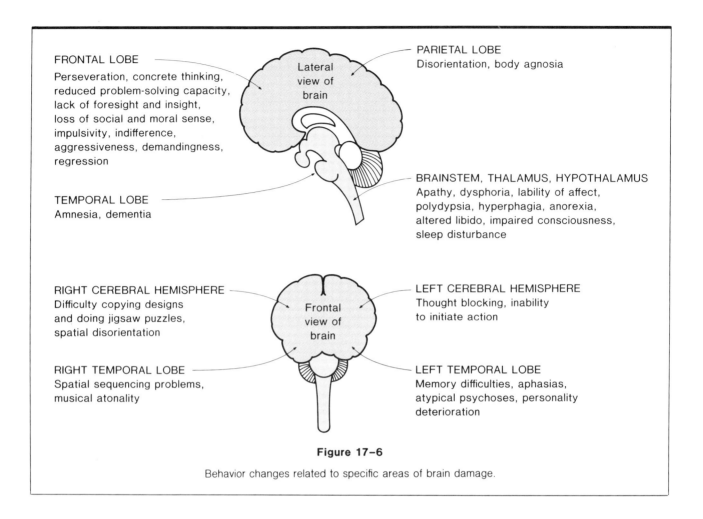

FRONTAL LOBE
Perseveration, concrete thinking, reduced problem-solving capacity, lack of foresight and insight, loss of social and moral sense, impulsivity, indifference, aggressiveness, demandingness, regression

TEMPORAL LOBE
Amnesia, dementia

PARIETAL LOBE
Disorientation, body agnosia

BRAINSTEM, THALAMUS, HYPOTHALAMUS
Apathy, dysphoria, lability of affect, polydypsia, hyperphagia, anorexia, altered libido, impaired consciousness, sleep disturbance

Lateral view of brain

RIGHT CEREBRAL HEMISPHERE
Difficulty copying designs and doing jigsaw puzzles, spatial disorientation

RIGHT TEMPORAL LOBE
Spatial sequencing problems, musical atonality

LEFT CEREBRAL HEMISPHERE
Thought blocking, inability to initiate action

LEFT TEMPORAL LOBE
Memory difficulties, aphasias, atypical psychoses, personality deterioration

Frontal view of brain

Figure 17–6

Behavior changes related to specific areas of brain damage.

clude anorexia, weight loss, nausea, vomiting, and diarrhea. A classic sign is a bluish hyperpigmentation of skin and buccal mucosa. Hypoglycemia, electrolyte disturbances, and hypotension complicate adrenal crises. Treatment depends on the cause of the decrease in adrenal steroid output (whether it is bacterial or fungal infection, surgical removal, hemorrhage, or systemic disease such as amyloidosis or scleroderma) and the extent of the damage that has occurred before detection.

Amyotrophic Lateral Sclerosis   Amyotrophic lateral sclerosis, or Lou Gehrig's disease, is a degenerative neurological disease of unknown etiology, with an adult onset, that affects the pyramidal tracts of the spinal cord and results in abnormalities of motor function. Cranial and spinal lower motor neurons may be affected, leading to muscle weakness, atrophy fasciculations, and diminished tone of the facial musculature and proximal extremities. Although cases of mental changes are somewhat rare, there are a significant number of reported disturbances of mood, affect, social behavior, and reality testing associated with the

disease. Nursing interventions are generally supportive.

Bacterial Infections   Acute bacterial infections of the central nervous system in the form of meningitis, encephalitis, and brain abscess produce classic physical signs as well as acute mental changes characteristic of delirium. There is a sudden onset of fever, headache, and stiff neck as well as confusion, disorientation, disturbed consciousness, and sometimes wild behavioral deviation. Chronic infections, such as those associated with brucellosis, tuberculosis, or syphilis, on the other hand, have a gradual onset and may be detected only because of the associated emotional or behavioral changes such as depression, insomnia, or psychosis. Successful treatment depends, in either case, on prompt identification of the offending organisms so that the appropriate antibiotic therapy can be instituted.

Cerebral Vascular Disease   Atherosclerosis, hypertension, thrombosis, hemorrhage, and autoimmune and/or collagen vascular disease may all produce varying degrees of altered cerebral functioning. Atherosclerosis presents as progressive impairment of memory, orientation, intellectual efficiency, and judgment, as well as emotional lability in an older person, frequently with a history of hypertension, diabetes, and angina. With thrombosis, hemorrhage, or embolism, the dramatic physical changes dominate the clinical picture. Coma or convulsions are more common central nervous system effects than psychosis. A collagen vascular disease such as periarteritis nodosa or systemic lupus erythematosus (SLE), on the other hand, more commonly presents with organic psychosis. Such symptoms may respond to the steroids used to treat the overall illness or may require additional use of antipsychotic medication (see Chapter 23).

Cushing's Disease   An excess of adrenal cortical hormones such as that associated with glandular tumor, hyperplasia, or iatrogenic administration of cortisone-type drugs produces a syndrome known as Cushing's disease. Clients may exhibit euphoria, heightened sense of well-being, or mania, with or without psychosis. Physically, the clients characteristically have a round face, thick neck, obese trunk, and accumulated fat on the shoulders, arms, and legs. Hirsutism, thin, easily bruised skin, and purple striae on the thighs and abdomen are common. The diagnosis is made by measuring the levels of steroids excreted in the urine, which are elevated when the disease is present. Depending on the cause, treatment may be surgical removal or stopping the administration of exogenous agents.

D was an eighteen-year-old woman who had been treated in the medical clinic for two years for systemic lupus erythematosus. On several occasions she had been quite ill, suffering kidney involvement necessitating hospitalization. Eventually, however, she would respond to prednisone treatment and recover. Her life was a shambles, however. She was forced to drop out of school because of long absences due to sickness. Because of her overall weakened condition, she could not keep up with her friends, who were attending parties, discos, etc.

D's main source of nurturance and gratification was her family. She had had an especially close relationship with her father. Then suddenly he was killed in a car accident coming home from work. For two weeks D was profoundly depressed. Then, rather suddenly, she shook off her depression and seemed almost elated, contacting friends, buying new clothes and records, and staying up very late at night. Within two weeks she needed

admission to the medical service as her physical condition had deteriorated. Her dose was raised from thirty to fifty milligrams of prednisone per day. Her renal status improved as a result, but she became more manic. D was transferred to psychiatry, where the treatment team faced three alternative conclusions: (1) that D's lupus had evolved to affect the central nervous system, as it does in advanced cases; (2) that the treatment for the lupus (the prednisone) was causing an organic affective syndrome; or (3) that D was suffering from a manic episode precipitated by the death of her father.

It was considered unwise to reduce the steroids, due to the severity of D's kidney condition. The team elected to attempt to deal with D's loss and to manage her behavior with drugs when necessary. D soon became a major ward figure. Although she remained manic, she was well liked by the ward staff members, who felt attached to and involved with her. After six months, however, D's physical condition deteriorated. She was transferred to the intensive care unit, and she died. A definitive diagnosis was never made, but the treatment team members felt that their interventions had lessened D's burden during her final months.

Diabetes Mellitus   Diabetes may cause changes in mental functioning. Some reported symptoms include fatigability, irritability, and impotence. There are diagnostic curves for the glucose tolerance test, and treatment is in the domain of the internist.

Hepatic Encephalopathy   Damage to liver cells for any reason can cause organic brain changes. This is essentially an example of an endogenous toxin, in this case ammonia, affecting cerebral functioning. Liver disease (such as alcoholic cirrhosis), severe hepatitis, or common bile duct stones can lead to hepatic failure. Physical signs of liver disease include telangiectasia, ascites, esophageal varices, caput medusae, flapping tremor of hands, and jaundice. Mental status changes range from confusion and apathy to disorientation and psychosis, with coma as a preterminal event.

Huntington's Chorea   A hereditary disease with an onset in adult life (ages twenty-five to fifty), Huntington's chorea is a syndrome of progressive mental deterioration and a jerking movement of the face and limbs. In its incipient stages, the organic mental changes are reflected either in mood disturbances or in impulsive, erratic, or irresponsible behavior. Only in the later stages does the dementia develop. In addition to choreiform movements, the client has speech difficulties and an ataxic, drunken gait. The family history may confirm the diagnosis, since Huntington's is passed to half the children of an affected parent (it has a dominant mode of inheritance).

R was a twenty-six-year-old man who first came to the attention of a psychiatric clinic as a result of a court referral. He had had a history of delinquent behavior during adolescence, including stealing, truancy, and drug abuse. In his twenties, R became involved in petty crime, which led to several arrests. Court social service agencies had seen him on numerous occasions but were convinced he was incorrigible. Most recently R had been the only one caught when a group held up a local grocery store, as he was slow to perceive that the police had been alerted. He was referred for psychiatric exam because he seemed strangely unconcerned about his arrest and appeared quite "nervous" to the magistrate.

R's family history revealed that he never knew who his father was and had been raised by an elderly grandmother because his mother worked. In an interview with the mother, however, the psychiatrist discovered that the father had not left but had been confined in a mental hospital when R was two years old and eventually died there when R was 10. This was a long-kept family secret.

The psychiatrist observed that R was unable to do arithmetic calculations, had a poor memory, and manifested nervousness with facial grimaces and tics and some involuntary shoulder shrugging. The tentative diagnosis was Huntington's chorea.

This case illustrates that, even when there is an organic illness, social and environmental factors may appear to account for the psychiatric disturbance. Mental health workers are more likely to respond to the psychological aspects of a client's history and ignore physiological elements.

Hyperthyroidism   Psychiatric symptoms can be the most notable abnormalities in a thyrotoxic client. These may include restlessness, tremulousness, agitation, and acute delirious states. Because it is a hypermetabolic state, hyperthyroidism causes physical changes in many organ systems, making diagnosis easier. Warm moist skin, accelerated heart rate, increased appetite, weight loss, heat intolerance, exophthalmos, myopathy, and a palpable thyroid constitute the classic syndrome. Laboratory tests such as basal metabolic rate (BMR) and protein-bound iodine (PBI) confirm the diagnosis.

Hypothyroidism   The decreased thyroid functioning of myxedema may also alter mental status. Usually the myxedematous client shows slow emotional responses, impaired memory, and slow calculation ability. In severe cases a dementia may develop. Physical changes classically include: thickened, dry skin; coarse, sparse hair; hoarse voice; cold intolerance; bradycardia; edema; hyporeflexia; and deafness. Treatment involves thyroid hormone replacement.

Idiopathic Spontaneous Hypoglycemia   This syndrome is often mistaken for a purely functional psychiatric condition. Idiopathic spontaneous hypoglycemia is hereditary and not necessarily related to stress. A client can experience marked changes in behavior and mood and appear acutely intoxicated as the blood sugar falls below sixty milligrams percent. Carbohydrate ingestion rapidly relieves the symptoms.

Jacob-Crutzfeldt Disease   A type of presenile dementia called Jacob–Crutzfeldt disease may be caused by a slowly developing viral invasion of the pyramidal and extrapyramidal tracts. Onset can occur in the third decade of life. The dementia is characterized by memory loss, reduced intellectual functioning, speech difficulties, deterioration of social appropriateness, and perceptual problems such as blindness and hallucinations. The neurological changes are so-called long tract signs, such as muscle wasting, hyperreflexia, clonus, and positive Babinski's reflex.

Korsakoff's Syndrome   Korsakoff's syndrome is a condition resulting from prolonged use of alcohol. Its direct cause is a deficiency of the vitamin thiamine from the poor dietary habits of some chronic alcoholics. The classical signs of Korsakoff's syndrome are global memory loss and striking confabulation. In DSM-III, Korsakoff's syndrome is called Alcohol-induced Amnestic Disorder.

Multiple Sclerosis   Also known as disseminated sclerosis, this degeneration of cerebral tissue is characterized by diffuse neurological symptoms, due to demyelination of nerve fibers in many areas of the nervous system. The symptoms tend to wax and wane rather than progress steadily. It is rare for frank psychosis, delirium, or dementia to occur, but emotional instability is commonly encountered and may well have an organic component. There is no treatment for the disease itself, only for its symptoms.

Neoplasms   Intracranial tumors of any variety can produce mental changes ranging from exaggeration of preexisting personality traits to dementia or delusions. Frequently, the type of mental symptom helps localize the tumor in the brain. For example, apathy or the progressive loss of intellectual functions suggests frontal lobe pathology, while memory loss, fear, depersonalization, déjà vu (paramnesia), derealization, temper outbursts, and olfactory hallucinations are indicative of a temporal lobe lesion. Body image changes, ignoring part of the body, loss of sense of direction, and visual hallucinations usually indicate a parietal lobe problem. Flashing lights correlate with occipital tumors. Diagnostic physical findings usually relate to each location as well, when tumors reach significant size. Treatment is surgical.

Neurofibromatosis This condition, also known as von Recklinghausen's disease, affects the skin and the central nervous system. It is inherited through dominant genes. Although there are gross neurological and dermatological findings, such as nodules, polyps, nevi, café au lait spots, sensory loss, and nerve deafness, the first signs may be altered behavior—hyperirritability, erratic behavior of abrupt onset, or even florid psychosis. The condition usually leads to increased intracranial pressure and seizures.

Parathyroid Hyperfunction Tumors of the parathyroid, both benign and malignant, and cellular hyperplasia cause excess production of parathyroid hormone. This elevates the blood calcium, which leads to manifestations of organic mental syndrome. There may be alterations in mood, such as depression, impairment of intellectual abilities, stupor, or psychosis. Some clients who complain of weakness, irritability, and bone pain may be mistaken as neurotic. Physically there are signs of calcium deposits in the conjunctiva and eyelids, as well as facial palsy, auditory impairment, and possibly hypertension. Treatment may involve surgical removal of a tumor.

Parathyroid Hypofunction Hypoparathyroidism may result from surgical removal of the parathyroid glands, either for the treatment of hyperfunction or accidentally (for example, in thyroid surgery), from dietary deficiencies of calcium or vitamin D, or from malabsorption in the intestines. In general, hypocalcemia leads to excitable central nervous system states that may manifest themselves as acute delirium, complete with agitation, disorientation, confusion, and hallucinations; mainly intellectual deterioration; odd or neurotic behavior; catatonia; or convulsions. Physical examination reveals hair loss, dry skin, deterioration of the teeth, cataracts, and signs of tetany—in other words, Trousseau's and Chvostek's signs. Treatment is ac-

complished by replacing parathormone, giving vitamin D, or giving calcium lactate.

Pellagra This condition is associated with "the three Ds": dermatitis, diarrhea, and dementia. Its cause is dietary deficiency of nicotinic acid, which can occur in alcoholics or in a population with very poor nutrition. In addition to the classical signs of dementia, symptoms include a swollen tongue, pathological sucking and grasping reflexes, decreased deep tendon reflexes (DTRs), rigidity, and pain corresponding to nerve pathways. Treatment is with nicotinic acid.

Pheochromocytoma Pheochromocytoma is a tumor of the adrenal medulla that causes excess norepinephrine production. It leads to anxiety and other personality changes that are organically determined. The physical signs of hypertension, pallor, sweating, and orthostatic hypotension strongly suggest the diagnosis. It can be cured by surgery.

Pituitary Hyperfunction Various types of tumors can cause increased secretion of pituitary hormones, and some of these lead to psychiatric signs and symptoms. They may be affective, behavioral, sexual (impotence, reduced libido), or perceptual/cognitive. Correct assessment is based on the presence of physical signs, especially bitemporal hemianopsia, dimished visual acuity, various endocrine organ malfunctions, including hypothalamic malfunction, and perhaps the rough, enlarged facial features and hands of the classic pituitary giant. Tumors can be ablated by X ray or surgery.

Pituitary Hypofunction A tumor, an infarction, bleeding, trauma, infection, irradiation, and surgery all can lead to undersecretion of pituitary hormone. If the condition occurs from hemorrhage and shock to a mother postpartum, it is referred to as Simmonds' disease. When a client is on steroid therapy for another condition, the pituitary may be suppressed and produce too little hormone. Clients complain of headache, appetite loss, low sexual drive, weakness, easy fatigability, irritability, and depression. They may become psychotic. Physically there is regression of sexual organs and secondary sex characteristics. The condition may be mistaken for anorexia nervosa.

Primary Degeneration of the Corpus Callosum This unusual hereditary degeneration, also known as Marchiafava's disease, occurs only in middle-aged Italian males. It seems to require a history of con-

| | | | Table 17–9 CLASSIFICATION OF TYPES OF EPILEPSY | | |
Type	Age of Onset	Signs and Symptoms	EEG Abnormality Between Seizures
Generalized			
Grand mal	One to fifteen years	Aura, unconsciousness, tonic-clonic seizure	20 percent abnormal awake 40 percent abnormal asleep
Petit mal	Five years	No aura, two-to fifteen-second lapse of consciousness, blinking, twitching	85 percent abnormal awake 90 percent abnormal asleep
Focal			
Jacksonian	Often posttraumatic	Begins in thumb or face, motor or sensory march of symptoms	30 percent abnormal awake 60 percent abnormal asleep
Psychomotor	Twenty years	Behavior and personality changes, lip-smacking	20 percent abnormal awake 80 percent abnormal asleep
Other	One to six years	Aura, focal movements or twitching related to localization	20 percent abnormal awake 80 percent abnormal asleep
Hypothalamic	Fifteen years	Rage attacks, emotional, sensory, and vegetative aura	8 percent abnormal awake 90 percent abnormal asleep

siderable intake of red wine, as well. The psychiatric symptoms are dramatic manifestations of paranoia, hypomanic behavior, or conversely, apathy progressing to dementia. Physically the motor system is impaired, there is aphasia, and convulsions occur.

Primary Degenerative Dementia: Alzheimer's Disease   These dementias involve atrophy of the cerebral cortex that can begin at a relatively young age (forty to sixty). Symptoms are characteristic of diseases affecting the cortex. Clients have problems with speech, motor coordination, recognition of familiar objects (even parts of their own bodies), and naming. Mental functions deteriorate slowly but progressively, leading to reduced intellectual capacity, impaired memory, loss of social sense, and apathy or restlessness. These may at first be mistaken for an involutional depression. Brain tests such as pneumoencephalograms reveal cortical atrophy. Seizures may complicate the picture.

Psychomotor Epilepsy   This form of epilepsy, affecting the temporal lobes, deserves special attention, since the signs of an attack are not as grossly evident as other grand mal types. Because it produces mainly bizarre behavior changes, it is commonly mistaken as a nonorganic psychiatric problem. Temporal lobe attacks may manifest themselves as aggressive outbursts, as psychotic episodes, as automatism, as trance or Amnestic Syndromes, or as affective states such as depres-

sion. Clients may report symptoms of visual, auditory, or olfactory hallucinations, derealization, or déjà vu. Sometimes attacks will be accompanied by observable lip smacking, incoherent speech, and involuntary purposeful movements. Electroencephalogram abnormalities are detectable in the temporal lobe. Clients may or may not have tumors. These fits, like other epilepsies, can be controlled with medications. Table 17–9 presents characteristics of the various types of epilepsy.

Subacute Combined Degeneration   Combined systems disease affects both motor and sensory systems of the central nervous system. Its cause is insufficient absorption of vitamin B_{12}, as in the disease pernicious anemia. The mental changes run the gamut of organically induced psychiatric syndromes, from irritability and negativism to paranoia, memory loss, and frank psychosis. Clients also complain of numbness and tingling in the extremities and pain in the legs. They exhibit loss of position and vibration sense, positive Romberg sign, spastic/ataxic gait, either hyper- or hyporeflexia, and prematurely grey hair. Genetic factors contribute to incidence, as the disease occurs more commonly in blue-eyed Scandinavian females than any other group, and runs in families. Treatment is with vitamin B_{12}.

Subdural Hematoma   A person who is suffering from bleeding around the surface of the brain may present a confusing clinical picture, and misdiagnosis may prove fatal. Especially when the onset is rather insidious, accurate recognition may be difficult. Bleeding may occur in an elderly person after a small injury to the head, and all that may be detectable is irritability, occasional memory lapses, and periodic mutism. The condition can progress, however, to loss of consciousness, coma, and death. Physical signs of a subdural hematoma include papilledema, unequal pupils, hemiparesis on the opposite side, increased DTRs, and positive Babinski's reflex. Electroencephalograms, X rays, brain scans, computerized axial tomography (CAT) scans, and possibly arteriography may be needed to establish and localize the lesion.

Sydenham's Chorea   People who have had rheumatic fever as children may develop Sydenham's chorea in their teens. It occurs more often in females. The mental symptoms, which can be dramatic in severe cases, may be the initial complaints. These range from apathy and irritability to what appears to be a manic episode. The physical signs are rapid shaking of the tongue, palate, and extremities, protrusion of the tongue, and facial grimacing. Onset of the syndrome may be provoked by pregnancy, and the condition may be mistaken for a bizarre conversion hysteria secondary to pregnancy during adolescence.

Tuberous Sclerosis   Epiloia or tuberous sclerosis is a disease of the myelin sheaths of nervous tissue in which lesions are scattered throughout the brain. Distinctive physical signs include skin lesions consisting of swollen sebaceous glands that appear over the nose and cheeks as bumps. In addition to intellectual retardation and seizures, clients may exhibit psychotic symptoms. Adolescents are frequently affected, and there appears to be a familial tendency.

Wernicke's Encephalopathy   When the thiamine deficiency of excessive alcohol use leads to lesions in the midbrain, the resulting syndrome is called Wernicke's encephalopathy. Classically, on physical examination there is paralysis of lateral gaze of the external ocular muscles, nystagmus, ptosis of the eyelids, tremor, ataxia, dysmetria, and visual problems. On mental status examination, the client may appear apathetic, indifferent, and disoriented, suffering memory loss, hallucinations, or confusion. Thiamine is therapeutic.

Wilson's Disease   Hepatolenticular degeneration or Wilson's disease is caused by deficient metabolism of copper, which then accumulates in the central nervous system, eyes, and brain. This is generally a familial disease. Dysfunction of the basal ganglia of the brain gives rise to extrapyramidal tract symptoms, such as muscular rigidity, flapping tremor of the arms, and masklike face. A greenish-brown ring around the cornea of the eye, the Kayser-Fleischer ring, confirms the diagnosis. Cirrhosis of the liver occurs. Behavior abnormalities may be dramatic, closely resembling schizophrenia. Chelating drugs, which bind copper and promote excretion, may alleviate some of the damage.

Intervention

Organic illness, specifically cerebral disease, can influence or induce psychological disruption in multiple dimensions. Figure 17–7 summarizes the main features of the processes potentially at work. Any plan for intervention must take into account each of the possible mechanisms of pathogenesis.

Typically, the medical community directs the bulk of its efforts at the structural and metabolic damage induced by the injury or illness. The procedures focus on diagnosis and medical/surgical treatment of this damage. Psychiatric professionals cannot afford to neglect this area when dealing with Organic Mental Disorders, as we noted above. Greater attention is now being paid to the influences exerted by more subtle physiological/psychological pathways, such as sleep regulation, sensory integration, and body image perception. With Organic Mental Syndromes, a considerable portion of the disturbance observed may be psychological; however, this tends to be neglected, especially in medical circles.

Limiting Physical Damage   Prompt diagnosis and treatment of organic insults are mandatory, if a treatment exists. In general, the factors that determine the extent of damage fall in both controllable and uncontrollable categories. Usually the insult or injury is what gives rise to medical attention, so that the level—for example, the amount of toxic substance ingested or the extent of damage due to trauma—is already an accomplished fact. In some cases, however, one of several factors in a multiple-disease process can be eliminated, relieving a portion of the cognitive or affective impairment. Such a situation might involve restoring electrolyte imbalance, increasing oxygenation, or providing glucose to an elderly person with a Primary Degenerative Dementia, for instance. The speed of an impairing organic process can sometimes be slowed by prompt, effective medical intervention, thus preventing some potential damage. In the case of trauma, for example, further damage due to brain edema might be

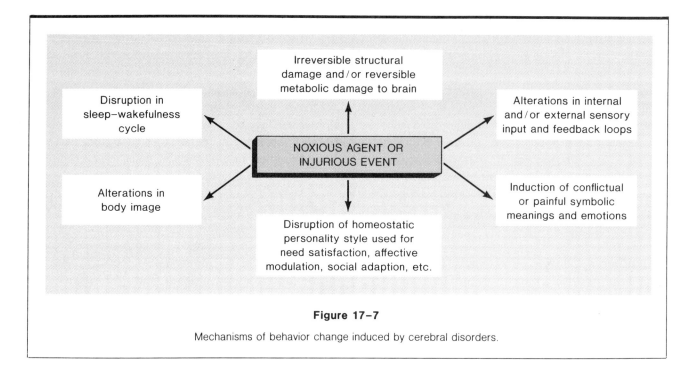

Figure 17-7

Mechanisms of behavior change induced by cerebral disorders.

avoided. Likewise, the length of time the pathology exists usually bears a direct relationship to the eventual deficits; thus, these can be reduced by prompt medical care.

The nurse, as the continuously observing arm of the treatment team, can play a major role in early detection. Careful assessment should be made of the mental status of all clients, in emergency rooms, medical wards, community centers, and nursing homes, each day or even each shift. Accurate recording of observations about clients in charts provides a cumulative record of the progression of any mental or physical process. If the notes are methodical, clear, and illustrative, the pathological process can be diagnosed more easily (see Chapter 8.)

Dealing with Psychological Concomitants   Not only does the injurious agent determine the extent of impairment, but also other conditions or situations affecting the individual tend to contribute to the final clinical picture. These include:

- Age
- Physiological vulnerability
- Personality style
- Sleep deprivation
- Chronic systemic disease
- Brain damage
- Current affective state

Some of these factors are fundamentally psychological. In particular, an individual's personality style and current emotional state can greatly influence the outcome of an organic illness. Highly controlling individuals can have terrible difficulties being sick and, therefore, feel relatively helpless and dependent. In their frame of reference, they are failing at the most basic of levels. People who are depressed or under stress are likely to be unable to mobilize the resources necessary to cope or likely to exhaust them rapidly and become overwhelmed by an illness. In such a case, the organic component may well produce a greater deficit, a more protracted course, and often a poorer outcome. To such people, illness represents just one more in a series of seemingly inevitable blows leading to further demoralization. Interventions by the psychiatric nurse to balance such unfavorable circumstances, at the level of the individual's symbolic processes, can be significantly beneficial. In medical settings, nursing homes, community health facilities, and mental health centers, a considerable proportion of the responsibility for such intervention may fall to the nurse.

Mr. M was a sixty-two-year-old male, president of a local bank, who was rushed to the medical center following the sudden onset of a severe left-sided headache and weakness of the right arm and leg, which had caused him to fall while running to a taxi. Mr. M was a very successful businessman whose life-long drive to the top of his profession was seldom slowed. He had suffered a myocardial infarction at age fifty-seven but fully recovered from it. At that time, it had been hard to get him to stay in the hospital for more than ten days, and he insisted on being back on the job one month after the attack.

In the intensive care unit, Mr. M's strength appeared to be coming back gradually, but he continued to have difficulty expressing himself. The hospital staff wanted to work Mr. M up for an evolving stroke versus transient ischemic attacks. Mr. M was very uncooperative about this, and verbally abused doctors and nurses alike. Although unsure of which hospital he was in, he accused the staff of just wanting to make more money for the hospital.

The hospital liaison psychiatric nurse brought in Mr. M's wife in an attempt to quiet him and enlist his cooperation. He immediately recognized her and became more settled and willing to listen. With the help of the liaison nurse, Mrs. M persuaded her husband to stay in the hospital. She assured him that she was quite able to manage in the home and that his job would undoubtedly be waiting for him when he was discharged.

Mr. M's reaction to the organic insult was based on his need to control his environment. This need was being thwarted both by his illness and by hospital personnel. Also underlying his behavior was considerable fear that he was gravely ill and perhaps even dying. Supportive interventions based on understanding these factors made Mr. M amenable to appropriate medical care.

Variables Affecting Client Response to Treatment   Certain variables of a psychological nature that nurses may be able to control can affect the processes associated with organic brain disease adversely or positively. These factors include:

- *The level of sensory input to clients.* In both health and sickness there appears to be an optimum level of sensory input for maintaining equilibrium. When the brain is impaired organically, equilibrium becomes increasingly precarious. Too great or too little sensory input can precipitate further cognitive, perceptual, and affective deterioration. The stimulus overload that is frequent in intensive care settings and the stimulus deprivation that may typify the rooms or wards of a hospital are both to be avoided.

- *The degree of social isolation experienced by clients.* When an already impaired person has little or no contact with caretaking personnel or family, the impairments tend to worsen. Clients with Organic Mental Syndromes need contacts with other human beings, especially well-known family members. The contacts may be rather simple and uncomplicated, but they must be frequent and reliable.

- *The unfamiliarity of the environment to clients.* The hospital stay can be a terrifying experience for the confused or disoriented person simply because of its strangeness. Due to the nature of organic impairments, such clients need a setting that is as readily recognizable as possible. The sick person often cannot be adequately maintained at home, but the hospital room might be furnished with some favorite items from home. Family members again can bridge the gap between home and hospital. Ideally, they might spend nights with the client in the hospital.

- *The interpersonal network available to clients.* All persons need a loving, reliable, and supportive social network around them, and this is especially true of sick people. The nurse may find fostering favorable interactions to be a simple or exceedingly complex task, depending on the preexisting relationships, the relative strength of the clients and those close to them, and the reactions of all involved to the distress of the illness. Interventions might range from simple explanations about the nature of the illness and suggestions about what might be helpful to full-fledged family therapy (see Chapter 21).

KEY NURSING CONCEPTS

✔ Many disorders presenting to the health team display a complex intermingling of physiological and psychological facets.

✔ Health care providers too often neglect the psychological needs of clients who present with physical symptoms, and ignoring these psychological components of illness can seriously undermine the effectiveness of medical treatment.

✔ Clients with diagnosis of Psychophysiological Disorder, Organic Brain Syndrome, or Mental Retardation are frequently considered undesirable treatment choices by mental health practitioners.

✔ Syndromes in which physical and psychological factors interact by means of "feedback loops" include ulcer, bowel disorders, cardiovascular disorders, asthma, arthritis, allergy, eating disorders, headache, and endocrine disorders.

✔ The humanistic symbolic interactionist approach of psychotherapy to clients who have psychophysiological disorders focuses on the communication aspect of their psychiatric symptoms: successful treatment necessitates discovering the meaning expressed through the client's symptom pattern.

✔ Prenatal, perinatal, postnatal, and sociocultural factors may cause Mental Retardation.

✔ Primary and secondary prevention are essential, though underdeveloped, intervention modes with the mentally retarded.

✔ Effective management of the retarded individual is based on flexibility and a treatment plan geared to changing problem areas during the life cycle.

✔ Psychological approaches to client's suffering Organic Brain Syndrome have received little attention from health care professionals.

✔ A large number of psychiatric conditions with organic etiology are almost totally reversible.

✔ Intervention in organic illness includes prompt limitation of physical damage and attention to psychological concomitants.

✔ Variables affecting client response to treatment include level of sensory input to the client, degree of social isolation, unfamiliarity of the environment, and the interpersonal network available to the client.

References

Abraham, K. *Selected Papers in Psychoanalysis.* London: Hogarth Press, 1927.

Alexander, F. *Psychosomatic Medicine: Its Principles and Application.* New York: W. W. Norton, 1950.

American Association of Mental Deficiency. *A Manual on Terminology and Classification,* Willimantic, Conn.: American Association on Mental Deficiency, 1961.

American Psychiatric Association. *Diagnostic and Statistical Manual of Mental Disorders.* 3d ed. Washington, D.C.: American Psychiatric Association, 1980.

Committee on Nomenclature and Statistics of the American Psychiatric Association. *DSM-II: Diagnostic and Statistical Manual of Mental Disorders.* 2d ed. Washington, D.C.: American Psychiatric Association, 1968.

Ferenczi, S. *Further Contributions to the Theory and Techniques of Psychoanalysis.* Compiled by J. Rickman. London: Hogarth Press, 1926.

Friedman, M. *Pathogenesis of Coronary Artery Disease.* New York: McGraw-Hill, 1969.

Friedman, M., and Rosenman, R. H. "Association of Specific Overt Behavior Pattern with Blood and Cardiovascular Findings: Blood Cholesterol Level, Blood Clotting Time, Incidence of Arcus Senilis, and Clinical Coronary Artery Disease." *Journal of the American Medical Association* 169 (1959): 1286.

Freud, S. "Fragment of an Analysis of a Case of Hysteria." In *Standard Edition of the Complete Works of Sigmund Freud.* London: Hogarth Press, 1953.

Lipowski, Z. L. "Organic Brain Syndromes: Overview and Clarification." In *Psychiatric Aspects of Neurological Disease,* edited by D. F. Benson and D. Blumer, pp. 11–35. New York: Grune and Stratton, 1975.

Piaget, J. *The Origins of Intelligence in the Child.* London: Routledge and Kegan Paul, 1953.

Rimon, R. "A Psychosomatic Approach to Rheumatoid Arthritis." *Acta Rheumatologica Scandinavica,* Supplement no. 13 (1969).

Selye, H. *The Physiology and Pathology of Exposure to Stress.* Montreal: Acta, 1950.

Spitzer, R. L.; Skodol, A. E.; Gibbon, M. G.; and Williams, J. B. W. *DSM-III Casebook.* Washington, D.C.: American Psychiatric Association, 1981.

Srole, L.; Langner, T. S.; Opler, M. K.; and Rennie, T. A. C. *Mental Health in the Metropolis.* New York: McGraw-Hill, 1962.

Further Reading

Bakan, D. *Disease, Pain and Sacrifice: Toward a Psychology of Suffering.* Boston: Beacon Press. 1971.

Baker, A. B., and Baher, L. H., *Clinical Neurology.* New York: Harper and Row, 1973.

Benson, D. F., and Blumer, D., eds. *Psychiatric Aspects of Neurologic Disease.* New York: Grune and Stratton, 1975.

Benton, A. L. *Behavior Change in Cerebrovascular Disease.* New York: Harper and Row, 1970.

Brain, W. R., and Wilkerson, M., eds. *Recent Advances in Neurology and Neuropsychiatry.* Boston: Little, Brown, 1969.

Brown, G. W., and Harris, T. *Social Origins of Depression.* London: Tavistock, 1978.

Bruch, H. *Eating Disorders: Obesity and Anorexia Nervosa and the Person Within.* New York: Basic Books, 1973.

Caplan, G., and Killilea, M. eds. *Support Systems and Mutual Help.* New York: Grune and Stratton, 1976.

Coelho, G. V.; Hamburg, D. A.; and Adams, J. E., eds. *Coping and Adaptation.* New York: Basic Books, 1974.

Dally, P. *Anorexia Nervosa.* New York: Grune and Stratton, 1969.

Dewan, J. G., and Spaulding, W. G. *The Organic Psychoses.* Toronto: University of Toronto Press, 1958.

Ellis, N. R., ed. *International Review of Research in Mental Retardation.* 6 vols. New York: Academic Press, 1966–1973.

Engel, G. L. *Psychological Development in Health and Disease.* Philadelphia: W. B. Saunders, 1962.

Gaitz, C. M., ed. *Aging in the Brain.* New York: Plenum Press, 1972.

Glaser, G., ed. *EEG and Bahavior.* New York: Basic Books, 1963.

Hansell, N. *The Person-in-Distress: On the Biological Dynamics of Adaptation.* New York: Behavioral Publications, 1976.

Harrison, T. R.; Adams, R. D.; Bennett, I. L., Jr.; Resnick, W. H.; Thorn, G. W.; and Wintrobe, M. M., eds. *Principles of Internal Medicine.* New York: McGraw-Hill, 1974.

Haywood, H. C., ed. *Socio-cultural Aspects of Mental Retardation.* New York: Appleton-Century-Crofts, 1970.

Hirt, M. L., ed. *Psychological and Allergic Aspects of Asthma.* Springfield, Ill.: Charles C Thomas, 1965.

Katz, E., ed. *Mental Health Services for the Mentally Retarded.* Springfield, Ill.: Charles C Thomas, 1972.

Kissen, D. M., and LeShan, L. C., eds. *Psychosomatic Aspects of Neoplastic Disease.* London: Pitman and Sons, 1964.

Koch, R., and Dobson, J. C., eds. *The Mentally Retarded Child and His Family.* New York: Brunner-Mazel, 1970.

Levi, L., ed. *Society, Stress and Disease.* London: Oxford University Press, 1971.

Lief, H. I.; Leif, V. F.; and Lief, H. R. *The Psychological Basis of Medical Practice.* New York: Harper and Row, 1963.

MacBryde, C. M., and Blacklaw, R. S. *Signs and Symptoms.* Philadelphia: J. B. Lippincott, 1970.

Mendels, J., ed. *Biological Psychiatry.* New York: John Wiley, 1973.

Michael, R. P. *Endocrinology and Human Behavior.* London: Oxford University Press, 1968.

Pasnau, R. O. *Consultation-Liaison Psychiatry.* New York: Grune and Stratton, 1975.

Philips, T., ed. *Prevention and Treatment of Mental Retardation.* New York: Basic Books, 1966.

Plum, R., and Posner, J. B. *The Diagnosis of Stupor and Coma.* Philadelphia: F. A. Davis, 1966.

Price, J. H., ed. *Modern Trends in Psychological Medicine.* London: Butterworth, 1970.

Rowland, C. V., ed. *Anorexia and Obesity.* Boston: Little, Brown, 1970.

Sarason, S. B., and Gladwin, T. *Psychological and Cultural Problems in Mental Subnormality: A Review of Research.* Provincetown, Mass.: Journal Press, 1958.

Scheinberg, P. *Modern Practical Neurology.* New York: Raven Press, 1977.

Shader, R. I. *Psychiatric Complications of Medical Drugs.* New York: Raven Press, 1972.

Stanbury, J. B.; Wyngaarden, J. B.; and Friedrickson, D. S., eds. *The Metabolic Basis of Inherited Disease.* 3d ed. New York: McGraw-Hill, 1972.

Steenbach, R. S. *Pain: A Psychophysiological Analysis.* New York: Academic Press, 1968.

Stoelinga, G. B.; Van Der Werff, B. A.; and Ten Bosch, J. J., eds. *Normal and Abnormal Development of Brain and Behavior.* Baltimore: Williams and Wilkins., 1971.

Strain, J. J., and Crossman, S. *Psychological Care of the Medically Ill: A Primer in Liaison Psychiatry.* New York: Appleton-Century-Crofts, 1975.

Teitelbaum, H. A. *Psychosomatic Neurology.* New York: Grune and Stratton, 1964.

Tizard, J., and Grad, C. *The Mentally Handicapped and Their Families.* London: Oxford University Press, 1961.

Walker, A. E.; Caveness, W. F.; and Critchley, M., eds. *The Late Effects of Head Injury.* Springfield, Ill.: Charles C Thomas, 1969.

Walker, S. S., III. *Psychiatric Signs and Symptoms Due to Medical Problems.* Springfield, Ill.: Charles C Thomas, 1967.

Weiner, H. *Psychobiology and Human Disease.* New York: Elsevier, North-Holland, 1977.

Wells, C. E. *Dementia.* Philadelphia: F. A. Davis, 1971.

Whitty, C. W. M., and Zangwill, . L., eds. *Amnesia.* New York: Appleton-Century-Crofts, 1966.

Wortis, J., ed. *Mental Retardation and Developmental Disabilities, An Annual Review.* New York: Brunner-Mazel, 1973.

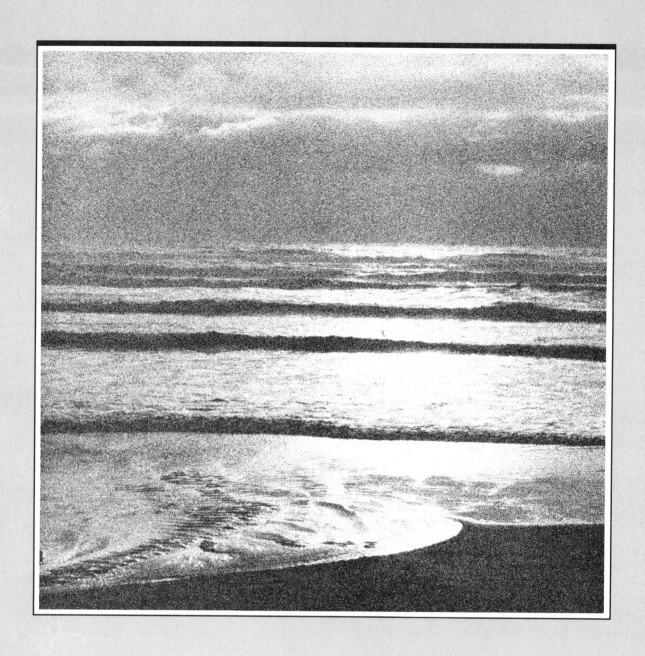

PART FIVE

Intervention Modes

PSYCHIATRIC NURSING IS A *practice discipline. While it cannot occur without application of theory, it is more than a purely intellectual enterprise. In Part Five we deal with the dominant modes of treatment used by psychiatric nurses with clients of all ages. In Chapter 18 we build on the theoretical foundations of group dynamics and group processes to explain and illustrate the nurse's role in group therapy. We outline and illustrate the intervention modes most frequently used in the mental health care of children, including play therapy and behavior modification in Chapter 19. In Chapter 20 our focus is on problems and approaches relevant to the turbulent period of adolescence. We introduce the nurse to family dynamics, family therapy, and marital counseling in Chapter 21. Numerous case examples and nursing care plans are presented. A wealth of useful material and information in the rapidly growing field of psychogerontology is given in Chapter 22, with particular attention to the nurse's roles. In Chapter 23 we acknowledge that much psychiatric care still occurs within the framework of a medical mode and that the most current research findings support a biological factor in psychiatric problems. Chapter 23 on biological therapies therefore collects for the nurse all information relevant to the wide range of biological treatments that often act in conjunction with nursing therapy. In Chapter 24 we recognize that all psychiatric nursing does not occur with labeled psychiatric clients in identified psychiatric settings. We discuss the role of the liaison psychiatric nurse consultant in the general hospital and the psychosocial concepts applicable in nonpsychiatric milieus. Finally in Chapter 25, we summarize and critique a wide range of modern healing therapies, some of which have roots in folk culture, religious practices, and the holistic health movement.*

18

Strategies of
Group Intervention

CHAPTER OUTLINE

Frameworks for Group Analysis
    The Johari Awareness Model
    FIRO: The Interpersonal Needs Approach
    The Authority Relations/Personal Relations
    Approach
    The Therapeutic Problem Approach
    Small Group Assessment
Interactional Group Therapy
    Advantages of Group over Individual Therapy
    Qualified Group Therapists
    The Curative Factors
    Types of Group Leadership
    Creating the Group
    Stages in Therapy Group Development
    The Here-and-Now Emphasis
Other Group Therapies and Therapeutic Groups
    Analytic Group Psychotherapy
    Psychodrama
    Sociodrama
    Multiple Family Group Therapy
    Self-help Groups
    Remotivation and Reeducation Groups
    Client Government Groups

    Activity Therapy Groups
    Groups of Clients with Pathophysiological
    Dysfunction and Families
    Community Client Groups
    Groups with Nurse Colleagues
Key Nursing Concepts

LEARNING OBJECTIVES

After reading this chapter, students should be able to

- Describe four frameworks for the assessment and understanding of therapy groups
- Assess small groups in terms of their functional, structural, and interactional characteristics
- Relate the egalitarian cotherapy approach to humanistic psychiatric nursing practice in interactional group therapy
- Describe the process of creating and maintaining a group
- Identify the stages in therapy group development
- Discuss the application of here-and-now activation and process illumination to psychotherapy groups
- Describe other related group therapies and therapeutic groups

CHAPTER 18

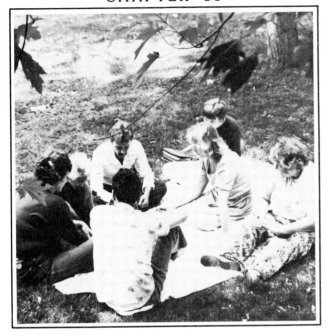

> *Much as architects design buildings to withstand the stresses and strains created by humanity and nature, members of psychotherapy groups are carefully selected to maximize the quality of the interpersonal relationships.*

Groups influence a person's psychological well-being. Mental well-being can be preserved, maintained, and restored through interaction with others in productive groups. The group intervention mode is one means by which psychiatric nurses can provide humanistic care for their clients. Therapy through the group process gives clients the opportunity to seek validation, give and receive interpersonal feedback, and test new and different ways of being that may increase their quality of life.

The psychiatric nurse, in the role of group leader/facilitator/therapist, may function autonomously or in collaboration with other members of the mental health team. Effectiveness depends not on the helping person's background discipline but rather on the match between the abilities and characteristics of the helper and the needs of clients.

This chapter discusses four frameworks for assessment of group processes (based on Chapter 9) and various methods of group intervention. It emphasizes the strategies in freely interactive verbal group therapy.

FRAMEWORKS FOR GROUP ANALYSIS

Operational frameworks for group analysis provide the means for understanding the dynamic processes that go on in groups. Frameworks help the group leader know where the group is, predict in what direction it might move, and identify the potentials within the group that might be facilitated or developed. The four models discussed below are useful guides against which to compare a group. Perceptions of a group should not be forced to fit any model but should emerge through the process of comparison.

The Johari Awareness Model

The Johari Awareness Model, often called the Johari Window, is a theoretical tool used to represent the total person in relation to other people. It is illustrated in Figure 18–1. The relationship of this heuristic device to individual awareness is discussed in Chapter 3. Its relationship to intragroup and intergroup awareness makes it an appropriate model to discuss here. We suggest a review of the components of the Johari Window described in Chapter 3 before you attempt to understand the model for a group framework.

Joseph Luft and Harry Ingham (1955), the creators of the Johari Awareness Model, maintain that interpersonal interaction, in a group setting, for example, is facilitated when people have sufficient knowledge about one another's actions, motivations, and feelings. Group members can use this knowledge to understand the significant events in a group more clearly.

Major elements in this awareness model are its assumptions that humans respond to groups and that change or learning can follow opportunities for new interaction. The primary principle of change in relation to the Johari Window is: A change in one quadrant will affect all other quadrants. Certain other general principles of change that derive from the Johari Window are particularly suited to the understanding of small group behavior. These principles are:

- A large open quadrant facilitates working with others. Therefore, more of the resources and abilities of group members can be brought to bear on the group task when members have large Q1 areas.

Figure 18–1

The Johari awareness model. (Adapted from *Group Processes: An Introduction to Group Dynamics* by Joseph Luft by permission of Mayfield Publishing Company [formerly National Press Books]. Copyright 1963, 1970 by Joseph Luft.)

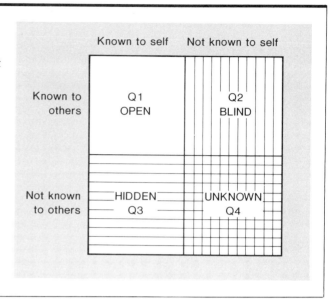

- The open quadrant can be enlarged, and awareness increased, by learning about group processes as they are being experienced.

- How a group confronts the unknown quadrant is influenced by the group's value system.

Intragroup Relations   In a new and immature group, Q1 is small, because free and spontaneous interaction does not occur in new groups. As the group matures, Q1 expands and Q3 shrinks accordingly. This means that members are becoming freer to be themselves and to perceive others as they really are. An atmosphere of increasing trust, risk taking, and self-disclosure begins to form. An enlarged area of free activity means that the group uses more energy to work on the group task than to maintain or defend the hidden or avoided area of Q3. Q2 also diminishes as members learn more about themselves. Q4 changes

more slowly and to a lesser degree, because it represents an area in which unknown behaviors and motives reside. Figure 18–2 compares the degrees of openness in immature and mature groups.

A group can also be understood and diagrammed according to the Johari Windows of the individual members.

Sam was a person with limited freedom. Although he was polite, he appeared to be superficial and constricted. He devoted large amounts of energy to walling off the behavior and motivations of Q2, Q3, and Q4 by intellectualizing. Laura was a group member whose great inner resources allowed her to develop a very large area of free activity. In contrast, Debbie was what Luft has termed a plunger. Debbie's spontaneity and "openness" lacked discretion and created distance in her relationships with other group members. Van and Maria,

Figure 18–2

The immature versus mature group. (Adapted from *Group Processes: An Introduction to Group Dynamics* by Joseph Luft by permission of Mayfield Publishing Company [formerly National Press Books]. Copyright 1963, 1970 by Joseph Luft).

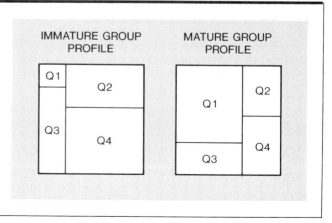

Figure 18–3

Awareness configurations in a specific group.

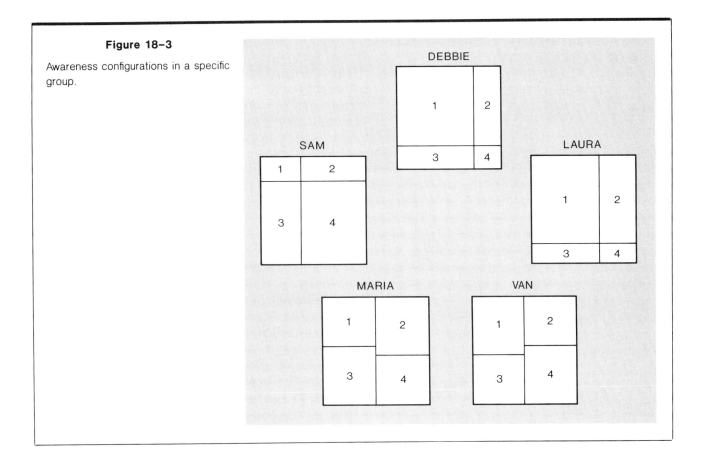

the other two members of this group, tended not to take many risks in their interactions with others, although their moderate openness indicated flexibility.

The Johari Window configurations of this group are illustrated in Figure 18–3. Sam's Johari Window shows a greatly reduced and constricted open quadrant. His behavior and feelings are likely to be limited in range, variety, and scope. His interactions tend to be conventional, and he is likely to be threatened by group behaviors that go beyond the bounds of convention. Laura's Johari Window represents a person whose interactions are characterized by great openness to the world. Much of her potential has been developed and realized. Debbie's Johari Window is that of the inappropriately transparent person who deals with others by disclosing too much. The Johari Windows of Maria and Van show moderately large open areas although Q2, Q3, and Q4 are equally large.

The awareness configurations raise an interesting question: What behaviors might be predicted in a group with members such as these? Obviously this group needs to resolve several problems. An "underdiscloser" like Sam reveals too little, thus reserving

control for himself. He tends to quell spontaneous reactions in order to double-check. He may be one of the last to acknowledge the development of trust. Debbie's failure to control her overdisclosures means that her relationships with others in the group will be either too smothering (because of being too close) or too demanding (because she imposes herself on others without considering their intimacy needs). She may trust everyone because she has not learned to discriminate among relationships. Her behavior forces others to take responsibility for defining the nature of the relationship. They are likely to feel threatened by her early spontaneous disclosures, which they may experience as overwhelming. Problems of trust, intimacy, and risk taking may arise in her interactions with these members.

Laura, because of her high degree of self-awareness, will be less preoccupied with defensiveness and distortion than other members. She will be able to accept the differences in others and serve as a model for them. Maria and Van, whose awareness configurations demonstrate they have progressed to moderate openness, will continue to grow in this direction with minimal discomfort to themselves and other group members.

Intergroup Relations A group can also be viewed as a whole entity in interactions with other groups. Q1 includes the open, available information that is known to the group as well as to others. Q2 is the area that others outside the group see but the group itself does not. Q3 has to do with the secret, hidden things that the group keeps to itself. Knowledge may be hidden purposefully to enable the group to manipulate other groups. A group of businesspeople who hide the flaws in a property they put up for sale illustrate this. Groups keep things hidden for other reasons as well, such as being ashamed of some activity or attitude or finding an event or belief hard to explain because it refers to idiosyncratic occurrences known only to the members. Hidden things form the *lore* of the group. Q4 includes behavior and motives that are unknown to the group and to outsiders as well. A covert and unrecognized split among the members with regard to the group goals would be one example. Difficulties in *effective* group functioning could result from such an unrecognized split.

FIRO: The Interpersonal Needs Approach

The Fundamental Interpersonal Relationship Orientation (FIRO) is a popular approach developed by William Schutz (1958a; 1958b). Some of his ideas were generated during his work for the Department of the Navy. The Navy was concerned with interpersonal problems experienced by the crews of nuclear submarines during their long-term cruises beneath the polar ice cap. While some crews functioned effectively and were satisfied with one another, others performed ineffectively and voiced their dissatisfactions. Schutz set out to learn how to predict which people were compatible with which other people. Theoretically, nuclear submarine crews could be composed of compatible individuals who would be more likely to perform effectively together and would find their lengthy enforced togetherness, if not totally pleasurable, at least tolerable.

The basic assumption of Schutz's theory is that people need people. In addition, people need to establish some equilibrium between themselves and the people in their environment. This equilibrium is determined by the interaction of certain interpersonal needs, and it appears to be synonymous with interpersonal compatibility.

Three Basic Interpersonal Needs An interpersonal need is one that can be satisfied only through relationships with people. Schutz postulated that every individual has three interpersonal needs: inclusion, control, and affection.

INCLUSION The interpersonal need for inclusion may be defined as the need to establish and maintain relationships with others that offer interactions and associations satisfying to the individual. A satisfying position in terms of inclusion includes:

• A psychologically comfortable relation with people somewhere on a continuum that ranges from initiating or originating interaction with all people to not initiating interaction with anyone. In other words, this dimension is *expressed* toward others.

• A psychologically comfortable relation with people in regard to wanting others to initiate interaction somewhere on a continuum that ranges from always initiating interaction with you to never initiating interaction with you. In other words, this dimension is *wanted* from others.

To put this another way, *expressed inclusion* is the ability to take an interest in others to a satisfactory degree, and *wanted inclusion* is the ability to allow other people to take an interest in you to a satisfying degree to yourself.

Connotative terms that point to a positive inclusion relation are: associate, interact, mingle, communicate, belong, companion, comrade, attend to, member, togetherness, join, extrovert. At the other end of the scale are terms that connote lack of inclusion, such as: exclusion, isolate, outsider, outcast, lonely, detached, withdrawn, abandoned, ignored. This need determines whether a person is outgoing or prefers privacy.

CONTROL The interpersonal need for control may be defined as the need to establish and maintain a satisfactory relation between oneself and other people with regard to power and influence. A satisfactory position in terms of control includes:

• A psychologically comfortable relation with people somewhere on a continuum that ranges from controlling all the behavior of other people to not controlling any behavior of others

• A psychologically comfortable relation with people in regard to their control behavior on a continuum that ranges from always wanting to be controlled by them to never wanting to be controlled by them

To put this another way, *expressed control* is the ability to take charge to a satisfactory degree, and *wanted control* is the ability to establish and maintain a feeling of respect for the competence and responsibleness of others to a satisfying degree to yourself.

Connotative terms for primarily positive control are: power, authority, dominance, influence, control, ruler, superior officer, leader. At the other end of the scale are terms that connote lack of control, or negative control: rebellion, resistance, follower, anarchy, submissive, henpecked, Milquetoast.

AFFECTION   The interpersonal need for affection may be defined as the need to establish and maintain a satisfactory relation between the self and other people with regard to love and affection. A satisfactory position in terms of affection includes:

- A psychologically comfortable relation with others somewhere on a continuum that ranges from initiating close, personal relations with *everyone* to originating close, personal relations with *no one*

- A psychologically comfortable relation with people in regard to their affection behavior on a continuum that ranges from wanting *everyone* to originate close, personal relations toward you, to wanting *no one* to originate close, personal relations toward you.

To put this another way, *expressed affection* is being able to love other people or to be close and intimate to a satisfactory degree, and *wanted affection* is having others love you or to be close and intimate with you to a satisfactory degree.

Connotative terms for an affection relation that is primarily positive are: love, like, emotionally close, positive feelings, personal, friendship. At the other end of the scale are terms that connote lack of affection or negative affection: hate, dislike, cool, emotionally distant.

The dimensions of the FIRO theory are illustrated in Figure 18–4.

Group Development   The interpersonal needs theory asserts that any group, given enough time, moves through three interpersonal phases—inclusion, control, and affection, in that order—that correspond to the three basic interpersonal needs.

INCLUSION PHASE   The first or inclusion phase is concerned with the problem of *in or out*. People attempt to find their place within the group and are concerned with learning whether they will be acknowledged as individuals or left behind and ignored. Because these concerns give rise to anxiety, this phase is dominated by behavior centered around the self. Overtalking, withdrawal, exhibitionism, and sharing other group experiences and biographies are some examples.

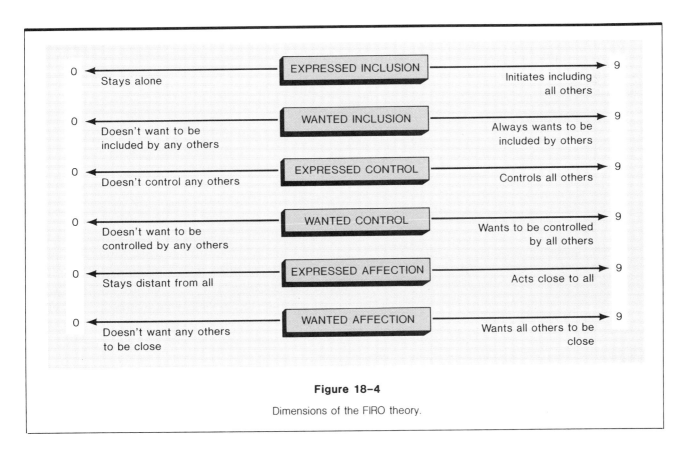

Figure 18–4

Dimensions of the FIRO theory.

Frequently, *goblet issues* predominate. These are issues of minor importance to the group that help people get to know one another and test each other. They are a vehicle for sizing up people. Goblet issues may revolve around the weather, the World Series, rules of procedure, and so on.

CONTROL PHASE   The second or control phase is concerned with the problem of *top or bottom*, which becomes salient after problems of inclusion have been resolved. Concern about decision-making procedures predominates, and the problems that emerge involve the sharing of responsibility and the distribution of power and influence. This phase is dominated by competitive behavior. There are struggles for leadership and about the structure, rules of procedure, and methods of decision-making. Members are attempting to establish comfortable positions for themselves in terms of responsibility and influence.

AFFECTION PHASE   The third or affection phase is concerned with the problem of *near or far,* and it follows satisfactory resolution of the preceding two phases. Individual members are now faced with the problem of becoming emotionally integrated. Concerns about not being liked by, being too close to, or not being close enough to others become relevant. The behavior in this phase is generally characterized by high emotion—positive feelings, jealousy, hostility, and pairing are some examples. Schutz (1958a) describes this phase as one in which, like porcupines, people attempt to get close enough to receive warmth, yet avoid the pain of sharp quills.

INTERWEAVING OF PHASES   None of these phases is distinct, since all three problem areas are present at all times, even though only one predominates. Schutz (1958a, p. 130) uses a tire-changing analogy, what he calls *tightening the bolts,* to describe the sequence of the phases:

> When a person changes a tire and replaces the wheel, he first sets the wheel in place and secures it by tightening the bolts one after another just so the wheel is in place and the next step can be taken. Then the bolts are tightened further, usually in the same sequence, until the wheel is firmly in place. Finally each bolt is gone over separately to secure it.

The leader helps the group work on all three interpersonal need areas in similar fashion, returning to and working over each area to a more satisfactory level than was reached the last time.

Applying the Theory   *Clearing the air* by making covert interpersonal difficulties overt is a major step in applying the FIRO theory. Although this step is initially uncomfortable, the final result is rewarding. Interpersonal difficulties that can be made overt are:

- Withdrawal or silence by members
- Inactivity and unintegrated behavior by members
- Overactivity and destructive behavior by members
- Power struggles between members
- Battles for attention among members
- Dissatisfaction with the leadership
- Dissatisfaction with the amount of recognition a member receives for contributions
- Dissatisfaction with the amount of affection and warmth demonstrated in the group

A group that is relatively compatible can function smoothly with minimal discussion of its problems. Groups in which the interpersonal problems are extremely minor can usually ignore them (or, if problems exist between two members, work them out outside the group) without hampering group effectiveness. A group that is basically incompatible has to spend much more time and energy resolving its interpersonal problems so that it can function effectively.

The interpersonal needs approach of Schutz is based on the belief that the way to attack problems within groups is by investigating what is going on among the individuals in the group and attempting to improve their interpersonal relations.

The Authority Relations/Personal Relations Approach

Two major areas of internal uncertainty or stress in groups, according to the theory developed by Warren Bennis and Herbert A. Shepard (1956), are dependence (authority relations) and interdependence (personal relations). The first area has to do with group members' orientations toward authority—the handling and distribution of power within the group. The second area has to do with group members' orientations toward one another. A central belief of this approach is that the principal obstacles to valid communication (and hence to effectiveness) in a group derive from the orientations toward authority and intimacy that members bring to the group.

A new group is highly concerned with authority and

Table 18-1 PHASE 1 OF GROUP DEVELOPMENT (DEPENDENCE—POWER RELATIONS)		
	Subphase 1 Dependence–Submission	Subphase 2 Counterdependence	Subphase 3 Resolution
1. Emotional modality	Dependence—flight.	Counterdependence—fight. Off-target fighting among members. Distrust of staff member. Ambivalence.	Pairing. Intense involvement in group task.
2. Content themes	Discussion of interpersonal problems external to training groups.	Discussion of group organization; i.e. what degree of structuring devices is needed for "effective" group behavior?	Discussion and definition of trainer role.
3. Dominant roles (central persons)	Assertive, aggressive members with rich previous organizational or social science experience.	Most assertive counterdependent and dependent members. Withdrawal of *less* assertive independents and dependents.	Assertive independents.
4. Group structure	Organized mainly into multi-subgroups based on members' past experiences.	Two tight subcliques consisting of leaders and members, of counterdependents and dependents.	Group unifies in pursuit of goal and develops internal authority system.
5. Group activity	Self-oriented behavior reminiscent of most new social gatherings.	Search for consensus mechanism: voting, setting up chairmen, search for "valid" content subjects.	Group members take over leadership roles formerly perceived as held by trainer.
6. Group movement facilitated by:	Staff member abnegation of traditional role of structuring situation, setting up rules of fair play, regulation of participation.	Disenthrallment with staff member coupled with absorption of uncertainty by most assertive counterdependent and dependent individuals. Subgroups form to ward off anxiety.	Revolt by assertive independents (catalysts) who fuse subgroups into unity by initiating and engineering trainer exit (barometric event).
7. Main defenses	Projection, denigration of authority.		Group moves into Phase II.

Source: W. Bennis and H. A. Shepard, "A Theory of Group Development." From *Human Relations*, Vol. 9, No. 4, 1956, published by the Tavistock Institute of Human Relations, London, and the Research Center for Group Dynamics, Ann Arbor. Used by permission of Plenum Publishing Corporation, New York.

power. Earlier experiences with authority influence and partially determine members' orientations toward other members. Bennis and Shepard have called this Phase I. Table 18-1 summarizes the major developmental events in Phase I.

As the group develops, it moves away from its preoccupation with authority toward a preoccupation with personal relations. This constitutes the second major phase in group development, called Phase II. Its major developmental events are summarized in Table 18-2.

Relevant Aspects of Member Personality   Bennis and Shepard view members as either conflicted or unconflicted around the dependence and personal aspects of group life. A *conflicted* member is one whose posture toward dependence or intimacy may be viewed as inflexible, rigid, or compulsive. These mem-

Table 18-2	PHASE II OF GROUP DEVELOPMENT (INTERDEPENDENCE—PERSONAL RELATIONS)		
	Subphase 4 Enchantment	Subphase 5 Disenchantment	Subphase 6 Consensual Validation
Emotional modality	Pairing—flight. Group becomes a respected icon beyond further analysis.	Fight—flight. Anxiety reactions. Distrust and suspicion of various group members.	Pairing, understanding, acceptance.
Content themes	Discussion of "group history," and generally salutary aspects of course, group, and membership.	Revival of content themes used in Subphase 1: What is a group? What are we doing here? What are the goals of the group? What do I have to give up to belong to this group? (How much intimacy and affection is required?) Invasion of privacy versus "group giving." Setting up proper codes of social behavior.	Course grading system. Discussion and assessment of member roles.
Dominant roles (central persons)	General distribution of participation for first time. Overpersonals have salience.	Most assertive counterpersonal and overpersonal individuals, with counterpersonals especially salient.	Assertive independents.
Group structure	Solidarity, fusion. High degree of camaraderie and suggestibility.	Restructuring of membership into two competing predominant subgroups made up of individuals who share similar attitudes concerning degree of intimacy required in social interaction, i.e., the counterpersonal and overpersonal groups. The personal individuals remain uncommitted but act according to needs of situation.	Diminishing of ties based on personal orientation. Group structure now presumably appropriate to needs of situation based on predominantly substantive rather than emotional orientations. Consensus significantly easier on important issues.

Table continues on next page

bers persist in the adoption of certain roles despite the situation. Conflicted members are responsible for communicative confusion within groups. An *unconflicted* member, also called an *independent,* is better able to assess situations and alter roles or behavior as appropriate.

There are two ways in which persons can be conflicted around authority relations. Members who are comforted by rules of procedure, agendas, and rely on the decisions of others (who are viewed as experts) are said to be *dependent.* Members who are uncomfortable with structure and authority are *counterdependent.* Counterdependents manifest their dissatisfaction with authority by opposing it regardless of its style or

intent. Nothing the authority or leader does is acceptable. Failure to design an agenda is viewed by the counterdependent as evidence of the authority's lack of ability. Paradoxically, designing an agenda may be viewed as too controlling. The counterdependent takes a "damned if you do, and damned if you don't" stance toward authority.

Members can be conflicted around personal relations in two ways as well. People who direct uninterrupted efforts toward reaching a high degree of intimacy with all other group members are termed *overpersonal.* When members expend great amounts of energy in avoiding intimacy and maintaining distance they are said to be *counterpersonal.*

Table 18-2 continued			
	Subphase 4 **Enchantment**	**Subphase 5** **Disenchantment**	**Subphase 6** **Consensual Validation**
Group activity	Laughter, joking, humor. Planning out-of-class activities such as parties. The institutionalization of happiness to be accomplished by ''fun'' activities. High rate of interaction and participation.	Disparagement of group in a variety of ways: high rate of absenteeism, tardiness, balkiness in initiating total group interaction, frequent statements concerning worthlessness of group, denial of importance of group. Occasional member asking for individual help finally rejected by the group.	Communication to others of self-system of interpersonal relations; i.e., making conscious to self and others conceptual system one uses to predict consequences of personal behavior. Acceptance of group on reality terms.
Group movement facilitated by:	Independence and achievement attained by trainer-rejection and its concomitant, deriving consensually some effective means for authority and control. (Subphase 3 rebellion bridges gap between Subphases 2 and 4.)	Disenchantment of group as a result of *fantasied expectations of group life.* The perceived threat to self-esteem that further group involvement signifies creates schism of group according to amount of affection and intimacy desired. The counterpersonal and overpersonal assertive individuals alleviate source of anxiety by disparaging or abnegating further group involvement. Subgroups form to ward off anxiety.	The external realities, group termination, and the prescribed need for a course grading system comprise the barometric event. Led by the personal individuals, the group tests reality and reduces autistic convictions concerning group involvement.
Main defenses	Denial, isolation, intellectualization, and alienation.		

Source: W. Bennis and H. A. Shepard, ''A Theory of Group Development.'' From *Human Relations,* Vol. 9, No. 4, 1956, published by the Tavistock Institute of Human Relations, London, and the Research Center for Group Dynamics, Ann Arbor. Used by permission of Plenum Publishing Corporation, New York.

Persons unconflicted in terms of either the authority relations or the personal relations in the group are responsible for major movements in the group's development toward valid communication. These unconflicted members who move the group on to the next phase are called *catalysts.* They reduce the internal uncertainty or stress in the group. Actions of these unconflicted members that move the group forward into the next phase are called *barometric events.* Figure 18-5 presents a grid of these aspects of member personality.

Relationship to Group Strategies   The Bennis and Shepard model demonstrates group development along a continuum from the emphasis on power to the emphasis on affection. The activities of Phase I are concerned with such things as social class, ethnic background, and personal and professional interests. Concern with personality and reaction to feelings, such as warmth, anger, love, and anxiety, arise in Phase II. Bennis and Shepard believe that group therapies should be based on an adequate understanding of the group dynamic barriers to communication.

The Therapeutic Problem Approach

The final approach to the analysis of groups that is considered in this chapter is one that describes group development—specifically, therapy group develop-

Figure 18-5

Member personality categories.

	CONFLICTED	UNCONFLICTED
AUTHORITY RELATIONS	Dependent Counterdependent	Independent (catalyst)
PERSONAL RELATIONS	Over personal Counterpersonal	Independent (catalyst)

ment—in six discrete phases. E. A. Martin and William F. Hill (1957) formulated this theory of group development from the basic assumption that distinct and common growth patterns exist in therapy groups and can be described, observed, and predicted. The major therapeutic problem encountered is the focal point for describing each phase. In this model, transitional stages between the developmental plateaus indicate potentials for movement from one phase to another. The six phases of therapy group development, according to Martin and Hill, are:

- Phase I. Individual unshared behavior in an imposed structure
- Phase II. Reactivation of fixed interpersonal stereotypes
- Phase III. Exploration of interpersonal potential within the group
- Phase IV. Awareness of interrelationships, subgrouping, and power structure
- Phase V. Responsiveness to group dynamic and group process problems
- Phase VI. The group as an integrative-creative social instrument

Like the other approaches discussed above, this theory sees groups passing along a developmental continuum from minimal to optimal effectiveness. Groups differ in the length of time they spend in any phase and the specific problems they face. Most groups disband before reaching the sixth, or ultimate, phase of development.

Phase I—Individual Behavior   The group in Phase I is best described as an aggregate of social isolates held together loosely by vague perceptions of the therapist and his or her role. Imposed structure, such as regularity of meeting time and place, consistency of

membership, and a group seating arrangement, encourage groupness, slight though it may be. Because of a lack of interpersonal, group-relevant structure, esprit de corps and cooperative ventures are latent but not yet realized.

Groups of clients with disintegrated interactional patterns are characterized by primarily autistic, or at least highly private, behavior. They are likely to manifest little concern about the leader. Groups of clients with disturbed personal coping patterns are characterized by behavior that is individualistic and egocentric but mutually compatible, even though it fails to be group-relevant. Concern about the therapist may be ever-present among these clients.

There is little justification for calling the aggregate of individuals in Phase I a group.

Transition from Phase I to Phase II   The major characteristic of the first transitional phase is that the therapist emerges as the leader of the group and is publicly acknowledged by the members. Autistic behavior diminishes. It is replaced by an *asyndetic* mode of interaction, a form of interpersonal interaction in which elements in a statement by one speaker function as a cue for the next speaker. A third, fourth, or fifth speaker may similarly be cued by the preceding speaker. It is a chain reaction that seems highly autistic, in that the material evoked by the cues is highly personal and does not enhance or elaborate the productions of the earlier speaker. There is some group relevance, however, in that the remarks indicate that members have paid at least some attention to each other. They thus establish social contacts of an oblique nature. The therapist can help the group move on to the next phase through modeling behavior that is not asyndetic but rather recognizes the members as social beings.

Phase II—Fixed Stereotypes   In the second phase, members' perceptions of one another are based on previously learned stereotypes. Although members publicly acknowledge one another's existence, the acknowledgment is in terms of "ghosts" of earlier interpersonal experiences. These stereotyped perceptions or ghosts fail to acknowledge the uniqueness of each member. A member may be called a "redneck," "sweet," or "macho," based not on how the person really is but rather on the stereotype assigned to that individual. The leader is frequently typecast in some sort of omniscient role, described as "a real brain" or "El Presidente," and dependence on the leader emerges. It is the socialization aspects of this phase that provide therapeutic value.

Transition from Phase II to Phase III   Social stereotypes break down during this transitional period, as members openly express resentment of being stereotyped and insist on their own rights and views. Appraisals of one another become more realistic. The members' idiosyncratic perceptions of the leader begin to give way to a group view. The therapist assists the group by helping members become more aware of the discrepancies in their views of the therapist. Leaders who play a role and maintain distance by being less human perpetuate rather than break down the typecasting phenomenon.

Phase III—Exploration of Potential   This phase is characterized by active emotional exchange geared to giving group members recognition as individuals. Although many asyndetic processes and autisms still occur, the group begins to deal with the here-and-now events in the group and with their perceptions of one another. A group norm appears that places high value on individual importance. It may be demonstrated by the devotion of one or more entire sessions to the problems or personality of one member or by a rapidly shifting give-and-take. Because the individual is of paramount importance, membership is valued, and absences, tardiness, or dropping out are grave concerns. In this phase, members learn to give emotional feedback to one another and become more aware of their effects on one another. The experience of being valued reduces anomie and facilitates self-worth. Martin and Hill (1957) caution the therapist against being caught up in the fervor of confession. They suggest that therapists refrain from becoming one of the gang through self-disclosure, since this may thwart the therapeutic goals.

Transition from Phase III to Phase IV   At the third transition point, the group suffers from ennui,

finding the dissection of one another's psyches boring and repetitious. The excitement and novelty of exploration abate, and group discussions turn to consideration of the relationships that have developed among group members. The therapist can help the group transcend this "same old faces and same old problems" feeling by making members aware of their boredom and encouraging their exploration of the relationships among members.

Phase IV—Awareness of Interrelationships
Growing awareness of certain relationships between and among members surfaces during Phase IV. Pairing relationships and hierarchical relationships are among those that emerge. Member skill at identifying relationship dynamics encourages them to consider their attempts to structure specific relationships with the therapist. "Teacher's pets" and "junior therapists" may be identified at this time. The group becomes polarized, as opinion leaders and emotional attitude leaders begin to surface and subgroups are established around them. Consequently, rivalries also develop, and subgroups struggle for power. The therapist's task is to help the members identify subgroup leaders and supporters and consider the potential consequences of a power struggle. According to Martin and Hill (1957), most therapy groups do not move beyond the third or fourth phase.

Transition from Phase IV to Phase V   A high state of tension exists within the group, and there is decreasing tolerance for the tension in the transition stage. Members may attempt, usually unsuccessfully, to replace subgroup operation with a total group orientation. To help the group attain a level of total group orientation, the therapist should make the group aware of the source of its dissatisfaction and provide helpful techniques, such as role playing, to identify and highlight the subgroup problems that have emerged.

Phase V—Responsiveness to Group Dynamics   Individual and subgroup problems become reinterpreted as group problems in the fifth phase. The group becomes process-oriented and attuned to the group dynamics. It demonstrates its awareness of silences, difficulty in getting started, taboo topics, and similar phenomena. The group seems to be concerned about learning how it functions, and the therapist can help by providing expertise in the description and comprehension of dynamics and processes. Because it is difficult for a group to remain for long at this sophisticated level of operation, regression to earlier behaviors is common.

Transition from Phase V to Phase VI   After experiencing process analysis as a rewarding endeavor, the group will attempt to remedy or take care of unwanted or undesirable features that came to light in the analysis. However, the desire to remedy does not always ensure the ability to remedy. The group finds itself frustrated in its problem-solving attempts and may need to rely on the skills of the therapist.

Phase VI—The Group as Social Instrument
The sixth phase constitutes the ideal phase of group life. The group becomes superbly effective at engaging in cooperative problem solving, diagnosing process and dynamics, making acceptable and appropriate decisions. In short, this group is characterized by competence. Leadership is fully distributed among the members, and the therapist becomes a resource person. Martin and Hill (1957, p. 28) describe the members of such groups as "masters of their fate."

Small Group Assessment

Any or all of the four operational frameworks described above can be helpful in the assessment of small groups. It is also helpful in the assessment of small groups to consider the following factors, identified by Compton and Galaway (1979, pp. 252–253):

1. Functional characteristics
   a. How group came to be
      (1) Natural group
      (2) Group formed by outside intervention
   b. Group's objectives
      (1) Affiliative, friendship, and social groups—satisfaction derived from positive social interaction, tendency to avoid conflict and stress identification
      (2) Task-oriented groups—created to achieve specific ends or resolve specific problems, emphasis on substantive rather than affective content
      (3) Personal change groups—emphasis on psychological and social content, dynamics of interpersonal behavior
      (4) Role enhancement and developmental groups—recreational, educational, and interest clusters, emphasis on rewards and gratifications of participation, observation, learning, and improved performance

   c. How group relates to contiguous groups, how it perceives itself and is perceived as conforming to or departing from outside values
2. Structural factors
   a. How members were selected; how new members gain entry
   b. Personality of individual members
      (1) Needs, motivations, personality patterns
      (2) Homogeneity–heterogeneity
      (3) Age of members
      (4) Factors of sex, social status, culture (see entries under individual assessment, above)
      (5) Subgroups—reasons for being, purposes they serve
      (6) Nature and locus of authority and control
         (a) How leadership roles develop
         (b) How decisions are made
3. Interactional factors
   a. Norms, values, beliefs
   b. Quality, depth, and nature of relationships
      (1) Formal or informal
      (2) Cooperative or competitive
      (3) Free or constrained
   c. Degree to which members experience interdependence as expressed in individual commitments to group's purposes, norms, and goals

Interactional Group Therapy

There is great diversity and flux in the field of group therapy. Many types of groups are found in mental health settings or in communities at large. Persons may be members of encounter groups, sensitivity training groups, gestalt groups, or transactional analysis groups, psychodrama groups, psychoanalytic groups, nonverbal groups, body movement groups, nude swimming therapy groups, etc. This list is certainly incomplete—a wide and bewildering array of group approaches is available to the willing. Chapter 25 discusses some of these "new therapies" in depth.

Certain common principles seem to apply to all therapeutic groups, although specific methods and techniques may vary according to the purpose of the group or the skills and theoretical orientation of the therapist. Irvin Yalom (1975) uses the term *interaction-*

al group therapy to describe a process of group therapy in which member interaction plays a crucial role. The common principles that apply to interactional group therapy are discussed below.

Advantages of Group over Individual Therapy

The advantages of group therapy stem from one major factor—the presence of many people, rather than a solitary therapist, who participate in the therapeutic experience. Specifically, group therapy provides:

- Stimuli from multiple sources, enabling distortions in interpersonal relationships to be revealed so that they can be examined and resolved
- Multiple sources of feedback
- An interpersonal testing ground that enables members to try out old and new ways of being in an environment specifically structured for that purpose

Qualified Group Therapists

In some mental health agencies, the belief seems to run rampant that all staff members, by virtue of their employment status, can lead groups. And this is exactly what seems to happen in some agencies. Mental health professionals may believe, in error, that group therapy is less complex and therefore "easier" than individual therapy, for example, because the presence of greater numbers of people makes interactions between therapist and client less intense. While it is true that the intensity of interactions between any one member and the therapist may be less intense because interactions are dispersed among others, it *does not follow* that anyone can be an effective group therapist.

To be effective, the group therapist should have the following special preparation:

- Education in small group dynamics
- Education in group therapy theory
- Clinical practice with groups
- Expert supervision of the clinical practice (with ongoing supervision and/or consultation, depending on level of expertise)

The ANA Standards (see Appendix A) identify the group psychotherapy role as appropriate for clinical specialists prepared at the master's level. Competent

therapists report that it is also valuable to be a member of a therapy or sensitivity training group, before becoming a group leader.

The Curative Factors

Yalom (1975) contends that eleven interdependent curative factors or mechanisms of change in group therapy help people. These factors are the framework for an effective approach to therapy, because they constitute a rational basis for the therapist's choices of tactics and strategies. They are identified and defined in Table 18–3.

Types of Group Leadership

Groups can be led by a therapist working alone or by cotherapists working together in a variety of ways. Leaderless groups are another possibility. Each approach is described and evaluated in the sections that follow.

The Single Therapist Approach   Groups led by a single therapist are common. They have an economic advantage in that only one therapist need be involved. A disadvantage is that the therapist cannot compare analyses of the group process with a cotherapist or get instant feedback or validation from a peer. On the other hand, therapists working alone do not have to direct their energies toward creating and maintaining a relationship with a colleague.

Recorders or observers may be used to help the solitary therapist be aware of the multiple complexities of any one group session. Nonparticipant observer/recorders are especially useful when they give the therapist feedback and focus on the nonverbal aspects of the session. If they are truly to be nonparticipants, recorder/ observers must be very careful not to react on a nonverbal level to the content or process of the session.

The Cotherapy Approach   It is becoming more common to see groups led by two therapists who share responsibility for leadership of the group to varying degrees. The two models seen most often are the junior–senior and the egalitarian styles of cotherapy.

THE JUNIOR–SENIOR POSITION   In the junior–senior approach, the therapists have unequal responsibilities toward the group. The senior member of the team is usually the more experienced, or more highly educat-

Table 18-3 CURATIVE FACTORS OF GROUP THERAPY	
Factor	**Definition**
Therapist:	
Instilling of hope	Imbuing the client with optimism for the success of the group therapy experience
Universality	Disconfirming the client's sense of aloneness or uniqueness in misery or hurt
Imparting of information	Giving didactic instruction, advice, or suggestions
Altruism	Finding that the client can be of importance to others; having something of value to give
Client:	
Corrective recapitulation of the primary family group	Reviewing and correctively reliving early familial conflicts and growth-inhibiting relationships
Development of socializing techniques	Acquiring sophisticated social skills, such as being attuned to process, resolving conflicts, and being facilitative toward others
Imitative behavior	Trying out bits and pieces of the behavior of others and experimenting with those that fit well
Interpersonal learning	Learning that one authors his or her interpersonal world and moving to alter it
Group cohesiveness	Being attracted to the group and the other members with a sense of "we"-ness rather than "I"-ness
Catharsis	Being able to express feelings
Existential factors	Being able to "be" with others; to be a part of a group

ed, of the two. Besides having major responsibility for the success of the group, the senior therapist is responsible for training the junior member of the team. This approach is commonly used in agency settings, because it provides in-service training of new personnel and nonprofessionals under the guidance and watchful eye of an experienced group leader. However, relationship problems frequently surface when the roles of the

leaders are not clear, or when one or both leaders are unable, or unwilling, to remain in the designated roles. The members of the group may also be unclear about the subordinate/superordinate roles and unsure of how to deal with and respond to leaders of unequal abilities and responsibilities.

THE EGALITARIAN POSITION In the egalitarian approach to cotherapy, two therapists of relatively equal skill, ability, and status share equally in responsibility for the group. This method is also used for training, with both cotherapists working under clinical supervision. It is preferable to the junior–senior approach for many reasons, which are set forth in Table 18–4. The egalitarian position is not without certain potential disadvantages, however. These are listed in Table 18–5. Overall, the advantages of the egalitarian approach outweigh its potential disadvantages. Cotherapists who arrange for supervision or consultation for themselves will find that potential disadvantages can be turned in their favor. Identification and analysis of disadvantages that arise can lead to learning and behavior change in the cotherapists.

Nurses considering an egalitarian cotherapy relationship with one another need to engage in preliminary work to determine whether such a relationship is feasible for them. Exploration should include a discussion of each therapist's theoretical approaches, intervention styles, past experiences with groups, background, and personality characteristics. The therapists should consider and resolve such issues as how and when feedback is to be given, how disagreements between them are to be handled in the session, and the general conditions under which they will work together.

Decisions on client selection, length and number of sessions, time, and place are made together. Decisions of an emergency nature made by one therapist in the absence of the other should be based on mutually agreed procedures for just such contingencies.

Obviously, egalitarian cotherapists must establish and maintain clear channels of communication. Not only must they expend a great deal of time and energy in preparation for the group experience, but they must also plan for pre- and postsession meetings, joint analysis of data, and joint supervision or consultation.

The Leaderless Approach There is increasing interest in leaderless groups in two common forms—the occasional or regularly scheduled leaderless meeting as part of the structure of a group that is basically led by a therapist, and the leaderless group structured in some programmed format, usually through audiotapes.

Table 18–4   ADVANTAGES OF EGALITARIAN COTHERAPIST APPROACH

Advantage	Rationale
Facilitates group development	Two therapists of similar abilities can monitor and facilitate group development better than one alone.
Facilitates dealing with heightened affect	One therapist can relate more directly to the member experiencing heightened affect, while the other therapist assumes responsibility for assisting the group members with their responses. When one therapist is involved in an interaction with a member or members, the other can take an observer stance, helping those involved to become more aware of the interaction and their participation in it.
Enhances therapists' personal and professional development	Egalitarian cotherapists can provide one another with corrective feedback and help one another analyze group process and plan intervention strategies.
Provides a synergistic effect	This is another way of saying "two heads are better than one." It is likely that two persons working together will make better decisions than one person working alone. The synergistic effect is similar to that of making decisions by consensus.
Provides an opportunity for modeling	Group members observe the acceptance and respect for one another that egalitarian cotherapists demonstrate. The therapists tolerate difference and disagreement between them in an atmosphere of mutual trust.
Reduces dependence	Because leadership is shared, the problem of dependence is somewhat dissipated.
Promotes appropriate pacing	Cotherapists check one another's timing, thus allowing the process to emerge. The presence of a cotherapist provides a respite from being continually "on guard" in relation to group process.

Table 18–5   POTENTIAL DISADVANTAGES OF EGALITARIAN COTHERAPIST APPROACH

Potential Disadvantage	Rationale
Creates conflict if therapists have different orientations	Although there is room for uniqueness and difference, radically different styles and/or beliefs about group therapy between cotherapists may hinder therapeutic work within the group.
Requires extra energy and time	Each therapist must spend time and energy maintaining an effective working relationship with the other, since the quality of the relationship between them determines their effectiveness in the group setting.
May make members feel overloaded	If the style of the therapists turns out to be "two-on-one" (both working at once with one group member), members may feel overwhelmed or "overtherapized."
May suffer from the fact that the therapists share blind spots	Therapists who are very similar in style and personality may have the same blind spots and fail to give one another corrective feedback.
May provide the opportunity for misleading modeling	The model the therapists provide may be negative if their relationship is tense, mistrustful, closed, competitive, or threatening.

Leaderless meetings in a therapist-led group should not be scheduled until the group has become cohesive and has established productive norms. Then the process can foster a sense of autonomy and responsibility. However, therapists should identify and examine their rationale for planning leaderless meetings. The repercussions of leaderless meetings are varied and complex and require an experienced group therapist to deal with them.

Other leaderless groups may be structured totally around following directions in a booklet and on tape. Encounter group or sensitivity training tapes are common. For example, members listen to a tape explaining the exercises assigned for that session. The members participate as instructed on the tape and spend the remainder of the session discussing the exercise and their reactions to it. The mechanistic steps involved in this procedure contrast strangely with the humanistic intent of the experience, however.

Creating the Group

The effectiveness of a group depends heavily on the conditions under which it is created. Much as architects design buildings to withstand the stresses and strains created by humanity and nature, therapists design groups with certain functions and characteristics in mind.

Selecting Members   Selecting the members is one of the most important functions of the therapists, since the quality of the interpersonal relationships among the members constitutes the core of successful group treatment. This is one of the major differences between group and individual therapy.

INCLUSION CRITERIA   It is more difficult to identify the characteristics of people who make good candidates for group therapy than those of people who do not make good candidates. We know that a person's motivation for therapy in general, and group therapy in particular, is of primary importance. Inclusion in a therapy group should also be at least partially determined by the effect a prospective member will have on the others, in terms of the prospective member's ability to bring the curative factors into play. Inclusion is also determined by the balance, in terms of behavior or characteristics, a prospective member will bring to the group. Will the person's subdued presentation prevent a member with similar behavior from being marginal and alone in the group? Does the person's age, occupation, or sex match another's so that the member will no longer be singled out as different or deviant? The factor that appears to be most important, however, is that members be homogeneous in terms of their vulnerability or ego strength. Highly vulnerable members will retard the progress of the less vulnerable, and vice versa.

EXCLUSION CRITERIA   There have been a number of studies of group therapy dropouts. Dropouts significantly reduce the effectiveness of a group. They tend to have a demoralizing effect on the remaining group members. The act of dropping out is perceived by members as a comment on the value or worth of the

group. For this reason, therapists should gear selection to avoid taking on members who are likely to terminate prematurely. Irvin Yalom (1975) identified several reasons given for premature termination. They are detailed in Table 18-6. Yalom's research has also demonstrated that people who drop out are likely to have at least some of the following characteristics:

- They use denial to a significant extent
- They somatize frequently
- They are less well motivated than those who continue
- They are less psychologically oriented than those who continue
- They are lower in socioeconomic status than those who continue
- They are less effective socially than those who continue
- They have lower IQs than those who continue

It is also not uncommon to find that group therapy dropouts are persons who used the group for crisis resolution. They drop out once the crisis has passed.

The Selection Interview   The pregroup interview session has two major purposes: selecting the members and establishing the initial contract. Cotherapists should always interview potential members jointly, and both should make all decisions regarding membership. The interview session gives members and therapists the opportunity to be exposed to one another. In a sense, it is a time for participants to size one another up. The therapists should accomplish the following tasks in the selection interview:

- Determine the motivation of the potential member
- Determine the presence and extent of any exclusion criteria
- Identify the presence of any external crisis that may have propelled the person into treatment
- Encourage the client to ask questions about the group
- Correct erroneous prejudgments or misinformation the client has about group therapy
- Inquire about any major pending life changes that may prevent the client's full and continued participation in the group

Table 18-6 CLIENT REASONS FOR PREMATURE TERMINATION OF GROUP THERAPY	
Reason	**Rationale**
External factors	
Physical reasons	Distance, commuting, transportation, or scheduling problems may arise.
High external stress	An extremely stressful life may make it difficult or impossible for a client to expend energy participating in the group.
Group deviance	Members who differ significantly from others may wish to terminate; however, deviance that is unrelated to the group task is irrelevant.
Problems of intimacy	Isolated and withdrawn persons, or those with a pervasive dread of self-disclosure, are threatened by group therapy.
Fear of emotional contagion	Members may find they become highly upset on hearing the problems of others.
Early provocateurs	Members may create a nonviable role for themselves in the group; they plunge in with behavior that provides the main focus, are furiously active, then wish to withdraw
Problems in orientation to group therapy	If pretherapy tasks have not been properly undertaken, the member may not be realistically prepared for the group.
Complications arising from subgrouping	Subunits that split up the group may disrupt therapeutic work if not understood and handled appropriately.
Complications arising from concurrent individual and group therapy	The member's two therapies may work at cross-purposes; members may "save" their affect and experiences in the group for exploration in an individual session

- Inquire about what hurts; what the client sees a need to work on
- Establish and clarify the initial group contract

During this period, therapists and members have a chance to decide whether they can work together in the specific group under consideration. Clients as well as therapists can choose whether they will participate or not.

The Group Contract   The group contract identifies the shared rights and responsibilities of therapists and members. It is an agreed set of rules or arrangements for the structure and functioning of the group. It may be written or verbal, and it should cover the following elements:

- Goals and purposes of the group
- Time and length of meetings
- Place of meetings
- Starting and ending dates
- Addition of new members
- Attendance
- Confidentiality
- Roles of members and therapists
- Fees

GOALS AND PURPOSES   The purpose of the group must be clear to all persons involved. In interactive group psychotherapy, the purpose is to effect enduring behavioral and character change. The interactive group psychotherapy experience takes place largely in the here-and-now.

Goals may be long-term or short-term and are both group-oriented and individualized. While some goals may be identified as early as the selection interview, others may be added as they emerge during the life of the group. Goals may be altered as appropriate.

TIME, LENGTH, AND FREQUENCY OF MEETINGS   Time of meetings may be mutually determined by the participants. The length and frequency of meetings should be determined by the therapists after consideration of the clients' needs. Most outpatient clients find one eighty-to ninety-minute session per week useful. Shorter periods may not allow adequate time for discussion. Longer periods are generally beyond the endurance and alertness levels of both members and therapists. Inpatient groups are generally held more than once per week and frequently last for fifty to sixty minutes, although they may be longer or shorter depending on the anxiety and tolerance levels of the particular clients.

PLACE OF MEETINGS   The physical environment is important and influences the interaction among members. It is best to choose a pleasant room with comfortable chairs, preferably placed in a circle. The room should be private and free from external distractions.

STARTING AND ENDING DATES   If the group has a predetermined life span and the inclusive dates are known, members should be told the dates. Groups without fixed termination dates usually plan termination individually as each member is ready to move away from the group.

ADDITION OF NEW MEMBERS   Open groups accept members after the first session; closed groups begin with a certain number of members and do not add new members. Open groups maintain their size by replacing members who leave the group. They may continue indefinitely or have a predetermined life span. Closed groups are more common in settings where stability of membership is likely. Such settings include residential facilities of various types, long-term psychiatric inpatient settings, and prisons. A major problem with the closed group is that it runs the risk of extinction as members leave the group for various reasons.

ATTENDANCE   It is important that members make a commitment to attend every session. Absences hinder the establishment of cohesion and have a dampening effect, especially when perceived as evidence that a member lacks interest or that the group is not attractive and valuable to its members. Stability of membership and high attendance have been demonstrated to be critical factors in the successful outcome of group therapy.

CONFIDENTIALITY   Some rules regarding confidentiality should be established, and clients' concerns about which people will have access to information concerning them should be explored. Many therapists like to use tape recorders in order to have their work evaluated afterward by supervisors. They must obtain the clients' agreement to use of a tape recorder.

Rules about confidentiality and access may be determined by the therapists' employing agency. In some instances, therapists may be required to make regular notes concerning each member's participation. Therapists may also wish to establish with group members guidelines on confidentiality that allow the therapists

to share content with professionals when clients are dangerous to themselves or others. A good rule of thumb is: *Promise only what you can safely deliver.* Members should also be held accountable to maintain the confidentiality of the group.

ROLES OF MEMBERS AND THERAPISTS   Therapists and clients should reach an understanding about the responsibilities of participants. Humanistic psychotherapy involves the full and informed participation of the client in the therapeutic process. Participants should share their expectations about the behavior and functions of clients and therapists and should clearly understand the modes for participation.

FEES   Fees should be determined in advance and arrangements for payment made. Most mental health agencies have a sliding fee scale determined by the client's income and ability to pay. Clients should know whether fees will be charged for missed sessions.

Stages in Therapy Group Development

There is comfort in being able to predict, to some extent, the behavior of members at specific points in the group's life. Therapists organize predictions around stages or phases in the therapeutic experience, hoping to be forewarned of or prepared for expressions of behavior. They must bear in mind, however, that human experiences are dynamic and fluid and do not always progress as neatly as predicted.

The Schutz, Bennis and Shepard, and Martin and Hill frameworks, presented earlier in this chapter, give clear indications of how group life develops, and they will not be repeated here. This section focuses on the characteristics of member behavior and therapist interventions in the beginning, middle, and termination phases of interactional group therapy. As members' problems in living are revealed, the group life becomes richer and more complex. Therefore, there is no "cookbook" method that a therapist can follow to meet each and every contingency. Table 18–7 is presented simply as a guide, to identify some of the more common characteristics of member behavior and therapist interventions that tend to occur at various points in the life of the group.

The Here-and-Now Emphasis

The core around which interactional group therapy revolves is the here-and-now. According to Irvin Yalom (1975, pp. 121–22), the here-and-now work of the interactional group therapist occurs on two tiers:

	Table 18-7 CHARACTERISTIC MEMBER BEHAVIORS AND NURSING INTERVENTIONS IN PHASES OF GROUP THERAPY		
Member Behavior	**Nursing Interventions**	**Member Behavior**	**Nursing Interventions**
Beginning Phase		Self-disclosure increases	Encourage exploration and move to problem solving
Anxiety is high	Move to reduce anxiety; avoid making demands until group anxiety has abated	Members are more aware of interpersonal interactions in the here-and-now	Encourage members to participate in observing and commenting on here-and-now; make process comments
Members unsure of what to do or say; need to be included	Be active and provide some structure and direction; suggest members introduce themselves; work to sustain therapeutic rather than social role; include all members and encourage sharing but limit monopolizing	Additions and losses of members evoke strong reactions	Prepare members for additions and losses where possible; provide opportunity to talk about addition and loss experience
Members unclear about contract	Clarify contract; give information to dispel confusion or misunderstandings	Ability to maintain focus on one topic increases	Encourage exploration of topic area in depth
Members test therapists and other members in terms of trustworthiness, value stances, etc., often through goblet issues	Capitalize on opportunity to "pass" tests by proving trustworthy and by being open to and accepting the values of others	*Termination Phase*	
		Feelings about separation may run gamut (anger, sadness, indifference, joy, etc.)	Provide adequate time in as many sessions as necessary to work through affective responses; be sure members know termination date in advance; help members leave with positive feelings by identifying positive changes that have occurred in individual members and in group
Beginning attempts at self-disclosure and problem identification are made	Focus on related themes; begin exploration; begin to focus on here-and-now experiences in session	Members may feel lost and rudderless	Explore support systems available to individual members; bridge gap where possible (to another agency, another therapist, etc.); keep in focus task of resolving loss
Members have sense of "I"-ness, little sense of "we"-ness	Encourage involvement with others through curative factor of *universality*		
Middle Phase			
Sense of "I"-ness is replaced by "we"-ness	Encourage cohesion; provide opportunity for expression of warm feelings		

1. Focusing attention on the member's feelings toward other group members, the therapists, and the group

2. Illuminating the process (the relationship implications of interpersonal transactions)

Thus, group members need to become aware of the here-and-now events—that is, *what* happened—and then reflect back on them—that is, *why* it happened. Yalom has called this the self-reflective loop.

The first task of the therapist is to steer the group into the here-and-now. As the group progresses and becomes comfortable with awareness of the here-and-now, much of the work is taken on by the members. Initially, however, the therapist actively steers group discourse in an *ahistoric* direction. In other words, events in the session take precedence over those that occur outside or have occurred outside.

If the group is to engage in interpersonal learning, the therapist must illuminate process. This is the second task of prime importance. The group must move beyond a focus on content toward a focus on process—that is, the "how" and the "why" of an interaction. The process can be considered from any number of perspectives. The perspective chosen should be determined by the mood of the group at that particular time and what its needs are. The group must recognize, examine, and understand process. The task of illuminating it belongs mainly to the therapist.

Process commentary is anxiety-producing, because there are so many injunctions against it in social situations. For example, commenting on someone's nervousness at a cocktail party is generally taboo. Not only is it uncomfortable for the person whose nervousness is being observed, but also it puts the process commentator in a high-risk situation. The comment may well be taken as criticism, or viewed as inappropriate to the social context, and the commentator then will be vulnerable to retaliation from others.

Focus on the here-and-now experience differentiates interactive group psychotherapy from many other group therapies or therapeutic groups. The following section discusses some of these other approaches. Sensitivity, encounter, marathon, and other growth groups are discussed in Chapter 25.

OTHER GROUP THERAPIES AND THERAPEUTIC GROUPS

Analytic Group Psychotherapy

Analytic group psychotherapy stems from psychoanalysis and shares its goal of personality reconstruction. In this process, there is an intensive analytic focus on the individuals within the group. It has sometimes been described as treatment of the one in front of an audience of the many. Dream material and fantasies are explored within the group, and the technique of free association is used. The interpersonal interactions of the members are of secondary importance and are explored in terms of how they demonstrate unresolved conflicts in the individual members' earlier relationships.

Psychodrama

Psychodrama is chiefly concerned with problems unique to the individual. It provides a medium through which catharsis can be achieved on both the nonverbal action and gesture level and the verbal level. In psychodrama groups, members act out real or imagined situations, while alter egos (other members) attempt to add what they think the actor may be feeling or thinking. The participants are encouraged to change roles. The practice of role reversal offers them the opportunity to "get into the other person's skin." The psychodramatist (therapist) is called a "director" whose responsibility is to direct the drama toward the goal of achieving catharsis and reaching for insight.

The psychodramatic stage may be quite complex. It sometimes consists of a series of tiers where different parts of the drama are acted out. Complex lighting and mood music may also be used to achieve the desired effect.

Sociodrama

Sociodrama stems from psychodrama and uses many of the same techniques, but it differs from psychodrama in its essential purpose. In sociodrama, the emphasis is on the commonalities in the social roles of people and not problems unique to the individual. It can be defined as an action-oriented laboratory for observing verbal and nonverbal communication and for studying and solving problems in interpersonal relationships (Kneisl 1968). Any therapeutic benefits that participants may derive from it are secondary to the primary goal.

The sociodramatic environment is a safe place for experimentation in solving problems of interpersonal relationships. In it, members have the opportunity to experience group problem-solving and decision-making processes, to give and receive feedback, and to improve their skills and gain insights.

The technique of sociodrama is also used by educators in a variety of settings. It is commonly used when the educational goal has to do with taking on a role performance. Educational programs for teachers and nurses frequently incorporate sociodrama.

Multiple Family Group Therapy

In multiple family group therapy, a number of families meet together as a group. The number of families included in the group is determined by the number of persons in each family. This approach enables families to compare and contrast their concerns and interactional patterns with those of other families. The therapist in multiple family group therapy should be skilled in both group and family therapy. Family therapy skills are outlined in Chapter 21.

Self-help Groups

Self-help groups are sometimes called self-directed groups or lay groups in the literature. The major operating principle in self-help groups is that the help given to members comes from members. A professional mental health worker is viewed as unnecessary. In fact, many of these groups (Alcoholics Anonymous and organizations for drug addicts, such as Synanon) were developed because of the failure of programs planned and implemented by professionals. Some, such as women's consciousness-raising groups, are truly leaderless. In many of the others, leaders are former members. Alcoholics Anonymous and Synanon are relatively well known examples of the latter.

Self-help groups abound in several areas of concern. Some others are:

- Recovery Incorporated, Schizophrenics Anonymous, and Neurotics Anonymous, concerned with mental illness

- T.O.P.S., Weight Watchers, Diet Workshop, and Fatties Anonymous, concerned with obesity

- Gamblers Anonymous and Gam-Anon, concerned with compulsive gambling

- Five-Day Plan and Smoke Watchers Anonymous, concerned with smoking

- Child Abuse Listening Mediation, Inc. (C.A.L.M.) and Parents Anonymous, concerned with child abuse

- Daughters of Bilitis, Mattachine Society, and a variety of gay liberation groups, concerned with homosexuality

- La Leche League, concerned with breast feeding

- Al-anon and Al-a-teen, concerned with the families of alcoholics

- Daytop and Phoenix House, concerned with drug addiction

Self-help groups are proliferating rapidly. Groups for divorced, widowed, or single persons, for parents of runaways and troubled adolescents, for parents who abuse their children, and for the recently bereaved are becoming a common part of the scene in most major cities throughout the world. Client clubs for persons having had a colostomy, ileostomy, laryngectomy, mastectomy, or amputation are also popular.

The role of the nurse in self-help groups is that of a resource person. Nurses need to be informed about such groups so that they can refer potential members to groups appropriate to their needs or to provide consultation when invited to do so.

Remotivation and Reeducation Groups

Remotivation and reeducation groups were developed to help persons who had undergone long-term institutionalization become less isolated and more socially adept. Long-term institutionalization produces apathy and isolation. Clients ready for release are often unaware of accepted norms or socially appropriate behavior and therefore ill-equipped to live outside a totally protected environment. Remotivation and reeducation groups help prepare these people to live beyond the confines of the institution. The groups bring members up to date with contemporary society. They can be led effectively by people with minimal preparation in group work. In many psychiatric hospitals, this role falls to the psychiatric aide who is trained in the five structured steps that form the basis for sessions. Nurses are more likely to supervise than to lead remotivation groups. The five steps in a remotivation group are:

1. *The climate of acceptance* (5 minutes): The leader extends appreciation to the group for coming to the session. Each client is greeted warmly and individually by name, and new members are introduced. Additional brief comments directed toward each person individually help make person-to-person contact. The purpose of this first step is to establish a comfortable, relaxed atmosphere.

2. *A bridge to reality* (15 minutes): The reading of poetry provided the bridge to reality when the remotivation technique was first developed. More recently, quotations or news items have been used as the basis for discussion in this second step. During this period of time, the leader should make sure that each member has participated or has been encouraged to participate.

3. *Sharing the world we live in* (15 minutes): This step provides time for discussion of the topic introduced in the bridge to reality. Planned questions help keep the group focused on the topic. Props can be used to stimulate interest. The key in this step is the careful planning of questions and props.

4. *An appreciation of the work of the world* (15 minutes): This step promotes the connection between the members and work in relation to themselves. This discussion flows from the third step as the leader directs the group toward considering work related to the planned topic. The discussion may center around how a certain commodity is produced or how a specific job is done. It may also include a discussion of members' job preferences and past job experiences.

5. *The climate of appreciation* (5 minutes): The leader expresses enjoyment of the group and indicates the plans for the next session. It provides the members with a sense of continuity, with something to look forward to, and with a warm feeling about having attended.

Client Government Groups

Most therapeutic milieus have numerous group activities. One of the commonest is some form of client government. Client governments take many forms, but in most cases staff and clients meet together once or twice a week to discuss and resolve day-to-day issues on the ward. Generally, these are key principles in client government:

- The client government should actually make and enforce most of the ward rules.
- The client government should organize and execute most of the routine ward tasks.
- No staff member should attempt to solve a problem if it can be delegated to the client government.

Among the problems the client government considers are the tidiness of the ward, late-night use of the television, whether or not to have a Christmas tree, and individual clients' disruptive behavior. To make client government work, staff members must consciously refrain from making unilateral decisions that override client prerogatives. Needless to say, this strategy produces power relationships unlike those in the traditional medical model, in which it is believed that

doctors and nurses are the experts and clients do not know what is best for them. Client government does not require that staff sit silently by, however. Rather, staff members should offer their perspective on the issues while agreeing to abide by the group's decision. Obviously, client government raises many thorny issues. Decisions about the granting of leave or the issuing of medications have legal implications that sometimes make client government infeasible. In many cases the real decisions on these subjects are made in a substructure of separate staff meetings. It is often preferable for staff members to discuss issues that present problems for them in the open forum of the client government meeting. Otherwise, clients have no way of knowing how the system really operates, how decisions are made, or what their place is in the overall structure. A client government that is not being covertly undermined:

- Has a constitution with bylaws, holds regular meetings, and elects officers
- Votes on complaints and suggestions and presents the outcome to hospital authorities as the collective wishes of the group rather than of one individual
- Organizes ward rules
- Recommends changes in ward rules
- Arranges, organizes, conducts, and assumes responsibility for social activities
- Originates, plans, and carries through a variety of special activity programs, such as mural painting or writing and editing a newspaper
- Forms committees and elects leaders to engage in any program of hospital betterment approved by hospital authorities (Hyde and Solomon 1950, p. 207)

Proponents of client government as a strategy of milieu therapy argue that it is a logical and effective way of permitting clients to provide themselves with a more creative and wholesome hospital life. Ideally, instead of experiencing hospitalization as combination of idleness, inactivity, boredom, and regimentation, they will learn democratic living and acquire more versatile social skills. The success of this approach, however, depends on the willingness of hospital administrators and psychiatric professionals to be receptive to clients' ideas and suggestions. If they do not accept as valid the clients' definitions of their hospital experience, nothing can be accomplished.

Client government has many advantages. It offers:

- A way of making life in a mental hospital resemble life in the external community
- A way of controlling deviant behavior with group pressure
- Group support for very disturbed clients
- A way of increasing recreational activities
- An opportunity for clients to understand administrative policy and help formulate it
- A way of increasing clients' self-esteem
- An opportunity for clients to express annoyances and resentments
- A channel of communication between clients and staff members and ways of improving morale through the free interchange of ideas and feelings and of uncovering and working out tensions between staff and clients

The psychiatric staff nurse often serves as a resource person to client government groups, attending meetings to discuss issues of concern to clients and/or staff.

Activity Therapy Groups

Activity therapies use manual, recreational, and creative techniques to facilitate personal experiences and increase social responses and self-esteem. Some of them, such as occupational and recreational therapies, are discussed in Chapter 3. While nurses may participate, activity therapies are generally the province of health and recreation specialists specifically educated to perform these roles.

Some activity therapies, such as the creative arts therapies discussed below, are organized and conducted in groups. Although there are specifically educated creative arts therapists, their numbers are small (see Chapter 3). Nurses may participate in these groups or use their principles to reach beyond the ordinary realm of verbal communication with clients.

Poetry Therapy Groups   The goal of poetry therapy groups is to help members get in touch with feelings and emotions through the use of poetry. Poems that are read aloud provide the stimulus for understanding and catharsis. They are selected as the therapeutic medium because they are powerful but not explicit avenues of communication. It is not necessary to be able to write poetry to be a member or leader of a poetry therapy group, although some members or leaders may be stimulated to write poems of their own.

Art Therapy Groups   Painting offers many people a comfortable opportunity for social exchange. In art therapy groups, the art produced by each member gives the art therapist a personal insight into the artist's personality. The art is produced during the session and is used as the basis for discussion and for exploring the members' feelings.

Music Therapy Groups   Music therapy consists of singing, rhythm, body movement, and listening. It is designed to increase the group members' concentration, memory retention, conceptual development, rhythmic behavior, movement behavior, verbal and nonverbal retention, and auditory discrimination. It is also used to stimulate the member's expression and discussion of affect.

Dance Therapy Groups   Dance as a therapeutic mode combines movement and verbal modes. In dance, members find it easier to express nonverbally the feelings and emotions that are a part of them but have been difficult to realize and communicate by other means. The person's inner sense is often reflected in body movements, and dance therapists work to help members integrate their experiences on the verbal level as well as the nonverbal one.

Bibliotherapy Groups   In bibliotherapy, literature is the means for achieving a therapeutic goal. The purpose of a bibliotherapy group is to assimilate the psychological, sociological, and esthetic values from books into human character, personality, and behavior. Literature provides the stimulus for the members to compare events and characters with their own interpersonal and intrapsychic experiences.

Groups of Clients with Pathophysiological Dysfunction and Families

Groups composed of medical-surgical clients are increasingly common, as psychiatric nurses move into general hospital settings offering liaison and consultation services to clients and hospital staff (see Chapter 24). Group work is useful for chronically ill or disabled persons, preoperative and postoperative clients, clients with regulative medical problems (such as diabetes, cardiac disease, or kidney disease), dying clients, the aged, and clients with psychophysiological disorders, among others.

Such groups generally focus on the stress of hospitalization and illness and have as their goal the reduction of stress. Groups may be composed of clients alone, family members alone, or a combination.

Community Client Groups

As psychiatric nurses move into community settings, they become more and more involved with different kinds of community groups. These settings include schools, youth centers, residential facilities for delinquent youths, for runaways, and for unwed mothers, industries, neighborhood centers, churches, prisons, summer camps, single-room occupancy boarding houses, transitional facilities (halfway houses), and

apartments for the elderly. The clients may also be persons who have direct contact with these groups, such as teachers, youth counselors, prison guards, police officers, and camp counselors.

Groups with Nurse Colleagues

There is increasing interest among nurses who work together in forming discussion and counseling groups to help reduce their job-related stress and to help them deal with problems of interpersonal relationships in more satisfying ways. Nurses in various intensive care and other high-pressure settings identify with increasing frequency the need for group work services that the psychiatric nurse can provide. The psychiatric nurse may also identify the need and offer this opportunity to colleagues.

KEY NURSING CONCEPTS

✔ Groups significantly affect the person's psychological well-being.

✔ Nurses can provide humanistic care to clients in a variety of settings through the mode of group intervention by offering them opportunities to seek validation, give and receive interpersonal feedback, and test new and different ways of being that may increase their quality of life.

✔ Nurses need a sound basis in small group dynamics and an operational framework for group assessment. To function as a therapist, nurses also need a background in group therapy theory and supervised clinical practice with groups.

✔ Four helpful operational frameworks for group analyses include the Johari Awareness Model, the FIRO Interpersonal Needs Approach, the Authority Relations/Personal Relations Approach, and the Therapeutic Problem Approach.

✔ According to the Johari Awareness Model, when people have sufficient knowledge about one another's actions, motivations, and feelings they can use this knowledge to more clearly understand the significant events in a group.

✔ A basic assumption of the Interpersonal Needs Approach is that groups move through three interpersonal phases: inclusion, control, and affection.

✔ The Authority Relations/Personal Relations framework asserts that the principle obstacles to communication in groups stem from the orientations of the group members toward authority and intimacy.

✔ The Therapeutic Problem Approach assumes that therapy groups have distinct and common growth patterns that can be described, observed, and predicted.

✔ A commonality among all four frameworks is the notion that group development occurs in identifiable stages and has implications for member behavior and therapist intervention.

✔ Curative factors, or mechanisms of change which constitute a rational basis for the therapist's choices of tactics and strategies, are unique to the group therapy process.

✔ Groups can be led by a single individual, by two therapists working together, or through a leaderless approach.

✔ The most advantageous leadership style in interactional therapy groups is the egalitarian cotherapy approach in which leadership is shared by two therapists of relatively equal skill, ability, and status.

✔ The egalitarian style also provides an important opportunity for the group leader's personal and professional development.

✔ The early design and construction of a group has the most significant impact on its future success and effectiveness.

✔ Critical considerations in designing a group are the selection of members and the establishment of a group contract.

✔ In interactive groups, member interaction plays a crucial role in characterologic change, which is achieved through the use of the here-and-now to illuminate group process.

References

Bennis, W., and Shepard, H. A. "A Theory of Group Development." *Human Relations* 9 (1956): 415–437.

Compton, B. R., and Galaway, B. *Social Work Processes.* 2d ed. Homewood, Ill.: Dorsey Press, 1979.

Hyde, R. W., and Solomon, H. C. "Patient Government: A New Form of Group Therapy." *Digest of Neurology and Psychiatry,* April 1950, pp. 207–218.

Kneisl, C. R. "Increasing Interpersonal Understanding through Sociodrama." *Perspectives in Psychiatric Care.* May–June 1968, pp. 104–109.

Luft, J. "The Johari Window: A Graphic Model of Awareness in Interpersonal Relations." In *Group Processes,* 2d ed., pp. 11–20. Palo Alto, Calif.: National Press Books, 1970.

Luft, J., and Ingham, H. "The Johari Window: A Graphic Model of Interpersonal Awareness." *Proceedings of the Western Training Laboratory in Group Development,* University of California, Los Angeles, Extension Office, August 1955.

Martin, E. A., Jr., and Hill, W. F. "Toward a Theory of Group Development." *International Journal of Group Psychotherapy* 7 (1957): 20–30.

Schutz, W. C. "Interpersonal Underworld." *Harvard Business Review* 36 (1958): 123–135. (a)

————. *The Interpersonal Underworld: FIRO.* Palo Alto, Calif.: Science and Behavior Books, 1958. (b)

Yalom, I. D. *The Theory and Practice of Group Psychotherapy.* 2d ed. New York: Basic Books, 1975.

Further Reading

Amdur, M. A., and Cohen, M. "Medication Groups for Psychiatric Patients." *American Journal of Nursing* 81 (1981): 343–345.

Benton, D. W. "The Significance of the Absent Member in Milieu Therapy." *Perspectives in Psychiatric Care* 80 (1980): 21–25.

Bogdanoff, M., and Elbaum, P. "Role Lock: Dealing with Monopolizers, Mistrusters, Isolaters, Helpful Hannahs, and Other Assorted Characters in Group Psychotherapy." *International Journal of Group Psychotherapy* 28 (1978): 247–261.

Davis, L. E. "Racial Composition of Groups." *Social Work* 24 (1979): 208–213.

Farhood, L. "Choosing A Partner For Co-Therapy." *Perspectives in Psychiatric Care* 13 (1975): 177–179.

Frank, J. D., et al. "Behavioral Patterns in Early Meetings of Therapeutic Groups." *American Journal of Psychiatry* 108 (1952): 771–778.

Getty, C., and Shannon, A. M. "Co-therapy as an Egalitarian Relationship." *American Journal of Nursing* 69 (1968): 767–771.

Guttmacher, J. A., and Birk, L. "Group Therapy: What Specific Therapeutic Advantages?" *Comprehensive Psychiatry* 12 (1971): 546–556.

Hellwig, K., et al. "Partners in Therapy: Using the Co-Therapy Relationship in a Group." *Journal of Psychiatric Nursing* 16 (1978): 42–44.

Kelly, H. S., and Philbin, M. K. "Sociodrama: An Action-oriented Laboratory for Teaching Interpersonal Relationship Skills." *Perspectives in Psychiatric Care,* May–June 1968, pp. 110–115.

Kibel, H. D. "A Schema for Understanding Resistances in Groups." *Group Processes* 7 (1977): 221–236.

Kneisl, C. R. "Parent, Adult, Child: Identifying Ego States in Group Therapy." In *ANA Clinical Sessions,* pp. 315–325. New York: Appleton-Century-Crofts, 1968.

Light, N. "The 'Chronic Helper' in Group Therapy." *Perspectives in Psychiatric Care* 12 (1974): 129–134.

Loomis, M. E. *Group Process for Nurses.* St. Louis: C. V. Mosby, 1979.

McGee, T. F. "Therapist Termination in Group Psychotherapy." *International Journal of Group Psychotherapy* 24 (1974): 3–12.

Moline, R. "The Therapeutic Community and Milieu Therapy: A Review and Current Assessment." *Community Mental Health Review* 2 (1977): 1–13.

Moreno, J. L. "Psychodramatic Production Techniques." *Group Psychotherapy* 4 (1952): 243–273.

Peters, C., and Grunebaum, H. "It Could Be Worse: Effective Group Psychotherapy with the Help-rejecting Complainer." *International Journal of Group Psychotherapy* 27 (1977): 471–480.

Rabin, H. M. "Preparing Patients for Group Therapy." *International Journal of Group Psychotherapy* 20 (1970): 133–145.

Rouslin, S. "Relatedness in Group Psychotherapy." *Perspectives in Psychiatric Care* 11 (1973): 165–171.

Ruffin, J. E. "Racism as Counter-transference in Psychotherapy Groups." *Perspectives in Psychiatric Care* 11 (1973): 173–178.

Samuels, A. "Use of Group Balance as a Therapeutic Technique." *Archives of General Psychiatry* 11 (1964): 411–420.

Schutz, W. C. "On Group Composition." *Journal of Abnormal and Social Psychology* 62 (1961): 275–281.

————. "The Leader as Completer." In *Small Group Communication,* edited by R. Cathcart and L. S. Samovar, pp. 390–395. Dubuque, Iowa: William C. Brown, 1974.

Toker, E. "The Scapegoat as an Essential Group Phenomenon." *International Journal of Group Psychotherapy* 22 (1972): 320–332.

Weiner, M. F. "Termination of Group Psychotherapy." *Group Process* 5 (1973): 85–96.

Whitaker, D. S. "A Group Centered Approach." *Group Process* 7 (1976): 37–57.

Whitaker, D., and Lieberman, M. A. *Psychotherapy through the Group Process.* New York: Atherton Press, 1967.

Williams, R. A. "Contract for Co-Therapists in Group Psychotherapy." *Journal of Psychiatric Nursing* 14 (1976): 11–14.

Yalom, I. D. "Problems of Neophyte Group Therapists." *International Journal of Social Psychiatry* 15 (1966): 52–59.

19

Mental Health Counseling with Children

by Pamela Burton

CHAPTER OUTLINE

Need for Child Psychiatric Services
Levels of Prevention
   Basic Prevention
   Secondary Prevention
   Tertiary Prevention
The Developmental Model as a Basis for Assessment and Intervention
Emotional Disturbances
   Pervasive Developmental Disorders
   Other Childhood Disturbances
   Role of the Nurse in Residential Treatment
Intervention
   Basic Goals of Treatment
   Assessment
   Health Assessment Outline
   Communication Skills
   Conveying Acceptance
   Setting Limits
   Countertransference
Specific Treatment Modes
   Treatment Facilities
   Therapy: An Overview
   Play Therapy
   Group Therapy
   Art Therapy
   Brief Therapy
   Family Therapy
   Behavior Modification
   Milieu Therapy
The Hospitalized Child
   Anaclitic Depression
   Separation Anxiety
   Castration and Mutilation Fantasies
   Psychological Care of the Pediatric Client
Key Nursing Concepts

LEARNING OBJECTIVES

After reading this chapter, students should be able to

- Discuss the role of the children's psychiatric nurse and relate this role to the need for child mental health services
- Identify key points and problems of each developmental stage up to adolescence
- Describe basic treatment goals in mental health work with children and identify nursing skills needed for their achievement
- Explain the characteristics of major treatment modes used with children
- Comprehend the psychological care of the pediatric client

CHAPTER 19

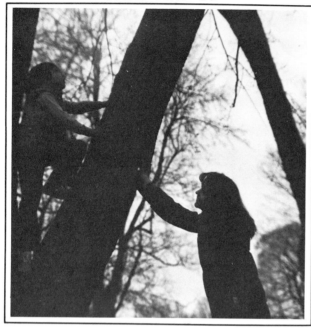

The child, as Wordsworth said, is father of the man. To understand adult growth, development, and pathology, we must understand primary, secondary, and tertiary prevention with children.

Child psychiatric nursing, like adult psychiatric nursing, is a specialty role. However, nursing generalists also work with children—in hospitals, in the community, in clinics, and in offices. The topic of child psychiatric nursing is relevant for these generalists—and for nurses who work with adult clients as well. Understanding normal growth and development and childhood psychopathology helps nurses understand adult psychological growth and development and psychopathology. The child, as Wordsworth said, is father of the man. To understand the adult client, we need to start with the child.

NEED FOR CHILD PSYCHIATRIC SERVICES

In the United States, only a fraction of the children who need mental health intervention receive it. According to the Joint Commission on Mental Health of Children, 1,400,000 children and adolescents need professional psychiatric help (1969, pp. 5–6). Current resources in the mental health field, particularly the resource of child psychiatric clinicians, cannot meet this demand for services.

The fundamental goal of all mental health services and interventions is to prevent mental illness and to encourage optimal mental health. The use of a developmental model for assessment helps meet this goal. Many developmental problems go unnoticed until the child enters school. Yet during the first five years, development is extremely rapid, and children are particularly vulnerable to both physiological and psychological trauma. According to the Joint Commission report, estimates indicate that 20 to 30 percent of chronic handicapping conditions could be prevented by comprehensive health care to age five. The report urges that highest priority be given to the development of "comprehensive mental health, pediatric, and supportive services for children under three, and that a major effort should be made to provide systematic care during the neonatal and postnatal stage (Joint Commission 1969, p. 33).

The development and implementation of this type of program depends largely on the availability of necessary personnel. Child mental health professionals, who cannot even meet current demands for service, will be needed in far greater numbers. Psychiatric nurses with expertise in child psychology are in a position to help meet this need.

LEVELS OF PREVENTION

The Joint Commission report advocates a network of mental health services designed to meet the developmental needs of the total child. These services are organized on three levels of prevention. At each level there is scope for the practice of child psychiatric nursing.

Basic Prevention

The goal of basic prevention is to ensure that the developmental needs of the child are met. Basic prevention would include comprehensive prenatal care, day care and preschool programs, nutritional programs, and guaranteed adequate housing, food, income, and transportation. At this level of prevention the children's psychiatric nurse can:

- Provide classes for prospective and expectant parents that include information on infant growth and development and assessment of parenting skills (for specific information on this particular approach to primary prevention, see Chapter 13)
- Offer child-centered divorce counseling
- Teach parenting and child growth and development classes through community agencies and schools
- Provide consultation to pediatric wards and day care centers

Secondary Prevention

Secondary prevention is designed to detect early warning signs, thus decreasing the disability rate by shortening the duration of the disorder. At this level, the psychiatric nurse has a role as a primary therapist in child guidance clinics, providing individual and group counseling for children, parents, and families. Working within the school system, the nurse could provide crisis intervention, as well as anticipatory guidance and information about parenting and child development. Alternatively, the psychiatric nurse is qualified to provide consultation to schools and school nurses. Systematic, developmental assessments and referrals by school nurses would contribute significantly to prevention at the secondary level. Another excellent example of secondary prevention in child mental health is provided by a new and exciting specialty within child psychiatry called infant psychiatry. Infant psychiatrists diagnose and treat emotional problems in very young children in the belief that intervention in the formative months can avert the development of grave psychiatric disturbances both in childhood (e.g., autism) and in later life.

Tertiary Prevention

Ideally, tertiary prevention provides the rehabilitation that prevents a disorder from becoming permanent. Its purpose is to allow the child to function at the optimal level of wellness. Services at the tertiary level could be designed on the basis of the child's level of functioning, rather than the medical model of diagnostic labels. It is on the tertiary level of prevention that psychiatric nurses have traditionally worked. In residential and day care programs for emotionally disturbed children,

they function as milieu therapists, group leaders, parent counselors, and occasionally as primary therapists.

As the nursing profession continues to examine expanded roles for nurses, more nurses are beginning to work with children in roles at all levels of prevention. The options—both current and future—are exciting.

THE DEVELOPMENTAL MODEL AS A BASIS FOR ASSESSMENT AND INTERVENTION

A sound working knowledge of growth and development is the foundation for all assessments and interventions. Nurses must understand normal growth and development in order to differentiate between pathological reactions and the disturbances intrinsic to normal developmental progression. Therefore, before considering problems associated with different developmental stages, the reader is encouraged to study Table 19-1, which presents the key points of normal developmental progression, using the concepts developed by Gesell (1940, 1946) for benchmarks in development and Erikson's (1950) basic tasks.

EMOTIONAL DISTURBANCES

What causes emotional disturbances? Theories of etiology range from the belief that they are all caused by unconscious or conscious maternal rejection to the belief that they are all caused by biochemical or physiological factors. Most clinicians are now steering a middle course that emphasizes the interaction between children and their environment. In the interactional view, emotional disturbance is caused by a dysfunctional interaction between a constitutionally susceptible child and a psychologically incompatible environment.

Emotional disturbances are not distinct clinical entities. This is particularly true in childhood. The Joint Commission (1969, p. 253) has formulated the following definition of emotionally disturbed children:

An emotionally disturbed child is one whose progressive personality development is interfered with or arrested by a variety of factors so that he shows impairment in the capacity expected of him for his age and endowment:
(1) for reasonable accurate perception of the world around him
(2) for impulse control

				Manifestations of Unsuccessful	Benchmarks in
Stage	Basic Task	Dynamics	Methods Used	Accomplishment	Development
Oral stage (approximately birth to 1 year)	To achieve basic trust versus mistrust	Infants learn to distinguish "me" from "not me" by forming an object attachment to primary caregiver, while realizing that they are separate. As the caregiver consistently and quickly meets their needs for comfort, food, and nurturance, infants develop a sense of trust in the world and the "not me" others who inhabit it.	1. *Oral exploration:* sucking, biting, spitting, mouthing. Used to examine environment, express feelings, obtain food. 2. *Crying* and other preverbal vocalizations used to communicate with others. 3. *Gratification:* obtained when biological needs are met, and infant and caregiver both experience fulfillment. 4. *Exploration:* infants use eyes, arms, and legs, as well as mouth, to explore environment, thus making it familiar rather than frightening.	1. Inability to trust, and so to form meaningful relationships with others. 2. Individual remains psychologically extremely dependent. 3. Individual becomes compulsive eater or drinker in attempt to reduce anxiety and satisfy needs for love and security.	*1 day to 1 month* Malus crawling movements Responds to heat *1 month* Makes a fist Tonic neck reflex Follows object to midline Coos and gurgles *2 months* Follows object 180° Social smile present Suck, grasp reflexes *4 months* Will reach for object *5 months* Can roll over *6 to 8 months* Sitting Crawling Uses raking grasps *9 months* Can intentionally release objects *10 months* Exhibits pincer grasp *10 to 14 months* Walking Use of three to four words

Table 19–1   NORMAL DEVELOPMENTAL PROGRESSION

Table continues on next page

Table 19–1 continued

Stage	Basic Task	Dynamics	Methods Used	Manifestations of Unsuccessful Accomplishment	Benchmarks in Development
Anal stage (approximately 1 to 3 years)	To achieve autonomy versus shame and doubt	The achievement of a sense of autonomy is closely linked with the muscular maturation necessary to control elimination. The child now has a choice. This choice is exercised by holding on or letting go. The ideal outcome of this stage is a sense of self-control without loss of self-esteem. Successful resolution of the previous stage gives the child a sense of initiative.	1. *Exploration:* The toddler, like the infant, continues to explore, experiment, and manipulate the environment. The ability to walk allows the child wider exploration of the surroundings. With masturbation, children explore their own bodies. 2. *Language:* Used for verbal communication of needs, feelings, and desires. 3. *Control:* Body is used to give or withhold part of self (bowel movement) in order to control others or to express feelings. This is important in helping the child to learn how to give, take, and choose. Willingness to delay gratification at the request of others can bring an increased sense of control and satisfaction. This is an important step in the socializing process.	1. Lowered self-esteem and feelings of doubt and shame that arise out of an unsuccessful resolution of the anal stage can result in a. Extremely negativistic behavior b. Passive-aggressive behavioral patterns c. Obsessive or compulsive neurosis d. Sadistic or masochistic tendencies	*1½ years* Scribbles Knows ten words Can build two-cube tower Has bowel training capability *2 years* Can build six-cube tower *2½ years* Can name six body parts Talks in three-word sentences and uses pronouns *3 years* Can match four colors Can copy a circle Can ride a tricycle
Oedipal stage (approximately 3 to 6 years)	To achieve a sense of initiative versus guilt	This stage is so named because the child normally experiences feelings of rivalry toward the parent of the same sex, while desiring the attention of the parent of the opposite sex.	1. *Fantasy:* The initiative developed at this stage depends partly on the ability to engage in fantasy play, through which children explore their identity. 2. *Exploration:* As mental and locomotor capabilities expand, the child explores self and environment using new skills. The dimension of planning is added to exploration. 3. *Developing a sense of self:* Through exploration, children learn about their	1. A sense of guilt rather than initiative or a sense of guilt linked to the sense of initiative. 2. Confused sex role identification. 3. Faulty superego development.	*3½ years* Can walk on a line Will take turns Talks to self and others *4 years* Can copy an X Can throw overhand *4½ years* Can copy a square

Table continues on next page

Table 19–1 continued

Stage	Basic Task	Dynamics	Methods Used	Manifestations of Unsuccessful Accomplishment	Benchmarks in Development
		Successful resolution of the previous stage, and the resulting sense of autonomy, give the child the skills and confidence needed to develop a sense of initiative.	family and sex roles and how to associate with peers. All this helps children develop a sense of self. They then begin to observe their own actions and thoughts. This is the beginning of the adult superego.		*5 years* Can copy a triangle Can tie knots in string *6 years* Can tie shoes Can ride two-wheeler Can copy a diamond Can print name Can make single function similarities
Latency stage (approximately 6 to 12 years)	To achieve a sense of industry versus inferiority	In this stage the beginnings of conscience and identification with the culture as represented by adults that started in the Oedipal stage are refined by a repression of libidinal drives and Oedipal desires with a concomitant strengthening of the ego. This allows the child to relinquish the "family romance" of the Oedipal stage and look outside the family for recognition.	1. *Exploration:* The child's world now includes the neighborhood and school, which offer the opportunity to learn and try out new skills and values. This expansion of the child's world also allows the child to try out roles and values in various social and authoritative situations, thus learning things such as acceptance of responsibility for own behavior, appropriate responses to situations, and acceptance of reasonable restrictions and demands. 2. *Peer relationships:* Through peer relationships, the child learns skills such as cooperation, compromise, and competition. 3. *Mastery:* The child earns recognition by mastering skills and tasks that result in the production of things. This leads to a sense of industry and accomplishment.	1. Feelings of inferiority and inadequacy, if child despairs of skills or status among peers. 2. Conflicts in sexual identification. 3. Fixation at this stage may result in a continuation of "chum" love and incapacity to direct love toward a member of the opposite sex.	*7 years* Knows days of week Can make simple opposite analogies *8 years* Can count five digits forward Can define some abstract terms such as *brave* and *nonsense* *9 years* Knows seasons, rhymes *10 years* Can count four digits backwards Can define more sophisticated abstract terms such as *pity* and *grief*

(3) for satisfying and satisfactory relations with others
(4) for learning
(5) any combination of these

All assessments of emotional disturbance must be evaluated within the framework of normal growth and development since behavior that is part of normal growth and development at one age may be a symptom of pathology at another age. For instance, persistent enuresis would be of concern in a ten-year-old, but not in a two-year-old.

Pervasive Developmental Disorders

Autism   The autistic child presents a special challenge to the psychiatric nurse. Unlike the schizophrenic child, who has withdrawn from interaction with others, the autistic child has never engaged in interaction. This lack of interaction can be baffling and frustrating if the nurse does not have a theoretical understanding of autism.

CHARACTERISTICS   Early Infantile Autism was first described by Kanner (1943). Kanner lists the following characteristics of the autistic child:

• *Lack of involvement with others.* From infancy, the child is unresponsive and uninterested in others. Parents of autistic children will say that the baby shows no reaction to being held or cuddled and does not seem to care about them or anyone else. One mother of an autistic child said holding her baby was "just like holding a sack of flour."

• *Lack of verbal communication.* Some autistic children never use speech at all. Others may repeat words or phrases endlessly (echolalia) or perform other verbal exercises. However, they do not use speech to convey meaning. This failure to employ speech for communication has both interpersonal and intrapsychic implications. Interpersonally, lack of verbal communication further isolates the autistic child from others. Intrapsychically, it impedes development of the ego. The use of speech to verbalize perceptions increases ego strength and allows the child to engage in reality testing. This, in turn, helps the child to learn to distinguish between fantasies, wishes, and thoughts on the one hand and reality on the other. Because autistic children cannot use speech to determine what is real and what is not, they do not move from primary process thought to secondary process thought. Thus they remain cap-

tive to thought processes usually abandoned in toddlerhood.

• *Preoccupation with inanimate objects.* Although they are seemingly unable to become involved with people, autistic children are fascinated by objects. Often they use objects, like words, in a repetitive manner. For instance, they may watch a record player spin around and around or turn lights on and off for hours.

• *Ritualistic behavior.* Preservation of routine and sameness is extremely important to autistic children. They possibly receive from this sameness some of the security they cannot get from interpersonal relationships. Autistic children order their lives strictly. Every commonplace activity has a rigid ritual attached to it. Every object must stay in the same place. A chair out of place or failure to follow a bedtime ritual can set off panic and rage in the autistic child.

All of the characteristics listed above are apparent in the following description of severely disturbed children on a residential unit.

These children showed serious and persistent psychotic behavior at all times of functioning. They were extremely sensitive to even apparently minor disappointments and frustrations. Their reaction was often profound withdrawal or destructive rage toward themselves and others—head-banging, kicking, biting, and tearing clothing. Their manneristic behavior included such isolated activities as rocking, twiddling objects, masturbating, aimless pacing and running, flapping arms and hands, and standing in one particular area in a fixed position. They often repeated certain acts over and over, such as retracing steps or touching, licking, or smelling certain objects. They had many difficulties in eating, sleeping, and elimination. . . . Their communication was usually nonverbal, distorted, and difficult to comprehend [Boatman 1971, p. 59].

ETIOLOGY OF AUTISM   There is controversy about the relative importance of heredity and environment in the etiology of autism. It is uncertain. The autistic child is thought to be regressed to, or fixated at, the earliest developmental stage before the child differentiates "me" from "not me." The causative factors are variously thought to be:

• *Environment only.* Infant is tabula rasa and all disturbance is directly attributable to the environment (primarily the parenting).

- *Heredity only.* For genetic, biochemical, or other pre-determined reasons, some infants will be psychotic regardless of the environment.

- *Combination of environment and heredity* plus *the interaction between them*. A susceptible infant, less-than-optimal parenting, and negative interaction between parent and infant will combine to produce disturbance.

Autistic children are not retarded. Though difficult to test, they are generally believed to be of well-above-average intelligence. Unfortunately, the psychopathology of Autism severely restricts the manner in which these children can use their intelligence. Most of their energy is invested in the defensive behaviors necessary to control their anxiety.

Childhood Onset Pervasive Developmental Disorder   As with the autistic child, the child suffering from a Childhood Onset Pervasive Developmental Disorder is severely disturbed. This disturbance, unlike a Specific Developmental Disorder, affects many basic areas of psychological development. Children now classified as victims of Pervasive Developmental Disorders may have been formerly labeled symbiotic-psychotic or childhood schizophrenic. The onset of this full syndrome is identified later than Autism, usually after thirty months and before twelve years. There are no delusions, hallucinations, incoherence, nor a marked loosening of associations, but the child displays an obvious and long-lasting impairment in social relationships, such as inappropriate clinging or a lack of affective response. The child also displays at least three of the following symptoms:

- Sudden excessive anxiety manifested by symptoms such as unexplained panic attacks, free-floating anxiety, or catastrophic reactions to everyday occurrences

- Constricted or inappropriate affect

- Resistance to change in the environment or ritualistic behavior

- Oddities of motor movement, such as peculiar posturing

- Abnormalities of speech

- Sensitivity to sensory stimulation that is either excessive or less than normal

- Self-mutilation

(American Psychiatric Association 1980(b), pp. 52–53)

Treatment for the Severely Disturbed Child
The severely disturbed child requires intensive psychotherapy and often milieu therapy available in residential or day care programs. Therapy is usually indicated for parents also. Psychiatric nurses can work on a primary level of prevention by assessing parenting skills of prospective parents and teaching them these skills. (See Chapter 13.) On a secondary level of prevention, psychiatric nurses can learn and teach others the early signs of childhood psychosis, making appropriate referrals. The earlier the intervention, the better the prognosis. On a tertiary level of prevention, psychiatric nurses work with severely disturbed children and their families in child guidance clinics and residential and day care settings. The decision to remove these children from their homes is not made lightly. The children in residential treatment settings are those considered severely disturbed.

Other Childhood Disturbances

Reactive Attachment Disorder of Infancy   The primary symptom or characteristic of a Reactive Attachment Disorder of Infancy (sometimes referred to as "failure to thrive") is a lack of emotional and physical development or growth in the infant over a period of time. A physiological etiology, such as heart, central nervous system, or kidney abnormalities, must be ruled out. Therefore, hospitalization and evaluation of physiological functioning are essential. If no physiological etiology can be isolated, the problem may be due to psychologically inadequate caretaking. During hospitalization, a nurturing plan is developed for the infant, using specifically assigned personnel and involving the caretaker parent. If the infant grows and develops with nurturing, it is usually concluded that a Reactive Attachment Disorder of Infancy exists, with problems of parenting as a causative factor. Frequently, psychotherapeutic and child-protective interventions are necessary.

Disorders with Physical Manifestations   A *refusal of food* on the part of the infant can be due to a Reactive Attachment Disorder, rigid feeding schedule, psychological stress, incompatible formula, or physiological causes such as pyloric stenosis. Pediatric evaluation is necessary, especially if the child is not gaining or is losing weight. A physiological etiology or incompatible formula should be ruled out, then the feeding style of the caretaker evaluated. Consider such things as whether the baby is on demand feeding, and whether the caretaker is sensitive to the infant's needs or communications about holding, hunger, and satiation. A serious feeding disturbance, in which the infant does not grow or develop over a period of time, may indicate a Reactive Attachment Disorder of Infancy, and the child should be hospitalized for evaluation.

Colic involves crying that usually is confined to one part of the day and starts after a feeding. It commonly begins in the first to the third month and may be caused by sharp intestinal pains produced by gas, possibly due to periodic tension in the infant's immature nervous system. Intervention consists of reassuring the parents and giving them information about the condition. Hot water bottles, rocking, rubbing the back, or a pacifier may soothe the infant.

Sleeping disturbances, in which the infant resists being put down to sleep or going to sleep, can be an indication that the infant wants more parental attention. This pattern can be formed during a period of colic or of illness, or it can be related to anxiety. If it is an attention-getting strategy, parental lack of response for a few nights usually breaks the pattern. If an emotional disturbance is suspected, evaluation of the infant–caretaker interaction and possible psychotherapeutic intervention is indicated. For guidelines to evaluate the infant–caretaker interaction, see Chapter 13.

Encopresis, or soiling, in the older child is rarely physiological but is the child's expression of anger or hostility. It is usually directed toward the parent with whom the child is experiencing conflict. Interventions include medical evaluation, then assessment and intervention in the child–parent relationship. Therapy may be indicated for both child and possibly parents.

Enuresis ordinarily refers to wetting while asleep (nocturnal enuresis), though some enuretic children wet themselves during the day also. Enuresis is a symptom, not a diagnosis or disease entity. The child under four years old is usually not considered enuretic. Causative factors are thought to be faulty toilet training (especially if the child wets during the day also) or psychological stress. Physiological etiology, such as genito-urinary (GU) tract infections or CNS disease, is rare.

Many approaches to enuresis have been tried, with varying degrees of success. These include Trofranil, fluid restriction, behavioral intervention (in which a buzzer wakes the child who is starting to wet), and psychotherapy. Educating parents in bladder-training techniques and attitudes can help solve the problem on a primary level. It is important when working with enuretic children or their parents to help the child overcome feelings of shame and guilt. These feelings are often exacerbated by well-meaning but misguided parents.

Constipation may be caused by a faulty diet, or the child may be withholding due to one or two hard, painful bowel movements. Psychological causation occurs when the child withholds from the parents to express anger or opposition or is passing through a very independent developmental stage. Interventions include evaluation of the child's diet and the consistency of the stools. Fecal softener can be prescribed if necessary. In all cases, the nurse should help the parent avoid making an issue of constipation with the child. Enemas are contraindicated. If the child is withholding and is toddler age, the parents should be encouraged to not force rigid toilet training on the child. (Most children are more cooperative about toilet training at eighteen to twenty-four months.)

Behavioral Disorders *Oppositional Disorders* include a pattern, for at least six months, of disobedient, negativistic opposition. The onset is after three years and before eighteen years. The general symptoms include violations of rules, temper tantrums, provocative behavior, argumentativeness, and stubbornness; but with no violation of the basic rights of others or of major age-appropriate societal norms or rules (American Psychiatric Association 1980(b), p. 41).

Excessive rebelliousness can include frequent temper tantrums, fighting, destruction of toys and other objects, and consistent oppositional behavior. This should not be confused with the expression of negativism that is normal at around two years of age, which is a necessary (although trying) developmental stage. Excessive rebelliousness usually indicates a frightened child. Inconsistency in handling the child, the setting of rigid limits, or the parents' refusal or inability to set limits all can create insecurity and fear in the child. The nurse should offer the parent counseling, if necessary. When working with the child, the nurse needs to be receptive and sympathetic while establishing and maintaining firm limits.

Conduct Disorders or *behavior problems* may be how older, latency-age children express their conflicts. This includes nonproductive behavior that is repeated despite threats, punishments, or rational argument and that usually leads to punishment. Persistent stealing and truancy are examples. The child is expressing and communicating conflicts through behavior, rather than verbally. Counseling or therapy for the child by a psychiatric nurse or other mental health worker can allow the child to resolve the basic conflict, thus making the problem behavior unnecessary. Conduct Disorders in the child can be aggressive (in which the basic rights of others are violated) or nonaggressive.

Attention Deficit Disorder with Hyperactivity   The child with an Attention Deficit Disorder with Hyperactivity is often attempting to control anxiety and can attend when interested or relaxed. Some psychologists speculate that hyperactive children do not fit smoothly into their environment, but the problem may be with the environment rather than with the child. In other words, the school environment requires a high degree of conformity; is the child who does not fit the mold necessarily emotionally disturbed?

Many children are incorrectly labeled hyperactive. The American Psychiatric Association, in the DSM-III, has delineated the following criteria for this diagnosis:

A. Inattention   The child demonstrates at least three of:

1. Fails to finish things started

2. Often doesn't seem to listen

3. Is easily distracted

4. Has difficulty concentrating

5. Has difficulty sticking to play activities

B. Impulsivity   At least three of:

1. Often acts before thinking

2. Shifts excessively from one activity to another

3. Has difficulty organizing work

4. Needs a lot of supervision

5. Often calls out in class

6. Has difficulty awaiting turn in games or group situations

C. Hyperactivity   At least two of:

1. Excessively runs about or climbs on things

2. Has difficulty sitting still

3. Has difficulty staying seated

4. Moves about excessively during sleep

5. Is always ''on the go''

(American Psychiatric Association 1980(a), pp. 43–44).

In addition, onset must be before seven years, the symptoms must have lasted at least six months, and the condition must not be due to another mental disorder. The child suffering from an Attention Deficit Disorder without Hyperactivity would display the same symptoms, except signs of hyperactivity.

Treatment for the child with an Attention Deficit Disorder with Hyperactivity is controversial. Sometimes Ritalin is prescribed, which for some clinicians raises the issue of whether an individual should be medicated in order to fit more smoothly into the environment. Therapy can help the child decrease anxiety and increase self-esteem, thus reducing the symptoms.

Anxiety Disorders   Anxiety Disorders in children can take the form of Separation Anxiety, Avoidant Disorders, and Overanxious Disorder (generalized anxiety not related to separation concerns). Of course, all children, like all adults, are subject to anxiety occasionally, and the symptoms must be of at least six months' duration for a diagnosis of *Anxiety Disorder* to be made.

Excessive Conformity includes a lack of spontaneity, anxious desire always to please all adult authority figures, timidity, refusal to assert needs, and passivity. The child may also seem preoccupied with past performance, be very concerned about competence, and be very self-conscious and susceptible to embarrassment (American Psychiatric Association 1980(b), p. 37). These children have established very rigid control in an attempt to handle fears. Harsh toilet training can produce an overly compliant child. These children need help as much as rebellious children, but they get it less frequently because their behavior is not a ''problem'' for parents or teachers.

Excessive Conformity can lead to compulsive, ritualistic, or obsessive behavior later. The psychiatric nurse needs to be able to identify these children then to work with the child and parents to encourage self-expression in the child. Psychotherapy may be necessary to help the child deal with repressed anger.

Excessive Fears are usually caused by anxiety. The child will be frightened even in nonthreatening situations. Nightmares and other sleep disturbances occur. The child may display an excessive need for reassurance, unrealistic worries about future events, and noticeable tension. This anxiety can be induced by many things, such as parental failure to set appropriate limits, physical or psychological abuse, or illness. (Imaginary worries are common at around four, so a four-year-old who is suddenly afraid of the dark, or dogs, or sirens is not necessarily suffering from Excessive Fears.)

Intervention includes, if possible, identifying and dealing with the factors that are producing the anxiety. Offer the child calm reassurance. Night lights and open doors can help allay night fears. With the hospitalized child, the nurse needs to be aware of and work with the fears common to the child's age group.

Regression includes resumption of activities, such as thumb sucking, soiling and wetting, or baby talk, that are characteristic of earlier developmental levels. The child is attempting to regain a more comfortable previous level of development in response to a threatening situation, such as a new baby or hospitalization experience. The nurse should counsel parents not to make an issue of the behavior but to offer the child emotional support and acceptance, though not approval, of the regressive behavior. It is also helpful to reassure the parents that such regressions are temporary, particularly when parents can continue to be supportive and accepting of the child.

Withdrawal or Avoidant Disorder is expressed by reduced body movement and verbalization, lack of close relationships, detachment, timidity, and seclusiveness. Withdrawal is defensive behavior through which the child controls anxiety by reducing contact with the outer world. Like the overcompliant child, the withdrawn child is frequently not identified as needing help, because this behavior is not a "problem."

The withdrawn child should be offered positive reinforcement when the child is more active. Techniques designed to help these children assert themselves and experience success at certain tasks can be helpful. Occasionally, parents of the withdrawn child are extremely overprotective; in this case, the nurse needs to work with the parents also. Therapy may be useful to work through anxiety and provide the child with an opportunity to form a trusting relationship with another.

"School Phobia" is actually not a phobia, but an acute anxiety reaction related to separation from home and major attachment figures. The child displays a sudden and seemingly inexplicable fear of going to school and/or complains of many physical symptoms on school days. If the child is allowed to stay home, the dread of returning to school usually increases. The child and parent should have psychiatric intervention quickly (before the problem becomes worse) to help the child separate from the parent. In addition to a reluctance or refusal to go to school; Separation Anxi-

ety Disorder can also manifest itself by: reluctance to go to sleep; avoidance of being alone in the house; unrealistic worries about the safety of major attachment figures and/or that untoward events will separate the child from the major attachment figure; nightmares about separation; sadness or apathy when not with the major attachment figure; and signs of excessive distress (for children under six, this must be of panic proportions to qualify as a symptom of Separation Anxiety Disorder) when anticipating separation from major attachment figures (American Psychiatric Association 1980(b), pp. 34–35). The duration of the disturbance must be at least two weeks for the child to be diagnosed as suffering from a Separation Anxiety Disorder.

Specific Developmental Disorders   Children who show failure or difficulty in learning at school are labeled "learning disabled." These disorders can be Developmental Reading Disorders, Developmental Language Disorders, Developmental Arithmetic Disorders, or a Mixed Specific Developmental Disorder (where there is more than one specific developmental disorder, but none is predominant). The disorders may be caused by many factors or combinations of factors. These include anxiety, poor sensory or sensorimotor integration, dyslexia, and receptive aphasia. Most children who fail at school experience feelings of inferiority, discouragement, and loss of confidence.

A comprehensive evaluation is essential. Ideally, this would include assessments by a pediatric neurologist, a mental health worker such as a psychiatric nurse or psychiatrist, a teacher trained especially to work with children with these disorders, and possibly an occupational therapist trained to work with sensory integration. Treatment is then based on the specific problem or problems.

Mental Retardation   The diagnostic criteria for Mental Retardation include an IQ of 70 or below on an individually administered IQ test (or for an infant, a clinical judgment of intellectual functioning that is significantly below average), concurrent deficits or impairments in adaptive behavior (age being taken into consideration), and onset before eighteen years of age (American Psychiatric Association 1980(b), pp. 25–26). There are four subtypes of Mental Retardation which are listed in Table 17–3. Partly because evaluation measures now in use with infants do not give numerical values, the possibility of Mental Retardation, except when it it profound, is more difficult to evaluate in younger children.

Treatment for the mentally retarded child has as its primary goal the optimum level of functioning possible for the individual child. Obviously, this will be determined to a large extent by the severity of the retardation. Except with the more severe forms of the condition, a supportive environment with the emphasis placed on what the children can achieve, rather than on their limitations, can do much to ameliorate the restrictions imposed by Mental Retardation. Chapter 17 discusses Mental Retardation in detail.

Schizoid Disorder of Childhood   The child suffering from a Schizoid Disorder of Childhood is an isolated child with a very limited ability to form social relationships. Unlike children with an Avoidant Disorder who desire social participation but are inhibited by anxiety, children with a Schizoid Disorder apparently prefer isolation and a lack of social involvement with peers. The child may develop a desire for increased socialization during adolescence or may become even more withdrawn leading to an Adult Schizoid Personality Disorder.

Role of the Nurse in Residential Treatment

The role of the nurse in the residential treatment of autistic and other severely disturbed children is not clearly defined. Many residential treatment institutions staff their units with child care workers under the direction of a psychiatrist or a psychologist or both. This is less expensive than hiring nursing staff. In residential treatment settings that do employ nurses, the nursing role is defined by the treatment philosophy of the unit or institution. The treatment philosophy is usually defined primarily by the medical staff, so indirectly it is the medical staff, rather than the nursing staff, who define the role of the nurse. This role can range from providing milieu, group, individual, and family therapy to doing only strictly traditional nursing and maintenance tasks. Despite this lack of continuity in the nursing role and function, all nurses who work with autistic and other severely disturbed children try to meet certain basic goals. These are listed below. The nursing care plan that follows illustrates how some of these goals are accomplished.

Nursing Goals   In working with autistic and severely disturbed children, some nursing goals are:

- Meet the child's basic needs to reduce tension and decrease the need for defensive behavior
- Help the child form a relationship with another person (a personal object relationship)
- Help the child develop a sense of self-identity
- Offer the child an opportunity to regress and relive previous developmental stages that were unsuccessfully resolved
- Help the child learn to communicate effectively
- Prevent the child from hurting self or others
- Help the child maintain physical health
- Help the child form relationships with others
- Promote reality testing by the child

Sample Nursing Care Plan   The nursing care plan in Table 19–2 is for a 5½-year-old in a residential treatment setting who exhibited many of the classic autistic characteristics. These included lack of verbal communication, isolative behavior, occasional attempts to hurt himself, disturbed peer and adult relationships, and failure to respond to physiological needs. Long-term goals established by the nursing staff were

- To help Allan develop a sense of trust
- To help Allan form satisfying relationships with others
- To help Allan develop a sense of self and begin to function independently

Short-term goals were

- To help Allan form a personal object relationship with a significant adult and form attachments to other significant adults
- To help Allan engage in and enjoy peer interaction
- To help Allan develop play and self-care skills
- To help Allan communicate verbally and nonverbally
- To help Allan learn to recognize and respond appropriately to his physiological needs
- To prevent Allan from hurting himself or others

The nursing care plan (Table 19–2) identifies the specific nursing interventions that were formulated to meet these goals.

Table 19-2   NURSING CARE PLAN FOR AN AUTISTIC CHILD

Goals	Current Status Assessment	Nursing Interventions
1. To help Allan form a personal object relationship with a significant adult	Since admission last month, Allan has made tentative approaches to Ms. L more than to any other staff member. He has also demonstrated responsiveness (verbal acknowledgment, eye contact, physical contact) to Ms. L.	Ms. L will be assigned as Allan's primary nurse. Ms. L will be given a consistent schedule, so Allan will know when she will be here. Scheduling will be arranged so Ms. L will have one hour a day to spend just with Allan.
2. To help Allan form attachments to other significant adults and engage in peer interaction	Interactions with adults are usually short. In them the adult follows Allan, since Allan cannot usually stay with an attentive adult.	Observe and record the sequences of interaction. Acknowledge his leaving. Follow him. Being pursued seems to be a significant part of establishing a relationship for Allan. If he is part of a structured group, expect and help him to stay with the group. Tell him when he will have time alone with an adult.
	Approaches to adults are tentative. Allan is not able to approach adults with confidence.	Always respond to Allan's tentative approaches without waiting for him to follow through. Respond in a warm and caring manner. If he is on the periphery of a group, verbally recognize and acknowledge him. Make space for him to join.
	Allan engages in isolated activities, choosing these over interaction with others.	Observe and record context and sequence of isolation. Some isolated play is a subtle offer of interaction, such as rolling a ball. Respond to his invitation if possible. If not, acknowledge him verbally. At times the isolation is a studied effort to avoid appearing or being left out. Invite him to join activities, making it clear that he is welcome. At times it may be appropriate to join Allan in an isolative activity, such as rocking.
	Unstructured interactions with peers are limited to brief, nonverbal exchanges.	Allow him to approach all other children if he does so in a safe manner. Be attentive, ready to protect either child if necessary. Verbalize and facilitate attempts to interact if necessary, but first allow for spontaneous play. Record the sequence.
3. To help Allan develop play and self-care skills	Allan seldom demonstrates self-care skills. Has demonstrated his ability (if not willingness) to dress himself, brush his teeth, and wash himself in the tub.	During washing and dressing, allow him time to do things for himself. Demonstrate expectation that he will do these things for himself. Praise him matter-of-factly when he does demonstrate self-care skills.

Table continues on next page

	Table 19–2 continued	
Goals	**Current Status Assessment**	**Nursing Interventions**
	Allan seldom demonstrates play skills. Most play is limited to isolative and repetitious manipulation of objects.	Primary nurse to spend one-to-one time with Allan every day to work on development of play skills.
		When introducing a new play activity, gradually involve Allan. For example, if finger painting:
		1. Demonstrate to him use of finger paints
		2. Put his hand on top of yours as you paint
		3. Put his hand on paper with your hand on top to guide him
		4. When he is ready, have him finger paint without assistance
		Praise him for attempts to play and use play materials.
	In structured play, Allan usually reacts negatively when an established routine is varied or new activities are introduced.	Verbally prepare him for changes.
		Allow him to get upset and verbally acknowledge his feelings, but help him try the activity. Direct physical assistance may be necessary.
		If possible, have the new activity be fun.
		When appropriate, verbalize his difficulties in allowing himself to have fun.
4. To help Allan communicate verbally and nonverbally	Allan uses speech infrequently and inconsistently. Speech is limited to words or short phrases. Does not use speech to indicate needs, feelings.	Record all words he speaks, noting situation, appropriateness, clarity, context.
		Respond to verbalization. Meet desire or need expressed as quickly and completely as possible.
		Respond to nonverbal cues with verbal interpretation. For example, if he points to the candy jar and looks at you, respond "You would like me to give you some candy."
	Nonverbal indications of needs, desires are frequently unclear. Facial and behavioral expression of emotion may be mixed or inappropriate.	Tell him what you don't understand.
		If nonverbal communication is ambiguous, verbalize ambiguity. Example: "You smiled when I asked you if you wanted to go out, but you just took your shoes off."
		Observe and record context in which unclarity took place.
		Note whether attempts to clarify increase or decrease his nonverbal clarity.
5. To help Allan learn to recognize and respond appropriately to his own physiological needs and urges	Allan does not defecate at regular and frequent intervals. Retains feces.	Verbalize his bodily needs, but don't make an issue of it.
		Stress comfort, not performance.
		Observe and record all bowel activity.
		Allow him privacy to defecate in the shower or bath area. He may be more comfortable defecating in the tub filled with warm water than on the toilet.
		Offer the toilet before the shower or bath.
		Frequently offer fluids. His favorites are grape juice and cola.
		Encourage as much exercise as possible.

Table continues on next page

	Table 19–2 continued	
Goals	**Current Status Assessment**	**Nursing Interventions**
	Allan does not urinate at regular and frequent intervals. Frequently does not respond to bodily need to urinate.	Observe and record urinary frequency. Respond to indications that he needs to urinate by offering to go to the bathroom with him. He occasionally indicates this need by touching his genital area or saying ''ba-roo.'' Offer the bathroom at appropriate intervals throughout the day.
	Allan eats selectively in small amounts, with little apparent pleasure.	Offer all foods at meals, but allow him to choose. Encourage and help him to prepare foods he likes. He will usually eat French toast, granola, eggnogs, flavored yogurt. Keep a supply of these in the kitchen. Do not expect him to share food. Give candy-coated multivitamin daily.
6. To prevent Allan from hurting himself or others	Allan hurts himself when he is angry, frustrated, or scared.	Be aware that his attempts to hurt himself are often subtle. For instance, he may rub his head against the wall, put his fingers in a door about to be closed, or lean against the radiator. Always acknowledge and stop his attempts to hurt himself as soon as possible. Express concern for him and recognize his feelings of anger, fear, or frustration. If he continues to hurt himself after verbal interventions, this may indicate that he is in distress. A continuous partial or complete restraint may be indicated. Observe and record sequence.
	Allan sometimes bites intervening adults.	Do not allow him to bite. Attempts to bite may be met with a firm ''No biting!'' Recognize that his attempts to bite are sometimes attempts to set up situations in which he will be punished or rejected. Do not punish or reject him. Observe and record whether he seems to be biting on purpose.
	Allan sometimes hurts other children.	Intervene if necessary, but allow some aggressive and self-protective behavior. Observe and record the sequence and result. Verbalize for him the sequence and other possible alternatives. Example: ''Joey took the ball you were rolling. That made you mad, and you shoved him down. You could have gotten the other ball. Or you could have played with Joey and the ball.'' Help the children resolve the conflict.

INTERVENTION

Basic Goals of Treatment

Each child is a unique individual with individual needs, strengths, and weaknesses. However, some basic goals of treatment apply generally when working with children. They include helping the child to:

- Work through earlier developmental stages that were unsuccessfully resolved
- Develop a realistic self-concept
- Develop healthy interpersonal relationships

General Treatment Plans   General treatment plans to meet these goals include:

- Modifying the child's intrapsychic processes
- Altering peer group interactions
- Altering interfamily functioning
- Modifying the child's adjustment to school
- Totally changing the environment, i.e., removing the child to an inpatient setting

Interdisciplinary Approach   Input from different disciplines usually produces a more accurate and holistic assessment. The teacher can furnish information about the child's age-comparable development, social skills, and learning style. The psychologist can validate assessments by testing the child's cognitive and intrapsychic functioning. Other professionals—learning disability specialists, speech therapists, occupational therapists, social workers, and psychiatrists—all have valuable contributions to make. Whenever possible, the collaborative and collegial approach in assessment, diagnosis, treatment planning, and evaluation is the method of choice.

Damon, eight years old, was referred to the child guidance center because he was having difficulties in school. Testing showed him to be well above normal intelligence, yet his teachers reported he was failing because he never finished his assignments. Because of his acting-out behavior, the teacher thought Damon's difficulties in school were due to emotional problems. She suggested the child guidance center to his parents. Before plans were made to start Damon in individual

therapy, a comprehensive assessment was done at the center. It revealed visual learning disabilities that had been making classroom work incredibly difficult for Damon. His acting out was his response to his frustration and bewilderment at having such difficulty doing tasks that seemed easy for most of his classmates. With special tutoring, Damon rapidly improved his school performance, and his acting-out behavior stopped.

In Damon's case therapy was not indicated. If the assessment had revealed interpersonal or intrapsychic conflicts that therapy could help Damon to resolve, therapy rather than, or in addition to, special tutoring would have been recommended. Different types of therapy are explored in the section on specific treatment modalities.

Nursing Skills   Specific nursing skills used to meet the basic goals of treatment include

- Assessment
- Communication skills
- Conveying acceptance
- Setting limits
- Establishing rapport
- Self-awareness

Assessment

The assessment of the current functioning of the child is the first step in treatment. The importance of a good assessment cannot be overstressed, for the assessment is the foundation on which all subsequent interventions rest. (See Chapter 8.) The first step in the assessment is the collection of a *data base*. This data base will vary depending on the presenting complaint, the availability of information and resources, and the nurse's own judgment. In general, however, the data base will consist of the things presented in the following health assessment outline.

Ideally, the assessment involves the child and both parents. After an initial introduction, the parents should be seen without the child to obtain referral, family, and history data. In some cases, it may be helpful to see the parents individually. The child is then seen individually to assess current functioning and the child's own perception of the problem. Finally the family can be seen together to discuss findings and recommendations. Using this format, the assessment will take about two hours.

The nurse may not have the opportunity or facilities to conduct this kind of assessment. Sometimes, too, the assessment must be modified to suit a particular situation. For instance, this much information would not be necessary to formulate intervention plans for a child hospitalized for a tonsillectomy. However, the following health assessment outline is presented as a general guide.

Health Assessment Outline

1. *Physical Health*

   a. Child

     (1) Current: Child should have had a physical recently to identify any physical problems and rule out an organic basis for the presenting problems. The nurse doing the assessment needs a copy of the physical or a report from the physician or nurse practitioner who performed the physical. The nurse should obtain permission from the parents before requesting this information from a colleague.

     (2) History: The child's health history may also be obtained from the pediatrician if the child has had regular medical care. If not, ask the parents about the usual childhood diseases, any major illnesses, hospitalizations, allergies, and the child's general state of health. Pregnancy and birth data should also be obtained from the parents. Ask questions such as

       (a) How was the pregnancy? Any problems?

       (b) Was the pregnancy planned?

       (c) How did you feel about it?

       (d) How was the delivery?

       (e) Were there any problems with labor or delivery?

       (f) How much did the baby weigh?

       (g) Were there any problems after the baby was born?

   b. Family

     (1) Current and history: Ask parents about the general state of health of all family members and serious or chronic illnesses (past and present).

2. *Family Composition*

   a. History and current functioning

     (1) Marital status and age of parents: Is the family intact? Previous marriage? If a single parent family, does the other parent have contact with the child? How long have parents been married?

     (2) Siblings: Number and age of siblings. If it is a blended or restructured family, ask about other parents of siblings.

     (3) Socioeconomic class: Ask parents about place and length of employment. Ask whether residence is rented or owned, and how large it is.

     (4) Families of origin: Determine if maternal and paternal grandparents are alive. If they and other extended family are in area, are they involved with the nuclear family? Also try to get some idea of the parents' relationship to their own parents. This can be done through the use of nondirective questions such as

       (a) Are you close to your parents now?

       (b) How was your childhood?

       (c) What kind of person was your mother?

       (d) Would you tell me a little about your father?

3. *Referral Data*

   a. Specific information: The nurse doing the assessment needs to know who made the referral and specifically why it was made. For instance, "Eight-year-old Shannon was referred to this clinic by the Fernwood School, where he was brought to the attention of the school psychologist by his teacher, who reports aggressive, acting-out behavior and poor academic performance of six months' duration." Both the presenting problem and the duration of symptoms should be included.

   b. Subjective perception of the problem

     (1) By parents: To obtain the parents' perceptions, ask questions such as

       (a) What do you see as the problem?

       (b) What are you particularly concerned about?

       (c) What would you like me to do for your child?

(d) How would you like your child to change?

(e) What strengths or positive things do you see in your child?

If the referral was made by someone other than the parents, such as the school, ask if the parents agree with the statements in it and if the child's behavior is different at home.

(2) By the child: During the play interview, try to get the child's perception of the problem by asking questions such as

(a) Can you tell me why you're here?

(b) Is there anything worrying you?

(c) How are things at school? at home?

(d) What do you like to do best?

(e) Do you have friends at school? at home?

Frequently the child is quite anxious and will answer, "I don't know" to all questions. It is important to verbalize the problems by saying something like "You've been having trouble at school lately, and your mother brought you here to see if we can figure out how to help."

4. *Developmental Data*

a. History (obtained from parents)

(1) Major physiological milestones: Ask when child sat up, walked, talked, was toilet trained, could ride a bicycle.

(2) Psychosocial milestones: Ask how child responded to primary caretakers in infancy; to toilet training. Ask whether child has friends. What things does child enjoy doing? The nature of these questions will be determined by the age of the child. For instance, the nurse wouldn't focus on the absence of cooperative peer relationships of a two-year-old, as this ability does not develop until later.

5. *Current Functioning of the Child.* This is assessed by interview and direct observation of the child. An office with play materials is the best setting. The parents should not be present during this part of the assessment, so the child will feel more free to reveal conflicts and problems.

a. Appearance: This includes a description of the child's size, appearance, and dress. Avoid vague generalities such as "appropriate dress."

b. Affect: Affect refers to the child's feelings or mood. It can be assessed throughout the interview. Assess both the various affects displayed and how appropriate the affect is to the topic discussed or the play in which the child is engaged. For instance, a smiling and happy affect would be appropriate if the child was describing a favorite activity. It would be inappropriate if the child was discussing failure in school. Take into account the child's possible anxiety, which may influence affect.

c. Orientation: Orientation refers to the child's awareness of time, place, and person. This can be assessed by asking the child questions such as name, address, birthdate, age and grade of siblings, where the child is now, and so forth. Keep developmental age in mind. A child of six who does not understand the concept of time would not necessarily be disoriented, since time concept often is not clear until eight or nine.

d. Perception: Perception refers to the ability to receive and interpret sensory information. This can be assessed throughout the interview by evaluating how the child uses the senses. Once again, developmental age must be considered. Exploring toys with the mouth would be appropriate for an infant but not for a six-year-old.

e. Verbalization and play: By examining verbalization and play, the nurse can assess the child's major concerns or preoccupations, the child's perception of the specific problem (if any), and the child's use of fantasy. Some children verbalize freely. This provides information about their social and cultural environment, their ability to relate, their interests, and so on. Other children verbalize little or not at all. Here the primary source of information will be play, which the nurse must interpret.

Five-year-old Allison had been referred for evaluation due to regressive behavior and frequent nightmares. Her parents thought the onset of symptoms coincided with their divorce six months before. The following dialogue took place between Allison and the psychiatric nurse interviewing her in the playroom:

NURSE: *Allison, do you know why you're here?*

ALLISON: *No.*

NURSE: *Why do you think your parents wanted you to see me?*

ALLISON: *I don't know.*

NURSE: *How have things been for you lately?*

ALLISON: *Okay.*

NURSE: *You think things have been okay, and you don't know why your parents brought you.*

ALLISON: *(No verbal response—looks at floor.)*

NURSE: *Your parents have told me that they're worried because they think you're unhappy right now. You've been acting different at home and having nightmares, and your parents brought you here so we can try to figure out how we can help you.*

ALLISON: *(No verbal response—refuses eye contact.)*

NURSE: *What do you think about that?*

ALLISON: *Nothing.*

Allison then went over to the dollhouse. For the next fifteen minutes she played out stories that revolved around the abandonment of a child, thus through her play communicating many of her fears, feelings, and perceptions.

---

f. Fantasy: Children's fantasies usually reveal their concerns, preoccupations, experiences, and perceptions. By observing their play, the nurse can often assess their fantasies. Another method is to ask children what they would wish for if they could have three things come true. Drawings, especially if the child is willing to comment on the drawing, offer another way to identify fantasies.

g. Self-concept: Self-concept includes both object relations and identifications. The nurse should assess how the child relates to the nurse, how the child interacts with the parents, and how the child separates from the parents. Information gathered from play, verbalizations, and fantasy should also be assessed for self-concept. Having the child draw family and self-portraits usually gives further information about self-concept.

After Allison had finished playing with the dollhouse, the nurse gave her paper and colored felt-tip pens and asked her to draw her family. Allison drew two large figures, very far apart, and a small figure in the lower right-hand corner. When asked, she identified the figure on the far left as Daddy and the other large figure as

Mommy. The last figure, isolated in the right-hand corner, Allison identified as herself. The nurse commented that the child in the corner looked kind of alone. Allison responded by saying, "She was bad, maybe." The nurse was careful to follow Allison's lead and continued to refer to the figure as "she" rather than "you," saying, "Maybe she was bad, and that's why she's alone." Allison answered, "Yes. Or maybe they don't want her." The nurse pursued this with Allison and, using her drawing as a vehicle, was able to allow Allison to express many of her fears and fantasies.

---

h. Neuromuscular skills and integration: Throughout the assessment, the nurse should assess the child's developmental neuromuscular skills and integration. Activities such as throwing a ball, picking up small objects, or grasping a pencil may be used to assess this area. Any suspected deviations from the developmental norm should be medically evaluated.

The information obtained from the health assessment guide furnishes the data base or raw material from which the assessment is formulated. The assessment, in turn, is the basis for everything that follows. Figure 19–1 illustrates the relationships among the components of nursing intervention.

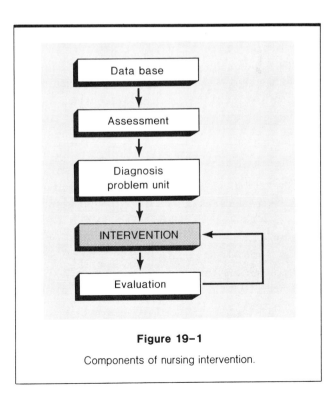

Figure 19–1

Components of nursing intervention.

Individual Differences and Environmental Stresses   After the data base has been obtained, the assessment is made. Normal growth and development varies with the individual. These variations must be assessed before an "abnormal" label is slapped on the child. In general, we expect to find more than one deviation from the usual developmental progress in the disturbed child. We also expect to observe any deviation more than once when making the assessment.

It is also important to differentiate between the child's reactions to internal intrapsychic factors and the child's reactions to environmental stresses. Environmental stresses might include

- Divorce or separation of parents
- Birth of a new sibling
- Multiple caretakers
- Hospitalization
- The loss of a significant other through death or illness
- Poverty
- Racism

In developmental assessment, the focus is on healthy development. The nurse asks, "What is healthy about this child? In what areas—social, psychological, physiological, intellectual, psychosexual—is this child's behavior age appropriate?" Any developmental delays noted are evaluated within the context of the child's strengths. The child's development is then evaluated again within the context of the family and the culture. This approach is designed to help children function at their optimal level of wellness. It differs from the traditional medical model, which focuses on illness and the treatment of symptoms and disease.

Communication Skills

Effective communication with children requires the same basic skills as effective communication with adults (see Chapter 6). These include active listening, reflection of feelings, and paraphrasing. With younger children, nonverbal communication is an important means of sending and receiving messages. The infant, and some psychotic children, rely solely on nonverbal communication.

Nathan, a six-year-old psychotic client in a residential treatment unit, was an elective mute. In the dining room during dinner, the nursing student was puzzled by

Nathan's behavior. He would hold some food in his mouth for several minutes and then spit it out on his plate, only to put it back in his mouth. The nurse also noted that Nathan seemed very upset when another child grabbed for something on his tray. After watching, puzzled, for several minutes, the nurse said to Nathan, "I'm wondering if you're doing that to make it last longer." Nathan looked at the nurse, who added, "There's plenty of food. You can have as much as you want. It's okay to swallow that; there's more." Nathan cautiously finished most of his chocolate milk, seeming very anxious and then reassured when the nurse quickly filled his glass again before it was completely empty. With the nurse's help, he was then able to finish the meal.

Sending Nonverbal Messages   Children who do not communicate verbally can be especially frustrating to the nurse who seeks verbal feedback from the client about "how I'm doing." Children—especially disturbed children—are quick to pick up uncertainty and anxiety, which the nurse may communicate nonverbally without realizing it. With good supervision, nurses can learn to pick up and interpret their own nonverbal messages. Knowing how to do this is important, since all communication is a two-way street. Supervisory conferences then offer these nurses an opportunity to explore their expectations, frustrations, fears, and ideas.

Play as Communication   Play is the child's primary method of expression. It is also an important method of resolving conflict. At times play is largely nonverbal. The child may communicate partly or entirely through body movements, activity level, choice of toys, and affect.

Jamie, eight years old, had been coming to the playroom with the nurse-therapist weekly for three months. He rarely talked to the nurse. He spent most of the playroom time playing with the toy barnyard and animals. In this play, the animals were always involved in situations of great danger and unpredictability. No matter what the animals did in the play, they always ended up being killed due to some frightening and unforeseen event. Jamie's expression during this play was angry and his body seemed tense. Although Jamie had not verbalized to the nurse his anger and fear about his very chaotic home life, the nurse was able to use the play as a means of communication from Jamie. The nurse verbalized to Jamie her interpretations of his play and possible feelings. Eventually, Jamie was able to verbalize some of his feelings, while he continued to play them out.

Primary Process Thought   Nurses who work with young children, or children whose developmental age is younger than their school age, should remember that primary process thinking influences how these children interpret communications. A three-year-old who is told, "You're mad and upset because Mother had to leave you here in the hospital" may interpret this as "Mother left me here because I am mad." Here again, a sound working knowledge of normal growth and development is invaluable. When communicating verbally with children, use simple sentences, words, and concepts that the child can understand. For instance, a nurse who tells the three-year-old, "Mommy will be back after you go to bed and wake up and eat breakfast" will probably be more readily understood than one who says, "Mommy will return at 10 A.M. tomorrow."

Conveying Acceptance

Acceptance can be a powerful therapeutic tool. It is based on knowing—and accepting—where the child is. This sounds simple, but cultural and personal values, biases, and anxieties often get in the way. It is easy to use cliches like "act your age" or "big boys shouldn't cry" if one feels uncomfortable about the child's attitudes or behavior. The message to the child is clearly "I don't accept you as you are right now, and I will withhold my approval until you conform to how I think you should be." This is counterproductive. It is important to accept the child no matter how one feels about the child's attitudes. This doesn't mean that one necessarily likes the attitudes, or that one wouldn't prefer a change. The nurse can accept where someone is at a given time while still believing that the person can grow and change.

Tod, a six-year-old boy in a day care program for disturbed children, became extremely aggressive whenever there was a change in his regular routine. Because he often hurt one of the other children, his nurse had started physically restraining Tod by holding him during these times. While holding him, the nurse told Tod, "It's not okay to hurt. You need me to help you not do it, and I will help you. I think someday you'll be able to do it by yourself."

Letting the Child Set the Pace   One aspect of acceptance that many adults find difficult when working with a child is letting the child set the pace. It's easy to intercede when a child is doing a simple task very slowly, but this intercession robs the child of a sense of completion and accomplishment. Letting the child set the pace may also conflict with the nurse's need to protect the child. Certainly there are times when adult intervention is necessary, either for safety or for expedience. There are also many times when adult intervention is not necessary but is forced on the child anyway. For hospitalized children, who are already struggling with a sense of helplessness and loss of control, having the chance to do things for themselves and thus be in control can be very important.

Five-year-old Carrie had been hospitalized for an infection that required antibiotic injections. She was terrified of the shots and would resist so strenuously that it took two nurses to hold her while a third gave the injection. After a few days of this, the evening nurse took a syringe, a vial of distilled water, and some alcohol wipes into Carrie's room. He told Carrie, "I know how scared you are of the shots. Sometimes it helps kids if they can play with the stuff we use to give them." Carrie was reluctant at first, and the nurse did not pressure her, telling her that it was okay if she didn't want to play "shot," and that if she needed to scream and be held down for her shots, that was okay too. With this adult acceptance of her needs, Carrie was able to express, play out, and master some of her fears about the injections. The nurse reported this during change of shift, and the rest of the staff continued to reinforce Carrie's sense of control by involving her as much as possible in the injections. They gave her some choice of injection site, let her use the alcohol wipe herself, and gave her a syringe without a needle to play with. Carrie was still very frightened by the injection and frequently cried, but she no longer needed to be held. This gave her a sense of control over herself and some control over the environment and significantly reduced her anxiety.

Starting Where the Child Is   When explaining procedures, discussing fears, or giving any information to a child, it is important to start where the child is. Don't offer the explanation without first finding out what the child's perceptions, fears, or fantasies are. With this information the nurse can deal with the real issues for that individual child. Most adults have had the experience of being so anxious they literally "didn't hear" what was said to them. Children selectively inattend in the same way. Acceptance is part of effective communication with children.

The accepting nurse ascertains, then tries to meet, the child's needs on whatever level the child chooses to present. This helps the child get in touch with self and validates his or her worth as an individual. If necessary, the child can revert to an earlier developmental level and work through frustrations or unmet needs. The nurse places no value judgment on the level the child chooses.

Seven-year-old Marie was hospitalized for a medical problem shortly after the birth of a sibling. The nurses were concerned about Marie's withdrawal, refusal to interact with or respond to anyone, and infantile behavior. On the fourth day of Marie's hospitalization, a consultation from the mental health nurse was requested. The nurse found Marie sucking her thumb and making infantlike sounds to herself. The nurse verbalized this to Marie, saying, "Sometimes it feels good to act like a baby." Marie did not respond verbally, but for the first time she made eye contact with the nurse, who added, "Sometimes when kids are scared, they need to be babies again for awhile. Would you like me to rock you for awhile?" Marie nodded, and the nurse carried Marie to the rocking chair and rocked her for twenty minutes. During this time, Marie continued to suck her thumb while curled in a fetal position in the nurse's lap. After this, Marie was able to begin to express her concerns and fears through play. The nurses encouraged this and continued to accept the occasional times Marie reverted to infant behaviors, responding by saying, "I guess you need to be a baby for a while right now." The nurse also explained Marie's behavior to Marie's concerned parents. Within a week, Marie had stopped her infantile behavior and was able to use play effectively to express and master her concerns, as well as to verbalize some of her fears.

Through the use of acceptance, the nurse did four things in this interaction with Marie.

1. *She accepted Marie where she was.* Chronologically, Marie was seven, but she needed to be a dependent infant at this time.

2. *She helped Marie explore ways to meet her needs.* The nurse did this by helping Marie meet her dependency needs and resolve conflict through play.

3. *She helped Marie gain a sense of control and mastery.* By accepting Marie's needs and her way of expressing them, the nurse allowed Marie the opportunity to resolve her conflicts in her own way. The nurse could have offered Marie reassurance instead, telling her that everything would be okay, that her parents still loved her, and so on. This would not have been as effective as helping Marie to resolve her concerns by herself and in her own way.

4. *She helped Marie gain a sense of accomplishment and self-esteem.* Because an adult who remained accepting of her helped Marie recognize and resolve her conflict and fears by herself, Marie's self-esteem was enhanced, and she gained a sense of accomplishment from her ability to meet her own needs.

Setting Limits

If one accepts the child completely, should one set limits? Yes. Setting limits does not mean that one doesn't accept the child. On the contrary, establishing clear limits is the most effective way to give the child a sense of trust and security. It enables the child to regress or explore, supplies external ego control if the child needs it, and fosters a sense of trust between child and adult. Conforming to limits is a fact of life for both children and adults. Children are made to conform by adults. With the development of the superego, children begin to internalize the limits first imposed on them by others. As adults, they are expected to impose limits on themselves, if they are to be socially and culturally accepted. The necessity to conform to limits is a fact of life, so limit setting with disturbed children serves as reality reinforcement in addition to helping establish trust and security.

The nature of the limits depends partly on the institutional setting. For instance, most institutions require children to be up at a certain time, to come to meals, to attend group activities, and so forth. Some general limits are applicable anywhere: Children are not allowed to hurt themselves, to hurt anyone else, or to destroy property.

Impersonal Language   When enforcing limits, it is important to convey a nonjudgmental attitude. One technique is to use impersonal language whenever possible. For instance, "The furniture stays on the floor" sounds like a statement about how things are. "You mustn't throw that chair" sounds like a judgment about the child's behavior.

Accept the Child's Feelings Do not attempt to limit how the child feels. Accepting how the child feels, even when limiting the actions that arise out of these feelings, gives the child a sense of acceptance as well as the security of firm limits.

Eight-year-old Eddie became very angry when the nurse told him that, due to doctor's orders, he could not go to the outside play area with some of the other ambulant children. Eddie raised his fists to the nurse, who said quickly, "You can't hit me, but you can hit this clown doll." As Eddie punched the Bobo doll, the nurse let him know she recognized his feelings by saying, "Boy, you are really mad. You're so mad at me right now that you're really punching Bobo." "I hate you!" Eddie responded. "You hate me," the nurse responded. A few minutes later, she added, "I guess it's pretty hard not to be able to go out." "I can't do anything here," Eddie said. "It's like I'm a baby." Eddie and the nurse were then able to talk about Eddie's feelings and to figure out ways his needs could be met within the necessary medical restriction.

In this limit-enforcing interaction the nurse has

- Acknowledged Eddie's needs
- Stated the limit clearly
- Indicated acceptance of Eddie's feelings
- Enforced the limit verbally, offering an alternative outlet for his anger

Letting the Child Express Anger and Frustration If the nurse had said, "Don't you dare hit me!" or had let Eddie hit her, it is doubtful that Eddie would have shared his feelings of loss of control. By allowing the child to express anger and frustration, the nurse accepted Eddie's needs and feelings although she set limits on his behavior.

General Guidelines Strategies depend on the situation and the individual child. Here are some general guidelines:

- State the limit clearly.
- Be aware of your feelings about the limit. A child will pick up any ambivalence.
- Don't be angry or punitive when setting limits.
- Set and enforce limits consistently in nonpersonal ways.

- Indicate your acceptance of the child's feelings.
- Offer alternatives, such as verbal expression and other outlets.

Countertransference

When working with children, particularly disturbed children, it is important to realize that many of your own childhood feelings may be reactivated. You may then unwittingly react to a child in response to some childhood conflict of your own, rather than reacting to the reality of the present situation.

This phenomenon is known as *countertransference*. It also occurs when working with adult psychiatric clients, but less often. Nurses should be aware of the possibility of countertransference reactions and should discuss them with an instructor or preceptor when they arise. This can turn a potential liability into a means of increasing self-awareness and understanding.

SPECIFIC TREATMENT MODES

Treatment Facilities

The specific treatment mode selected will depend on the needs of the individual child, the goals set for the treatment, and the availability of financial, personal, and professional resources. Some of the standard treatment facilities for disturbed children are child guidance centers, residential treatment settings, and day care treatment centers.

Child Guidance Center The child guidance center is a clinic where the child or the family or both are seen on an outpatient basis. The emphasis is frequently on the family as the unit of treatment, rather than on the individual child. The child's emotional difficulties are perceived as the product of disturbed interpersonal relationships in the home. The professional staff in a child guidance center could include: clinical psychologists; psychiatric social workers; marriage, family, and child counselors; psychiatrists; and clinical nurse specialists. Some multidisciplinary clinics may offer more holistic services using learning disability specialists, special education teachers, occupational therapists, or speech therapists.

Residential Treatment Setting The residential treatment setting is necessary if the child is so disturbed that intensive inpatient treatment is necessary, or if the home environment is so detrimental that the child must be removed from it at least temporarily. Most residential treatment settings have school facilities. Children may live in small dormitories or cottages with resident counselors or in hospital-style wards. The staff manipulate the milieu to offer the children a therapeutic environment as well as individual or group therapy. The staff at a residential treatment center usually includes psychiatrists, specially trained aides, teachers, registered nurses, clinical nurse specialists in child psychiatry, and clinical psychologists. (See the section on the role of the nurse in residential treatment earlier in this chapter.)

Day Care Treatment Center The day care treatment center falls somewhere between the child guidance center and the residential treatment setting. Children do not live at the day care center, but they spend a lot of time there. Usually, a combination of special education and therapy is offered.

Which Setting for Which Therapy? Certain therapies work best in certain settings. Milieu therapy is connected with residential treatment. Brief therapy is done on an outpatient basis. Play therapy, behavior modification, art therapy, group therapy, and family therapy can be provided in any of the treatment settings described above. They are also provided by private mental health practitioners. Many treatment centers and private practitioners follow an eclectic approach to treatment, using many different types of therapy to meet the needs of the child and the family. The goal of all therapies and all treatment settings is to meet the mental health needs of the client; selection of the most appropriate therapy and setting is an important part of meeting these needs.

Therapy: An Overview

The following sections discuss different kinds of therapy. Broadly speaking, however, all therapies fall into one of three classifications. They can be

1. Cognitive, focusing on specific problems and their solution
2. Supportive or emotional, focusing on providing a relationship with a warm, sympathetic, and accepting adult

3. A combination of both cognitive and supportive. In this case the therapist actively supports the child while helping him or her solve specific problems

Play Therapy

The treatment modality most widely used with children is play therapy. Play therapy lets children use their natural medium of expression to resolve conflicts. The play therapist adds the further resource of an accepting, understanding adult.

Functions of Play Play has many functions. Children use it to

- Master and assimilate past experiences that they had no control over
- Communicate with the unconscious
- Communicate with others
- Explore and experiment while learning how to relate to self, the world, and others
- Compromise between the demands of drives and the dictates of reality

Play therapy offers the child a safe place to explore all of the uses of play, thus dealing with conflictual material, developing a healthy self-image, and learning about self in relation to the therapist. In short, play therapy offers the opportunity for growth under stable conditions.

Seven-year-old Randy had been an only child until the birth of his sister four months ago. Since then, he had become a behavior problem in school, frequently disrupting class and being very aggressive toward the other children. During the intake interview at the child guidance clinic, his mother told the nurse therapist that at home Randy was quiet and seemed almost sad. Both parents were concerned and felt their attempts to help Randy were ineffective.

Randy began weekly play therapy sessions. During the third session, he picked up a doll and began hitting it. When he realized that the therapist was not going to censure his behavior, he continued to hit the doll and curse it, telling it how bad it was. The therapist remarked that Randy seemed pretty mad at the doll. Randy nodded emphatically. Then he buried the doll in sand, saying, "There, now you're dead, and I'm glad." The therapist continued to let Randy set the pace by reflecting what he said, rather than verbalizing the obvious interpretation that Randy wished his sister dead. During the next several sessions, Randy continued to hit, swear at, and kill the doll. The therapist remained accepting, acknowledging and reflecting his feelings. Gradually, Randy dropped the doll play during the sessions and spent most of the hour exploring other toys. His mother reported that his problem behavior in school had ceased, and that he seemed "like himself again" at home.

Role of the Play Therapist   The role of play therapist is not a passive one, but it is essentially nondirective. The child sets the pace and does the work. The therapist contributes personally as an accepting and understanding adult whose goal is to foster the child's development of self. The relationship between the child and therapist is a new experience for the child, one that does not translate effectively outside the play therapy situation. The therapist accepts these children fully as they are, yet maintains the belief that they can change and grow. As they begin to trust the relationship, children can use it as a context for trying out new ways of behaving and relating to themselves and others.

Dynamics of Play Therapy   The acceptance the therapist gives these children can help them evolve a new self-image. Fearful and passive children may be able to try out some assertive or aggressive behavior. Consistently aggressive children may explore new ways to meet their needs. Children who perceive themselves as worthless may eventually accept the therapist's message that they are valuable, worthwhile people. In some cases, it may be a matter of educating the child to the possibility of different interactive patterns. It is difficult for young children to think of theoretical alternatives. They may believe that a dysfunctional family interactional pattern is the only possible one. Given a new pattern, they can explore new behavior. As their conflicts begin to be resolved and as confidence and trust evolve from the therapeutic relationship, their tension decreases, and they can expand their new awareness outside the therapeutic relationship.

Five-year-old Lisa had been referred for play therapy because of her tantrums and clingy, demanding behavior in school. The history given by her mother included early, very rigid weaning from the bottle and maternal intolerance of any form of infantile oral exploration. During the third play session, Lisa picked up the baby bottle from the toy shelf and asked the therapist what it was for. The therapist replied that it was for anything Lisa wanted it to be for. Lisa giggled nervously and said that she was a big girl and everyone know that only babies used bottles. During the next several sessions, she ignored the bottle while consistently breaking limits and acting "bad" to test the therapist's acceptance and the playroom situation. The therapist consistently enforced the limits of not hurting self or the therapist or breaking the toys, while she continued to give Lisa a sense of being accepted and valued. Having tested the therapist's acceptance in less threatening ways, Lisa could then risk using the bottle. Gradually, with the therapist's continuing support, Lisa worked on resolving her unmet infancy dependency needs. She spent several sessions curled up on the therapist's lap, sucking on the bottle. After several months, Lisa gradually lost interest in the bottle, using her playroom time for more age-appropriate play. Her teacher reported that Lisa's tantrums had almost entirely ceased, and that she seldom exhibited her former clingy and demanding behavior.

Setting for Play Therapy   Ideally, play therapy is done in a well-equipped playroom. Toys might include dollhouse and furniture, puppets, dolls, blocks, art materials (Play-Doh, clay, paper, crayons, paints, marking pens), toy animals, telephone, cars and trucks, play kitchen, musical instruments, toy soldiers and guns, checkers and other games, and clothes for make-believe. (This kind of equipment is not strictly necessary. The nurse who is helping the fearful child overcome a terror of injections by letting the child handle the injection paraphernalia is also doing play therapy.) The toys stay in the playroom, and children use them there. In the initial session, the therapist tells the children that the playroom is for them to use as they please during the time they are there, and sets the limits (usually the minimal ones of not hurting self or therapist or breaking equipment). Usually, therapists will try to find out children's perceptions of what's going on by asking them why they are there. Therapists will offer briefly their own understanding for the referral (i.e., you're having trouble in school). How things proceed from there is largely up to the child. Most children are eager to use the playroom situation and the presence of an accepting, consistent, and understanding adult to resolve conflicts and try out different ways of relating to self and others.

Group Therapy

Group play therapy with children follows basically the same ground rules as individual play therapy. However, there are two major differences. The first is the need to select group members that can work together as a group. The second is the fact that the therapist or group leader needs group skills.

The children's play group follows the same process as an adult group. This process consists of four phases—the beginning or exploratory phase, the transition phase, the working phase, and the termination phase.

Process of Group Therapy

THE BEGINNING PHASE   During the beginning phase, the leader can expect children to test the new experience. They may ask questions about the group and leader. They may make rules. They may engage in acting-out behavior to test limits, in superficial conversation, or in behavior that indicates anxiety (such as giggling). During the beginning phase, the leader is directive and provides the structure necessary to reduce anxiety and facilitate group process. Together with the group members, the leader establishes group goals, rules, and limits. The leader usually structures the time by providing activities for the group.

THE TRANSITION PHASE   This is a very difficult phase for both the group members and the leader. As the children move from the superficial and safe beginning phase towards the working phase and the beginning of self-disclosure, anxiety and testing behavior will increase. There will be frequent reversions to the more superficial beginning phase and much testing of the leader for acceptance and trust. This testing behavior can be upsetting to a leader who is not aware that it is a normal and necessary part of the group process. Group members may test by being demanding, provocative, hyperactive, or infantile. During this phase, the leader needs to continue to demonstrate acceptance of both the individual group members and the group as a whole, while still setting and maintaining limits. As in individual play therapy, the limits apply to behavior, not to feelings or verbalizations. The leader should support any group members who risk self-disclosure. During this phase, the group seems scattered. There is little cohesive group activity. It is usually helpful to provide structured activities and some external organization.

THE WORKING PHASE   As the group moves into the working phase, the leader can usually be less directive and active. During this phase, anxiety decreases as trust and cohesiveness increase. The leader will have less need to enforce limits as the children grow more self-disciplined, sharing, and cooperative. This is a pro-

ductive phase, during which self-disclosure and group activity and cohesiveness increase. During this phase, the leader acts as a role model and a facilitator of group process.

THE TERMINATION PHASE   The termination phase usually begins when the leader brings up the subject of ending the group. As a general rule, children's groups should last at least three months. The termination date should be established at the beginning of the group. It should be brought up again far enough in advance for the group members to work through termination issues. The time this takes will vary with the age of the group members, but the termination phase should begin at least three sessions before the final session. During the termination phase, children usually regress to behaviors associated with the transition phase. There may be testing and acting-out behavior. Group members exhibit unwillingness to terminate by increased dependence on the group leader and requests to continue the group beyond the established time for ending. The role of the leader during this phase includes open acknowledgment and discussion of termination. The group members should be helped to evaluate their own growth. Some group leaders like to have the last session be a special one that includes refreshments. (For a more complete discussion of group dynamics and group therapy, see Chapters 9 and 18.)

Choosing Group Members

The choice of group members is crucial to the success of the group. One of the major differences between individual and group therapy is that in group therapy peers, as well as the group leader, provide role models who demonstrate alternative ways of behavior. One obvious criterion for choosing group members is that each child should be able to learn from peers and peer interactions. The group could include immature, withdrawn, overcompliant, and aggressive children and children who have poor peer relationships due to socialization problems. It could exclude psychotic or psychopathic children, children with strong sibling rivalry, extremely aggressive children, and children who are experiencing extreme stress.

The total composition of the group should also be considered. A group composed entirely of passive, withdrawn children will not be able to use each other as role models. Neither will a group composed entirely of aggressive, acting-out children. The group should include children of different personality types. They should all be approximately the same age and size. It is usually a good idea to include one or two children who are less disturbed than the others. These children can add balance to the group. The group experience can be useful for these children as they learn to relate to others different from themselves. Group size varies from three to six children. Generally, preschool groups are smaller and are not segregated by sex.

Art Therapy

Art can be an important vehicle for self-expression and communication. Children frequently find it less threatening than verbalization or play. Art can also be used in a directive way to accomplish a specific goal. For example, therapists can use art to evaluate children's feelings and perceptions about themselves. Art can also be used as a cathartic experience.

Eight-year-old Ethan had been hospitalized four days previously for a herniorrhaphy. Physical postoperative recovery was uneventful, but he was withdrawn and uncommunicative. Ward personnel referred him to the psychiatric nurse consultant. During the initial interview, she was unable to elicit anything from Ethan directly. He refused to talk and ignored the playroom toys. The next

day, the nurse brought paper and felt tip pens. She gave them to Ethan, remarking, "Sometimes it's hard to talk about things. I thought you might draw a picture of yourself or the hospital or anything you want to for me." Ethan accepted the art materials and drew a detailed picture that included a tiny boy with a large bandage over his entire torso in one corner of the paper. Large, angry adults surrounded the boy. The nurse commented, "That boy looks very little. I guess he's pretty scared." Ethan agreed and added, "He was bad, so they cut him up." The nurse and Ethan continued to talk about his feelings and experiences, using the picture as a vehicle. The next day, Ethan was able to voice some of his concerns directly to the nurse.

Uses of Art Therapy   For the nurse, art therapy is a useful assessment tool. When children draw, they usually draw themselves and their subjective reality. Having children draw themselves, their family, their school, or themselves when they are angry, sad, or happy can furnish valuable material for evaluation.

In addition to evaluation, art therapy can be used to facilitate group process and focus activity. Pounding on clay, tearing newspaper, or drawing on very large pieces of paper are strategies for relieving tension or anger or focusing overactivity. In a group setting, art

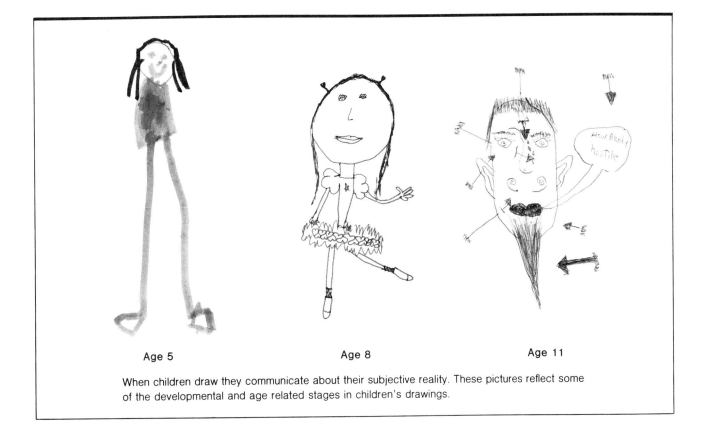

Age 5   Age 8   Age 11

When children draw they communicate about their subjective reality. These pictures reflect some of the developmental and age related stages in children's drawings.

projects can be used to increase group cooperation and cohesiveness and as a vehicle for insights if the project is something like a group collage of a world you would all like to live in, or a picture of the group.

Art Materials   The choice of art materials will depend on the setting, the specific art project, and the age of the child. Children under four need large pieces of paper, large crayons, felt pens, finger paints, and clay or Play-Doh. For the older child, tempera paints, brushes, pencils, crayons, finger paints, clay, collage material, and paper of various sizes should be available. The specific choice of materials depends on the setting, the project, and the child or group of children.

Stages in Children's Art   The scribbling stage begins at two and ends about four. Although the scribbles produced at this age are not representational, they usually have meaning for the child. Often they clearly express emotions such as anger or happiness. The preschematic stage begins at four and ends at seven. Drawings may still include some scribbling, but they are representational and include forms and images as well. In the schematic stage (seven to nine), children draw their own subjective reality—the world as it is to them. Perspective is highly individualized rather than objectively realistic. At about nine, drawings become more realistic and detailed. Subject matter often extends beyond the child's immediate world. All children's art is expressive and a communication about the child, whatever the stage of the art. However, the nurse who is familiar with the normal sequence of stages can use the child's art for developmental as well as emotional assessment.

Brief Therapy

The demand for child psychiatric services is appallingly greater than the supply. Brief, focused therapy helps to make these services available to more of the community. Brief therapy is a pragmatic approach. If it works, resources—therapist time, client time, and money—have been conserved. If it doesn't work, more complex therapy can be instituted.

Rationale and Methodology   Brief therapy is quite unlike play therapy. It is focused, directive, and active. The therapist, with the child and parents, first identifies a specific problem or problem area and then directs and helps the child and family find ways of solving the identified problem. Brief therapy is symptom, rather than insight, oriented.

Brief therapy is particularly effective at the level of primary prevention. Often children's disturbances start out as relatively simple behavioral problems. These problems are exacerbated by the reactions of parents, teachers, and other adults. A vicious circle develops as the behavioral problem intensifies and affects other areas of the child's functioning. Since these problems are provoked by adult reactions, brief therapy usually involves the parents. The therapist helps the parents to explore the interactional nature of the problem and to learn how they may be unwittingly perpetuating it. If the interactional pattern is broken, the problem behavior often changes.

Seven-year-old Dawn C and her parents came to the mental health clinic because her parents "couldn't stand her temper tantrums any longer." The psychiatric nurse who did the intake decided to see Dawn and her parents together for brief family therapy. The problem behavior was clearly Dawn's temper tantrums. Asked how they responded to the tantrums, Mrs. C replied that they usually tried reasoning with Dawn but frequently resorted to yelling and spanking. The nurse asked Dawn why she threw tantrums. Dawn said, "To get what I want." The nurse asked what that was. Dawn said she wanted different things at different times. Mr C added that it seemed to him maybe she wanted attention. During the next sessions, the nurse explored this with the family, giving them specific assignments that included downplaying the tantrums by matter-of-factly having Dawn stay in her room until she was through. Together, the nurse and family also figured out some ways Dawn could get the attention she wanted from her parents in more constructive ways. Over a two-month period, Dawn's tantrums almost entirely ceased, as she tried out new and more effective ways to obtain the parental attention she needed. When she did throw a tantrum, she received no reinforcement, and this encouraged her to seek attention in other ways.

Effectiveness   Because family involvement and cooperation are usually necessary for brief therapy to succeed, its applicability is limited. Intact families who are willing to make a real effort to change and are not hostile to therapy are the best candidates for this approach. Brief therapy is effective in dealing with maturational crises, such as the onset of puberty; situational crises, such as school entry or illness or death in the family; and behavioral problems, such as drug abuse, truancy, or temper tantrums. The specific technique varies with the situation and the clients. Some examples would be behavior modification, use of drugs, individual therapy, family therapy, parent counseling, or combinations of these techniques.

Brief therapy is health oriented. The child's and the family's strengths are first identified. Then the therapist helps the family use them to solve both current and future problems. Brief therapy does not even attempt to resolve all the problems a family may face. It attempts to enhance the family's problem-solving abilities. It leaves the family better prepared to deal with future problems and problems not dealt with directly during the therapy.

Family Therapy

When treating the disturbed child, it is crucial to consider the family. Even if family therapy per se is not feasible or is not the treatment of choice, the therapist must see the child not just as an individual but as part of a family with complex interactional patterns.

The Family as a System   A child may be identified as the "sick one" when the family dynamics themselves are dysfunctional. Sometimes the child's "illness" is all that is holding the family together. In this case, the entire family (including the identified client) needs to have the child remain ill. If the nurse doesn't pick up on this, all therapeutic efforts will be futile. The child is part of a family system. If the system changes, the chances are good that the child will change, too. (See Chapter 21 for an in-depth discussion.)

Eleven-year-old Rudy S had been referred to the mental health clinic by his family physician because he had made an attempt to commit suicide. During the intake interview, Rudy's parents said he was "really sick, very depressed and crazy." They added that Rudy had been sick for several years, but it was getting worse. Questioned about siblings, they said that Wanda, Rudy's eight-year-old sister, was "no trouble at all and a very good student." The therapist recognized that Rudy was being labeled as the identified client and requested family sessions, at least initially. The family agreed reluctantly, stressing that it was only to "help Rudy."

In the course of therapy, it was revealed that Mr. S was an alcoholic who had tried unsuccessfully for years to quit drinking. Mrs. S had threatened since Rudy's infancy to leave him if he didn't quit, but felt they should stay together for the children. Mrs. S also had a long history of depression, frequently spending days at a time lying on the couch. It became evident during the family sessions that Rudy got "sicker" and threatened suicide in response to threats of family disintegration—

specifically when his father was on a drinking binge and his mother was threatening to leave or was very depressed or both. The parents responded to Rudy's illness by drawing together to try and help him, thus keeping the family intact. Wanda tried to keep the family intact by never causing any trouble. She was an abnormally passive and fearful child. In the course of long-term family therapy, and couples therapy for the parents, the family began to deal with and resolve some basic issues and conflicts, making a change in family dynamics possible. As a result, Rudy was able to stop his unconscious, desperate attempts to maintain family homeostasis, and Wanda was able to risk letting go of her overcompliant role.

The Family Therapist   Family therapy is not for the beginning therapist. It is too complex. The client or patient is the family, and families are complicated. The acknowledged and unacknowledged rules, roles, and communication patterns of the family must be delineated and used to help the family understand its own interaction process. The family therapist may draw on systems, role, communications, psychoanalytic, interpersonal, and change theories in the course of treating one family. The family therapist must be skilled at communication and observation. These skills are pinpointed and discussed in Chapter 21.

Behavior Modification

Behavior modification therapy is based on the principle that behavior is determined by its consequences. Therefore, behavior can be altered by altering consequences. Behavior modification is not concerned with growth and development, except in the sense that the undesirable behavior must first be evaluated developmentally. For instance, it would be unrealistic to attempt to toilet train a child who was physiologically unable to achieve sphincter control, or to stop a four-month-old child's thumb sucking.

Goal and Techniques   Behavior modification is not concerned with intrapsychic conflicts. It focuses on one piece of behavior, which is labeled the symptom. The goal is to change or remove the symptom. This is done systematically by

- Identifying and specifying the behavior to be changed, developed, or modified, i.e., stopping temper tantrums
- Recording behavior, including frequency, and circumstances

- Determining what conditions maintain the behavior, i.e., the child is given candy to stop throwing tantrums
- Determining how to change these conditions and use reinforcements to decrease the unwanted behavior and increase desirable behavior

Reinforcement   Most parents are very effective at developing and maintaining desirable behaviors through the use of positive reinforcement. Usually, the positive reinforcement takes the form of praise. Behaviors to be eliminated can be dealt with by positive reinforcement, negative reinforcement, or lack of reinforcement. Positive reinforcement can be given when the behavior does not occur. For instance, if Johnny avoids doing homework, he is given a nickel for each night he completes it. Negative reinforcement is given when the behavior does occur. Johnny might lose his tv privileges each time he did not do his homework. Lack of reinforcement means giving neither positive nor negative reinforcement—that is, ignoring the behavior. Obviously, the use of this technique depends on how well the parents can tolerate the behavior. Frequently, positive and negative reinforcement are combined.

Requirements for Effective Behavior Modification   Behavior modification could be called the therapy of logical consequences. Its success or failure depends primarily on the motivation and consistency of the parents. Behavior modification is very effective for many "problem" behaviors, and it is fairly simple to do, but it requires commitment and energy. The reinforcements, or consequences, must be consistent. If they aren't, the whole purpose is defeated, and things may be worse than ever, since an intermittently reinforced behavior is the most difficult kind to change.

Milieu Therapy

This technique takes its name from the milieu, or environment, in which it is practiced. It consists of providing the severely disturbed child with a controlled and consistent environment and healthy interpersonal relationships that are therapeutic in themselves. Milieu therapy may be practiced in a residential, day treatment, or inpatient treatment center. It is used in addition to other treatment modalities (such as individual therapy), not in place of them.

Five-year-old Joshua had been admitted to the residential psychiatric ward the previous year. History, including failure to verbalize, revealed psychotic symptoms as early as the first year. The nursing staff found Joshua demanding to care for because of his persistent attempts to hurt himself and other children, his fecal and urinary incontinence, and his consistent oppositional behavior.

One afternoon, Joshua's primary nurse returned from lunch to find Joshua obviously very upset. The nurse thought it might be due to a change that had been made in his schedule. Joshua, like most severely disturbed children, reacted with fear and anger to any change in routine. The nurse sat on the floor next to Joshua and began to verbalize her interpretation of his feelings. At that, Joshua darted up and kicked the child closest to him. The nurse restrained Joshua, who immediately began screaming and became rigid. The nurse carried Joshua to an unoccupied room and sat down on the floor, holding him so that he was against her but restrained. Joshua continued to scream and try to get away. The nurse continued to hold him. When his screams subsided, she said, "Joshua, you seem mad and scared. Maybe you're scared because things were different and I wasn't here. I guess you might be mad at me because I wasn't here. It's okay to be mad. I'm going to help you not hurt yourself or anyone else." Joshua acknowledged this by making eye contact. Then he began screaming and flailing around again. When he stopped for a minute, the nurse said, "I'll hold you as long as you need me." Joshua immediately started screaming again, occasionally stopping for a few seconds to make eye contact with the nurse, who continued to reassure him with phrases such as "I'm still here." After twenty minutes, Joshua was able to return to the living room.

In this interaction with Joshua, the nurse

- Acknowledged his feelings and her acceptance of them
- Encouraged appropriate affective development by verbally linking his feelings (anger, fear) to causes (change, abandonment)
- Provided external ego control for Joshua when he was unable to provide it for himself
- Prevented Joshua from hurting himself or her while still indicating her acceptance of him, thus giving him some security

Providing Structure   Milieu therapy provides structure for the child's daily life. Within this structure, peers are available for identification or acting out, and many adults are available for role models. From the adult staff, the children receive a sense of being accepted and the opportunity to choose adults who meet their individual needs.

Differences in Milieu   The nature of the milieu depends on the treatment center and its theoretical interpretation of emotional disorders. Some centers believe that intrapsychic disturbances are caused by impaired parenting. These centers emphasize relationships between the child and a significant adult on the staff. Other centers focus on the behavioral and social causes of emotional disorders. These centers use behavior modification techniques to teach the child how to make it in the outside world. The important thing is that the milieu be consistent with both the philosophy of the center and the philosophy of the individual staff members. Staff members also need opportunities to work out the guilt, resentment, and hopelessness that inevitably arise when one works closely with severely disturbed children. Otherwise they will be unable to provide the consistent, accepting atmosphere necessary to milieu therapy.

Relationship within the Milieu   Within the milieu the relationship between a child and a staff member is used as a therapeutic tool. To a large extent, the staff individually and collectively create and maintain a therapeutic milieu. The relationship between staff members and disturbed children can encourage affective development in the children and help them develop a sense of continuity of identity. Effective psychiatric nurses use themselves as important therapeutic tools.

Larry, a staff nurse at a small residential treatment center that used milieu therapy for disturbed children, was assigned as primary nurse for six-year-old John. John appeared very withdrawn and unresponsive, and rarely spoke. At a joint treatment planning session, Larry, along with the other professional staff members (including the psychiatrist who would be seeing John in daily play therapy sessions), identified goals for John, which included encouraging appropriate affective development.

For his work with John, Larry pursued this goal by spending the first several weeks sitting quietly by John and helping him start to identify different emotions and differentiate between himself and others. This usually took the form of a running commentary, such as "Amanda is sad, John. Amanda is crying. John is not crying." or "Whitney is mad, John. Whitney is hitting the

wall." or "John is hiding his face. I wonder if John is feeling sad?" Larry tried to be consistently nonthreatening to John, not trying to force eye contact or any other response from him, but building trust by being dependably there with him and continuing to comment on feelings and affect, including occasionally his own feelings. Two months after John's admission, Larry was greatly encouraged when, after telling John one day that it was time for him, Larry, to leave and he wouldn't be back for two days, John scowled and said "No! John mad."

THE HOSPITALIZED CHILD

Hospitalized children of any age are under great stress and need psychiatric nursing interventions. Traditionally, pediatric wards emphasize the physiological care of the child, which can result in excellent medical care with little or no psychological care. It has been demonstrated in both clinical and research settings that hospitalized children need emotional, as well as physical, care. The nurse on the staff of the pediatric ward and the psychiatric nurse-consultant (see Chapter 24) are in a position to meet these emotional needs.

Anaclitic Depression

Research studies, notably those of Bowlby (1960) and Spitz (1946), have established the profound and often irreversible effects on infants of long-term hospitalization and concomitant maternal deprivation. Infants separated from the mother (or other primary caregiver) during the first year of life, due to prolonged hospitalization of the child or placement in an institution such as an orphanage, frequently became withdrawn, apathetic, and emaciated. Although they received adequate physical care, these infants frequently died.

Separation Anxiety

Separation Anxiety is one of the major psychological stresses on the hospitalized child. Although it is less severe than Anaclitic Depression, the child who experiences Separation Anxiety needs psychiatric nursing intervention. Bowlby (1960) and Robertson (1958) distinguish three stages in the Separation Anxiety experienced by hospitalized children.

Protest   This first stage lasts from a few hours to several days. Children in this stage still consciously need mother and expect that their efforts to regain her will succeed. They still hope that mother will meet their needs as she has in the past. Need for mother and terror at losing her produce an anxiety that sharply reduces the child's perceptual field. Behavioral manifestations of this stage include loud crying, screaming, tossing around in bed or crib, focusing eagerly on any sight or sound that might be the mother, and rejecting the attentions of others.

Despair   In this stage the child still consciously needs mother but no longer expects that efforts to regain her will succeed. Crying is now intermittent or monotonous, replacing the screams of rage and terror characteristic of the protest stage. The despairing child is apathetic and listless and does not interact with the environment.

Detachment   In this stage children use the defense mechanism of repression to deal with their intense anxiety. They repress their need of the mother, often to the point of not seeming to recognize her when she visits. At this stage the child does not cry when mother leaves and does interact with the environment. The child in Anaclitic Depression is in the final stages of the detachment phase.

Children who have reached the detachment phase are often erroneously believed to have adjusted to the hospital situation. Actually, these children have lost faith in their parents' love and ability and willingness to protect them. This loss of faith has obvious implications for their readjustment on returning home. It may also affect how they will handle terminations and separations for the rest of their lives.

Two-year-old Maddy G was being released after several weeks in the hospital for orthopedic surgery. The psychiatric nurse-consultant had helped Maddy deal with the anxiety aroused by separation from mother and home by engaging her in play therapy, involving Maddy's mother as much as possible in the nurturing aspects of Maddy's care, and having regular nurses care for Maddy. On the day of Maddy's release, the psychiatric nurse spent some time with Maddy's mother explaining the separation anxiety process and providing Ms. G with anticipatory counseling about possible problems that might come up at home.

A week later Ms. G told the public health nurse visiting Maddy, "Thank heavens the nurse in the hospital warned me what I might expect! Maddy has been impossible, so demanding and babyish. If I hadn't known ahead of time this might happen, I wouldn't have had the slightest idea how to handle it." The public health nurse asked Ms. G how she was handling Maddy's regressive behavior. Ms. G replied that, on the advice of the psychiatric nurse-consultant in the hospital, she was trying to accept Maddy and her need to "be babyish" and was helping Maddy express her feelings by verbally acknowledging and accepting her anger toward her mother, her fears of being left again, and her need to regress. Ms. G added that the psychiatric nurse had really helped by offering specific things she could say to Maddy, such as "I guess you're pretty mad at me right now, and I guess you are pretty mad that I left you in the hospital," when Maddy was having a tantrum, or "It looks like you need to be a baby for awhile now. That's okay. Later you won't need to be a baby," when Maddy was doing something regressive, such as wetting her pants. Ms. G added, "Things are getting back to normal now, but it feels good to talk about it." The public health nurse offered Ms. G positive reinforcement for the use she had been able to make of the anticipatory counseling given by the child psychiatric nurse.

The Hospitalized Toddler   Hospitalized toddlers are a high-risk group. They are vulnerable because their ego is still evolving and as yet is not highly integrated or sophisticated. For the toddler, the parents still fill superego functions. Their presence is important because it furnishes external controls to bolster the toddler's poor impulse control.

The toddler's primary process thinking increases this vulnerability. Toddlers cannot understand the need for hospitalization. The toddler sees the parents as omnipotent and therefore able to control the situation. Since they can control the situation, they must have chosen to let the hospitalization happen. At first the toddler feels angry, especially at the primary caregiver. In the projection characteristic of primary process thought, it is a short mental step from anger at mother to conviction that mother is angry, that hospitalization is punishment, and that the child has somehow caused the event.

Castration and Mutilation Fantasies

Fears of mutilation are especially prevalent in the four-to-seven-year-old hospitalized child. These fears are present in all hospitalized children to some extent, particularly when surgical treatment is necessary, but the four-to-seven-year-old needs special reassurance. These children need to know that intrusive procedures will not permanently damage their bodies. They need to know that neither they nor anyone else is to blame for the hospitalization. And they need to know what the intrusive procedures are designed to do.

Case Study and Sample Care Plan   The following case study and care plan illustrate the interventions designed by the nurse to alleviate the castration and mutilation fears of a hospitalized child.

Five-year-old Che had been admitted to the hospital for surgical hypospadias repair. Despite preoperative reassurance about the surgery, and reassurance that his penis would still be all there, Che was agitated after the operation. He cried and was frequently observed clutching his penis with an anxious expression. After repeated attempts by the pediatric nurses and his mother to reassure him had failed, the mental health nurse-consultant talked with the staff and Che's mother and had a diagnostic play session with Che. Che's play during this session revealed his conviction that he had been permanently mutilated. It also revealed his confused feelings that he was somehow responsible and was being punished. His anger toward his mother for not preventing the frightening experience was also apparent from his behavior in the diagnostic play session.

CHE: *(Lines up most of the toy soldiers so they are pointing aggressively at one lone soldier.)*

NURSE: *What's happening?*

CHE: *They're going to get him. (Moves soldiers to surround single soldier.)*

NURSE: *All of those soldiers are going to get that one little soldier.*

CHE: *Yeah. Then they're going to cut him up. He'll never be back together.*

NURSE: *I guess he must be pretty scared.*

CHE: *He was bad, so they'll cut him up. (Knocks lone soldier down.)*

NURSE: *They are cutting him up because he was bad?*

CHE: *Yeah, and he'll still be alive, but he'll always be cut up. (Moves a large tank by the lone soldier, whom he stands up again to face the rest of the soldiers.)*

NURSE: *You say he'll always be cut up. What's happening now?*

CHE: *This big tank could help the soldier.*

NURSE: *It could help?*

CHE: *It could make all these others go away. (Moves tank out of sight.) But it won't. So he gets cut again.*

NURSE: *The tank could have helped the soldier not get cut again, but it didn't. How does the soldier feel?*

CHE: *He hates that tank now.*

Following this diagnostic play session, the psychiatric nurse-consultant worked up a care plan with the ward personnel. This care plan is shown in Table 19–3.

Psychological Care of the Pediatric Client

The psychiatric nurse specialist and the pediatric nurse often work with physically ill pediatric clients. Mental health interventions with these clients are usually on a primary or secondary level of prevention. These interventions can avert the possible serious psychological consequences of hospitalization. The psychological care plans shown in Tables 19–4 to 19–7 give the main objectives and interventions for the hospitalized child. These tables appear on the following pages.

Table 19-3 CARE PLAN FOR A CHILD WITH MUTILATION FANTASIES		
Nursing Intervention	**Rationale**	**Expected Outcome**
1. Assign one nurse to Che as consistently as possible.	To furnish Che with some stability in a situation that is confusing for him, and to allow him the opportunity to form a positive attachment to a staff member.	This stability will help reduce Che's general anxiety.
2. Help Che deal with his feelings, including mutilation and castration fantasies, by encouraging him to play them out. Furnish play materials to help him do this. Nurse-consultant to see Che daily for half an hour to engage in play and encourage play at other times.	To give Che an opportunity to communicate his concerns. To help him gain a sense of mastery over and assimilation of a frightening and stressful situation over which he has had no control. Play will allow Che to relive frightening events in an active role, rather than in the passive and helpless role he has been thrust into as a pediatric client. This will help him assimilate the experiences and master his anxieties.	Communicating his fears and gaining a sense of mastery and assimilation from the play experiences will help Che resolve his feelings of anger, guilt, and helplessness and his fears of mutilation.
3. Find out how much Che understands about his hospitalization and surgery. Then use the boy doll (with genitals), drawings, and other visual aids to correct misconceptions and explain the condition and surgical repair to Che. Encourage questions and give him verbal reinforcement for any understanding he demonstrates.	At five Che is capable of understanding simple anatomy and physiology. Visual aids will help. When he understands the real nature of his surgery and the reason for it, Che's frightening fantasies will decrease. Mastery of this material will also enhance Che's self-esteem.	Che will understand his condition and the surgery. This will decrease his feelings of helplessness and guilt and his fears of mutilation.
4. Encourage mother to continue regular visits. Explain Che's feelings, including his anger toward her, and the reasons for these feelings. Encourage her to accept Che's feelings and to support him. Offer her positive reinforcement for doing so. Allow for her expression of possible anger, guilt, or confusion. If Che's anger takes the form of pretending to ignore his mother, reassure her of her importance to Che and encourage her to remain actively involved.	It is important for Che to know that his mother still loves him and will not be destroyed or withdraw her love if he is angry with her. This is also a difficult time for Che's mother. She needs support, instruction, and encouragement both for herself and so she can help Che more effectively.	
5. Encourage Che to participate in his own care.	At five, Che has just learned how to care for himself. Having to relinquish this care to others reinforces his feelings of helplessness, powerlessness.	Che will participate in his own care and will not regress in self-care activities. This will enhance his self-esteem.

**Table 19–4   PSYCHOLOGICAL CARE PLAN: HOSPITALIZED INFANT
(BIRTH TO APPROXIMATELY ONE YEAR)**

Nursing Care Objectives	Nursing Interventions	Nursing Care Objectives	Nursing Interventions
To help infant develop trust	1. Assign one nurse and one relief staff member to care for infant. 2. Arrange parental rooming-in, if possible. 3. Provide infant with a maternal substitute if parent does not room-in. 4. Encourage parent to participate in care as much as possible. 5. Have parent present during assigned nurse's first interactions with infant to facilitate infant's trust in the nurse.		3. Provide tactile stimulation by holding, cuddling, rocking infant. 1. Nurse assigned to infant needs to work closely with parents, giving them recognition and helping them to stay involved in infant's care. 2. Offer parents the opportunity to express their needs and feelings. 3. A psychiatric nurse clinician or other mental health worker could meet this need. The ward staff members should offer parents the opportunity to talk and should accept their possible frustration, anger, or fears.
To provide infant with pleasurable sensory and tactile stimulation	1. Provide cuddly toys and visual stimulants, such as mobiles. 2. Provide auditory stimulation, such as music, singing, talking.	To support parents so they can continue to meet infant's needs	

Table 19-5 PSYCHOLOGICAL CARE PLAN: HOSPITALIZED TODDLER (APPROXIMATELY ONE TO THREE YEARS)			
Nursing Care Objectives	**Nursing Interventions**	**Nursing Care Objectives**	**Nursing Interventions**
To avoid disrupting the parent-child relationship, which the toddler needs in order to accomplish the separation-individuation process	1. Have parent room-in if possible. 2. Involve parent in child's care as much as possible. 3. Explain the dynamics of separation anxiety and the toddler's vulnerability to parents. If parents do not understand why the child is clingy or appears to ignore them during visits, they may visit less often. 4. Provide parents with support, so they can continue to support child. Specifically, parents need the opportunity to verbalize feelings, concerns, fears, and anger.	To help the child deal with the fear of abandonment	mommy will be back tomorrow at nine," say, "After you go to bed, wake up in the morning, and eat breakfast, mommy will be back." 1. Try to incorporate some of the child's home routines into the hospital care to give the child a sense of stability about some aspects of daily life. 2. Have parents leave transitional objects from home with the child. 3. Promote the continuity of the parent-child relationship (see first objective), stressing to parents the importance of regular visiting if parents are not rooming-in. 4. Give the child opportunity to use play to help resolve fears and conflicts. If child is nonambulatory and cannot go to the ward playroom, furnish child with toys and companionship.
To help the toddler meet needs for control	1. Whenever possible, offer a choice, for example, a choice of foods. Do not offer a "choice" concerning necessary medical procedures that the child in fact has no choice about. 2. Be honest and consistent. 3. Encourage verbal and symbolic expression of conflicts to help the child assimilate and master frightening events and feelings.	To prepare the child for medical or surgical procedures	1. Give the toddler the opportunity to play with as much as possible of the equipment used in his or her care, such as syringes without needles. 2. Tell the younger toddler about a procedure just before it is to be done. Tell older toddlers several hours ahead, or earlier if considerable preparation is involved. 3. Be honest about whether the procedure will hurt. 4. Be clear with the child that necessary medical procedures will be carried out, and that the child doesn't have a choice about them. 5. Encourage child to express objections to and anger about being subjected to painful or frightening procedures and having no control over them. Expression may be verbal or symbolic (through play). Indicate acceptance of child's feelings by saying, for instance, "I guess you're pretty mad at me because I gave you that shot. It's hard to have to get shots."
To help parents and child separate when necessary	1. Have parents tell child when they will return. 2. Have parents leave immediately after they tell child they're going. 3. Stay with child for awhile after parents leave. Let parents know you will do this to help child to cope with their leaving. 4. Give parents recognition and support for being able to separate from child. 5. Stress that it is important for parents to return when they tell child they will. Also stress the importance of not lying to the child ("Mommy's just going to the store. I'll be right back") or leaving without letting child know. 6. Make sure child knows when parent will return. Toddlers do not understand time well, so relate visits to daily activity. For instance, rather than saying, "Your		

Table 19-6 PSYCHOLOGICAL CARE PLAN: HOSPITALIZED OEDIPAL AGE CHILD (APPROXIMATELY THREE TO SIX YEARS)			
Nursing Care Objectives	**Nursing Interventions**	**Nursing Care Objectives**	**Nursing Interventions**
To help the child meet the developmental task of achieving a sense of initiative versus guilt	1. Provide the child with some stability by assigning one nurse and one relief staff member to the child.		Encourage questions and give positive reinforcement for curiosity and for child's ability to understand answers.
	2. Explain to parents the importance of regular visits. These give children the confidence in continued parental support and love that they need to continue to explore themselves and the environment.	To help the child deal with mutilation and castration fantasies	1. Before explaining the child's condition, find out how the child understands it. If the child will not verbalize his or her ideas, the nurse may be able to assess them during a play session.
	3. Be aware that the Oedipal-age child is absorbed with guilt and blame and egocentric thinking. When appropriate, stress to these children that no one (including themselves) is to blame for their illness. One strategy to convey this, if the child does not verbalize or otherwise directly communicate concern, is to say, "Sometimes kids think they get sick because they're bad or someone is punishing them. That's not true."		2. Be aware that Oedipal-age children tend to believe their entire body is vulnerable. This is especially important in pre- and postoperative teaching. Stress that the surgical procedure will be (or was) limited to one specific part of the body.
	4. Give the child the opportunity to use play and play materials to help resolve feelings of guilt. Many children will play out fantasies they won't verbalize. For instance, the child might have a doll or toy animal be sick because "he's bad." Play times are opportunities for the nurse to assess the child's possible feelings of guilt or blame or both and offer reassurance.		3. Give the child the materials and the opportunity to play out, and thus help resolve, mutilation fears.
			4. Offer clear explanations of the child's condition and treatment.
	5. Encourage these children to participate in their own medical and personal care. This gives them a sense of control, confidence, and mastery.	To prepare the child for medical or surgical procedures	1. This age group can understand simple anatomy and physiology, so offer specific explanations, rather than general ones such as "We are going to fix your eyes."
	6. Praise the child for exploring and participating in self-care.		2. Find out how much the child understands about the condition and the treatments both before and after you have explained them. Then clarify misunderstandings and deal with possible fantasies of guilt and mutilation.
			3. Use visual aids. These should include body outline drawings, dolls, and actual equipment used in treatment, such as intravenous tubing, dressings, and drains. Encourage the child to handle and play with equipment.

		Table 19–7	PSYCHOLOGICAL CARE PLAN: HOSPITALIZED LATENCY AGE CHILD (APPROXIMATELY SIX TO TWELVE YEARS)	

Nursing Care Objectives	Nursing Interventions	Nursing Care Objectives	Nursing Interventions
To help the child use the hospitalization to achieve a sense of industry by promoting exploration and mastery of skills	1. Find out how much these children understand about their condition. Then actively involve them as you teach them about it. 2. When teaching, use a more sophisticated, scientific approach than is used with younger children. Include medical terminology. Give verbal recognition of understanding and learning. 3. Encourage questions and curiosity. 4. Make actual equipment available to child for exploration. Give verbal recognition if the child is able to use the equipment.		injections, in a group setting. Use actual equipment and encourage participation.
		To help the child deal with possible fears of death	1. Be aware that a fear of death is common at this age. 2. Encourage verbal expression of fears and symbolic expression through play. The child may not express the fear directly but may tell stories about children who died. 3. Be very clear when teaching about which part of the child's body will be involved. Stress that no other body part will be involved. 4. Let child know that many other children have been treated successfully at the hospital for the same condition. 5. Express confidence in the child's physician and in other health workers.

Interactions with peers	1. Peer relationships are important in this age group, so encourage peer interaction by strategies such as
	
	  a. Making available a playroom that includes games, interesting equipment or models, and other toys that promote group play.
	
	  b. Involving the nonambulant child by wheeling the bed into the playroom or by arranging the room so that other children can come in to play.
	
	  c. Offering the child in isolation more direct contact with the nurse.
	
	  d. Teaching about common experiences, such as
		To prepare the child for medical and surgical procedures	See first part of this section and section on preparation of Oedipal-age child for specific techniques. Be alert for the possibility of regression due to the stress of hospitalization. This stress may arouse fears, such as fear of separation or mutilation, normally associated with a younger age group. Hospitalization is usually less traumatic for the latency age child, since these children separate more easily from parents and home, are interested in trying out new roles and exploring new situations, and are more reality oriented and better able to reason than the younger child. If the nurse uses these characteristics in helping the child to cope with the hospitalization, it can be a positive experience for the child.

KEY NURSING CONCEPTS

✔ Child psychiatric nursing is a specialty role performed by nurses prepared at the graduate level.

✔ There is a great shortage of child mental health intervention services in the United States.

✔ Many mental health problems stem from trauma in the first five years of life.

✔ The interactional view holds that emotional disturbance is caused by a dysfunctional interaction between a constitutionally susceptible child and a psychologically incompatible environment.

✔ General intervention goals for disturbed children include working through unsuccessfully resolved development stages, development of a realistic self-concept, and development of healthy interpersonal relations.

✔ A holistic approach to assessment, diagnosis, treatment, and evaluation of child mental health services encourages input from many different disciplines.

✔ Basic prevention in mental health services for the child is designed to ensure that developmental needs are met.

✔ Secondary prevention is designed to detect early warning signs of mental health problems.

✔ Tertiary prevention provides rehabilitation in an effort to decrease the likelihood of chronic disability.

✔ Nurses need to know normal growth and development in order to differentiate between normal and pathological reactions.

✔ Emotionally disturbed children show impairment in perception of the world, relations with others, and learning.

✔ Nursing skills used to meet the basic goals of treatment include assessment, communication skills, conveying acceptance, setting limits, establishing rapport, and self-awareness.

✔ Effective communication with children requires the same basic skills as with adults.

✔ Modes of therapy for work with disturbed children may include play therapy, group therapy, family therapy, behavior modification, and milieu therapy.

✔ Three stages of Separation Anxiety experienced by hospitalized children include protest, despair, and detachment.

✔ The pediatric staff nurse and the psychiatric nurse-consultant are in key positions to identify and attend to the hospitalized child's psychological needs.

References

American Psychiatric Association. *Diagnostic and Statistical Manual of Mental Disorders*, 3d ed., Washington, D.C.: American Psychiatric Association, 1980(a).

American Psychiatric Association. *Quick Reference to the Diagnostic Criteria from DSM-III (Mini-D)*. Washington, D.C.: American Psychiatric Association, 1980(b).

Boatman, M. J. "A Historical Description of the Program." In *Inpatient Care for the Psychotic Child*, edited by S. A. Szurek; I. N. Berlin; and M. J. Boatman, pp. 50–65. Langley Porter Child Psychiatry Series, vol. 5, Palo Alto, Calif.: Science and Behavior Books, 1971.

Bowlby, J. "Separation Anxiety." *International Journal of Psychoanalysis* 41 (1960): 89–135.

Erikson, E. *Childhood and Society*. 2d ed. New York: W. W. Norton, 1950.

Gesell, A. *The First Five Years of Life*. New York: Harper and Row, 1940.

———. *The Child from Five to Ten*. New York: Harper and Row, 1946.

Joint Commission on Mental Health of Children. *Crisis in Child Mental Health, Challenge for the 1970's*. New York: Harper and Row, 1969.

Kanner, L. "Autistic Disturbances of Affective Contact." *Nervous Child* 2 (1943): 217–250.

Robertson, J. *Young Children in Hospital*. London: Tavistock Publications, 1958.

Spitz, R. "Hospitalism." *Psychoanalytic Study of the Child* 2 (1945): 53–74.

———. "Hospitalism: A Follow Up Report." *Psychoanalytic Study of the Child* 2 (1946): 313–342.

Further Reading

Axline, V. *Play Therapy*. New York: Ballantine Books, 1947.

Barker, P. "The Aims and Nature of the Inpatient Psychiatric Treatment of Children." In *The Residential Psychiatric Treatment of Children*, edited by P. Barker, pp. 27–47. New York: John Wiley, 1974.

Barten, H., and Barten, S. *Children and Their Parents in Brief Therapy*. New York; Behavioral Publications, 1973.

Brazelton, T. B. *Infants and Mothers*. New York: Delta Publishing, 1969.

———. *Toddlers and Parents*. New York: Delta Publishing, 1974.

Cramer, J. B. "Psychiatric Examination of the Child." In *Comprehensive Textbook of Psychiatry III*, vol. 3, edited by A. M. Freedman, H. I. Kaplan, and B. J. Sadock, pp. 2453–2461. Baltimore: Williams and Wilkins, 1980.

Critchley, Deane L. "Mental Status Examinations with Children and Adolescents, A Developmental Approach." In *The Nursing Clinics of North America, Symposium on Child Psychiatric Nursing*, edited by Evelyn M. McElroy. vol. 14, No. 3, pp. 429–441. Philadelphia: W. B. Saunders, September, 1979.

Despert, J. L. *The Inner Voices of Children*. Photography by D. Pallottelli. New York: Brunner/Mazel, 1975.

DiLeo, J. H. *Young Children and Their Drawings*. New York: Brunner/Mazel, 1970.

———. *Children's Drawings as Diagnostic Aids*. New York: Brunner/Mazel, 1973.

Fagin, C. *Nursing in Child Psychiatry*. St. Louis: C. V. Mosby, 1972.

———. *Readings in Child and Adolescent Psychiatric Nursing*. St. Louis: C. V. Mosby, 1974.

Freedman, A., and Kaplan, H., eds. *The Child: His Psychological and Cultural Development*. 2 vols. New York: Atheneum Publishers, 1972.

Freud, A. *Normality and Pathology in Childhood*. New York: International Universities Press, 1965.

Haworth, M. R. ed. *Child Psychotherapy*. New York: Basic Books, 1964.

Howells, J., ed. *Modern Perspectives in Child Psychiatry*. New York: Brunner/Mazel, 1971.

Kanner, L. "Early Infantile Autism." *American Journal of Psychiatry* 103 (1946): 242–246.

Lidz, T. *The Person*. Rev. ed. New York: Basic Books, 1968.

Mahler, M. "Autism and Symbosis: Two Extreme Disturbances of Identity." *International Journal of Psychoanalysis* 39 (1958): 77–83.

Moustakas, C. E. *Psychotherapy with Children*. New York: Harper and Row, 1959.

Petrillo, M., and Sanger, S. *Emotional Care of Hospitalized Children*. Philadelphia: J. B. Lippincott, 1972.

Pothier, P. *Mental Health Counseling with Children*. Boston: Little, Brown, 1976.

Rosenthal, A. J. "Brief Focused Psychotherapy with Children and Families." In *Basic Handbook of Child Psychiatry*, edited by J. Nozlipitz. New York: Basic Books, 1980.

Simmons, J. E. *Psychiatric Examination of Children*. Philadelphia: Lea and Febiger, 1974.

Sullivan, H. S. *Conceptions of Modern Psychiatry*, edited by H. S. Perry and M. L. Gawel. New York: W. W. Norton, 1953.

Thomas, A.; Chess, S.; and Birch, H. *Temperament and Behavior Disorders in Children*. New York: New York University Press, 1968.

Williams, P. D. "Preparation of School-age Children for Surgery." *International Journal of Nursing Studies* 17(1980): 107–119.

20

Mental Health Counseling with Adolescents

by Carol Bradley

CHAPTER OUTLINE

The Normative Process of Adolescence
   Physical and Sexual Development
   Mental Development
   Social Development
   Emotional Development
Developmental Theories
   Freud and the Reemergence of the Oedipal Conflict
   Erikson and the Life Cycle
   Sullivan and the Need for Interpersonal Intimacy
   The Theories in Summary
The Role of the Nurse
   In the Outpatient Setting
   In the Hospital Setting
Specific Issues and Problems
   Seduction of the Nurse
   Communication
   Testing and Limit Setting
   Anxiety and Resistance
   Anger and Hostility
   Scapegoating
   Sexual Behavior of the Adolescent
   Dietary Problems
   Drug Use and Abuse
   Juvenile Delinquency
   Suicide
Dealing with Families of Adolescent Clients
Key Nursing Concepts

LEARNING OBJECTIVES

After reading this chapter, students should be able to

- Compare and contrast the physical, mental, social, and emotional development of adolescents to that of people at other life stages
- Relate the developmental theories of Freud, Erikson, and Sullivan to the adolescent
- Describe the role and function of the nurse in treatment settings for adolescents
- Identify the issues and problems specifically related to the humanistic nursing care of the adolescent client
- Describe the role and function of the nurse in working with the families of adolescent clients

CHAPTER 20

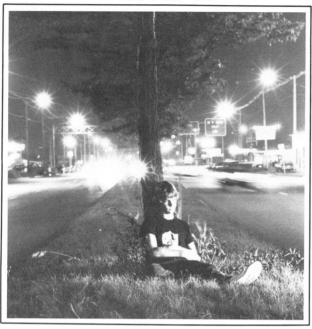

Adolescence is a stormy period in life—a time when conflicting ideas and feelings intensify on all fronts. The struggle for identity is its central task.

The chapter considers various treatment modalities emphasizing the therapeutic community. Special consideration is given to specific behaviors that are unique to adolescents and that frequently pose difficulties for the nurse.

THE NORMATIVE PROCESS OF ADOLESCENCE

Let's take a closer look at the person who is approaching adolescence and embarking on a relatively normal process of growth and development.

Physical and Sexual Development

Children approaching puberty have had several years to grow accustomed to their body size and build. The physical changes that characterized the first ten to eleven years of life have diminished to a dormant or latent state, and the individual has been able to focus on the task of developing and experimenting with various social skills. But with the onset of puberty (around twelve to fourteen years of age), spectacular physical and sexual changes occur. A boy may grow four or five inches in a single year. Over the course of a summer vacation, a girl may reach menarche and begin to develop breasts. Although the pubertal changes have actually been going on for some time, they seem sudden to the adolescent. The timing and the extent of these changes are unpredictable. The degree to which the adolescent can adapt to them and to the upsurge in sexual capacity is equally unpredictable.

As adolescents attempt to adjust to physical changes, their behavior and attitudes change. Up to now the child has been preoccupied with developing into a fully social being. The young adolescent becomes obsessed with changes in body image, peer group acceptance, and development of individual identity. Experimentation in every facet of life is the norm, yet conformity and peer approval is a daily (if not hourly) preoccupation. Interest in makeup and dress plays an important part in the adolescent's search for

What is adolescence? Some sources define it simply as the time of physical and psychosocial development between the ages of twelve and twenty. Others have described it as a period of "normal psychosis." Still others see it as an attempt by a tyrannical subculture to overtake adult America. It is not necessary to accept verbatim either of these last two definitions in order to understand their implications. Most people recognize the immense stress that occurs during adolescence and the importance it holds for the adult's future.

Adolescence is not just a time of physical and sexual growth. It is a stormy period in life, an interruption between the docility of the latency years and the acclimation of adulthood. Adolescence is a time when the individual is confronted with conflicting ideas and feelings, when inconsistency and disharmony are the norm. In comparison to adult behavior, the adolescent's incongruous activity does seem to warrant professional attention. In fact, a steady state during this period of reawakening and redefining could be considered deviant.

Trying to understand the adolescent is a challenge to anyone. For the nurse who chooses to work with adolescents, the challenge offers considerable rewards.

This chapter examines the role of the nurse in the interpersonal relationship with adolescent clients. The psychosocial developmental theories of Freud, Erikson, and Sullivan provide the nurse with a basis for making accurate assessments and appropriate interventions.

Table 20-1 PHYSICAL CHANGES DURING PUBERTY		
Characteristic	**In Males**	**In Females**
Maturation of genitals and accessory reproductive organs	Acceleration of growth of penis and testes Development of breasts, which is usually transitory and subsides Occurrence of seminal emissions	Development of skin and tissue surrounding vulval region Rapid increase in growth of uterus and ovaries Development of breasts Ovulation and beginning of menses
Development of the secondary sex characteristics	Development of pubic hair Appearance of axillary hair and facial hair approximately two years after development of pubic hair Rapid increase in growth of larynx, resulting in "breaking" of voice	Development of pubic hair approximately two years prior to menarche Appearance of axillary hair approximately two years after onset of pubic hair Increase in growth of larynx, less pronounced in females
	Axillary sweat glands becoming functional in both sexes Appearance of acne common, especially in males	
	Increased pigmentation of skin, particularly darkening of areola in males Loss of scalp hair toward end of puberty	Increased pigmentation of skin, particularly darkening of areola (although to lesser extent than in males, except during and after pregnancy)
Development of the skeleton	Dramatic acceleration of growth in both height and weight, beginning at approximately 12½ to 13 years; pubertal spurt greater than in females	Acceleration of growth in both height and weight, beginning approximately at 10½ to 11 years, pubertal spurt less than in males
	Generally, growth of skeleton begins with feet and hands, followed by calf and forearm, followed by hips and chest, and finally by shoulders	
	Shoulders grow more than pelvis	Pelvis becomes wider, shallower, and roomier than in male
Development of teeth	Acquisition of full dentition by the end of puberty	

a congenial role. Often these preoccupations assume an unconventional nature. Table 20-1 summarizes the physical changes that occur during this time. Nurses who can recollect their own experiences and reactions during this tumultuous time will better appreciate the adolescent's dilemma.

Mental Development

People make great strides on all intellectual fronts during the adolescent years. They gain in intellectual capacity and power. They exhibit increasing progress in forming concepts, understanding time, generalizing, and abstracting. Like a child, the adolescent lives in the present, but unlike the child, also lives in the future in the realm of the hypothetical. Jean Piaget notes that

the adolescent's conceptual world is full of informal theories about self and about life (see Flavell 1963). These theories include idealistic plans for the individual's and society's future. This egocentrism in adolescence motivates the individual toward a naive idealism, dedicated to the reshaping and perfecting of reality. It is not unusual to hear an adolescent making grandiose plans to reorganize the structure of the federal government or to eradicate poverty.

Social Development

The individual's relationship to others of the same age becomes increasingly important during adolescence. Becoming competent in social skills, developing bonds of mutual trust, attaining peer acceptance, and establishing a unique form of communication all become tantamount to achieving success and happiness. Attempts to do this take many forms. These include formulating esoteric words or terms understood only by companions, forming exclusive groups or cliques, sharing a multitude of secrets, and generally establishing ways to identify the adolescent's own group as unique. It is particularly important to be recognized as separate from the world of the adult. In developing this sense of belonging, adolescents ward off the fear of loneliness and rejection. They are secure in the belief that their newfound feelings and images are acceptable to the group, and therefore acceptable to themselves. Establishing close ties and identifying with the group make it easier for adolescents to cope with their physical changes, sexual urges, social adjustment, and competitive feelings.

During late adolescence, normal individuals begin to establish an intimate relationship with someone of the opposite sex, in an eager attempt to fuse the facets of their own developing identity with that of another. These social attempts with the group and with another individual create alternating excitement and fear, skillfulness and awkwardness, elation and despair.

Emotional Development

Nurses need more than a cognitive awareness of the adolescent's emotional development. They must understand the adolescent's conflicting feelings and their importance in order to establish the interpersonal relationships so vital to successful work with adolescents.

This period of conflict and disharmony is an emotionally labile time, when numerous doubts, uncertainties, and fears surface. The fourteen-year-old who was happily listening to her favorite song on the radio five minutes ago may now be uncontrollably sobbing about a fantasied love loss because she hasn't yet received an expected telephone call. However, her feelings of loss are as real as if her boy friend had actually rejected her. The nurse who has difficulty with mood changes, or who views inconsistencies as abnormal, will most certainly be ineffective in dealing with the adolescent at all levels, from casual conversation to immediate limit setting. The nurse who knows something about psychosocial development will understand more about adolescent behavior and can evaluate and remove obstacles to successful relationships with adolescent clients.

DEVELOPMENTAL THEORIES

The developmental theories of three notable experts yield considerable insight into the struggle to attain adulthood. The theories presented in this chapter are those of Sigmund Freud, Erik Erikson, and Harry Stack Sullivan. Other chapters, such as 10, 11, 19, and 22, discuss these developmental struggles as they are lived in other age groups.

Freud and the Reemergence of the Oedipal Conflict

Of the three masters of developmental theory, Freud spends the least amount of time on the adolescent period. His interest is focused on the Oedipus complex, which develops between about two-and-a-half and six years of age but has by no means vanished by adolescence. In fact, Freud states that the object relations that comprise this phase of life are highly significant to both normal and abnormal mental development (Freud, S., 1924).

During the latency period that precedes puberty, some regression of sexual development occurs. This regression is both physically and organically determined. However, at the time of puberty, the Oedipus complex reappears with all the intensity of adolescent lust. Again the parents—the original objects of sexual desire—become the libidinal objects. At this point children must free themselves from these objects and discover a foreign object of love. The son must become reconciled with his father or free himself from his father's domination, as the case may be. At the same time he must free himself from sexual desire for his mother. For the daughter the situation is reversed. Freud asserts that failure in either case cripples the personality. Neurotic adults who have been unable to accomplish this release of feeling have remained "attached" to their parents.

Anna Freud furthers this exploration into the adolescent's psychological strivings (Freud, A., 1966). She describes the ego-defensive processes in adolescence and the specific defense activities that are used to ward off unacceptable impulses. As in the early infantile period, a relatively strong id confronts a relatively weak ego. The docile period during latency gives way to an increase in the id or instinctual impulses on all fronts. Aggressive impulses are intensified to the point of complete unrestraint. Habits of cleanliness and order give way to pleasure in dirt and disorder. Oral and anal interests reemerge into consciousness. The adolescent's ego becomes dedicated to preserving the character it developed during the latency years and uses various defenses to accomplish this end. The following list summarizes these methods.

- Asceticism: This mechanism prohibits the expression of instinct, thereby keeping the id within limits. The individual mistrusts enjoyment. When the instinct says, "I will," the ego retorts, "Thou shalt not." The danger is that this may begin with instinctual wishes but gradually extend to the most ordinary social or physical needs. For example, the individual may shun all entertainment or social interaction and refuse to engage in harmless activities such as dancing.

- Intellectualization: This mechanism favors active mastery and allows the discharge of aggression into displaced form. As adolescent thinking takes on a more abstract quality, the individual can discuss philosophical issues, speculate on insoluble problems, and, indeed, fantasize about many unreal events. The adolescent derives gratification from this process and turns toward the instinctual threats in an attempt to deal with the id impulses.

- Object love and identification: The characteristics of the two preceding defenses come together in this third type. In this defense method, as in asceticism, adolescents isolate themselves from the family and from the superego. And as in intellectualization, adolescents turn toward the instinctual threat in an attempt to deal with it in an idealized way. Thus, they may form attachments to individuals of the same age or to older persons as substitutes for the abandoned parent objects. They may also become involved in groups. In all three cases they gain access to a full and exciting outer life. This counteracts the feelings of emptiness, isolation, and loneliness caused by pulling away from the parents.

Erikson and the Life Cycle

While Freud concentrates on the Oedipal conflict and the resolution of libidinal feelings toward the parents, Erikson focuses on the resolution of conflicts throughout the life cycle. Erikson is most notably associated with the term *identity* as it applies to individuals and their development (Erikson 1968). He defines identity as the result of a process of simultaneous reflection and observation, a process of increasing differentiation, which grows more inclusive as we become aware of the increasing number of others significant to ourselves. This process begins with the first meeting between the mother and baby and culminates in a normative crisis during adolescence. Identity formation is preceded by the resolution of conflicts in what Erikson calls the *life cycle*—stages through which each individual must progress in the attempt to attain psychosocial maturity.

Erikson explains the necessity of resolving the conflict so that the person may emerge from each crisis with an increased sense of inner unity. He states, "We are not the inevitable products of genes and early childhood experiences, although they strongly influence us. In adolescence, we begin to make a series of decisions that reflect what is possible as well as what once happened" (Coles 1970, p. 75). Thus, within each stage of development, there is an ascendance, a crisis, and, ideally, a solution.

The development of a sense of identity entails a preoccupation with self-image. It also entails a connection between future role and past experiences. In the search for a new sense of sameness and continuity, many adolescents must repeat the crisis resolutions of earlier years in order to integrate these past elements and establish the lasting ideals of a final identity. According to Erikson, these crisis periods or stages are reviews of the adolescent's sense of trust, autonomy, initiative, and industry, in that order.

A Sense of Trust   In the first stage, the adolescent must look for ideas and objects in which to believe or to whom the adolescent may prove trustworthiness. Simultaneously, however, the adolescent fears too strong a commitment and so expresses this need for faith in boisterous and doubtful mistrust.

The "oral character" is a term used to portray the individual with unresolved conflicts of this stage (Erikson 1968, p. 102). Such persons may fear "being left empty" or simply "being left." They may display their insatiable needs simply, as with overeating. In more severe cases, they may make hostile or sarcastic remarks as an ineffectual way of getting what they need from others. They both desperately need and fear trusting relationships, since they have not received satisfaction from them in the past.

Jimmy is an obese boy of twelve who was referred to the school nurse-counselor because of his boisterous classroom behavior. His parents were first separated when he was an infant, at the time when development of trust is so important. Although his mother has attempted to understand him and encourage a change in his behavior, she has received nothing but insults and sarcasm in return. Jimmy manifests all the unresolved feelings of this stage. These feelings are expressed in verbal pessimism, sarcasm, insatiable gratification of oral needs, and mistrust of others.

A Sense of Autonomy   In the second stage, the adolescent must learn to perform or decide independently. This involves a venture into one of the available or necessary methods of service. Examples could be volunteer work at a hospital or participation in a church-related program. It must involve some free choice for the adolescent, however. Again, adolescents fear being forced to engage in activities that would result in ridicule or self-doubt. They prefer to perform possibly embarrassing activities voluntarily, and in the presence of adults, rather than under compulsion, and in the presence of peers.

Steven is a pert, independent boy of thirteen. His parents are divorced. In discussing them, Steven says, "Then my parents were divorced—thank goodness! My father has been much happier since she left. She was quite difficult to get along with." Although Steven boasts about his father and the attention he receives from him, the grade counselor views Steven as a neglected child whose father cares only about his achievements in school and elsewere. Steven denies having any friends and says his greatest joy is in winning a chess game from his father. He tries hard to perform optimally—at any task—and is given to intellectualization in discussions with the nurse-counselor. He seems to have to prove himself continually to gain the sense of autonomy so important to his self-esteem.

A Sense of Initiative   The third stage originates in childhood when children are no longer concerned with *how* to walk but rather what they can do with that ability. They then experiment with what they *may* do rather than what they *can* do. The task in the third stage is to free the adolescent's initiative and sense of purpose for adult tasks that will fulfill the adolescent's range of capabilities. In the third stage, the individual seems unrestrained by any limitations to the self-image. Ambition knows no bounds.

At fourteen, Shirley is striving to attain a sense of initiative. At present she is testing her imagination by mentally casting herself in various life roles. One day she is avidly reading about a career in nursing. The next day she has plans to become a dancer and appear on Broadway. She shows much initiative in group work and in instituting activities that will contribute to her aspirations.

A Sense of Industry   In the fourth stage, a sense of industry demands that the adolescent choose a career that not only promises financial success but also provides the satisfaction of performing well. The very reason that many young people postpone or even shun work is to avoid entering a field that would not yield these satisfactions. They may also wish to avoid being coerced into such work.

Matthew is a very interesting boy of sixteen who is striving for a sense of industry. He is representative of other youths his age who must find themselves before they can begin seriously considering their life's work. He has moved from truancy to drugs to stealing and has now begun to reevaluate his life and what he hopes to gain from his experiences. He says that he now wants to "start anew" and work diligently toward a career as a policeman or as a probation officer.

Completing the Process of Identity Formation   In order to complete the process of identity formation, the ego must integrate psychosexual and psychosocial factors and newly added identity elements with those already in existence. In other words, the process of identity formation evolves from the ever-changing ego synthesis and resynthesis that occurs throughout childhood. Identity formation is influenced by the individual's developmental needs, capabilities, consistent role models, identifications, and successful defenses and sublimations. This struggle for identity imposes many conflicts. Erikson states, "Conflict touches every minute of every day. There is a decided disbelief in the possibility that time may bring change, and yet also . . . a violent fear that it might" (Coles 1970, p. 78).

Sullivan and the Need for Interpersonal Intimacy

Sullivan's theories are both similar to and different from Freud's and Erikson's. Like Freud, Sullivan attaches fundamental importance to the role of the parents, especially the mother or substitute figure, in infancy and childhood. However, he does not see this role as a sexual one, even in the broad sense in which Freud conceives of sexuality. Thus, the Oedipus complex with its implications assumes little if any importance in Sullivan's theory of adolescent development (Sullivan 1953).

Sullivan's theory resembles Erikson's in one respect: in both, each step in the developmental process is preceded by the successful realization of the previous step. Here the similarity ends, however, for the nature of the stages and the objects of each successful venture are very different in Sullivan's theory.

For Sullivan, maturity is determined by the extent of interpersonal relations with others. The term *interpersonal* is broadly interpreted to include "fantastic personifications"—people who are real in themselves but who actually represent other significant people in one's past (Sullivan 1953, pp. 247–48).

Sullivan poses seven stages of personality development.

1. Infancy, which lasts until the development of articulate speech
2. Childhood, which lasts until the need for playmates develops
3. The juvenile era, which lasts until the need for an intimate relationship develops
4. Preadolescence
5. Early adolescence
6. Late adolescence
7. Adulthood

The stages of preadolescence, early adolescence, and late adolescence are discussed below. These three stages are the ones that directly concern the nurse who deals with adolescent clients.

Preadolescence and the Chum Relationship

Preadolescence is an exceedingly important but chronologically brief period. It begins with the need for an intimate relation with another person of comparable status. This entails a new type of interest in a particular member of the same sex, who becomes a chum or a close friend. In the company of their chums, preadolescents are more and more able to talk about things that they had learned not to talk about during the juvenile era.

This birth of the need for a chum represents the beginning of love. Having a chum helps the preadolescent develop real sensitivity to what matters to another person. Besides collaborating in moving toward a common goal, chums also supply one another with satisfactions. They take on one another's successes in the maintenance of prestige, status, and all the things that represent freedom from anxiety, or the diminution of anxiety. This phase is especially significant in correcting autistic, fantastic ideas about oneself or others. Sullivan believes that the development of the chum relationship is what saves many seriously handicapped people from otherwise inevitable serious mental disorder.

Sullivan sees no similarity between love and sexual contact. Love is a manifestation of the need for interpersonal intimacy. Intimacy, in this sense, is that situation which involves two people in a closeness, not necessarily sexual, that permits validation of all components of personal worth. This requires a type of collaboration in which these two people compare symbols, information, and data about life and the world, formulating behavioral adjustments to promote their mutual satisfaction and security. This differs from the consensual validation of the juvenile era, in which habits of compromise and cooperation are established. In the juvenile era, one learns to repress meanings and ideas that are less likely to maintain status and prestige or to limit anxiety.

Early Adolescence and the Heterophilic Relationship
Preadolescence ends with puberty. At first, nothing seems to be drastically altered. The last significant maturation of which the adolescent is aware is the orgasm, which is manifested as part of the lust dynamism. Sullivan perceives no close relationship between the need for intimacy and lust as an integrating tendency, except that both characterize individuals at the early adolescent stage of development.

As early adolescence begins, the object of intimacy changes. Now one seeks a *heterophilic* relationship. That is, one begins to seek someone different from oneself as opposed to someone very similar. If no significant impediment to maturation exists, the change from preadolescence to adolescence is influenced by the appearance of the genital drive—the growing interest in a measure of intimacy with the opposite sex.

Late Adolescence and Satisfactory Genital Activity   Late adolescence is marked by the achievement of satisfactory genital activity. According to Sullivan, this last developmental accomplishment is somewhat difficult to attain because of the many religious, social, and political taboos in American society. Therefore, unsatisfactory genital activity is the presenting difficulty in the lives of many thwarted individuals.

The Theories in Summary

The ideas of these three masters of developmental theory offer insights into the adolescent's quest for maturity. Although Freud offers little explanation for adolescent growth other than the reemergence of the Oedipal conflict, the significance of the parental figures in this context cannot be ignored. Sullivan agrees with Freud that the parental figures are important but disagrees about the sexual nature of their role.

Erikson and Sullivan hold similar views concerning the stages of development. Erikson focuses on conflicts that must be resolved throughout life. Both Erikson and Sullivan view the completion of each stage as necessary to optimal development. Therefore they agree that abnormalities arise whenever a stage is not completed. For example, Sullivan believes that failure to move from a similar to a different object of intimacy may lead to overt or covert homosexual tendencies. Abnormalities also arise whenever a crisis is not resolved (a case in point is Erikson's oral character).

Erikson and Sullivan disagree about the ultimate goal of development. Erikson believes this goal to be the formation of identity. He is therefore primarily concerned with the origin of identity in the adolescent period. For Sullivan, the ultimate goal is satisfactory genital activity.

Intimacy also plays an important role in the developmental theories of both Erikson and Sullivan. Attempts to attain intimacy, sexual or otherwise, are significant in Erikson's identity formation. The results of these attempts can lead to isolation or superficiality in personal relationships if individuals cannot resolve the psychological strain caused by the interplay among their conflicting feelings. Intimacy and sexual closeness are less closely related in Sullivan's theory. Sullivan even asserts that in the beginning stages of development, sexual activity is not considered. He defines intimacy

as a situation that involves closeness and a validation of the other's worth. At the point when the genital drive appears, the change from a similar to a different object occurs.

As for love, Freud defines it as a sublimated sexuality (see Brown 1961, p. 173). Sullivan believes that love evolves only if one feels as strongly about the love object's welfare as one does about one's own. The object of Sullivan's love is a person. The object of Freud's sexuality is the release of a physical tension. Erikson does not even seriously consider love in the adolescent years. He believes that adolescent love is merely a projection of one's diffused self-image onto another in an attempt to define one's identity.

Table 20–2 summarizes information about these theories that may be used to assess the adolescent's maturational level. Regardless of the theory one chooses to use in practice, the value and relatedness of the others cannot be overlooked. The similarities as well as the contrasts among them offer nurses insights into the many complex facets of adolescent psychosocial development.

THE ROLE OF THE NURSE

Given a knowledge and understanding of adolescence, the nurse can help maintain the adolescent client's health and well-being and identify abnormal or problem-causing behavior during this difficult period.

In the Outpatient Setting

As a Community Health Nurse   In the school, clinic, or community health agency, the nurse has excellent opportunities to observe the adolescent engage in the normal activities of daily living. The nurse will have frequent occasions to counsel adolescents in the usual problems that confront them daily and to advise school or clinic staff members in their encounters with adolescents. Moreover, the nurse who knows how to deal with normal adolescent problems will also be adept in identifying obstacles to effective resolution of emotional problems and suggesting further treatment.

Many studies have indicated a direct correlation between problems of early school life and the incidence of subsequent juvenile delinquency (Glueck and Glueck 1972, pp. 85–88; Andry 1971, pp. 95–96; Redl 1951, p. 53; and Glueck and Glueck 1950, pp. 257–58). Un-

Table 20–2   COMPARATIVE CHART OF PSYCHOSOCIAL DEVELOPMENT OF ADOLESCENCE

Chronological Age	Freudian Stage or Phase	Means of Gratification	Freud's Object Relations	Erikson's First Six Stages of Man	Sullivan's Stages of Personality Development	Objects of Interpersonal Relationships
Birth to one year	Oral	Mouth: sucking, mouthing, biting	Mother or mother substitute	Trust versus mistrust		
One year to two and one-half years	Anal	Anus: expelling and retaining feces		Autonomy versus shame, doubt		
Two and one-half years to six years	Oedipal or phallic	Genitals: masturbating, looking, exhibiting	Twofold attitude toward both parents: eliminate jealously hated father and take his place with mother, or vice versa	Initiative versus guilt	Juvenile	Playmates
Six years to twelve years Latency				Industry versus inferiority	Preadolescence (eight and one-half to twelve years approximately)	Close friend or chum of same sex
Puberty and adolescence	Capacity for orgasm	Return to genital masturbation and reawakening of Oedipal conflict	Oedipal conflict reawakened	Identity versus role confusion Intimacy versus isolation	Early adolescence (puberty to voice change) Late adolescence (patterning of genital behavior)	Member of opposite sex with appearance of genital drive Intimacy grows through achievement of satisfactory genital activity

fortunately, the school nurse's role in the early recognition and treatment of predelinquent individuals has been minimized or has gone unrecognized. There are several reasons for this. First, school administrators and teachers tend to view the school nurse as a person who deals only with physical sickness and medical emergencies. They may not be aware that the nurse can also help a verbally abusive or disruptive student.

Second, administrators tend to limit the nurse's activities to the school itself. They may see no need for the nurse to make home visits to meet with the sick student's family or to view problems firsthand. Finally, many school districts lack time and money to provide for counseling families or individuals in a more formal setting. As the role of the independent nursing practitioner expands, and as legislation for third-party reimbursement for independent practice becomes a reality, nurses will be better able to fulfill the role of nurse–counselor within the schools.

Meanwhile, the nurse who is already employed in the school setting or community agency can seize every opportunity to provide an active school health program and to educate school administrators and faculty to the importance of preventive care. For example, Fredlund says that the nurse in a viable school health program can provide preventive counseling not only to troubled adolescents in school, but also to their preschool siblings during routine home visits (Fredlund 1974). She also emphasizes that nurses should establish productive relationships with teachers, help other faculty members encourage parent–teacher conferences, take an active part in developing the curriculum, and help adolescents on probation or parole return to school.

As a Nurse–Counselor   The psychiatric nurse has many opportunities to organize individual, group, or family counseling sessions. Nurses can function within a variety of treatment roles, depending on their experience and capabilities. They can sometimes provide formal psychotherapy, depending on their credentials and experience and on the existing protocol within the agency of employment. A nurse should practice in this capacity only with certification as a primary therapist, or with adequate supervision by a certified individual. Nurses can also use their skills and knowledge to identify clients who need counseling and determine the most appropriate and effective means for changing the clients' behavior.

As an Individual Therapist   The nurse may decide to counsel the student on an individual basis. Sometimes the nurse can establish a trusting alliance and can facilitate communication with the student. On the other hand, the adolescent may be too threatened to talk openly with the nurse in this intimate setting. Some adolescents view the nurse as an authority figure and will resist all efforts to communicate. The nurse may make more headway with this mode of treatment when it is used in conjunction with group counseling.

As a Group Therapist   Usually, it is most effective to work with adolescents in a group. Because the values, acceptance, and recognition of peers are so important during adolescence, the group can provide the support the student needs to deal with presenting problems and to effect change. In addition, involving the adolescent's peers helps dilute the conflict with adults that may exist in one-to-one work.

As a Family Therapist   Meetings with family members may be indicated if the adolescent's role within the family seems to be compounded by the problems presented in the school or agency setting. The nurse should consider it an important part of the problem-solving process to organize initial interviews with parents and family members. The information gathered during these meetings can be used to determine whether the problems stem from difficulties posed by the larger system (the family), and, if so, whether family therapy is indicated. If the nurse is not skilled in assessing the need for family therapy or in providing this service, the family should be referred to a competent family therapist. Chapter 21 provides specific information on family therapy.

The nurse may identify a need for all of the above therapies in dealing with an individual's problem. In some cases, an informal discussion with the nurse is all that is warranted. In other cases, the nurse may identify problems that require considerable attention. Sometimes a period of unsuccessful treatment is necessary in order to determine that outpatient therapy is ineffective, and that hospitalization is indicated. In these circumstances, it is essential to establish a trusting relationship with the client and the parents in order to make such a recommendation.

In the Hospital Setting

Admission into a hospital or other residential treatment facility may be indicated

- If the adolescent lacks sufficient ego strength to cope with inner impulses
- If the degree of destructive or antisocial behavior escalates to a point beyond the normative limits
- If the adolescent cannot form meaningful, stable relationships within the immediate environment

The existence of any one of these criteria warrants counseling or professional treatment. The combination of two or more is likely to make treatment on an outpatient basis virtually ineffective.

There are many advantages of hospitalization for the disturbed adolescent:

- It provides additional structure within which to handle the physically destructive elements of the adolescent's behavior
- It removes the individual from the stresses of a disturbed family environment
- It offers opportunities for supporting existing ego strengths and for promoting whatever ability the client has for forming relationships

Adolescents are sometimes institutionalized because their ideas are strange or threatening to their families, or because the responsible authorities seek to punish the adolescent's unacceptable behavior. The results can be disastrous. Therefore, it is important that accurate assessments be made and that early treatment, when indicated, be implemented. The nurse has a valuable role within the community setting in making such assessments, undertaking appropriate interventions, and educating parents, teachers, and school officials to recognize such needs.

The Value of the Therapeutic Milieu   Many authors have described the importance of the therapeutic milieu, indicating the strong influence of the treatment environment on the treatment outcome. A brief review of the literature over the past fifty years reveals the gradually broadening focus from the sole importance of the individual's psychopathology to the increasing influence of the environment. For example, Alfred Stanton and Morris Schwartz (1954) established that the significance of the milieu is equivalent to that of individual therapy. In fact, the therapeutic milieu itself can provide the primary treatment as well as support or complement the other therapies. The importance of staff–client interactions, communication, and interpersonal relationships, and the interplay of group processes and dynamics cannot be overestimated. Numerous studies offer examples of these factors.

Stanton and Schwartz also discovered (1949) that a parallel process occurred in the behavior of clients and staff—when staff disagreed among themselves, so did clients. The resolution of conflict among staff members diminished the disturbances in the client population.

Harry Stack Sullivan (1931) investigated the idea of staff attitudes and interactions when he created a therapeutic milieu at the Sheppard and Enoch Pratt Hospital in Towson, Maryland. He observed that schizophrenics did not behave in a psychotic manner in a ward staffed by sympathetic people. Ernst Simmel (1937) was the first to apply psychoanalytic principles to hospital organization. At the Tegel Sanitarium in Germany, Simmel tried using increasing, carefully dosed frustration sequences, involving a period of indulgence followed by frustration. The purpose of this approach, which came to be known as anaclitic therapy, was to encourage the gradual replacement of the pleasure principle with the reality principle. At the Menninger Clinic in Topeka, Kansas, psychoanalytic principles were systematically applied to the management of clients. Following a careful diagnosis of the client's unconscious emotional needs, explicit instructions were given to the staff regarding their attitudes and behavior toward each client. Using these attitude prescriptions, the staff provided for the discharge of aggressive (destructive) and erotic (constructive) instinctual drives (Menninger 1939).

Communication and interpersonal relationships became the focus for other studies of the milieu. Milton Greenblatt and his associates Richard H. York and Esther Lucille Brown (1955) studied the factors that differentiated custodial from therapeutic client care. They found that in a therapeutic milieu, staff members interacted more frequently and were more facilitative when communicating with clients, applied therapeutic pressure based on sound rationale, and allowed clients greater freedom and control over their lives.

Interpersonal relationships were the focus of the staff at Chestnut Lodge. Frieda Fromm-Reichmann (1950) emphasized the effects of staff attitudes and interpersonal relationships on the client's behavior. Rather than prescribing staff attitudes like Menninger, however, she permitted attitudes to vary from person to person. Then she identified troublesome attitudes and approached them as if they were personal problems, to be brought to light in supervision.

Finally, some studies emphasize the significance of group roles, processes, and dynamics. While posing as a client in a psychiatric hospital, William Caudill (1958) gathered information that enabled him to delineate the effects of culture, or organized values, customs, and norms, on client care. Erving Goffman (1961) explored the characteristics of the mental hospital as a total institution and the process of institutionalization. In Goffman's framework the mental hospital was a *"forcing* house," much like a prison, for changing persons. He described a series of abasements, degredations, and humiliations of the self that were imposed on hospitalized clients and detailed the privileges and punishments meted out by the staff as a basic means of social control over the inmates. Holly Skodol Wilson (1982) undertook a similar analysis of Soteria House, a residential community for the alternative treatment of schizophrenics. Although the staff professed a philosophy of client freedom, there was actually a tacit infracontrol structure to maintain some degree of social order. The *"physical presence"* of sufficient numbers of people who themselves were in control was the major method of maintaining social control of resident clients. Problems of staff member management were addressed through a *"fairing process,"* and problems with outsiders were prevented by strategies for *"limiting intrusion."*

As the emphasis gradually changed from a focus on the individual's psychopathology to the effects of environmental factors influencing treatment, the role of the nurse changed from custodial to therapeutic and rehabilitative. Gwen Tudor (1952) reported a classic study based on interpersonal processes, demonstrating that nurses are essential in the therapeutic process that promotes emotional growth in the client. She identified the existence of the problem of mutual withdrawal between clients and staff members and developed a specific nursing intervention with a sociopsychiatric base—a unique contribution, at that time, to psychiatric nursing and to understanding the importance of milieu factors. Maxwell Jones (1968), who developed the theory of the therapeutic community, recognized the important role of nurses as change agents within the social systems of mental hospitals (1978).

The Development of the Therapeutic Community

Although the underlying concepts and practices of "the therapeutic community" development extend back several hundred years, the term, as applied to a specific type of psychiatric treatment carried out in a hospital milieu, is of relatively recent origin. The term "therapeutic community" was described originally by Maxwell Jones in 1953. Jones recognized the social environment of the inpatient setting and designed a theoretical and operating mode for psychiatric inpatient treatment. Jones described the value of the socioenvironmental and interpersonal influences in the treatment program of a therapeutic community as follows:

It would seem that in some, if not all, psychiatric conditions there is much to be learned from observing the patient in a relatively ordinary and familiar social environment so that his usual ways of relating to other people, reaction to stress, and so on can be observed. If at the same time he can be made aware of the effect of his behavior on other people and helped to understand some of the motivations underlying his actions, the situation is potentially therapeutic. This we believe to be the distinctive quality of a therapeutic community. Clearly there is the possibility of any interpersonal relationship being therapeutic or antitherapeutic. It is the introduction of trained staff personnel into the group situation together with planned collaboration of patients and staff in most, if not all, aspects of the unit life which heightens the possibility of the social experience being therapeutic (1968, p. 11).

Harry Wilmer (1958) went further in contrasting the value of the therapeutic community to the more traditional mental health hospital setting. Wilmer notes that the basic departure from the traditional setting stems from the therapeutic community's view of staff–client roles and relationships. The traditional view maintains that clients are sick; consequently, staff attitudes are based on the expectation of sick behavior. In fact, Wilmer states, it is even possible that certain clinical syndromes or characteristic patterns of behavior in a hospital environment are actually a response to this expectation. In contrast, the therapeutic community assigns to clients the role of responsible members of a social group with expectation that their behavior will conform as nearly as possible to the norms of society.

The therapeutic community approach suggests that the client is encouraged to be an active, independent collaborator and participant in his treatment. The milieu is directed toward finding the optimal balance between freedom, protection, and self-expression, unlike other settings: e.g., the orthodox authoritarian milieu directed toward control. As a result, the therapeutic community creates an environmental milieu that

reproduces as nearby as possible the types of interpersonal communications and actions that exist in the outside world from which the patient has come and to which it is hoped he will be able to return as a useful member. Staff-patient and patient-patient relations take their form, like the relations of persons in the outside world, from common members in the social group and the mutual responsibility that attends this membership. (Wilmer 1958, p. 9)

Thus, the primary value of the therapeutic community lies in the opportunities it provides as a corrective social climate in which the client can recreate and resolve irrational fears and/or other obstacles to constructive social relationships.

In considering adolescents' needs for peer acceptance, their overwhelming uncertainties and fears, and their ever-changing behavior and attitudes about identity, it should be readily apparent that the adolescents' chances for success in inpatient treatment are increased by a peer group setting. Much has been written about the value of the therapeutic milieu in dealing with adolescent problems, including the problems of drug abuse and similar destructive activities (Amini and Salasnek 1975; Amini, Salasnek, and Burke 1976; Zilberg and Burke 1979). The peer group setting provides social interaction and living-learning situations without which psychotherapy of the adolescent may be sterile and ineffectual. The nurse can maintain the therapeutic nature of this environment by providing a physically safe environment, establishing interpersonal relationships with clients, intervening in potentially harmful interactions among clients, and offering more satisfying alternatives to destructive behavior.

A Therapeutic Community The Youth Service (Unit B) of the Langley Porter Psychiatric Institute in San Francisco provides an example of the value of the therapeutic milieu and the importance of the nurse's role within this setting. The Youth Service is a therapeutic community that provides twenty-four-hour care to a maximum of fourteen clients. The program is offered to young men and women ranging in age from fourteen to twenty-five. The average age is between fourteen and eighteen.

The treatment focus of the Youth Service is primarily psychoanalytic. Clients are involved in both individual and group therapies. They explore their behavior through individual sessions, community meetings, family therapy, small group therapy, psychodrama, the school program, recreational therapy, and vocational counseling. The aim is to identify the meaning their behavior holds for them, and to work through the conflicts that act as obstacles to their success and happiness.

The clients present behavioral or Personality Disorders. They are usually referred through the court system, after having committed illegal acts such as drug abuse or burglary, or by their families, following antisocial behavior beyond their parents' control. Acutely disturbed or psychotic adolescents are generally not accepted into the program because of the exploratory nature of the therapy and the open-door policy of the

ward. Generally, the door is open during the day, and clients are granted varying degrees of privilege in coming and going.

The nursing staff, consisting of psychiatric nurses and psychiatric technicians, play a vital role within the therapeutic community and in the clients' lives. They provide the twenty-four-hour, around-the-clock management of the ward. They assume primary responsibility for the maintenance of the therapeutic milieu. And they have ongoing direct contact with the clients, with whom they establish meaningful one-to-one relationships. They are active in all group therapies and occasionally assume the role of primary therapist as well.

Many of the clients' conflicts result from a lack of nurturing during the crucial early period of life. Therefore these clients are contending with more than the usual emotional upheaval created by adolescence. They come to the Youth Service with maladaptive ways of dealing with anger and depression. Generally they find it difficult to establish healthy relationships. It becomes the task of the entire staff, particularly the nursing staff, to attempt to understand their behavior and help them resolve the underlying conflicts. The nursing staff are the persons most often engaged in the stormy process of getting close to clients, setting limits for them, and working through their immediate problems.

Several rules have been identified as providing a nonthreatening atmosphere in which treatment objectives can be attained.

- There should be no acts or threats of physical violence between clients or between clients and staff.
- There should be no sexual intercourse between clients or between clients and staff.
- While in treatment, clients should refrain from the use of all drugs, including alcohol.
- Clients should attend all meetings.

Enforcing these rules to the limit presents many problems. Given the nature of adolescents, particularly disturbed adolescents, a great deal of testing occurs around rules. Indeed, strict adherence to rules is not the prime objective in successful treatment. Rather, it is the struggle around rules that provides nursing staff and clients with external evidence of the adolescent's internal struggle and forms a basis for the beginning of problem solving within the relationships. This process entails considerable acting out of past experience, as clients repeat earlier patterns of relating to others and attempt to use previously maladaptive measures to overcome obstacles to satisfaction.

The Concept of Acting Out   The concept of acting out is complex. The term has been used to describe a variety of behaviors, ranging from antisocial, destructive acts to unconscious impulses expressed in action rather than in symbolic words or symptoms. Acting out may, and often does, include destructive actions and seemingly undefinable behaviors. The term describes a recreation of the client's life experiences, the relationships with significant others, and the resultant unresolved conflicts.

These are all components of what is commonly referred to as the client's "life script," which unfolds as the client relates, reacts, and behaves in accustomed ways. Through observation of and interaction with the client, the nurse can uncover the meanings that various behaviors and actions hold for the individual. As an example, the child who has assumed the "Black Sheep" role in the family will seek to recreate that familiar role in relation to others outside the home, particularly in the inpatient setting. The following clinical example illustrates one girl's relationship with her parents as replayed with the nursing staff on an inpatient unit.

Liza is fourteen years old. She has been on the unit for six days. She is an attractive, engaging young person who has been friendly with both staff and clients. Liza has been on the periphery of several rule-breaking incidents but has not been directly involved. She has begun to establish close ties with Jim, a male nurse, and engages in frequent lengthy discussions with him about her innermost feelings and fears. One evening she candidly talks to him about the callous way in which she was treated by one of the other nurses, a woman, in regard to a gynecological problem. Liza says with undisguised fear and embarrassment that she is afraid the situation will repeat itself. She expresses great respect for Jim's knowledge and style and asks him to attend to any subsequent problems himself rather than report her dissatisfaction with Jane, the other nurse.

The implications for treatment are many. The most important factors for Jim to consider are what meaning Liza's behavior has for her and what the most therapeutically effective way to deal with the situation

would be. The client's presenting problems and the expectation that the client will act out previous conflicts and life scripts have provided Jim adequate information on which to base an appropriate intervention. The client's attempt to seduce the nurse, and the need for nurses to examine their own behavior and motivations, are discussed in detail later in this chapter.

Jim recognizes the "pull" from Liza to feel that only he can adequately handle the situation. He remembers that Liza's home situation is chaotic. Liza's mother and father frequently fight over who is the better parent. Jim surmises that Liza also plays a part in these fights. The present situation seems to indicate that he is about to be played off against Jane, just as Liza perhaps plays one parent against the other. Jim responds by reiterating his concern for her dilemma and suggesting that Liza speak with Jane about the situation.

In this situation it is clear that the client is attempting to recreate her home situation, using two of the nurses to reenact the roles of her parents. Had Jim been seduced into playing the father's role in the script, he would have furthered the process and recreated the conflict on the ward. The ideal solution is for staff to interrupt this pathological process by substituting a healthier way of resolving the problem. Thus Jim does not react with compliance or with anger to Liza's attempts. Instead he recognizes the significance of her behavior and deals with the situation in a concerned yet healthy way, suggesting a resolution to the immediate problem that demonstrates respect for both Liza's and Jane's abilities to resolve the conflict.

Such situations are commonplace on an adolescent service. They require nursing staff to evaluate the client's psychodynamics and psychopathology as well as their own inner feelings and behavior. But these situations are not limited to the inpatient setting. This fact alone obliges nurses to be alert in observing and assessing verbal and nonverbal communication and to understand their own feelings and behavior in order to make accurate evaluations and appropriate interventions.

A Residential Treatment Program   The Kansas Boys Industrial School is a good example of a residential treatment program that emphasizes the behavioral aspects of the boys' progress. Clients who are committed to the Boys School have been judged delinquent in juvenile court, tend to be impulsive and nonreflective, and usually resort to antisocial behavior when overwhelmed by their feelings.

The treatment program includes group and individual counseling, group psychotherapy, specially selected educational classes, and family therapy. The average length of stay is fourteen months, and the population ranges from 160 to 250. The institution maintains external control of the boys while it helps them learn to control their own behavior and impulses. Whenever a boy seems to be losing self-control, he is helped by reducing the number of his relationships and minimizing the demands placed on him.

This program offers clients several advantages. First, it helps the boys understand which of their previous behaviors have been inappropriate and self-destructive. Second, it encourages them to identify and develop their strengths and assets. Third, through the use of sports and other activities, it teaches them to redirect some of their aggressive energy into more appropriate channels. Last and most important, it gives them the opportunity to establish positive and stable relationships with healthy adult figures.

Both the Kansas Boys Industrial School and the Youth Service of Langley Porter Psychiatric Institute illustrate the effectiveness of the group setting in dealing with the behavior problems of disturbed adolescents and in helping them change their lives.

SPECIFIC ISSUES AND PROBLEMS

Seduction of the Nurse

The intimate nature of the nurse's involvement with these clients, the narcissism inherent in this age group, and the nurse's all-accepting attitude in working with the adolescent all make it easy for the nurse to be seduced into relating in a nontherapeutic way. As a point of clarification, narcissism in this age group is caused by the child's withdrawal from the parents and their value system. This withdrawal leads to a general self-centeredness and overevaluation of the self characterized by heightened self-perception, decreased ability for reality testing, and extreme self-absorption. The result is that the objects or individuals to whom adolescents turn become all-important and perfect in their eyes. Nurses may be strongly tempted to respond accordingly.

The dangers inherent in this situation are not simply the two possible extremes—total submission to temptation and participation in a sexual relationship with the client, or strong denial of temptation by maintaining a rigid, unapproachable stance that makes it impossible to establish a meaningful, trusting relationship. Neither of these extremes is unknown, but the greatest danger is actually intrinsic to the role of the helping professional. It is tempting to respond to the adolescent's idealized view, to be the "savior" who succeeded with this difficult person where everyone else has failed, to feel superior to the imperfect parents, the harassed school teacher, the skeptical juvenile judge, or the other staff on the unit. However, the nurse should not give in to such temptations. Complications will most certainly develop that at best will temporarily compromise the nurse's effectiveness and at worst will render the treatment program completely ineffective.

Nurses who work intensively with adolescents often face situations in which their own unresolved feelings are aroused. They must choose whether to act on these impulses or to explore their origin. Of course, one is not always conscious of these unresolved feelings. It would be absurd to expect nurses to be totally aware of the meaning of their behavior at any given moment. On the other hand, the skilled clinician is usually acquainted with the issues or conflicts that have caused problems in the past. In doubtful cases the knowledgeable nurse will seek consultation from such a clinician. The clinician can help the nurse assess the situation and understand what part the nurse may have played in initiating it. Nurses who wish to explore their personal conflicts further may then seek counseling or therapy.

On the Youth Service many forums are provided for the purposes of self-evaluation and feedback. These include the nurse's own ongoing supervision, a monthly meeting for all nursing staff to discuss difficult situations and conflicting feelings, and a weekly staff meeting in which all disciplines evaluate interpersonal obstacles to optimal treatment. Given the nature of their work, the staff—particularly the nursing staff—undergoes considerable stress as accepted ideas and values are constantly challenged and explored. A recent research study evaluated the levels of stress perceived by the Youth Service staff. In describing the events that produced stress, the staff reported experiencing only low to moderate stress in what seemed to be high-stress situations (Campbell 1977, pp. 60–62). This raises the question of the extent to which staff members use denial in dealing with stressful issues and suggests how much denial may be necessary in working with disturbed adolescents on a daily basis.

Communication

Communication with the adolescent is an art in itself. Nurses must have both verbal and nonverbal skills. They must anticipate and understand the client's use of unconventional language and profanity. The nurse who learns the skills of interviewing and the use of nonverbal cues and messages can use them comfortably and naturally in communicating with the adolescent (see Chapter 6).

Adolescents give many nonverbal cues to the specific emotional struggles, underlying confusion, or simply transitory moods that they are experiencing. A glance around their rooms or a brief study of their dress can tell the nurse more than several direct questions would elicit. Sometimes adolescents give obvious cues. A client who wears a coat around the unit is perhaps planning to run away. Other less obvious behaviors, which are often outside the client's conscious awareness or control, can also yield vital information. A sudden escalation of horseplay among the boys around bedtime is an example. The nurse would probably be correct in identifying this behavior as an expression of anxiety related to struggles around sexual identity and fears of homosexual feelings. Interactional theory holds that the adolescent boy's newfound sexual feelings and changing body image provide unfamiliar ways of relating to members of his own sex. As a result, he regresses to preadolescent behavior, which served him well in handling close feelings up to now, but which now proves inappropriate. In this instance, firm limit setting is in order. The nurse should avoid interpreting the behavior or paying undue attention to the specifics. Testing and limit setting are discussed later in this chapter.

Adolescents seek to create a language all their own. This takes some understanding and acceptance. In seeking their identity, adolescents establish a form of communication unique to the group. To gain acceptance into the adolescent world, the adult must accept this need to employ ambiguous (to the adult) yet specific (to the adolescent) terms to express themselves. In many cases, the nurse must communicate with adolescents by using their own jargon.

This jargon often includes obscene and profane words. This is particularly true of disturbed adolescents, who have an especially difficult time expressing

anger and fear appropriately. The words employed often reveal the nature of the emotional conflict. For example, a young male adolescent grappling with his sexual identity and aggressive feelings may resort to sexually graphic words when he feels anxious or afraid. The nurse may sometimes find it productive to use similar words to give explanations or to clarify communication. Understandably, some nurses have difficulty tolerating profane or sexually graphic language. However, nurses need to evaluate their clients' underlying reasons for using such language so that they can help clients understand their feelings. Only then can they encourage clients to use more appropriate means of expression. Needless to say, if clients sense that the reason the nurse wants them to speak more appropriately is only to make the nurse more comfortable, the end result will not be satisfactory.

Testing and Limit Setting

As young adolescents attempt to adjust to the upheaval in their emotional lives and begin to emancipate themselves from parental figures, a good deal of testing is to be expected. This is normal. However, the meaning that testing holds for the disturbed adolescent is a more complicated matter. As the clients in the Youth Service demonstrate, adolescents who lack early nurturing have difficulty with interpersonal relations. In most cases, the parents were emotionally unable to provide parenting. In a few cases, they chose not to impose their values on their children. In either case, the children never developed the internalized values that cause conflict and lead to crisis in adolescence. This causes identity diffusions, which in turn result in emptiness, a lack of basic trust, and difficulties with intimacy on any level (Amini and Salasnek 1975). In the treatment setting, testing for these clients seems to consist of making limitless and absolute demands. Although the limits the staff impose on these clients' behavior are frequently met with cries of injustice, the clients often really seem to be asking for limits as an indication of caring (Burke 1970).

Julie had been on the unit only two days. During that time she had seen several of the older clients run away from the unit, commonly known as going AWOL, and had witnessed the staff members' attempts to encourage those remaining on the ward to deal with whatever feelings they were experiencing. Toward the end of her second evening, Julie abruptly jumped up from a *conversation with a nurse and ran toward the open door. The surprised nurse immediately followed, running down the stairs after her. A smiling Julie was waiting at the bottom step when the nurse arrived, quite breathless and thoroughly confused, and began her barrage of questions. Julie quickly answered, "I just wanted to see if you cared enough to come after me."*

In this situation no further action was necessary.

Sometimes the client may use annoying or destructive behavior to test the nurse. At these times, firm limit setting without further interpretation or exploration may be indicated. In other instances, the client may not be testing the nurse but be reacting to some real threat or uncomfortable situation.

Joanne was quietly playing pool by herself when she noticed her therapist talking to a new female client. Her volatile nature gave way to jealousy and rage, and she immediately began to hit the billiard balls off the table, making a lot of noise and startling everyone around her. The nurse who had been observing her witnessed the change in her behavior and understood the reaction. Without questioning Joanne's apparent anger, she stepped up to the table and challenged her to a game, which Joanne immediately accepted. Since Joanne prided herself on her pool-playing ability, she quickly channeled her energy and competitive feelings into the game and won. She then sought out her therapist and happily announced her victory.

Had the nurse not understood what had triggered Joanne's outburst, she might have become angry with her for making noise. She might have seen this as a form of testing and might even have begun to set limits on Joanne's privilege of playing pool. This would certainly have produced a helpless and even angrier Joanne, who would probably have escalated her behavior. Since the nurse was perceptive and adept in handling such situations, the results were more satisfying to both parties. Because of the nurse's action, Joanne was able to save face by winning at pool and was not forced to feel more helpless.

Table 20–3 lists some guidelines for dealing with testing and limit setting. (This nursing care plan and the others in this chapter evolved from the work of the Youth Service nursing staff at Langley Porter Psychiatric Institute, San Francisco.)

Anxiety and Resistance

Anxiety takes many forms and can have many different causes. Anxiety generally arises from an inner conflict. It can exist as a conscious state or as a symptom of an unconscious state. Normal adolescents frequently feel anxious as they experience change and inner turmoil in adapting to a new identity.

The anxiety evidenced by the disturbed adolescent in treatment can indicate many other things. The changes required of the disturbed adolescent are much more threatening than those required of the normal adolescent. If treatment is to be successful, clients must look at the meaning of their behavior and must change many of their earlier interactional patterns. This can be frightening. For example, it is more comfortable to play the role of the "bad seed" or "bad kid," with its known pitfalls and expectations, than to attempt a change that entails many uncertainties and unknowns. Clients feel threatened and anxious when the nurse does not act in accord with the familiar life script because they must then find other ways of handling the situation. They must also deal with the anxiety. Frequently this anxiety will be channeled into a game of "cops and robbers" as the client once again assumes a familiar role and maintains the negative or unhealthy image. The anxiety that results from the unfamiliar roles will be dissipated by further testing and acting out. The nurse should not take this as an indication that therapy is not working. It may simply indicate that the client needs to move ahead more slowly with insightful discoveries and needs the nurse's support in doing so.

Sometimes nurses find it difficult to allow adolescents to grapple with their anxieties and fears. At other times, the nurse may not recognize the client's behavior as a symptom of anxiety or depression.

Kathy was the quietest and most aloof client on the ward. She had isolated herself from the other clients during the week that followed admission and avoided conversing with staff members outside of meetings. One evening she seemed especially receptive to the new nurse, Ellie, who was able to interest her in a sewing project. Ellie, who was a new graduate, felt pleased that Kathy had responded warmly to her during their time together. The next day Kathy did not speak to Ellie and seemed to avoid her at all costs. Later Ellie noticed that the dress Kathy had been sewing was torn into shreds and stuffed into the wastepaper basket. Ellie interpreted this quite personally. She felt deeply hurt and rejected. In

Table 20–3 NURSING CARE PLAN: TESTING AND LIMIT SETTING		
Problem	**Outcome**	**Nursing Orders**
Difficulty with trust Has difficulty in trusting others and in establishing close relationships with authority figures or peers.	Will be able to establish trusting relationships Will establish a trusting relationship with both staff members and clients, resulting in voluntary, reciprocal expression of feelings. Will articulate positive feelings toward another person; e.g., "I liked going to the park with you yesterday." Will initiate activity with another. Will be able to ask for assistance or a favor; e.g., "Will you help me put up the hem of this dress?"	Attempt to establish positive relationship with client on one-to-one basis, offering expression of feelings and expecting same. Be clear and concise in stating your intentions, setting limits, and so on. Answer any questions she asks (e.g., "What are you going to put in the report about me?") in a similar fashion. Seek her out, offering time alone with her, yet allowing her to go at her own pace with the relationship. Encourage group activities with other patients. She especially enjoys Scrabble, guitar playing, baseball, and other sports. Provide opportunities for following up on her interests in improving cooking and sewing skills. Observe interactions with other staff and clients, pointing out the nature and process of destructive exchanges with them, e.g., "It seems that Sue was trying to be friendly in asking you to play Scrabble and you snapped at her. How come?"
Poor impulse control and testing with antisocial behaviors Engages in inordinate amount of testing with antisocial behaviors (drugs: "downers" and alcohol, primarily; verbally abusive of staff; violent behavior). Constantly sets up situations that provoke anger or rejection from staff.	Will curb testing and impulsive behavior Will learn to express feelings in more acceptable ways and ask directly for what she needs in a relationship. Will choose to exert own controls without staff intervention. Verbalizes how behavior serves as an expression of anxiety, anger, and so on, e.g., "I felt like getting stoned before family meeting, but I realized that I was really scared about being mad at my sister. Being stoned would have not only kept me from confronting her, but I would have felt guilty as well."	Anticipate angry or potentially explosive situations, allowing time for her to talk about it, or at least acknowledge existence of present situation, e.g., "I think you're trying to get me angry now by throwing those things around the room. I would rather talk about what's happening between us." Set firm limits on behavior while she can still hear them, before behavior escalates out of control. Expect that she will control her actions. Confiscate any drugs or alcohol found on ward. Help her to see correlation between destructive behavior and feelings, e.g., "You were angry at Ellen when she refused to go jogging with you. Does that have something to do with your wanting to get loaded now?" Reinforce good behavior and give feedback at times when she uses control, e.g., "I liked the way you handled John's provocative behavior today. You were cool when you told him that you were angry without storming around." Spend time with her when she is not acting out. Do not wait for negative behavior to give her attention.

Table 20-4   NURSING CARE PLAN: ANXIETY AND RESISTANCE

Problem	Outcome	Nursing Orders
Difficulty with intimacy and trust Tends to flee when he begins to feel close to others. Has left two other treatment programs when he began to establish relationships with others, and when he began to experience changes from treatment. Avoids situations that would encourage intimacy or close feelings. Uses disruptive behavior or excessive talk to undermine discussion of feelings that he needs to avoid or deny.	Will be able to tolerate feelings of closeness Will establish trusting relationship with staff and with peers. Will be able to verbalize reciprocal expressions of liking or feeling close to others. Will not take flight in response to problems and will verbalize why he is tempted to do so, e.g., "I wanted to leave the group today on the outing. I guess I was uncomfortable because we had talked about my depression. I never talk about my feelings to anyone." Will recognize his need to distance others or control them with talkativeness, e.g., "I'm so anxious now that I just feel like babbling."	Encourage him to stay put when close or uncomfortable feelings arise. Point out to him what his purpose is in physically leaving difficult situations. Provide a nonthreatening, consistent atmosphere in which to verbalize and explore his feelings, e.g., his discomfort. Offer walks with him in lieu of AWOL. Gradually increase the amount and degree of his participation with others. He can tolerate attending sports activities but dislikes movies with an intensely emotional theme, e.g., walked out of *Love Story* and immediately went AWOL from group. Tell him how you are feeling when he attempts to put you off with talkativeness or with disruptive behavior, e.g., "This means a lot to me, and I get annoyed when you keep changing the subject or being disruptive when others are talking. Do you know what that's all about for you?" Suggest he listen to others and consider what they have to say. Encourage others to tell him how they feel when he interrupts them or makes light of their comments. Allow him space when his anxiety is great.

---

her discussion with her supervisor Ellie showed her disappointment and anger. Her supervisor observed that, although the good time and feelings that Ellie and Kathy had shared the evening before were genuine, Kathy had not experienced many such times before with her parents or other adults. She suggested that Kathy was probably angry with Ellie for pointing up what she, Kathy, had missed. The supervisor suggested that Ellie be patient with Kathy. Perhaps later Ellie could reestablish the bond, and they would be able to talk about what had happened.

Fortunately, Ellie did not act on her angry feelings. Instead she sought advice. Ellie's supervisor recognized that Ellie wanted badly to do well and needed positive feedback. She also realized that Ellie did not understand the nature of giving to emotionally disturbed adolescents. Had Ellie not sought advice, she might have acted on her angry feelings, further alienating Kathy and causing herself more anger and frustration. With-

out an understanding of Kathy's actions, Ellie would have continued to expect kindness in return for kindness and would have been keenly disappointed.

Table 20-4 lists some helpful guidelines for handling a client's anxiety and resistance to treatment.

Anger and Hostility

How effectively we deal with expressions of anger and hostility will depend on how effectively we handle our own angry or hostile feelings. Nurses who are uncomfortable with expressions of anger or hostility, or who view them as negative or as something to be avoided at all costs, compromise their own effectiveness. In some situations a disturbed adolescent's ability to express anger directly to another person can be a sign of success in treatment.

Expressions of anger and hostility are common on an adolescent ward. Verbal expressions usually take the form of profanity. Depending on the degree to which the client is experiencing and expressing these feelings, the nurse may choose any one of a variety of interventions. These range from doing nothing other than observing the client's behavior to physically restraining someone who is attempting some destructive action. The choice of interventions also depends on the nurse's own experiences with such feelings, the nurse's knowledge and understanding of this client's life experiences with anger, and the external limits imposed by the agency.

Steve had expressed great interest in building a model airplane. He had saved up his money and had taken a long time to choose "just the right one" at the hobby shop. After spending most of the afternoon constructing and painting it, he was interrupted by a phone call from his mother. She told him that she would not be able to attend the family meeting that week, giving a number of specious-sounding reasons. This was the third consecutive week that she had missed. Each time she gave questionable reasons for being unable to attend. Steve was disappointed and angry. He slammed down the receiver, yelling obscenities in response to the nurse's questions, and ran into his room. There he began to destroy the plane by throwing it repeatedly on the floor.

In the preceding example, Steve was not hurting himself or another. Although he did destroy property, the plane belonged to him, and he was free to do with it as he chose. The nurse resisted any impulse to stop Steve from damaging his plane. Since it was of significant value to him, he later regretted having taken out his aggressions on it. However, the situation provided Steve with an opportunity to explore his actions, and he later asked the nurse why he would destroy something that he valued so much after his mother had disappointed and angered him. The parallel between this situation and hurting himself with drugs right after he had argued with his mother was only too apparent.

Incidents in which the nurse bears the brunt of a client's anger or hostility do not offer such obvious solutions. Disturbed adolescents may not think twice about addressing a female nurse as "bitch" and coupling such a greeting with a request for a favor. Adolescents direct insults and hostile remarks at nurses for many reasons, most of which have little to do with the nurses as people but a lot to do with them as adults or authority figures.

There are as many suggestions for intervention as there are people who will be involved in such ex-

changes. In assessing the situation, nurses should consider the meaning behind the client's behavior, their own relationship with this client, their own immediate feelings, and the end result desired. For example, if the client calls the nurse "bitch" the first time they meet, the nurse may interpret this as a form of testing. She may choose to respond immediately with a bewildered look at this unwarranted display of hostility. Later, the nurse may approach the client, expressing a naive curiosity as to the origin of the hostile feelings: "Hey, I don't understand what happened between us a few minutes ago. We just met, and you're calling me a bitch. What's that all about?" This simple question conveys two messages. First, it indicates to the client that the nurse is not accustomed to this kind of salutation. Second, it indicates that the nurse is more interested in the motivation for the remark than she is in curtailing its use.

On the other hand, if the client resorts to name calling only when angry or under stress, the nurse may decide to ignore the words and deal only with the feelings involved. For example, if a client has angrily left an ongoing family meeting, and then calls the nurse who attempts to talk with him a bitch, the nurse can probably assume that the anger is displaced. It is probably a result of overwhelming feelings experienced during the meeting. The nurse may elect simply to say, "I know you're not angry at me right now. It seems like the meeting is pretty heavy, though. Do you want to talk about why you don't want to be in there now?" In neither situation is the name calling intended as a personal affront. However, the way the nurse handles it will determine both the outcome of the immediate situation and the nurse's chances for furthering the relationship with the client.

This brings up a subject that is not considered in most nursing textbooks—anger felt and expressed by the nurse toward the client. Texts in general nursing focus on the client's need for understanding and good care. It is not acceptable for the nurse to display negative feelings toward the client. In the nursing care of adolescents, however, a constant all-giving and all-accepting attitude on the part of the nurse, particularly during times of testing, would not only be nontherapeutic but illogical and dishonest as well. Testing behavior is then at an all-time high, and adolescents need honest feedback. The adolescent will sometimes escalate the provocative behavior to evoke just such an angry reaction from the nurse. For nurses to pretend that they are not angry in such a situation is as undesirable for treatment as it would be for them to pretend that they were fond of the client. Honesty with one's feelings is a prime prerequisite in establishing and maintaining meaningful and productive relationships with adolescent clients. This does not mean that nurses should give vent indiscriminately to all their thoughts or impulses. They should be aware of their own reactions and use good judgment in handling them (see Chapter 3).

Scapegoating

Scapegoating is common in many groups, particularly adolescent groups. It occurs in three stages.

1. Frustration generates aggression.
2. Aggression becomes displaced on relatively defenseless others.
3. Through blaming, projecting, and stereotyping, this displaced aggression is rationalized and finally justified (Allport 1954, p. 350).

Thus the members of a group tend to attack the scapegoated individual because they are afraid to attack the person on whom their feelings are actually focused.

Adolescents readily identify peers who are "different" and project on them their own fears and insecurities about their changing images. Moreover, MacLennan and Felsenfeld discovered that adolescents use scapegoating to test operations. In the group they studied, adolescents attempted to "feel out" the leader, to test his style, his objectives, and his patience. Essentially they scapegoated the leader and combined with each other in what the therapists called "collaborative resistance." In so doing, they developed a group identity and cohesiveness that would otherwise have been difficult to achieve (MacLennan and Felsenfeld 1968, pp. 86, 94).

Scapegoating, then, can be therapeutic or nontherapeutic. At any rate, scapegoating does occur within the group, and the nurse will need to know what to expect and how to deal with it. The client identified as the scapegoat will be the object of much teasing and many hostile remarks. The nurse should refrain from attempting merely to rescue the scapegoat, since this may augment the other clients' anger and frustration and encourage an escalation of the hostility. The nurse would do better to ask the group to focus on what is going on, to acknowledge the anxiety or other uncomfortable feeling that preceded the scapegoating incident. If possible, the nurse should anticipate the occurrence of scapegoating in times of stress and attempt to circumvent the process before it gets out of control.

The nurse should also be aware that identified scapegoats share some responsibility for their predicament by presenting themselves to the other clients in a different or provocative stance. In some instances the scapegoat of choice has an inner need to be punished and meets the group's urgent need to punish as well. The nurse can be valuable to these clients by helping them to explore whatever function this role serves for them. Suggestions for doing this are given in Table 20–5.

Sexual Behavior of the Adolescent

Jersild (1978, p. 109) says, "Sexual development is a meeting ground of the biological, psychological, and moral influences that shape an adolescent's life." The nurse should not underestimate the importance of the adolescent's experimentation and attitude in sexual matters. Likewise, nurses should evaluate their own attitudes and feelings about sexual issues as they relate to their own past experiences and current activities. Conflicts in such matters or residual resentments left over from the past will certainly affect their decisions or interaction with the client regarding sexual matters. Again, while it is not necessary that the nurse resolve all these issues, it is highly desirable to be aware of areas of conflict that make it difficult to view a situation objectively or set rational limits.

The adolescent will use sexual behavior as a means of acting out other conflicts and as a testing ground for the nursing staff's feelings and attitudes.

This was the third time Barbara, a nurse, had gone into Laurie's room to check on two clients, Laurie and Bill, who were an identified couple on the ward. Although there was a rule against clients having sexual intercourse with each other, Laurie and Bill had been discovered in the act each evening Barbara was on duty. Barbara found these discoveries disconcerting. She began to wonder whether she was the only staff member who checked on clients, since no one else had reported any sexual activity. She decided to bring the subject up in the next nursing care plan meeting to find a more effective way of dealing with the situation.

Imagine Barbara's surprise when the group agreed that Barbara was actually partly responsible for Laurie and Bill's acting out! While they supported Barbara, they evaluated the problem and gave Barbara feedback regarding her nonverbal messages. It seemed that her frequent checking on clients conveyed her expectation that they were up to something. Barbara acknowledged that she expected that sort of behavior from them and was quite afraid of discovering them in the act of

---

Table 20-5   NURSING CARE PLAN: THE CLIENT AS SCAPEGOAT

Problem	Outcome	Nursing Orders

Difficulty with socialization: Is frequently scapegoated
 	
  Isolates self from peer group or remains on periphery of activities.
 	
  Spends inordinate amount of time with staff.
 	
  Deals with own anger with other clients by remaining silent and passive, not responding when addressed, and generally doing provocative things to encourage them to scapegoat client (e.g., dresses in a bizarre fashion; rebuffs peers' attempts to socialize; sits apart from group in chair when others are gathered together on the floor).
 	
  Is unduly suspicious of the motives of others and projects rejecting feelings onto them.
	Will participate in group activities and will lessen need to be scapegoat for group
	
	Will accept offers to engage in activities with peers and will initiate offers.
	
	Will recognize pattern of being "different" and feeling outcast, e.g., "I want them to like me, but I never want to do the things they want to do."
	
	Will spend less time with staff and feel more comfortable with peers
	
	Will be able to express anger and negative feelings in more direct ways
	
	Will be able to check out beliefs about others, identifying their motives for seeking contact with client and dealing more directly with own suspicious ideas.
		Encourage participation in group activities and offer opportunities for one-to-one exchanges with other clients.
		
		Discourage monopolizing of staff members' time, pointing out how this isolates client from peers.
		
		Give feedback on how client's behavior affects others. Encourage peers to say how they feel when client rejects them, e.g., when client refuses to play pool with them.
		
		Intervene when peers are being sadistic toward client, pointing out the process rather than simply rescuing client.
		
		Encourage role modeling of healthy figures of client's sex on ward.
		
		Encourage direct expression of feelings when client begins to act out anger or rejection passively.
		
		Help client check out motivations for staff members' or peers' behavior when client suspects rejection or hostile intentions.

---

intercourse. The group helped Barbara to see that her own expectations were being met. Laurie and Bill were doing exactly what she expected them to do—maybe even wanted them to do. Laurie and Bill were following their scripts of being "bad" and expressing their hostility to Barbara. When Barbara heard how other staff members spent time with the couple to encourage them in indirect ways to join the larger group activities, and compared her own behavior to that of her peers, it became apparent to her how obvious her anxiety and unconscious messages actually were! She then began to question her own attitudes about sexual matters and to explore why she feared discovering the couple engaged in sexual intercourse.

Until adolescents master their anxieties and fears about their sexual identity and gain control over sexual urges, they will exhibit a variety of behaviors and attitudes that may confuse or trouble the nurse. The following sections focus specifically on five related issues: masturbation, nocturnal emission, latent homosexuality, promiscuity, and pregnancy (also see Chapter 12).

Masturbation   Masturbation is a normal sexual activity for people of all ages, from the beginning of sexual awareness to senescence. If the nurse has a relatively healthy attitude toward masturbation, it is not likely to cause problems unless the client masturbates in inappropriate places or uses masturbation to express hostility. There may be times when the nurse will be confronted with an adolescent boy who fondles his genitals when he is anxious or feels threatened. Understanding his behavior as an indication of anxiety, the nurse may elect to ignore the gesture and explore the nature of his anxiety with him. At other times, the boy may make a masturbatory gesture to convey contempt or hostility to the nurse. In this case it would be ludicrous to feign indifference in response. The nurse's reaction will depend on all the previously mentioned factors, such as his or her relationship with the client and the behavior that preceded the gesture. Generally, however, it would be wise to comment on the client's gesture, for example, by mentioning it as an attempt to "put me uptight," and then to allow the client the opportunity to express verbally what he is feeling. It is unlikely that this intervention will produce a tumultuous outpouring of feeling resulting in immediate resolution. However, it does allow the nurse to acknowledge both the client's and the nurse's own feelings, perhaps paving the way for a more appropriate exchange in the future.

Nocturnal Emission   Nocturnal emissions, commonly referred to as "wet dreams," are involuntary. They occur while the subject is asleep. Many boys have experienced nocturnal emissions before the age of fifteen. A large percentage of them have probably experienced ejaculation brought about by masturbation or sex play with others before they experience nocturnal emission. Those who have not may not understand that nocturnal emission is a normal part of their development. They may be unduly concerned and find it difficult to approach the nurse, especially a female nurse, with questions about it. An astute nurse may note evidence of nocturnal emission on the client's linens. The best policy in this case is to say nothing to the client but to inform the nursing staff in case the client indicates later that he needs to discuss it. Ongoing sex education classes for adolescent clients are highly desirable. These classes prepare the adolescent for the normal developmental process, thus alleviating some of the inherent anxieties. They also provide a regular forum for questions.

Homosexual Feelings and Experiences   During preadolescence, people normally choose a member of the same sex with whom to experience intimate or loving feelings. This does not necessarily mean that a sexual relationship will ensue, although it often does. Homosexual activity may continue into the adolescent years. Generally, however, adolescents begin to view homosexual feelings as a threat to the development of their identity. As a result, they may ward off such feelings by engaging in frantic sexual activity with a member of the opposite sex. This is particularly true for boys. It is normal for the adolescent boy to be afraid of his own passive wishes and to label them homosexual. This is normal because he has probably been brought up to relate to physical displays of strength or aggressive displays of power. Thus, an incident in which he feels threatened or powerless would produce feelings of sexual impotence, a fear of castration, a feeling of dependency or weakness, and a greater fear of homosexuality. The adolescent in treatment may resort to acting out these feelings. Or he may attempt to reaffirm his masculinity with inappropriate displays of ag-

gression or destructive behavior. The nurse should anticipate such behavior and provide other ways for the adolescent to demonstrate his masculinity, perhaps by organizing a game of football or tennis, if he is fairly proficient at these skills, or engaging him in some other activity in which he excels. The point is to reestablish the adolescent's feeling of competency and control. Without such intervention his feelings of impotence will escalate to the point where he will most certainly act them out in a negative way.

At the other extreme are adolescents who engage in predominantly homosexual activities. Many of these individuals find relationships with the opposite sex threatening and continue to seek intimacy and solace with people like themselves. Some feel more comfortable with companions of the same sex and are satisfied with these relationships. Others use their homosexual affiliation to express and act out hostility directed against their parents and their parents' values.

Since nurses who work with adolescents may encounter any or all of these situations, they must attempt to understand the meaning of given clients' homosexual activities or life-style. The clients may need to explore their feelings and anxieties openly. Open discussion with an understanding yet knowledgeable professional may resolve many of the conflicts inherent in the choice between homosexual and heterosexual life-styles. Many professionals believe that homosexual behavior in any age group is abnormal, and that particularly during adolescence conflictual feelings about sexual identity may be acted out before the identity conflict is resolved. This group advocates psychotherapy as the only answer to help such people deal with the conflictual feelings and to resolve the conflicts.

Clients who use homosexuality to express hostility toward their parents will undoubtedly act out with the staff as well. The nurse would be wise to remain objective and relatively nonjudgmental with these clients, allowing them to deal with the feelings of anger or depression that may result from addressing the conflict.

Although adolescence is a very young age at which to make lifelong decisions regarding homosexual relationships, some may decide on homosexuality as a satisfactory alternative. These people will not experience conflictual feelings about such relationships. They also will not need to flaunt them or to act out with the staff in an angry or hostile way. Nurses then may have to deal with their own negative feelings about such a life-style. It is important that nurses consider what these relationships mean to the clients and respect the clients' rights to make life-style choices for themselves.

Table 20-6 NURSING CARE PLAN: HOMOSEXUALITY AS AN EXPRESSION OF HOSTILITY		
Problem	**Outcome**	**Nursing Orders**
Use of homosexual relationship to express hostility (at parents via the staff) Identifies girl friend, Felice, off the unit, as sole friend and confidante, rejecting other people's attempts to be friendly with her. Goes out of her way to express affection for Felice in inappropriate ways in presence of others, e.g., engages in passionate kisses and fondling in front of staff. Initiates topic of sexual experiences with Felice during group meetings with peers, ignoring peers' protestations or accusing them of not being "liberated." Consistently asks for unacceptable passes with Felice and goes AWOL when refused; says no one understands her, no one wants her to be loved.	Will gain insight into need for relationship, decreasing the need to express hostility indirectly Will cease to use homosexual activities in blatantly hostile manner. Will establish relationships with others. Will be able to express hostility and anger at parents and staff directly. Will be able to plan acceptable passes with Felice and use relationship in a constructive way, if possible.	Seek her out and attempt to engage in appropriate activities, using areas of strength or activities that interest her (e.g., she enjoys candle making). Initiate contact around this and help her to obtain materials. Attempt to establish close, trusting relationship with her, recognizing her value as an individual and not focusing on the struggle between her and others. Attempt to include Felice in appropriate activities with group, recognizing her importance for the client and demonstrating acceptance of Felice's positive traits. Set limits on passionate displays as with heterosexual relationships, expressing how you feel during them, e.g., "Your behavior makes me uncomfortable, and I don't want to take you out if you and Felice are going to continue fighting with me about this." Encourage peers to express how they feel about her, both when she behaves acceptably and when she behaves unacceptably with Felice. Point out the struggle she sets up with the passes. Refuse inappropriate passes, encourage appropriate visits, and give clear messages that you are concerned about her and what her relationship means. Encourage her to participate in individual and family therapy sessions to deal more directly with the underlying conflicts.

Table 20–6 contains some helpful suggestions for relating to the client who uses homosexuality in a hostile way.

Heterosexual Behavior Heterosexual activity is normal and desirable during adolescence. However, the nurse who works with either normal or disturbed adolescents will sometimes see them engage in sexual activities that do not seem healthy or growth-producing. For example, the adolescent girl who seeks punishment rather than true pleasure in her sexual exploits will display them in an overt, exhibitionistic way in a place where a particularly moralistic person will discover her and give her the reprimands she desires. She may be testing her mother's values in an attempt to resolve her own inner conflicts about this. Adolescents in an inpatient treatment setting where sexual intercourse is forbidden will engage in sexual intercourse where a staff member will be sure to discover them. The experience may reinforce their image of sexual behavior as "bad" behavior. Or it may simply provide a means of acting out their defiance of the rules, thereby earning the familiar "bad kid" label. The incident involving the nurse Barbara and the clients Laurie and Bill is an excellent example.

Pregnancy The etiology of adolescent pregnancy includes social and family expectations and unconscious motivations. Some teenage girls are quite pleased with the state of motherhood and suffer no emotional consequences from the decision to become a mother. However, generally speaking, a conscious, deliberate decision for pregnancy at this age is manipulative. The goal may be to escape a difficult family situation, to express hostility toward parents, or to act out a life script in which the daughter is seen as "bad." In cases where the adolescent failed to receive adequate nurturing as a child, she could be acting out dependency needs in an attempt to give the baby the love and caring she herself did not receive.

The nurse should be sensitive to motivational factors in dealing with emotionally deprived adolescents. It is important to use the educational tools and interpersonal relationships that exist to help adolescent girls understand their needs and motivations in becoming pregnant. It is also important to provide teenagers of both sexes with knowledge about sex and birth control. Too often parents and professionals alike tend to deny the adolescent's sexual activity until an unwanted pregnancy occurs and it is too late to discuss the meaning or possible consequences of sexual behavior.

Chapter 13 provides valuable information on the process of parenting, including a section on adolescent parents. The nurse can be helpful to the adolescent in providing much needed information on parenting skills.

Dietary Problems

Food Fads and Diets   The eating habits and preferences of disturbed adolescents can reveal a lot about the nature of their inner turmoil. A comparison between the inpatient's diet and that of a normal adolescent may show little difference in variety, but it will probably reveal a great difference in quantity. Adolescents who have been deprived of early nurturing tend to eat more than normal adolescents and will probably place a higher value on mealtimes and on their "share" of the food. The nurse may notice that adolescents consume more milk than usual during periods of stress or anxiety. Generally speaking, girls will want to follow food fads or unreasonable dietary regimens in order to become slim and attractive. This usually gives the nurse an opportunity to engage in health teaching about food and exercise and to express a cooperative interest in their developing feminine identity.

Obesity   In the American culture slimness is admired, and many adolescent girls will go to great lengths to fit into that size five dress. By the same token, the obese adolescent often feels unattractive and unpopular. In both "normal" and disturbed adoles-

cents the need to overeat may have deep-rooted psychological implications. Adolescents may eat compulsively in an attempt to compensate for the love and nurturing that they did not receive as children. They may also turn to obesity as a defense against intimacy with the opposite sex. While they keep this emotional distance, they frequently use excuses such as, "I would be popular if I weren't so fat," or "When I lose weight, I'm going to learn to dance." The nurse should recognize these defenses for what they are but generally should not challenge them until the obese adolescent has progressed far enough to look at their meaning. Other adolescents may tease and ostracize their obese peer. When this happens, the nurse can support the client while, in as nonthreatening a way as possible, asking what the obesity does for him or her. Obviously, the nurse should constantly encourage the client to understand the implications of obesity and should constantly try to further a healthier sexual identity for the client. However, the nurse should be careful not to let this persistence take on the same character as teasing from the adolescent's peers.

Anorexia Nervosa   Anorexia Nervosa is not nearly as prevalent as obesity. The clinical picture is of a person, usually a young woman, who is obsessed with the idea of being thin and who consistently restricts food intake to the extreme of dangerous emaciation. At other times, she may indulge in enormous eating binges, alternating them with periods of fasting. Generally speaking, inpatient treatment within the therapeutic milieu in conjunction with behavior therapy yields positive results. The nurse plays an important part in planning and implementing dietary and behavioral regimens during the client's hospitalization. The nursing care plan in Table 20–7 was provided by the nursing staff of the Inpatient Treatment and Research Service (ITRS) at Langley Porter Psychiatric Institute. It is an excellent illustration of the nurse's role in the behavioral treatment of Anorexia Nervosa.

Drug Use and Abuse

Experimentation with drugs among the adolescent population is widespread. In one study as much as 96 percent of the adolescent subjects reported using drugs, including alcohol, at least once (Lettieri 1975, p. 112). Adolescents give many reasons for using drugs: to experiment, to get high, to "get inside my head," to have fun, to understand more about life. Although the general public may disagree about whether drugs are

	Table 20-7	NURSING CARE PLAN: ANOREXIA NERVOSA	
Problem	**Outcome**	**Nursing Orders**
Ambivalence about food Takes a very long time to eat. Attempts to hide food (under napkins, in pockets, and so on) to avoid eating. Hoards food to gorge self later. Attempts to maneuver staff and other clients (by talking, crying) to take the focus off eating.	Will have adequate dietary intake for weight gain Behaviors associated with food ambivalence will cease.	Client is first in line for meals and has thirty minutes to eat. Give one-to-one supervision during meals and observe closely for any indication of hiding food. Client sits with staff member who is supervising at a table separate from other clients. Do not encourage client to eat during the thirty minutes. Keep other clients away from the table.
Does not make appropriate food choices.	Will be eating a standard nutritional diet.	Staff member will pick up tray from dietary personnel, checking diet slip to make certain all items are there, including milk and dessert. No omissions or substitutions.
Leaves part or all of the meal uneaten.	Will eat all of the meal to avoid negative reinforcement for not eating.	After thirty-minute mealtime, pick up tray without speaking. Check the tray for uneaten food, looking under plates and napkin. Any food remaining on tray after thirty minutes will be blended and tube fed. Limit fluids to 500 cc. at one time.
Attempts to vomit food after eating.		Client is to be in dayroom for thirty minutes with one-to-one supervision after meals; no bathroom privilege at this time. Client is to be supervised by staff in bathroom.
Will exercise to burn calories.		Set limits on physical activities. Client is not to take part in activities that involve exercise not prescribed in doctors' orders. Chart activity level on the ward (pacing, standing, isometrics). Client is to be weighed Tuesday, Thursday, and Saturday in hospital gown and pajamas at 7 a.m.

Table continues on next page

harmful, the fact remains that using drugs is acceptable to most adolescents—at least on an experimental level.

How can the nurse determine when drug use becomes drug abuse? Generally, the adolescent who abuses drugs, including alcohol, exhibits at least one of the following characteristics:

• The adolescent's performance at school or work increasingly deteriorates.

• The adolescent is frequently caught high or in the act of getting high by parents or other authority figures.

• The adolescent increasingly resorts to drugs in times of stress or boredom.

• The adolescent has seriously deficient interpersonal relationships and can relate only when under the influence of drugs.

• The adolescent may lose interest in interpersonal re-

| Table 20–7 continued | | |
Problem	Outcome	Nursing Orders
Anger at staff over loss of autonomy as a result of regime restrictions	The regime will remain constant while anger and feeling of ineffectuality are acknowledged.	One staff member will work with physician to establish regime and weight goals before these are presented to client. One staff member will be present while the regime is presented to client. Make certain that regime is presented clearly and in full detail. Answer client's questions at the time of the initial presentation. No staff member will answer questions or respond directly to comments about the regime once the physician and nurse have explained it. Direct the client to the doctor for any discussion of regime. Do not converse with client about food or weight. Acknowledge client's anger when it is verbalized but do not deal with issues of weight or food. In all aspects of regime staff must be extremely consistent. Refer any staff member's questions about the regime to team or client's nurse.
Cathexic, malnourished, and dehydrated Has dry skin and hair, skin breakdown over bony prominences, and unstable vital signs.	Will be adequately hydrated; skin integrity will be maintained; vital signs will be clearly monitored as an aid in evaluating health status.	Discourage daily bathing. Provide lanolin cream after bathing and twice a day. Massage skin over bony prominences twice a day and teach patient to do likewise frequently throughout the day. Carefully monitor vital signs and blood pressure.

lationships altogether, preferring to be high alone rather than to be with others.

Nurses are most effective when they can discern what the particular drug or high does for the client. A boy with a poor self-image and low self-esteem may say that it makes him "feel like a man." A particularly shy or introverted girl may say that it makes her "outgoing and friendly." The nurse may discover that being high helps to rid disturbed adolescents of angry or depressed feelings. Indeed, in the treatment setting the client will frequently resort to smoking marijuana or "popping" uppers or downers in an attempt to escape uncomfortable feelings. The nurse who harbors feelings of disdain or envy for the drug user cannot establish a therapeutic relationship with the client. Only by

viewing drug abuse as a symptom of a broader illness can the nurse be effective in dealing with adolescents.

Nurses who have contact with adolescents, especially in school or community settings, would be well advised to familiarize themselves with the general effects of various drugs and the first aid treatment for each. Table 20–8 provides a handy guide for quick reference (see also Chapter 15).

Juvenile Delinquency

Many adolescent boys and girls have committed offenses that, in the strictest legal sense, are delinquent acts, such as stealing a steak from the market or being truant from school. From a legal point of view, both acts are delinquent. However, the social context and

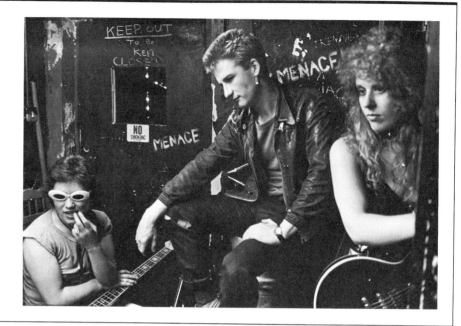

To these adolescent punk rockers, attaining peer acceptance and establishing a unique form of communication are particularly important in order to be recognized as separate from the world of the adult.

life experiences of the participants affect the meanings such behavior holds for them. In some cases "delinquent" behavior may be seen as laudatory by some participants. For example, if the person stealing from the market is a son in a starving family, he may be seen by family members as supplying them with food and appreciated as a rescuer or savior. On the other hand, the owner of the store sees the act as a malicious one that causes a personal monetary loss. Similarly, if the school truant is a daughter in a lower-class family that does not value school attendance, she is not violating a family norm and may, indeed, be engaged in domestic activities or paid work that the family values. To the probation or truant officer, her behavior may indicate poor progress and a lack of initiative, warranting the imposition of other external limits on her to enforce school attendance. Nurses need to recognize the effects of social contexts on the meanings of behavior, so that they can evaluate an adolescent's behavior on the continuum from "normal" to "delinquent." Another key factor is whether the behavior constitutes a repeated pattern.

For the adolescent offender to become a juvenile delinquent, several things must take place.

- The offense must be one that would be punishable if it were committed by an adult

- The offender must be apprehended.

- The offender must have a victim or an accuser.

- The offender must appear in court (Jersild 1978, p. 409).

For various reasons, ranging from the offender's socioeconomic status to the number of violations, the incident may never be officially recorded. However, the offender is sometimes not only prosecuted but punished. In many cases the basis for the delinquent act is an underlying emotional problem. These problems require treatment, not punishment. Offenders who are punished may well repeat the act, either "justifiably," for the sake of revenge, or simply because the problem was not resolved. Unfortunately, the general public and some professionals seem more interested in punishing the juvenile offender than in tackling the problem itself.

The nurse who works in a community agency and has frequent contacts with uninformed or vengeful adults can help educate them about the connection between juvenile delinquency and emotional problems. The nurse can also offer alternative solutions to the customary punishments.

Suicide

The incidence of suicide rises dramatically after the onset of puberty. In 1977 there were only two reported suicides in the five-to-nine age group. There were 188 in the ten-to-fourteen age group. In the fifteen-to-nineteen age group there were 1871 (U.S. Department of Health and Human Services 1977, pp. 7–150).

Most suicides or suicide attempts are preceded by verbal or action threats, a statement of intent or a suicidal gesture. However, this is less true of adolescents,

Table 20–8   GENERAL DRUG USE GUIDE FOR QUICK REFERENCE

Name	Slang Name	Route of Administration	Desired Effects or Reasons for Taking Drug	Objective Symptoms	Untoward Symptoms and Long-term Effects	Symptoms of Overdose	First Aid
Alcohol	Booze	Orally: liquid	Relaxation; euphoria; disinhibition; social custom and conformity	Variable: irritability; reduction in neuromuscular control (affecting speech, gait, coordination); varying behavioral symptoms ranging from release of inhibitions, congeniality, and increased self-confidence to increase in depression with macabre affect; warm, flushed skin; drowsiness	Nausea, vomiting, diarrhea; habituation and addiction; irreversible brain and liver damage; gastritis, ulceration, hemorrhage; severe withdrawal symptoms; death (with blood levels above 600 mg./100 ml. or after long-term abuse with complications); crosses placental barrier, affecting infant Withdrawal symptoms in adult (in order of succession): tremors ("shakes"); weakness, profuse perspiration, headache, anorexia, nausea, abdominal cramps; retching and vomiting; flushed face; intense craving for alcohol or sedative; acute alcoholic hallucinations; seizures; agitated delirium	Irregularity of behavior and reduction in neuromuscular control, increasingly leading to stupor and coma. On rare occasions, may exhibit outburst of irrational, combative, and destructive behavior, known as pathological intoxication or acute alcoholic paranoid state	Acute alcohol intoxication: strong coffee, warm shower followed by cold shower, forced activity, and induced vomiting have been used. Generally, if vital signs are stable, no special measures are indicated. Alcohol coma: is a medical emergency. Danger is death from respiratory depression. Maintain patent airway. Transport for emergency medical treatment. Pathological intoxication: use restraints and transport for medical emergency treatment.

Table continues on next page

Table 20-8 continued

Name	Slang Name	Route of Administration	Desired Effects or Reasons for Taking Drug	Objective Symptoms	Untoward Symptoms and Long-term Effects	Symptoms of Overdose	First Aid
					Fetal alcohol syndrome: prenatal onset; growth deficiency and developmental delay; numerous systemic complications secondary to birth defects. Withdrawal symptoms in infant, beginning with drowsiness and irritability		Withdrawal and delirium tremens: hospitalize for regimen of intravenous fluids and electrolytes, observation of vital signs, and general care.
Amphetamines	Wake-ups, pep pills, uppers	Orally: pill, capsule; subcutaneously; intravenously	Euphoria; relief of fatigue; increase in alertness; loss of appetite	Variable: remarkable alertness; pressure of speech; irritability; dry mouth; restlessness; agitation; hyperactivity; rapid flight of ideas; mood swings; loss of appetite; weight loss; aggressiveness; increase in pulse and blood pressure; dilated pupils; needle marks and tracks with intravenous use	Restlessness; irritability; habituation; insomnia; weight loss to malnutrition; unexplainable fear; possible hallucinations; paranoid psychosis; nausea and vomiting; twitching muscles; seizures; hyperpyrexia. Withdrawal symptoms: psychic depression; lethargy; apathy; somnolence; lack of initiative; pressure to take amphetamines; suicidal ideation	Dizziness; tremor; irritability; confusion; hostility and assaultiveness; auditory and visual hallucinations; panic states; chest pain and palpitations; headache; cardiac arrhythmias; flushed skin; hypertension; vomiting; abdominal cramps; excessive sweating; hyperthermia; shock; convulsions; death	"Bad trip": talk the person down, reduce the stimuli, and reduce the fever. If large amount has been ingested and person is alert, induce vomiting. Attempt to control hyperthermia as soon as detected to avoid associated convulsions. With severe physical or behavioral symptoms, immediately seek emergency treatment.

Drug	Slang names	How taken	Effects sought	Long-term symptoms / dangers	Symptoms of overdose	Treatment
Benzedrine	Bennies, cartwheels					
Dexedrine	Dexies, Christmas trees					
Methedrine	Crystal, speed, meth					
Barbiturates	Barbs, goofballs, candy, peanuts, pink ladies, block-busters, downers	Orally: capsules or pills; intravenously	Relaxation or sleep; euphoria; disinhibition; "rush" after intravenous injection; as antidote to ill effects of other drugs	Irritability; weight loss; habituation and addiction; severe withdrawal symptoms; cellulitis and vascular complications after intravenous use; medical dangers inherent with any nonmedical use of hypodermic needles; overdose with many users	Variable: relaxation; sometimes euphoria; drowsiness; impaired judgment, coordination; muscle relaxation. Pupils may be dilated, but if used in combination with opiates may be pinpoint	Withdrawal: stay with the person and watch for indications of suicidal intent. Seek medical attention.
				Withdrawal symptoms in adult: anxiety; sleep disturbances; restlessness; irritability; postural hypotension; tremors, muscular weakness; delirium; seizures, hyperpyrexia	Slurred speech; staggering gait; sustained nystagmus; slowed reactions; lethargy; progressive respiratory depression evidenced by shallow and irregular breathing; coma; death	Overdose: keep the person awake and moving to reduce chance of coma. May give activated charcoal to delay gastric absorption. Apply general supportive measures, such as maintaining airway and adequate respirations. Keep warm. Do not use stimulants, because they can cause additional hazards. Transport as soon as possible for emergency medical treatment.
				Withdrawal symptoms in infant: high-pitched cry; tremors; restlessness; disturbances in sleep; hyperreflexia; hyperphagia; diarrhea; vomiting; seizures		Withdrawal: almost invariably requires hospitalization. Transfer for emergency treatment, especially with more advanced symptoms.
Amytal	Rainbows, blue heavens, blue devils					
Nembutal	Yellow jackets, dolls, abbotts, blockbusters, nemmies					
Phenobarbital	Phennies, purple hearts					
Seconal	Reds, red birds, red devils, pinks					
Tuinal	Rainbows, tuies					

Table continues on next page

Table 20-8 continued

Name	Slang Name	Route of Administration	Desired Effects or Reasons for Taking Drug	Objective Symptoms	Untoward Symptoms and Long-term Effects	Symptoms of Overdose	First Aid
Cocaine	Coke, snow, big C	Intranasally ("sniffing"); subcutaneously; intravenously	Euphoria; to get high; sexual stimulation	Variable: same visions and hallucinations as the amphetamine user but for shorter periods of time	Hallucinations; paranoid thoughts; toxic psychosis; scars and abscesses if injected; depression and apathy after a high	Same as for amphetamines	Overdose or toxic psychosis: transport to medical emergency setting immediately.
Glue, gasoline, solvents		Inhalation	To get high; euphoria; relief from depression; increase in sensory awareness	Variable: euphoria; impaired coordination and judgment; mood change; slurred speech; impulsive destructive behavior. Effects are brief	Anorexia; tinnitus; sneezing; coughing; nausea and vomiting; diarrhea; chest pain; muscular and joint pain; visual or auditory hallucinations; unconsciousness. Some substances can severely damage liver or kidneys	Unconsciousness; hypoxia. Death may occur if person becomes unconscious and continues to sniff fumes from plastic bag around mouth and nose that maintains airtight seal.	Overdose: Give immediate artificial respiration with subsequent cardiopulmonary resuscitation (CPR) as indicated. Transfer for medical evaluation.
Hallucinogens			"Mind expansion"; self-exploration; increase in visual images and sensory awareness; increase in creativity and insight	Unusual sensations and changes in self-perception; occasionally hallucinations; feelings of euphoria and excitement; rapid mood swings; flight of ideas; sense of observing while participating; sense of tremendous	Anxiety; nausea; chills, tremors, shivering; impaired coordination; rapid mood swings; can precipitate or intensify an existing psychosis; depression. Constitutes a "bad trip" if panic reaction occurs with feelings of fear, loss of control,	With large doses or combinations of drugs, seizures or coma may complicate existing anxiety-provoking feelings.	"Bad trip": person needs nonthreatening environment with subdued and pleasant stimuli. Find out from user or friends nature and quantity of drug and time ingested. Maintain understanding yet firm approach without critical or judgmental

LSD	Sugar, acid, trip, big D	Orally: liquid, capsule, pill (or sugar cube)	insight. Usual effects are sympathomimetic, including pupil dilation and increased blood pressure and paranoid mistrust and suspiciousness. Combinations of drugs may lead to depressed level of consciousness, seizures, or threatening delusional behavior	attitude. Approach consists of talking down the person and should include friends or other comforting people. This may take eight to twenty-four hours. Provide orientation and diversion. Continuity is essential. Do more than periodically check on the person. Overdose: with overdose or evidence of other complication, including decreased level of consciousness, use supportive measures to maintain airway and immediately transfer to emergency treatment setting. Use of tranquilizing drugs should be avoided if possible.
Mescaline	Big chief, mese, pink wedge	Orally: capsule, chewing plant		
Peyote	Cactus, bad seed, moon, button			
Psilocybin	Mushrooms			

Table continues on next page

Table 20–8 continued

Name	Slang Name	Route of Administration	Desired Effects or Reasons for Taking Drug	Objective Symptoms	Untoward Symptoms and Long-term Effects	Symptoms of Overdose	First Aid
Heroin	Smack, "H," horse, junk, shit	Intranasally ("snorting"); orally; intravenously	Euphoria; "thrill," "kick," or "flash" likened to sexual orgasm with intravenous use	Foggy period of mental clouding and little inclination toward physical activity; look of sublime contentment with loss of anxiety, worry, sexual desire, appetite; needle tracks; scarred veins; inflammation and edema of nasal mucosa (if snorted)	Itching and decreased blood pressure after intravenous use; habituation and addiction; minimal or absent sexual desire; hepatitis; sepsis; shock; pulmonary edema; allergic reactions; crosses placental barrier, affecting infant Withdrawal symptoms in adult: anxiety; runny nose; dilated pupils; cramps, diarrhea, vomiting, shaking, chills; profuse sweating; sleep disturbances; aches and pains Withdrawal symptoms in infant: irritability; hyperactivity; tremulousness; vomiting; poor food intake; diarrhea; fever; high-pitched cry; seizures	Depressed level of consciousness; depressed respiratory rate; pupillary constriction (unless in combination with other drugs or during anoxic state); pale, cool, clammy skin with cyanotic tinge	Overdose: immediate support for vital functions is imperative. Institute CPR and transfer to emergency treatment. Withdrawal: person with beginning symptoms should be seen by physician for medical regimen of methadone or other drugs for symptoms, including control of gastrointestinal symptoms, anxiety, and sleep problems. Person with severe symptoms will need immediate emergency treatment with methadone, phenobarbital, and other drugs to alleviate symptoms.

| Marijuana | Pot, dope, joint, grass, mary jane, boo, charge, hay, jive, sweet lucy, tea, weed, reefer | Inhalation (smoking); orally | Euphoria; to get high; relaxation; social custom or conformity; disinhibition; relief from anxiety or depression; increase in visual and sensory awareness; increase in pleasure during sexual activity | Variable: possible impairment of judgment and coordination; disorientation to time; sense of well-being and tranquility; euphoria; increase in appetite (munching); increase in pulse; increased awareness of environment | Few symptoms reported: panic reaction with feelings of loss of control or sense of dying; acute depression; toxic psychosis | Same as untoward reaction with feelings of loss of control or depression; may experience nausea and vomiting with oral ingestion | Panic reaction: use the technique of talking down described under hallucinogen and amphetamine use. Acute depression and psychosis: usually subsides when THC (psychoactive compound in marijuana and hashish) is metabolized. Overdose: Same as above. |

unless they have a history of long-standing problems and behavior change. Often adolescent suicides occur without warning. Frequently, they are triggered by a seemingly trivial incident—a fight with a boy friend or a quarrel with parents. The suicide is a sudden, impulsive reaction to a stressful situation.

Which adolescents are likeliest to commit suicide? A study of the psychodynamics of the suicidal adolescent and the nature of the preceding psychopathology provide some answers to this question. Finch and Poznanski (1971, p. 4) list three criteria that tend to predict suicide in adolescents.

1. There is a long-standing history of problems that can usually be traced back to childhood years.

2. There is a period in adolescence when the identified problem is escalated. This gives rise to coping difficulties greater than those normally associated with adolescence.

3. There is a chain-reaction dissolution of the adolescent's meaningful social relationships.

Kurt Glaser has outlined some more specific factors that may be used to detect potential suicides in children and adolescents (Glaser 1976, pp. 89–92). The following list of warning signals can help nurses assess the seriousness of an act and determine the most appropriate means of treatment:

• Suicidal tendency: Is expressed in various ways, ranging from a casual statement to the actual, completed suicide. The method of expression used is not a reliable indicator of the severity of the conflict. The statement "If I don't get what I want, I'll kill myself" may be simply a casual remark, or it may be a plea for help that will be followed by a more serious threat or by the actual suicide.

• Suicidal gesture: Is a more serious warning signal than a statement and may be followed by a suicidal act. It is carefully planned so as to attract attention without seriously injuring the subject. The purpose of the gesture is to influence others and to manipulate the situation. A superficial scratch across the wrist, if it goes unheeded, may be followed by a more dramatic display.

• Suicidal threat: Is more serious than the casual statement and is accompanied by other behavior changes. These may include mood swings, temper outbursts, a decline in school or work performance, character-

ological changes, sudden or gradual withdrawal from friends, or other significant changes in attitude.

• Suicidal attempt: Is a strong and desperate call for help. It is often the final call, for unlike the suicidal gesture it involves a definite risk. The outcome frequently depends on the circumstances and is not under the person's control. For example, someone who takes a heavy overdose of sleeping pills may or may not be discovered in time.

Prevention and treatment of adolescent suicide can be implemented in the following six steps:

1. Accept the warning signals as appeals for help from the client.

2. Obtain a careful history from the parent or the client or both. This history should elicit evidence of mood change, increased temper outbursts, changes in school or work performance, withdrawal from friends, or other changes in attitude toward the environment. Do not rely on evidence of depression alone, since a chronically depressed person may suddenly become cheerful after having made the decision to commit suicide. Depression is not a reliable indicator in adolescents anyway, due to their mood swings. Instead, use somatic equivalents of depression, such as insomnia, loss of appetite, fatigue, and decreased libido.

3. Assess the nature of the stressful situation that triggered the suicidal episode. This gives an indication of the client's tolerance for stress: the milder the stress, the weaker the defenses and coping mechanisms and the greater the chance of recurrence.

4. Evaluate the nature and depth of the inner conflict and the degree of disharmony that exists in the family living situation or equivalent environment. Include an evaluation of the resources available to the client and the willingness of these resources to help.

5. Inform the parents. The primary aim in prevention is to open lines of communication between the nurse or other professional and the client, and later between the parents and the client, so that conflicts may be expressed in words rather than in action.

6. Remove the client from the source of anxiety. Obtain outpatient therapy for the nonhospitalized adolescent whenever possible, since hospitalization may exacerbate feelings of isolation, helplessness, and inadequacy.

DEALING WITH FAMILIES OF ADOLESCENT CLIENTS

Being a parent of a "normal" adolescent is difficult, at best. As the child grows into adulthood with all its perplexing questions and problems, the parents will normally worry about their child's safety and well-being. They may feel rejected because they are no longer needed in quite the same way as they were before. Since many parents of relatively normal adolescents share this plight, they can usually find receptive listeners who will give them comfort and support.

The problems of the parents of emotionally disturbed adolescents are more complicated. Many such parents have a strong sense of failure, because their children did not turn out "right." Their feelings of guilt, frustration, and helplessness are likely to increase if their child is institutionalized. They have probably felt confused and resentful when experts offered them smug and guilt-provoking advice. Unlike the parents of normal adolescents, they probably have no one in whom to confide, either because they lack the support and understanding of others, or because their own self-incriminating feelings prevent them from seeking out confidants.

The nurse should show compassion and understanding for the parents' dilemma without blaming them or their offspring. Parents will be more receptive to family therapy and to exploring their part in the adolescent's problems if they sense that the nurse will support them, too. Earlier in this chapter we mentioned that any tendency to feel self-righteous or superior to the disturbed adolescent's parents would be an obstacle to effective treatment. Such feelings are readily communicated to parents and can only validate their fear of blame and increase their reluctance to participate in therapy with their child. The adolescent's chances for resolving the underlying conflicts and for maintaining a healthy life will be virtually nil if the family system remains unchanged.

Parents, school, and agency staff must understand the objectives and goals of treatment in order to appreciate the progress the client has made and avoid reinforcing the client's previously maladaptive behavior. The following incident illustrates the problems that arise when parents and school authorities, particularly those who must deal directly with behavior problems in the classroom, lack psychological sophistication.

Jeremy, a thirteen-year-old boy, was referred to the school nurse because he was introverted and isolative. He made no contact with either his peers or teachers and rarely spoke unless addressed directly. After he had spent three months in group and individual therapy sessions with the nurse, Jeremy began to come to the grade counselor's office of his own accord to talk about his depression and the problems he had been having in his family. Both the grade counselor and the boy's family believed this to be an indication that his difficulties had worsened, and they began to complain to the nurse about his illness! Not only were Jeremy's parents and counselor ignorant of the goals of treatment and the behaviors expected to come with change, but apparently they were also uncomfortable with the changes in Jeremy's behavior and with the implications of these changes for their relationships with him.

The client's siblings may experience many different feelings. Sometimes they share in the parents' guilt and shame. On the other hand, they may be quite pleased and relieved that the "troublemaker" is out of the family and hospitalized. The nurse should extend the same degree of understanding to the siblings as to the parents and should help them see how each member of the family contributes to the problem. Often another member of the family, usually a sibling, will assume the role of the "bad" or "sick" person in the family, since the identified "bad" person is no longer at home. The nurse should be aware of this tendency. Nurses who are involved in family therapy sessions can more easily perceive this pattern and take direct steps to deal with it.

The diverse nature of families with their individual backgrounds, problems, strengths, goals, and habits suggests equally diverse modes of treatment. A unique method is used at the Ska Children's Village, on an island south of Stockholm. Here juvenile delinquents come with their families for group therapy and rehabilitation. Everyone in the village has approximately fifteen hours a week in group therapy. Everyone is expected to participate in the outings and management of the village. And all are encouraged to talk over their problems with one another. Obviously, everyone's problems are confronted: although the children's behavior is the initial reason for referral, the adults' problems with alcohol, drugs, wife beating, and broken homes are tackled as well. The degree of success is hard to determine. Although the women and children seem to benefit most in opening up lines of communication, the transition back to city life and routine problems after a stay at the village takes its toll.

Chapter 21 provides useful information for nurses who work with families.

KEY NURSING CONCEPTS

✔ The normative process of adolescence includes rapid physical and sexual development, intellectual gains, emotional change, and social awareness. It is a stormy time of conflicting ideas and feelings.

✔ Nurses need to be aware of the social contexts and the meaning of behavior in order to evaluate an adolescent's behavior.

✔ Significant psychosocial developmental theories have been formulated by Sigmund Freud, Erik Erikson, and Harry Stack Sullivan; these theories provide the nurse with a basis for making accurate assessments and appropriate interventions.

✔ Nurses work with adolescents in the outpatient setting as a community health nurse; nurse-counselor; individual, group, or family therapist; and in hospital and residential treatment program settings.

✔ The nurse can maintain a therapeutic milieu by providing a physically safe environment, establishing interpersonal relationships with clients, intervening in potentially harmful interactions among clients, and offering more satisfying alternatives to destructive behavior.

✔ Key factors in working effectively with adolescents include the adequacy of the therapeutic milieu and the nurse's ability to establish interpersonal relationships and to explore the adolescent's own feelings and life experiences.

✔ Specific issues and problems frequently related to psychiatric nursing care of adolescents include the adolescent's attempts to seduce the nurse into relating in a nontherapeutic way, the client's use of unconventional language and profanity, testing and limit setting, anxiety and resistance, anger and hostility, scapegoating, adolescent sexual behavior, dietary problems such as obesity and anorexia nervosa, drug use and abuse, juvenile delinquency, and suicide.

✔ The nurse plays a central role in counseling parents and families of adolescent clients.

References

Allport, G. W. *The Nature of Prejudice*. Boston: Beacon Press, 1954.

Amini, F., and Salasnek, S. "Adolescent Drug Abuse: Search for a Treatment Model." *Comprehensive Psychiatry* 16 (1975): 379–389.

Amini, F.; Salasnek, S.; and Burke, E. L., "Adolescent Drug Abuse: Etiological and Treatment Considerations." *Adolescence* 11 (1976): 281–299.

Andry, R. G. *Delinquency and Parental Pathology*. Rev. ed. London: Staples Press, 1971.

Brown, J. A. C. *Freud and the Post-Freudians*. London: Penguin Books, 1961.

Burke, E. "Patient Values on an Adolescent Drug Unit." *American Journal of Psychotherapy* 24 (1970): 400–410.

Campbell, C. "Perception of Stress by Staff Members in an Adolescent Milieu." Unpublished research. San Francisco: Youth Service, Langley Porter Institute, 1977.

Caudill, W. *The Psychiatric Hospital as a Small Society*. Cambridge: Harvard University Press, 1958.

Coles, R. "Profiles: The Measure of Man, II." *New Yorker*, November 14, 1970, pp. 59–138.

Erikson E. *Identity: Youth and Crisis*. New York: W. W. Norton, 1968.

Finch, S. M., and Poznanski, E. O. *Adolescent Suicide*. Springfield, Ill.: Charles C Thomas, 1971.

Flavell, J. H. *The Developmental Psychology of Jean Piaget*. New York: Van Nostrand Reinhold, 1963.

Fredlund, D. "Juvenile Delinquency and School Nursing." In *Child and Adolescent Psychiatric Nursing*, edited by C. M. Fagin, pp. 154–60. St. Louis: C. V. Mosby, 1974.

Freud, A. *The Ego and the Mechanisms of Defense,* rev. ed. New York: International Universities Press, 1966.

Freud, S. "The Passing of the Oedipus-Complex." *Collected Papers* 2 (1924): 269–276.

Fromm-Reichmann, F. *Principles of Intensive Psychotherapy.* Chicago: University of Chiacgo Press, 1950.

Glaser, K. "Suicide in Children and Adolescents." In *Acting Out: Theoretical and Clinical Aspects,* edited by L. E. Abt and S. L. Weissman, pp. 87–99. 2d ed. New York: Jason Aronson, 1976.

Glueck, S., and Glueck, E., eds. *Unraveling Juvenile Delinquency.* New York: Commonwealth Fund, 1950.

———. *Identification of Predelinquents.* New York: Intercontinental Medical Book, 1972.

Goffman, E. *Asylums: Essays on the Social Situation of Mental Patients and Other Inmates.* Chicago: Aldine Publishing, 1961.

Greenblatt, M.; York, R. H.; and Brown, E. L. *From Custodial to Therapeutic Patient Care in Mental Hospitals.* New York: Russell Sage Foundation, 1955.

Jersild, A. T. *The Psychology of Adolescence.* 3d ed. New York: Macmillan, 1978.

Jones, M. *The Therapeutic Community: A New Treatment Method in Psychiatry.* New York: Basic Books, 1953.

———. *Beyond the Therapeutic Community: Social Learning and Social Psychiatry.* New Haven: Yale University Press, 1968.

———. "Nurses Can Change the Social Systems of Hospitals." *American Journal of Nursing* 78 (1978): 1012–1014.

Lettieri, D. J., Ed. *Predicting Adolescent Drug Abuse.* Washington, D.C.: Government Printing Office, 1975.

MacLennan, B. W., and Felsenfeld, N. *Group Counseling and Psychotherapy with Adolescents.* New York: Columbia University Press, 1968.

Menninger, W. C. "Psychoanalytic Principles in Psychiatric Hospital Therapy." *Southern Medical Journal* 32 (1939): 348–354.

Redl, F., and Wineman, D. *Children Who Hate.* Glencoe, Ill.; Free Press, 1951.

Simmel, E. "The Psychoanalytic Sanitarium and the Psychoanalytic Movement." *Bulletin of the Menninger Clinic* 1 (1937): 133–143.

Stanton, A. H., and Schwartz, M. S. "The Management of a Type of Institutional Participation in Mental Illness." *Psychiatry* 12 (1949): 13–26.

———. *The Mental Hospital.* New York: Basic Books, 1954.

Sullivan, H. S. "The Modified Psychoanalytic Treatment of Schizophrenia." *American Journal of Psychiatry* 87 (1931): 977–991.

———. *The Interpersonal Theory of Psychiatry.* New York: W. W. Norton, 1953.

Tudor, G. E. "A Sociopsychiatric Nursing Approach to Intervention in a Problem of Mutual Withdrawal on a Mental Hospital Ward." *Psychiatry* 15 (1952): 193–217.

U.S. Department of Health and Human Services. *Mortality,* Part B. II. Washington, D.C.: Government Printing Office, 1977.

Wilmer, H. A. *Social Psychiatry in Action: A Therapeutic Community.* Springfield, Ill.: Charles C Thomas, 1958.

Wilson, H. S. "Presencing: Social Control of 'Schizophrenics' in an Antipsychiatric Community." In *Current Perspectives in Psychiatric Nursing: Issues and Trends,* vol. 1, edited by C. R. Kneisl and H. S. Wilson, pp. 164–175. St. Louis: C. V. Mosby, 1976.

———. *Deinstitutionalized Residential Care for the Severely Mentally Disordered: The Soteria House Approach.* New York: Grune and Stratton, 1982.

Zilberg, N. J., and Burke, E. L. "Inpatient vs. Outpatient Treatment of Delinquent Drug-Abusers: An Outcome Study." Paper presented at the 87th Annual Convention of the American Psychological Association, New York City, September 1979.

Further Reading

Abt, L. E., and Weissman, S. L., eds. *Acting Out: Theoretical and Clinical Aspects.* 2d ed. New York: Jason Aronson, 1976.

Amini, F., and Burke, E. "Acting Out and its Role in the Treatment of Adolescents: An Object Relations Viewpoint." *Bulletin of the Menninger Clinic* 43 (1979): 249–259.

Blos, P. *On Adolescence: A Psychoanalytic Interpretation.* New York: Free Press, 1962.

Bourne, P. G., ed. *Acute Drug Abuse Emergencies.* New York: Academic Press, 1976.

Bruch, H. *The Importance of Overweight.* New York: W. W. Norton, 1957.

———. *Eating Disorders.* New York: Basic Books, 1973.

———. *The Golden Cage: The Enigma of Anorexia Nervosa.* Cambridge: Harvard University Press, 1978.

Burke, E., and Amini, F. "A Significant Aspect of Acting Out and Its Management on an Adolescent Ward: 'Jailification.'" *Adolescence* 16 (1981): 33–37.

Coles, R. "Profiles: The Measure of Man, I." *New Yorker,* November 7, 1970, pp. 51–131.

Donovan, B. T. *Physiology of Puberty.* London: Edward Arnold Publishers, 1965.

Easson, W. M. *The Severely Disturbed Adolescent.* New York: International Universities Press, 1969.

Edelson, M. *Ego Psychology, Group Dynamics, and the Therapeutic Community.* New York: Grune and Stratton, 1964.

Erikson, E. H. *Childhood and Society.* 2d ed. New York: W. W. Norton, 1963.

————. *Youth: Change and Challenge.* New York: Basic Books, 1963.

Fagin, C. M., ed. *Child and Adolescent Psychiatric Nursing.* St. Louis: C. V. Mosby, 1974.

Fort, J. *The Pleasure Seekers: The Drug Crisis, Youth and Society.* Indianapolis: Bobbs-Merrill, 1969.

Friedenberg, E. Z. *The Vanishing Adolescent.* New York: Dell Publishing, 1959.

Friedman, A. S.; Sonne, J. C.; Speck, R. V.; Barr, J. P.; Jungreis, J. E.; Boszormenyi-Nagy, I.; Lincoln, G.; Cohen, G.; Spark, G.; and Weiner, O. R. *Therapy with Families of Sexually Acting-Out Girls.* New York: Springer Publishing, 1971.

Hofmann, F. G., and Hofmann, A. D. *A Handbook on Drug and Alcohol Abuse.* New York: Oxford University Press, 1975.

Kantor, D., and Lehr, W. *Inside the Family.* San Francisco: Jossey-Bass, 1975.

Luke, B. "Maternal Alcoholism and Fetal Alcohol Syndrome." *American Journal of Nursing* 77 (1977): 1924–1926.

Marcus, I. M., and Francis, J. J. *Masturbation: from Infancy to Senescence.* New York: International Universities Press, 1975.

Melton, J. H. "A Boy with Anorexia Nervosa." *American Journal of Nursing* 74 (1974): 1949–1951.

Mullahy, P. *Oedipus: Myth and Complex.* New York: Grove Press, 1955.

Robbins, L. L. "The Hospital As a Therapeutic Community." In *Comprehensive Textbook of Psychiatry*, vol. 3, edited by H. J. Kaplan, A. M. Freedman, and F. J. Sadock, pp. 2362–2368. Baltimore: Williams and Wilkins, 1980.

Satir, V.; Stachowiak, J.; and Taschman, H. A. *Helping Families to Change.* New York: Jason Aronson, 1975.

Sinclair, D. *Human Growth after Birth.* 3d ed. London: Oxford University Press, 1978.

Smith, D. E., and Gay, G. R. *It's So Good, Don't Even Try It Once.* Englewood Cliffs, N.J.: Prentice-Hall, 1972.

Smith, D. E.; Bentel, D. J.; and Schwartz, J. L., eds. *The Free Clinic: A Community Approach to Health Care and Drug Abuse.* Beloit, Wis.: Stash Press, 1971.

Sugar, M., ed. *The Adolescent in Group and Family Therapy.* New York: Brunner/Mazel Publishers, 1975.

Wesson, D. R., and Smith, D. E. *Barbiturates: Their Use, Misuse, and Abuse.* New York: Human Sciences Press, 1977.

Wolf, M. S. "A Review of Literature on Milieu Therapy." *Journal of Psychiatric Nursing and Mental Health Services* 15 (1977): 26–33.

Mental Health Counseling with Families

CHAPTER OUTLINE

Will the *Real* Family Please Stand Up?

    The Traditional Nuclear Family

    The Single Parent Family

    The Blended Family

    Alternative Family Forms

Developmental Tasks Confronting Families

The Family as a System

Family Characteristics and Dynamics

    Roles

    Power

    Behavior

Defining Family Therapy

The Family Movement in Historical Perspective

Approaches to Family Therapy

Qualifications of Family Therapists

Relational and Communicational Intricacies in Families

    The Self-fulfilling Prophecy and Life Scripts

    Family Myths, Life-styles, and Themes

    Coalitions, Dyads, and Triangles

    Pseudomutuality and Pseudohostility

    Deviations in the Parental Coalition

    Scapegoating

    Paradoxes and Double Binds

The Treatment Unit and the Treatment Setting

The Components of Family Therapy

    Family Assessment

    Contract or Goal Negotiation

    Intervention

Criteria for Terminating Treatment

The Nursing Process in Family Counseling

Family-oriented Preventive Psychiatry Programs

Couples Therapy

    Developmental Tasks Confronting Couples

    Types of Therapy

    Focus of Therapy

Key Nursing Concepts

LEARNING OBJECTIVES

After reading this chapter, students should be able to

- Identify the existing diverse forms of family life
- Identify the developmental tasks that confront couples and families
- Describe the family comprehensively in terms of the relationships, associations, and connections that occur in a dynamic, interacting whole
- Describe the relational and communicational intricacies in families as they relate to functional families and families in difficulty
- Relate the major components of family therapy to humanistic psychiatric nursing practice
- Identify primary, secondary, and tertiary prevention approaches that may be used to provide for family mental health
- Describe some of the important factors in the counseling of couples

CHAPTER 21

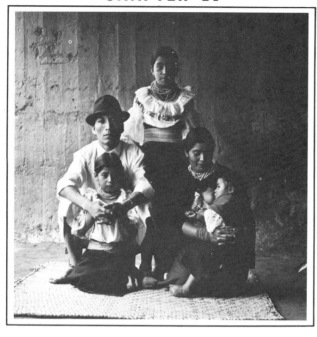

The family is the context in which people develop their first relationships with other people. How they view the larger social world outside the family is molded by the events that happen within families and that influence the development of the individual.

Nurses encounter families in many areas of their practice—in the emergency room, the intensive care unit, the school, the cancer hospital, the community health setting, and the mental health setting, among others. Assessment of families in trouble, and intervention on their behalf, must be based on an understanding of how families grow and interact and how family coping patterns develop. This chapter describes those processes and offers strategies for intervention into dysfunctional marital dyads or family systems.

WILL THE *REAL* FAMILY PLEASE STAND UP?

Today's family is:

- Mom, dad, and 2.4 kids
- A couple with eight kids—three of hers, three of his, and two of theirs
- A thirty-two-year-old electrical engineer and his three foster children

- A divorced woman and her infant child
- A widowed man, his two children, and his parents
- A grandmother raising her two grandchildren
- Two lesbian mothers and their children
- Two couples sharing an apartment neither could afford alone
- Three gay men who live and work together on a collaboratively owned vegetable farm
- Four couples and their children in a remote commune

Identifying the "real" family has become an issue because of arguments over whether the family is suddenly changing or even dying. Professional meetings carry such titles as "The Family—Can It Be Saved?" A White House Conference on the Family, originally scheduled for December 1979 to ring out the 1970s and herald the 1980s onto the social scene, was rescheduled for 1981, after the presidential election. It had become too political, too controversial. Essentially, a battle arose between two groups—those who wanted it called "The White House Conference on *the Family*" (the nuclear family), and those who wanted it called "The White House Conference on *Families*" (recognizing the existing diversity in family life).

Is it true that the family is dying out? Actually, perpetual transformation or change is the one permanent quality of the family. A myriad of family forms have appeared, disappeared, reappeared, and coexisted within and across cultures. Families have been defined by blood relationships, tribes, households, kinship systems, clans, and language alliances. They have been called *blended, extended, conjugal,* and *communal.* The American family is changing, but not dying: it is simply becoming different.

The Traditional Nuclear Family

The *traditional nuclear family* is a two-parent, time-limited, two-generation family consisting of a married couple and their children by birth or adoption. Despite its name, it is a relatively recent development in human history. It evolved as societies became more urban and industrialized in the move away from agrarianism. It is time-limited because, in most instances, the members of the younger generation begin their own families soon after they are twenty years of age.

Soon after its development, the traditional nuclear family became known as the *isolated nuclear family.* Ties to the *extended family*—all persons related by birth, marriage, or adoption to the nuclear family— were weakened. This diminished the basic support system that formerly surrounded families. The isolated nuclear family had less contact with the adults' *families of origin* (the families from which they came).

The nuclear family is the family structure about which people speak when they are concerned with "strengthening the family." This narrow definition of family, however, does not recognize and consider the wide variety of family constellations that exist in contemporary society.

The Single Parent Family

A *single parent family* is also two-generational and occurs when a lone parent and offspring live together as a nucleus. It is a more common family form than most people believe. James A. Levine (1978) notes that one in six children under eighteen—or 17 percent of all children—lives in a single parent family. In some communities, the number is even higher. While it is common knowledge that numerous single parent families exist in the inner-city areas of large, metropolitan centers, their existence in well-to-do suburban communities is acknowledged less often.

After two months of third grade in a large suburban school, eight-year-old Joshua told his father of feeling strange and different because he was from a single parent family. A review of the class list sent home by the teacher surprised both Joshua and his dad. They found that nineteen of the thirty-two children in Joshua's class also lived in single parent homes. The community in which Joshua lived had a 75 percent divorce rate, and most of his classmates in single parent families lived with their mothers.

While most single parent families result from death or divorce, increasing numbers of women are bearing children with the intention of rearing them alone. Single women and men are also adopting children with increasing frequency, something that was not done or even permitted only a few years ago. And more often than ever before, single parent families, like Joshua's, are being headed by men.

Levine (1978) cites the prediction of Paul Glick, a senior demographer with the U.S. Census Bureau, that fully 45 percent of the children born in 1977 will live in single parent families at some time before they reach eighteen years of age.

The Blended Family

The *blended family* has been defined as the joining of nuclear families that are missing adult members to form a new nucleus (Satir 1972). Blended families usually come about through remarriage after divorce or after the death of a spouse. Various types of blended families exist. The loosest structure is a weekend blending that occurs when the children from one parent's previous marriage visit that parent's later family for a brief time. In a more permanent blend, the children from a previous marriage live with one parent and a later spouse, forming the new nucleus. A third type of blended family is one in which the children from previous marriages of both spouses are included in the same household. A "mine, yours, and ours" variety also includes children who are the offspring of the new marriage.

Alternative Family Forms

Alternative families consist of persons with or without blood or conjugal (marriage) ties who live and interact together in order to achieve common goals. Two or more adults, of the same or opposite sexes, and their children, or adults without children, may choose to live together. Unlike the family constellations described earlier, alternative families may be one-generational, consisting of adult members of a single generation.

Communal arrangements, in which many people band together, are found both in sophisticated metropolitan centers and in more remote agricultural areas. The commune is further defined by how members have negotiated the privileges and responsibilities associated with their roles, material possessions, economic concerns, sexual expressions, and parenting activities. The Israeli kibbutzim are among the best known of the communes. Another type of communal arrangement is that of the religious cult. Cults are discussed thoroughly in Chapter 26.

Households of homosexual (gay) people are another alternative family form. Gay people who live together in the same household are choosing to be open about their life-style. This life-style is not yet recognized as an acceptable alternative by all segments of society, and gays still face restrictions that often prevent them from adopting children or gaining custody of children from

their previous heterosexual marriages that ended in divorce.

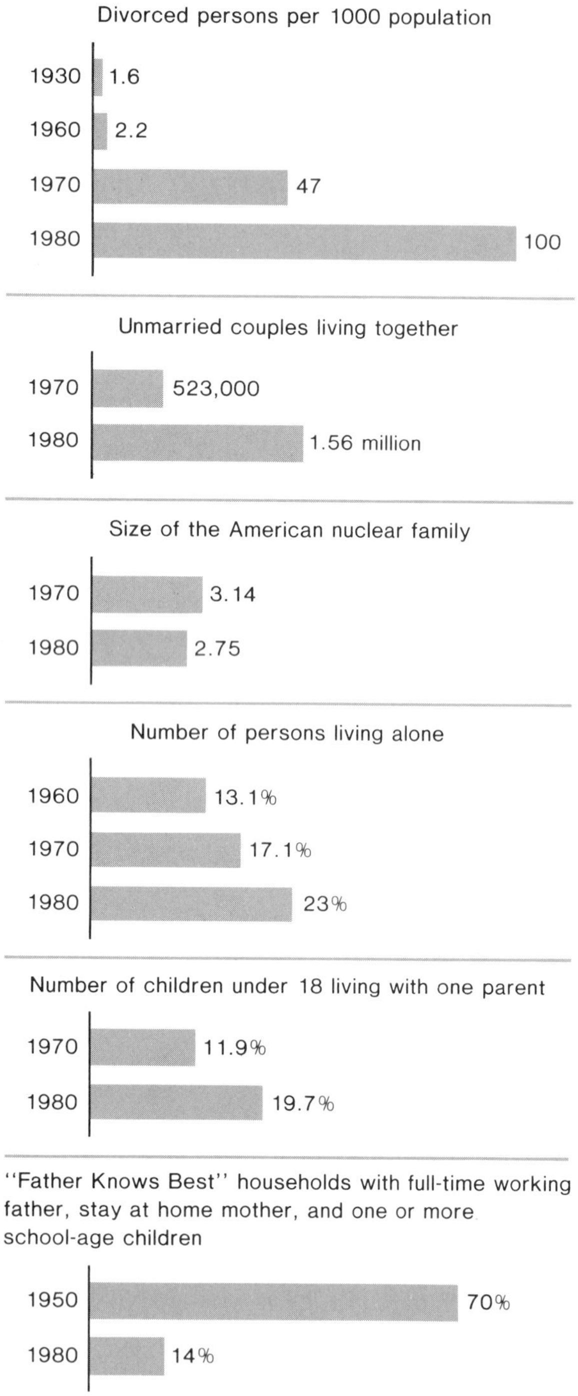

Even the well-known phrase, "You can choose your friends but you can't choose your relatives," is becoming obsolete according to Lindsey (1982), who has written a book on chosen kin. In her view, two factors in contemporary life are important. The first is economics. Because many singles and the elderly can no longer afford to live alone, there is a trend toward communal, familial living among these groups. The second is geography. Because the average American moves once every three years, an individual who lives in the East may have family on the West Coast. Friends become kin chosen to recreate the extended family. Figure 21–1 illustrates how American family life-styles are changing.

DEVELOPMENTAL TASKS CONFRONTING FAMILIES

Just as individuals and groups are confronted with developmental tasks (see Chapters 10 and 18), so are families. The family sociologist Evelyn Duval (1971, p. 5) lists the following developmental tasks of American families:

- *Physical maintenance*—providing food, shelter, clothing, health care.
- *Resource allocation (both physical and emotional)*—meeting family expenses; apportioning material goods, space, and facilities; and apportioning emotional goods, such as affection, respect, and authority.
- *Division of labor*—deciding who does what in relation to earning money, managing the household, caring for family members, and so on.
- *Socialization of family members*—guiding members in mature patterns of controlling aggression, elimination, food intake, sexual drives, sleep, etc.
- *Reproduction, recruitment, and release of family members*—giving birth to or adopting children, rearing them for release from the family at maturity, incorporating new members, and establishing policies for including others, such as in-laws, stepparents, and friends.
- *Maintenance of order*—administering sanctions to ensure conformity to family and/or societal norms.

Figure 21–1

Changing family life-styles in America.

- *Placement of members in the larger society*—interacting with the community, school, church, and economic and political systems to protect family members from undesirable outside influences.

- *Maintenance of motivation and morale*—rewarding members for achievements; developing a life philosophy and sense of family loyalty through rituals and celebrations; satisfying personal needs for acceptance, encouragement, and affection; meeting personal and family crises.

These developmental tasks are a considerable undertaking. It is the families who do not succeed very well at accomplishing them who come to the psychiatric nurse's attention most often.

THE FAMILY AS A SYSTEM

In a general systems theory framework, a family can be seen as a system of interrelated parts forming a whole. A family system includes not only the family members but also their relationships, their communication with one another, and their interactions with the environment.

Because a system functions as a whole, its parts are interdependent, and a change or movement in any part of the system affects all other parts. For example, an accomplishment by one member of the family affects all the other members in the family system. Dysfunction in one member also changes the whole system. This concept of *wholeness* is important in understanding families. It means that counseling one family member will change all members in some way.

Another important characteristic of a system is that it strives to maintain a dynamic equilibrium, or balance, among the various forces that operate within and on it. This process is referred to as *homeostasis*. All systems need to balance themselves within a range of functioning in which the work of the system can be accomplished. The mental image of a seesaw may help show what happens in the attempt to achieve balance. Too much weight on one end will bring it to the ground. It is no longer in balance. However, before that point, balance can be achieved at any of several points, even though the seesaw is not perfectly horizontal. When a family member behaves in a way not prescribed within the family system, other members will react with attempts to minimize the disruption, always trying to maintain a steady state. Don D. Jackson

(1957) introduced the concept of *family homeostasis* based on his observations that the families of psychiatric clients often experienced Depression or Psychophysiological Disorders when the client improved. He postulated that these behaviors of family members and the psychological disruptions of the client were homeostatic mechanisms that operated to bring the disturbed system back into its delicate balance. When a family has to use most of its energy to maintain balance, little energy is left for the growth of the family or its individual members.

Elements in the system may also be parts of another system. Billy may be simultaneously the oldest child in the family, a catcher for the junior league baseball team, and a member of the debate team. Billy's family is a member of other larger systems as well—the extended family, the city, the nation, etc. The family itself has *subsystems*, such as dyads (Billy and his father), triads (Billy, his brother, and his sister), or other groups of members who are linked together in some special association.

Systems can also be viewed as *open* or *closed*, although these are actually the extremes of a continuum. Some family systems are more open than others, while some are more closed. Openness requires a system to be flexible in adapting to the changes demanded by the environment. Adaptation takes energy to maintain homeostasis in the face of outside information or new input. Families whose systems are more closed tend to shut out or distort information from the environment in order not to upset their balance.

Family systems have *boundaries* as well. Boundaries define who participates in the system. They also tell family members the extent of differentiation permitted (among members and between members and outsiders), the amount or intensity of emotional investment in the system, the amount and kind of experiences available outside the system, and particular ways to evaluate experiences in terms of the family system (Hess and Handel 1967, p. 21). Boundaries may be clear, rigid, diffuse, or conflicting. These critical factors in family systems will be referred to throughout this chapter.

FAMILY CHARACTERISTICS AND DYNAMICS

Whether they are functional or dysfunctional, families have certain specific characteristics and dynamics in operation. The functional family is distinguished from the dysfunctional one by the amount and quality of the energy used to maintain the family system.

Roles

Members of a family must determine how to accomplish the family developmental tasks listed earlier in this chapter. They do so by establishing roles, patterns of behavior sanctioned by the culture. Don D. Jackson (1965) has postulated that families set roles by operating as a rule-governed system—an ordered format designed so that members may be aware of their positions in relation to one another. Although a family system engages in a multitude of behaviors, a relatively small set of rules is sufficient to govern family life. Roles are assigned according to family rules. Families decide which roles will exist within the system, socialize members into the roles, and then expend energy maintaining members within their roles.

When members are unable or unwilling to perform assigned roles, the family experiences stress. For example, the roles of mother and father have long been stereotyped in American society. Mothers were the family nurturers and caretakers, while fathers were the family decision-makers and wage earners. These roles are not completely satisfying in all American families, and many women and men have moved to negotiate their roles differently. The trend in society is now toward families with two working parents and families in which fathers share, or assume, the nurturing role. James Levine (1978) notes that both parents work in 46 percent of husband–wife families with children under eighteen, and that fathers in a small, but steadily increasing, number of families have chosen to stay home part- or full-time. For the health of the family system, roles often must be negotiated in other than stereotyped ways. When the roles are not negotiated satisfactorily, family disequilibrium results.

Power

Most families have a hierarchical power structure in which the adults wield power, usually in an authoritarian manner. The power structure is often developed in this way because it creates a safe environment in which young children can grow and develop, and because it is easy to operate. However, stress develops when disagreements exist about who holds the power.

Tom, the seventeen-year-old son in the M family, continually used the family car without permission.

Although some serious arguments ensued between Tom and his father, no restrictions were placed on Tom's behavior, and the car keys continued to hang on a key rack in the front hall. Tom's paternal grandfather, who lived with the M family, took Tom's side in his arguments with his father. Grandfather M adopted a fond "boys will be boys" stance. One evening when the family car was in an auto repair shop for some minor work, Tom "borrowed" his grandfather's new car. Tom was involved in a collision about an hour later. Although no one was injured, Grandfather M's car had to be towed away, extensively damaged. Later that night, the adults of the M family managed to come together to agree on a stance that they could mutually support.

Once the adults in the M family were able to openly acknowledge their internal power struggle and come to an agreement on what rules were to be set and by whom, the system was less stressed. Grandparents residing with a family are not the only causes of disagreements. Disagreements between husband and wife about who holds the power are also common. In some dysfunctional families, there is chronic discord about power.

When children mature and become capable of assuming greater responsibility for their own functioning, power is often diffused among all members of a family system in a more democratic fashion. Certain families do not allow power to be redistributed, however, thus interfering with the individual development of the members who have less power.

Behavior

In the systems view of a family, the family interaction system has four important qualities. The first, *wholeness*, was discussed earlier in this chapter. It refers to the interrelationship of all the elements in the system.

Synergy, the second characteristic, refers to the fact that the whole is greater than the sum of its parts. In other words, combined efforts produce a greater effect than the sum of individual actions. Two young children at play in their mother's cosmetics exemplify the effects of synergy. They encourage one another gleefully and enthusiastically to open and use the various jars, pots, and tubes they have discovered. Before long, the children and the environment have been thoroughly decorated. To their angry mother, each child blames the other, believing that without the other they would not have been in trouble. The effects of synergy can also be seen in families distinguished by open affection. Open affection stimulates more open affection, which cycles back into the system to stimulate even more of this particular distinguishing characteristic.

Circularity and *feedback* also characterize family system behavior. Each member engages in behavior that influences the other members. The process has been characterized as an uninterrupted sequence of interchanges (Watzlawick, Beavin, and Jackson 1967). The usual way people think about relationships does not allow for circularity. In a teenage daughter's view, for example, if her mother would only trust her, they would get along better. The mother's view is that the problem lies with the teen's uncooperativeness. Both mother and daughter are stopping the circular process by seeing one behavior as a cause and the other as an effect. The concept of circularity views each person's behavior as both cause and effect at the same time. Mother and daughter are caught up in a cycle, as they monitor and influence one another. Circularity, feedback, and mutual influence are discussed at length in Chapter 6.

DEFINING
FAMILY THERAPY

Nurses in the past have worked with families and family problems in many different settings. Most often nurses encountered family members while in a health teaching role—that is, while caring for the diabetic client, the client who has undergone major surgery, or the client who has had a myocardial infarction, the nurse taught the client's family how to care for that person physically and what life-style changes the illness might impose on the family. The family therapy role, however, is still a relatively new one for nurses.

Family therapy is a different way of viewing problems. In general, family therapists believe that the emotional symptoms or problems of an individual are an expression of emotional symptoms or problems in a family. Therefore, family therapists view the family system as the unit of treatment. Their concerns are basically with the relationships *between* the family members, not with the intrapsychic functioning of Mom, Dad, Kevin, or Susan.

Various therapeutic strategies have emerged from these shared beliefs. Family therapists do not have as fixed a set of procedures for intervention as psychoanalysts do. However, certain intervention strategies and therapeutic postures seem to flow naturally from the

basic beliefs family therapists hold. These strategies and postures are discussed later in this chapter.

THE FAMILY MOVEMENT IN
HISTORICAL PERSPECTIVE

Professionals doing psychotherapy were bound by commitment and theoretical orientation to the practice of one-to-one work with clients until the early 1940s. In those early years, Freud's psychoanalytic theory was the dominating force in psychotherapeutic work with clients. The child guidance movement, which began in the forties, is credited with including the client's family in the thinking and activities of therapists. However, family thinking at this time was an extension of psychoanalytic theory. Generally, the child was seen by the psychiatrist and the family by the social worker. Child guidance workers saw no reason to work with the child and the parents or other family members together.

The psychoanalytic theory of personality development continued to be tremendously influential in the 1940s. While most theorists and clinicians were aware of the effects of family relationships, they resisted active involvement of the family in treatment. To do so would have been viewed as a violation of the sacred analyst–client relationship.

In the early 1950s some therapists began to experiment somewhat clandestinely with family therapy. Jay Haley (1962) notes that therapists who were seeing families did not talk or write about their work. They had to refrain from alienating the psychiatric establishment, which considered family members irrelevant to the nature and treatment of psychopathology. Because these therapists earned their living in the mental health field, they cautiously avoided incurring the wrath of their professional groups. When persons develop new ideas that threaten the comfortable status quo, it is not uncommon to find that they are ostracized by their colleagues.

The family therapy movement gained momentum and began to be acknowledged openly by the mid-1950s. Some theorists and clinicians began to publish their views, experiences, and research and learn of the work of others.

Since that time, the family therapy movement has flourished. There are now several different schools or approaches, each with its own style.

APPROACHES TO FAMILY THERAPY

Rather than identify family therapy approaches by the names of the family therapists who developed them, we will briefly discuss the approaches as Jones (1980) suggests. Jones categorizes the research and literature on family therapy into seven major approaches.

1. The integrative approach is represented by the work of Nathan Ackerman (1958). Ackerman emphasized the need to take individual as well as family dynamics into account. Although his approach is the only one that does not rely heavily on systems concepts, it does bridge the gap between the psychoanalytic approach and the "maverick" approaches of those who focus on interpersonal and transactional phenomena.

2. The psychoanalytic approach is based directly on Freudian psychoanalytic theory and conforms to an illness model of family therapy. In this model it is believed that one or more disturbed marital partners account for the dysfunctions experienced in the family. An emphasis is placed on the reconstruction of the personality of the disturbed mate(s). The names of Boszormenyi-Nagy and Framo (1965) are linked with the psychoanalytic approach.

3. In the Bowen approach, the family is thought of as a system combining both emotional and social relationships. Bowen (1960, 1978) has developed his approach into specifics that can be easily taught. Some of his concepts, such as family triangles and multigenerational transmission processes, are discussed later. This approach is an extremely popular one, probably because it is so specific.

4. The structural approach describes the family as an open system governed by rules or boundaries that define who participates with whom, and how (Minuchin 1974). There are two types of dysfunctional patterns—enmeshment and disengagement—both of which are discussed later. The goal of the family therapist in this approach is to transform the family structure in the interest of creating clear boundaries.

5. The interactional approach is called a communicational approach in some of the literature. The unit of analysis for therapy is the behavior and communication among and between family members. These concepts were developed in the fifties and sixties through research on the possible relationship between the double-bind concept and schizophrenia and on dysfunctional communication in families (see Jackson 1968a, 1968b, 1957; Bateson et al. 1956; Lidz et al. 1958; Haley 1971, 1976; and Satir 1967, 1972). Many of these concepts are discussed later in this chapter.

6. The social network approach includes the persons—friends, neighbors, relatives, fellow workers—with whom the family in crisis has a social relationship (Speck 1967). Social network therapy is a sort of extended group therapy with the goal of bringing together as many people of a family's social network as possible. It takes place in the home and involves large groups of people (from 40 to 100 is not uncommon). It has been found particularly helpful in crisis and disaster situations and has been compared to the tribal meetings for healing purposes that occur in other cultures (Speck and Attneave 1973).

7. The behavioral approach is based on Skinnerian theories of learning. It consists of adapting principles and techniques of behavior modification for use with families. One of the most prominent authors and theorists concerned with the behavioral approach to family therapy is Gerald Patterson (1976).

QUALIFICATIONS OF FAMILY THERAPISTS

Family therapists should be specially educated in the practice of family therapy and strongly committed to a belief in the importance of the family. Increasing numbers of psychiatric nursing clinical specialists are being prepared in graduate programs that provide both theory and supervised clinical practice in this specialized area. While undergraduate nursing programs focus on the importance of relating to families in all settings, they (rightfully) do not prepare nurses as family therapists.

RELATIONAL AND COMMUNICATIONAL INTRICACIES IN FAMILIES

People negotiate their views of themselves and others on the basis of their perceptions. Perceptions also influence how people interact with one another on both content and relationship levels. In a family system, each person's behavior is contingent on the behavior of the others. This creates some interesting and intricate turns in family relationships.

Functional families allow for individuation and growth-producing experiences. Rigidity within a family system makes it difficult for the family to adapt to change and easier for the family to become dysfunctional. Some of the relational intricacies described below exist in all families, but dysfunctional families handle them differently from functional families. Other factors arise only in family systems that are dysfunctional.

Although some of the factors discussed below may be easily categorized as communicational, it is important to recognize their relational aspects. Other communication factors (discounting, disconfirming, disqualifying, symmetry, complementarity, congruity, and incongruity) are discussed in Chapter 6.

The Self-fulfilling Prophecy and Life Scripts

William W. Wilmot (1975, p. 119) gives the following example of a self-fulfilling prophecy in action.

Let's assume for a moment that you are sitting at home watching television, when there is a knock at the door. Three large men in white uniforms burst into the room shouting, "There he is, get him!" As they wrestle you to the floor, you scream violent protest (in between biting and kicking). When they have you under control, they show you a court order committing you to a mental institution because of your aggressive and violent behavior against your relatives, though you know your relatives are committing you unjustly. Once in the institution you are released from the restraint. You demand to see the director, pleading that it is all some horrible mistake. When he comes to your ward, you explain the circumstances. He says, "There now, it's all right. A lot of us think we are something we are not." The more you protest, the less convinced he becomes, so you protest more vigorously. As you shake him and scream, "I am not violent," the attendants slap a straightjacket on you. The prophecy is fulfilled.

In families, self-fulfilling prophecies are often seen in the guise of family life scripts. Claude Steiner (1974, p. 51) calls a *script* "the blueprint for a life course." It is a plan decided not by the fates, but by experiences early in life. In Steiner's words (p. 54), "Human beings are

deeply affected by and submissive to the will of the specific divinities of their household—their parents—whose injunctions they are impotent against as they blindly follow them through life, sometimes to their self-destruction." People with life scripts are following forced, premature, early-childhood decisions. Steiner notes that, while not everyone has a script, script-free living is the exception rather than the rule.

There is an endless variety among life scripts. The Miss America script is written for the five-year-old girl whose parents enroll her in the Little Miss New York State (or Kansas or Colorado) competition. There are My Son the Doctor, Delinquent, Alcoholic, and Drug Addict scripts. A person with a script, either "good" or "bad," is terribly disadvantaged in terms of autonomy or life potentials. Unless people recognize what the script is, and take steps to change it, they are prevented from living to the fullest human potential.

Family Myths, Life-styles, and Themes

Family myths, life-styles, and themes help families maintain balance by permitting them to resist change. According to Antonio J. Ferreira (1963, p. 457), "each family group has a life of its own and develops its own myths." *Family myths* are well-integrated beliefs, shared by all family members, about each other and their positions in family life. The beliefs are unchallenged, even though family members may have to resort to distortions to maintain the myth. The family myth is related to the family's inner image—how the family appears to its members. For example, one family myth was that the father had the ability to make wise decisions. Individual members in this family participated to maintain the myth of the father as a Solomon by gearing interactions with him in such a way that he appeared to make high-level family decisions single-handedly.

The concepts of family theme (Hess and Handel 1959) and family life-style (Deutsch 1967) are related in their focus on the family's ways of relating to the outside world. The *family theme* is the family's perception of its development and history. One family had a theme constructed around second-generation grandparents of Austrian descent, who were able to provide their oldest son with a law school education through their hard work. This family conceived of persons on welfare as "lazy," thus reaffirming its view of the value of working hard and becoming educated. Determining the salient themes in a family's life helps us see how the fates of individual members are shaped by those themes and the pressures with which each person must contend.

The *family life-style* has to do with the family's biased perception of the outside world and its automated means of coping with this world. Family life-styles are designed to uphold particular images of the family—as the most popular, talented, financially successful, nonconformist, or whatever. The life-style is the front or facade the family strives to present to others.

Coalitions, Dyads, and Triangles

Of all the forms of communicative exchange, dyadic communication is the most common. In fact, a family begins with a dyad, the marital couple. These two become, in Virginia Satir's (1967) words, the architects of the family. The natural alliance, or coalition, of this dyad presents a united front to the world—to deal with one member, people have to deal with them both. However, if one partner does not actively support the other, severe strain results.

The presence of a third person always has an effect on an existing dyad. When the marital couple gives birth to a child, the relationship becomes a triadic one. A triad is not a stable social situation, since it actually consists of a dyad plus one. Shifting alliances characterize triads—mother and father may unite to discipline the child, mother and child may unite to argue for a family vacation, or father and child may join forces to go fishing together. These triadic relationships are shown in Figure 21–2. The illustration demonstrates Theodore Caplow's (1968, p. 42) notion that "the most significant property of the triad is its tendency to divide a coalition of two members against the third." The process of forming a triad is called *triangulation*. Triangulation becomes dysfunctional when issues are solved in families by shifting the intimacy among members, rather than by working the actual issue through. Such coalitions always result in someone feeling "left out." Triangulation is a major concept in the Bowen approach to family therapy.

Coalitions arise basically to affect the distribution of power. By joining forces, two persons can increase their influence over a third. A husband and wife frequently pair up to discipline their child better. However, the child may also attempt to pair up with one parent to avoid discipline. In families with a number of children, typical coalitions involve children closest in age, or children of the same sex.

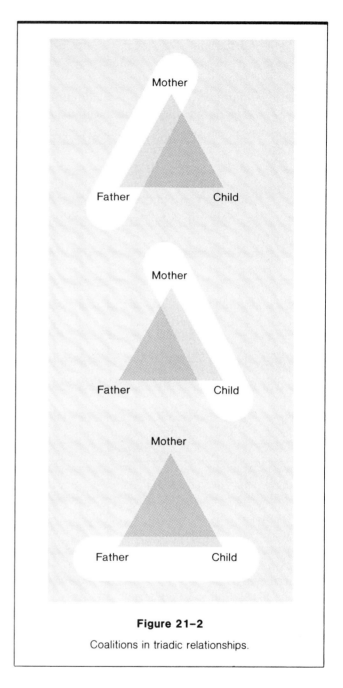

Figure 21–2

Coalitions in triadic relationships.

Pseudomutuality and Pseudohostility

A family in which *pseudomutuality* occurs functions "as if" it were a close, happy family. According to Lyman Wynne and his associates (1958), who use the interactional approach to family therapy, this pattern of relating has the following characteristics:

- Persistent sameness in the structuring of roles

- Insistence on the desirability and appropriateness of the role structure, despite evidence to the contrary

- Intense concern over deviations from the role structure or emerging autonomy
- Marked absence of spontaneity, enthusiasm, and humor in participating together

In these families, the members do not form intimate bonds with one another as individuals. Instead, an inordinate amount of energy is expended in maintaining ritualized and stereotyped ways of behaving and relating. There is a sort of desperate struggle to maintain harmony. Wynne and associates (1958) gave a perfect example in one mother who said: "We are all peaceful. I like peace if I have to kill someone to get it." Such a family requires its members to give up their sense of personal identity.

Pseudohostility exists in families in which there are chronic conflict, alienation, tension, and inappropriate remoteness among the members. As in pseudomutuality, the problems of family life are denied in an attempt to negate the hostility among the members. Family members view their differences as only minor ones. Both pseudomutual and pseudohostile family environments are stifling milieus.

Deviations in the Parental Coalition

In some families, problems develop from the parents' inability to form a satisfying coalition in terms of intimacy and control. Several common deviations are examined in the sections below.

Schism   Theodore Lidz and his associates (1957), who also advocate the interactional approach, have identified two types of families with parental coalition problems. They result from marital schism and marital skew. *Schismatic* families are those in which the children are forced to join one or the other camp of two warring spouses. It is hypothesized (Lidz, Fleck, and Cornelison 1966) that the constant fighting in these families is a defense against intimacy or closeness. In schismatic families, the spouses devalue and undercut one another. This makes it difficult for the children to want to be like either of them. The devaluation thus interferes with the development of a clear sexual identity by the children. Lidz and his associates also believe that marital schism is linked with schizophrenia in female children.

Skew   *Skewed* families are those in which one spouse is severely dysfunctional. The other spouse, who is usually aware of the dysfunction of the partner, assumes a passive, peacemaking, submissive stance in order to preserve the marriage. The passive partner is caught between effectively responding to the view of "reality" of the outside world and abrogating this view within the home, accepting the dysfunctional mate's view. On the surface, a skewed couple may appear to be complementary. Their relationship is actually lopsided and unsuited to many basic family tasks, however. This pattern has been linked with schizophrenia in male children.

Enmeshment   Other family patterns are enmeshment and disengagement, as described by Salvador Minuchin (1974), who advocates a structural approach to family therapy. *Enmeshed* families are characterized by a fast tempo of interpersonal exchange. Interactions within the family are of high intensity and are directed more toward issues of power than toward issues of affection. In enmeshed families, the mothers are often found to be overcontrolling and become anxious over the possibility of losing control over the children. The mother appears to be trying to prevent herself from becoming helpless. Adult males are often absent in these families, or, if present, are controlled in much the same way the children are.

Disengagement   *Disengaged* families move to the other extreme from enmeshment—abandonment. Family members seem oblivious to the effects of their actions on one another. They are unresponsive and unconnected to each other. Structure, order, or authority in the family may be weak or nonexistant. Assuming control and guidance increases the mother's anxiety, and she may feel overwhelmed and depressed. In these families, a child often assumes the parental role.

Scapegoating

Scapegoating is a social process that has been written and talked about since the time of the ancient Greeks. A *scapegoat* is defined by Sherry Johnson-Soderberg (1977, p. 154) as "a person, race, institution, or sex that bears the blame, prejudices, displaced aggression, irrational hostility, and projected feelings of others." In families, a disturbed member may play the role of family scapegoat, thus acting out the conflicts in the system and stabilizing it.

According to Nathan Ackerman (1971) the following constellation of roles occurs:

- The *scapegoat,* or victim, who best symbolizes the conflicts
- The *family persecutor,* who uses a special prejudice as the vehicle of attack
- The *family healer,* who intervenes to neutralize the attack and rescue the victim

Ezra F. Vogel and Norman W. Bell (1967) note that the emotionally disturbed child often serves as a scapegoat for conflicts between the parents, performing the valuable function of keeping the unit together. The parents implicitly encourage the child's behavior so that scapegoating can be maintained. The child, on the other hand, carries out the role of a "problem." Children are not the only persons who are scapegoated. Adults, or whole groups of people, may also be scapegoated.

Paradoxes and Double Binds

A *paradox* is a self-contradictory communication. A popular paradox is the message appearing on the bumpers of some cars—"THIS IS NOT A BUMPER STICKER!"

Paradoxes are common in everyday communication. Dan Greenburg (1964) offers the following one:

"Florence, what have you done to your hair? It looks like you're wearing a wig."
"I am—all my hair fell out!"
"Oh, listen, it looks so natural I'd never have known."

The client who says to the nurse: "Tell me what to do, so I can be independent," places the nurse in a paradox. The nurse who says: "I think you should find a new job, but it's not my place to say so," places the client in a paradox.

The double bind is a complex series of paradoxes. The example of a double-bind situation classically cited is from Gregory Bateson and his associates (1956, p. 259):

A young man who had fairly well recovered from an acute schizophrenic episode was visited in the hospital by his mother. He was glad to see her and impulsively put his arm around her shoulders, whereupon she stiffened. He withdrew his arm and she asked, "Don't you love me anymore?" He then blushed, and she said, "Dear, you must not be so easily embarrassed and afraid of your feelings." The client was able to stay with *her only a few minutes more and following her departure he assaulted an aide and was put in the tubs.*

The conditions necessary to produce the double bind are present in this example:

- Two persons, one of whom is the victim (the young man)
- A repeated experience, so that the double bind becomes a habitual expectation
- A primary negative injunction, carrying a threat of punishment (mother stiffens)
- A secondary injunction conflicting with the first injunction, but at a more abstract level. Like the primary injunction, the second threatens punishment ("Don't you love me anymore?")
- A tertiary negative injunction prohibiting the victim from escaping from the field ("Dear, you must not be so easily embarrassed and afraid of your feelings.")

It is theorized that repeated exposure to double binds in families produces Schizophrenia. The evidence, however, is not totally convincing (Jones 1977; Schuham 1967). While people labeled schizophrenic are victims of double binds, not all victims of double binds are, or become, schizophrenic. Most of the classic and early research on the double bind was carried out by Bateson and his colleagues, now associated in the interactional approach to family therapy.

THE TREATMENT UNIT AND THE TREATMENT SETTING

Most family therapists recommend that all persons in the family constellation participate in the assessment phase of family therapy. Not all agree on what persons comprise the family constellation or the treatment unit. Some include all members of the nuclear family; others include members of the extended family; and still others, large numbers of people in the family's social network. Different coalitions may be seen together at different times to accomplish specific purposes. For example, the mates are often seen together for the first few sessions.

Children four years of age and younger are often omitted from ongoing family therapy sessions. They may misinterpret, or be frightened by, the dialogue. In addition, small children tend to be disruptive. Satir (1967), however, makes it a point to bring all the children into therapy for at least two sessions in order to see how the family as a whole operates.

Family therapists often reverse the traditional territorial control of the professional by engaging the family system in therapy in its own milieu—the home. There are several reasons these therapists see families on their own ground:

- The interactions of the family system are more natural in their usual environment.

- Customary roles are more spontaneously played out on home ground.

- Family members reluctant to participate in therapy tend to be less so in the home than in a formal office or mental health agency setting.

While it is common to hold sessions in the home, family therapy may also take place in the professional's office setting.

THE COMPONENTS OF FAMILY THERAPY

Family therapy consists of three major components—assessment, contract or goal negotiation, and intervention.

Family Assessment

According to Henry Grunebaum (1970, pp. 57–58), the following factors are essential in family assessment:

- Identification of the family life issue, its effects on family functioning, and the affect that accompanies it. Is the issue: the basics of life, such as food, shelter, or money; the entry of a third person; the exit of the children from the household; illness; etc.?

- Identification of the assets, liabilities, and capabilities of the family in terms of resolving the issue and coping with the accompanying affects. What are the nature and effectiveness of the members' defense mechanisms, cognitive capacities, and communicative abilities?

- Identification of the willingness and ability of family members to undertake therapeutic tasks. Is the family willing to participate? Is it able to change?

Compton and Galaway (1979, pp. 251–252) suggest that a thorough family assessment should consider the following factors:

1. *Family as a social system*
   a. Family as responsive and contributing unit within network of other social units
      (1) Family boundaries—permeability or rigidity
      (2) Nature of input from other social units
      (3) Extent to which family fits into cultural mold and expectations of larger system
      (4) Degree to which family is considered deviant
   b. Roles of family members
      (1) Formal roles and role performance (father, child, etc.)
      (2) Informal roles and role performance (scapegoat, controller, follower, decision-maker)
      (3) Degree of family agreement on assignment of roles and their performance
      (4) Interrelationship of various roles—degree of "fit" within total family
   c. Family rules
      (1) Family rules that foster stability and maintenance
      (2) Family rules that foster maladaptation
      (3) Conformity of rules to family's life-style
      (4) How rules are modified; respect for difference
   d. Communication network
      (1) How family communicates and provides information to members
      (2) Channels of communication—who speaks to whom
      (3) Quality of messages—clarity or ambiguity
2. *Developmental stage of family*
   a. Chronological stage of family
   b. Problems and adaptations of transition
   c. Shifts in role responsibility over time
   d. Ways and means of solving problems at earlier stages

3. *Subsystems operating within family*

    a. Function of family alliances in family stability

    b. Conflict or support of other family subsystems and family as a whole

4. *Physical and emotional needs*

    a. Level at which family meets essential physical needs

    b. Level at which family meets social and emotional needs

    c. Resources within family to meet physical and emotional needs

    d. Disparities between individual needs and family's willingness or ability to meet them

5. *Goals, values, and aspirations*

    a. Extent to which family members' goals and values are articulated and understood by all members

    b. Extent to which family values reflect resignation or compromise

    c. Extent to which family will permit pursuit of individual goals and values

6. *Socioeconomic factors*

    a. Economic factors—level of income, adequacy of subsistence; how this affects life-style, sense of adequacy, self-worth

    b. Employment and attitudes about it

    c. Racial, cultural, and ethnic identification: sense of identity and belonging

    d. Religious identification and link to significant value systems, norms, and practices

Family assessments may be accomplished in a variety of ways. Some suggestions are given below. Others are discussed in the later section on intervention.

Taking a Family Life Chronology   Virginia Satir (1967) suggests that the family therapist should structure at least the first two sessions of therapy by taking a family life chronology. Her rationale is based on the following factors:

• The family therapist enters a session knowing little more than who the "identified patient" (IP) is and what symptoms that person manifests. The therapist does not have clues about the meaning of the symptoms, how the pain that exists in the marital relationship is expressed, how the mates have attempted to cope with their problems, or what models have influenced each mate's expectations about being a mate or parent.

• The therapist knows that the family has a history but does not know what that history is—what events have occurred and which members were influenced (directly or indirectly) by those events.

• Family members are fearful about embarking on family therapy. Structuring early sessions with a family life chronology helps decrease the threat. Members can answer relatively nonthreatening questions, and they tend to relax as the therapist demonstrates ability to take charge and keep things under control.

• Family members are often despairing when they enter therapy. The therapist's structure tells the family that there are specific directions to take in order to accomplish goals. The questions also provide family members with the opportunity to review successes as well as failures.

• The family life chronology is a nonthreatening way to change the focus from a "sick" family member to the family system and marital relationship.

• Taking the chronology gives the family therapist the opportunity to be a model of effective communication and provides the framework within which change can take place.

The specific structure of the family life chronology recommended by Satir is illustrated in Figure 21–3.

Family Genealogy or Time Line   Walter Toman's family constellation theory (1976), which uses generational transmission concepts, is a useful basis for constructing a family genealogy or time line. Since the production of *Roots* on television, families have found this to be a particularly interesting task.

From the study of families in detail, it becomes apparent that patterns are spread over generations. At first Bowen believed that a schizophrenic child could be produced after psychological impairment in three generations. He now believes that the level of impairment in Schizophrenia is not produced until eight to ten generations have passed. An intrinsic difficulty in analyzing generational transmission is that only a minute slice of a family generation—3 generations out of at least 4,000—can be studied. Few people are able to do what radiation biologist Dr. Joseph K. Gong, of the State University of New York at Buffalo, can. He can trace his paternal ancestry in China back to 2255 B.C.—an incredible 4,000 years and 131 generations.

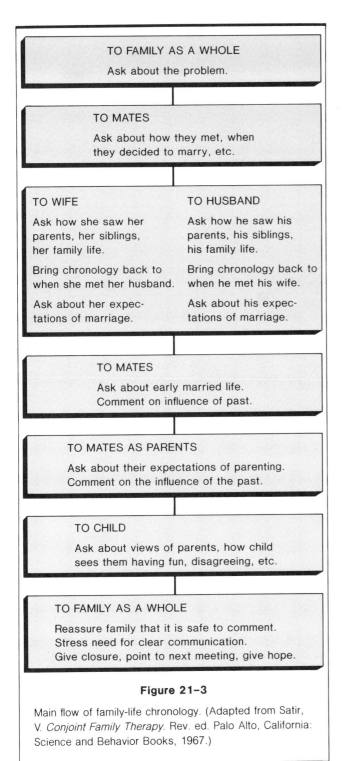

Figure 21–3

Main flow of family-life chronology. (Adapted from Satir, V. *Conjoint Family Therapy*. Rev. ed. Palo Alto, California: Science and Behavior Books, 1967.)

Each generation, according to Laing (1972, p. 77), projects onto the next the following elements:

- What was projected onto it by prior generations
- What was induced in it by prior generations
- Its response to this projection and induction

This process, which Laing calls *mapping*, is endless. Since it is impractical and impossible to understand the effect of 4,000 earlier generations on a family, the time line can serve a therapist and a family as a more limited means for understanding the family's roots.

The time line is highly effective as a visual representation. The therapist who draws it on a long, narrow piece of paper that is taped to the wall during the family's sessions can use it time and time again as the family therapy progresses. Colored lines can be used to differentiate individual family members. Colored flags, pins, or asterisks can identify and call attention to significant events in the family history. Births, deaths, marriages, and leave takings should be noted. The family therapist can use any of several family-tree or genealogical tracings for the family time line. One method is illustrated in Figure 21–4.

The Structured Family Interview   A structured family interview (Watzlawick 1966) has elements similar to Satir's family life chronology. In addition, it asks family members to participate in demonstrating the system's operation. The structured interview is composed of the following segments:

- *The main problems:* Each member is asked separately to identify what he or she considers the main problems in the family. The therapist assures the family member that the answer will not be divulged. Family members are then brought together to discuss this topic. The therapist leaves the room after telling the family members that their conversation will be recorded and they will be observed through a one-way screen. This task undermines the myth that the IP is the only "problem" in the family and paves the way for future work.

- *Planning something together:* The family is asked to plan something together, as a family, in the five minutes during which the therapist leaves the room. The important things in this task are whether and how a decision was reached. The content of the task, while revealing, is of secondary importance

- *How the mates met:* This task is for the mates only. With the children in another room, the mates are asked how, out of all the millions of people in the world, they got together. The parents share their views of the past and reveal their predominant patterns of interacting in the present.

- *The meaning of a proverb:* The parents are asked to discuss the meaning of the proverb "A rolling stone

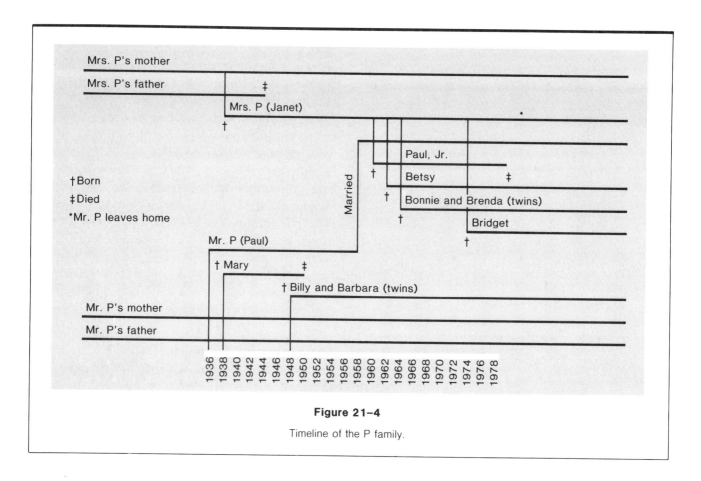

†Born
‡Died
*Mr. P leaves home

Figure 21-4

Timeline of the P family.

gathers no moss." At the end of five minutes, they are to call the children in and teach them the meaning of the proverb. This proverb has two valid but *mutually exclusive* interpretations—that *moss* (roots, stability, friends, etc.) is valuable, or that *rolling* (not stagnating, being alert, moving) is desirable. This task reveals how the mates handle disagreements and how they explain things to their offspring.

• *Blaming:* The entire family and the therapist are together for this task. The father sits to the left of the therapist followed at his left by the mother and the children, from the oldest to the youngest, in a clockwise direction around the table. Each family member is asked to write down, on a three-by-five card, the main fault of the person to the left. (The youngest child writes what he or she sees as the main fault of the father.) The therapist writes two cards, which state "too good" and "too weak." The therapist collects the cards and reads them out loud, beginning with the two she or he has authored. The therapist then asks to which two family members these cards apply. The other cards are read aloud in random order, and the authors are not revealed. This task reveals such processes as scapegoating, favoritism,

and self-blame. This assessment tool may actually serve a therapeutic function and be used as an intervention technique if it helps family members achieve spontaneous understanding of the patterns and relationships in their family.

Contract or Goal Negotiation

The negotiation phase of family therapy is begun by identifying what each member would like changed in the family. When each family member and the therapist have identified what they see as important goals, work begins on negotiating a set of attainable goals that everyone is willing to work on. Compromise is needed to achieve a working goal. At this time, the family therapist may also identify the means—tasks, strategies, etc.—that will be used to reach the negotiated goals.

Written and verbal contracts for work with individuals and groups have been discussed in Chapters 7 and 18. Chapter 7 also illustrates written contracts in current use. They may be adapted for use with families. A structured and specific marriage contract is discussed and illustrated later in this chapter.

Intervention

Therapy for a family system involves understanding and use of the here-and-now, of the basic processes that occur in the system. General guidelines for using the here-and-now process with families are given below. Some of the wide variety of specific strategies and tasks are also discussed.

Role of the Family Therapist   Virginia Satir (1967, pp. 160–176) offers the following guidelines for the role of the family therapist:

1. Creating a setting in which members can risk looking at themselves and their actions
   a. Reducing their fears
   b. Giving direction
   c. Helping them feel comfortable and hopeful about the therapy process
   d. Accepting the "expert" label and being comfortable in the role
   e. Structuring questions to gain important data

2. Being unafraid but open
   a. Framing questions to help members be less afraid
   b. Validating members' assumptions and questioning personal assumptions
   c. Eliciting the facts about planning processes, loopholes in planning, perceptions of self and others, perceptions of roles, communication patterns and techniques, sexual feelings and activities
   d. Responding with a belief in the integrity of the members

3. Helping members see how they look to others
   a. Sharing observations of how members manifest themselves
   b. Teaching members how to share their observations with one another
   c. Playing back tape recordings (or video tapes)

4. Asking for and giving information in a matter-of-fact, nonjudgmental, light, congruent way
   a. Verbally recreating situations (with imagination) in order to collect pertinent facts
   b. Being easy about giving and receiving information and thereby making it easier for family members to do so

5. Building self-esteem
   a. Making constant "I value you" comments
   b. Labeling assets
   c. Asking questions that family members can answer
   d. Emphasizing that the therapist and family members are equals in learning from therapy
   e. Responding as a person whose meaning or intent can be checked on
   f. Noting past achievements
   g. Accentuating the family's "good" intentions but "bad" communication
   h. Asking each family member what he or she can do to bring pleasure to another family member
   i. Being human, clear, and direct (and recognizing that warmth and good intentions are not enough in themselves)

6. Decreasing threat by setting rules for interaction
   a. Seeing to it that all members participate
   b. Making it clear that interruptions are not tolerated
   c. Emphasizing that acting out or making it impossible to converse is not allowed
   d. Making sure that no one speaks for anyone else
   e. Helping everyone speak out clearly so that each can be heard
   f. Using humor appropriately
   g. Connecting silence to covert control

7. Decreasing threat by structuring sessions
   a. Announcing concrete goals and a definite end to the therapy or deadlines for reevaluation
   b. Viewing the family as a family and not taking sides
   c. Seeing units or subsystems of the family alone to accomplish specific work or because this is feasible or practical (e.g., other members are not available), with the knowledge and understanding of all members

8. Decreasing threat by reducing the need for defenses
   a. Discussing anger and hurt openly, thus decreasing fears about showing anger or hurt

b. Interpreting anger as hurt

c. Acknowledging anger as a defense and dealing with the hurt

d. Showing that pain and the "forbidden" are safe to look at

e. Burlesquing basic fears—painting a picture exaggerated to the point of absurdity—to decrease overprotectiveness and feelings of omnipotence

9. Decreasing threat by handling loaded material with care

   a. Using careful timing

   b. Moving from the least loaded to the most loaded

   c. Switching to less loaded material when things get hot (to another subject or to the past rather than the present)

   d. Generalizing about what a therapist expects to see in families (hurt, anger, fear, fighting, etc.)

   e. Relating feelings to facts (events, circumstances)

   f. Using personal idioms, slang, profanity, or vulgarity when appropriate, and avoiding pedantic words and psychiatric jargon

   g. Preventing closure on episodes or complaints; assuring that things will become clearer as learning continues

10. Reeducating members to be accountable

    a. Reminding members of their ability to be in charge of themselves

    b. Identifying global pronouns

    c. Dealing openly with tattletales, spokespersons, and acting-out members

    d. Highlighting problems of accountability in the relationship with the therapist

11. Helping members see the influence of past models on their expectations and behavior

    a. Reminding members that they are acting from past models

    b. Openly challenging expectations

    c. Highlighting expectations by helping members verbalize the unspoken

    d. Highlighting expectations by exaggerating them

12. Delineating family roles and functions

    a. Recognizing roles by calling the parents "Mom" and "Dad" when referring to them as parents and "Jane" and "Bill" when addressing them as individuals or as husband and wife

    b. Including members in history taking in the order of their entrance into the family

    c. Questioning members about their roles

    d. Teaching explicitly about role responses and role choices

13. Completing gaps in communication and interpreting messages

    a. Clarifying the content and relationship aspects of messages

    b. Separating comments about the self from comments about others

    c. Pointing out significant discrepancies, incongruities, or double-level messages

    d. Spelling out nonverbal communication

Structured Family Tasks and Therapeutic Techniques Structured family tasks are used for joint assessment and intervention purposes. They provide historical data and, in some cases, relate the data to present behavior. They offer family members the opportunity to collaborate actively in changing the family system.

SCULPTING Sculpting is a technique in which a client builds a living sculpture, based on his or her perceptions. Family members physically place one another in locations or positions that best represent their perceptions of one another. This live family portrait has the advantage of condensing and projecting into a visual picture the essence of one member's experience in the family (Papp, Silverstein, and Carter 1973, p. 197). Triangles, alliances, and conflicts are choreographed and thus made available for analysis. This often reveals hidden aspects of the family's inner life.

FAMILY ALBUM PHOTOSTUDY Rae Sedgwick (1978) suggests photostudy of the family album as a means of providing tangible, longitudinal evidence to raise questions, validate or invalidate hunches, and developmentally examine the individual and the family. Sedgwick suggests that the family picture album is one of the most obvious, and most overlooked, tools for understanding family dynamics. The photographs and the

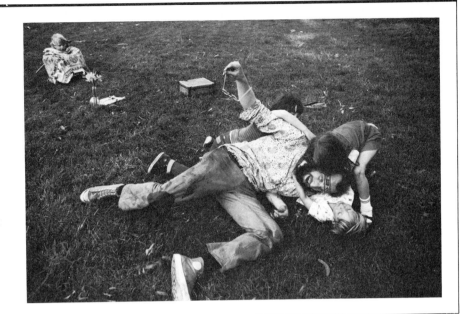

In this family sculpture, the child at the left has choreographed her sense of isolation from her father and siblings.

process of selecting them give insights into decision making, themes, interaction patterns, patterns of development, and power and influence relationships within the family. The therapist and family discuss and analyze the photographs together.

Other interesting family tasks suggested by Sedgwick (1976) include: writing a family autobiography; comparing and contrasting family members with one another and with selected families from the neighborhood, the school, or the church; drawing a family picture; writing a family news article or a family epitaph; dispelling a family myth; weaving a family dream; or writing a family play. Such tools are helpful in examining histories, prophecies, scripts, and myths. They are limited only by the imagination and ingenuity of the therapist.

ROLE PLAYING, GAMES, AND SIMULATED FAMILY EXPERIENCES In her practice, Virginia Satir (1967) uses role playing with families. The simulated family experience is used to teach families about themselves. Family members may simulate each other's behavior or their conceptions of it. They may also play themselves in a simulated situation. Videotape feedback helps family members become acquainted with their own behavior. In addition, systems games and communication games (Satir 1967, pp. 187–88) are used to help families communicate more effectively and congruently. These role-playing experiences are also effective educational tools in the preparation of family therapists.

CRITERIA FOR TERMINATING TREATMENT

Satir (1967, p. 176) has developed criteria for determining when to terminate family therapy. Termination is appropriate when family members can

- Complete transactions, check, and ask
- Interpret hostility
- See how others see them
- Tell one another how they appear
- Tell one another their hopes, fears, and expectations
- Disagree
- Make choices
- Learn through practice
- Free them from harmful influences of past models
- Give clear messages

THE NURSING PROCESS IN FAMILY COUNSELING

The following case study of the Wilson family (Black, 1982) demonstrates a humanistic psychiatric nursing approach to family counseling. It shows how a nurse applied an understanding of family process and dynamics (elaborated on in this chapter) and used the covert rehearsal phase of the symbolic interaction model (illustrated in Figure 6–7) and general communication principles (Chapter 6) along with principles of relationship building (Chapter 7). When you read it keep in mind the nursing process components (Chapter 4).

CASE EXAMPLE:
JOHN DAVID AND THE WILSON FAMILY*

John, a graduate student in psychiatric-mental health nursing, is assigned to work with the Wilson family during his final clinical placement. The arrangement is made by his instructor in cooperation with the family clinic of the local community mental health center. The family is selected by the staff team that John has joined as a member. The team includes a social worker, a psychiatrist, a psychologist, and a clinical nurse specialist. On each of his clinical days, John attends the daily team meeting in which the group shares their progress in working with their families, exchanges insights, and provides each other with mutual support as family problems are worked through. John's instructor attends several of the meetings on John's clinical days.

The intake report provides the team with information on which to base John's assignment. Mr. and Mrs. Wilson applied to the center as a result of a referral made by a local police official. Ross Wilson, their ten-year-old son, had been brought home by an officer following his fifth runaway episode in as many weeks.

At the request of the team, the intake worker makes a first appointment for John to meet with Ross and his parents at the center. Ross's younger brother and sister are left at home with their aunt. They can be expected to share in the benefits resulting from favorable behavioral and role changes brought about in a significant part of the family system. The assignment of this particular family to John is made mainly because the dysfunction seems to be of recent origin and essentially located within the triangle formed by Ross and his parents. This limits the complexity of the interrelationships that John will be called on to deal with.

Initiating the Relationship

John prepares himself for his first interview with the family by engaging in an inner rehearsal. He anticipates that the parents will be anxious and embarrassed at having to explain their problem to yet another stranger. Their anxiety will be compounded by the prospect of being required to incorporate an outsider into the family's functional system. This, John reasons, might be offset to

From Black, K., Short-term Counseling: A Humanistic Approach for the Helping Professions, pp. 200–205. Copyright © 1983 by Addison-Wesley Publishing Co., Inc., Menlo Park, Calif.

some extent by the fact that a state of psychologic crisis tends to create an unusual openness in its victims to accepting outside help.

John sees his immediate task as twofold: (a) to build the foundation of a relationship of mutual trust with the client family and (b) to work with them in defining the problem or problems that precipitated the present family crisis. Recognizing that his sensitivity to his clients' feelings will enable him to express genuine concern and a sincere desire to help, he also determines to keep the meetings family centered throughout. He plans to clarify his own role as catalytic but peripheral to the family's identification and implementation of new methods of coping. By these measures he hopes to reinforce the family's potential to function as a complete, interdependent system of mutual support.

Ross proves, on acquaintance, to be the least self-conscious of any in the group. He is an outgoing child, not overtly concerned about his problem behavior, but obviously eager to please his parents in other ways. When John issues a general invitation to all three to fill him in on the details of the problem that brought them to the center, all three participate about equally in the response. The parents tell of their worry over what might happen to Ross during his absence from home. Ross speaks sheepishly, but with a touch of pride, about having been repeatedly picked up in various public places by uniformed police officers late at night. John reflects the parental concern as inevitable under the circumstances, then to Ross his fascination with the police uniform.

Ross responds boastfully that his father also has a uniform and drives a truck. This leads to a description of the family's general lifestyle and, from that, to the particular events connected with the runaway episodes. The remainder of the first meeting and most of the next is taken up with the family's story. At first, John keeps it moving comfortably with only an occasional continuing response.

It develops that Mr. Wilson, who is employed to drive locally for a department store, is becoming increasingly discontent with the duties the job entails. At this point in the narrative, he and Mrs. Wilson engage in an argument that is a replay of one that, they admit, frequently breaks out at home. The husband says that he wants to transfer to a long-distance assignment, whereupon his wife complains to John that her husband's transfer would leave her with night and day responsibility for the home and family much of the time. Also addressing John, Mr. Wilson raises his voice in angry frustration at not being given an opportunity to explain how much better off the family would be if he could only take a better-paying job.

Mindful of the principles he has studied, John is alert to the danger of being triangled into the family conflict. He relects Mrs. Wilson's apprehension directly to her and

Mr. Wilson's anger to him, and he gently calls their attention to the fact that they are reliving feelings aroused in the past in the midst of the group's present information-gathering task.

With only an occasional outburst centering on the same theme, the sequence of events that typically precedes and follows Ross's leaving home is elicited as follows:

1. The argument about Mr. Wilson's proposed transfer begins in the course of a work-day evening meal.

2. Mr. Wilson shouts in frustration; Mrs. Wilson voices her fears and finally leaves the room in tears with the two younger children to put them to bed.

3. Ross remains with his father, who tells him of the joys of long-distance trucking.

4. On returning, Mrs. Wilson scolds Ross and her husband for lack of consideration for her and sends Ross to do his homework.

5. Mr. and Mrs. Wilson are uncommunicative with each other and with Ross for the next day or two.

6. One evening soon after, Mrs. Wilson prepares her husband's favorite dishes for supper. When Ross is again banished to do his homework, it is obvious to him that his parents are averse to having him present during their reconciliation.

7. Ross wanders off instead of going to school the next morning.

8. The police bring him home late in the evening.

9. His mother cries and scolds Ross, his father whips him with a belt, and he is sent to bed without any supper.

10. At supper the next evening, Mr. Wilson casually asks Ross where he went and what happened on the day that he missed school. He listens to the account with interest. Mrs. Wilson does not participate and, before long, suggests that Mr. Wilson would probably like to run away from the family too.

The argument about the transfer begins again.

John recognizes that Ross, without being fully aware of it, picks up the metacommunicative approval and empathy in his father's questions about his escapades and identifies with his father's desire to see new places. Although Mrs. Wilson has come close to recognizing the command aspect of her husband's transactions, her feedback conveys criticism rather than understanding. With John's help, the three family members are able—the parents grudgingly at first—to identify the meanings that are thinly covered in their pattern of interaction.

Team discussion corroborates John's opinion that the family pattern currently displays a typically dysfunctional family triangle: a repetitive cycle of conflict, distance, and closeness; scapegoating to a minor degree; and the feedback cycle that Weakland describes. These insights

are not communicated to the family. The team is in agreement that the maladaptive pattern will be broken up and reassembled as family members move to assume the group task of defining their goals and accepting responsibility for each other in a unified effort at planning and implementation.

Assessment and Planning

At his third meeting with the family, it is evident to John that Mr. and Mrs. Wilson have done some homework between meetings. Mr. Wilson announces that, although Ross's running away from home is in no way excusable, he and his wife feel that their quarreling has made the child's home too hellish at times for him to want to stay there. Mrs. Wilson adds that the two younger children have been unusually fractious in the worrisome home atmosphere. She perceives her own impatience as both causing and resulting from the family's general state of disorder. Not to be outdone, Mr. Wilson says then that because his job is his own responsibility, he will see what he can do about it without bothering anyone else.

John observes, while Mr. Wilson is speaking, that Mrs. Wilson is becoming flushed and Ross is beginning to squirm. John briefly reinforces the starts the parents have made toward defining their feelings about their present situation. He then points out in matter-of-fact terms the body language he noted, and he makes the connection between it and Mr. Wilson's statement about solving a significant family problem alone. Mrs. Wilson says emphatically that the problem concerns all of them and that she would like to have some say in how it is solved. Her husband concedes that she has that right, and they begin to discuss the pros and cons of the transfer.

This time, the parents address one another rather than attempting to involve John. Their argument is less heated than at the previous meeting. When they tend to move to positions at extreme ends of the issue, John helps them identify gray areas and calls attention to connections between judgmental opposites. Tendencies to blame or to dwell on the past are diverted into making plans to cope with present and foreseeable circumstances.

Ross's first attempt to contribute to the discussion is disregarded until John breaks in to reflect its underlying feeling. It shows that the boy is beginning to identify more evenly now and is trying to find ways of supporting his mother's point of view as well as his father's. John's response, although directed to Ross, serves to remind the parents that Ross's feelings are a significant factor in the problem as a whole. Thereafter they try, sometimes with John's help, to integrate Ross's comments into their overall assessment.

During the remainder of this meeting and the next, the family group is involved in action planning that is divided between the improvement of family relationships and a solution to the question of Mr. Wilson's transfer. The problem of Mrs. Wilson being left to cope alone while her husband is out of town brings a response from Ross that signifies that, as the man of the house, he is quite able to protect her. It also leads to an assessment of resources outside the immediate family. Grandparents, an uncle, and two aunts who live nearby are identified as being closely concerned with the family's welfare. The parents admit that the relatives' interest in the children has recently been neglected.

As discussion proceeds, John continues to be aware of the importance of modeling clear and accurate communication in his own statements. He also gives and elicits feedback when necessary to clarify the contributions of the other three participants. Generalizations that the parents tend to make on the basis of untested assumptions are exposed and called into question, and interdependent, supportive interactions are strongly reinforced. Frequent summary evaluations of progress serve to reassure, as well as reinforce, the family as an effectively functioning unit.

Implementation

By the fifth meeting, a compromise plan has been reached on the question of the transfer. Implementation of the plan is clearly a family responsibility. The family agrees that Mr. Wilson will postpone making a change until both of the younger children attend school for a full-day session. Mrs. Wilson feels that she will be better able to cope with intercurrent difficulties when they are in someone else's care for a few hours a day. Mr. and Mrs. Wilson resolve to keep in closer touch with the relatives on whom Mrs. Wilson can depend for moral support. Ross promises to stay near his home and to spend some of his free time each day with the younger children.

Evaluation and Termination

John is able to utilize evaluation both as an ongoing impetus to the process of intervention and as a learning experience for himself. The three Wilsons soon participate with pleasure in the reviews, which highlight the steps of their progress in family collaboration as well as in problem solving. At staff team meetings, John reports each day's interaction with as much verbatim content as he can remember, and he joins the other team members in an evaluative exchange of questions, interpretations, and suggestions.

The team discusses the matter of termination midway in the series of six meetings. Progress to date gives every indication that the family will soon be functioning at a somewhat higher level than they achieved before lapsing into dysfunction. The shared predicton is that, if they agree to termination by the sixth meeting, it will be effected at that point without referral or planned followup.

Much of the fifth meeting is taken up by the members of the now-functional triangle in telling John how well

things are going at home. John periodically expresses his observation of their sensitivity to each other's feelings and their supportiveness of one another. As the meeting ends, he indicates that they are now working together so effectively that there is little need for any help he can give. They assent willingly to his suggestion that the sixth meeting be the last and that it be used as a general windup. When his mother remarks that the children's aunt will be relieved to hear that her babysitting chore is nearly over, Ross suggests that the other two children come along for the last meeting so that John can meet them.

With the two children aged five and six present, the sixth meeting turns out to be a little boisterous. John notes that Ross now identifies with his parents in monitoring the behavior of the younger children in keeping with his parents' commands. When he takes the others to explore a courtyard that can be seen from the window of the meeting room, the parents thank John for all his help, saying that they wish they had known sooner of the work of the family clinic. John uses this opportunity to reinforce their consciousness of new-found strength in their unified approach to problems, adding that there are sure to be more problems as time goes on. He assures them of the continuing availability of the clinic as a community resource. Ross proffers a gruff thank you when the children gather to add their farewells to those of their parents.

FAMILY-ORIENTED PREVENTIVE PSYCHIATRY PROGRAMS

According to William M. Bolman (1972), since the family is the most strategic social unit, preventive psychiatric services should be oriented toward it. Table 21–1 identifies primary, secondary, and tertiary prevention approaches that may be used to provide for family mental health.

COUPLES THERAPY

Couples therapy is the more contemporary term for what used to be known as *marital therapy*. The later term acknowledges the existence of interactional dyads not necessarily based on marriage. Couples may seek counseling when difficulties between the couple are specific to their relationship.

Table 21-1   PREVENTIVE APPROACHES FOR FAMILY MENTAL HEALTH

Target Population	Goals	General Approach	Specific Examples
1. Families in crisis due to the loss of a member (death, desertion, chronic hospitalization).	Provision of flexible support according to the event, how perceived and managed, and the resources and the life-style of the surviving family fragment.	Primary and secondary preventive, high-risk and communitywide approaches.	Group meetings in hospital of parents of fatally ill children; expanded emergency room coverage; neighborhood information centers; walk-in clinics for problems of living; some mental health clinics.
2. Families under stress due to a handicapped parent (mental illness, retardation, alcoholism, or other chronic disorder).	Identification and support as needed for these families as in 1, above.	Primary and secondary preventive, high-risk approaches for children; tertiary preventive, communitywide approaches for parents.	Public health nurse makes regular home visits to family of alcoholic; family medical clinics; mental-hospital-based services; homemaker services for mentally ill mothers.
3. Families under stress due to internal imbalance or disorder (schism, double bind, skew, pseudomutuality, and other types of marital discord).	Assistance either in correcting the imbalance or in minimizing the impact on the children.	Primary or secondary preventive, high-risk approaches for children; secondary or tertiary preventive, communitywide approaches for parents.	Marital counseling; family therapy, parents' groups, individual therapy; legal guardian ad litem for children in divorce actions; legal aid for low-income families through neighborhood law offices.
4. Families under stress as a result of vulnerability to normal developmental changes (birth of a child, school entry, puberty, climacteric, retirement).	Sensitivity to the variety of family stresses or crises that may result, leading to earlier recognition and intervention as needed, often via very short-term crisis-oriented therapy.	Primary and secondary preventive, high-risk, communitywide, and milestone approaches.	Many of the above programs, especially neighborhood and/or comprehensive health, mental health, and social welfare services. Awareness of the opportunities for stress and crisis assistance is more important than the specific program setting.
5. Families living in areas lacking necessary biopsychosocial supplies (police protection, housing, quality education, etc.), in areas such as urban slums, depressed rural areas, migrant workers' camps, Indian reservations, and housing projects.	Provision of these basic necessities through community development approaches.	Primary, secondary, and tertiary preventive, high-risk approaches.	Community development approaches originating through schools, churches, social agencies, neighborhood service centers, family life educators, mental health centers, etc.

Table continues on next page

		Table 21–1 continued		
Target Population	**Goals**	**General Approach**	**Specific Examples**
6. Families caught in the cycle of intergenerational poverty.	Provision of multiple and flexible opportunities for attaining desired personal, social, and economic goals.	Primary, secondary, and tertiary preventive, high-risk approaches.	Same as in 5; also a variety of antipoverty programs, such as Headstart, Upward Bound, and Job Corps, and agencies such as Mobilization for Youth, and Community Progress, Inc.
7. Disorganized families characterized by multiple and complex problems (emotional disorder, social dependence, poverty, chronic physical illness, child neglect or abuse, alcoholism and other addictions) and multiple needs (personal, social, medical, economic).	Use of a problem-centered versus a discipline-centered approach to diagnose the total range of causative factors, identify those most accessible to change, and plan a step-by-step program.	Primary, secondary, and tertiary preventive, high-risk approaches for adults and children.	All programs in this section may be relevant. Again, the point of view or approach is more important than the program. Several additional possibilities include twenty-four-hour emergency homemakers, and other emergency care for children needing substitute parenting.
8. Families with potentially stressful role handicaps (childlessness, adoptive parenthood, foster-parenting, working mothers, and student families, such as medical and other graduate students).	Awareness of the potential for stress or crisis so that early recognition and supportive help are available.	Secondary preventive, high-risk, and communitywide approaches.	Groups for adoptive or foster parents, groups for adoptive children; reliable day care centers.

Source: W. M. Bolman, ''Preventive Psychiatry for the Family: Theory, Approaches, and Programs,'' *American Journal of Psychiatry* 125 (1968): 464–65. Copyright 1968, the American Psychiatric Association. Reprinted by permission.

Developmental Tasks Confronting Couples

Ellen M. Berman and Harold I. Lief (1975) have added to Erik Erikson's theory of psychosocial development (see Chapter 10) by identifying adult developmental tasks and stages as they relate to the marital life cycle. Their tasks for each stage are outlined in Table 21–2.

Types of Therapy

There are basically four types of therapy for couples. *Collaborative therapy* is individual therapy for each

partner by two therapists. *Concurrent therapy* is individual therapy for each partner by the same therapist. Neither one is truly *couples* therapy. Both fit into the one-to-one mode. *Conjoint therapy* occurs when the couple is seen together by a single therapist or by cotherapists. Male and female cotherapists are particularly effective as models in conjoint therapy. *Couples group therapy* is group therapy engaged in by several couples who meet with a therapist or cotherapists. The latter two modes can be more appropriately termed couples therapy.

Table 21-2 TASKS AND STAGES IN THE MARITAL LIFE CYCLE		
Stage	**Age**	**Tasks**
I	Eighteen to twenty-one	Pulling up roots; developing autonomy; shifting commitment from family of origin to a new relationship; testing power and intimacy; experiencing conflicts over in-laws; fragile marital boundaries are threatened.
II	Twenty-two to twenty-eight	Developing intimacy and occupational identification; stresses over parenthood and uncertainty about choice of marital partner; intimacy is deepening but ambivalent; patterns of conflict resolution over power issues are established; work, friends, and potential lovers challenge the marital boundaries.
III	Twenty-nine to thirty-one	Restlessness; conflicts about work versus marriage, parenthood, and increasing distance from partner; reevaluation; partners vie for power and dominance; compensatory "fortress-building" or extramarital involvement.
IV	Thirty-two to thirty-nine	Settling down; deepening commitments; long-range goals established; conflicts over productivity of partners; boundaries closed, as dominance and decision-making patterns and powers are firmly established.
V	Forty to forty-two	Mid-life transition; search for a "fit" between aspirations and reality; past is reviewed and new future goals are established; conflicts over individual success, staying in the marriage; increased fantasies about other relationships.
VI	Forty-three to fifty-nine	Restabilization and reordering of priorities; "empty nest" syndrome appears; intimacy with partners changes; boundaries are fixed.
VII	Sixty and over	Aging, illness, and death must be dealt with; marital conflicts and fears center on loneliness and sexual failure; stable plateau of intimacy; marital boundaries solidify; physical environment is critical for maintaining ties with the outside world.

Source: Compiled from E. M. Berman and H. I. Lief, "Marital Therapy from a Psychiatric Perspective: An Overview," *American Journal of Psychiatry* 6 (1975): 583–592.

Focus of Therapy

Couples therapy focuses on the relationship between the individuals and the similarities and differences between them that comprise the rules (Jackson 1965) on which the relationship is based. Norman Sheresky and Marya Mannes suggest in a radical guide to wedlock (1972) that partners explore the rules together *before* marriage occurs. These authors urge that marriage vows be written in the form of a legal contract and that rules be made in the open before trouble occurs.

The following is an example of a premarital contract from their work (1972, pp. 36–37):

ARTICLE III
Future Expectations

(a) Donald and Ina have discussed fully where they propose to reside during the course of their marriage. They agree that considerations relating to the location of their respective families should play no part in such determination. They agree their primary consideration shall be proximity to Donald's place of business. That factor should govern regardless of where Ina may be employed and regardless of whose earnings are greater.

(b) Neither party to this Memorandum holds any formal religious beliefs that should in any way interfere with the marriage. Neither insists on, or has even expressed any preference concerning, the other's adherence to any particular religious belief. Neither will, without the consent of the other, impose any religious belief upon any children of the marriage.

(c) It is the parties' present intention that Ina continue to work, health permitting, until such time as she may become pregnant. The parties have no exact intentions concerning the employment of Ina after the birth of any child or children, although Ina has expressed the feeling that simply caring for children would not be sufficiently stimulating to her. Donald's inclination at the present time is that he would prefer for Ina to discontinue any full-time employment if she had a child, but he would not insist upon it.

Both parties agree that any subsequent employment of Ina after the birth of a child should be such that it would permit her to spend reasonable periods of time with the child and that it should not entail any evening or weekend hours.

Sheresky and Mannes contend that such a marriage contract would go a long way toward preventing certain unsuccessful marriages and the resulting crisis of divorce.

KEY NURSING CONCEPTS

✔ The family is the context in which people develop their first relationships with others. How one views the world is molded by the events that happen within the family.

✔ Family forms in the United States are changing and becoming more diverse; a wide variety of family constellations exists in contemporary society.

✔ The family can be viewed as a system in terms of the relationships, associations, and connections that occur in a dynamic, interacting whole.

✔ The family system includes not only family members but their relationships, communications, and interactions with the environment.

✔ A change or movement in any part of the family system affects all other parts of the family system.

✔ The family seeks to maintain a dynamic balance, or "homeostasis," among various forces that operate within and upon it.

✔ Just as individuals and groups are confronted with developmental tasks, so are families.

✔ The functional family is distinguished from the dysfunctional one by the amount and quality of energy used to maintain the family system and to achieve the developmental tasks.

✔ Family therapists believe that emotional symptoms or problems of an individual are an expression of emotional symptoms or problems in a family. In family therapy work, the family system is the unit of treatment.

✔ Nurses work with families and family problems in many settings. In order to function as a family therapist, the psychiatric nurse needs graduate level preparation.

✔ Specific relational and communicational intricacies occur and affect the functioning of the family and its members. These include life scripts; family myths, life-styles, and themes; coalitions, dyads, and triangles; pseudomutuality and pseudohostility; marital schism and skew; enmeshment and disengagement; scapegoating; and double-binds.

✔ Contemporary approaches to family therapy include the integrative approach, psychoanalytic approach, Bowen approach, structural approach, interactional approach, social network approach, and the behavioral approach.

✔ The milieu for family therapy often is the family's own home.

✔ Major components of family therapy include assessment, contract negotiation, and intervention.

✔ It is best for all family members to participate in the assessment phase of family therapy.

✔ The family therapist may use structured family tasks and therapeutic strategies for both assessment and intervention.

✔ The family therapist helps family members look at themselves in the here-and-now and recognize the influence of past models on their behavior and expectations.

✔ Preventive approaches toward attaining or maintaining mental health should be oriented toward the family as the basic social unit.

✔ Couples therapy may be instituted when difficulties between a couple are assessed to be specific to their relationship.

References

Ackerman, N. W. *The Psychodynamics of Family Life.* New York: Basic Books, 1958.

———. "Prejudicial Scapegoating and Neutralizing Forces in the Family Group with Special Reference to the Role 'Family Healer.'" In *Theory and Practice of Family Psychiatry*, edited by J. G. Howells, pp. 626–634. New York: Brunner/Mazel, 1971.

Bateson, G.; Jackson, D. D.; Haley, J.; and Weakland, J. H. "Toward a Theory of Schizophrenia." *Behavioral Science* 1 (1956): 251–264.

Berman, E. M., and Lief, H. I. "Marital Therapy from a Psychiatric Perspective: An Overview." *American Journal of Psychiatry* 6 (1975): 583–592.

Black, K. *Short-term Counseling: A Humanistic Approach for the Helping Professions.* Menlo Park, Calif.: Addison-Wesley, 1983.

Bolman, W. M. "Preventive Psychiatry for the Family: Theory, Approaches, and Programs." In *Family Therapy*, edited by G. D. Erickson and T. P. Hogan, pp. 377–401. Monterey, Calif.: Brooks/Cole, 1972.

Boszormenyi-Nagy, I., and Framo, J., eds. *Intensive Family Therapy.* New York: Harper and Row, 1965.

Bowen, M. "A Family Concept of Schizophrenia." In *The Etiology of Schizophrenia*, edited by D. D. Jackson, pp. 346–372. New York: Basic Books, 1960.

Bowen, M. *Family Therapy in Clinical Practice.* New York: Jason Aronson, 1978.

Caplow, T. *Two against One: Coalitions in Triads.* Englewood Cliffs, N.J.: Prentice-Hall, 1968.

Compton, B. R., and Galaway, B. *Social Work Processes.* 2d ed. Homewood, Ill.: Dorsey Press, 1979.

Deutsch, D. "Family Therapy and Family Life Style." *Journal of Individual Psychology* 23 (1967): 217–223.

Duvall, E. *Family Development.* Philadelphia: J. B. Lippincott, 1971.

Ferreira, A. J. "Family Myth and Homeostasis." *Archives of General Psychiatry* 9 (1963): 457–463.

Greenburg, D. *How to Be a Jewish Mother.* Los Angeles: Price, Sloan, and Stern, 1964.

Grunebaum, H. U. *The Practice of Community Mental Health.* Boston: Little, Brown, 1970.

Haley, J. "Whither Family Therapy?" *Family Process* 1 (1962): 69–100.

———. *Problem Solving Therapy.* San Francisco: Jossey-Bass, 1976.

———, ed. *Changing Families: A Family Therapy Reader.* New York: Grune and Stratton, 1971.

Hess, R. D., and Handel, G. *Family Worlds: A Psychosocial Approach to Family Life.* Chicago: University of Chicago Press, 1959.

———. "The Family as a Psychosocial Orientation." In *The Psychosocial Interior of the Family*, edited by G. Handel, pp. 10–24. Chicago: Aldine Publishing, 1967.

Jackson, D. D. "The Question of Family Homeostasis." *Psychiatric Quarterly Supplement*, part 1 (1957): 79–90.

———. "Family Rules: Marital Quid Pro Quo." *Archives of General Psychiatry* 12 (1965): 589–594.

———, ed. *Communication, Family, and Marriage.* Palo Alto, Calif.: Science and Behavior Books, 1968. (a)

———, ed. *Therapy, Communication, and Change.* Palo Alto, Calif.: Science and Behavior Books, 1968. (b)

Johnson-Soderberg, S. "Theory and Practice of Scapegoating." *Perspectives in Psychiatric Care* 15 (1977): 154–159.

Jones, S. L. "The Double Bind as a 'Tested' Theoretical Formulation." *Perspectives in Psychiatric Care* 15 (1977): 162–169.

———. *Family Therapy: A Comparison of Approaches.* Bowie, Md.: Robert J. Brady, 1980.

Laing, R.D. *The Politics of the Family.* New York: Vintage Books, 1972.

Levine, J. A. "Real Kids vs. 'The Average' Family," *Psychology Today*, June 1978, pp. 14–15.

Lidz, T.; Cornelison, A. R.; and Terry, D. "The Intrafamilial Environment of the Schizophrenic Patient: Marital Schism and Marital Skew." *American Journal of Psychiatry* 114 (1957): 241–248.

Lidz, T.; Cornelison, A.; Terry, D.; and Fleck, S. "Intrafamilial Environment of the Schizophrenic Patient, VI, The Transmission of Irrationality." *Archives of Neurology and Psychiatry* 79 (1958): 305–316.

Lidz, T.; Fleck, S.; and Cornelison, A. *Schizophrenia and the Family.* New York: International Universities Press, 1966.

Lindsey, K. *Friends or Family.* New York: Beacon Press, 1982.

Minuchin, S. *Families and Family Therapy.* Cambridge, Mass.: Harvard University Press, 1974.

Papp, P.; Silverstein, O.; and Carter, E. "Family Sculpting in Preventive Work with 'Well Families.'" *Family Process* 12 (1973): 194–204.

Patterson, G. *Living With Children: New Methods for Parents and Teachers.* Champaign, Ill.: Research Press, 1976.

Saluter, A. S. *Marital Status and Living Arrangements: March 1980.* U.S. Census Bureau, 1981.

Satir, V. *Conjoint Family Therapy.* Rev. ed. Palo Alto, Calif.: Science and Behavior Books, 1967.

————. *Peoplemaking.* Palo Alto, Calif.: Science and Behavior Books, 1972.

Satir, V.; Stackowiak, J.; and Taschman, H. *Helping Families to Change.* New York: Jason Aronson, 1975.

Schuham, A. I. "The Double-Bind Hypothesis a Decade Later." *Psychological Bulletin* 68 (1967): 409–416.

Sedgwick, R. "Family Mental Health: A Sociopsychological Approach." In *Current Perspectives in Psychiatric Nursing: Issues and Trends,* vol. 1, edited by C. R. Kneisl and H. S. Wilson, pp. 190–200. St. Louis: C. V. Mosby, 1976.

————. "Photostudy as a Diagnostic Tool in Working with Families." In *Current Perspectives in Psychiatric Nursing: Issues and Trends,* vol. 2, edited by C. R. Kneisl and H. S. Wilson, pp. 60–69. St. Louis: C. V. Mosby, 1978.

Sheresky, N., and Mannes, M. *Uncoupling: The Art of Coming Apart.* New York: Viking Press, 1972.

Speck, R. V. "Psychotherapy of the Social Network of a Schizophrenic Family." *Family Process* 6 (1967): 208–214.

Speck, R. V., and Attneave, L. *Family Networks.* New York: Pantheon Books, 1973.

Spiegel, J. P. "The Resolution of Role Conflict within the Family." In *The Patient and the Mental Hospital,* edited by M. Greenblatt; D. Levinson; and R. Williams, pp. 545–564. New York: Free Press, 1957.

Steiner, C. *Scripts People Live.* New York: Grove Press, 1974.

Toman, W. *Family Constellation.* 3d ed. New York: Springer Publishing, 1976.

Vogel, E. F., and Bell, N. W. "The Emotionally Disturbed Child as the Family Scapegoat." In *The Psychosocial Interior of the Family,* edited by G. Handel, pp. 424–442. Chicago: Aldine Publishing, 1967.

Watzlawick, P. "A Structured Family Interview." *Family Process* 5 (1966): 256–271.

Watzlawick, P.; Beavin, J. H.; and Jackson, D. D. *The Pragmatics of Human Communication.* New York: W. W. Norton, 1967.

Wilmot, W. W. *Dyadic Communication: A Transactional Perspective.* Reading, Mass.: Addison-Wesley, 1975.

Wynne, L.; Ryckoff, I. M.; Day, J.; and Hirsch, S. I. "Pseudo-mutuality in the Family Relationships of Schizophrenics." *Psychiatry* 21 (1958): 205–220.

Further Reading

Barry, M. P. "Feedback Concepts in Family Therapy." *Perspectives in Psychiatric Care* 7 (1969): 58–67.

Cain, A. "The Therapist's Role in Family Systems Therapy." *The Family* 3 (1976): 65–74.

Getty, C., and Humphreys, W., eds. *Perspectives on the Family: Stress and Change in American Family Life.* New York: Appleton-Century-Crofts, 1981.

Goldenberg, H., and Goldenberg, I. *Family Therapy: An Overview.* Monterey, Ca.: Brooks/Cole, 1980.

Grace, H. K., and Knafl, K. A. "Family Beginnings: The Dynamics of Role Making." In *Current Perspectives in Psychiatric Nursing: Issues and Trends,* vol. 1, edited by C. R. Kneisl and H. S. Wilson, pp. 176–189. St. Louis: C. V. Mosby, 1976.

Haller, L. L. "Family Systems Theory in Psychiatric Interventions." *American Journal of Nursing* 74 (1974): 462–463.

Knafl, K. A., and Grace, H. K. "Negotiative Processes in the First Year of Marriage." In *Current Perspectives in Psychiatric Nursing: Issues and Trends,* vol. 2, edited by C. R. Kneisl and H. S. Wilson, pp. 123–134. St. Louis: C. V. Mosby, 1978.

Lewis, J. M.; Beavers, W. R.; Gossett, J. T.; and Phillips, V. A. *No Single Thread: Psychological Health in Family Systems.* New York: Brunner/Mazel, 1976.

Mealey, A. R. "Sculpting as a Group Technique for Increasing Awareness." *Perspectives in Psychiatric Care* 15 (1977): 118–121.

Meister, S. B. "Charting a Family's Developmental Status: For Intervention and for the Record." *Maternal Child Nursing* (January–February 1977): 43–48.

Rogers, C. *Becoming Partners: Marriage and Its Alternatives.* New York: Dell Publishing, 1972.

Sedgwick, R. *Family Mental Health: Theory and Practice.* St. Louis: C. V. Mosby, 1981.

Skolnick, A., and Skolnick, J. H. *Family in Transition.* 3d. ed. Boston: Little, Brown, 1980.

Smoyak, S., ed. *The Psychiatric Nurse as a Family Therapist.* New York: John Wiley, 1975.

Weis, D. P. "Children's Interpretation of Marital Conflict." *Family Process* 13 (1974): 385–393.

22

Mental Health Counseling with the Aged

by Priscilla Ebersole

CHAPTER OUTLINE

Philosophical Perspective of Aging
Parameters of Old Age and Mental Health
Mental Health in Old Age
  Criteria for Mental Health in Old Age
Understanding the Aged
  Lifelong Habits and Strengths
  Physical and Neural Changes
  Needs of the Aged
  Developmental Tasks of Aging
  Nurses' Attitudes toward Aging
Stresses Characteristic of Aging
  Fear of Aging
  Loneliness
  Loss
  Meaninglessness
  Physical Deterioration
  Stigma
  Sexuality
  Relocation
  Abuse and Neglect
Reactions to Problems of Aging
  Disturbed Behaviors
  Disruptive Patterns
  Disintegrative Patterns
  Cognitive Function
Common Evidence of Psychic Distress
  Stress Anxiety

  Depression
  Substance Abuse
  Suicide
Family Reactions to the Psychically Distressed Aged
Intervention Strategies
  Family Support Therapy
  Individual Psychotherapy
  Brief Psychotherapy
  Crisis Intervention
  Psychotropic Drugs
  Group Work
  Family Support Groups
  Networking
  Confidants
  Reminiscing
  Supporting the Dying and the Grieving
Key Nursing Concepts

LEARNING OBJECTIVES

After reading this chapter, students should be able to

- Identify characteristics of normal aging
- Describe several areas significant to the emotional adaptation of the aged
- Describe several sources of emotional problems common to the aged

CHAPTER 22

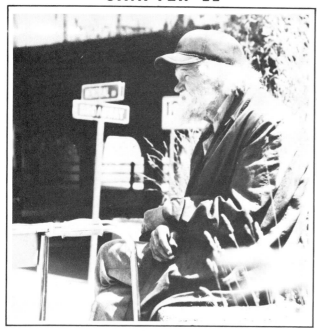

Percy Joe confronts us with our own aging. With elders like him we can reflect on the past, gain the beginnings of wisdom, and develop awareness of adaptability, courage, and humanity.

- Develop awareness of common reactions to problems of aging
- Identify evidence of psychic distress in the aged
- Identify specific therapeutic strategies of intervention useful in restoring the mental health of the aged
- Provide support to the aged experiencing disturbed, disruptive, or disintegrative reactions

PHILOSOPHICAL PERSPECTIVE OF AGING

The aged among us reflect the past and show us what we will become. Interactions with them can be mutually enriching, providing us with the beginnings of wisdom and giving them a sense of purpose. In less technological and media-oriented societies the aged have always been reservoirs of knowledge, and now they are especially needed for their understanding of adaptability, their courage, and their deeper awareness of humanity.

The psychiatric nurse will interact professionally most frequently with elders who have strained the limits of adaptability, and lost their sense of purpose and confidence in the meaning and value of living. Nowhere else in nursing is the impact of symbolic interac-

tionism so clear. The disturbed elderly reflect an internalized cultural devaluation of their place in society. The disruptive elderly are those who resist assignment to a junkyard of worn-out and discarded beings. Disintegrative patterns arise most frequently in the aged who are physiologically, socially, and psychologically frail. Their integrative capacities have broken down under long-term or intensely stressful situations. To work with them in a restorative, nurturing, or protective capacity is to confront our own aging. Some students are frightened, angered, or dismayed by the realization that they too are vulnerable to the passage of time and the inequities of life. This chapter is designed to offer insights and skills particularly helpful in the mental health counseling of the aged.

PARAMETERS OF OLD AGE AND MENTAL HEALTH

Young people find it hard to identify with old age and age avoidance may continue until even those who are 80 or more have been known to call themselves "middle-aged." In our culture old age seems to be equated with lack of social relevance or work force participation. Therefore, retirement from the work force at 65 has been the traditional transition to "old." If the retirement age rises, our definition of old may change. In our youthful, rapidly changing culture, old is bad; but we must remember that in traditional cultures old people are revered as keepers of the stability. All these factors must be considered when we decide who is old and why they may or may not adapt well to old age.

About 11½ percent of the people in the United States are over sixty-five. This percentage will steadily increase to a record number in 2020 when the children of the "baby boom" will comprise the aged population. Clearly the "problems of aging" will continue to demand more attention.

MENTAL HEALTH IN OLD AGE

Of the 100 million persons fifty years old and over, most receive medical attention, only a few receive mental health services, and even fewer have any intensive psychotherapy or counseling directed toward psychic conflict resolution and personality growth. Among the many reasons for this are:

- A generally negative attitude among professionals about the growth potential of those of fifty and over
- Federal funding limitations on mental health services
- The complexity of issues presented as emotional disorders of aging
- The pragmatic, stoic, or fatalistic attitudes of many aged persons
- The distrust of psychological schools of thought by those who grew up in the early Freudian era
- The great diversity of adaptation levels of the aged, which makes it difficult to delineate conclusive criteria indicative of mental health or mental illness

Criteria for Mental Health in Old Age

Mental health in old age is affected by a conglomerate of needs, relationships, attitudes, values, survival skills, and cohort expectations. Mental health cannot be measured by a few socially valued parameters of a given time and culture. We believe that mental health in old age is based on ability to fulfill appropriate roles, accept new challenges, adapt to losses and age-related changes, remain flexible, and interact with others in gratifying ways. Most old people do these things most of the time. This chapter is concerned with identifying, understanding, and helping those who do not.

UNDERSTANDING THE AGED

Lifelong Habits and Strengths

The aged are diverse and tend to become more unlike each other the older they become. Experience has shaped each of them in unique ways and their values, attitudes, and personality characteristics become more pronounced with age. Many of the aged say they feel much freer to be themselves than when they were younger. Their strength lies in their unique coping strategies. They are survivors and adapters, having lived through more fundamental changes in culture and technology than any previous generation on earth.

Physical and Neural Changes

Physiologically, the aged are less resilient and slower to recover homeostatic balance after interruptions. Body tolerances are decreased, and the margin of normal function narrows. Chronic problems predominate over acute illness processes. Major organs function less efficiently, so enzyme and hormone production is decreased. The kidneys, liver, and pancreas are about half as effective at seventy as they were at twenty. Pulmonary and cardiac capacity decreases depending on lifetime dietary, exercise, and smoking patterns. All older persons are less energetic than when they were young.

Due to the changes experienced in the aging process certain issues become very important to the maintenance of mental health. These are chiefly related to environmental and interpersonal negotiations. The gradual loss of sensorial efficiency may diminish the impact of events and the perceptual organization of environmental stimuli. Therefore, the aged function best in situations that are familiar and allow time for processing new events and expectations. There is a slow but consistent decline in sensory acuity after middle age, and auditory efficiency begins to deteriorate in young adulthood. Neurologic, psychologic and physiologic changes attributed to normal aging are usually compensated by life experience and self-awareness, so most old persons adapt very well when in an ego enhancing milieu. Clearly, territorial security and predictability enhance mental health and adaptation.

Needs of the Aged

Maslow's hierarchy of human needs is an extremely valuable guide for assessing the psychological reactions and adaptations of the aged. From the perspective of the symbolic interactionist, needs are indicated in Table 22–1.

Those unfamiliar with Maslow's need hierarchy may want to review this theory in Chapter 10. In mental health nursing, assessment of need deficiency assists in planning appropriate nursing interventions. Among the aged, disintegrative life patterns often emerge from se-

Table 22-1 NEEDS OF THE AGED		
Interactional Need	**Human Need**	**Personal Need**
Freedom from stereotyped expectations; support of individuality	Self-actualization	Values and commitment
Recognition; specific praise	Self-esteem	Valued roles in society
Sharing, love, intimacy	Belonging	Persons and groups of significance to the individual
Protection, nurturance	Safety and security	Environmental predictability
Information, reassurance, technical assistance	Basic biointegrity	Comfort and confidence in one's survival capacity

vere deprivation in any of the first four levels of needs. Figure 22–1 relates the nursing process to basic needs among the aged.

Developmental Tasks of Aging

Each stage of life encompasses certain tasks that must be accomplished in order to progress to the next stage. The last stages of life have not been studied as carefully or frequently as the earlier ones. Some research seems to emphasize only tasks of adaptation to losses, deprivations, illness, and death. While these are necessary adjustments, overemphasis may convey the notion that successful old age is only a time to withdraw gracefully from full living. Old age can be dynamic—a time to become fully oneself, experience uniqueness, and strive for individuality (Jung 1961). Internal experiences, dreams, fantasies, and memories are increasingly important as sources of understanding and enrichment. Social interaction, recognition, and status are filtered and modified by a strong sense of self and personal integrity.

Peck (1968) has used Erikson's (1963) criterion of integrity versus despair as the basis for identifying three subsidiary late life tasks:

1. Establishing body transcendence for body preoccupation
2. Establishing ego identity for work role preoccupation
3. Establishing ego transcendence for ego preoccupation

These three tasks are listed in order of accomplishment; that is, one must progress beyond body fixation

and ego fixation before mortality can be placed in the perspective of the human condition as an avenue of transcendence.

Body Transcendence   Body preoccupation is necessary when we are ill, and monitoring our body functions helps us maintain good health, but constant hypochondriacal focus on the body is a self-defeating activity because it leads to increasing self-absorption and repels the very attention it is meant to attract. Nurses will listen to much hypochondriacal complaining from the disturbed elderly, and they must allow time for this stage in a developing relationship. It may be the only means of relating available to the client for a time. When this occurs, the nurse will:

- Recognize the underlying need for attention
- Attend to the total individual rather than the "organ recital"
- Help the client identify times and patterns of body preoccupation
- Explore unmet needs
- Help the client understand the connection between unmet needs and hypochondriacal reactions

Body transcendence will develop as confidence returns.

Ego Identity   The next task involves helping clients view their existence as comprised of more than the many roles they have occupied. Roles are social constructs with certain expectations related to the maintenance of social structure and order. To the degree that the aged are seen as unimportant in a society they will find no substantial, positive roles. The role of spouse

PROBLEMS	SYMPTOMS		NEEDS	INTERVENTIONS
Social clocks Self-fulfilling prophesies Routinized life	Apathy Rigidity Boredom Ennui	Self- actualization	Self-expression New situations Self-transcendence Stimulation	Creative pursuits Meditation Reflection Fantasy Teaching / learning Relaxation
Social devaluation Lack of role Meaninglessness Little autonomy	Delusions Paranoia Depression Anger Indecisiveness	Self-esteem	Control Success To be needed	Reminiscing Control of money Activate latent interests Allowed to help others Identify legacy
Displacement Losses	Depression Hallucinations Alienation Loneliness	Belonging	Territory Friends Family Group affiliation Philosophy Confidante	Significant objects Pets, plants Soap opera families Touch group participation Listening Fictive kin
Sensory losses Limited mobility Translocation	Illusions Hallucinations Confusion Compulsions Obsessions Fear / anxiety	Safety and security	Safe environment Sensory accoutrements Mobility	Familiar routines Spaced stimulation Explanations Environmental cues
Homeostatic resilience Poor nutrition Medications Income Subclinical disease (Birren) Pain	Confusion Depression Fear Anxiety Disorientation	Biologic integrity	Food Shelter Sex Rest Body integrity Comfort	Adequate resources Knowledge of medications Conservation of energy Napping Small, frequent meals Choice of food

Figure 22–1

Nursing process and Malsow's hierarchy of needs among the aged. (Adapted from Priscilla Ebersole and Patricia Hess, *Toward Healthy Aging.* St. Louis: C. V. Mosby, 1981.)

will disappear, the role of parent or grandparent will lose its importance, and the role of worker or homemaker may no longer be possible or may become less meaningful. In American society old people usually hold the roles of major health care consumers and recipients of social services. These are both passive roles and don't contribute much to the ego identity of the aged.

Lacking relevant role models or cultural expectations, and, thanks to technology, living longer than they had planned or even wished to, old people may find themselves sinking into apathetic disengagement. The disengagement theory (Cummings and Henry 1961) that caused such a furor among gerontologists was based on a functional assessment and the belief that while society naturally excluded the aged from a meaningful role, the aged simultaneously withdrew from active involvement. Both of these moves were judged natural and mutually desirable.

What norms and expectations have we for a 94-year-old man? What does he expect of himself? What are the developmental tasks by which we measure his adaptational success? These questions are not easily answered. If he is one of the elite, exceptionally healthy, witty, and intelligent, he is viewed as an anomaly. If his body and his wits have been eroded by time, he is generally considered a nuisance. If he depends on others for survival services, he is a "case" or a "problem." To his family he may be a worry or an excessive drain on their time and energy. What social contribution validates his existence and earns approval and approbation? Often he receives approval for what he does not do rather than what he does. Successful social adaptation may be viewed as not complaining, not demanding, not expecting, not seeking, not drinking, not becoming disorganized or disoriented.

New, active, nonwork roles must be sought and cultivated by and for the aged. What are their dreams, hopes, attitudes, values, and fantasies? How do they describe themselves? What do they enjoy doing? What philosophies sustain them? Who are their heroes or heroines? What traditions give their lives meaning? With time to explore the inner self, an old person can become aware of being much more than a bookkeeper, a homemaker, a wife, a lawyer, or whatever role was habitually used as a basis for self-definition and evaluation. A nurse may ask older clients to list all their roles and all the things they do that are unrelated to their defined roles. The Johari Window exercise is another method for focusing on the total self. (See Chapter 3.) Those with special skills may have the role of consultant, counselor, teacher, or leader. But since the aged have managed to survive longer than others, their most important role may be to socialize youth to old age, just as parents socialize children to adulthood. The aged demonstrate history, adaptability, and survival skills. All old people are not wise but they teach through their mistakes and their successes. Rapid social changes highlight the importance of continuity provided by the elders in a community.

Ego Transcendence   The third task of aging is to put one's life experience in the context of a larger perspective. The prospect of death is not endurable unless life can be seen as having some meaning. Ego preoccupation occurs when one defies or rejects the possibility of personal death. Helping an individual confront mortality and transcend it may be a difficult task. One helpful method is to discuss legacies, history, and the impact of a person's life. Religious beliefs, creative works, descendents, contributions to society, talents, and special skills often allow individuals to see ways they will survive beyond themselves. Those with unfinished business may not be ready for transcendence. Religious conflicts, neglected relationships, thwarted creativity, lost opportunities, and wasted talents may need to be aired and dealt with before people can fo-

cus on their unique life space and fit it into the history of humanity.

The most successful interactions occur when the nurse and the aged person are able to maintain a whole-life perspective. Appraising the here and now is appropriate when expectations are clear and roles are easily defined. For the elderly, however, examining their life patterns as they fit within history may be far more useful and revealing. Feedback and interactional exchange based on the individual's total life experience will create respect for survival capacity, understanding of life span events, and awareness of the uniqueness of each life. Appraisal of courage, endurance, survival capacity, and limits of personal control may be more revealing than the more common appraisal of present activities, affect, relationships, and cognition.

Idiosyncratic Adaptations   The unusual and eccentric elderly—insisting on their own individuality and adamantly refusing to bend to the whims of social, political, or cultural forces—may be the most mentally healthy. In the course of a hundred years the mentally healthy person has been portrayed as stoic, hedonistic, sensual, pragmatic, patriotic, defiant, verbal, silent, assertive, compliant, self-reliant, and other-oriented. Often whether people are judged mentally healthy in old age depends on their income and status. Who are (or were) some of the eccentric elderly? Mother Teresa, William O. Douglas, Melvin Belli, Groucho Marx, Ghandi, Einstein, and Churchill are outstanding examples. Perhaps retaining the strength of your convictions is the first criterion of mental health. Nurses need to look first for an individual's unique adaptations to the passage of time before assuming that disruptive behaviors are unhealthy. The aged who have extremely individualistic life-styles may be quite satisfied and live very well without much feedback and external affirmation. Maslow would call these elderly "self-actualized." Those who have lived long with a well-developed sense of self are less vulnerable to interactional feedback of a positive or negative nature than those who are younger or less self-assured.

Nurses' Attitudes toward Aging

To claim yourself fully you must embrace your aged self. This is done most readily when prior experiences with the aged have been gratifying and warm. The interactionist perspective allows us to see ourselves in the aged around us. When we are frightened, we are

---

Table 22–2   QUESTIONS TO PROMOTE PERSONAL REVELATION AMONG THE AGED

1. What are your areas of daily gratifications? (Awareness of the present provides daily satisfaction.)
2. Who provides you with the greatest comfort and support? (Confidantes and intimates are essential to mental health.)
3. What experiences have had the most profound influence on you? (The past continues to influence our present abilities and expectations.)
4. What has been your most difficult experience and how did you handle it? (One's capacity for survival builds self-esteem.)
5. What unfulfilled hopes do you have? (Hope is essential to survival.)
6. What is your greatest problem right now? (Mutual problem-solving creates an alliance of concern and promotes growth.)

Table 22–3   SOURCES OF ATTITUDES TOWARD THE AGED

Health status
Occupation
Educational background and training
Political persuasion and influence
Laws
Religious views
All influences of early childhood
Language
Media:
  News
  Advertising
  Recreational viewing and reading
Genetic predispositions
Financial status
Geographic environment:
  Urban vs. rural, etc.
Sex differences
Context of exposure; e.g., Aged seen only when sick or dying
Cultural perspectives:
  Progressive vs. cyclic
Peer relationships (especially significant in adolescence)

Source: Developed by Priscilla Ebersole in collaboration with Saul Cohen and Loyd Kepferle.

---

afraid for our own future; when we are callous, we have shielded ourselves from viewing our future; when we are overwhelmed, we have forgotten the uniqueness of each personality and our own potential.

Attitudes toward aging generally improve with knowledge, but an affectual involvement is even more important. The most important thing nurses can do in this respect is to maintain contact with well-adapted, vital old people. This contact will allow them to avoid the skewed institutional view of aging as only illness and deficiency.

A first experience in psychiatric care of the aged should be an interaction based on discovery. A client who is able to communicate clearly may respond to some of the questions in Table 22–2.

The nurse is not only a nonjudgmental listener but an active participant sharing hopes, joys, and thoughts with clients in a human encounter. Students often ask, "Is it appropriate for me to talk about myself?" Of course it is, and particularly with the aged, who may share their insights from a long-life perspective. But nurses must be careful not to allow their needs to override the needs of the client.

In addition to developing relationships with aged people, nurses must examine their attitudes toward aging and the sources of those attitudes. See Table 22–3.

The aged themselves seem to have a derogatory image of aging. Old people are often known to say, "I don't want to be around those old fogeys." A 76-year-

old volunteer was heard saying, "those old codgers are at the end of their road." Most older people feel younger than their chronological age and will define themselves as middle-aged while considering others of the same age "old." Literature concerning how old people assess and accept their own aging shows that most old people feel mentally younger than their chronological age by at least 17 years (Plawecki and Plawecki 1981). The older they become—barring illness and severe deterioration—the greater the time lag between real and felt age. This time lag phenomenon begins in early adulthood. Older people often prefer the company of middle-aged persons. The implications of these findings are that the aged may respond better if age-condescending or patronizing behaviors can be eliminated. In addition, felt age should be part of basic information obtained since it may be more relevant to care planning than chronologic age.

STRESSES CHARACTERISTIC OF AGING

Many stresses characteristic of aging create disturbed, disruptive, or disorganized reactions. Common stresses and the cognitive, affectual, and behavioral reactions to them are discussed below.

Fear of Aging

Fear of aging occurs particularly as the aged see their cohorts deteriorate and die in unpleasant surroundings often with disabling illnesses. Most old people are more afraid of the circumstances of their death than of death itself. They fear being alone when they die, being in prolonged pain, or cognitive deterioration. This fear may make old people reluctant to be around their peers. In long-term care there is a common status hierarchy in which the most functional elders avoid and insult those with lower functional capacity. Fear of contagion by association often prevents the socialization and peer support nurses may hope to promote.

Loneliness

Much has been written about the loneliness of old people. It is generally assumed that the number of losses the aged experience must result in loneliness. Younger people must remember, however, that loss is as integral a part of life as birth. Most old people say they are no lonelier than when they were younger (Harris 1975). Loneliness is a condition that knows no age barriers and as Moustakas states: "Loneliness is as much organic to human existence as the blood is to the heart" (1961, p. 34). During periods of stress or loss, feelings of loneliness may become particularly acute. Those who are in poor health and lack adequate housing and transportation are most subject to episodes of loneliness. Loneliness is not a generic condition but arises from many sources and is expressed in many ways. See Figure 22–2.

Loss

Loss goes hand in hand with aging. There are always more endings than beginnings. Losses that occur simultaneously or one upon another strain the coping capacity of most individuals. Time is the essential healer, but some old people are in a state of chronic grief as their losses occur so frequently that they never fully recover before being assaulted by another loss. When working with any aged person, the nurse must assess the na-

ture, frequency, and number of losses in order to assess the potential effect and time needed for recovery. Some of the things commonly lost by the old are:

- Home
- Mobility
- Spouse
- Health
- Peers
- Siblings
- Work role

- Strength, energy, vitality
- Driver's license
- Hearing
- Sight
- Cherished possessions
- Income
- Pets

Meaninglessness

The impetus for life is the search for meaning. In youth daily demands may be so absorbing that meaning is seldom questioned. The aged have more available time and a distinct need to ponder the meaning of life as they have lived it and the meaning of the time remaining. To those who have not mastered the psychologic tasks of aging, existence may seem pointless. Being needed by someone provides gratification throughout life. Many elders feel unnecessary or, worse, that they are an unwanted burden and would be better off dead.

The nurse attempting to deal with this state of meaninglessness must first believe there is meaning in life as long as life persists. We cannot impose meanings on another but we can help them explore, through "life-review" and legacy identification, whatever has motivated them in the past and what remains to be done. Often small things are sustaining.

Olga J. was inspired to survive so she could attend her granddaughter's wedding. Martha L. felt it was important to record her thoughts for her grandchildren. Walt A. made complaining about his inadequate care his mission. He established client councils to seek better conditions in the convalescent hospital where he lived. Catherine G. didn't know why she lived so long but accepted her survival as part of God's plan for her. That was sufficient.

Physical Deterioration

A major source of emotional problems in old people is physical deterioration. Sometimes it is the first confrontation with personal vulnerability. Those with a lifelong concern with their health may feel betrayed when their body defaults in spite of their efforts, and

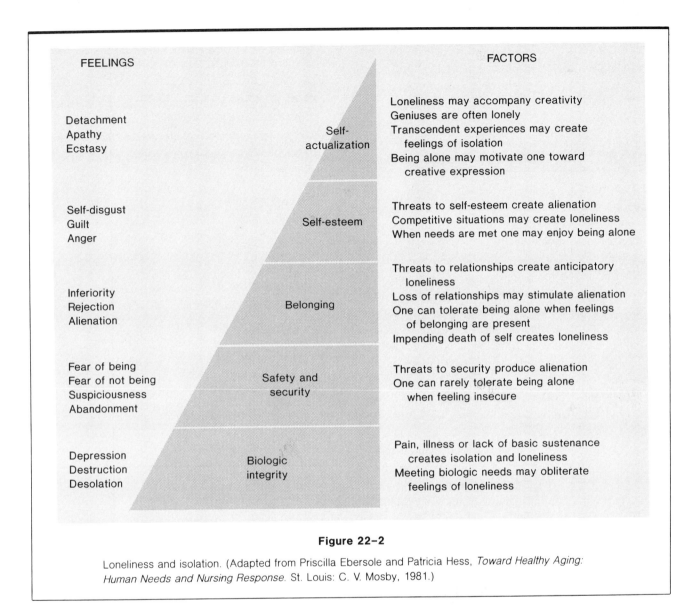

Figure 22-2

Loneliness and isolation. (Adapted from Priscilla Ebersole and Patricia Hess, *Toward Healthy Aging: Human Needs and Nursing Response.* St. Louis: C. V. Mosby, 1981.)

they may become angry or resigned. The grief process related to the lost image of a perfectly functioning body is similar to that of the young mother who bears a defective child and must mourn the loss of her expected perfect infant.

Psychiatric nursing of the aged often involves extensive attention to physical problems. Many of the elderly develop disorganized emotional responses based on physiologic disturbance. (See Chapter 17.) When function cannot be restored, comfort measures and warm, consistent relationships may ease the elderly person's psychic distress.

Stigma

Visible deterioration often has more emotional ramifications than the invisible disorders that the aged experience. The stigma associated with certain disabilities

and conditions alienate the individual and increase the sense of isolation and feelings of being invalid. So much of personal worth in our society is derived from presentation of self. "Each person evaluates his image through the eyes of culture, era, trends, reflections from important others, and mirrors" (Ebersole and Hess 1981). When most in need of acceptance and understanding, the aged person with missing dentures, stroke paralysis, aphasia, skin eruptions, and odors of illness may repel others. All nurses have their own particular revulsions and must come to terms with them before attempting to care for those exhibiting the offensive condition. Whatever impairs the nurse's ability to relate to an individual will decrease effectiveness and erode the individual's self-esteem.

In most cases a nurse can assist by grooming, improving unsightly conditions, and banishing offensive odors. There is never a reason for the smell of urine to linger on an individual, for the body or clothing to be foul smelling and stained with feces, for hair to be matted and tangled, or for fingernails to be long and torn. Attention to such visible and reversible problems will have immediate positive effects on self-image.

Sexuality

Sexual expression remains important to most people throughout their life span. Barring illness or widowhood, earlier levels of interest in sexual expression remain consistent throughout life with a gradual decline in frequency of sexual intercourse beginning in middle-age. Pleasure in the many expressions of sexuality can effectively compensate for any decreases in performance capacity. Older women often express a need to be held and touched; older men may need reassurance about their sexual adequacy since it is often tied to their feelings of success in other aspects of life.

Elders are not sexless beings but many have adopted this idea and report no sexual activity in their lives (Ludeman 1981). Cultural conditioning, media presentations of youth and sexuality, attitudes of adult children and peers, illness, and widowhood may all make it difficult for the aged to view themselves as fully functional sexual beings. In an effort to overcome these negative perceptions of sexuality, gerontologists have often overcompensated and promoted sexual attitudes and activities that were not acceptable to the aged. When working with the aged, it is most helpful to learn what they want and what they think is possible. Factual information should be given regarding physiologic changes in capacity and the availability of sexual counseling, but it is more important to explore the client's attitudes and feelings about sexuality in earlier years. The guidelines in Table 22–4 will assist the nurse in conducting sexual assessment of the aged and Chapter 12 provides additional information related to human sexuality. These questions should be used in the course of conversation and with sensitivity to responses indicating discomfort. Some older people consider sexuality a very private matter. If they do not wish to discuss it, that is their prerogative.

Nurses need to curb the tendency to view the sexual expressions of older persons as "cute," amusing, or disgusting. These attitudes are often derived from the nurse's unresolved struggles with sexuality. "Dirty old men" and, with increasing frequency, "dirty old ladies" are the inventions of those who would restrict sexuality to the young.

Table 22–4   GUIDELINES FOR ASSESSING THE SEXUAL NEEDS OF THE AGED

1. When you were growing up, did people you knew discuss sex and romance?
2. How do you feel about discussing it now?
3. What do you think about romance at this stage in your life?
4. What were you told about sex when you were a child?
5. Do you think it is a very important part of life satisfaction for people of all ages?
6. How important has sexual activity been in your life?
7. What were you told about masturbation?
8. What does sexuality mean to you?
9. Does your present living situation give you opportunities to express your sexuality?
10. What values and morals influence your feelings about sex now?
11. How are your needs of intimacy being met now?

Clark M. was 92 years old when he proposed marriage to an 80-year-old woman in a nursing home. He used the intercom to announce his intentions. The staff were supportive and helped them hold a wedding. The children of the couple thought they were foolish or "senile" and had some concerns about the prospect of a diminished inheritance.

Many elders do not wish to marry but would like opportunities for sexual release and recognition as sexual beings. Some have been conditioned in their youth to abhor masturbation. A nurse needs to discuss sexuality with older persons and find out how their need for intimacy can be met most appropriately within their value system. If their needs cannot be met, the nurse must recognize this and realize it may be experienced as a serious deprivation.

Research findings indicate that a sex education program provided by older adults for other elders, their families, and nursing home staff members creates more positive attitudes, increases knowledge, and improves behaviors toward sexuality (White and Catania 1980).

Relocation

Familiar objects, available services, and a comfortable setting make the adjustment to old age easier. *Translocation shock* is a term applied to the reactions elders have when uprooted, often without adequate preparation or their consent. When this must occur due to illness or inability to cope with the daily demands in the familiar environment, it is imperative that the nurse make every effort to simplify adjustment to the new setting by providing maps, directions, information, and instructions. Bringing personally significant items to the new setting often eases the transition. It is most important to engage the translocated person in decisions about the new environment. This practice restores a sense of control. Even in an acute hospital, decisions about placement of equipment and necessary items can be adapted to the personal desires of the client.

Catherine G. had lived in a small cubicle in a convalescent hospital for nine years and still exerted autonomy over her environment. Her clock and radio were within easy reach. The curtains were pulled two thirds closed on the bed and window so she could see others coming and still maintain her privacy. A roll of toilet paper was always on the upper right corner of her bed. Her cane lay by her side. The bathroom door was opened just enough so she could reach the knob and hold onto the foot of the bed with her other hand. All of these were her choices and added to her sense of security and control—important aspects of mental health.

Close relationships with friends, family, and staff members exert a positive influence on aged persons undergoing a relocation crisis (Wells and Macdonald 1981). Those who have any of these significant relationships maintain self-esteem and life satisfaction and avoid physical and mental deterioration. The sustaining importance of quality relationships supports staff involvement with aged persons on a personal level.

Abuse and Neglect

Attitudes toward aging, fear of aging, and frustration contribute to abuse or neglect of the aged. Certainly our national policies perpetuate neglect of the aged in many spheres. For example, while massive efforts have been made to alter structures, communication modes, and supportive services for disabled persons, many disabled old people do not have a wheelchair, 40 percent of the hearing impaired have never had audiometric testing, and the vast majority of the disabled aged are confined to regimented institutional settings.

Self-abuse and self-neglect is also a problem. Many old people forget to eat, over- or undermedicate themselves, and withdraw into a self-made prison. They have incorporated the belief that to be old is to be a useless burden on family and society. This attitude reduces their incentive to live and care for themselves properly.

One in ten old people interviewed in a chronic illness center had suffered abuse or neglect by a family member (Lau and Cosberg, 1978). There may be many more who do not admit to having such problems because they fear retribution or the possibility of a worse living situation. Some feel a strong sense of family loyalty or believe they deserve the treatment they are getting. Abuse of the aged has only recently been brought to the public attention and the data available are extremely limited. Most of the theories regarding cause and effects have been extrapolated from knowledge about child abuse (see Chapter 19). We do know that the older and more dependent people become, the more likely they are to be abused, especially if they are female.

A major problem in discussing abuse of the elderly is the lack of clear definition of what constitutes abuse. The law can describe abuse in general terms or it can depict specific, explicit forms of abuse. However, such definitions often focus on physical abuse while neglecting psychological issues. It is important to recognize the various forms of psychological abuse to which the elderly are subject, since such abuse may be as damaging as a physical assault. Abuse of the elderly may take any of the following forms (Block and Sinnott 1979):

- Physical abuse, including direct beatings, lack of food, lack of medical care, and lack of supervision
- Psychological abuse, including verbal assault, threat, fear, and isolation
- Material abuse, including theft or misuse of money or property
- Violation of rights, including forced removal from home, or forced entry into nursing home when individual is not dangerous to self or others

Investigations in the last few years have found that abuse of the aged occurs as frequently as, or more often than abuse of children or spouse. Yet, few professionals are willing to believe or report such occurrences. The idea of abusing frail, dependent elders is so abhorrent that it is easy to lose sight of the abuser's position. Abusers are often strained beyond their coping capacity having made superhuman efforts to care for an elder with little support from family, friends, or society. In exasperation and frustration the abuser may lash out at the most obvious source of the problem—the elder.

When severe abuse is discovered, it is imperative to remove the elder from the situation immediately to prevent retaliation by the abuser. Legal action is often necessary. Some states have mandatory reporting laws and fines for professionals who do not comply. At present, however, there are few protocols for effective and comprehensive handling of abuse cases and even fewer available alternative placements.

The presence of abuse must be considered in any of the following situations:

- Overmedication or deprivation of life-sustaining medications

- Falls and injuries, particularly bruises on face, arms, legs, and buttocks

- Malnutrition

- Extended periods of neglect or restraint evidenced by contractures; pressure sores; and long, curved finger- and toenails

- Agitation when certain persons appear: family, friends, or caretakers

It is also important to be aware that most elders will not report abuse for the following reasons:

- Fear of retaliation from the abuser

- Fear that the alternative living situation would be less desirable than the present one

- Loyalty to the abuser

- Belief that they deserve the treatment they are receiving

- Lack of contact with anyone who can assist them

The following services should be available:

- Counseling for the abused

- Counseling for the abuser

- Alternative housing when needed

- Legal procedures that would assure instant removal of the aged from a dangerous situation

- Services to relieve the stress of families caring for the aged before uncontrollable tensions build up

Nurses may institute support groups and locate resources for families caring for aged members and attempt to reduce the stress experienced in such situations. Home visits are also desirable to assess the adequacy of the situation and institute a supportive relationship.

REACTIONS TO PROBLEMS OF AGING

The presenting affect, behavior, and thoughts of the aged who are experiencing emotional stress due to the problems discussed earlier will be influenced by personality, magnitude and persistence of the problem, general health, cognitive capacity, and personal support systems. Their reactions will be categorized according to the degree of disturbance created for them and for others.

Many of the reactions of the aged that might be considered disturbed in youth are quite reasonable in old age. For example, compulsive behaviors afford a sense of security and maintain feelings of autonomy and control as well as provide patterns for marking empty time. Suspiciousness is wise considering how frequently the aged are victimized or forced into situations without their knowledge or consent. It also helps them maintain a sense of power and importance, defending against apathy and inadequacy. Denial of aging is also adaptive for elders, allowing them to avoid internalizing the negative "ageism" of society. Even the social isolate, who seems maladapted in youth, is often better in old age when he or she has less to lose (Butler and Lewis 1981).

Disturbed Behaviors

Disturbed patterns in the aged usually arise from long-standing problems in adaptation or an overload of present stresses and are frequently exhibited by depressive affect and compulsive behaviors. Thoughts may be obsessional and ruminative. Psychic conflicts may be more firmly defended as one ages. Repression certainly continues into old age and in addition many persons have developed a conscious capacity for distracting attention from painful events of the past. Both the unconscious defenses and the conscious distractions serve one well until energies are depleted by illness or crises. Then unresolved issues erupt and add to the stress experienced.

Jake S., a hard-driving man of many abilities, felt quite gratified and successful. He viewed therapy as appropriate only for the inadequate or inept. After his retirement and the loss of his spouse he became painfully aware that he had never developed good relationships with his children. To make up for years of neglect he began attempting to become involved in their lives. Of course they were annoyed and unresponsive. He began to ruminate over his failure as a father and vacillated between anger and oversolicitousness with his adult children. In his pain he finally sought counseling. The counselor helped him understand the following:

- *His own father had been a remote, frightening figure and had died when he was young. His fathering role had been underdeveloped.*
- *When his children were young the Great Depression consumed his energies. Survival was his foremost concern at that time.*
- *In his present grief over major losses he felt a genuine need for support.*
- *His children could not and would not compensate for his losses.*
- *Cultivation of friendships among peers who shared the same historic pressures and present stresses could be very gratifying.*

The sources of disturbed emotions include: mourning, guilt about realistic issues, death or future anxiety, and a rage directed at the unfairness of life or toward specific individuals (Butler and Lewis 1981). Abuse, stigma, feelings of meaninglessness, physical deterioration, and fear of aging will produce disturbed reactions. They are disturbing problems.

Disturbing emotions may result in increased dependency, often magnified by the behavior of caretaking persons. Isolation and withdrawal are other methods of coping with disturbance. Listlessness may cover thoughts, feelings, and desires and therefore become a protective mechanism for many. Apathy and lethargy, resulting from extended isolation and withdrawal, perpetuate a meaningless existence. Depression is an undercurrent in all these situations and must be recog-

nized and dealt with by nurse and client. Nurses need to be aware that initial assessment of the aged client may be clouded. Old people who are feeling inadequate tend to express favorable attitudes in surveys as a means of denying problems or of giving the image of successful coping (Carp and Carp 1981). Speculating on the life-preserving quality of hope, we might say it is a method of maintaining spirit.

Disruptive Patterns

Disruptive patterns occur as a behavioral response to unmet needs or from an idiosyncratic perceptual organization. They are often evidenced by suspiciousness, anger, apathetic withdrawal, or substance abuse.

Otto R. had been reasonably content living in an urban ghetto, spending his social security allotment on liquor and women and then begging when his money ran out. He often called his niece in a distant city for additional money. She became irritated and worried about him and enlisted the assistance of a social service agency. Within months Otto was under conservatorship based on his inability to care for himself and was taken to a "convalescent" hospital. He was angry and obstreperous. He managed to create havoc in the facility by throwing food in the dining room, stuffing towels in toilet bowls, and sneaking out to beg in a nearby shopping center. He was declared unmanageable and was transferred to a locked facility. There he became subdued and totally apathetic. Rapid deterioration and death ended his struggle to cope with the well-intentioned interventions of others.

Otto R. might have responded well to interventions if others had recognized:

- His strong independent nature
- His need for occasional female companionship
- His nutritional needs
- His long-standing pattern of marginal involvement in society
- His enjoyment of alcoholic beverages

Appropriate interventions in his life-style might have included:

- Infrequent public health nurse visits with Otto R. to demonstrate some interest and availability

- Contact with his hotel manager regarding services available when Otto wanted or needed them

- A discussion with Otto regarding meal sites and senior center card rooms

- A discussion with Otto about problems he recognized in his life-style and assistance in modifying within Otto's value system.

Disintegrative Patterns

Disintegrative patterns in the aged arise most frequently from physiologic disturbance. The psychologic disturbances so often responsible for disintegrative or psychotic reactions in the young are less frequently manifested in the old. (See Chapter 16.) When psychotic conditions occur, nurses must first rule out organic origins. (See Chapter 17.) The most prevalent psychotic conditions of old age are Paranoia, Major Depression Episode with psychotic features, and Primary Degenerative Dementia.

Disintegrative emotional reactions may arise from impaired grief, unrealistic ruminative guilt, overwhelming anxiety, panic arising from severe need deprivation, and unexpressed rage. Severe physical deterioration or cognitive impairment are the source of many disintegrative patterns. Disintegrative reactions such as confusion, disorientation, wandering, paranoia, illusions, and depression are most often the result of temporary or permanent organic disorders. However, paranoia, delusions, and hallucinations of overwhelming proportions may arise from a functional or nonorganic base. Old people may appear temporarily psychotic when overwhelmed with losses, following surgeries or accidents, or when deprived of caring human interactions.

Ester was brought by the police to the emergency room. She had been wandering about the airport, mumbling and occasionally calling someone. In the emergency room she continued to mumble and search through her purse feverishly. She did not respond to efforts of hospital staff to communicate with her. Her son's name was found in her purse, and he was contacted. He revealed that she had not been eating or sleeping and had talked incessantly about finding her husband, who died six months previously.

Sensory limitations, environmental deprivations, body system malfunction, and isolation from interactional exchange all make the elderly more vulnerable to disintegrative interpretations of reality. Therefore, restoration of body function, sensory aids, a structured and moderately stimulating environment, and caring interactions are basic to recovery. It is important for elderly people to be treated on psychic and practical daily living levels. Therapy is rarely successful without practical supports for basic functioning and skills education. Some disturbed and disintegrative reactions experienced by the aged are perceived by caretakers as disruptive patterns. Extreme dependency, agitation and wandering, confusion and disorientation, and paranoia tend to disrupt the milieu and create anger or disgust in others. Nurses need patience, peer support, and professional collaboration to deal effectively and compassionately with their own reactions and the needs of the elderly.

Cognitive Function

Cerebral integrative capacity is critically important to life satisfaction at any age. Older people are too often assumed to be impaired with little or no cause. This section examines normal and abnormal cognitive function in late life.

Normal Changes   Some cognitive changes occur normally in the process of aging. Everyone begins losing functional cerebral cells early in youth and continues to do so throughout life. Fortunately, we are endowed with many more than we can possibly use. It is estimated that 10 to 20 percent of the very old have some cognitive impairment due to loss of cerebral cellular functions but this is not an expectable consequence of aging.

The differences in cognition that can be anticipated with age have been studied more than any other aspect of gerontology. Recent findings have demonstrated the invalidity of many testing procedures used to determine intelligence and learning capacity of the old. The present state of knowledge about cognitive function in old age is summarized as follows:

- Verbal skills tend to increase

- Spatial perceptual organization diminishes

- Retrieval of data in long-term memory is slower

- New information is learned more slowly

- Creativity remains high in subjects who have demonstrated it earlier in life
- More caution is exerted in decision-making tasks

Older learners are inclined to perform best when

- Material is relevant to their needs
- The learning situation is comfortable and non-threatening
- Sufficient time is allowed
- They are in good health
- The method and amount of prior educational experience is considered
- Beliefs and values do not conflict with the new material

Some common problems in attempting to teach the aged include lack of consideration to

- Cohort learning styles
- Sensory deficits
- Boundaries of life experience
- Comfort
- General health
- Situational anxiety

From a practical viewpoint, the nurse will avoid burdening the troubled elder with irrelevant information and advise against unnecessary testing. Psychological tests should be administered, when necessary, in brief segments and by qualified persons. Most older people have not been "psychologized" and many skip multiple choice questions when they do not clearly agree with any answer. They have learned through experience that most situations are complex and subject to multiple interpretations.

Impaired Cognitive Function   Cognitive dysfunction is the most devastating aspect of aging. The alteration of judgment, memory, affect, and effective living skills in a society where humans are valued for their intelligence and performance is a fate worse than death and, for many, becomes a living death. Cognitive impairment may be the result of untreated hypertension, vital organ deterioration, cerebrovascular disease, drugs, compromised cerebral oxygen, infectious disease, excessive prolonged strain, fatigue, or psychologic deprivation or overload.

CONFUSION   Confusion is the most common emotional, behavioral, and cognitive reaction to stressors in old age.

A mild confusional tendency and disturbed behavior may simply indicate sensory impairment, a lack of structure, insufficient environmental cues (clocks, calendars, etc.), or lack of attention to such cues. A deprived, boring environment will often induce a state of confusion. Preoccupation with fears, losses, or threats to security and independence may also appear as confusion. More pronounced confusional states leading to disruptive behaviors often follow translocation, environmental overload, and acute grief.

The most devastating confusional states, including severe disorientation, occur with severe overtaxing of physiologic homeostatic mechanisms by injuries, toxic conditions, metabolic deficiencies, impaired cerebral metabolism (enzymatic or circulatory), and disease processes. In other words, anything that taxes the limits of homeostatic resilience may result in temporary disintegrative patterns, confusion, and disorientation (Wolanin and Phillips 1981).

DISORIENTATION   Disorientation is the inability to state the time and date, the present location, and the name of the person you are relating to or speaking about. Before assuming disorientation in any realm, determine the presence or absence of environmental cues. Often the lack of clocks, calendars, and other cues makes it difficult for a client to determine time and place. For example, a group of hospitals use the same laundry service and it is not uncommon for towels and sheets to be imprinted "St. Joseph's" when, in fact, the hospital may be "Providence." Likewise, orientation to a person may be hindered by the sheer numbers of people who enter the client's room in an average day. If individuals do not know the year or month or where home is and firmly believe you are a relative (if you are not), it is pretty safe to assume that they are disoriented.

Disorientation about past events or present expectations must also be thoughtfully assessed. Do clients remember the names of siblings or the date of their own birth? These facts are normally fixed firmly in memory. While the present may be very confusing, the past should be fairly clear.

A common method used to determine mental status is the Kahn-Goldfarb mental status questionnaire.

MENTAL STATUS QUESTIONNAIRE FOR COGNITIVE IMPAIRMENTS

To estimate impairment, ask the following questions:

1. Where are we now? (Place orientation)
2. Where is this place located? (Place orientation)
3. What month is it? (Time orientation)
4. What day of the month is it? (Time orientation)
5. What year is it? (Time orientation)
6. How old are you? (Memory)
7. When is your birthday? (Memory)
8. Where were you born? (Memory)
9. Who is the President of the United States? (General information and memory)
10. Who was President before him? (General information and memory)

None to two errors indicate no, or mild, impairment. Three to eight errors indicate moderately advanced impairment. Nine to ten errors indicate severe brain dysfunction.

The test should be given in a comfortable atmosphere by an individual with whom the person feels comfortable. The anxiety of a test situation may block responses.

Environmental cues must be available in the setting; e.g., clocks and calendars. The test should be given two or three times if the responses are not accurate. In these cases you may want to try another time of day and another setting.

From R. L. Kohn and A. Goldfarb, *American Journal of Psychiatry*, 117(1960):326, American Psychiatric Association.

CONFABULATION   The interviewer must be aware that older people with well-developed verbal skills may avoid direct answers to questions by using confabulation. Confabulation is the art of filling in imaginary information to cover memory gaps. Older people do this to maintain self-esteem and save face when they are aware of failing mental capacities.

DEMENTIA   Permanent personality disorganization is much less frequent than generally supposed or diagnosed and is accompanied by irreversible loss of cerebral cellular function. This is often called Primary Degenerative, or Senile, Dementia and is usually the result of a poorly understood, progressive, and irreversible condition called Alzheimer's disease (see Chapter 17). The number of people who develop this condition increases appreciably after age 80 to an estimated 10 to 20 percent of the aged population. Specific changes occur in cerebral cells that are microscopically visible and accurately diagnosed only on autopsy. This condition simulates some of the cerebral cellular changes that occur in normal aging, but the changes are more profuse and overwhelming. The progressive decline in memory, judgment, affect, coordination, and organized behavior patterns follows a steady course and generally ends in death in about two years. With excellent care some survive as long as ten years.

TRANSIENT ISCHEMIC ATTACKS   Another type of personality disintegration may occur gradually with a series of Transient Ischemic Attacks (TIAs or "little strokes"). These are the result of atherosclerotic obstruction of adequate cerebral circulation or vascular spasms interrupting the flow of blood to the brain. The specific attacks may be transient or asymptomatic. Personality change becomes noticeable later, chiefly exhibited by deterioration of appearance and manners.

Major cerebrovascular accidents, or strokes, also cause disintegration of personality but in time and with therapy many persons recover full or partial function. One psychological ramification is the "time bomb" effect. Those who have had strokes are uneasy, wondering when the next one will occur.

INTERVENTIONS FOR COGNITIVE DYSFUNCTION AMONG THE AGED   When you have thoughtfully determined the degree and presence of cognitive dysfunctions, begin to orient the person to essential information in a relaxed way using the following guidelines:

ORIENTATION GUIDELINES FOR WORKING WITH CONFUSED ELDERLY

- Add as many visual cues to the setting as you can. When vision is impaired, consistent auditory input is essential. Check hearing aids and eyeglasses for effective function.

- Make the environment as predictable as possible by anticipatory planning and a safe, routine, printed schedule. When changes must be made, introduce them slowly and rehearse expected performance with the individual involved.

- Arrange for a thorough physical and neurological exam to rule out organic bases of confusion. Remember, however, that too many intrusive or diagnostic procedures in a short time will increase confusion.

- **Assess the stresses** experienced recently and within the last two years (see Chapter 11).

- If sensory deprivation or lack of stimulation is the problem, add color, texture, flavor, and noncompetitive activity to the daily schedule. If an overload of new expectations and adaptations has occurred, increase environmental stability, reduce expectations, and promote rest and continuity of supportive personnel.

- When confusion is extensive and organically based, reduce expectations to those that can be accomplished and give consistent, immediate praise for any degree of success. This must be done by all personnel and long-term, consistent efforts are essential.

- Establish a relationship that conveys the value of the client regardless of functional capacity.

- Develop a solid personal peer support system. Those who understand the disappointments and struggles of nursing are in the best position to listen to each other. Sharing feelings, anger, exasperation, and humor helps the nurse continue in a very difficult task.

COMMON EVIDENCE OF PSYCHIC DISTRESS

Stress Anxiety

Stressors are perceived events and stress anxiety is the affective, physiologic, cognitive, and behavioral response. In old age the response to stressors is often global. The whole being responds symptomatically with agitation, confusion, or the "freeze reaction." The freeze reaction is seen in the aged who lack the energy to fight or flee (Jarvik and Russel 1979). Freezing is not giving up; it is maintaining a state of "vigilant watchfulness." This state is often incorrectly assessed as apathy, neutrality, or acceptance. It may be uniquely adapted to the stressors of the aged that have long-term effects on life-style.

Overload Anxiety accompanies an overload of stressful events. It is important to remember that "overload" is individually variable depending on frequency, duration, personality, general health, and the nature and availability of support systems. When work-

ing with an anxious elderly person, one must explore the impact of stressors and the adaptive capacity available to the individual at that time. Stressors are generally less frequent in old age, but they are of greater consequence than in youth. Illness, relocation, death of significant others, loss of mobility, economic depletion, severe sensory impairment, and loss of driver's license are sources of stress far more common and devastating to the old than to the young. Fear of victimization plagues most of the elderly. Though they are less likely than younger people to be the victims of criminal attack, the consequences may be much more severe. The accompanying stress anxiety may be physically and psychologically debilitating and precipitate increasing withdrawal and alienation from the neighborhood and community. One elderly lady in New York had not been farther than the corner grocery in thirteen years. This kind of fear might be reduced by neighborhood coalitions that provide escort service and check on each other.

Boredom Another stressor, not exclusive to old age, is a lack of sufficient stress to maintain interest. A boring, barren, unchallenging life situation may be as personally devastating as one that is overly demanding. There is also a need to distinguish between the effects of noxious and pleasant stimuli when assessing stressors. Neurophysiologic evidence shows that the central nervous system mechanisms for pleasant and unpleasant inputs are clearly separate (Stagner 1981). This is an important distinction, but it is difficult to separate negative and positive stressors and demonstrate the different types of reactions and coping responses. Holmes and Rahe's (1967) life change units are a useful measure of stress impact. They help people become aware of their stress load, but they are not sufficiently discriminating to predict response.

Assessment of stress in aging should include:

- The positive or negative consequence of the stress (affective component)
- The individual's prior experience with such stress (novelty component)
- The magnitude of the stress (impact)
- The chronicity of the stress (time element)
- The person's comfort zones (sustaining element)
- Coping resource repertoire (habituation range of responses)
- Personality type (Dionysian/Apollonian)

Table 22–5 POLARITY OF DIONYSIAN/APOLLONIAN PRINCIPLES	
Dionysian	**Apollonian**
Magic	Rational
Dreams	Prestige
Visions	Duty
Illusions	Material
Faith	Plan
Supernatural	Lawful
Hope	Pragmatic
Sacred	Secular
Idealism	Realism
Metaphysical	Physical
Intrinsic	Extrinsic
Intuitive	Evidence
Passion	Discipline
Subjective	Objective
Belief	Fact
Sensation	Thought
Universal	Individual
Innovation	Tradition
Aesthetics	Ethics
Ephemeral	Tangible

Source: Priscilla Ebersole and Patricia Hess, *Toward Healthy Aging*, St. Louis: The C. V. Mosby Co., 1981; developed from R. Benedict, *Nursing Response: Patterns of Culture*, New York: Houghton Mifflin Co., 1934.

This last element has rarely been considered. Personality typology has been popular for only three decades, and many older persons may not even have considered that they have a personality type. Two personality types, the Apollonian and Dionysian, originally defined by Nietzsche are helpful in understanding why some people cope better than others when in similar external circumstances. Dionysians are reactive and value sensations. Apollonians are practical, orderly, and intellectual in the classic sense. Apollonians tend to fare better when dealing with external surroundings in which they feel a sense of control. Dionysians manage better in deprived situations, since they can sustain themselves with inner experience, but they may feel acute grief at the loss of sensate experience.

See Table 22–5 for qualities of Dionysians and Apollonians.

Depression

Depression is a familiar reaction of the aged. Estimates of the incidence of Depression among the aged are from 20 to 60 percent of the population. It is an accompanying symptom in most of the problems of aging and in many ways successful aging involves the ability to tolerate periods of depression.

The severity of depressive states in the aged is affected by decreasing secretions of mood-influencing neurotransmitters and increasing life changes. Assessing the severity of Depression is complicated by the lack of adequate and precise diagnostic criteria. The Zung depression scale (Zung 1964) is widely used but also criticized because it was not derived from norms for the aged and primarily reflects reactions that may be indices of physiologic slowing or subclinical disease rather than Depression. Constipation, insomnia, fatigue, anorexia, retarded thoughts and movements—the classic signs of Depression—may not be indicative of Depression in old age. To complicate the problem further, the symptoms of profound Depression in the aged are frequently misdiagnosed as Organic Brain Syndrome. Nurses must be aware of this hazard. A trial period of antidepressant medications may be helpful in these cases (Cavenar et al. 1979).

Hypochondria   In the elderly, hypochondria may signal the presence of Depression; but a preoccupation with one's body does not always indicate Depression. Full and comprehensive physical examinations are necessary when the client persistently complains of body discomfort (see Chapter 8).

The relationship between Depression, somatic complaints, and physical illness in older persons is not necessarily congruent. In a study by Stever (1980) physicians' ratings of health were not significantly related to Depression, but somatic complaints—particularly of fatigue—were positively and significantly correlated to Depression. In Stever's sample of healthy depressed elderly clients, somatic symptoms were reported less frequently than lack of hope, inactivity, uselessness, and problems with decision-making and doing things. Thus the generally accepted belief that Depression in the aged is exhibited by hypochondria was not supported by this study. However, the sample members were voluntarily seeking help for Depression and were aware of its presence. This additional information may account for the unexpected finding.

Substance Abuse

Medications The aged are particularly prone to the intentional and unintentional abuse of prescription and over-the-counter medications. They may have five or six physicians treating their various ailments and prescribing drugs without knowledge of drugs already prescribed. The aged are seldom given sufficient education about drug actions and interactions.

Jake S. was given Quinidine to take four times daily for his "heart." When he would develop anginal pains, he would take an extra Quinidine.

Marie G. noticed her legs were swollen at night. Going to the doctor was an effort and drugs are expensive, so she borrowed a "water pill" from a neighbor.

Martha R. never throws any drugs away and therefore saves money by treating herself from the warehouse of drugs she has collected over the years.

Jake S. consumed a full bottle of Nyquil each evening because he couldn't tolerate "those sleepless nights."

Jennie H. used a bottle of milk of magnesia daily to "keep my system clean."

Walter L. was told by his physician that a brandy each evening would relax him and increase his peripheral circulation. He was seldom seen sober in the evenings after that.

Many people operate on the principle that if a little of something is good, then more must be better. For the aged who are alone and have little but pills and meals to mark the passing of days it is understandable that they begin to rely on those substances to give their lives meaning and structure.

Alcohol Retirement, grief, loneliness, and pain are often the factors that trigger alcohol abuse in old age. The problem of elderly alcoholism is increasing, not only among the dejected remnants of humanity in the streets and slums, but in the homes of the middle and upper class elderly who can't tolerate the decreased activity and status of their "golden years." Managers

of luxurious retirement centers and adult communities are becoming alarmed at the increased visibility of alcoholism among their residents.

The National Institute for Alcohol Abuse states that two-thirds of the senior population uses alcohol and 15 percent of those become alcoholics. Programs are emerging for elderly alcoholics using ex-alcoholic senior volunteers to tour senior centers, hospitals, and retirement homes discussing their experiences. There is a great need for this kind of outreach and education about alcoholism among the elderly, who may not seek treatment for what they consider a moral rather than a medical problem.

Suicide

Prolonged depressive bouts or overwhelming problems that seem insoluble may lead the aged to suicide. Most often their attempts are lethal. Clues to potential suicide may or may not be present, though suicide among the aged is more likely to be carefully planned than impulsive. For discussions of suicide, see Chapters 5 and 11.

Various studies indicate that factors such as bereavement, illness, depression, retirement, and Organic Brain Disorders account for the high rate of suicidal behavior in aged men though there is no sudden increase in suicide after sixty-five. The rate of male suicide increases continuously from age fifteen onward. Female suicide rates are highest between ages forty-five and fifty-four. Suicidal behavior in the aged includes covert as well as overt methods though statistics do not reflect this. The aged who refuse to eat or take life-sustaining medications may be attempting suicide. Substance abuse is also seen as subliminal suicide. Nurses must attempt to establish interpersonal connections with the suicidal aged, particularly those in the early stages of bereavement. Yet, suicide is the final statement of autonomy for some of the elderly and may be the most desirable option open to them. Ethical reflection is especially necessary when working with such clients.

FAMILY REACTIONS TO PSYCHICALLY DISTRESSED AGED

Families are the most frequent providers of care for the disturbed, disruptive, and mentally impaired elderly. In addition to the personal, financial, and psychological burdens of such care, family caregivers are often unable to find support from physicians or agencies. Elderly mentally impaired persons often minimize or deny problems and may present a far more integrated performance to a physician than they can sustain at home (Reifler et al. 1981).

Mary L., a very depressed and forgetful older lady, would not get out of bed. She would moan all night and keep her husband awake. He complained to other family members and the family physician but received no sympathy or assistance as she would become more alert and animated in their presence. The depth of her depression was not visible to those who were not with her on a daily basis.

Companions are much more apt to be accurate in their assessment of problems than the client or the physician. Successful intervention in these cases often requires a minimum of four multidisciplinary home visits and a multifaceted evaluation of the total situation as perceived by client, family, and professional. Some of the most crucial variables are:

- Housing and suitability of living situation
- Dietary history and lab tests to reveal dietary deficiencies
- Reports from client and family regarding self-care activities
- Complete physical exam of client
- Psychiatric evaluation of emotional and mental responses
- Financial matters
- Adequacy of transportation
- Schedule of daily activities and interests
- Family stressors
- Level of interference in family function due to client's illness

Premature or inappropriate institutionalization may be averted by a thorough assessment and provision of family support, including practical advice and some form of respite care for the family, such as day care for the client. When clients continue to deny the existence of problems, they may be induced to participate for the sake of the family. It is not necessary that they agree with the family about their problems.

Mary L. was given a tricyclic antidepressant before bedtime. Subsequently she slept better, her husband slept better, and she began to work through her depression slowly. With the most troubling problem (sleeplessness) solved, the couple could function as a unit again. Realizing that she responded much better to the physician and family members than to her husband, the children began visiting more frequently and the physician requested weekly visits from the public health nurse.

Reactions to the problems of aging are often devastating to the individual and family. A concerned nurse will function as an advocate for all affected persons, sustaining the integrity of the individual's most critical support system—the family. Often family support therapy is necessary (see Chapter 21).

INTERVENTION STRATEGIES

Intervention strategies applicable to the care of the aged include all those that are used for younger persons. Modified goals and expectations may be dictated by availability of time, money, and appropriate personnel more than by the actual needs of the elders.

Family Support Therapy

Family support therapy includes family members and the aged individual. Brink (1976) gives the following principles as guidelines for these sessions:

- Clear goals and time limitations must be mutually established.
- Practical interventions are more helpful than attempts at personality reconstruction.
- Maintaining established family patterns with as little interference as possible produces best results.
- The family member least willing to attend should receive the first attention. Often the older person does not see a problem and is attending unwillingly.
- All parties must receive equal attention in the course of the session.
- It is helpful to ask each member to keep a daily diary of activities and frustrating events. This allows the therapist to identify specific problems that can be modified.

- Counselors should clearly define their role and limitations when working with a family.
- Contingency plans and anticipatory guidance reduce the family's stress when crises occur. For instance, if the family is unable to move toward the most desirable goal, what optional plans are feasible?

Individual Psychotherapy

The aged are grossly underrepresented in individual psychotherapy, though it is estimated that 14 to 20 percent of them have functional psychiatric disturbances. The lack of geropsychiatrists, medicare and medicaid restrictions, and negative attitudes of therapists prevent many aged from receiving needed psychotherapy. Some therapists believe it is a waste of time and resources to treat the aged who have little time left to benefit from their efforts. A humanist might counter that, with less time remaining, the quality of that time becomes more important.

Brief Psychotherapy

Because of previously mentioned problems, many therapists rely on brief psychotherapy with older people. Sessions may be weekly, of fifteen minutes to an hour in duration, over a period of six to fifteen weeks. The following principles guide these sessions:

- Immediately and mutually establish specific goals.
- Promote positive transference between therapist and client.
- Encourage active involvement and sharing by the therapist.
- Promote self-esteem through supportive feedback, empathy, openness, and acceptance.
- Pay attention to total life context and provide practical support.

Improvement in social adaptation and psychologic function has been reported for as many as 80 percent of the aged treated in brief psychotherapy. Even those with cognitive impairment have benefited.

Crisis Intervention

Crisis intervention strategies with the elderly are similar to those used in any situation (see Chapter 11). Some guidelines are given below.

CRISIS INTERVENTION STRATEGIES WITH THE AGED

- Identify crisis the client is experiencing.
- Maintain routine, and support usual habits that give a sense of security (e.g., familiar setting, cup of tea).
- Review and clarify cognitive perception of the disruptive event.
- Encourage reminiscing in order to learn client's characteristic behavior, level of self-esteem, past coping patterns, and unique needs.
- Encourage expression of feelings to reduce anxiety and restore a sense of control.
- Do not dismiss any complaint as unimportant.
- Identify available supports for the client.
- Write down or repeat important information as necessary.
- Recognize the ruminative tendency during crises as necessary for restored function. Support this process by indicating to client that it is a stage in the resolution of crises.
- Leave the client with some tangible benefit and a sense of hope (e.g., a phone number to call for assistance or a plan of action).

Psychotropic Drugs

Many of the elderly are overtreated with medication in lieu of psychotherapy or other therapeutic interventions. Drugs are certainly a helpful adjunct when used judiciously, but they are often used indiscriminately. The overuse of psychotropic medications in the care of the aged has been widely documented. A national sample of 6,200 adults over 65 showed psychotropic drug use was exceeded only by use of medications for heart disease and hypertension (Watson et al. 1980). More than 10 percent of this sample had taken psychotropics within two weeks prior to the interview. Unmarried older adults in poor health were most likely to use psychotropic drugs. Females used them more than males and use declined for both sexes with increased age.

The emotional needs of the elderly will remain unmet as long as drugs are the main mode of treatment. In addition, many drugs used to treat disorders of the aged may create mental and emotional disturbances. Some of the common offenders and symptoms are noted in Table 22–6 (also see Chapter 23).

Table 22–6 GERIATRIC SYMPTOMS OF DRUGS COMMONLY USED	
Drugs	**Symptoms**
Hypoglycemics and hypotensives (phenothiazines, antidepressants, narcotic analgesics, antiarrhythmic drugs, antihypertensives)	Nervousness, apprehension, irritability, disorientation, dizziness, syncope
Cortisone	Severe depression
Digitalis	Arrhythmias, confusion, agitation, disorientation, dizziness, apathy, depression, headache, hallucinations
Central nervous system depressants (major and minor tranquilizers, sedatives, hypnotics, alcohol, methyldopa, antidepressants, narcotic analgesics, reserpine)	Lethargy, memory problems, perceptual disorders, delusions, agitation, panic, confusion
Anticholinergics (atropine, major tranquilizers, antidepressants, anti-parkinsonian drugs)	Confusion, blurred vision, agitation, disorientation, impaired memory
Propranolol	Nightmares
Quinidine	Vertigo, tinnitus, headache
Procainamide	Manic behavior, giddiness, psychosis, hallucinations, depression
Lithium toxicity	Blurred vision, slurred speech, ataxia, tremors

Data from: B. Todd, "Drugs and the Elderly: Could Your Patient's Confusion Be Caused by Drugs?" *Geriatric Nursing* 7 (May/June 1981): 219–220.

Drugs must always be given cautiously and in reduced dosage. Circulation, detoxification, and excretion are impaired in the aged, so drugs have more lasting and often idiosyncratic effects. Physicians and nurses need special education in geriatric pharmacology, particularly regarding drug incompatabilities and interactions, since the average old person takes six drugs daily. It is not possible to cover all the specific drug problems in this chapter, but Table 22–7 highlights some that are of major concern when giving psychotropic drugs.

Because of the prevalence of alcoholism among the aged, we include Table 22–8 to help nurses recognize problems occurring due to alcohol and drug interactions.

Be sure medications are not being used to disguise, suppress, or avoid dealing with psychic or interpersonal problems. They are sometimes given to the aged to restore the tranquillity of caretakers rather than clients.

Group Work

Chiefly because of the lack of available trained personnel and the need of many aged for therapy and increased socialization, group work has been the most frequent mode of intervention with the aged. Groups have been created and promoted for any imaginable problem of aging and to support those functioning on the lowest and highest levels. Burnside (1978) has edited an excellent resource book for nurses wishing to institute group strategies with the aged. It includes plans for self-help, recreational, remotivational, reality orientation, reminiscing, resocialization, and many other types of groups. Most of these are oriented toward clients in long-term care situations, but they can be modified to fit varied settings. Table 22–9 gives guidelines for three group strategies. See also Chapter 18. Groups can be one means of building a social network. Reactivating social skills and sharing information about resources can increase life satisfaction on both interpersonal and practical levels.

Family Support Groups

Families caring for aged members or those who have found institutionalization necessary need the support of families in similar situations. Such groups may be quite specific, such as those organized for the families of institutionalized persons, stroke and cancer victims, Alzheimer clients, or more general problems. Many families need help to deal with the guilt accompanying institutionalization of a parent. Mutual problem solving, shared reactions, ventilation of feelings, and edu-

Table 22-7 PRINCIPLES OF ADMINISTERING PSYCHOTROPIC DRUGS TO THE AGED	
Nursing Responsibilities	**Nursing Concerns**
1. Accurate observation of need should guide decisions regarding drugs. Inexact impressions are dangerous.	1. Tranquilizers in conjunction with diuretics increase the incidence of hypotension, confusion, and incontinence.
2. Educate clients and observe for potentially hazardous side effects.	2. Hypnotics increase the incidence of incontinence, confusion, and falls.
3. Use minimum amounts of medication and increase dosage only when necessary.	3. Tricyclics may cause urinary retention and cardiac complications.
4. Give sufficient time to assessing response to a drug rather than prematurely switching to another.	4. Minor tranquilizers increase problems of mobility in persons with an unsteady gait.
5. Confer with physicians regarding specific reason for selecting and prescribing a certain drug.	5. Cumulative reactions, including tardive dyskinesia, are more frequent occurrences among the old taking major tranquilizers.
6. Alert physicians to the total drug profile of an individual—including over-the-counter drugs that are habitually used and alcohol intake. Hazardous interactions are frequent.	6. Depression, confusion, and paradoxic agitation may be due to psychoactive drug intake.
7. Encourage periodic lab tests to monitor cumulative toxicity.	7. Reduced smooth muscle mobility and mucoid secretions that occur in normal aging are increased by the use of major tranquilizers.
8. Encourage physicians to discontinue all but life-sustaining medications for the first week of hospital stay. Medications may be the source of symptoms.	8. Tranquilizers (major and minor) and hypnotics may lower body temperature to dangerous levels in the aged who are prone to hypothermia.
9. Use interpersonal contact and comfort measures before resorting to the use of hypnotics or minor tranquilizers.	9. Many psychoactive drugs increase intraocular pressure and reduce visual accommodation. This is dangerous for persons with glaucoma and those with already poor visual accommodation.
10. Accurately record drugs given and reactions.	10. The aged are more vulnerable to Lithium and tricyclic toxicity due to impaired renal filtration and clearance.

cation about aging will help families remain involved in the lives of their aged members.

Networking

Networking is a current and popular concept that means we establish and tap a network of services and individuals to meet our needs. A network involves some reciprocity. Primary networks are personal, intimate, and affectual. Secondary networks usually involve acquaintances or service providers and are used to obtain specific assistance. We need both types just as a tree needs a tap root (primary) for nourishment and superficial roots (secondary) for support. The aged rely most heavily on primary networks when possible and may not have developed an adequate secondary network. When working with disturbed, disruptive, or decompensated aged, it is important to determine the quality and stability of the networks, to use them appropriately, and to reinforce them.

Some aged are unaware of the existence of a supportive network, saying such things as, "I'm all alone, I don't have anyone." The nurse will need to explore this statement fully in order to establish the existence of a potential support group. Some of the following may be unrecognized people in a person's network: barber/hairdresser, grocer, bus driver, minister, auto mechanic, telephone operator, bank clerks, physician, nurse, bartender, landlord. Making a list of the persons one contacts in a month is a helpful beginning. Searching out the existing network and planning how it can best be used and reinforced is very helpful to the aged. Another method of assistance is network support. All members of an individual's network are brought together to give each other support, share concerns, and solve problems together. Some of the most effective

Table 22-8 ALCOHOL AND DRUG INTERACTIONS

Class	Generic names	Specific problems	Antagonistic	Additive	Supra-additive	Cross-tolerance	Unpredictable	Untoward, life-threatening
Analgesics	Aspirin (ASA), acetaminophen	Delayed clotting time, gastrointestinal bleeding, fecal blood loss, hemorrhage					X	
Anesthetics	Chloroform, ether	Deep narcosis, excessive recovery time; more needed initially to induce sleep		X	X	X		
Antialcohol preparations	Disulfiram	Increase blood pressure, facial flushing, tachycardia, headache, nausea, dizziness, fainting						X
Antianginal drugs Antihypertensives	Nitroglycerin, methyldopa, hydralazine, guanethidine, reserpine, peripheral vasodilators	Hypotension, faintness, loss of consciousness		X				
Anticonvulsants	Phenytoin	Accelerated metabolism, normal dosage inadequate				X		
Antidepressants	Monoamine oxidase (MAO) inhibitors	Hypertensive crisis—particularly with Chianti wine and beer			X			X
	Tricyclics: desipramine, amytriptyline	Increased susceptibility to convulsions, hypotension	X	X				
Antidiabetics / hypoglycemics	Tolbutamide, chlorpropamide, acetohexamide, tolazamide	Severe hypoglycemia, unpredictable fluctuations in serum glucose levels, increased rate of metabolism of drug					X	
Antihistamines	Diphenhydramine	Reduced performance ability, increased sedation, operation of machinery hazardous		X	X			
Antimicrobials / anti-infectives	Chloramphenicol, furazolidone, metronidazole, griseofulvin, isoniazid, quinacrine	Similar to disulfiram reactions (above), but milder					X	
Barbiturates	Secobarbital (Seconal), pentobarbital	Vomiting, severe motor impairment, unconsciousness, coma and death						X

Drug class	Examples	Effects			
Chloral hydrate		Profound vasodilation—sometimes 7 days after ingestion of alcohol; dysphoria, tachycardia	X		X
Major tranquilizers	Phenothiazines, thioridazine	Respiratory depression, increased seizure susceptibility, impaired hepatic function, hypotension	X	X	
Minor tranquilizers	Meprobamate, benzodiazepines, diazepam	Central nervous system depression, interferes with skills and alertness; despite literature to contrary, diazepam and alcohol combination is dangerous	X	X	
Narcotics	Hydromorphone, meperidine, morphine, propoxyphene	Central nervous system depression	X	X	
Stimulants	Caffeine, amphetamine	Variable effects on selected behaviors—depression, released inhibitions	X	X	X

Source: U.S. Department of Health, Education and Welfare, *FDA Drug Bulletin* 2(February-March, 1979):2.

Table 22-9 DIFFERENCES BETWEEN REMOTIVATION, RESOCIALIZATION, AND REALITY ORIENTATION		
Reality orientation	**Resocialization**	**Remotivation**
1. Correct position or relation with the existing situation in a community. Maximum use of assets	1. Continuation of reality living situation in a community	1. Orientation to reality for community living; present oriented
2. Called reality orientation and classroom reality orientation program	2. Called discussion group or resocialization to differentiate between a social function instead of a therapeutic need	2. Called remotivation
3. Structured	3. Unstructured	3. Definite structure
4. Refreshments and/or food may be served for identification	4. Refreshments served	4. Refreshments not served
5. Appreciation of the work of the world. Constantly reminded of who he is, where he is, why he is here, and what is expected of him	5. Appreciation of the work of the world. Reliving happy experiences. Encourages participation in home activities relating to subject	5. Appreciation of the work of the group stimulates the desire to return to function in society
6. Class range from 3 to 5, depending on degree/level of confusion or disorientation from any cause	6. Group range from 5 to 17, depending on mental and physical capabilities	6. Group size: 5 to 12
7. Meeting ½ hour daily at same time in same place	7. Meetings three times weekly for ½ to 1 hour	7. Meeting once to twice weekly for an hour
8. Planned procedure: reality-centered objects	8. No planned topic; group centered feelings	8. Preselected and reality-centered objects
9. Response of resident is responsibility of teacher	9. Clarification and interpretation is responsibility of leader	9. No exploration of feelings
10. Periodic reality orientation test pertaining to residents' level of confusion or disorientation	10. Periodic progress notes pertaining to residents' enjoyment and improvements	10. Progress ratings
11. Emphasis on time, place, person orientation	11. Any topic freely discussed	11. Topic: no discussion of religion, politics, or death
12. Use of portion of mind function still intact	12. Vast stockpile of memories and experiences	12. Untouched area of the mind
13. Resident greeted by name, thanked for coming, and extend hand shake and/or physical contact according to attitude approach in group	13. Resident greeted on arrival, thanked, and extended a handshake upon leaving	13. No physical contact permitted. Acceptance and acknowledgment of everyone's contribution
14. Conducted by trained aides and activity assistants	14. Conducted by RN, LPN/LVN, aides, and program assistants	14. Conducted by trained psychiatric aides

Source: Adapted by permission of *The Gerontologist/the Journal of Gerontology*, from E. Barns, A. Sack, and H. Shore, *The Gerontologist* 13(1973):513.

therapy is indirect and consists simply of reinforcing the strength of a network.

Confidants

Lowenthal and Haven (1968) found the presence of a confidant, or primary support person, was essential to the maintenance of mental health in old age. Morbidity is considerably reduced in elderly people who have even one supportive person available to them (Berkman and Syme 1980). Nurses are initially part of a secondary support system but often become part of the primary support system of an aged individual. The nature of nursing is to interact in intimate and affectual events, and therefore the superficiality of secondary relationships is quickly replaced by much more personal interactions. It is clear that the aged, who experience many losses in primary supports, need responsive caring interactions.

Reminiscing

The tendency all people have to recall and ponder past experience gives life meaning and continuity. Older people, having more past experiences, may draw on them more frequently. Reminiscing can be used:

- Diagnostically
- To build a relationship
- To determine coping strategies
- To maintain self-esteem
- To resolve emotional disturbances
- To establish meaning through a legacy

Diagnosis   When recalling past events, the present affectual state will influence what the client remembers. Therefore, present emotional tone can be derived from the nature of retrieved memories: hopelessness, depression, fear, pessimism, resignation, acceptance, optimism, joy, suspicion, and many other feelings and attitudes can be determined if the nurse listens carefully to the shared experiences.

Relationship Building   When building trust in a relationship, it is imperative to develop a sense of the person we are talking to. Asking about a client's past and significant events makes us participant observers of life as another has experienced it. This helps establish foundations of understanding.

Coping Strategies   To determine potential strength and coping capacity, nurses need to know how clients have handled crises and problems in the past. Asking about previous stressful times and resources used gives a basis for planning present care for an individual. Personal strength, sense of humor, and capacity for interest in others is apparent as we share memories of difficult times.

Maintenance of Self-esteem   In later years many persons lose sight of their accomplishments and capabilities—particularly during periods when they are disturbed, distressed, or grief-stricken. It is imperative for the nurse to assist the aged toward a whole life perspective by asking about successes, roles, fulfillments, products, skills, and so on.

Having established a relationship, determined coping strategies, identified present affectual state and attitudes, and confirmed strengths, it is possible to begin working on resolutions of emotional disturbance through the process of life review.

Life Review   The disturbed elderly are those who are disappointed with the lives they have lived and feel they are the pawns of fate or have mismanaged situations and opportunities. Regrets about wrongdoing or injustices may become a preoccupation of old age since there is no time to undo real or imagined failures. Those who believe themselves to be victims may be pessimistic and paranoid, but those who accept personal responsibility for a life of disappointment may be profoundly depressed.

The therapeutic task with an aged client is to facilitate and support the process of life review (Butler 1963). This is a process of reviewing painful and disappointing life events, ventilating feelings, sharing another's perspective, and modifying self-perception. Throughout life everyone evaluates themselves internally and from the feedback of others. Harsh judgments may need to be modified by intensive exploration of actions and events. Self-examination and revelation is a painful process.

Nurses engaging in this process can expect to participate in another's sorrow and grief. It is not easy, and it requires a large time commitment. However, it is one of the most efficacious of all interactions. The nurse's acceptance validates the goodness of those who judge themselves harshly. Those who are grieving lost opportunities can relinquish some grief, and the nurse can reinforce their courage with attention and feedback. Those with unresolved anger at life's inequities may regain a sense of control as they recognize their successes and accept personal responsibility as neither absent or total. Relationships may be repaired as the client and nurse rehearse ways to communicate with those who are alienated. The nurse may introduce alternative views of a situation, and exploration of the complexities of events may help the despairing elderly achieve a sense of integrity and accept their life as it was lived. The nurse need only listen, validate, explore, and give feedback. In the process the nurse and client become more fully human and accepting of the strengths and frailties of living beings.

Since life review is a critical component of adjustment and fulfillment in later life, professionals will need to stimulate and support the process. The following guidelines will be helpful.

Table 22-10 LEGACIES	
Tangible	**Intangible**
Homes	Courage
Money	Endurance
Property	Integrity
Collections	Wisdom
Art objects	Awareness/cognition
Belongings	Humor
Children, friends, family	Flexibility
Products	Curiosity
Contributions	Creativity
	Titles
	Positions
	Roles

GUIDELINES FOR LIFE-REVIEW THERAPY

- Alert aged people to the characteristics and normality of the life review process.
- Provide opportunities for aged people to recapitulate events in their lives, by asking such questions as: What has most influenced the course of your life? Who has most influenced the course of your life?
- Help aged people view their life experiences in a broader or different context, using such questions as: Can you think of other factors that contributed to those events? How would you have changed your life then? What factors influenced your course of action? What would you do differently now?
- Facilitate connections between past hopes, present events, and future expectations.
- Be aware that the process may be carried out sporadically over several months. It is a painful examination of the past and is sometimes avoided.

Legacies   Legacies are the substance and meaning of existence. They include tangible and intangible personal assets. Tangible assets form the substance of legacies and intangible assets create the meaning. See Table 22-10. Old people usually have both and it is important to identify and validate them.

Supporting the Dying and the Grieving

Mr. L. cried as he shared how his life had been empty, meaningless, and a failure. He was uneducated and had worked from childhood in menial hard labor. He had served in two wars and never married. No relatives survived him who would mourn his impending death. He had no belongings of his own and his last two years had been spent immobilized in a hospital bed. The depression and futility he felt were overwhelming. The nurse began to cry with him, then she took action. She developed a nursing plan around her assessment of his need to establish a legacy, to increase his self-esteem and reduce his isolation.

To reduce his isolation, the nurse

- *Moved his bed to the lounge each afternoon*
- *Obtained a small radio, calendar, and clock to give time structure and enjoyment through music*
- *Spent time with him daily*

To establish a legacy and elevate his self-esteem, the nurse

- *Began life review, focusing on his intangible assets: courage, patriotism, endurance, appreciation of music, and his influence on and help to others in the course of his life*
- *Encouraged him to express his disappointment and lost opportunities and tried to help him look at them in the context of his total situation at the time*

Table 22-11 GRIEF IN OLD AGE	
Characteristics	**Interventions**
1. Chronicity or grief overload arising from multiple, frequent losses	1. Identify number of losses and presence of grief and depression since the client may not recognize it. Encourage verbal review of the losses.
2. Regret for what cannot be undone	2. Review context of life situation that produces regret and/or guilt.
3. Premature grief for one's own death and separation from loved ones	3. Listen to expressions of grief, establish legacy, provide opportunities for intimate time with loved ones, singly rather than in groups.
4. Grief for the alteration of one's own personality and cognition through disease processes	4. Support individual and family in focusing on remaining strengths and exchanging caring gestures.
5. Grieving the loss of companionship with a mentally deteriorating aged spouse	5. Assist functioning spouse to establish or find a support group of persons in similar situation. Locate respite services for functioning spouse. Provide anticipatory guidance for handling problems of deterioration.
6. Survival anguish, particularly that of outliving one's children or siblings	6. Provide consistent support through grief process, paying particular attention to holidays and anniversary dates. Reduce survivor guilt by conducting life review and establishing legacy of the deceased.
7. Grief over the loss of body function or parts	7. Encourage person to mourn; do not avoid talking of the loss. Tell them grief process is normal and painful. Listen. Help them identify compensatory functions when acute grief subsides.

• *Told him how important he was to her and how much she had learned from him*

With increasing socialization and self-esteem through interpersonal contact, Mr. L. was able to accept his life as in many ways disappointing but no less full of meaning.

Supporting the dying and the grieving is an essential function of gerontological nursing. When support has been missing, the client may exhibit pathologic grief and despair and profound, immobilizing depression. Fortunately, it is never too late to grieve fully and become aware of the feelings and reactions that normally accompany grief. Depression, lack of concentration, lowered self-esteem, apathy, and inability to make decisions are often dismissed as the normal concomitants of aging rather than symptoms of unresolved grief. Table 22-11 enumerates the characteristics of grief in old age and lists interventions to assist the grief process.

Many situations that produce grief reactions have been discussed throughout this chapter, and any of the therapeutic strategies suggested may be appropriate modes of intervention depending on the individual. Psychotherapy and family and support groups assist the grieving. Reminiscing, life review, and legacy building are part of the process of dying. Nurses should review Lindemann's (1944) classic article identifying grief reactions and Kubler-Ross's (1969) stages of dying. It is a nursing privilege to spend time with the dying and grieving, encouraging verbalization of related feelings and sharing this most significant time.

The last days of life can be a time of resolution and psychological growth (Kubler-Ross 1975). Older people are only individuals who have lived a long time. Linear time is a western civilization obsession and so much of our difficulty relating to the aged appropriately comes from our notion of finite time and our collective neuroses about endings. Of course, the aged often share this cultural viewpoint. The end of personal time is inconceivable to most of us when young, and the task of later years is to find meaning in this human condition. Youth is the time of data accumulation and later life is the time for using knowledge to develop wisdom. The nurse's relationship with aging people transcends time as each participates in the experience of the other.

KEY NURSING CONCEPTS

✔ Most aged individuals remain vitally alive and mentally healthy.

✔ The disturbed elderly reflect an internalized cultural devaluation of their place in society.

✔ Interactions with aged individuals can help the nurse to confront his or her own aging.

✔ The nurse's positive attitude toward aging may be best facilitated by keeping contact with well-adapted, vital aged persons.

✔ Common stresses among aged individuals include fear of aging, loneliness, loss, meaningless-ness, physical deterioration, stigma, sexuality, relocation, and abuse and neglect.

✔ The definition of "old" is a changing, socially determined idea.

✔ Aged individuals receive only a small percentage of contemporary mental health services.

✔ Survivability, stamina, and a clear sense of self may be most indicative of mental health in old age.

✔ Maintenance of mental health in the aged is strongly related to environmental and interper-sonal negotiations.

✔ Three late-life tasks include the establishment of body-transcendence versus body preoccupa-tion, ego-identity versus role preoccupation, and ego-transcendence versus ego preoccupation.

✔ Idiosyncratic behavior in the aged individual may be a product of strong, mentally healthy adaptation; in fact, many of the reactions of the aged that might be considered disturbed in youth are reasonable in old age.

✔ Disturbed patterns in the aged usually arise either from long-standing problems in adaptation or an overload of present stresses.

✔ Disintegrative patterns in the aged most frequently arise from physiologic disturbance.

✔ Restoration of body function, sensory accoutrements, a structured and moderately stimulat-ing environment, and caring interactions are basic to recovery of disintegrative patterns in the aged.

✔ Confusion is the most common emotional, behavioral, and cognitive reaction to stressors in old age.

✔ Confabulation may be used by the older adult in an attempt to maintain self-esteem by covering memory gaps.

✔ Nursing intervention with the aged person who has a cognitive dysfunction is begun by orienting the person to essential information in a relaxed way.

✔ In the elderly, hypochrondriasis often signals the presence of depression.

✔ Suicidal attempts in the aged are likely to be planned and successful.

✔ Family members caring for an aged adult frequently need physical, emotional, and informa-tional support in order to cope successfully.

✔ Many elderly are overtreated with medication in lieu of psychotherapy or other therapeutic intervention.

✔ For the older adult participation in groups can be an important means of establishing a social network, maintaining social skills, and increasing self-esteem.

✔ The presence of a confidant, or primary support person, can be essential to the maintenance of mental health in old age.

✔ Reminiscing can be a significant therapeutic tool in counseling the elderly.

✔ Identification and recognition of the older adult's legacies through the process of life review can be an important therapeutic experience.

References

Berkman, L., and Syme, L. "Social Networks, Host Resistance and Mortality: a Nine-Year Followup Study of Alameda County Residents." *American Journal of Epidemiology* 109 (1979): 109–186.

Block, M., and Sinnott, J. *The Battered Elderly Syndrome.* College Park, Md.: University of Maryland Center on Aging, 1979.

Brink, T. "Geriatric Counseling: A Practical Guide." *Family Therapy* 3 (1976): 163.

Burnside, I., ed. *Working with the Elderly: Group Processes and Techniques.* North Scituate, Mass.: Duxbury Press, 1978.

Butler, R. "Life Review: An Interpretation of Reminiscence in the Aged." *Psychiatry* 26 (1963): 65.

Butler, R. N., and Lewis, M. I. *Aging and Mental Health: Positive Psychosocial Approaches.* 3d ed. St. Louis: C. V. Mosby, 1981.

Carp, F., and Carp, A. "It May Not Be the Answer, It May Not Be the Question." *Research on Aging* 3 (1981): 85–100.

Cavenar, J.; Malthie, A.; and Austin, L. "Depression Simulating Organic Brain Disease." *American Journal of Psychiatry* 136 (1979): 521.

Cummings, E., and Henry, W. *Growing Old.* New York: Basic Books, 1961.

Ebersole, P., and Hess, P. *Toward Healthy Aging: Human Needs and Nursing Response.* St. Louis, Mo.: C. V. Mosby, 1981.

Erikson, E. *Childhood and Society.* 2d ed. New York: W. W. Norton, 1963.

Harris, L. *The Myth and Reality of Aging in America.* Washington, D.C.: National Council on the Aging, 1975.

Holmes, T., and Rahe, H. "The Social Readjustment Rating Scale," *Journal of Psychomatic Response* 11 (1967): 213.

Javrik, L., and Russell, D. "Anxiety, Aging and the Third Emergency Reaction." *Journal of Gerontology* 34 (1979): 197.

Jung, C. *Memories, Dreams, Reflections.* New York: Alfred A. Knopf and Random House, 1961.

Kubler-Ross, E. *On Death and Dying.* New York: Macmillan, 1969.

———. *Death: The Final Stage of Growth.* Englewood Cliffs, N.J.: Prentice-Hall, 1975.

Lau, E., and Cosberg, J. *Abuse of the Elderly by Informal Care Providers: Practice and Research Issues.* Paper presented at 31st Annual Meeting of Gerontological Society, Dallas, Texas, 1978.

Lindemann, D. "Symptomatology and Management of Acute Grief." *American Journal of Psychiatry* 101 (1944): 101–148.

Lowenthal, M., and Haven, C. "Interaction and Adaptation: Intimacy as a Crucial Variable." *American Sociological Review* 33 (1960): 1.

Lundeman, K. "The Sexuality of the Older Person: Review of the Literature." *Gerontologist* 21 (1981): 203–208.

Maslow, A. *Toward a Psychology of Being.* New York: Van Nostrand, 1962.

Moustakas, C. *Loneliness.* Englewood Cliffs, N.J.: Prentice-Hall, 1961.

Peck, R. "Psychological Developments in the Second Half of Life." In *Middle Age and Aging,* edited by B. Neugarten. Chicago: University of Chicago Press, 1968.

Plawecki, H., and Plawecki, J. "Aging Each Other." *Journal of Gerontological Nursing* 7 (1981): 35–40.

Reifler, B.; Cox, G.; and Hanley, R. "Problems of Mentally Ill Elderly as Perceived by Patients, Families, and Clinicians." *Gerontologist* 21 (1981): 165–170.

Stagner, R. "Stress, Strain, Coping, and Defense." *Research on Aging* 3 (1981): 3–32.

Stever, J.; Bank, L.; Olsen, E.; and Javrik, L. "Depression, Physical Health, and Somatic Complaints in the Elderly: A Study of the Zung Self-rating Depression Scale." *Journal of Gerontology* 34 (1980): 683–688.

Todd, B. "Drugs and the Elderly: Could Your Patient's Confusion Be Caused by Drugs?" *Geriatric Nursing* 7 (May/June 1981): 219–220.

Watson, J.; Eve, S.; and Reiss, E. "Use of Psychotropic Prescription Medicines among Older Adults." *Gerontologist* 20 (1980): 220.

Wells, L., and Macdonald, G. "Interpersonal Networks

and Post-relocation Adjustment of the Institutionalized Elderly." *Gerontologist* 21 (1981): 177–183.

White, C., and Catania, J. "An Intervention Program for Sexual Attitudes, Knowledge, and Behavior with the Community Aged, Service Providers and Families." *Gerontologist* 20 (1980): 210.

Wolanin, M., and Phillips, O. *Confusion: Prevention and Care.* St. Louis: C. V. Mosby, 1981.

Zung, W. "Zung Self-rating Depression Scale." *Archives of General Psychiatry* 12 (1964): 62.

Further Reading

Baum, M., and Baum, R. C. *Growing Old: A Societal Perspective.* Englewood Cliffs, N.J.: Prentice-Hall, 1980.

Berry, W. *The Memory of Old Jack.* New York: Harcourt Brace Jovanovich, 1975.

Eisdorfer, C., and Friedel, R. *Cognitive and Emotional Disturbance in the Elderly.* Chicago: Year Book Medical Publishers, 1977.

Gaitz, C. M. *Aging and the Brain.* New York: Plenum Publishing, 1972.

Grollman, E. A. *Concerning Death: A Practical Guide for the Living.* Boston: Beacon Press, 1974.

Murray, R.; Huelskoetter, M. M.; and Driscoll, D. *The Nursing Process in Later Maturity.* Englewood Cliffs, N.J.: Prentice-Hall, 1980.

Rossman, I. *Clinical Geriatrics.* 2d ed. Philadelphia: Lippincott, 1979.

Stoddard, S. *The Hospice Movement: A Better Way of Caring for the Dying.* Briarcliff Manor, N.Y.: Stein and Day, 1978.

VSDHEW. *Readings in Psychotherapy with Older People.* Washington, D.C.: National Institute of Mental Health, 1977.

23

Biological Therapies

by Andrew E. Skodol

CHAPTER OUTLINE

Changing Roles for Nurses
    Negotiating Communication
    The Nurse as Client Advocate
Psychotropic Drugs
    Antipsychotic Drugs
    Antidepressant Drugs
    The Antimania Drug (Lithium)
    Antianxiety Drugs
    Hypnotic Drugs
Electroconvulsive Therapy
    Indications for Use
    Procedure
    Course of Treatment
    Complications
Narcotherapy
Radical Biological Therapies
    Psychosurgery
    Insulin Coma Treatment
Newer Organic Therapies
    Niacin Therapy

    Electrosleep Therapy
    Nonconvulsive Electrical Stimulation Therapy
    Hemodialysis
Key Nursing Concepts

LEARNING OBJECTIVES

After reading this chapter, students should be able to

- Explore the role of biological therapies within the humanistic interactionist perspective of mental health care
- Recall the properties, classification, use, and side effects of the major psychotropic drugs
- Identify the indications, contraindications, and major considerations in the use of biological therapies such as ECT, narcotherapy, insulin coma treatment, psychosurgery, and the newer organic therapies
- Discuss the role of the nurse in biological therapies

CHAPTER 23

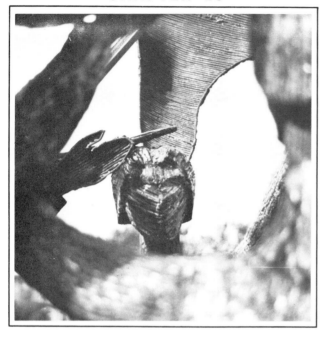

The increased reliance on biological therapies in psychiatric care provides the nurse with a unique opportunity to advocate and teach their use in meaningful and positive, rather than controlling, inhibiting, and dehumanizing, ways.

CHANGING ROLES FOR NURSES

The modern history of biological therapy in psychiatry is characterized by increasing reliance on the use of psychotropic medications and electroconvulsive therapies. Initially reserved for the most seriously disturbed or distraught, biological treatment is now used even for individuals with relatively minor conditions. The climate conducive to this trend has been created by progressively more sophisticated attempts by research neurobiologists to define the biological mechanisms of both normal and abnormal brain functioning.

The criteria used to measure the success of the biological model have been debated even within the medically oriented community. Whether the degree of deviation from the norm (i.e., symptomatology), amount of time hospitalized, level of functioning as reflected by employment history, or quantity and quality of social relations constitute valid measures of human functioning or potential is hotly contested in the literature. In an antimedical setting even more challenges would be raised.

It may appear paradoxical to present a chapter on biological therapies in a textbook of psychiatric nursing that explicitly challenges the appropriateness of the medical model for dealing with problems of human emotions. Nonetheless, in the practice of modern clinical psychiatry, whether in a hospital, clinic, or commu-

nity, biological therapies flourish. Thus, an understanding of their use and misuse must be integrated into any approach to psychiatric nursing. It would be as reductionistic and irrational for humanists to ignore or dismiss biological therapies arbitrarily as for medical psychiatry to neglect humanistic considerations. The task of the psychiatric nurse parallels the apparent paradox of this chapter: to integrate the appropriate use of biological treatments in a meaningful, positive way into the lives of clients.

Negotiating Communication

Revision of the psychiatric nurse's role in the biological therapies can be approached as an example of the application of symbolic interactionism. This, of course, assumes that nurses depart widely from the traditional nursing responsibilities regarding medication, electroconvulsive therapy (ECT), and coma therapies, for example. No longer would they consider it sufficient merely to measure and dispense medications or offer pre- and postoperative technical care to a client. A changed role further implies at least a partial reworking of the underlying theoretical assumptions that determine the nursing approach.

Neither chance nor devious manipulation resulted in the predominance of the medical model in the field of psychiatry. The special relationship that has developed between certain people in distress and a group of care givers seems to be a perfect example of a negotiated communication. Both doctors and clients have agreed to treat stressful life conditions and internal experiences as illnesses, symptoms, and diseases. However, many clinical examples illustrate the potentially inappropriate, and occasionally maladaptive, behavior patterns and identifications that can result from this steady state. For example, the clinging dependency characteristic of the client who attempts to adapt to stressful circumstances by assuming the "sick role" and the secondary gain (gratification) that frequently accrues to the client from this posture can pose considerable difficulties for family and therapist alike. Or the negative identity associated with the word *invalidism*, as applied to the chronically afflicted, can literally discount the experience of these human beings, further alienating them from their social networks. It is clear that we must renegotiate the meaning of being a psychiatric client.

The Nurse as Client Advocate

The psychiatric nurse may be in an especially advantageous position, in relationship to the biological therapies, to balance the strong tendency for the traditional doctor–client relationship to flourish. Nurse and client could develop an advocacy model that would maximize the effectiveness of appropriate biological treatment. There is a distinct need to discuss and renegotiate the negative, invalidating meanings attached to words such as *symptoms, illness, chronicity,* and *treatment,* with special attention paid to understanding and responding to meanings within the individual client's frame of reference.

An Example of the Need for Advocacy   This chapter cannot present all the possible models or examples of potentially useful social dialogues between client and nurse. As a concrete example, however, of the use of interactional and biological treatments as adjunct approaches, we will consider an issue of considerable relevance to clinical psychopharmacology. Lack of client cooperation in taking psychotropic medication constitutes the greatest and most frequently overlooked threat to positive clinical response. From the "cuckoo's nest" of Ken Kesey's novel (1962), to the real state hospitals, outpatient clinics, and private practices, clients do not take their medications. It is exceedingly common to find in such cases that the psychiatrist and the client have failed to reach an understanding about how medication will be used or even that this course will be undertaken. More than any other factor, this failure is responsible for relapse and readmission—the so-called revolving door syndrome.

It should come as no suprise that, when asked their reasons for "noncompliance," clients describe special meanings—some shared, some idiosyncratic—that they attach to the instruction to take medication. To one client, the need for medications represents a severe blow to self-esteem, a jolt to the client's self-image as an autonomous, capable human being. To another, being viewed by others as unable to control one's own emotions or behavior is a particularly frightening, embarrassing, or depressing state. To yet others, an attempt by the doctor to use medications in the treatment may evoke uncomfortable memories of other powerful figures who attempted to exert influence over them, perhaps in cruel and sadistic ways, perhaps selfishly, without regard to their wishes or feelings. To some clients, the introduction of medications symbolizes chronicity. The doctor has given up hope of helping them and is consigning them to the status of incurables. Addiction is another common fear, even if the client has been given substantial reassurance to the contrary. Medication is also an overt assault on the secondary gain derived from the "sick" role. This can be a source of considerable resistance from a client who feels hopeless to find an alternative satisfying or gratifying role in the family or social group.

The issue of client compliance with treatment is important not only for psychopharmacology but also for the other biological therapies and perhaps for all psychiatric or even all medical treatments. How the designated client chooses to respond to the intervention of the treating person is neglected all too often. Knowledge about biological therapies and skill in negotiating the therapeutic contract can make the nurse invaluable in this area.

Psychiatric nurses have expressed great interest in teaching clients to understand the nature of their treatment, especially when medications are involved, and have exerted leadership in integrating client education about drugs into the overall care plan for psychiatric clients. Janet Smith and her nursing colleagues have developed a series of drug information cards for each of the major classes of psychotropic drugs (Smith 1981). Smith hypothesized that clients often fail to follow their medication regimens after discharge from the hospital because they do not understand why they need the drugs or what side effects might occur and how they might deal with them. Therefore the drug cards give:

- The name of the drug
- The prescribed dosage
- The therapeutic action
- The possible side effects
- The precautions the client can take to avoid, minimize, or alleviate the side effects

The Nurse's Salutary Position   The meanings attached to treatment in the psychiatric setting are complex and nearly always individual. There are no prescriptions for dealing with the hopes, wishes, and fears of clients. There is no shortcut to approaching clients in an advocacy role, attempting to understand and work with each one's individual concerns. The modern psychiatric nurse has the opportunity to become a specialist in this area of communication, since the psychiatrist is less likely to be able to cast aside the medical orientation sufficiently to meet clients halfway.

This chapter presents basic knowledge on the biological therapies, primarily from a medical point of view, since the model of symptoms, diagnoses, and prognoses is most commonly applied in biological treatment. We emphasize, however, that the nurse should not be overwhelmed by the relevance of the medical model. In the field of psychiatry, no treatment approach yet discovered is definitive and sufficient for any group of clients defined according to any classification scheme. This is also true for biological treatment.

PSYCHOTROPIC DRUGS

By far the most significant of all biological therapies, for clinical purposes, is the use of psychotropic drugs. These medications that literally "act upon the mind" are now among the most widely prescribed in all of medicine, not only psychiatry. The beneficial effects on emotional states of virtually all the early important drugs were discovered fortuitously. Thus the historical orientation of psychopharmacology is geared to symptom relief. On the other hand, no other single approach has been more fruitful than pharmacology in leading to discoveries about the etiologies of the mental disorders. The mechanisms of action of the psychotropic drugs have provided "windows" on the brain's functioning. Thus, in addition to having universally widespread clinical utility, these medications have helped unlock the mysteries of the biological basis of emotional life. An example is the discovery that certain drugs can induce and remit Depression by their consistent pharmacological effect on the *neurotransmitters* (the chemical substances responsible for the conducting of nerve impulses through the brain). Table 23–1 summarizes these relationships for drugs that affect Depression. On the basis of these observations, inadequate amounts of norepinephrine have been postulated as critical mechanisms in the development of certain kinds of Depressive Disorders.

The issue of diagnostic accuracy arises before consideration of psychopharmacological treatment, or any biological therapy for that matter. Although that topic is beyond the scope of this chapter, valid and reliable assessment of the client's condition is a prerequisite for effective psychopharmacological management (see

Table 23–1 EFFECTS OF DRUGS ON NOREPINEPHRINE SECRETION AND DEPRESSION

Type of Drug	Effect
Drugs that increase the effective amount of the norepinephrine (NE) available for nerve impulse transmission at the synaptic membrane	
Tricyclic antidepressants—inhibit the reuptake pump that brings NE back into the presynaptic cell where it is more rapidly degraded and less available to conduct impulses	Reduces depression
Monoamine oxidase (MAO) inhibitors—inhibit intracellular destruction of NE by the enzyme monoamine oxidase	Reduces depression
Drugs that lower the NE in the brain	
Reserpine—reduces storage of NE in granules in cells, where it is protected from degradation	Induces depression
Alpha-methyl-dopa—interferes with NE synthesis by displacement	Induces depression

Source: From Davis, "Central Biogenic Amines and Theories of Depression and Mania," in W. E. Fann; I. Karacen; A. D. Pokorny; and R. L. Williams, eds., *Phenomenology and Treatment of Depression* (New York: Spectrum Publications, 1977), p. 23.

Chapter 8). Interspersed through the body of this chapter are brief tables to alert nurses to important aspects of diagnosis or client assessment. All drug treatment approaches try to match particular syndromes with indicated drug regimens. No psychotropic agents have limitless potential for *even* symptomatic relief.

There are many confusing and ambiguous classification schemes for the psychotropic medications. Hollister (1973), whose system we will use here, classifies the medications according to their major symptomatic effects:

- Antipsychotics
- Antidepressants
- Antimania agents
- Antianxiety agents

Table 23–2	MEDICAL ILLNESSES PRESENTING A PSYCHOTIC SYNDROME
Type of Illness	**Example**
Exogenous substance	Steroid-induced OBS
Infectious	Viral encephalitis
Neurologic	Neoplasms
Cardiovascular	Hypertension
Endocrine	Thyroid disease
Metabolic	Diabetes
Collagen	Systemic lupus erythematosus

Source: Compiled from R. I. Shader, *Manual of Psychiatric Therapeutics* (Boston: Little, Brown and Co., 1975), pp. 64-65.

Antipsychotic Drugs

Background   The discovery of the first and most important antipsychotic drug, chlorpromazine (Thorazine), is a prime example of the role chance has played in the history of psychopharmacology. This drug was initially synthesized as an antihistamine and was not tried as a tranquilizer with schizophrenic persons until 1952. Its effects on the behavior, thinking, affect, and perception of schizophrenic persons was so profound that knowledge of its properties was rapidly disseminated and it became widely used within three or four years. Chlorpromazine's effects on the hospital practice of psychiatry were staggering. Its use reversed a steadily increasing census in United States mental institutions, and it has led to a progressive decrease in the mental hospital population ever since. One might say that chlorpromazine gave birth to the modern notions of psychiatric treatment—unlocked wards, milieu treatment, occupational and recreational therapy, and halfway houses. The entire field of community mental health is intimately linked to its discovery, because it enabled clients to return to their homes.

Major Effects   The beneficial effects of the antipsychotic medications in all functional psychotic states have been demonstrated beyond question, using multiple and varied criteria to measure improvement. The manifestations of disintegrative patterns affected by these drugs include delusional thinking, confusion, motor agitation, and motor retardation. In addition anti-

psychotic drug treatment causes a decrease in formal thought disorder, blunted affect, bizarre behavior, social withdrawal, hallucinations, belligerence, and uncooperativeness.

The most common disintegrative condition treated with the antipsychotic drugs is the group of symptoms traditionally labeled Schizophrenia. The proper manner for evaluating the so-called schizophrenic client and the diagnostic criteria in DSM-III appear in Chapter 16. The problem of assessment is complicated by the fact that many physical diseases can cause Organic Brain Syndromes with features like those of Schizophrenia. Examples of these are listed in Table 23–2 (see also Chapter 8). Suffice it to say that all clients manifesting a psychotic syndrome should have a thorough medical history and physical examination to rule out treatable medical illnesses. An example of the consequences of not doing so is presented in the following case.

Vera, an eighteen-year-old female, was brought to the psychiatric emergency area by her parents, one week after she had graduated from high school, because of a four-day history of bizarre behavior. She was staying inside, behaving erratically, and "talking nonsense" to her parents and her two siblings. She had done quite well in high school, had friends, dated, and was planning to attend the local community college in the fall. There was no history of abnormal behavior in the past. Drug use was also denied by her parents.

On examination the client was extremely agitated, ran around the waiting area, and screamed. She appeared frightened, and although her speech was basically incoherent the nurse could detect Vera's fears of being harmed by invisible people. Her furtive glances about the room suggested she was hearing voices. She was admitted with a diagnosis of "Acute Psychotic Episode, with Schizophrenia and Toxic or Organic Conditions to be ruled out." She was medicated with haloperidol 5 mg. intramuscularly.

One hour later, when the client had become quiet and routine vital signs were taken, her temperature was 102.5 degrees. The medical consultant was called, and Vera was given a workup for a fever of unknown origin. Without further medication Vera remained somnolent. The following day she lapsed into coma. A diagnosis of viral encephalitis resulting in an Organic Delusional Syndrome was made. Forty-eight hours after admission, Vera died.

Choice of Specific Drug   Although there are a great many antipsychotic medications on the market and claims are made for the greater efficacy of one

			Potency (Mg. Equivalent to 100 Mg. Chlorpro-	Usual Dosage Range	Side Effects		
Class	Generic Name	Trade Name	mazine)	(Mg./Day)	Sedative	Extrapyramidal*	Anticholinergic*
Pheno-thiazines							
Aliphatic	Chlorpromazine	Thorazine	100	150–1500	Very strong	Moderate	Strong
Piperadine	Thioridazine	Mellaril	100	150–800	Moderate	Minimal	Moderate
Piperizine	Trifluoperazine	Stelazine	5	10–60	Weak	Strong	Weak
	Fluphenazine	Prolixin	2	3–45	Weak	Strong	Weak
	Perphenazine	Trilafon	10	12–60	Weak	Strong	Weak
Butyro-phenones	Haloperidol	Haldol	2.5	2–40	Weak	Strong	Weak
Thiox-anthenes	Thiothixene	Navane	5	10–60	Weak	Strong	Weak
	Chlorprothixene	Taractan	100	40–600	Strong	Moderate	Strong
Dihydro-indolones	Molindone	Moban	10	15–225	Weak	Moderate	Weak
Dibenzo-xazepines	Loxipine	Loxitane	20	10–100	Moderate	Strong	Moderate

Table 23–3 ANTIPSYCHOTIC DRUGS

* Extrapyramidal and anticholinergic side effects are discussed later in this chapter.

over another, especially by the respective drug companies, controlled studies have failed to demonstrate substantially different antipsychotic effects among the drugs. The choice of a particular medication, then, usually depends on knowledge of the various pharmacological properties and side effects, the client's or a family member's history of drug response, and the psychiatrist's experience with various compounds. Important client variables are past successes with specific drugs, history of allergies, and history of serious or intolerable side effects. Certain side effects can often be used beneficially with clients, as we will discuss below. A certain amount of trial and error is expected in each clinical application.

Table 23–3 summarizes the characteristics of the major antipsychotic drugs. As the list of these drugs is extensive and growing, it makes sense for each member of the treatment team to become familiar with just a few representative drugs, their predictable effects, and their common side effects. The characteristics covered in the table are discussed in sequence in the sections that follow.

CLASS It is relevant that there are now five distinct chemical classes of antipsychotic medications commonly available and used in the United States. One class, the phenothiazines, can be broken down into three different types of medications. This provides a broad choice in terms of side effects and potential client responsiveness. A client who is unresponsive to one class may well respond to another that circumvents a problem in absorption, accumulation at neurotransmitter receptor sites, or metabolism.

POTENCY Table 23–3 indicates that there is wide variability among these medications in milligram per milligram potency. This fact has most relevance when treating clients who require large doses. A potent medication is then best.

DOSAGE Dosage ranges vary widely among clients. Medications must be titrated against the psychotic target symptoms and the appearance of side effects. Most approaches to management start with a relatively low dose (equivalent to 25 to 50 mg. orally or 25 mg. intramuscularly [IM] of chlorpromazine) to test for adverse effects for one to two hours. Then the medication is typically given in a starting dose of 300 to 400 mg. chlorpromazine (or IM equivalent) per day, and gradually increased by 25 to 50 percent a day until maximum improvement is noted or intolerable side effects are encountered.

The treatment setting frequently influences the drug regimen. In a crowded hospital emergency room, hourly doses of medication will be given until a client is sedated. In more completely staffed, private inpatient units, a client may be observed drug-free for a couple of weeks before medication is instituted. It is interesting to note, however, that in terms of long-term outcome and length of eventual remission, neither approach can claim documented superiority.

Certain clients, who are extremely agitated, violent, severely withdrawn, or catatonic, require significant doses during the first few days of treatment, delivered by injection to ensure the most rapid onset of relief. Chlorpromazine 50 to 100 mg. IM may be used, particularly if sedation is required. The nurse must be aware that this is an irritating drug; injections must be deeply intramuscular in either the buttocks or upper arms, and sites must be rotated. Substantial IM doses of the more potent antipsychotics, such as haloperidol 10 mg. or trifluoperazine 10 mg., may be given to agitated clients. This approach frequently avoids some of the more troublesome side effects while bringing behavior and cognitive processes into control.

Because the antipsychotic medications have a rather long biological half-life and many of them have significant sedative effects, there is little reason to give divided doses of medication after the initial days of treatment. It is recommended that the drugs, particularly the sedative ones, such as chlorpromazine, be given in substantial doses at bedtime. In addition to promoting sleep, decreasing the chances that the client will forget to take a dose once out of the hospital, and saving nursing time in the hospital, this method saves money, since large-dose capsules or tablets cost less than an equivalent amount of medication prepared in smaller doses.

It is important to recognize that, owing to peculiarities in absorption and metabolism, some clients who appear unresponsive to ordinary doses of all classifications of antipsychotic drugs will respond to high doses. Apparently refractory clients warrant trials at two to four times the normal doses, and certain clients, under ideal monitoring conditions, may require doses thirty to sixty times the normal amount. The data on such high-dose treatment are far from conclusive, however.

After maximum clinical improvement has been obtained, antipsychotic drugs are generally gradually reduced. Continuing to give a client modest doses of an antipsychotic medication following a psychotic episode has been demonstrated to lower the chance of a relapse of symptoms and to protect against rehospitalization. Psychotherapy for clients traditionally labeled schizophrenic may not be particularly effective without the use of maintenance medications in conventional treatment settings, but it does improve psychosocial functioning in clients who are also taking maintenance medications. It is generally felt that clients should be kept on doses of antipsychotics sufficient to suppress symptoms for three months to one year following an acute episode. After such an interval, the particular client's course and life situation must be considered and treatment individualized. Some clients will recover from a psychotic episode completely within six months. These clients, with so-called Schizophreniform Disorder, should not receive long-term maintenance drug treatment. For other individuals who have already experienced recurrent episodes and demonstrate a deteriorating course, it is clearly advantageous to prevent relapses with drugs if possible.

Because of the long-term toxic effects of antipsychotics, *"drug holidays"* are generally recommended as a part of maintenance treatment. This might mean that medications are taken every other day or five days a week with weekends off. No significant increases in relapse rates have been observed with these intermittent schedules.

Decision to Use a Drug   No studies indicate that combining different antipsychotic drugs is more effective than using appropriate doses of a single effective agent. In addition, large studies using traditional outcome measures have demonstrated that the best of social therapies are not substitutes for medications in managing disintegrative patterns. Psychotherapy and social and rehabilitative work may enhance the results beyond medication alone, but, by today's standards, withholding antipsychotics could be considered malpractice, unless defended by a specific alternative therapeutic rationale. Such rationales have been put into practice, for example, in certain experimental residential treatment settings. The work of Wilson, Mosher, and Menn at Soteria House in California suggests that unconventional psychosocial approaches to some highly selected individuals traditionally considered schizophrenic can lead to improvement despite the absence of intervention with medication.

Generally the principles that govern antipsychotic drug use today are:

- The drugs are given to treat target symptoms of Schizophrenia or other psychotic disorders.
- Initial treatment may require parenteral doses. These are changed to oral pill or concentrate forms as the behavior disturbance subsides.
- Total dosages are tailored to individual needs; wide variations exist among clients.
- Divided doses are changed to a single dose primarily at bedtime, as soon as is practical, to maximize use of the drug's sedative properties.
- Most clients with a chronic course require maintenance doses for sustained improvement.

Three special considerations involving the use of antipsychotic medication deserve mention.

1. *A unique route of administration.* The phenothiazine fluphenazine (Prolixin) is available in long-acting intramuscular injectable forms that behave like sustained-release capsules. The medication is gradually released over a long period of time—two to three weeks. Long-acting Prolixin is available in an enanthate or a decanoate preparation, the difference being that the vehicle substance of the decanoate type releases the medication even more slowly than the enanthate. The main advantages of the long-acting injectable forms are that they largely circumvent a client's ambivalence about taking medication and eliminate the need for constant pill taking. The treatment team must also be aware that the client's civil liberties must be honored, and truly involuntary treatment can be performed only according to due process, as required by a particular state's mental hygiene laws. The psychiatric nurse in a community setting may frequently have occasion to administer the long-acting Prolixin. Usually, a dose of regular Prolixin is injected first, to rule out the possibility of allergic reactions. Such reactions can be devastating if discovered after a two- to three-week supply of medicine has been irreversibly given. If no adverse reactions are noted within one hour, the long-acting form is injected (25 mg. equals 1 cc., which is equivalent to 5 mg. per day in oral form), usually in the upper, outer quadrant of the buttocks.

2. *The medication requirements of certain age groups, specifically the elderly and children.* In elderly persons, the agitation often associated with Organic Mental Syndromes is markedly responsive to phenothiazines. Other sedatives, such as the barbiturates and the benzodiazepines, may further compromise cerebral functioning (further depress the level of awareness and concentration), and thus worsen such syndromes. Doses of phenothiazines are generally reduced for the geriatric population. Stelazine 5 to 20 mg. per day or Haldol 1 to 6 mg. per day might constitute adequate treatment.

Antipsychotic medications are effective in treating childhood psychoses and in managing the behavior problems associated with Mental Retardation. The general principle of reduced dosage is again applicable. The upper limit of the usual daily dosage for children under twelve might be 200 mg. per day of Thorazine or Mellaril or 20 mg. per day of Stelazine. Amounts of individual intramuscular injections must also be curtailed to 25 to 50 mg.

3. *Evaluating the potential side effects of the antipsychotic medications.* Their continuous contact with the clients gives nurses an advantage over physicians, who may be seeing a client only every other day or, at best, at the same time every day. Both the dangerous and the more uncomfortable side effects frequently have a rapid onset and need attention promptly.

The side effects of antipsychotic medications that nurses must recognize can be divided into the following general classes:

- Autonomic nervous system
- Extrapyramidal
- Other central nervous system
- Allergic
- Blood
- Skin
- Eye
- Endocrine

AUTONOMIC NERVOUS SYSTEM EFFECTS   The antipsychotics all possess anticholinergic and antiadrenergic properties. That is, they interfere with the usual transmission of nerve impulses by acetylcholine and epinephrine, in both central and peripheral nerves. The most common side effects encountered are the anticholinergic effects. These include dry mouth, blurred vision, constipation, urinary hesitance or retention, and, under rarer circumstances, paralytic ileus. Although clients usually adjust to minor side effects, such as dry mouth, it is helpful for the nurse to suggest that

				Preparation	
Generic Name	**Trade Name**	**Usual Dose**	**Tablet**	**Elixir**	**Injectable**
Benztropine	Cogentin	1–2 mg. BID or TID	Yes	No	Yes
Trihexyphenidyl	Artane	2–5 mg. TID or QID	Yes	Yes	No
Biperiden	Akineton	2–4 mg. TID or QID	Yes	No	Yes
Procyclidine	Kemadrin	5–10 mg. TID or QID	Yes	No	No
Diphenhydramine	Benadryl	25 mg. TID or QID	Yes	Yes	Yes

Table 23–4   ANTIPARKINSONIAN DRUGS

Source: Adapted from W. S. Appleton and J. M. Davis, *Practical Clinical Psychopharmacology* (Baltimore: Medcom, Inc., 1973), p. 79. © 1973 The Williams & Wilkins Co., Baltimore.

they rinse their mouths with water, chew sugarless gum, or eat sugarless candy to help relieve this symptom.

Postural hypotension is a common antiadrenergic effect. The primary danger here is injury from a fall. Clients receiving parenteral medications, such as chlorpromazine IM, must have their blood pressure monitored, sitting and standing, before and a half hour after each dose. Clients should be advised to rise from a supine position gradually and to sit back down if they feel faint. Support stockings may be indicated. This problem is much less significant with oral administration of the drugs.

EXTRAPYRAMIDAL EFFECTS   Another common and sometimes frightening group of adverse reactions results from the effects of antipsychotics on the extrapyramidal tracts of the central nervous system, which are involved in the production and control of involuntary movements. These reactions can be broken down into four types, each with distinguishing clinical characteristics and times of onset after the initiation of drug therapy.

The earliest and most dramatic reactions are the *acute dystonic reactions.* These occur in the first days of treatment, sometimes after a single dose of medication. They involve bizarre and severe muscle contractions usually of the tongue, face, or extraoccular muscles, producing *torticollis, opisthotonos,* and *occulogyric crises.* These reactions can be physically painful and are almost always frightening to the individual. They are readily reversible with one of the antiparkinsonian agents—benztropine 1 to 2 mg. or diphenhydramine 25 to 50 mg. intravenously (for immediate relief), intramuscularly (for rapid action), or

orally (for relief within hours). Table 23–4 summarizes useful information about the antiparkinsonian agents.

The *parkinsonian syndrome,* named because of its striking resemblance to true Parkinson's disease, commonly occurs after a week or two of the therapy. The hallmark signs include masklike facies, resting tremor, general rigidity of posture with slow voluntary movement, and a shuffling gait. This syndrome, too, is treatable with the antiparkinsonian agents listed in Table 23–4. Oral medication is usually sufficient, since urgency is seldom a consideration in the management of this syndrome.

A third reversible extrapyramidal syndrome is known as *akathisia.* This characteristically is a motor restlessness perceived subjectively by the client and experienced as an urge to pace, a need to shift weight from one foot to another, or an inability to sit or stand still. Generally akathisia is a later complication of drug treatment, occurring weeks to months into the course of therapy. Nonetheless, it responds to oral antiparkinsonian agents as well.

Accurate observation of the course of therapy by the psychiatric nurse can be of great significance in the prompt recognition and proper interpretation of these syndromes. If care is not taken the appearance of the parkinsonian client can be misinterpreted as increasing withdrawal, emotional blunting, apathy, and lack of spontaneity, symptoms that are sometimes seen in the deteriorating schizophrenic client. This interpretation leads to an increase in the dosage of antipsychotic medication, thus worsening the syndrome. Similarly, akathisia can be confused with psychotic agitation, and this error also prompts an increase in medication. For a comparison of the two conditions, see Table 23–5. Clients with akathisia require a reduction in the dosage

Table 23-5   COMPARISON OF AKATHISIA AND AGITATION OR PSYCHOTIC RELAPSE

Akathisia	Agitation or Relapse
Motor restlessness predominates, verbal complaints minimal	Verbalization prominent
Condition is outside voluntary control	Condition controllable
Condition is worsened by medication increase	Condition improved by raising dosage
Reduction of phenothiazine relieves symptoms	Reduction of phenothiazine worsens symptoms
Condition is responsive to antiparkinsonian agents	Condition is unresponsive to antiparkinsonian agents

Source: Adapted from W. S. Appleton and J. M. Davis, *Practical Clinical Psychopharmacology* (Baltimore: Medcom, Inc., 1973), p. 57. © 1973 The Williams & Wilkins Co., Baltimore.

Table 23-6   SYMPTOMS OF TARDIVE DYSKINESIA

Body Area Affected	Symptoms
Facial-lingual	Chewing, tongue protrusion, blinking, lip smacking, tongue tremor, spastic grimaces, sucking, wormlike movements on tongue surface
Neck-truncal	Spastic torticolis, torsian movements of trunk, retrocolis, hip rocking
Extremities	Choreoathetoid movements

Source: Adapted from R. I. Shader, *Manual of Psychiatric Therapeutics* (Boston: Little, Brown and Co., 1975), p. 93. © 1975. Used by permission of Little, Brown and Co.

of phenothiazines or other offending agents and/or treatment with an antiparkinsonian drug. The nurse can save the client many uncomfortable and worrisome days by being aware of the frequency with which these syndromes complicate treatment and by reporting any suspicious sign or symptom to the physician, while reassuring the client of the reversibility of the syndrome in almost all cases.

Whether clients should be treated prophylactically with antiparkinsonian agents, in view of the relatively high incidence of these syndromes, is open to debate. Some argue that the use of antiparkinsonian agents eventually leads to relatively higher antipsychotic doses and thus increases the probability of serious side reactions. Another argument is that antiparkinsonian agents have toxicity of their own and thus should be used only to counteract extrapyramidal syndromes, not to guard against their possible emergence. Moreover, a great many clients never develop the syndromes even in the absence of prophylaxis. Suffice it to say that, if the likelihood of an extrapyramidal reaction is high (if, for example, the client has a history of them) and the possible consequences significant (that is, the client may discontinue medication or drop out of treatment altogether), antipsychotic and antiparkin-

sonian agents are frequently initiated simultaneously by the treatment team.

The last extrapyramidal syndrome to emerge in the course of treatment is also the most severe, since it can be largely irreversible. This is *tardive dyskinesia*, a disorder characterized by involuntary movements of the face, jaw, and tongue resulting in bizarre grimacing, lip smacking, and protrusion of the tongue. In addition there may be jerky choreiform movements of the upper extremities, slow writhing athetoid movements of the arms and the legs, and tense, tonic contractions of the neck and back. The symptoms are categorized in Table 23-6. The syndrome frequently comes on after years of antipsychotic drug treatment, although it can occur earlier. It usually occurs after a maintenance dose is discontinued or reduced, and it can be masked—but not treated—by reinstituting the medication or the dosage or by switching to another drug. There is no known cure for the syndrome. The recommended manner of intervention is to stop all medication to see if the syndrome will spontaneously remit. This course of action must be weighed against the client's need for medication and the likelihood of relapse into psychosis. Reserpine, deanol, and several other drugs have been used experimentally to treat tardive dyskinesia, with equivocal results. The difficulty of identifying the syndrome is illustrated in the following case.

Caroline was a twenty-seven-year-old married woman who carried a diagnosis of chronic Schizophrenia, had been hospitalized once at age twenty-four, and was managed on moderate doses of antipsychotics: chlorpromazine 400–600 mg. per day or haloperidol 10-15 mg. per day. Approximately a year after her discharge, her psychiatrist noted that Caroline was becoming increasingly agitated, was having difficulty concentrating, and would rock in her chair. She felt better when she stood up and stretched or walked. At first, psychotic decompensation was suspected, and, following the client's suggestion that it worked best for her, she was placed on fluphenazine enanthate. The symptoms cleared transiently, but about two weeks later they returned and were much worse. The dose of enanthate was doubled to 50 mg., and again the symptoms disappeared for several days but then returned even more severely. By this time the client had to pace continually, her gait was unsteady, and her legs seemed to twitch and jerk uncontrollably, causing her to lose her balance. To ambulate she had to hold on to chairs and even the walls. At this point the psychiatrist diagnosed akathisia due to phenothiazines and prescribed first benztropine, then trihexyphenidyl, then diphenhydramine in substantial doses and by every available route, but there was no improvement. All phenothiazines were stopped, but the syndrome continued. When sitting, Caroline rocked vigorously on her hips, her arms and legs had choreoathetoid movements, and her neck was twisted to one side. Her face seemed uninvolved. To rule out tardive dyskinesia or an organic neurological abnormality, Caroline was admitted to a neurology ward where, almost miraculously, the syndrome cleared up in three days without treatment. Electroencephalogram, brain scan, spinal tap, echoencephalogram, and general medical tests were normal. She was transferred to psychiatry, and the symptoms returned.

At this point the client was put on deanol, an experimental drug for tardive dyskinesia, up to 1,000 mg. per day, but without effect. She was given then a physostigmine test for the syndrome, but the results were equivocal. She was discharged from the unit still symptomatic.

Caroline was managed for eight months without antipsychotic medication, while her therapy focused on the incredible difficulties the symptoms created in her marriage. Much of her household work had been assumed by her husband, and sex was unrewarding if not impossible. The symptoms gradually disappeared, with no obvious explanation. Establishing the diagnosis between tardive dyskinesia and a type of conversion disorder could not be done. Unfortunately, during the drug-free interval, the client began to exhibit disintegrative patterns again and the psychiatrist felt she needed

antipsychotics. Thioridazine was used. After six months of this treatment Caroline had not developed any similar motor syndrome.

OTHER CENTRAL NERVOUS SYSTEM EFFECTS   Other central nervous system side effects to note are sedation and reduction of seizure threshold. Since antipsychotic drugs vary in their sedative effects, if this side effect is troublesome, it can be managed by changing to a less sedating agent. Seizures are not a contraindication for the drugs, but they do require close client observation.

ALLERGIC EFFECTS   The principal allergic manifestation of the antipsychotics is cholestatic jaundice, which arises with chlorpromazine treatment. This occurs much less commonly than in the early days of psychopharmacology, and it is usually a benign and self-limited condition.

BLOOD, SKIN, AND EYE EFFECTS   Among the other side effects, agranulocytosis (that is, a marked decrease in granulated white blood cells, or leukocytes) is the most serious. It is both potentially fatal and, fortunately, extremely rare. Usually the person gets an infection and deteriorates rapidly or begins to bleed spontaneously. It requires emergency medical attention. Skin eruptions, photosensitivity leading to severe sunburn, blue-grey metallic discolorations over face and hands, and pigmentary changes in the eyes are all potential side effects from chlorpromazine. Clients are generally advised to avoid prolonged exposure to sunlight or to use a sunscreen agent such as Uval when out of doors. These conditions usually remit. One serious eye change that is permanent is retinitis pigmentosa, which may occur in persons on doses of thioridazine exceeding 800 mg. a day. This reaction may lead to blindness. Therefore doses exceeding 800 mg. per day are contraindicated.

ENDOCRINE EFFECTS   Lactation in females and gynecomastia and impotence in males lead a list of endocrine changes that can occur with antipsychotic drug treatments. The nurse should be alerted to any changes in body function reported by clients receiving such drugs.

Table 23–7 summarizes the side effects of the antipsychotic class of medications. Table 23–8 highlights the effects of interactions of other drugs with antipsychotics.

The following drug information card outlines the instructions a nurse should give to a client taking antipsychotic agents.

ANTIPSYCHOTICS

(Thorazine, Mellaril, Stelazine, Prolixin, Trilafon, Haldol, Navane, Moban, Loxitane)

Action: This medication will help you to relax, think more clearly, and keep your thoughts together.

Side Effects / Precautions:

1. You may experience drowsiness, blurred vision, dry mouth, or constipation while taking this medication.

2. Do not use alcohol or other depressant drugs while taking this medication. Any use of alcohol or other drugs should be discussed with your doctor.

3. Do not drive a car until you are sure the medication does not make you drowsy.

4. You may experience dizziness or lightheadedness. Get up from a lying position slowly, as standing quickly can cause dizziness. In the morning when you awaken, sit up in the bed for one full minute before standing.

5. If you develop a sore throat without other cold or flu symptoms, this should be reported to your doctor.

6. You may experience periods of muscle stiffening or muscle restlessness. These symptoms should be reported to your doctor.

7. Your skin may be extremely sensitive to the sun. If you are going to be outside, be sure your skin is covered or use a sun-screening preparation containing PABA (para amino benzoic acid). The following products contain PABA: Pabanol (Elder Company), Pre Sun (Eastwood Pharmaceuticals).

8. This medication may rarely cause females to miss menstrual periods. If this occurs, notify your doctor.

9. It is important to take this medication exactly as directed by your doctor. Do not stop taking the medication or change the dosage without contacting your doctor. If you forget a dose during the day, you may take that dose later in the day.

10. Notify your doctor if you are constipated or have difficulty passing urine. Use of a stool softener, such as dioctyl sodium sulfosuccinate, or Colace, may be beneficial if you are constipated.

11. Do not take antacids (Maalox, Mylanta, etc.) within an hour of taking this medication.

Your drug is _____

Your dosage is _____

Adapted from J. E. Smith, Improving Drug Knowledge in Psychiatric Patients. *Journal of Psychiatric Nursing and Mental Health Services*, Vol. 9 (April 1981), pp. 16–18.

Etiological Considerations A final consideration is the potential etiological significance of the effectiveness of all the antipsychotic medications on disturbances labeled Schizophrenia. Bringing together the facts that antipsychotic drugs cause a parkinsonian syndrome, that Parkinson's disease is a result of a central nervous system dopamine deficiency, and that antipsychotics bring relief to schizophrenic symptoms, it has been postulated that Schizophrenia is an illness caused by dopamine excess in specific regions of the brain and that the drugs exert their effects by blocking dopaminergic receptors. There is a considerable body of evidence from experimental biochemistry that is consistent with such a theory of Schizophrenia. The theory is still speculative, but it is noteworthy that it developed from an understanding of the action of drugs used to reduce symptoms.

Antidepressant Drugs

Background The major antidepressant drugs, like the antipsychotics, were discovered accidentally. In the case of imipramine (Tofranil), the first of the tricyclic antidepressants, investigators were actually searching for more effective antipsychotics similar to chlorpromazine. Iproniazid, a monoamine oxidase (MAO) inhibitor, was discovered after practitioners noticed that tuberculous clients became less depressed when regularly treated with a similar drug, isoniazid. The antidepressants have shed considerable light on the biochemical mechanisms of the brain in both normal and abnormal emotional expression.

The initial distinction to be understood, in the psychopharmacology of Depression, is between true antidepressants and stimulants or euphoriants. The tri-

Table 23-7   SIDE EFFECTS OF ANTIPSYCHOTIC MEDICATION

Effect	Chlorpro-mazine (Thorazine)	Halo-peridol (Haldol)	Loxipine (Loxitane)	Molindone (Moban)	Thiori-dazine (Mellaril)	Thiothixine (Navane)	Trifluoper-azine (Stelazine)
Akathisia	Occasional	Frequent	Occasional	Frequent	Occasional	Occasional	Frequent
Allergic skin reactions	Occasional	Rare	Rare	Rare	Not reported	Rare	Rare
Anticholiner-gic effects	Frequent	Not reported	Rare	Occasional	Frequent	Occasional	Frequent
Blood dyscrasia	Occasional	Occasional	Not reported	Rare	Rare	Rare	Rare
Cholestatic jaundice	Occasional	Rare	Not reported	Not reported	Rare	Rare	Rare
Dystonias	Occasional	Frequent	Rare	Occasional	Occasional	Occasional	Frequent
Impotence	Occasional	Not reported	Not reported	Not reported	Occasional	Not reported	Occasional
Parkinsonism	Occasional	Frequent	Frequent	Occasional	Occasional	Occasional	Frequent
Photosensi-tivity	Occasional	Rare	Not reported	Not reported	Occasional	Rare	Occasional
Postural hy-potension	Frequent	Occasional	Rare	Rare	Frequent	Occasional	Rare
Retinitis pig-mentosa	Not reported	Not reported	Not reported	Not reported	Occasional	Not reported	Not reported
Sedation	Frequent	Not reported	Occasional	Rare	Frequent	Frequent	Not reported

cyclic compounds and the monoamine oxidase (MAO) inhibitors are not stimulants and will not induce euphoria in normal persons. Rather, in a single dose, they have a sedative effect. Amphetamines and methylphenidate (Ritalin), on the other hand, are stimulants but not antidepressants in the pharmacological sense. They can induce an increased sense of well-being in certain individuals, but they do nothing to combat Depression on a lasting basis. The antidepressants actually appear to correct a deficiency in certain types of depressed clients. This fact may have etiological significance.

Clinical Considerations in Use   The most important clinical consideration about the use of medications in the treatment of Depression is that antidepressant drugs are not effective in all cases of depressed mood. Evidence from research and clinical practice indicates that only a proportion of Depressive Disorders respond to this class of drugs. Table 23-9 describes the conditions and the indicated treatments. Thus, accurate diagnosis is necessary to ensure maximum effec-

tiveness. In general, persons for whom antidepressants are indicated usually suffer from characteristic symptoms: a severely depressed mood; loss of interest; inability to respond to normally pleasurable events or situations; a depression that is worse in the morning and may lessen slightly as the day goes by; early morning awakening (and the inability to fall asleep again); marked psychomotor retardation or agitation; significant anorexia and weight loss; and excessive or inappropriate guilt. DSM-III calls this *Melancholia*. In fact, the symptoms of Melancholia are the features of a Depression that most reliably predict response to drug therapy. A significant, and commonly overlooked, clinical consideration is that antidepressants have a delayed reaction onset. Thus, a client will not show lessening of depressed mood until a week to ten days following the institution of an adequate dose of tricyclics, for example.

Tricyclics   By far the most important and most commonly used class of antidepressant drugs is the tricyclics. These compounds are close in chemical struc-

Table 23–8 DRUG INTERACTIONS WITH THE ANTIPSYCHOTICS

Agent	Effect
Alcohol and/or barbiturates	Speeds the action of liver microsomal enzymes so antipsychotic is metabolized more quickly; potentiates CNS depressant effect
Tricyclic antidepressants	Can lead to severe anticholinergic side effects; antipsychotics can raise the plasma level of the antidepressant, probably by inhibiting metabolism of the antidepressant
Hydrochlorthiazide and hydralazine	Can produce severe hypotension
Guanethidine	Antihypertensive effect is blocked by chlorpromazine, haloperidol, and thiothixene
Cigarettes	Heavy consumption requires larger doses of antipsychotic
Meperidine	Respiratory depression is enhanced by chlorpromazine
Anticonvulsants	Seizure threshold may be lowered by antipsychotic requiring adjustment of anticonvulsant
Levodopa	Antiparkinsonian effect may be inhibited by antipsychotics
General anesthesia	Antipsychotic may potentiate effect of anesthetic

Source: From "Antipsychotic Medications" by E. Harris, copyright © 1981, American Journal of Nursing Company. Reproduced with permission from *The American Journal of Nursing*, Vol. 81, No. 7 (July 1981), p. 1320.

ture to the phenothiazines and have many similar side effects but profoundly different effects on mood, behavior, and cognition. Tricyclic antidepressants are not antipsychotic agents when given to so-called Schizophrenic persons and may, in fact, aggravate a disintegrative pattern or precipitate overt symptoms in a client with latent disintegrative behavior. The phenothiazines, on the other hand, do exert some antidepressant activity. Imipramine (Tofranil) and amitriptyline (Elavil) are the two prime representatives of tricyclic antidepressants. Desipramine (Norpramin, Pertofran),

nortriptyline (Aventyl), and protriptyline (Vivactyl) are compounds prepared in simpler forms, similar to the conversions made in normal metabolism, that are reported to reduce the incidence of side effects. Familiarity with Tofranil and Elavil usually implies an understanding of the basic principles of antidepressant pharmacology, however, and covers most clinical situations. Therefore the psychiatric nurse can focus attention primarily on these two. Table 23–10 summarizes the basic data on the major antidepressant drugs.

DOSAGE What constitutes an adequate dose of tricyclics is a matter of debate, but most clinicians agree that the bulk of responsive clients with a Major Depression need doses of 150 to 250 mg. per day. Some may respond to as little as 75 mg. and some require 400 mg., but these are exceptional doses.

Ordinarily, a client is started on 25 mg. of a tricyclic three times a day for two days, and the dosage is increased by 25 to 50 percent every other day, if no intolerable side effects are encountered, until 200 or 250 mg. is reached. Common clinical practice is to use Tofranil in the presence of motor retardation and Elavil with agitated clients because it has a more sedative effect. Once the client's dosage is established, it can be converted to a single bedtime dose. This practice frequently precludes the need for another medication for insomnia. Since the onset of action of the drug takes seven to ten days, the waiting period then begins. Although full improvement may take as long as four weeks, a gradual lessening of the symptoms will become apparent in those who are going to eventually respond.

After remission of the symptoms, clients who are put on a reduced maintenance dose (perhaps 50 percent of the acute dosage) show less likelihood of relapse. Therefore most clients are continued on treatment for six months to one year following a Major Depressive Episode. Clients who have had repeated episodes may require more prolonged drug maintenance or should be considered for lithium carbonate treatment because of its prophylactic effects on recurrent Major Depression and the depressive episodes of Bipolar Disorder.

Most depressive clients who do not respond to tricyclic antidepressants suffer from a form of illness that is not of the melancholic type. These may include so-called neurotic or characterological depressions, termed *Dysthymic Disorder* in DSM-III. Other clients do not reach or maintain effective blood levels of the drugs even when given adequate daily doses, because

Table 23–9   TYPES OF DEPRESSION AND INDICATED TREATMENTS

Type of Depression	Distinguishing Characteristics	Type of Treatment				
		Tricyclics	**MAO Inhibitors**	**Amphetamines**	**Electro-convulsive Therapy**	**Psycho-therapy**
Grief reaction	Follows major loss. Shock and disbelief (denial) give way to sadness, crying, irritability, anger. Acceptance and some equanimity usually develop within two months.	Not indicated	Not indicated	Not indicated	Not indicated	Possible to use
Pathological grief	Follows major loss. Prolonged grieving, excessive guilt, withdrawal from friends and activities, somatic symptoms, anniversary reactions.	Not Indicated	Not Indicated	Not Indicated	Not indicated	Indicated
Adjustment Disorder	Follows blow to self-esteem. Sadness, discontent, feelings of worthlessness, lack of initiative, hypersomnia, hyperphagia.	Not indicated	Not indicated	Possible to use	Not indicated	Indicated
Major Depression with melancholia	May be related or unrelated to life events. Positive family history common. Loss of interest, inability to respond to pleasurable stimuli, worse in A.M., early morning awakening, severe weight loss, guilt, psychomotor disturbance.	Indicated	Possible to use	Not indicated	Not indicated	Possible to use
Severe Depression	Major depression with psychosis or severe suicidal risk.	Possible to use	Possible to use	Not indicated	Indicated	Indicated

| | | | Starting | Effective | |
| | Generic | Trade | Dose | Dose Range | Maintenance |
Class	Name	Name	(Mg./Day)	(Mg./Day)	(Mg./Day)
Tricyclics	Imipramine	Tofranil	75	150–300	150
Dibenzazepines	Amitriptyline	Elavil	75	150–300	150
	Desipramine	Norpramin, Pertofran	75	150–250	150
Dibenzocycloheptenes	Nortriptyline	Aventyl	40–75	40–100	100
	Protriptyline	Vivactyl	15	15–60	30
Dibenzoxepins	Doxepin	Sinequan	75	75–300	150
MAO inhibitors	Tranylcypromine	Parnate	20	20–60	20
	Isocarboxazid	Marplan	10	20–60	20
	Phenelzine	Nardil	15	45–90	45
Central nervous system stimulants	Dextroamphetamine	—	5	5–30	—
	Methamphetamine	—	2.5	2.5–20	—
	Methylphenidate	Ritalin	10	10–60	—

Table 23–10   ANTIDEPRESSANT DRUGS

Source: Compiled in part from L. E. Hollister, *Clinical Use of Psychotherapeutic Drugs* (Springfield, Ill.: Charles C Thomas, Publisher, 1973), p. 97.

of idiosyncrasies in their metabolic processes. At present, tricyclic blood levels can be measured in many centers and doses increased until an effective blood level is obtained.

SIDE EFFECTS   Many of the common side effects of the tricyclic drugs are autonomic, due to the anticholinergic characteristics of the medications. These would include dry mouth, blurred vision, constipation, palpitations, and urinary retention. Clients with glaucoma must be treated with caution. Some allergic skin reactions have been observed. Tricyclics also cause changes in the normal electrical conduction of the heart, which is particularly significant in treating persons with a history of cardiovascular disease, especially heart block. Sudden death has occurred during tricyclic treatment. Clients with known heart disease and most elderly clients thus require electrocardiograms before initiating tricyclic therapy, and periodically during the course of treatment. Several other central nervous system effects may occur, including tremor, twitching, paresthesias, ataxia, and convulsions. Table 23–11 presents the common side effects of antidepressant medications, along with suggested nursing interventions.

OVERDOSE EFFECTS   One aspect of tricyclic treatment that deserves attention is the consequences of an overdose, which are rather serious. Significant overdoses may cause delirium, hyperthermia, convulsions, and even coma, shock, and respiratory failure. A lethal dose of an antidepressant such as amitriptyline is estimated at between 10 and 30 times the usual daily therapeutic dose. Drug intake deserves close attention, since many of the clients treated with these drugs are severely suicidal. Serious overdosage is a medical emergency and may require heroic resuscitative measures. When the nurse reports delirium and peripheral autonomic symptoms of anticholinergic poisoning due to mild overdosage, the psychiatrist can intervene with intravenous or intramuscular physostigmine (0.2 or 0.4 mg.), an anticholinesterase that will reverse the delirium and other symptoms at least transiently.

Problems in the use of antidepressants are illustrated in the following case study.

Donald was a thirty-three-year-old, single, male X-ray technician who was brought to the mental health center

Table 23-11 SOME COMMON SIDE EFFECTS OF ANTIDEPRESSANT MEDICATIONS

Side Effect	Intervention	Side Effect	Intervention
Anticholinergic		*Psychiatric*	
Dry mouth	Encourage frequent sips of water. Suggest lemon juice and glycerine mouth swabs, dietetic or nonsucrose sour ball candies, or a commercial oral lubricant.	Anxiety, restlessness, irritability	Advise physician, as dose may need to be decreased or increased or time of administration changed; medication may need to be changed to one that produces more sedation, such as amitriptyline; sedatives and or antipsychotics may be required.
Constipation	Encourage intake of bran, fresh fruits and vegetables, and prunes. Maintain adequate fluid intake. Suggest stool softeners or laxatives. Withhold medication and advise physician, as urecholine may be needed to prevent paralytic ileus when constipation is severe.	Hypomania	Withhold medication and inform physician, as antidepressant may be unmasking a Bipolar Disorder.
Urinary retention and delayed micturition	Monitor intake and output. Check for abdominal distention. Withhold medication and advise physician if client unable to void; catheterization and/or urecholine may be required.	Mental confusion, psychotic behavior	Discontinue drug; physostigmine (antidote for severe anticholinergic side effects).
		Neurologic	
Blurred vision	Assure client this is temporary. Suggest eye consult if this persists beyond medication adjustment (about 3 weeks).	Drowsiness	Advise client initially not to operate hazardous machinery. Administer medication at bedtime. If persistent, advise physician, as medication may need to be changed to a less sedative antidepressant.
Diaphoresis	Encourage adequate fluid intake (preferably noncaloric) to replace lost fluid. Observe for symptoms of electrolyte imbalance.	Lowering of seizure threshold	Observe seizure precautions during initial treatment. Advise physician if seizure occurs, as adjustment of anticonvulsant in clients with seizure disorders and/or discontinuation of antidepressant may be warranted.
Atropine psychosis	Withhold medication and advise physician, as medication must be discontinued.		
Cardiovascular		Fine tremor and/or ataxia	If severe, stop medication and advise physician, change in dose or medication may be needed.
Tachycardia	Monitor pulse for rate and arrhythmias. Withhold medication and notify physician if resting pulse rate is faster than 120.	*Endocrinologic/ Metabolic*	
		Decreased or increased libido	Assure client that this is usually transitory. If persistent or interfering with compliance, advise physician, as change in medication and/or dose may be indicated.
Orthostatic hypotension	Record blood pressure with client sitting and standing; withhold medication and notify physician if systolic blood pressure drops more than 20 to 30 mm.		
		Ejaculatory and erection disturbances	Advise physician if this interferes with compliance, as medication or dose may need changing.
Arrhythmias and T-wave abnormalities	Monitor pulse for irregularities. Provide for routine electrocardiogram (ECG) and serial ECGs if client has history of conduction defects.	Weight gain	Monitor weight. Counsel client to eat nutritionally balanced adequate diet.

Adapted from ''Antidepressant Drug Therapy,'' by M. D. DeGennaro et al., copyright © 1981, American Journal of Nursing Company. Reproduced, with permission, from *American Journal of Nursing*, Vol. 81, No. 7 (July 1981), pp. 1306–1307.

by police. The officers had broken into Donald's apartment as he was preparing to attempt suicide. He had been upset over a recent argument with his girl friend. She had told him she was uncertain that they should become engaged. Donald had turned to alcohol, which he often did during difficult times, and he then decided to inject himself with potassium chloride, which he had obtained from his hospital after a similar disagreement some weeks ago. Fortunately Donald made a last telephone call to his girl friend alerting her to his plan, and the police were able to intervene.

Donald described himself as having been depressed for several months, and said that the argument had merely been the last straw. He claimed he slept late many mornings, ate and drank excessively, and was preoccupied with thoughts of suicide, especially when he felt marriage to his girl friend was not possible.

The crisis team was concerned about the lethality of his suicide plan and thus decided to "try everything." They placed him on Elavil 50 mg., raised to a total daily dose of 200 mg. within the first week, and made plans to see him twice weekly in crisis intervention psychotherapy. They explained to the client that there probably was a biological cause for his depression and that the medication would be of great benefit.

The following day, at the first session after the emergency visit, the treating therapist was struck by the client's remarkable improvement. Donald claimed that the crisis team had saved his life, that already he and his girl friend were making up, and that he was sure the Elavil was lifting his spirits. The six months of psychotherapy that followed were troubled by Donald's insistence that he had little control over his mood or responsibility for it because of his biochemical deficits. He was reluctant, therefore, to examine his internal states and his motivations for feeling and acting.

Donald's mood, in fact, continued to vacillate according to the ups and down of his relationship. He revealed himself to be a dependent man with low regard for himself as an individual, but he would become angry if the therapist suggested this.

The use of Elavil in this Depression was premature, most likely unwarranted (since the Depression was situational), and an obstacle to psychotherapy, because the decision to use medication and its meaning were presented to the client without first exploring his attitude toward them, let alone elucidating the proper clinical criteria for prescribing a tricyclic drug.

MAO Inhibitors   Some clients who do not respond to tricyclic antidepressants may respond to the other major class, the monoamine oxidase (MAO) inhibitors.

Table 23–12 SUBSTANCES CAUSING HYPERTENSIVE CRISES WITH MAO INHIBITOR TREATMENT		
Foods to Avoid		**Drugs to Avoid**
Cheddar or other aged cheese	Coffee	Amphetamine
	Licorice	Dextroampheta-mine
Beer	Pickles	
Wine (particularly Chianti)	Sauerkraut	Methylampheta-mine
Chicken liver	Smoked salmon (lox)	Ephedrine
Yeast products		Dopamine
Broad beans	Snails	Phenylpropano-lamine
Pickled herring	Raisins	
Chocolate	Figs	Caffeine
Yogurt	Soy sauce	Epinephrine

Source: Compiled in part from W. S. Appleton and J. M. Davis, *Practical Clinical Psychopharmacology* (New York: Medcom Press, 1973), pp. 114–115.

These drugs generally are not as effective as tricyclics and are somewhat slower to act, sometimes requiring a month or two of treatment before improvement shows. Iproniazid (Marsilid) is considered the most effective, with phenelzine (Nardil) and tranylcypromine (Parnate) slightly behind. (Iproniazid is not available in the United States, however.) Table 23–10 presents the basic data on the MAO inhibitors. What complicates the decision to use MAO inhibitors is that they are associated with several very severe side effects. Hepatic necrosis, commonly fatal, and hypertensive crises leading to intracranial bleeding are among the most threatening. This latter reaction, heralded by symptoms of severe headache, stiff neck, nausea, vomiting, and sharply increased blood pressure, follows the ingestion of foods that contain the amino acid tryramine and of sympathomimetic medications. The foods and drugs that are to be avoided during treatment are listed in Table 23–12. Clients taking tricyclics and MAO inhibitors conjointly have also occasionally had severe reactions, with fever, convulsions, and even death. Therefore, a seven- to ten-day washout period is recommended between these types of medications. Under experienced guidance and control, however, they can be prescribed simultaneously. The principles for use of both tricyclic and MAO inhibitor antidepressants are:

- Drug treatment does not preclude psychotherapy, electroconvulsive therapy, or behavioral treatments if they are also indicated.
- Tricyclic treatment should be given first unless there are contraindications, clinical indications for MAO inhibitors, or a past history of tricyclic antidepressant unresponsiveness.
- The usual therapeutic range is 150 to 300 mg. per day. Dosages may be variable and may be limited by significant side effects.
- A response is seen two or three weeks after the therapeutic dose is reached.
- Clients with recurrent Major Depressive Episodes with melancholia may require long-term maintenance treatment, although doses are usually lower than those needed in acute episodes.

The following drug information cards outline the health teaching guidelines a nurse should give to a client taking antidepressants.

TRICYCLIC ANTIDEPRESSANTS

(Elavil, Tofranil, Norpramine, Triavil, Sinequan)

Action: Antidepressant

Side Effects/Precautions:

1. You may experience a dry mouth, blurred vision, constipation, or drowsiness while taking this medication.
2. It may take up to 3 or 4 weeks before you begin to feel less depressed, but it is essential that you continue to take this medication as directed by your doctor, even though you do not feel any positive effect.
3. Avoid the use of alcohol and other depressant drugs while taking this medication, unless directed by your physician.
4. Do not drive a car until you are sure the medication does not make you drowsy.
5. You may be lightheaded or dizzy when standing up. Standing up slowly will help to prevent this. In the morning when you awaken, sit up in bed for one full minute before standing.
6. Notify your doctor if you become constipated or have difficulty passing urine. Use of a stool softener such as dioctyl sodium sulfosuccinate (Colace), may be beneficial if you are constipated.

Your drug is _____

Your dosage is _____

From drug cards written by Janet E. Smith RN, MSN.

MAO INHIBITORS

(Parnate, Nardil)

Action: Antidepressant

Side Effects/Precautions:

1. It is essential that you continue to take this medication as directed by your doctor, even though you do not feel any positive effect. It may take up to 3 or 4 weeks before you begin to feel less depressed.
2. You may be lightheaded or dizzy when standing up. Standing up slowly will help to prevent this. In the morning when you awaken, sit up in bed for one full minute before standing.
3. Do not use alcohol while taking this medication.
4. Some foods contain a substance (tyramine) that may cause a serious increase in your blood pressure while taking this medication. Do not eat the following:

Beer	Pods of broad beans (fava
Canned figs	beans)
Chianti wine	Raisins
Cheese	Bananas or avocados
Chocolate	Sherry
All types of liver	Sour cream
Meat tenderizer	Soy sauce
Pickled herring	Yeast extracts

5. Do not use large amounts of caffeine in any form (coffee, tea, cola).
6. Many medications used in combinations with MAO inhibitors can increase your blood pressure. These include other types of antidepressants, cough and cold preparations, and sedatives. Do not take any over-the-counter products without consulting your doctor or pharmacist. Tell any doctor you visit that you are taking an MAO inhibitor.
7. Notify your doctor if you become constipated or have difficulty passing urine. Use of a stool softener such as dioctyl sodium sulfosuccinate (Colace) may be beneficial if you are constipated.

8. Report any of the following symptoms to your doctor: headache, stiff neck, nausea, or dizziness.

9. Your doctor or pharmacist may give you an ID card which states that you are taking an MAO inhibitor. Carry this with you at all times.

Your drug is _____

Your dosage is _____

From drug cards written by Janet E. Smith RN, MSN.

Other Drugs   Stimulants, such as amphetamines and methylphenidate (Ritalin), and the phenothiazines are less commonly used antidepressants. Stimulants are not a proven treatment. Phenothiazines may be particularly useful in the presence of agitation. Some clinicians and researchers believe that Major Depressive Episodes with psychotic features (delusional depressions) respond better to a combination of an antidepressant and an antipsychotic agent or to electroconvulsive therapy (ECT) than to antidepressants alone. Others simply recommend higher-than-usual doses of antidepressants.

Special Syndromes Treated with Antidepressants   Several special syndromes respond to antidepressants.

• Spontaneous panic attacks often leading to agoraphobia have been shown to respond much more effectively to imipramine (Tofranil) than to the usual drug treatments of anxiety.

• Syndromes characterized by high levels of anxiety associated with Depression, have often been treated with the tricyclic doxepin (Sinequan), which combines antidepressant and antianxiety effects. Triavil, a combination of perphenazine (Trilafon) and amitriptylene (Elavil), has also been used.

• The stimulant drugs amphetamine and methylphenidate have been used with success in the treatment of hyperactivity in children suffering from Attention Deficit Disorders.

Etiological Considerations   Studying the pharmacology of the antidepressants has led to a theory of the biochemistry of Depression. Basically, all the true antidepressants make the neurotransmitter substances *norepinephrine* (NE) and *serotonin* (5-HT) more avail-

able to the synaptic receptors in the central nervous system. Tricyclics block the reuptake of these substances into the neuron after their release, thereby postponing their degradation. MAO inhibitors interfere with the enzymes responsible for the actual breakdown of the neurotransmitters. Since both are antidepressants, these observations have led to the theory that NE and 5-HT shortages in the brain cause Depression, at least the type of depression that responds to drug therapy.

The Antimania Drug (Lithium)

Background   The psychopharmacological treatment of conditions labeled Mania has become virtually synonymous with lithium carbonate therapy in the United States in the past ten years. Many well-controlled clinical studies indicate unequivocally that lithium is the most effective agent for treating the vast majority of Acute Manic and Hypomanic Episodes. In addition, due to the absence of sedative side effects, the client feels much more related to the environment and able to function normally while under the influence of lithium.

Diagnosis   An accurate diagnosis of Mania is, as always, the most important factor in maximizing the effect of a positive clinical response. An outline of the DSM-III diagnostic criteria for a Manic Episode appear in Chapter 16.

Dosage   The management of an Acute Manic Episode involves rapid initiation of lithium, increased to substantial doses during the first week of treatment. Usually between 1,500 and 2,100 mg. per day are needed by the average-sized client in an acute period. Lithium is available only in oral form in 250 and 300 mg. capsules and tablets. Since lithium is an ion, its concentration can be measured in the blood. In the acute phase the blood level usually must attain a concentration of 1.0 to 1.5 mEq/l. After a week to ten days, as the symptoms subside, the dose can be decreased to 900 to 1,200 mg. per day, with the blood level maintained in the range of 0.7 to 1.2 mEq/l for continuing control.

The basic principles for antimania drug therapy are:

• Lithium is indicated and effective in the treatment of Acute Manic Episodes and in the prevention of recurrent Manic or Depressive Episodes.

Table 23-13 SIDE EFFECTS FROM LITHIUM CARBONATE THERAPY				
Organ System Affected	**Mild (Normal)**	**Moderate (May Be Normal or May Suggest Impending Toxicity)**	**Severe (Toxic)**	**Extreme**
Gastrointestinal tract	Nausea	Anorexia, vomiting, diarrhea, thirst	None	None
Neuromuscular system	Tremor	Muscle weakness, muscle hyperirritability, coarse tremor, ataxia	Hypertonic muscles, hyperactive reflexes, choreoathetoid movements	None
Central nervous system	None	Sedation, fatigue, giddiness	Blurred vision, slurred speech, vertigo, somnolence, confusion, stupor, focal neurological signs, seizures	Coma Death
Cardiovascular system	None	None	Pulse irregularities, hypotension, electrocardiogram abnormalties	Circulatory collapse
Miscellaneous	None	Polyuria, glycosuria, dehydration	None	None

Source: Compiled from D. F. Klein and J. M. Davis, *Diagnosis and Drug Treatment of Psychiatric Disorders* (Baltimore: Williams and Wilkins Co., 1969), p. 238; and R. I. Shader, *Manual of Psychiatric Therapeutics* (Boston: Little, Brown and Co., 1975), p. 110.

- Lithium is given in divided doses with increases in the daily dose until the blood level reaches 1.0–1.5 mEq/l in acute stages of the disorder. Blood levels must be monitored after each increase.

- Antipsychotic medications may be necessary early in the course of treatment for behavior control.

- Following symptom resolution, lithium is decreased for maintenance treatment to approximately half to two-thirds the acute dose. Blood levels are checked every two to three months or when there is reason to suspect a change.

Walt, a twenty-three-year-old musician, came for treatment after losing his job in a Broadway show. His producer had fired him because he was irritable and argumentative and seemed to refuse to concentrate on his pieces during rehearsals, instead roaming around the stage giving unsolicited advice to others. His wife had called the mental health center in desperation, claiming that Walt was pacing the apartment talking out of his head, and that he seemed totally unconcerned about losing his job. The day before he had been admitted and discharged against medical advice from a local hospital, where he had received chlorpromazine.

On observation, Walt exhibited pressured speech with grandiose ideas, an irritable mood, and an inability to sit in the chair in the interviewing room. His family history revealed that his father had lost many jobs and had now been taking lithium for the past five years. It was explained to the client that he had Bipolar Disorder with a genetic basis, and he was started on lithium carbonate 300 mg. BID. This was raised by 300 mg. every third day, with a blood level sample drawn and tested after each increase, until Walt was on 1,500 mg. per day and showed a level of 1.3 mEq/l. The client was asymptomatic one week later, without hospitalization, and returned to work.

Side Effects   Lithium has a significant number of side effects that can be troublesome and, in some cases, quite dangerous. They are detailed in Table 23-13. Significant side effects are usually correlated with blood levels of lithium above 1.5 mEq/l. Common side

Table 23-14 NURSING CARE PLAN FOR CLIENTS ON LITHIUM		
Problem	**Objective**	**Nursing Interventions**
1. Air, Food, Fluid Intake of food and fluid is impaired due to side effects affecting the gastrointestinal (GI) system.	1. To maintain balanced food and fluid intake	1. Obtain diet history to determine usual intake. 2. Monitor intake of foods containing sodium. 3. Teach clients to avoid fluctuations of sodium intake. 4. Monitor fluid intake. 5. Encourage at least six-eight glasses fluid per day.
	2. To support clients when they experience unavoidable side effects	1. Administer lithium spaced through the day (TID or QID). 2. Give with meals or with food in the stomach. 3. Give tea and crackers for nausea. 4. Teach clients to rinse mouth frequently and practice oral hygiene when they experience dryness of the mouth. 5. Observe for persistence and exacerbations of GI side effects.
2. Elimination Bowel and urinary elimination is altered due to side effects affecting the gastrointestinal system and kidney functioning.	1. To maintain balanced intake and output 2. To support clients when they experience unavoidable side effects	1. Monitor bowel and bladder output. 2. Observe for persistence and exacerbations of GI side effects.
3. Personal Hygiene and Body Temperature Physical hygiene needs and maintenance may be altered due to side effects.	1. To promote and maintain physical hygiene and skin integrity	1. Assess skin condition and hygiene needs. 2. Monitor symptoms of edema through measuring extremities with a tape measure. 3. Teach clients to elevate legs when edema is present. 4. Teach and assist clients to perform routine personal hygiene. 5. Monitor skin condition and observe for signs of dehydration, pruritus, or hypothyroidism.
Fluid and electrolyte balance may be altered due to changes in body temperature.	1. Limit alterations in body temperature. 2. Promote fluid-electrolyte balance	1. Assess body temperature. 2. Assist clients to choose clothes appropriate for weather conditions. 3. Teach clients to avoid exposure to extreme fluctuations in climate. 4. Monitor sodium intake.
4. Rest and Activity Rest and activity may be impaired due to side effects affecting various body systems.	1. To promote a balance of rest and activity 2. To support the client when he experiences unavoidable side effects	1. Assess rest/activity pattern. 2. Identify activity that may result in excessive perspiration. 3. Protect clients from exhaustion due to overactivity by providing a quiet room and limited stimulation. 4. Promote safety through teaching clients to avoid operating an automobile or smoking alone if they experience lethargy. 5. Assist clients to plan schedule for rest and activity.

Table continues on next page

Table 23–14 continued		
Problem	**Objective**	**Nursing Interventions**
5. Solitude and Socialization Skills needed for solitude and socialization may be impaired due to symptoms of the client.	1. To develop a balance of solitude/socialization patterns and skills	1. Assist clients to learn the effects and side effects of lithium carbonate. 2. Assist clients to learn difference between effects, side effects, and symptoms of their illness.

Source: From "Nursing Care of Patients on Lithium," by Susan Hunn, Cecile Miranda, Vivian Molyneaux, and Catherine Warshaw, *Perspectives in Psychiatric Care* Vol. 18, No. 5 (Sept.-Oct., 1980), pp. 218-219.

effects include tremor, nausea, thirst, and polyuria. Thyroid goiter has also been seen as a side effect. Severe lithium poisoning presents a potential medical emergency. Early signs include vomiting and diarrhea, lethargy, and muscle twitching. These may progress to ataxia and slurred speech. A serious situation exists when the client becomes semiconscious or comatose. At that point seizures may occur, and electrolyte imbalances may lead to cardiac arrest. This syndrome of severe toxicity ordinarily occurs only when the client has a lithium level of 2.0 to 3.0 mEq/l. The client may have overdosed or severely restricted food or salt intake (or taken diuretics) to induce this state.

Occasionally, very violent, agitated, or paranoid individuals with Mania will require phenothiazines at the beginning of their treatment. These can be started simultaneously with the lithium, raised to whatever level is required to control the disintegrative behavior, then gradually reduced, and eliminated after therapeutic lithium levels have been effective for approximately one week.

A nursing care plan for clients on lithium is presented in Table 23–14.

Prophylactic Uses   In addition to the management of the Acute Manic Episode, the use of lithium is established for the prophylactic prevention of recurrent Manic and Depressive Episodes in Bipolar Disorder. As mentioned earlier, lithium may be effective in prophylaxis against recurrent Unipolar Major Depressions as well. A schematic illustration of these diagnoses according to the American Psychiatric Association's Diagnostic and Statistical Manual (DSM-III) is given in Figure 23–1. Lithium is not an established treatment for Depression in the acute stages. The following drug information card outlines the health care guidelines a nurse should give to a client taking lithium.

LITHIUM CARBONATE

(Eskalith, Lithane)

Action: This medication maintains an even mood. It is used to treat Bipolar Disorder and to prevent recurrent Depressions.

Side Effects/Precautions:

1. Take this medication *exactly* as directed by your doctor. You must take the medication every day at the indicated time (e.g., morning and evening; morning, noon, and evening, etc.). If you skip a dose, *do not* double the dosage the next time you take your medication, but continue your regular schedule.

2. Be sure to maintain an adequate fluid intake, since you may urinate more than usual.

3. Do not take any other medication, including over-the-counter products, without consulting your M.D. or pharmacist. Do not take a diuretic (water pill) unless directed to do so by your doctor. Be sure to tell any other doctor that you visit that you are taking Lithium.

4. It is important to maintain a normal, well-balanced diet while taking this medication. Be sure you do not become dehydrated due to excessive heat or exercise. If you do sweat a great deal due to heat or exercise, you should try to replace some of the salt you have lost by

eating a salty snack like pretzels or potato chips. You may also take salt tablets if approved by your doctor.

5. When you first start taking this medication, you may experience excessive urination, mild nausea, or general discomfort. These symptoms will pass in a few weeks. If they persist, contact your doctor.

6. Contact your doctor if you have any of the following symptoms: diarrhea, vomiting, fine tremors of the hands, drowsiness, muscular weakness, or ringing in the ears.

7. Your doctor or pharmacist may give you an ID card which states that you are taking Lithium. Carry this with you at all times.

8. On the day that you have your lithium blood level drawn, do not take a dose of lithium for 8–12 hours prior to the blood test.

Your drug is _____

Your dosage is _____

From drug cards written by Janet E. Smith RN, MSN.

Antianxiety Drugs

Effects   The antianxiety agents—sedatives and hypnotics—have very similar pharmacological attributes. All, in fact, can be used in small or modest doses to relieve anxiety and in larger doses to induce sleep. Although they share the major clinical effect of tranquili-

Table 23–15 COMPARISON OF ANTIANXIETY AND ANTIPSYCHOTIC TRANQUILIZERS		
Effect	**Antianxiety Agents**	**Antipsychotic Agents**
Antipsychotic	No	No
Antianxiety	No	No
Sedative	No	No
Anesthetic	No	No
Addictive	No	No
Muscle relaxant	No	No
Antiemetic	No	No
Hypotensive	No	No
Anticonvulsant	No	No

Source: Adapted from R. I. Shader, *Manual of Psychiatric Therapeutics* (Boston: Little, Brown and Co., 1975), p. 2. © 1975. Used by permission of Little, Brown and Co.

zation or disinhibition of fear-induced behavior, their side effects, including their addictive potentials and overdose sequelae, make certain representatives of this class more suitable for routine use and others better to reserve for limited, special circumstances.

The antianxiety agents are sometimes referred to as "minor tranquilizers," but this is a misleading term, since their effects on anxiety are qualitatively, not quantitatively, different from those of the "major tranquilizers" or antipsychotic agents. Table 23–15 compares the two.

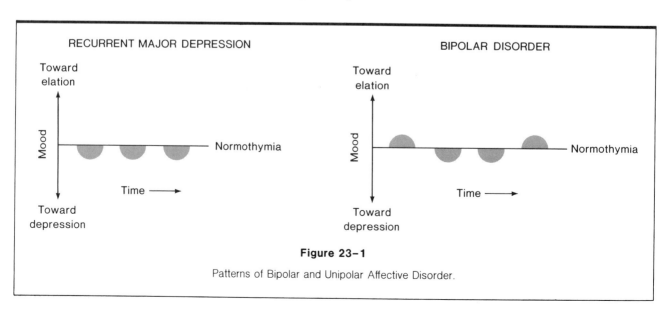

Figure 23–1

Patterns of Bipolar and Unipolar Affective Disorder.

Diagnosis   DSM-III describes motor tension, autonomic hyperactivity, apprehension expectation, and vigilance and scanning behavior as the hallmark symptoms of anxiety (see Chapter 14). It divides anxiety states into two types:

1. Panic Disorder, which is characterized by sudden, intense, and discrete periods of extreme fear accompanied by symptoms such as dyspnea, palpitations, chest pain, choking sensations, dizziness, derealization, paresthesias, hot and cold flashes, sweating, faintness, trembling or shaking, and a fear of impending doom.
2. Generalized Anxiety Disorder, which is manifested by steady, continuous, and persistent anxiety symptoms.

There is considerable evidence that Generalized Anxiety responds best to the benzodiazepine drugs but that Panic Attacks are rarely helped by these drugs. As was mentioned earlier in the chapter, Panic Attacks are very effectively suppressed with antidepressant drugs, especially the tricyclic imipramine.

The many medical conditions that may present symptoms of anxiety must be ruled out. A thorough history and physical exam are thus necessary prerequisites to antianxiety drug therapy (see Chapter 8). Among the medical conditions associated with anxiety symptoms are angina pectoris, allergic reactions, drug intoxications or withdrawal, caffeinism, temporal lobe epilepsy, hyperventilation, hypoglycemia, asthma, mitral valve prolapse, paroxysmal atrial tachycardia, pulmonary embolus, hyperthyroidism, hypoglycemia, pheochromocytoma, pain, hemorrhage, and electrolyte imbalance.

Meprobamate   Meprobamate (Miltown, Equanil) was the first antianxiety agent to gain popularity in the early 1960s. The result of controlled studies of the effects of meprobamate compared to placebos are generally favorable but not overwhelmingly convincing. This, and the addictive and fatal overdose potentials of the drug, led investigators to develop more effective and safer medications that have all but made meprobamate obsolete.

Benzodiazepines   The major class of drugs today in the management of anxiety is the benzodiazepines. This group, represented by chlordiazepoxide (Librium) and diazepam (Valium), accounts for a very high percentage of all the psychoactive medications prescribed in the United States by psychiatrists and medical practitioners alike. This fact usually evokes a mixed response in professional circles. The easy distribution of drugs for such a ubiquitous human phenomenon as anxiety fosters the development of a pill-oriented and pill-dependent society, say critics. Sympathizers focus on the proved effectiveness of the drugs, which help people achieve higher levels of functioning, more pleasurable experiences, and even more productive psychotherapies in some instances.

USE IN REDUCING ANXIETY   There is no question that chlordiazepoxide and diazepam offer a rather rapid, effective, and safe treatment for the emotional state commonly known as anxiety. In contrast to all other sedatives with proved effectiveness, the benzodiazepines have a low physiological addiction potential, have never been solely responsible for a fatality from overdose, and do not interfere with or accelerate the metabolism of medications taken concurrently.

The usual schedule for administering benzodiazepines begins with chlordiazepoxide, for example, 10 mg. three or four times daily or diazepam 5 mg. two or three times daily. Ordinary doses may range up to 25 mg. chlordiazepoxide or 10 mg. diazepam four times a day. The effects are evident within the first days of treatment. These medications are absorbed much more rapidly and completely from the gastrointestinal tract than from intramuscular injection and so are almost always administered orally. An exception is the use of intravenous diazepam to induce sleep before anesthesia or to manage status epilepticus. Peak levels of chlordiazepoxide are reached in the bloodstream two to four hours after oral ingestion and of diazepam in one to two hours.

One frequently unrecognized property of the benzodiazepines is their relatively long half-life (that is, their slow rate of metabolism). For chlordiazepoxide and diazepam, the half-life has been estimated at approximately twenty-four hours. This calls into question the use of divided doses and suggests that these medications, too, might be administered in single bedtime doses.

The major side effects of the benzodiazepines are related to their sedative qualities. Clients may complain of excessive drowsiness and must be cautioned against driving a car or operating other machinery in this state.

Other drugs used to treat anxiety but generally less effective include the antihistamines diphenhydramine

Table 23–16	ANTIANXIETY AGENTS		
Class	**Generic Name**	**Trade Name**	**Usual Dosage Range**
Benzodiazepines	Chlordiazepoxide	Librium	5–25 mg. TID or QID
	Diazepam	Valium	2–10 mg. BID or QID
Propanediols	Meprobamate	Miltown	400 mg. TID or QID
		Equanil	
Antihistamines	Diphenhydramine	Benadryl	25–50 mg. TID or QID
	Hydroxyzine	Vistaril	25–50 mg. TID or QID
		Atarax	

(Benadryl) and hydroxyzine (Vistaril, Atarax), propranolol (Inderal), and methaqualone (Quaalude), a synthetic, nonbarbiturate sedative. Methaqualone has been a leading drug of abuse, probably due to the intense feeling associated with peak blood levels. The basic data on all antianxiety drugs are presented in Table 23–16.

The drug information card given below outlines the instructions that the nurse should give to a client taking antianxiety agents.

ANTIANXIETY AGENTS

(Valium, Librium, Tranxene, Serax, Vistaril)

Action: Decreases anxiety

Side Effects/Precautions:

1. You may experience drowsiness or dizziness while taking this medication.

2. Avoid the use of alcohol or other depressant drugs while taking this medication. The use of alcohol or other drugs should be discussed with your doctor.

3. You may be lightheaded or dizzy when standing up from a lying or sitting position. If this occurs, sit down until the dizziness passes and then stand up slowly.

4. Do not drive a car until you are sure the medication does not make you drowsy.

5. Do not abruptly stop taking this medication unless directed by your doctor.

Your drug is _____

Your dosage is _____

From drug cards written by Janet E. Smith RN, MSN.

USE IN ALCOHOL DETOXIFICATION Another common use of benzodiazepines, especially Librium, is in the detoxification of individuals addicted to alcohol. Symptoms experienced during alcohol withdrawal include: coarse tremor; nausea and vomiting; malaise or weakness; sweating; elevated blood pressure; anxiety; irritability; and orthostatic hypotension. When alcohol withdrawal becomes severe, delirium may develop with clouding of consciousness, disorientation, memory impairment, perceptual disturbances (illusions or hallucinations), incoherence, insomnia, and agitation. Given adequate doses of benzodiazepines to induce sedation (usually starting at 150 to 350 mg. per day of chlordiazepoxide), alcoholic clients can be smoothly withdrawn by stepwise reductions in chlordiazepoxide dose over a one- to two-week period, without encountering alcohol withdrawal delirium or grand mal seizures.

Hypnotic Drugs

The pharmacological management of insomnia presents an interesting and challenging clinical problem. Many of the truly hypnotic drugs tend to have undesirable effects, including physiological addiction, fatal overdose potential, and dangerous interactions with other medications because of liver enzyme induction. The first principle of treatment is to assess whether the insomnia is related to one of the major mental disorders, such as Schizophrenia or Major Depression. If so, the insomnia can and should be treated as part of the larger problem, and sedative antipsychotics or antidepressants may be given at bedtime to accomplish this purpose.

Benzodiazepines In the management of simple insomnia without an associated major mental disorder, a

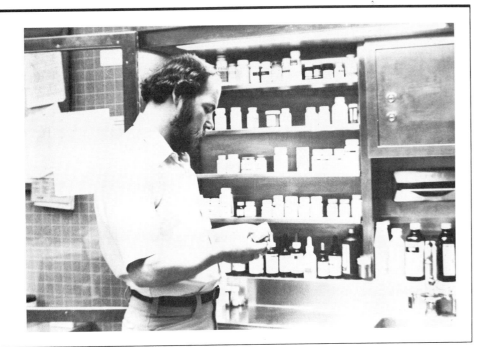

The nurses' role is crucial in the use of the most widely prescribed of all biological therapies, psychotropic drugs—medicines that literally act upon the mind.

benzodiazepine compound flurazepam (Dalmane) 15 or 30 mg. at bedtime is the drug of choice. This drug is as free of toxicity as others in its class and therefore is both effective and safe. It is the one sleeping medication that does not seem to interfere with REM (rapid eye movement) sleep and therefore can be used on consecutive nights for approximately a month.

Barbiturates   Barbiturates are commonly prescribed for their hypnotic effects. Their only advantage over the benzodiazepines is their low cost. Barbiturates, especially the short-acting types, such as secobarbital (Seconal), are powerfully addicting substances. They are frequently used in successful suicide attempts, because overdoses can cause severe central nervous system respiratory depression. Barbiturates suppress REM sleep, leading to the phenomenon of REM deprivation and REM rebound—that is, after a week or two of treatment, they help create the insomnia they were intended to control. Barbiturates also speed up the metabolism of anticoagulant and other drugs because they induce liver enzyme synthesis. This effect can be fatal. Long-acting barbiturates (phenobarbital) are very useful, however, in the detoxification of barbiturate addicts and the management of epilepsy.

Other Insomnia Drugs   Several nonbarbiturate hypnotics are also of questionable use. Among these are ethchlorvynol (Placidyl), which is fatal in doses only five times the usual therapeutic dose, and glutethimide

(Doriden), which is addicting and produces complicated, fluctuating, and difficult-to-manage states of consciousness following overdose. There seem to be no valid indications for the use of these two drugs. Chloral hydrate (Noctec) and methyprylon (Noludar) can be used under closely controlled conditions such as those of an inpatient psychiatric service.

The basic data on hypnotic agents are presented in Table 23–17.

ELECTROCONVULSIVE THERAPY

Electroconvulsive therapy (ECT) remains a useful treatment in a number of circumscribed situations for a limited number of specific clinical conditions. This is true despite the revolution in psychiatric biological therapy brought about by psychopharmacology. There are few subjects in psychiatry, however, that have provoked as intensely negative emotions on the part of the public or stirred up as much controversy within the profession. This has brought about the unfortunate situation in which a potentially valid treatment has in some states been taken out of the hands of the psychiatric treatment team and put under the control of legislators. Instead of determining the indications and contraindications for ECT based on controlled clinical research, popular opinion and special interest groups are dictating policy. The California experience indicates

Table 23–17   HYPNOTIC AGENTS

Class	Generic Name	Trade Name	Usual Dosage Range (Mg. at Bedtime)	Side Effects		
				REM Sleep Depression	Liver Enzyme Induction	Addictive Potential
Benzodiazepines	Flurazepam	Dalmane	15–30	No	No	Lower
Barbiturates (short-acting)	Secobarbital	Seconal	100	Yes	Yes	Higher
	Pentobarbital	Nembutal	100–200	Yes	Yes	Higher
Chloral derivatives	Chloral hydrate	Noctec	500–1,000	Probable	No	Higher
Others	Methyprylon	Noludar	200–400	Yes	?	Higher
	Glutethimide	Doriden	500–1,000	Yes	Yes	Higher
	Ethchlorvynol	Placidyl	500–1,000	?	?	Higher
	Methaqualone	Quaalude	150–400	Probable	?	Higher

Source: Compiled from R. I. Shader, *Manual of Psychiatric Therapeutics* (Boston: Little, Brown and Co., 1975), pp. 312–315.

that this mechanism for establishing principles of psychiatric practice is not desirable. In that state, the treatment was first totally outlawed, even for straightforward illnesses and persons voluntarily requesting it. Then criteria for its use were introduced that undoubtedly allow its use beyond its proved range of effectiveness. The dangers of ECT, to which criticisms were addressed, were largely phenomena of antiquated techniques or poor client selection.

Indications for Use

The primary indications for ECT are Major Depression with Melancholia especially in the presence of severe suicidal risk, and Acute Catatonic Excitements or Severe Catatonic Withdrawal, either of which may present life-threatening situations. In addition, a proportion of clients with Unipolar or Bipolar Affective Disorders or Acute Schizophrenia prove unresponsive to appropriate trials of psychotropic medications and can benefit from a course of ECT. Lastly, some clients suffering from Organic Mental Syndrome (OMS) with psychosis secondary to atherosclerosis or senility may show symptomatic improvement in behavior following ECT.

Symptoms that predict a good response to ECT are:

• Feeling of worthlessness
• Feeling of helplessness

• Feeling of hopelessness
• Anorexia
• Recent weight loss
• Constipation
• Reduced libido
• Early morning awakening
• Suicidal inclinations

Procedure

Since its introduction in 1938, the procedure for applying electroconvulsive therapy has evolved over the years into a fairly benign format. The media's graphic portrayals of the horrors of shock therapy are no longer accurate. The principal improvements are use of a short-acting intravenous barbiturate, methohexital (Brevital), to induce anesthesia before applying the electrodes, and of a muscle relaxant, succinylcholine, during the treatment. The client is no longer aware of the procedure, feels no sensation, has a mild anterograde amnesia that includes the trip to the operating room, and has only a barely perceptible convulsion. Rarely, if ever, does a client suffer any injury. Pretreatment spine films are no longer required at most centers.

Clients are generally not allowed to take anything orally (NPO) before treatment. They should empty their bladders and remove their dentures. Following administration of the anesthesia, the electrodes are attached with electrojelly to decrease skin resistance, the muscle relaxant is injected, and, just as paralysis is noted, the electrical stimulus is given. If the stimulus has been adequate (70 to 130 volts alternating current for 0.1 to 0.5 seconds), a convulsion can be observed that is characterized by a tonic phase lasting approximately ten seconds and a clonic phase of thirty to forty seconds. Sometimes the movements are so slight that only initial plantar flexion of the feet followed by jerking movement of the toes are perceptible. Gooseflesh also indicates that a convulsion has occurred. Subconvulsive treatments are ineffective; if no movement is noted, the stimulus is repeated. During the paralysis, and following treatment, clients require artificial support of respiration. They become conscious in a few minutes but will be confused for one hour or so, requiring close observation before return to the unit. Outpatients should be accompanied home.

The traditional nursing responsibilities in the ECT procedure are:

- The nurse generally checks the chart for relevant laboratory and physical examination data and for the signed consent form.
- The nurse makes sure that the client is NPO and encourages the client to void.
- The nurse checks that hairpins and dentures are removed, and that the client is dressed in pajamas or other loose clothing.
- The nurse takes the vital signs.
- After the treatment, the nurse observes the client for signs of respiratory difficulties, until the client is fully oriented, alert, and able to get out of bed.

A modern nursing approach integrates into the care of a client receiving ECT efforts to provide accurate and reassuring information about the procedure, attempts to alleviate fear, and explorations of any adverse meanings the client may attach to either the treatment or the underlying problems.

Course of Treatment

For Depression, a relatively short course of ECT often brings dramatic results. Clients may respond in three to four treatments (commonly given three times per week), but they should usually receive two or three more for a more complete effect. Acute Schizophrenia may also respond to a very few treatments but requires a more prolonged series—ten to twenty treat-

ments—to prevent immediate relapse. There are no guarantees against eventual relapse. Some clinicians have tried monthly maintenance ECT, especially for Depression. Maintenance antidepressant medications or prophylactic lithium carbonate is preferable, however, in recurrent Major Depression.

Complications

As mentioned earlier, fractures are no longer a complication of ECT. Memory impairment continues to be a problem, although most investigators have shown the impairment to be temporary. In recent years, unilateral ECT—that is, application of the electrical current only to the nondominant hemisphere of the brain—has been recommended due to a reduced incidence of confusion and memory impairment. Most studies, however, have not shown that unilateral ECT is as reliably effective in alleviating Depression as bilateral ECT. The only absolute contraindication to ECT is brain tumor (which may present as Depression), because the increases in intracranial pressure that normally occur during a convulsion may lead to brainstem herniation and cause the death of a client with a preexisting elevated pressure. The actual incidence of death resulting from treatment is very low in spite of the high percentage of elderly persons who receive ECT. Clients have been successfully treated with ECT who have cardiovascular disease (even recent myocardial infarctions), peptic ulcers, and glaucoma. Caution is indicated in applying ECT to such clients, however.

Mrs. S was a fifty-nine-year-old female with a history of one prior psychiatric hospitalization for Depression that responded to ECT. She was brought to the hospital by her daughter, because she seemed to sit in her chair staring most of the time. On the day of the hospitalization, her daughter had telephoned Mrs. S, but there was no answer. She went to her mother's house and found her mute and virtually unresponsive. In the hospital Mrs. S displayed severe motor retardation, a blank expression, and little communication, save the shaking of her head. She barely slept, ate almost nothing, and seemed to be unaware of her surroundings. Following a negative medical workup, Mrs. S's condition was diagnosed as Unipolar Depression. She was started on imipramine and raised to 200 mg. per day by the psychiatric resident. In spite of Mrs. S's previous positive response to ECT, the resident rejected this option and admitted being prejudiced against the treatment. On the ninth hospital day, Mrs. S had an episode of acute urinary retention and needed catheterization for several days. Imipramine was replaced by doxepin, but three weeks later Mrs. S was still severely depressed. At that point, the treatment team convinced the reluctant resident to give ECT. Mrs. S consented to the treatment. After four treatments, she was talking and joking with her fellow clients and the staff. She was discharged after two additional treatments, fully herself according to her family's impression.

NARCOTHERAPY

The use of intravenous barbiturates and stimulants to facilitate client expression of highly emotionally charged feelings remains in the psychotherapeutic armamentarium. Although ordinarily classified with the biological therapies, this method differs from the bulk of organic treatments in a fundamental way. It is not the agent itself that is of therapeutic value but a process akin to psychotherapy. This is a two-step process promoted by the agent. Step one is an *emotional catharsis.* The mere reliving or reexperiencing of the emotions associated with a traumatic event, which have been submerged deep in the unconscious, has a beneficial effect. The second step, known as *narcosynthesis,* consists of interpretations or other psychotherapeutic interventions by the therapist. These are more easily accepted by a client while under the drug's influence and thus perhaps more available for insight (the client is less resistant).

The drugs used for narcotherapy include thiopental sodium (Sodium Pentothal) .25 to 1.0 gm., amobarbital (Amytal) or methylphenidate (Ritalin) 20 to 40 mg. Mute psychotic clients may respond to barbiturates. Other obviously traumatized or amnestic clients may respond to either the sedative or the stimulant approach. There is also some diagnostic value in the approach, since intravenous barbiturates worsen Organic Mental Syndrome and thereby help distinguish it from a functional illness that may be mimicking neurological disease. Also, clients in catatonic stupors become more lucid following injection of barbiturates, while severely depressed and withdrawn clients fall asleep.

The major danger in the treatment is that of laryngospasm secondary to intravenous barbiturates.

There is no validity to the claim that thiopental sodium acts as a truth serum. Interviews with clients under the influence of the drug are not admissible as evidence in a court of law.

RADICAL BIOLOGICAL THERAPIES

Several rather dramatic approaches to the biological treatment of mental illness were developed over the years. Due to their radical nature and inherent risks, the search for more benign approaches continued. These treatments have been largely replaced, primarily by psychopharmacological agents. Occasionally, in the face of severely debilitating illness and repeated unresponsiveness to drug therapy or ECT, a more radical approach may have to be considered.

Psychosurgery

The practice of frontal lobe surgery for the treatment of Schizophrenia was developed in 1936 by Egas Moniz in Portugal. Although antipsychotic medications have now largely supplanted lobotomy in the treatment of clients with Chronic Schizophrenia, neurosurgeons have, over the years, refined their techniques to permit smaller and smaller destructive lesions to provide relief without undesirable widespread personality changes.

Modern psychosurgery, practiced primarily in Europe, consists of stereotaxic operations performed at various locations in the *limbic system,* which is known to be the center of emotional life in the brain. In addition to ablative lesions made with surgical instruments, implantation of radioactive materials and use of ultrasonic waves have been tried. Figure 23–2 illustrates the locations for psychosurgical intervention.

The desired effect of all psychosurgery is to diminish unpleasant affects. It has little impact on disintegrative symptoms, such as hallucinations and delusions, but the client clearly is no longer threatened, frightened, or distressed by them. The same blasé attitude, however, carries over to the rest of the client's life, especially when large areas of the brain are removed. Clients have little feeling for members of their families, their personal appearance, socially unacceptable behaviors, and their general future. These side effects are much diminished by the newer stereotaxic methods, however.

At the present time in the United States, psychosurgery is generally reserved for the severely ill after all other therapeutic measures have been attempted and failed. Some argue that very distressed but less severely ill clients, such as the so-called pseudoneurotic schizophrenic, may derive great benefit from surgical procedures, but these clients are not widely treated in

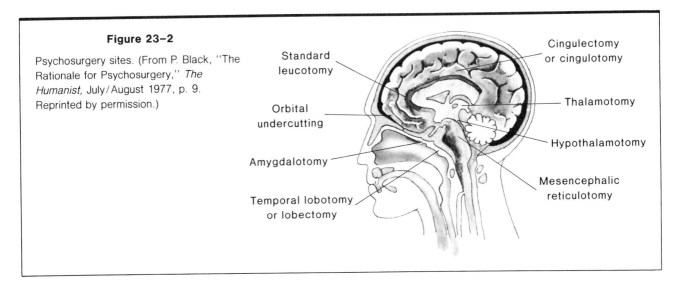

Figure 23-2

Psychosurgery sites. (From P. Black, "The Rationale for Psychosurgery," *The Humanist,* July/August 1977, p. 9. Reprinted by permission.)

Standard leucotomy

Orbital undercutting

Amygdalotomy

Temporal lobotomy or lobectomy

Cingulectomy or cingulotomy

Thalamotomy

Hypothalamotomy

Mesencephalic reticulotomy

this manner. A controversial issue is whether to treat persons labeled criminal or sexual psychopaths with psychosurgery. Such approaches are largely experimental and may involve more moral and legal questions than medical issues at this time (see Chapter 5).

Insulin Coma Treatment

Insulin coma treatment for Schizophrenia, discovered in 1933 by Manfred Sakel, was once deemed worthy of a Nobel Prize. This indicates the incredible human devastation represented by Schizophrenia and the helplessness the scientific community felt in combating it. Insulin coma treatment has been made obsolete by the antipsychotic medications.

Insulin coma therapy was a long, complex procedure, requiring up to 100 treatments over five or six months of hospitalization, using expensive operating-room facilities for each treatment, and raising the danger of many complications. Clients with cardiovascular, renal, respiratory, or other medical disease were treated at considerable risk. The treatment is no longer practiced at the major psychiatric centers, and may not be practiced anywhere in the United States. It is mentioned here primarily for historical interest and for those nurses who may encounter it. The customary nursing responsibilities for coma treatments are:

1. Pretreatment preparation—make sure the client
    a. Is NPO (nothing by mouth)
    b. Has voided
    c. Is dressed in pajamas
    d. Is stable in vital signs

2. Observations and interventions during procedure
    a. Observe for confusion and excitement
    b. Dry any excessive perspiration
    c. Give sips of water if thirsty and swallowing reflexes are intact
    d. Drain or suction saliva
    e. Observe vital signs for weak or irregular pulse, shallow respirations
    f. Position and support head and body to promote respirations

3. Posttreatment care
    a. Check vital signs
    b. Provide new gown and bedclothes
    c. Serve meal 1½ hours after treatment
    d. Insure two hours' bed rest
    e. Give sugar water and fruit juice
    f. Observe for adverse reactions

The complications that may arise from insulin coma treatment and the appropriate nursing interventions appear in Table 23–18. Complications should be reported immediately to the physician.

NEWER ORGANIC THERAPIES

At the other end of the continuum from the treatments that are becoming obsolete are a number of new approaches that show promise but have not yet been fully proved by repeated controlled tests. These de-

Table 23-18 COMPLICATIONS OF INSULIN COMA TREATMENT		
Nature	**Signs or Symptoms**	**Nursing Intervention**
Extreme excitement	Agitation, hyperactivity, confusion, belligerence, aggressiveness	Protect and reassure client
Laryngospasm	Respiratory difficulty	Pass airway
Aspiration	Respiratory difficulty, fever	Apply suction, begin postural drainage, lower temperature
Circulatory collapse	Weak, slow, irregular, rapid, or thready pulse, hypotension	Trendelenberg client, prepare cardiac resuscitation tray
Grand mal seizure	Tonic-clonic movements of extremities, biting tongue, incontinence	Place tongue blade in mouth, unbind limbs, protect client from injury
Posttreatment hypoglycemia	Weakness, drowsiness, ataxia, perspiration, hunger	Give 40-percent sugar solution or orange juice orally or call doctor for glucose injection

serve mention, however, since some may surface as valid biological therapies or even revolutionize the biological approach to some mental illnesses in the near future. Lithium carbonate was in this category several years ago.

Niacin Therapy

Large doses of niacin (vitamin B_3, or nicotinic acid) are the cornerstone of a recent popular approach to the treatment of Schizophrenia. This method is known as *megavitamin therapy* or *orthomolecular psychiatry* (see also Chapter 25). Various other combinations of vitamins (vitamin C, vitamin E) and special diets are also usually used. Although the originators of the treatment have claimed spectacular results, less biased investigators have been unable to demonstrate a significant superiority of this therapy to placebos in carefully controlled, *double-blind studies* (studies in which both the investigators and the subjects are not told which treatments are placebos). At the present time, megavitamins should not replace standard treatments, and there is considerable opinion that megavitamins may interfere with treatment when given simultaneously with conventional drug treatments.

Electrosleep Therapy

Electrosleep, which does not actually involve sleep at all, refers to a treatment that sends low milliamperage, pulsed, unidirectional current through electrodes placed over the client's ocular orbits and mastoid processes. Treatments last a half hour to an hour and are given daily in a series of five to ten sessions. The pro-

cess causes some tingling sensations but no untoward effects. Double-blind studies have indicated that it may relieve anxiety, insomnia, and depression in anxious and depressed neurotic outpatients. The treatments may worsen psychotic depressions, however. This mode appears to have some merit, but it needs replication of study results by a variety of investigators before it can be established as effective.

Nonconvulsive Electrical Stimulation Therapy

A new approach has been derived from conventional electroconvulsive therapy. It is well known that subconvulsive stimuli during ECT are associated with poor therapeutic response. Proponents of nonconvulsive treatment agree that this is true for clients for whom standard ECT is indicated. They argue, however, that a large group of clients for whom ECT is not indicated are responsive to nonconvulsive electrical stimulation. These include clients suffering from behaviors traditionally labeled Anxiety Neurosis, Phobic Neurosis, Depressive Neurosis, and Personality Disorders. As yet there are no controlled studies of this method, so judgment must be postponed.

Hemodialysis

Studies are underway to test the possible beneficial effects of dialysis on Schizophrenia. Dialysis, if effective, might remove a schizophrenogenic substance, such as a type of endorphin, from the brain. To date, however, there is no convincing proof that this treatment works.

KEY NURSING CONCEPTS

✔ Due to the flourishing of biologic therapies in modern clinical psychiatry, an understanding of their use and misuse is essential for the psychiatric nurse.

✔ The field of psychopharmacology holds the most promising medical approach for clients with emotional disorders, but the psychiatric nurse can integrate appropriate use of biological therapies in a meaningful, positive way into clients' lives.

✔ One classification system for psychotropic medications lists them according to their major symptomatic effects: antipsychotics, antidepressants, antimania drugs, and antianxiety drugs.

✔ The discovery and use of chlorpromazine for psychotic clients heralded modern psychiatric treatment and the field of community psychiatry.

✔ Lithium is considered the most effective agent for treating acute mania and hypomania attacks.

✔ The major clinical effect of antianxiety agents is tranquilization of fear-induced behavior.

✔ In the pharmacological management of insomnia it is important to evaluate whether sleeplessness is related to a major psychiatric disorder before recommending a pharmacologic intervention.

✔ Electroconvulsive therapy (ECT) has been a useful treatment for severe endogenomorphic depression.

✔ Narcotherapy is the use of intravenous barbiturates and stimulants to facilitate client expression of highly emotionally charged feelings.

✔ More radical biologic therapies for mental illness include psychosurgery and insulin coma treatment.

✔ Newer organic therapies include niacin therapy, electrosleep therapy, and nonconvulsive electrical stimulation therapy.

References

American Psychiatric Association. *Diagnostic and Statistical Manual of Mental Disorders,* 3d ed. Washington, D.C.: American Psychiatric Association, 1980.

Appleton, W. S., and Davis, J. M. *Practical Clinical Psychopharmacology.* New York: Medcom Press, 1973.

DeGennaro, M. D.; Hymen, R.; Crannell, A. M.; and Mansky, P. A. "Antidepressant Drug Therapy." *American Journal of Nursing* 81 (July 1981): 1304–1308.

Eisdorfer, C., and Fann, W. E., eds. *Psychopharmacology and Aging.* New York: Plenum Publishing Corp., 1973.

Fann, W. E.; Karacan, I.; Pokorny, A. D.; and Williams, R. L., eds. *Phenomenology and Treatment of Depression.* New York: Spectrum Publications, 1977.

Kaplan, H. I.; Freedman, A. M.; and Sadock, B. J., eds. *Comprehensive Textbook of Psychiatry/III.* Baltimore: Williams and Wilkins, 1981.

Greenblatt, M.; Solomon, M. H.; Evans, A. S.; and Brooks,

G. W., eds. *Drugs and Social Therapy in Chronic Schizophrenia.* Springfield, Ill.: Charles C Thomas, 1965.

Harris, E. "Antidepressants: Old Drugs, New Uses," "Lithium," "Antipsychotic Medications," "Extrapyramidal Side Effects of Antispychotic Medications," "Sedative-Hypnotic Drugs." *American Journal of Nursing* (July 1981): 1308–1334.

Hollister, L. E. *Clinical Use of Psychotherapeutic Drugs.* Springfield, Ill.: Charles C Thomas, 1973.

Kesey, K. *One Flew Over the Cuckoo's Nest.* New York: New American Library, 1962.

Klein, D. F., and Davis, J. M. *Diagnosis and Drug Treatment of Psychiatric Disorders.* Baltimore: Williams and Wilkins, 1969.

Klein, D. F., Gittelman, R.; Quitkin, F.; and Rifkin, A. *Diagnosis and Drug Treatment of Psychiatric Disorders: Adults and Children,* 2d ed. Baltimore: Williams and Wilkins, 1980.

Shader, R. I. *Manual of Psychiatric Therapeutics.* Boston: Little Brown, 1975.

Smith, J. E. "Improving Drug Knowledge in Psychiatric Patients." *Journal of Psychiatric Nursing and Mental Health Services* 19 (April 1981): 16–18.

Further Reading

Clark, W. G., and del Giudice, J. *Principles of Psychopharmacology.* New York: Academic Press, 1970.

DiMascio, A., and Shader, R. I. *Butyrophenones in Psychiatry.* New York: Raven Press, 1972.

Fink, M.; Kety, S.; McGaugh, J.; and Williams, T. A., eds. *Psychobiology of Convulsive Therapy.* Washington, D.C.; V. H. Winston, 1974.

Garattini, S.; Mussini, E.; and Randall, L.O., eds. *The Benzodiazepines.* New York: Raven Press, 1973.

Gershon, S., and Shopsin, B. *Lithium, Its Role in Psychiatric Research and Treatment.* New York: Plenum Press, 1973.

Greenblatt, M. *Drugs in Combination with Other Therapies.* New York: Grune and Stratton, 1975.

Greenspoon, L.; Ewalt, J. R.; and Shader, R. I. *Schizophrenia: Pharmacotherapy and Psychotherapy.* Baltimore: Williams and Wilkins, 1972.

Kalinowsky, L. B., and Hippius, H. *Pharmacological, Convulsive and Other Somatic Treatments in Psychiatry.* New York: Grune and Stratton, 1969.

Kalinowsky, L. B., and Hock, P. H. *Somatic Treatments in Psychiatry.* New York: Grune and Stratton, 1961.

Klein, D. F., and Gittleman-Klein, R. *Progress in Psychiatric Drug Treatment.* New York: Brunner/Mazel, 1975.

Rinkel, M., and Himwich, H. E. *Insulin Treatment in Psychiatry.* New York: Philosophical Library, 1959.

Shader, R. I., and DiMascio, A. *Psychotropic Drug Side Effects.* Baltimore: Williams and Wilkins, 1970.

Solomon, P. *Psychiatric Drugs.* New York: Grune and Stratton, 1966.

Warburton, D. M. *Brain, Behavior and Drugs: An Introduction to the Neurochemistry of Behavior.* New York: John Wiley, 1975.

24

Psychosocial Concepts in the General Hospital Setting

by Mary-Eve Mirenda Zangari

CHAPTER OUTLINE

Incorporating Psychosocial Principles in General Hospital Work
   A Holistic Concept of Illness
   Holistic Health Concepts
   Crisis Theory
   Preventive Aspects of Consultation
The Role of the Psychiatric Nursing Consultant
   History of Consultation in the Hospital Setting
   Types of Mental Health Consultation
   Guidelines for Mental Health Consultation
   Qualifications of the Consultant
   Building Relationships
   Negotiating the Consultation Contract
Clinical Situations Commonly Encountered
   The Demanding Client
   The Client in Pain
   The Dependent Client
   The Client's Family
   The Client in the Intensive Care Unit
   The Client Who Is Sexually Acting Out

The Noncompliant Client
The Dying Client
Key Nursing Concepts

LEARNING OBJECTIVES

After reading this chapter, students should be able to

- Relate the multicausational concept of illness to humanistic nursing practice
- Identify the need for a psychiatric nurse consultant in a general hospital setting
- Relate the concepts of crisis theory and preventive psychiatry to the hospitalized person's experiences
- Identify four types of mental health consultation
- Describe the role and functions of the psychiatric nursing consultant
- Discuss the interpersonal dynamics and nursing intervention in commonly encountered clinical situations

CHAPTER 24

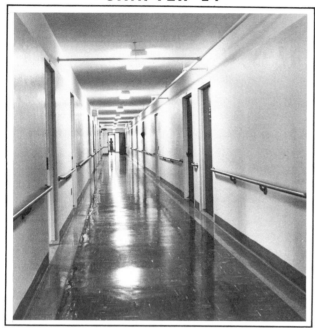

Hospitals can be cold and lonely places in which physical needs only are attended to. Psychosocial concepts must be incorporated into nursing practice in general hospital settings.

INCORPORATING PSYCHOSOCIAL PRINCIPLES IN GENERAL HOSPITAL WORK

In the past decade we have seen a gradual trend toward more humanistic values in the nursing and medical professions. Some of these changes have been reactions to public demand for more personalized health care. Other influences have come from research that indicated that disease is not a one-dimensional phenomenon but has multiple, interrelated antecedents. Consequently, we must now examine not only the bodies of clients, but also their environment, lifestyles, and psyches.

This chapter explains the theoretical basis for a holistic approach to caring for physically ill people and helps the nurse apply knowledge of psychiatric nursing principles to work with the general hospital client. To aid nurses in making this transfer, many hospitals have added psychiatric nurse consultants to their staff. This chapter not only describes this important role of psychiatric nurses but also helps nurses in general hospital settings learn how best to use a psychiatric nurse consultant. Clinical examples demonstrate how theory may be connected to practice.

A Holistic Concept of Illness

The relationship between the mind and the body has always been a subject for conjecture. Early man had a holistic approach to disease, making no distinction between physical and mental illness. From Socrates we have, "As it is not proper to cure the eyes without the head, nor the head without the body, so neither is it proper to cure the body without the soul." And from Hippocrates, "In order to cure the body it is necessary to have a knowledge of the whole of things." Then, during the Middle Ages, medicine became dominated by mysticism and religion. "Sinning" was thought to be the cause of disease. In reaction to this view, and in conjunction with the scientific discoveries of the Renaissance (autopsy and microscopy), the study of the psyche was completely divorced from the study of medicine. In the nineteenth century, the schism was deepened by further scientific advances. It was thought that all disease must be associated with structural cell changes. Hence, the disease and not the client was the focus. Now, in the twentieth century, we have come full circle, and the mind and body are again united. How they are united is still unknown, although many theorists have attempted to explain the nature of the relationship (see Chapter 1).

The Specificity Model One theory is the specificity model of Franz Alexander (1950). According to Alexander, specific types of emotional conflict cause anxiety in the individual. In defending against this anxiety, the individual regresses to an earlier psychological and physiological state of development. For instance they may regress to the oral receptive stage, in which they unconsciously wish to be fed by the mother. This results in gastric hypersecretion, and if the person has a vulnerable duodenal mucosa, peptic ulcer may result. The following case example illustrates how the specificity model is applied.

Miss S, a twenty-year-old nursing student, has been diagnosed with a small peptic ulcer, treatable with diet and medication. Because she mentioned that she was having difficulties at school, she is also referred to the psychiatry service, where she meets with a psychoanalytically inclined therapist. He asks Miss S about her childhood and discovers that she was cared for by her grandmother while both her parents were away at work during the day. Later, Miss S had to take care of a younger sister and brother after school and on weekends. The student says she never had a "real childhood" and doesn't ever remember her mother being there when she needed her. According to Alexander's model, the therapist would deduce that Miss S has a dependency conflict deriving from her early childhood. Current academic stress causes her to wish for a time when she was protected and nurtured by her mother. These unconscious feelings produce gastric hypersecretion, and eventually a peptic ulcer.

Other investigators made further attempts to relate specific personality characteristics to certain diseases. People with ulcerative colitis were found to be passive, conforming, and dependent. Those with hypertension had counterdependency striving. Diabetic people were passive, needed affection, and wished to be cared for. Women with dysmenorrhea were infantile and expressed hopelessness and self-abnegation. Cancer clients were found to be selfless and undemanding (Sachar 1975).

On closer scrutiny, the specificity theory is not very specific after all. Certain emotional states, such as dependency, appear to be common to all disorders. Furthermore, research does not indicate whether dependence is a cause or an effect of the disease process. Another criticism is that some of the relationships described above have been based on faulty physiological premises. For instance, ulcerative colitis is thought to be caused by an inability to express anger openly. Instead, the client's rage "explodes" in uncontrollable bouts of diarrhea. It was believed that the frequent evacuations caused inflammation of the bowel lining. However, recent research has shown that *before* the persistent diarrhea appears, small ulcerations are already forming in the bowel (Sachar 1975).

The Nonspecific Stress Model   A second theory is the nonspecific stress model of Gustav Mahl (1953) (see Chapter 17). Unlike Alexander, who focused on specific types of emotional conflict, Mahl theorized

that the psychosomatic process can be activated by any stressful event. The stress can be precipitated by an external physical event, such as an earthquake, or by a more subtle intrapsychic event, such as a fear of elevators. Whatever the source of the stress, the physiologic responses will be identical for everyone. These physiologic responses have also been studied by Selye (1950). They include gastric and cardiovascular hyperfunctioning and hormonal changes, such as increased adrenal steroid secretion. A person who experiences chronic stress may develop a biological symptom, the nature of which will be determined by organ susceptibility and early learning experiences involving pathologic responses.

This nonspecific model can be applied to the same case study that was used to illustrate Alexander's specificity model. Miss S, the nursing student, still has a small peptic ulcer, but with this model it is explained differently.

Miss S experienced the usual school stresses along with the rest of her classmates. But Miss S develops an ulcer because her stomach is particularly vulnerable to stress. She may naturally produce an excess of hydrochloric acid, or her stomach lining may have some congenital defect. Along with organ susceptibility, Miss S may have a parent who also had a peptic ulcer. She may have seen a parent react to stress with abdominal disturbances and learned to react in a similar manner.

This viewpoint is consistent with the clinical research data that have been gathered from studying subjects under stress. However, what this theory fails to take into account is the wide variability of individual perceptions of stressful events. Not all events evoke the same stress reactions in everyone.

The Individual Response Specificity Model   A third theory is the individual response specificity model formulated by Lacey, Bateman, and Van Lehn (1953). According to this model, individuals tend to show highly characteristic and consistent physiological responses to a wide range of stimuli. This contradicts the nonspecific model, which states that everyone responds in much the same way to stress. The individual response model speaks instead of "cardiac reactors," "gastric reactors," and "hypertensive reactors."

To illustrate this model, we return to Miss S with her peptic ulcer.

Table 24-1 PEPTIC ULCER EXPLAINED BY THREE DIFFERENT THEORIES			
Model	**Stimulus**	**Biological Responses**	**Emerging Symptom**
Specificity model	Stress evokes a specific unconscious psychic conflict, i.e., dependency needs	Regression to oral receptive stage; increase in secretion of hydrochloric acid	Peptic ulcer
Nonspecific stress model	Any environmental stress	General stress response: increased blood pressure, increased adrenalin secretion, and so on	Peptic ulcer results because stomach was most susceptible organ
Individual response specificity model	Any environmental stress	Individual is a "gastric reactor"	Peptic ulcer

Miss S always has indigestion when she becomes upset. However, Miss M, her roommate, never has indigestion. Instead, she frequently has migraine headaches.

This theory is compatible with the previously mentioned theories of organ susceptibility and early learning experiences. Because it encompasses much of the current research data, this theory has become increasingly popular. Table 24–1 explains peptic ulcer according to these three theories.

The Multicausational Concept of Illness   It is readily apparent that the preceding models do not illuminate the relationships between emotions and physical functioning. By taking some other factors into account, a more useful model can be developed. Some of these factors are presented in the research by Holmes and Rahe (1967), Mutter and Schleifer (1966), and Rahe and Arthur (1978). These studies show that physical illness is commonly preceded by stressful life changes, which indicates that emotions have a role in all disease processes. The studies further suggest that physical illness, like mental illness, is related to social class. Furthermore, individuals in similar social situations defined those situations differently and consequently had different reactions to the similar situations.

Several basic considerations emerge from these findings.

• The concept of separation of mind and body is not useful in understanding the total disease process.

• Stress comes in many forms—psychological, physiological, and sociological—and is a causative factor in all illness.

• Stress is perceived differently, depending on the specific individual and the specific context.

All of these factors point to a multicausational concept of illness. This is an ecological concept that is congruent with a humanistic philosophy. The multicausational concept of the disease process is illustrated in Figure 24–1 and in the following case history.

Peter G, five years old, was admitted for the fourth time in six months for an acute asthma attack. While Peter was being treated medically, his parents waited in the family room. Mrs. G sat crying and wringing her hands while Mr. G paced the floor with a strained expression on his face. A staff nurse was able to talk to them and trace the sequence of events leading up to Peter's admission to the hospital.

It was a Saturday afternoon, and Mr. and Mrs. G had been arguing about whether to send Peter to kindergarten in the fall. Two points of view had emerged. Mr. G was all for it. He wanted Peter to grow up quickly and leave his "babyish ways" behind. Mrs. G was against it. Peter was the baby of the family, and Mrs. G felt that her husband was always pushing him to do things too advanced for a five-year-old. Peter had awakened from his nap to hear his parents shouting at each other. The quarrel ended abruptly when Peter started to wheeze, and both parents rushed to his bedside, united in their concern for him.

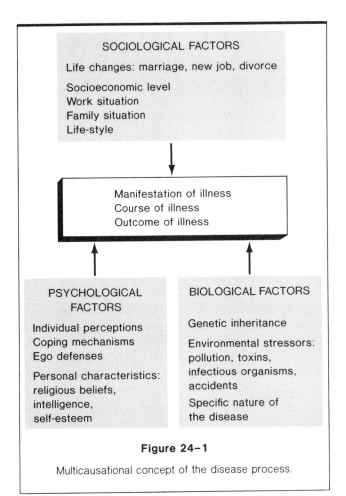

SOCIOLOGICAL FACTORS

Life changes: marriage, new job, divorce

Socioeconomic level
Work situation
Family situation
Life-style

Manifestation of illness
Course of illness
Outcome of illness

PSYCHOLOGICAL
FACTORS

Individual perceptions
Coping mechanisms
Ego defenses

Personal characteristics:
religious beliefs,
intelligence,
self-esteem

BIOLOGICAL FACTORS

Genetic inheritance

Environmental stressors:
pollution, toxins,
infectious organisms,
accidents

Specific nature of
the disease

Figure 24–1

Multicausational concept of the disease process.

What were the factors that brought on Peter's asthma attack at that particular time? The biological factors include Peter's physiological makeup. His mother had been a child asthmatic. She and Peter were both allergic to chocolate, eggs, feathers, and dust. Peter had inherited certain genetic features that made him susceptible to certain environmental stressors—in this case, the specific allergens. Sociological components of Peter's illness revolve around his family's functioning. Mr. and Mrs. G had different viewpoints on what Peter's role in the family should be. Their conflicts created a second source of stress for Peter. A third component is Peter's psychological state. A five-year-old child views the integrity of his family as extremely important, and parental conflicts may threaten his sense of security. Peter had discovered that his parents rallied together when he was ill.

In view of these contributing factors, the treatment plan for Peter would not end when Peter stopped wheezing. In order to reduce the number of such emergencies, a long-range treatment plan would be required. This plan should encompass the physiological,

psychological, and sociological components of Peter's asthma attacks.

Holistic Health Concepts

Hospital clients cannot be treated successfully by attending only to their physical needs. Since illness is multidetermined to begin with, treatment must address the same range of factors. This holistic approach is well illustrated by the Simontons' work with cancer clients. It has long been recognized that emotions play a part in the development and course of cancer. Following the holistic concepts of disease incidence, treatment, and recovery, the Simontons have developed a treatment program that consists of a traditional medical regimen plus a comprehensive mental health component. The latter includes: reading about holistic concepts of illness; learning relaxation techniques and creative mental imagery; identifying stresses; overcoming fears, anger, and resentment; and setting goals. Preliminary results of this program indicate that clients so treated survived up to twice as long as would have been expected, based on national averages (Simonton 1980). Subsequently, many centers throughout the country have set up similar programs; we eagerly await their research findings.

Since nursing itself is rooted in holistic health concepts, the nursing profession can be strengthened by the current interest in these ideas. The following is a listing of the main concepts in the holistic health philosophy.

- Positive wellness, not simply the absence of disease, is the goal of health care.

- Prevention of illness does not lie in the annual physical examination, but in the individual's daily habits.

- The causes of most illnesses are to be found in the individual's environment, life-style, and emotional makeup.

- Illness can be viewed as an expression of some imbalance in the individual's life, and can be a "teacher" and impetus toward health.

- Responsibility for health lies with the individual, not with a physician or other health professional.

- Health-restorative approaches should work in conjunction with the body's natural homeostatic mechanisms.

- Approaches to healing should focus on the *basis* of the problem, not on the symptoms.

- Western medicine is valuable but limited in its focus on pathology and its dismissal of alternative healing methods.

These holistic concepts, further discussed in Chapter 25, are part of the psychosocial base that must be incorporated into general hospital practice. Other components of the theoretical base are crisis theory and the related concept of preventive psychiatry, discussed below.

Crisis Theory

Hospitals are ideal places in which to see crisis brewing. The emergency room and the cardiac and intensive care units are designed specifically for clients who are experiencing an unexpected illness or accident. However, general medical and surgical floors, where clients are admitted by schedule, also include clients in states of crisis. Any hospitalization is extremely stressful. Clients are in a strange environment away from their customary supports of family and friends. They literally fear for their lives. Never knowing from minute to minute what to expect, they are subjected to all sorts of indignities. Usually no one informs them of procedures more than a few minutes ahead of time, and what is worse, they are the last to know the results of their many tests. In a large teaching hospital, the client has a specialist for everything and consequently may not develop a supportive relationship with any one doctor or nurse. These clients are constrained to lie passively in bed, while the parade of hospital personnel work on their various parts. In addition to this lack of customary support systems and the fear of bodily injury, they suffer a psychological reaction to hospitalization. Clients are expected to assume the *sick role* described by Parsons (1951). While occupying this role, they are exempt from responsibility and from their normal social role obligations. They are expected to depend on others, not to be self-directed. Essentially, clients can be left almost totally without their usual supports, including the coping mechanisms of their own self-system.

A nurse who recognizes a crisis is in a strategic position to affect its outcome because, according to crisis theory (see Chapter 11), a client in crisis is most receptive to intervention. When the crisis is a physical illness, crisis resolution is actually the process of recovery. This model is sometimes applied in treating clients

who have had myocardial infarctions. Researchers have found that the client's emotional state is crucial in determining the rate of recovery. Taking this into account, hospitals attempt to create a less impersonal critical care unit environment, to allow clients to follow their previous daily routines as closely as possible, and to understand the emotional state of a client in such a precarious position.

If the nurse's proximity to the client equips the nurse to handle a crisis, so, too, do the parallels between the nursing process and the crisis intervention model. The nursing process consists of assessing, diagnosing, planning, implementing, and evaluating (see Chapter 4). The parallel steps of the crisis model, according to Aguilera and Messick (1978, p. 19), are:

- Assessment of the individual and the problem
- Planning of the therapeutic intervention
- Intervention
- Resolution of the crisis and anticipatory planning

Part of the role of the psychiatric clinical specialist is to support the nursing staff in their work as crisis intervenors. This involves acting as a role model by performing crisis intervention in difficult situations, as well as providing in-service education for the staff. Unfortunately, nurses do not always realize their own potential. They may need to be helped to use their knowledge and influence for the client's benefit. The psychiatric clinician can provide the support and encouragement the staff nurses need to expand their capabilities.

It is not always clients and their families who are having the crisis. Ironically enough, staff nurses are often in a state of crisis themselves. When clients don't get well, when clients die, when clients complain, nurses are not able to "nurse." They see themselves as failing in their role of healer. This is an extremely important concept to understand if one is called in to consult during a hospital crisis. Obviously, nurses cannot be expected to intervene in a client crisis when they are having one of their own. Another task of the consultant, then, is to determine *who* is in crisis. Usually it will be some combination of client, client's family, and the nursing and medical staff. If it is determined that the crisis is shared by the nursing staff, the intervention begins there.

Consultation work with staff members can be

thought of as a means of preventing future client crises. With the help of the consultant, nurses often learn to gain support from the clinician and from each other. In this way, they can become crisis intervenors in their own right. Chapter 11 discusses the role of the nurse in crisis intervention in depth.

Preventive Aspects of Consultation

The theory of preventive psychiatry is closely related to crisis intervention theory, the classic work in both areas having been written by Gerald Caplan (1964). Crisis intervention aims at preventing a maladaptive resolution of the crisis, and at fostering growth at a crucial time when the client is eager for outside help. The final step in the crisis intervention process is anticipatory planning, which helps clients deal with events that are probably going to confront them in the future. When clients have an idea of what to expect, they are better able to prepare themselves. Anticipation and preparation are the basic ideas behind preventive psychiatry, the purpose being to prevent further crisis situations.

Prevention is usually defined on three levels. *Primary prevention* is the elimination of factors that cause or contribute to the development of disease. *Secondary prevention* is the early detection and treatment of disease. *Tertiary prevention* is the elimination or reduction of residual disability following illness.

When nurses do admission assessments, they are practicing primary prevention. By establishing a data base, the nurse becomes alert to potential problems the client may experience during hospitalization. The following clinical example demonstrates primary prevention in practice.

Mrs. K was eighty-five, a tiny, white-haired woman who had been admitted with a possible fractured hip. She was hard of hearing and appeared frightened and very hesitant to take off her many layers of clothing. From her daughter, who accompanied her, the nurses learned that Mrs. K lived alone and was very active. In fact, her daughter had trouble getting her to slow down. In admitting Mrs. K to her room, the nurse was careful to take her time and help Mrs. K adjust to the strange surroundings. She helped Mrs. K undress, taking special care of the clothing the client obviously valued, and assuring her that soon she'd be able to wear her own nightgowns. What was crucial in Mrs. K's treatment was

to allow her as much autonomy as possible and to explain carefully and patiently any restrictions she was to observe. She was not to be treated like a "little old lady." This would have been a blow to her self-esteem, which was already damaged by the hip injury. By giving this client extra time and attention, the nurse was anticipating the kinds of problems a hospitalization might pose for such an independent person who was suddenly being confronted with the fact that she was aging.

Primary prevention means being alert to potential problems that accompany any physical illness. Most clients have families who feel useless, afraid, helpless, and generally unsure of how to treat their sick relative. Including the family in the client's care plan makes them allies in the recovery process, instead of "outsiders" who are always "in the way." This principle is commonly adhered to in pediatric units. Although some degree of separation anxiety is inevitable, efforts are made to allow parents to spend as much time as possible with their sick child. In some cases rooming-in is thought appropriate. Conversely, when the parents are clients, it's important during long hospitalizations not to isolate them from their families. Frequent visits keep the family support system intact, an invaluable factor in recovery. In short, primary prevention forms the basis for many nursing actions, from carefully individualizing a client's care plan to explaining to clients that the hospital is usually short-staffed on weekends.

Secondary prevention, also a common task in nursing, is the process of looking for and recognizing early signs of a problem.

Mrs. D had left-sided hemiplegia and was aphasic. It was too early to determine what permanent damage the cerebrovascular accident had caused. However, she was showing signs of improvement daily. The client had a large family that visited frequently, hovering around the bed, whispering to each other, but not approaching the nurses for information. The staff were beginning to complain that the family interfered with the client's care, and the family were beginning to ask for permission for one of them to stay overnight with Mrs. D. At this point, the head nurse asked the psychiatric nurse clinician for assistance. A meeting was arranged with the family members, the head nurse, the client's primary nurse, and the psychiatric nurse clinician. Here the family were able to voice their fears that Mrs. D was going to die while they were away. They confessed they were in total confusion as to what was happening to Mrs. D, and talking among themselves only added to their fund of misinformation. The nurses were able to explain the situation and reassure the family that they would be kept informed of any changes. A plan was designed for a more coordinated visiting schedule, and family members who wished to do so were allowed to help with the client's daily care. In this way, a family that was showing signs of becoming overprotective and smothering was transformed into an integral part of Mrs. D's rehabilitation.

Once the problem has appeared, the principles of tertiary prevention become operative. Tertiary prevention begins when the staff call the psychiatric nurse clinician in the middle of a full-blown crisis, as the following clinical material illustrates.

Mr. J is dressed half in pajamas, half in street clothes and is heading for the elevator. He is an alcoholic who is frequently admitted to the unit in delirium tremens. The staff have just spent an exhausting week, keeping Mr. J restrained and working desperately to keep in his intravenous line and supply him with fluids. Now almost detoxified, he says he "needs another drink" and is headed for the corner bar. The doctors are unable to convince him to stay, and he leaves without signing an "against medical advice" form.

In this situation, the psychiatric nurse clinician helped the staff deal with their feelings of frustration and anger at the client. There may be no way to prevent this kind of incident, but the staff can be helped to realize that they are not at fault. This prevents them from becoming demoralized and acting out their frustration toward each other or toward other clients who remind them of their "failure" with Mr. J.

As the case examples illustrate, the psychiatric nurse clinician cannot carry out prevention single-handed. Part of the clinician's role is to provide opportunities for staff education that promote autonomous functioning. In most cases, the staff are capable of providing clients with the emotional support they need. The clinician's job is to tap the staff's potential, cultivate their interpersonal skills, render the total care plan effective, and provide support when the staff are in crisis. The following section will explain how these goals are met through the process of consultation.

THE ROLE OF THE PSYCHIATRIC NURSING CONSULTANT

History of Consultation in the Hospital Setting

Physicians were the first to practice *consultation-liaison psychiatry*—providing psychiatric consultation to clients in the general hospital—based on the previously discussed concepts of psychophysiologic medicine and preventive psychiatry. Liaison psychiatry originated in the late 1950s. Paralleling this trend, psychiatric nurses also began to act as consultants to their colleagues in medical and surgical settings. At first, the *liaison nurses* remained based on their psychiatric units, providing indirect assistance when it was requested. Later, they began to work directly with clients and their families (Nelson and Schilke 1976). Currently, psychiatric nurse clinicians perform both direct and indirect consultative functions. Consultation work, to be effective, should be based on sound judgment, and this in turn is grounded in theoretical knowledge of the consultative process. Again, the classic work in this area was done by Gerald Caplan (1964).

Types of Mental Health Consultation

Caplan defines *consultation* as the "interaction between two professional persons in regard to a current work problem with which the consultee is having some difficulty and which he has decided is within the consultant's area of competence" (Caplan 1964, p. 212).

The phrase "two professional persons" implies an egalitarian relationship between consultant and consultee. The nurse who requests the consultation is on a peer level with the clinician. Both have their individual areas of expertise, and both should recognize that the ultimate professional responsibility for the client lies with the consultee. (Note that the situation is different when the psychiatric clinician assumes the role of therapist to the client or the family. It should be clear that this definition refers to clinicians in their consultative role.)

Caplan goes on to define four types of consultation. These are: client-centered case consultation; program-centered administrative consultation; consultee-centered case consultation; and consultee-centered administrative consultation. Most of the consultant's functions fall into one or another of these categories, although there will be some overlap at times.

Client-centered Case Consultation   In this type of consultation, the client's problems are the immediate focus. Often a time factor is involved—the client is only in the hospital for a short time, and the problem must be dealt with *now*. The main concern is improving the client's status and eliminating any blocks to physical recovery. Some examples of client-centered case consultation follow.

Mrs. B was a seventy-five-year-old widow, very slight, who had been extremely fastidious about her personal hygiene. She was a client on a surgical unit where, following a diagnosis of cancer of the colon, a temporary colostomy had been performed. The cancer had been resectable, and plans were made to perform an anastomosis in four to six weeks. The prognosis was good. However, the client began to act increasingly bizarre. She refused to eat meals, to wash, or to change her nightclothes. She refused to allow the nurses to change the bed sheets, and she became increasingly withdrawn. Because of this behavior, the nurses asked the psychiatric nurse clinician to see the client. The clinician discovered a very frightened woman who had completely misunderstood the purpose of the proposed second surgery. Mrs. B thought that the doctors had to operate to take out the rest of the cancer and was convinced that she was "filled with cancer." Why else would someone need two operations? The nurses thought the client was aware of her good prognosis, while Mrs. B thought the nurses had given her up as a goner. When the new information was constantly reinforced, the client began to eat and returned to her former meticulous ways.

Mr. L, a sixty-five-year-old security guard, was admitted with newly diagnosed acute leukemia. Although his prognosis was very poor, he was started on chemotherapy and put into reverse isolation due to his extremely low white count. The staff nurses became concerned because Mr. L was extremely passive and smiled pleasantly and resignedly even during the most unpleasant procedures. Mr. L's only relative was a brother who tried to visit often but hesitated to spend much time with Mr. L because of the isolation setup. The psychiatric clinician determined that part of Mr. L's passivity was due to his extreme weakness, but that he was also very frightened of hospitals, doctors, and nurses. He had never been sick before, and now this illness put him into a state of shock. Mr. L was a very lonely man who was too weak and too frightened to protest. Along with the psychiatric nurse clinician and the intern, the staff nurses were able to plan a different approach to Mr. L's care.

It was decided that since Mr. L's condition was terminal, the oncology service would be asked to discontinue the reverse isolation. They readily agreed to do so, admitting that it was not really necessary. Mr. L's brother could now visit more frequently, and the nursing staff were able to spend more time with the client, who began to make his needs known to them. Mr. L died within the week, but his brother and the nursing staff were able to be with him.

The psychiatric nurse clinician does not always need to make a "diagnosis" of the client's problem. Sometimes consultation is a matter of validating the nurse's original judgment, as in Mr. L's case. The staff nurses were surprised at how readily the oncology service cooperated, once they made the suggestion.

Program-centered Administrative Consultation   In this type of consultation, the consultant is asked to help develop or improve a specific program. The programs can vary, as these next examples demonstrate.

The nurses who taught diabetic classes were reporting that they had trouble keeping the group's attention. They felt they needed some help in acquiring group skills. The consultant worked with the nurses for several weeks, giving them information on basic group dynamics. She also helped them improve their skills by having them role-play in small groups of their own.

Besides attending to client needs, consultants also use their skills in less direct ways.

One hospital planned regular in-service sessions for its head nurse and supervisor group. A major goal of nursing service at that time was to improve the staff nurses' ability to teach clients. It was thought that the place to begin was with the head nurses and supervisors, who would be role models for the rest of the staff. The consultant was asked to plan methods of working with this group. What resulted was a series of day-long work sessions that focused on effective teaching and learning techniques.

In this example, the consultant was instrumental in planning not only the *content* of the sessions, but also the methods for reaching the ultimate goal of better client-learning programs.

In program-centered administrative consultation, the clinicians use their knowledge to help plan orientation programs, in-service seminars, and client-teaching programs, to name only a few. Actually, there are innumerable opportunities in a hospital setting for clinicians to use their knowledge. Their input will be determined by the imagination and attitude of the hospital administration and nursing service.

Consultee-centered Case Consultation   The focus here is on the consultee—the nurse—rather than on the particular client with whom the nurse is experiencing difficulties. Although a specific client is the identified reason for the consultation, and the client will gain some benefit from the consultation, the main goal is to improve the nurse's overall functioning. Sometimes the nurse will be vague about the reason for the consultation, expressing dissatisfaction with the client's progress but not really sure how the consultant can help. The following example illustrates how consultees can be helped.

A nursing assistant complained to the psychiatric nurse consultant about the behavior of one of her clients—a forty-five-year-old woman with a metastatic breast cancer. This client, an attractive, wealthy woman, was losing her hair, becoming pitifully thin, and beginning to have uncontrollable bowel movements. According to the nursing assistant, the client whined constantly, refusing to take even minimal care of herself. What really irritated the nursing assistant was the client's insistence on wearing her own lacy nightgowns despite her frequent incontinence. After allowing the aide to ventilate her feelings, the clinician explored with her the client's probable state of mind. Once the aide moved beyond her own feelings of frustration, she was able to see more clearly that the client needed to maintain her individuality and self-esteem. After the consultation, the aide found it much easier to accept the client's behavior and no longer perceived it as personally antagonistic.

In this case, the aide needed help in understanding psychological factors and making meaningful connections. Consultees may also need assistance because they lack the skill to carry out a specific plan. If so, the consultant may want to plan a workshop on basic communication skills or interviewing techniques.

Consultees may also have difficulties because they have a deep personal involvement with a client.

A recent nursing graduate told the psychiatric clinician that she'd just lost her enthusiasm for work, and thought that maybe she wasn't cut out for nursing. Her first assignment had been a woman of her own age who was dying from Hodgkin's disease. She'd spent every day for two weeks caring for this client, becoming deeply involved with the family and even spending some off-duty time with the client. She had no energy left over for her other clients and felt isolated from them and the rest of the staff. The clinician discussed with the nurse the similarities between the client and herself and suggested that this was indeed a difficult first assignment. The new graduate confessed that she'd been afraid to ask for relief in caring for the client for fear the head nurse would disapprove. The clinician continued to work with this nurse, encouraging her to ask for assistance when she needed it from the other staff members and validating her need for some temporary distance from the client.

This type of consultative situation is not to be considered therapy, although the process in itself is therapeutic. The egalitarian relationship is maintained between consultant and consultee, and no attempt is made to delve into any of the nurse's personal problems that are not directly connected to the nurse–client relationship that originally prompted the consultation. More will be said about this point later.

A common problem in consulting with nurses is their lack of confidence and self-esteem. Nurses are often unaware of the enormous effect they have on clients, and they underestimate their communication skills, preferring to leave the task of "giving emotional support" to the psychiatric nursing specialist. As in the case example of Mr. L, who needed to be taken out of isolation, the nurse usually knows what the correct action is, but needs to be encouraged to take it. Some goals in consultee-centered case consultation are to overcome the nurse's fear of failure, fear of appearing different, and fear of acting assertively. A clinician can dissipate these fears by modeling the desired behaviors and treating nurse-consultees with professional respect.

Consultee-centered Administrative Consultation   Applied to the hospital setting, this type of consultation refers to helping nurses with problems that involve the hospital administrative or organizational structure. Consultants who wish to become involved in this type of consultation need a background in organizational theory and the concepts of planned change. Staff nurses who want to negotiate changes in hospital procedures or policy may request help in deciding where to target their efforts.

The nurses in a special protective care unit were concerned that the medical staff were using poor isolation technique and most probably were contributing to the spread of infectious organisms in the hospital. In this particular unit, the clinician held weekly client care conferences, and she began to note that the nursing staff spent a great deal of time complaining about the physicians' noncompliance with the unit's procedures. However, the staff were unable to work toward a solution. Here the clinician was useful in channeling their energy toward finding workable solutions. Instead of spending their time complaining, they planned ways to deal with the infection problem, first with the doctors on one-to-one terms, and then on a broader basis as a part of a nurse-initiated infection control committee.

Guidelines for Mental Health Consultation

It should be noted that Caplan developed the four categories of consultation for use in a community mental health setting. In a hospital setting, priorities are different, one does not have the luxury of time, and the client is more easily accessible for evaluation by the consultant. For these reasons, Caplan's guidelines have been adapted for the hospital setting.

- Mental health consultation is a process of interaction between two professionals with respect to a client or a program for clients.

- Ideally, the consultant has no administrative responsibility for the consultee's work. He or she is under no compulsion to alter the consultee's handling of the case.

- The consultee has no obligation to accept the consultant's ideas or suggestions.

- The basic relationship between the two is egalitarian. This allows the consultee to accept or reject what the consultant says and to incorporate any ideas the consultee feels are appropriate to the situation.

- Consultation can take various forms. These include individual and group consultation and work with staff as well as with clients, depending on the particular situation.

- The exact form of the consultation is made explicit in the contract—a verbal or written agreement between consultant and consultees.

- The goals of consultation are to help the consultees improve their handling or understanding of the current work problem and to generalize this learning to future similar situations.

- The consultative process is not therapy, but it can be therapeutic. By increasing a consultee's competence in the work situation, it will give the consultee an overall sense of accomplishment and self-worth (Caplan 1970, pp. 28–30).

Caplan suggests that the consultant usually need not personally visit the client for an evaluation. This helps preserve the egalitarian nature of the consultant–consultee relationship, giving the message that the consultee's report of the client is thought reliable. However, in certain cases direct intervention is most effective. These include times when the client needs support and the staff for one reason or another are unable to give it. For example, a client who is dying may have a nurse who is not ready to become involved. Then, too, some problems are very complicated and should be dealt with by an expert. For example, there are times when a client has so alienated the staff that they are not willing or able to care for that client effectively. The family who must learn to adjust to an invalid member may also need this expert help.

In any event, the consultant always works toward two ultimate goals: the welfare of the client and the continued growth of the staff nurse's supportive skills.

Qualifications of the Consultant

A psychiatric nurse clinical specialist has been defined by the American Nurses' Association as a registered nurse with a master's degree in psychiatric nursing. Some graduate programs are specifically geared to liaison nursing and provide clinical experiences in a general hospital setting. Other programs are oriented toward the community mental health center or the psychiatric inpatient unit. In any case, the consultant's education includes classroom and supervised clinical experiences in individual, group, and family therapy, since all these modes will be used in practice. Most graduate programs include courses in organizational theory in which the principles of power and influence and planned change are emphasized. A hospital is an incredibly complex organization, and the more ammunition consultants have, the better they can withstand the bureaucratic onslaught.

Consultants who have actual staff nursing experience in a nonpsychiatric general hospital setting have an invaluable advantage over the inexperienced clinician. They have first-hand knowledge of the day-to-day problems facing the staff nurse: what it is like to rotate shifts; having to work weekends; being the only registered nurse in charge of forty clients; dealing with complaints from X ray, dietary, and the operating room—and on top of it all, having clients say they would get better service for less money in a hotel down the street. It is definitely true that nursing educators and administrators gain respect by having "paid their dues." Consultants with staff experience start out with two advantages. They are *nurses*, and they share a common background of experience with their consultees.

A very important, but subtle, factor is that the consultant should *like* nurses and enjoy being a nurse. Too often, nurses go to graduate school to escape what they consider dull nursing duties, only to return to the hospital setting and encourage staff nurses to enjoy the duties they themselves are happy to avoid. This attitude will almost certainly come through in the course of consultation work. Consultants are ineffective unless they convey a genuine respect for the staff nurse's job.

A successful consultant, like a successful therapist, needs a solid theoretical and experiential base, along with confidence, competence, and concern.

Building Relationships

Ideally, consultants enter the hospital system in a staff rather than a line position. This means they are outside the chain of command and have no formal authority in the organizational hierarchy. Instead, their authority stems from their special knowledge and skills. There are several reasons for entering the system in this manner. First, it maintains an egalitarian relationship between consultant and consultee. It is clear that the consultee has ultimate control in managing the client problem. Also the consultative process, which aims for increasing self-awareness and gradual behavior changes, is most effective when the consultee enters the relationship voluntarily. As in therapy, an important factor is the motivation of the consultee. This mo-

tivation is optimal when the consultee initiates and maintains ultimate control over the relationship. An example of this important concept follows.

A head nurse asked one of the hospital supervisors to hold group meetings with the staff nurses of the intensive care unit because they were exhibiting "attitude" problems. This supervisor had previously been the psychiatric consultant for the hospital. However, she now held a line position. The group attendance was good, but the interaction remained stilted, and no real progress was made. Later it emerged that the staff believed that they had been pressured into attending group meetings because the head nurse said they had to go. They also felt intimidated by the consultant-supervisor, who had actually hired many of them originally and who still supervised their work. An experienced consultant would seriously hesitate to work with a group that had been formed under these conditions. These meetings were almost certainly doomed to failure.

One further reason why consultants should stay outside the power structure is that they need to remain as nonthreatening as possible. They should try to dissipate the common myths frequently circulated about psychiatric workers. The staff may fear that the clinician can read their minds and has been hired by administration to "shrink the staff." Consider the following instance:

A new consultant introduced herself to the head nurse on a hemodialysis unit. Before the clinician could say another word, the head nurse declared that on her unit they were already very aware of the emotional needs of their clients and held weekly staff meetings to plan client care. Of course, she added nervously, the clinician would probably be able "to pick out things that we're doing that we aren't even aware of."

It is important to dispel these notions from the beginning. Clinicians cannot perform magic, although at first the staff may demand that their most difficult clients be instantly "cured." Nor will they try to pry out secrets about the personal lives of their consultees. They have no special powers that they use to influence or to change people against their will. They should make it clear that they are eager to share whatever skills they do possess with the staff. All this is a gradual process.

It involves consistent role modeling, and it requires the clinician to become personally acquainted with as many hospital staff members as possible.

Paying Attention to Key People

In introducing themselves initially, new consultants pay attention to key people in the organization. These include supervisors, head nurses, other clinicians, heads of other hospital departments such as social work and client services, and the physician-psychiatric liaison team. In some cases, there is overlap among the various services, and future antagonism can be avoided if the consultant and other professionals clearly define their respective roles. These key people also provide access to their staff and subsequently to clients, making it crucial to have their acceptance and support. The new consultant, then, has the initial task of forming relationships with key people in the organization.

Setting up the Ground Rules

The second task is setting up the ground rules for consultation. This involves nothing less than establishing a basic philosophy about the consultation service. The ground rules are determined through input from the potential consultees, the administration, and the individual consultant, and by the needs of the clients in that particular setting.

In most hospitals, the psychiatric nurse consultation service is a relatively recent phenomenon, and therefore lacks a strong traditional framework like that found in the medical consultation process. Working out a philosophy for practice is an evolving task, one that takes many hours of individual contemplation and group discussion. It is important to recognize that each participant's conceptual framework directs what actually happens among consultees, clients, and the consultant.

For example, in one hospital where the director of nursing had little autonomy from the medical hierarchy, the nurse-clinician functioned under the direction of the psychiatrist-consultant. The clinician's primary role was to see clients on a one-to-one basis and formulate a diagnosis under the supervision of the psychiatrist. A secondary role was to attend nursing care plan conferences to explain the dynamics behind the client's particular maladaptive behavior, and discuss various psychotherapeutic and chemotherapeutic treatment approaches.

In a second hospital, where the department of nursing and the psychiatric nurse-clinician were organizationally separate from the medical service, a different scene evolved. The staff nurses called the clinician on a whenever-necessary basis. Sometimes the consultant would see the client for evaluation and sometimes not. In accordance with this institution's commitment to primary nursing, the clinician's role was secondary to and supportive of the primary nurse's role. Rather than intervene directly, the consultant worked through the existing relationship between the primary nurse and the client. The consultant's work in this hospital consisted of meeting with the nursing staff to discuss how the primary nurse could meet the emotional needs of the client as part of the overall care plan. The consultant also planned and implemented in-service and continuing education programs and workshops to improve the functioning of the nursing staff as a whole.

The process of forming a philosophy for practice as a consultant in a general hospital differs from the process in private practice. The consultant's individual philosophy is constantly modified by the goals and values of the institution. This is not to say that you compromise your ideals, but you remain aware of the reason and purpose behind each particular intervention. What evolves from these considerations is the *contract*.

Negotiating the Consultation Contract

The notion of contract is a crucial element in the consultative process. A contract can be a verbal agreement made over coffee or a formal written document signed by the participants. The essential element is that the contract clearly defines the expectations of all parties involved. Contracting involves *listening* to what is being asked of the consultant, as this example demonstrates.

On a Friday afternoon the psychiatric nurse consultant was called to a medical unit about a problem with Mrs. L. This client was a seventy-nine-year-old diabetic woman with a gangrenous left foot. Since admission she had been refusing all treatment, saying that she wanted to go home and die in peace. The doctors were discussing this possibility while Mrs. L lay in bed restlessly pulling at her intravenous and nasogastric tubes. Because of the possibility of a cardiac arrest, the physicians were hesitant to sedate her. Mrs. L managed to untie all forms of soft restraints, and after replacing her various tubes for the third time, the harried intern ordered leather restraints. It was at this point that the staff nurses called in the consultant.

The consultant listened to their description of the events and then asked the nurses what they had in mind. They had already arranged with the evening supervisor to obtain a private nurse for Mrs. L for the evening shift. The night shift would probably also be able to give Mrs. L almost constant supervision, so that the leather restraints would not be needed. There had been a continuing dialogue between the nurses and client's family, who understood why the restraints were necessary. The nurses also planned to consult the intern periodically for the purpose of ordering an appropriate sedative. In short, the staff nurses needed the consultant to obtain some leather restraints in case they became necessary (these were available only to the consultant), and to validate their plan of action.

In the above example, the consultant could have immediately visited the client herself to assess the situation. This premature act might have given the staff the message that the consultant did not trust their account of the problem. Instead, the consultant learned that the staff already had a viable plan. The consultant agreed to obtain the restraints and to be available for further consultation. The staff were left feeling confident about their ability to carry out their plan.

On another unit, the head nurse approached the consultant about intrastaff conflicts. This particular unit had the reputation of having clients with the most severe and complicated long-term problems. The staff nurses were known to the rest of the hospital as extremely competent and hard working, but among themselves there was much competition and very little cooperation or staff cohesion. This unit utilized team nursing, and the two teams had constant arguments about the assignment of clients and the use of temporary personnel sent from the nursing office on especially heavy days.

The consultant's first task was to talk with the staff nurses themselves to get their views. Did they think they had a problem? Did they define it in the same terms as the head nurse had? As expected, the staff were divided on their view of the conflict; however, everyone was willing to work with the consultant toward a solution. A beginning contract was made among the staff, head nurse, and consultant to meet initially one hour a week for six weeks, to find the source of the conflict and work out solutions. This proved to be an extremely complicated task. For starters, the staff consisted of nurses from many different backgrounds—baccalaureate, associate degree, and di-

ploma graduates. Competition existed around who could give the best client care and whose philosophy of nursing was the most relevant in this particular setting. Also, several of the nurses were having problems in their personal lives and were carrying their conflicts into the work situation. To make matters worse, the head nurse had requested a transfer to another unit, leaving the staff in confusion about their future leader.

After many tense sessions, a successful solution was found. Since the head nurse was leaving, and the staff consisted of four very competent nurses, none of whom was interested in becoming head nurse, it was decided to implement primary nursing. This would satisfy staff wishes to give direct client care and retain a degree of autonomy. It would also allow for individual differences in approach to client care. Of course this solution involved negotiation with the nursing administration, but the major points to be noted here refer to the consultation process. First, the contract was made with the staff nurses, not just with the head nurse. The consultant was responsive to staff needs, not just to the demands of their supervisor. The consultant abided by the terms of the contract. This called for a high level of expertise, because the conflicts were on so many different levels.

By focusing on the *work* situation, the consultant avoided turning the sessions into group therapy. It is extremely important that the consultant avoid this kind of involvement. For one thing, the contract did not call for group psychotherapy. It called for help in solving a work-related, client-oriented problem. Also the consultative process is not parallel to the normal course of therapy, the resistance and working-through stages of which include a dependency on the therapist. This is not to say that these dynamics are not present in any consultation group, but they should not be its primary focus. In this particular example, the staff spent time ventilating their resentment and discouragement about the difficult clients their unit received. They also voiced anger toward the head nurse, whom they perceived as deserting them. The consultant supported them all in their efforts to communicate with one another in a nonthreatening manner but consistently discouraged them from discussing any personal problems in these sessions. Such are the intricacies of the consultative process. It is essential to have a clear contract that can be referred to for guidance along the way.

Another advantage of the contract is that it focuses on goals and hence on evaluating the outcome of the process. Nurses are currently interested in accountability, and clinical specialists are no exception. They need more than subjective evidence of their success. Part of the consultative process is to keep records and to devise methods of evaluating one's interventions to ensure continued high quality practice (and to ensure continued funding!).

CLINICAL SITUATIONS COMMONLY ENCOUNTERED

The Demanding Client

Ruth was a resident of a home for the permanently disabled. She had been admitted to the hospital for a possible bowel obstruction. She was sixty-five and had lived most of her life in a wheelchair. Her body was misshapen from cerebral palsy, and she had no use of her legs or left hand. Recently she had developed arthritis in her right hand and could use it only for short periods each day. She had also been born with megacolon and was obsessed with the use of various laxatives. Ruth's appearance belied the fact that she was very intelligent, although humorless, as the staff soon found out.

According to the staff, Ruth was the "worst client they'd ever had." Ruth wanted to direct her own care in meticulous detail. She had to be bathed at a certain time and in a certain sequence, out of bed in time for breakfast and dressed by her own idiosyncratic method. It took two nurses one half hour to make her bed—they declared they needed a ruler to make sure the bedclothes hung precisely even. Medications were a real problem. Ruth had many p.r.n. medicines and constantly experimented with various combinations of laxatives, antispasmodics, and tranquilizers. No matter how one tried to please Ruth, she always found some fault with her nurse for the day, until finally she had been through the entire staff, and they all dreaded seeing her name on their assignment list.

The consultant could hardly believe that any one client could generate such hostility. She decided to work along with the staff nurse who had been assigned to Ruth that day. If anything, Ruth's behavior was worse than the staff had described. Since it seemed that she would be hospitalized for several more weeks, some plan had to be formulated. The consultant agreed to visit Ruth daily and to meet with the nurse who was giving Ruth her direct care. One nurse had volunteered to be responsible for coordinating Ruth's daily care and medications and to confer with the evening and night shifts.

In this case, the consultant's work was mainly supportive and educative. As she worked with Ruth, the consultant realized that her demanding attitude was a lifestyle that had been exaggerated by the current hospitalization. The nurse clinician helped the staff understand Ruth's behavior by looking at the underlying dynamics. Ruth had a distorted body image that reached back to her childhood, when she was confined to her bedroom and had to deal with body casts and braces. She had had to rely on others all her life and apparently had never resolved this dependency issue. To counteract her rage at being so helpless, she devised ways to control her environment by making incessant demands on others. In this way she vented her anger toward those with normal bodies. At the same time, she felt as if she had some degree of control over her surroundings. At one point, the clinician led the group of staff nurses through a guided fantasy of what it would be like to be in Ruth's position: to have an active energetic mind in an uncontrollable body. Ruth had behind her a lifetime of maladaption to her handicap, and it was not to be expected that she would change overnight. In fact, the current loss of functioning of her right hand constituted a crisis situation for Ruth. Behind Ruth's demands lay a myriad of feelings: anger, helplessness, frustration, jealousy, fear, and ambivalence.

In this intervention, the consultant found herself performing a *parallel process*. This means that she was fulfilling parallel needs for both the staff and the client. She would meet with Ruth and allow her to vent her feelings of anger and frustration—some of which were justified and some of which were distortions of reality—toward the staff and the world in general. She encouraged Ruth to use her coping mechanism of intellectualization to recognize how she distorted reality because of fear and frustration.

At the same time the clinician worked with the staff, allowing them to express their feelings about Ruth. These feelings were also justified. Here, the clinician worked toward helping the staff recognize their anger at the client—a very difficult task for most nurses. Once the anger has been identified, steps can be taken to control it. Otherwise nurse and client engage in a no-win battle over control. The clinician demonstrated that anger was acceptable between nurse and client. She taught the staff how to set limits without being punitive or feeling guilty. This is also a difficult task for nurses who often feel they must fulfill everyone's wishes without paying any attention to their own needs.

A dependent person *needs* to have limits set, and to be treated in a consistent and nonconflicted manner. Thus Ruth's nurse conveyed to her that she wanted to make her as comfortable as possible, but that she couldn't spend a half hour making and remaking the bed until she got it just right. It was okay for the nurse to tell Ruth when she was angry, to be clear about what had provoked the anger, and to demonstrate that this did not mean that she would abandon or punish her. The staff and the clinician hoped that Ruth would begin to learn how to handle her own anger.

A client as difficult as Ruth always arouses feelings that nurses usually find unacceptable in themselves. But before we can accept anger from a client, we must learn to accept it in ourselves and learn that it will not overwhelm us. Working with demanding clients involves looking behind the external behavior for the reasons that are always there, although not always obvious.

The Client in Pain

Probably every nurse remembers the first time we received an order to give an injection of sterile water for pain. Feeling guilty about carrying out such an order, we wondered why the client would "pretend" to be in pain. Who'd *want* to get injections, anyway?

The whole issue of pain and the use of medication to alleviate it is laden with myth and value judgments. We hear references to psychogenic pain versus "real" pain (see Chapter 14). In fact, pain is both an objective and a subjective experience. A nurse can observe pain behaviors like wincing, limping, or splinting. And a nurse can listen to a client's reports of feeling pain. How a client manifests pain depends on many factors. These include the client's background, previous experiences with pain, family's attitude toward the expression of pain, immediate environment, illness, and emotional state. The nurse's perception of a client's pain depends on the same factors. A nurse who thinks that people should suffer in silence will be intolerant of a client with a low pain threshold. It is important to realize that whether it is labeled psychogenic or physiological, the client *experiences* the same pain.

An accompanying factor is the emotional component of pain. Anxiety, depression, guilt, anger, and hostility can all be associated with the experience of pain and can, in fact, become indistinguishable from one another.

There is a familiar cartoon that shows a client sitting on a stretcher, his sleeve rolled up, his eyes shut tight-

ly, waiting for the nurse to give the injection. As she rubs the client's arm with alcohol, the client lets out a scream of pain and relief, only to discover that the worst is yet to come. The cartoon's point is that the expectation can be much more painful than the actual experience, and that one can actually *feel* the emotion of anxiety.

In the general hospital, the nurse will encounter pain in all its variations, from the post-cardiac-surgery client, to the cancer client with pathologic fractures, to the adolescent who has just had a tonsilectomy. Each client will have an individual response to particular stimuli. Therefore the nurse should evaluate each client's needs individually. Here is a case in point.

Mr. S had been a client on the oncology service for eight months. He had come to America from his home in Brazil when he discovered that he had a mandibular tumor. He had heard that the United States had the most advanced methods of chemotherapeutic and surgical treatment of cancer. During his eight months of hospitalization, Mr. S had undergone numerous courses of chemotherapy and four operations. Now he was ambulatory and self-sufficient. He had facial scars and a left-sided facial paralysis, but he could communicate clearly. His treatment had come to a standstill, and the doctors were planning discharge. However, Mr. S complained of constant severe pain that he reported kept him awake all night and prevented him from thinking about anything else. At this point the psychiatric clinician was asked to see Mr. S and help with the discharge planning.

The clinician did a comprehensive assessment of Mr. S's situation. This involved learning about his family background, his present relationship to his family, his plans for the immediate and distant future, and his perception of his illness. It also involved obtaining a detailed account of his pain experience.

Mr. S had left all his friends and relatives in Brazil. He was divorced and had a twelve-year-old daughter. In Brazil, he had held a university position, but he was not interested in returning either to his job or to his family. His reasons were not very clear, but he kept saying that he wanted to get a doctoral degree and a teaching position in the United States. He had written to several universities to inquire about their programs but had not made any definite plans. Apparently, money was no problem, but Mr. S repeatedly returned to the issue of his pain. This pain kept him from making progress—he couldn't rest until he knew whether the pain was from another tumor growing in his jaw. For this reason he felt he had to stay in the hospital for further tests.

A coordinated approach with the clinician as the client's primary contact was decided on. First, the clinician obtained information about Mr. S's medical status and asked the physicians to communicate clearly to Mr. S his present condition and his prognosis. He was told that there was no evidence of another tumor, that no further treatment was indicated at this time, and that they were willing to help him make plans for discharge. Next, the clinician carefully evaluated the client's pain behavior. Exactly where was the pain? When was it most severe? What medications helped most? What activities made it worse or better? Together with Mr. S, the staff nurses, and the physicians, the clinician implemented a plan whereby Mr. S could gradually be weaned off his present analgesics. This plan used the principles of behavior modification. The client was also taught how to meditate and use distraction and relaxation techniques. Underlying the entire plan was the relationship formed between Mr. S and the clinician. It was understood that Mr. S had developed a strong dependency on the hospital and indeed believed he could not survive outside its walls. The clinician aimed to reduce this dependency gradually, guiding Mr. S through the process of regaining his autonomy.

Mr. S's pain behavior was related to his fear of dying, his fear of rejection due to disfigurement, his fear that he had lost his status and role in his own country, and his fear of leaving the hospital. All these issues were considered in his treatment plan. This story has a happy ending. Mr. S returned to Brazil to his former position, needing only a nonnarcotic analgesic.

In complicated cases like this, the consultant may need to work directly with the client. However, the consultant still continues to include the nursing staff in planning and implementing the various interventions.

At other times, the consultant will need to help the staff deal with their own anxiety about the client's pain.

Mrs. J had terminal cancer and was receiving 100 mg. of Demerol intramuscularly every four hours for pain. Her buttocks were scarred and hardened—there didn't seem to be any place left to give another injection. Mrs. J dozed fitfully between medications but always awoke one half hour before the four hours were up, crying and moaning. The nurses began to avoid Mrs. J's room, going in only to give the medication and then leaving her with a hopeless pat on the shoulder. They told the clinician that they felt angry with Mrs. J, but that they didn't understand why.

This anger results from the frustration and anxiety that nurses feel when the client does not respond in the

desired way. Why won't this client feel better?! Anxiety on the part of the nurse can also take the form of apathy, depression, and avoidance of the client. All these behaviors are the result of the nurse's feeling of helplessness in the face of unrelenting pain. The clinician's role is to help the staff express and share their feelings, thus alleviating their guilt and apathy and freeing them to relate more fully to the client.

The Dependent Client

Some degree of dependency is a normal, necessary, and expected part of the person's new role as client. In order to be cured, clients allow us to take control of most of their bodily functions. They obediently open their mouths for the thermometer at six in the morning. They cooperate while we record everything they eat, drink, and eliminate. They answer questions in minute detail about their most intimate parts. Dependency and regression are aspects of their new role that allow clients to tolerate hospital life.

American culture values self-reliance and independence. But when we become ill, it becomes socially acceptable to ask for help. In fact, this is exactly what is expected. But sometimes the system backfires, and instead of giving up the sick role after the appropriate convalescent period, the client continues to act helpless. Whether or not clients return to their prior level of functioning depends on many factors. These include the length and severity of the illness, the client's personality, the client's family situation, and the attitude of the nursing staff, as illustrated in the following case.

Mrs. C was admitted to a neurology unit amid rumors that she probably had Guillain Barré syndrome, a rare disease that sometimes ends in total paralysis. The nurses were afraid to leave her bedside, expecting that at any moment she would stop breathing. After the official diagnosis had been made, Mrs. C was intubated and transferred to the intensive care unit, where she remained for four weeks. When she returned to the neurology unit, the nurses met a severely regressed young woman who needed complete and total nursing care. Mrs. C was off the respirator, and she was able to blink her eyelids. Otherwise she could move her limbs only with excruciating pain. Imagine the sensation one feels when one's leg has fallen asleep and one is trying to move it—that was only a fraction of what Mrs. C felt.

At first the nurses were awed and sympathetic. Mrs. C had survived. Now the staff's goal was to return her to her former role as a wife and mother. After several weeks, however, staff members became disillusioned. It seemed that Mrs. C did not always share the staff's grand design for her rehabilitation. She cried that getting out of bed was too painful. She couldn't possibly brush her own teeth. At times Mrs. C was too exhausted even to talk, and seemed scarcely better than she had been on admission.

The psychiatric nurse clinician began to meet with the staff to discuss Mrs. C's lack of progress. It was established that the nurses were anxious for her to improve because they wanted to deny the extreme severity of Mrs. C's illness. This woman had suffered a catastrophic event, and it reminded the nurses that sickness is often meaningless and uncontrollable. Staff members discussed their need to control her progress. In their heads, they had formulated a time chart on which to record Mrs. C's expected progress. It was very difficult to accept that the client didn't meet their expectations, because to them this meant that they were failures as nurses. It is interesting to observe that the nurses' need for control was actually aggravating the client's dependency. Mrs. C was to give up her dependency according to the nurses' schedule! This is like demanding that someone "be spontaneous!"

Another factor in this case was the prolonged period of immobility and complete helplessness that Mrs. C had experienced. Her regression had been severe, and she needed time to relearn how to function on her own. This was a fearful and bewildering period for Mrs. C and her family. For the first time, she contemplated how close she had come to death. Because Mrs. C had been mercifully unconscious for much of the time in the ICU, this period was analogous to a rebirth for her. Psychologically and physically she had to learn to live again.

Because the nurses were insightful and perceptive enough to recognize their part in the situation, and because Mrs. C had the desire to regain her former role, this case had a satisfactory ending. When the nurses were able to let go of their own objectives, Mrs. C gained the ability to progress at her own rate.

Other dependent clients are not as rewarding to work with as Mrs. C.

Mr. B was a middle-aged man on the neurosurgery service for evaluation of persistent back pain, a neurogenic bladder, and left-sided weakness. These disorders were the aftermath of numerous surgical procedures on Mr. B's back, gall bladder, stomach, rectum, prostate, and various other organs. He had acquired thick charts at all the major hospitals in the city.

He was a forlorn sight in his wheelchair, unshaven and wearing a ratty bathrobe. He was a most obliging examinee and would endlessly describe his medical history to anyone who would listen. Being sick had become Mr. B's permanent and only role. He had not worked for years and had no family except a brother with whom he lived. He had no friends and no outside interests. His obsession was his health—the present problem being to find the source of his back pain. Both the psychiatric service and the nurse clinician became involved with Mr. B. After studying the dynamics of Mr. B's behavior, they were confronted with the futility of using traditional psychotherapy in this case.

One meets many clients like Mr. B in all services of the general hospital. Although their symptoms may vary, the underlying dynamics are similar. These clients are extremely dependent and obsessed with their health. They perceive themselves as worthless, which accounts for their willingness to undergo painful procedures repeatedly. They are depressed. They feel both hopeless and worthless. At times, they are angry and suspicious and will call certain doctors "quacks," while at other times they perceive the doctors as all-knowing, magnanimous creatures. These clients receive little gratification from life except for the attention paid to them in hospitals and clinics. Their hostility is veiled by their helpless, passive appearance but is apparent in their resistance to becoming more independent. These clients essentially force people to take care of them.

A noncompliant client (one who will not be cured) can be viewed as seeking to retaliate against the "parent"-doctor. These clients wield a great deal of subtle power over physicians and nurses by setting up interactions in which the treatment always fails and the hospital staff can never do enough. Moreover, although the underlying dynamics make for interesting discussions of the clients' behavior, these clients seldom benefit from having the dynamics presented to them. These clients usually have little insight and can see no connection between their emotional state and their illness. Therefore, they are not motivated to seek psychiatric help. Psychotherapy that is initiated in the general hospital is supportive and probably does more to benefit the medical and nursing staffs.

One approach to the very dependent client is behavior modification. After a thorough assessment, the consultant and the nursing staff can design a behavior modification program. The consultant's main job will probably be to support the staff, who may become

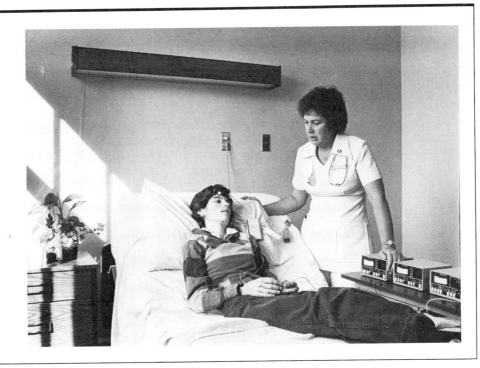

This liaison psychiatric nurse is caring directly for an anorexic woman who is hospitalized on a medical unit.

angry, frustrated, and depressed. Dependent clients are very draining, and the nurse gets little gratification from caring for them. The staff will need help in handling their feelings without letting them interfere with caring for the client. They will also need help in setting limits without being angry or punitive toward the client.

The two clients presented here represent the two ends of a spectrum. On one end is the client who makes a complete recovery after a devastating illness. On the other end is the client who seems to become progressively worse. The consultant is called on in extreme circumstances such as these, but consultants can also help by pointing out that all clients face, in some way, the issue of dependency.

The Client's Family

Hospital personnel speak of "the patient with breast cancer," as if that phrase defined the target of their treatment. It may be more appropriate and accurate to talk about "the family of the patient with breast cancer." This is because family members constitute a system, each part of which affects the functioning of all the other parts (see Chapter 21). Each family member fills a certain role, and if one member is hospitalized, that role is left vacant. The remaining members must make adjustments to compensate for the missing role. For instance, the father is usually the family breadwin-

ner. If he becomes ill and unable to work, the mother may have to support the family, and the children may have to give up their plans for college. If the mother's role is to nurture and give emotional guidance to her family, and she becomes ill, the family may feel abandoned, sensing that they have lost their support.

The illness of a family member constitutes a family crisis. It will be remembered that a crisis represents a turning point, the outcome of which can be adaptive or maladaptive depending on the contributing factors. The consultant is often called on when the nursing staff believe that the client's family are not making a positive contribution to their efforts to treat the client. That is what happened in the following case.

Mrs. W was recovering from a stroke that had left her aphasic and with right-sided weakness. Her treatment included physical therapy, speech therapy, and a weight-reducing, low-salt diet. The client, a widow, had been living alone at the time of the stroke. Luckily her daughter had found her collapsed on the kitchen floor and had brought her to the hospital.

Mrs. W's daughter and son visited her every night, bringing her presents of candy, fried chicken, and potato chips. They literally spoon-fed her and were horrified when the nurse suggested that Mrs. W show her family how she could feed herself. The nurses were angry, believing that the family were encouraging Mrs. W to remain dependent and spoiling her weight reduction regimen. The consultant was asked for suggestions on how to deal with them.

One evening during dinner, the consultant dropped in on Mrs. W and her family. She commented to the children that they showed great concern for their mother, and that it must sometimes be a strain to visit the hospital every night when they had families of their own. The son nodded agreement, but the daughter's eyes filled with tears and she asked to talk to the clinician alone. She began to tell her how guilty she felt about her mother's stroke. She had not visited Mrs. W for several weeks prior to the accident, saying she was too busy. When she finally had visited, it was to find Mrs. W unconscious. If only she'd been a better daughter! Now the barrage of food and attention became understandable. Mrs. W's children needed to assuage their guilt over what they believed to be neglect of their mother. The consultant made it clear that the staff did not view them as neglectful and indeed needed their help in rehabilitating Mrs. W. Plans were made to incorporate them into the client's care.

Another situation frequently encountered is that of the angry, demanding family. They complain about the nursing care, ask to talk to the supervisor, and may even ask to see the hospital administrator. This behavior is one way a family can cope with their rage and impotence. It is not acceptable to express anger toward the ill family member, although many spouses do experience anger. A wife is angered and frightened by her heavy new responsibilities and by the possibility of her husband's death. She cannot express this anger to her husband. Nor can she direct it toward the doctors, who seem to have the power of life and death. Often she takes her feelings out on the nurse, who is less threatening and more accessible. A husband whose wife is ill is also angry and frightened and feeling particularly left out in caring for his wife. He may overcompensate by keeping a close watch on the care the nurses are giving.

Clinicians can provide this kind of family with a safe place to express their anger, fear, and frustration. They can let these families know that their feelings are not unusual and that the clinician doesn't find them selfish or insensitive. The staff can also be helped to understand the meaning of the family's behavior. This often leads to a decrease in hostility and allows everyone to spend more energy on adaptive methods of coping.

The nursing staff are often instrumental in helping the family cope successfully.

Ella came in four times a week to visit her mother, Mrs. R. This client was eighty-seven and had suffered a severe stroke three months ago. She had been hospitalized all that time, awaiting placement in a nursing home. Ella was upset that she couldn't take her mother home, but she had a full-time job and realized that she couldn't give her mother the proper care. Mrs. R was fully bathed every morning by the nursing staff. Nevertheless, Ella always gave her mother a complete bath on each visit, checking her carefully for any sign of bedsores and finishing off with a cloud of dusting powder. Often one of the nurses would assist Ella with the second bath. The staff did not consider this a comment on their ability to give adequate care. Instead, they recognized the pleasure Ella received in caring for her mother. Mrs. R was eventually discharged to a nursing home.

Several months later the staff learned that Ella was a client on the psychiatric unit. Mrs. R had died, and Ella had reacted with a psychotic episode. One of the nurses went to visit Ella on the psychiatric ward. Ella immediately recognized her and embraced her warmly. Excitedly, she began to ask the nurse, "Didn't I take good care of my mother? She never had a sore on her body when she was here!" Then she told how the nursing home staff had refused to let her bathe her mother, and how one day she had discovered an ugly bedsore on Mrs. R's hip. Shortly thereafter, Mrs. R had died.

This example illustrates the powerful bonds that exist between family members. These bonds are strained when one member becomes seriously ill. Nurses can help maintain the integrity of the family unit, thus providing the client with this very crucial element of support.

The Client in the Intensive Care Unit

Throughout this chapter we have emphasized the importance of recognizing that the hospitalized client is under stress, and that this stress is both physiological and psychological in nature. Because the stress is multidetermined, we have stated that meeting the client's physical needs alone will not restore the client's equilibrium. In an intensive care unit—that is, in any specialized acute care area such as cardiac care or respiratory care—the stress is magnified many times because the client's life is acutely threatened. All efforts are directed toward keeping the client's body functioning, a task that involves using sophisticated machinery and highly trained personnel. It is understandable that amid these valiant efforts, the client's psychological state may well be overlooked. However, now that the intensive care unit is no longer a novelty, more attention is being paid to making it a more humane place for clients, their families, and the staff.

Clients in these units commonly develop an *ICU Psychosis*, or *Intensive Care Syndrome*. This diagnosis is not exact and may refer to any combination of the following: depression, withdrawal, anxiety, hallucinations, delusions, paranoia, and delirium. A typical case is described below.

Mr. W, a fifty-five-year-old man, was admitted with a possible myocardial infarction. After forty-eight hours in the unit, he began to call for the nurses constantly. He would clutch their hands and plead with them to stay at his bedside. He would cry when the technicians came to draw blood, or when he received injections. Mrs. W reported that her husband could not keep track of her visits and was very much afraid that he would be left in the hospital all alone. This behavior lasted twenty-four hours. At that point Mr. W was transferred out of the unit onto a general medical floor. His progress thereafter was uneventful, and there was no recurrence of any confused behavior.

The stresses on such a client can be divided into three categories: environmental, psychological, and physiological. The following list includes some stressors that belong in each category.

1. Environmental stressors
   a. Sensory overload from constant noise, lights, unfamiliar treatments
   b. Sensory deprivation from immobility, restraints, bandages
   c. Lack of familiar orienting cues such as clocks, calendars, windows, meals, radio, television
   d. Close proximity to other clients who are also very ill
   e. Constant attendance by physicians, nurses, and technicians
   f. Lack of personal belongings
2. Psychological stressors
   a. Fear of mutilation or death
   b. Little or no understanding of medical jargon or procedures
   c. Separation from family and friends
   d. Separation from familiar environment
   e. Depersonalization and physical exposure
   f. Powerlessness
   g. Pain
   h. Inability to release tension in accustomed fashion
3. Physiological stressors
   a. Metabolic changes
   b. Decreased cardiac output
   c. Neurologic status
   d. Fever
   e. Electrolyte imbalance
   f. Drugs
   g. Pain
   h. Length of time spent on pump or under anesthesia
   i. Sleep deprivation

All clients in acute care areas experience some of these stressors. What can be done to reduce the occurrence of an ICU psychosis? Obviously, the stressors themselves should be eliminated, if possible. Many intensive care units are now being remodeled to create a less frightening environment for the patient. When structural alterations are not feasible, other innovations can be made, such as adding color and pictures, arranging beds for maximum privacy, and turning lights down at night. In essence, any manipulation of the environment that will reduce stress and increase positive meaningful sensory input is helpful.

Clients and their families should be adequately prepared if circumstances permit. Clients who know what they can expect are much less frightened by the strangeness of the unit. Ideally, clients should meet some of the staff who will be caring for them. A familiar face is a welcome sight to someone who is recovering from anesthesia or waking from a fitful sleep.

Clients should be provided with consistent nursing personnel. This will diminish the process of depersonalization and isolation that always occurs to some degree in an intensive care unit. Family members can be encouraged to visit as the situation permits. An often overlooked feature is a room where family members can spend their many hours of waiting.

There is one other way to reduce client stress in the acute care areas. This is to attend to the frustrations and needs of the staff. Work in a high-pressure unit affects staff dramatically, causing a high turnover rate and sometimes intrastaff conflict. The nursing staff should identify ways in which they can support one another. This may range from weekly meetings with the psychiatric nursing consultant to regular intrastaff volleyball games. It is crucial that the staff have some means of dealing with the enormous pressures they face. Perhaps this is where the consultant can be most helpful—as a vital link in the chain of support.

The Client Who Is Sexually Acting Out

Sexual acting out is psychiatric jargon for sexual behavior sometimes seen in the general hospital. For example, male or female clients may make flirtatious comments, attempt to touch or hold a male or female nurse, boast about sexual experiences, or deliberately expose their genitals while bathing or changing. One sees a wide range of reactions toward this kind of behavior from the staff. Some nurses react by chastising clients verbally and then shunning them or reporting them to a supervisor or doctor. Other nurses simply ignore it, or do not notice it, or do not consider this kind of behavior important enough to comment on. Part of the reason for these varied responses to sexual behavior lies in the differences among clients and the perceptions and values of staff members. A young, attractive man who flirts with the female nurses may be acceptable, while a paunchy middle-aged man who exhibits the same behavior may be labeled a sex maniac. If a young woman client wears makeup and sexy nightgowns, she is criticized, while an elderly woman who habitually exposes herself is virtually ignored.

Another reason for staff members' varied responses is that regressive behavior in the hospital is expected and even encouraged. *Regression* means that the client role includes, among other things, loss of identity, especially one's sexual identity. Clients are dressed in flimsy hospital gowns, they are left lying naked under the sheets on a stretcher, and they are examined without much attention to discretion or modesty. Because the system encourages sexual regression, a client's acting out may not be seen as anything unusual.

A third factor to consider is the attitude of the individual nurse about his or her own sexuality (see Chapter 12). These personal values will determine how nurses view the client's behavior and how they will choose to interact with the sexually acting-out client. The following case history illustrates many of these factors.

Mr. H was a nineteen-year-old male who had been admitted for a crush injury of the right hand. He was a frequent drug abuser, lived in a slum area, and was unemployed. From the beginning, he was not a popular client. He complained constantly of pain and demanded narcotics by name and dosage. No amount of medication seemed to hold him for very long, and he began threatening to call his friends and have them bring in the drugs he needed. Indeed, some shady-looking visitors were often seen in Mr. H's room. This unpleasant situation reached crisis proportions when Mr. H hung a pornographic poster in his room. At this point the staff called the psychiatric nursing consultant, and a staff conference was arranged.

Everyone was noticeably unnerved by the situation and needed to verbalize individual reactions to seeing the poster. One nurse had demanded that he take it down immediately. This confrontation had ended in a heated argument between the nurse and the client, and the poster was back on the wall the next day. Another nurse had quickly averted her eyes and pretended not to have noticed it. Thereafter, she avoided entering his room. A third nurse, alone on the night shift, became very frightened when Mr. H asked to have his back rubbed. She spent a very uncomfortable eight-hour shift, feeling both afraid and guilty. The consultant accepted and understood all these reactions. However, none of them had proved a useful intervention.

The consultant now explored with the group some of the possible dynamics behind Mr. H's behavior. Mr. H was only nineteen, an age when one's sexuality is extremely important. But both his injury and the hospitalization were threats to his image of himself as an active sexual male. The clinician discussed several issues. She explained the depersonalization and desexualization of a hospitalized client. Added to this, she pointed out, is the powerlessness and dependence of the client role. Many clients, especially unpopular ones, also experience emotional and touch deprivation. Another important concept in understanding Mr. H was the insult to his body image. What was his perception of himself without the use of his right hand? Also, what sexual significance did his right hand have for him?

The staff responded readily to these ideas. They began to see Mr. H as someone who was trying to maintain some control and self-esteem in a situation that was very threatening to him. It was decided that the staff would talk to him on a one-to-one basis and state their true reactions to his poster: "Mr. H, I feel very uncomfortable being in your room since you hung that poster. I would appreciate it if you'd keep it in a more private place." Mr. H soon complied, and overall relationships improved rapidly as other suggestions were made. These included allowing Mr. H time to be alone with his girl friend; being more aware of his need for privacy; and giving him more control over his daily activities.

These new policies resulted in more open communication with the client in other areas as well. The nurses explained to Mr. H that they wanted to keep him pain-free, but that it was impossible to assess the effects of analgesics when he was suspected of taking drugs on his own. This medication issue remained a problem, but the nurses felt much less judgmental and were better able to tolerate Mr. H's behavior. This interaction with the consultant allowed the staff to explore some of their own values about sexuality. It also showed them how these values affected their ability to give optimal client care.

The following case example illustrates some further issues in dealing with the sexual concerns of clients.

Mr. M, a sixty-eight-year-old man, had been on the unit for four weeks. During this time he had received cancer chemotherapy, and he was now in a state of remission. The psychiatric nursing clinical specialist had not been consulted for this particular client, but while she was spending time on the unit, she noted some unusual behavior. Mr. M would pinch the nurses whenever they got near enough. They would respond by making a disapproving face that Mr. M couldn't see, or by completely ignoring him. He also made suggestive remarks which the staff also ignored. On one occasion, Mr. M approached the consultant, saying he wanted to kiss her for "good luck." The consultant thought it important to understand the meaning of his behavior. Reading his chart, she learned that he had been impotent for the last six months.

Because the consultant already had a good working relationship with the staff, she approached them with the data she had gathered, instead of waiting for them to consult her. A staff conference was held. At this conference the nurses discussed why they had not taken direct measures to deal with Mr. M's behavior. An important point was that the staff consisted mostly of newly graduated female nurses. Several nurses said they thought they were the only ones that Mr. M was bothering and felt that they personally had done something to provoke him. Others said they were afraid

that the doctors or nursing supervisors would laugh if they voiced their concerns. Another issue was documentation—they were uncertain whether such behavior should be noted in the client's chart. Was this information important? Would it be harmful to the client to document his behavior?

It became clear that the nurses were missing the meaning of Mr. M's behavior because they became uncertain and embarrassed when the behavior was overtly sexual. Looking further, they could see the behavior as a defense against the actual impotence Mr. M was experiencing. The consultant developed a therapeutic relationship with Mr. M, who subsequently ceased his sexual acting out but became depressed instead. He and the consultant began working their way through the natural grieving process he had to undergo in relation to having cancer.

As this example illustrates, it is important for nurses to understand that all client behavior has meaning. It also points again to the all-important task of exploring your own sexuality in order to understand the sexual behavior that clients present during hospitalization. Human sexuality is presented as a crucial component of self-actualization and self-expression in Chapter 12. Chapter 12 also includes guidelines for assessing the nurse's personal attitudes toward sex.

The Noncompliant Client

The noncompliant client is both poorly understood and poorly tolerated (see Chapter 23). Many people fall under this label: the man with a recent myocardial infarction who refuses to stay in bed; the new diabetic who won't test his urine; the hypertensive who forgets to take her medicine. These clients may verbally state their understanding of the prescribed regimen, but their behavior indicates an underlying problem. Research with outpatients indicates that at least one third of those studied did not follow their prescribed regimen (Gillum and Barsky 1974). Noncompliance is also common among inpatients, causing frustration for the nurse whose task it is to promote the highest possible level of client learning and functioning.

Mrs. Schwartz is a fifty-four-year-old woman who has been diabetic since age thirty. She is divorced, has no children, and lives alone in a small apartment. She works as a cashier in a parking lot. Over the years, she has controlled her diabetes with diet and later with insulin.

Recently she injured her left foot, but did not seek treatment for several weeks until her foot became black and swollen. Now she is hospitalized for a below-the-knee amputation of her left leg. Mrs. Schwartz is very aggressive and controlling. Because she has been diabetic for so long, she views herself as an expert, and taunts the younger nurses about their ignorance on the subject of diabetic teaching. Mrs. Schwartz does not comply with the hospital routine; instead she follows her own regimen of self-care which is not sound in principle.

There is always a reason for noncompliance, although neither the nurse nor the client may initially understand the dynamics involved. Many nurses respond to such clients with anger and impatience, which serves only to increase the distance between client and nurse. It is admittedly very difficult to watch self-destructive behavior that thwarts what we believe to be the correct therapeutic route. The nurse can reach an understanding of the client's behavior only through careful thought and observation.

In general, the factors that contribute to noncompliance can be summarized as follows (Gillum and Barsky 1974, Strauss 1975):

- *Psychological*—lack of knowledge; clients' attitudes, beliefs, and values; denial of illness and other defense mechanisms; personality type (rigid, defensive, etc.); very low or very high anxiety levels
- *Environmental and social*—lack of support system; other problems that distract from health care; finances, transportation, and housing
- *Characteristics of the regimen*—demands too much change from client; not enough benefit realized; too difficult, complicated; distressing side effects; leads to social isolation and stigma
- *Properties of the provider-client relationship*—faulty communication; client perceives provider as cold, uncaring, authoritative; client feels discounted and treated like an "object"; both parties engage in struggle for control

The example of Mrs. Schwartz illustrates many of the above factors. Her psychological profile includes long-standing rigidity. She is extremely independent and strong-willed. Presently, she has the added need for control to compensate for the loss of her leg. This client should not be expected to accept a new regimen from an unfamiliar hospital staff. The fact that Mrs.

Schwartz lives alone and has no family will contribute to her difficulty in learning new behaviors because she will have no one to *reinforce* her new behaviors. Also important is the nature of the regimen itself. If Mrs. Schwartz follows the regimen set out for her, will she see results quickly, and will those results be worth the effort of following the plan?

In addition, the nurse must examine the nature of the relationship with the client. Research points out that clients respond negatively to nurses and doctors who are cold, disapproving, rigid, and controlling. Mrs. Schwartz could easily engage with such a nurse in a battle for control. An added detriment would be a frequent turnover of nurses, none of whom feel responsible for the client, and hence do not form a stable relationship with her.

Contracting as an Approach to Noncompliance   The "contract" approach can deal with noncompliance as well as prevent its occurrence. A contrast is a mutual verbal or written agreement between client and nurse about their expectations of each other (see Chapter 7). It makes clear that they are equal partners with certain responsibilities toward established common goals. The contract makes expectations, goals, and responsibilities explicit (Zangari and Duffy 1980).

This approach can prevent noncompliance because it reduces faulty communication. The process of setting goals and assigning responsibility forces both nurse and client to make a clear commitment to each other. Contracting can also reduce control conflicts since the nurse who understands the concept fully will implement it with respect for the client as an equal participant in the health regimen. Zangari and Duffy (1980) explain how a nurse can use this concept with hospitalized clients. They present the theoretical basis for contracting, along with examples of how it can be accomplished.

Mrs. Schwartz's noncompliance can be dealt with through contracting. One nurse could be assigned to her for the duration of her hospitalization. This would foster mutual communication, commitment, and understanding. Nurse and client would explore the *client's* goals, which would undoubtedly include prevention of further complications. They could establish what steps to take to meet the goals.

As the steps are discussed, the nurse should acknowledge Mrs. Schwartz's self-care activities and ask her to review the basics of a diabetic regimen. Since the client's goal is to reduce complications, she should agree to review this material with the nurse. Mrs. Schwartz will probably respond to being treated like an individual, not like another client who "needs diabetic teaching." Ideally, in this atmosphere of mutual respect, the client can relearn some important principles without having to admit that she has been amiss in her own routine.

Even when the nurse understands the dynamics leading to noncompliance and takes measures to prevent it, the client may not always respond to her efforts. Then the nurse must deal with her own feelings of frustration. Resolution of this frustration will come only when the nurse accepts that clients are ultimately responsible for their own actions (see Chapter 5).

The Dying Client

Discussion of the dying client is presented last because all the behaviors previously described can be seen at various stages in the dying process. Kübler-Ross (1969) describes the five stages of dying: denial and isolation; anger; bargaining; depression; and acceptance. Her teaching has been invaluable, but some professionals have tended to use these stages as a shorthand method of working with dying people. They think that as long as they can recognize which stage the person is in, they have counseled the dying client.

In nursing education, continuing education courses, and various workshops, death and dying has become a popular topic. Everywhere we hear that we must "confront our own feelings about death" before we will be able to help the client. It is very difficult to find out exactly what that phrase means, or how to go about doing it.

The psychiatric clinical specialist deals with these issues at a grassroots level. The staff want to know what to say, how to act, what to expect. They will tell the consultant, "I like that client too much to be able to talk to her about dying, so every time she brings it up I just leave the room." The consultant's role is not to do the actual work with the dying client, but to support the nursing staff as they care for their dying clients.

Staff nurses often do not believe in their own ability to meet their clients' needs. But there are professionals outside nursing who see the nurse as an important source of strength. For example, Jourard says: "One

of the events which we believe inspires faith and hope in a client is the conviction that somebody cares about him. If this proves true, it implies that the quality of the nurse–client relationship is a factor in the client's recovery. Direct contact with a client somehow increases his sense of being a worthwhile individual person, and this experience inspires him" (Jourard 1971, p. 206). No consultant can take the place of the nurse who actually bathes a client's back or is there in the middle of the night with a glass of warm milk. The consultant's message to the nursing staff is: "Your relationship with your client is a powerful source of strength. I will help you learn how to use that strength when your client needs it."

The consultant will see parallel processes at work in clients, their families, and the nursing staff. Just as clients have varying reactions to dying, so nurses may completely withdraw from or become overidentified with a client. Nurses also experience stages of bereavement (see Chapter 11), especially when they have formed close relationships with clients. They will see these clients as family members and actually grieve along with them and their families. Could this be what is meant by "confronting our own feelings about death?" It seems that the only way to do this is to *share* the experience of a dying person—to participate in another's death.

Avery Weisman uses a beautiful phrase to describe this sharing. He calls it "safe conduct" (Weisman 1975, p. 241). Dying people say that one of their greatest fears is the fear of being left alone, and that just the presence of another human being is very comforting. How do we ensure our clients safe conduct? It is a simple and a difficult task. We spend time with them, we listen to them, we touch them, we accept whatever feelings they express, be they anger, hopelessness, denial, or fear. We assure them that they will not be alone when they die.

Yet we cannot possibly become so involved with all our clients. In fact, we may need to withdraw periodically to replenish our own resources. The key to being with dying clients is acceptance, and nurses who are able to accept that they cannot be all things to all people will be able to give fully of themselves when they are able. Consultation can be conceptualized as a chain of support that allows the nurse to participate in the part of life that includes a client's death.

KEY NURSING CONCEPTS

✔ Theories of humanism, holistic health, crisis, and preventive psychiatry all serve as a base for nursing practice in the general hospital setting.

✔ Psychiatric nurse consultants are useful in general hospital settings because all illnesses have emotional components. Hospitalization constitutes a crisis for the client, and complications can be minimized when attention is paid to the client's psychological state.

✔ The multicausational concept purports that individuals in similar social situations define those situations differently and therefore respond with different reactions.

✔ The hospitalized client is under both physiological and psychological stress. Because stress is multidetermined, meeting the client's physical needs alone will not suffice to restore equilibrium.

✔ The psychiatric nursing consultant may provide client-centered case consultation, program-centered administrative consultation, consultee-centered case consultation, and consultee-centered administrative consultation.

✔ In client-centered case consultation, the client's problems are the immediate focus.

✔ In program-centered administrative consultation, the consultant is asked to help develop or improve a specific program.

✔ In consultee-centered case consultation the focus is on the consultee nurse rather than any particular client.

✔ Consultee-centered administrative consultation refers to helping nurses with problems that involve administration or organizational structure.

✔ The psychiatric nurse consultant working in the general hospital should be prepared at the graduate level, have a solid theoretical and experiential base, and be able to interact effectively with clients, their families, and colleagues.

✔ Building egalitarian relationships, paying attention to key people, setting up ground rules, and negotiating the consultation contract are essential elements in the consultative process.

✔ In the general hospital setting the psychiatric nurse consultant may work with staff members, because they are subject to the same stresses that affect the client. Consultation with staff members can be thought of as a means of preventing future client crises.

✔ Important functions of the nurse consultant are to tap the staff's potential, cultivate their interpersonal skills, render the total care plan effective, and provide support when the staff is in crisis.

✔ In the general hospital the psychiatric nurse consultant is alert to potential problems that accompany any physical illness and practices primary, secondary, and tertiary prevention.

✔ Ideally, the consultants' authority stems from their special knowledge and skills rather than from formal authority in the organizational structure. The nurse who requests consultation and the nurse who provides it are on a peer level.

✔ In order to build helpful relationships the nurse consultant will pay attention to key people and set up ground rules for consultation.

✔ The contract for consultation should clearly define the expectations of all parties involved.

References

Aguilera, D., and Messick, J. *Crisis Intervention.* 3d ed. St. Louis: C. V. Mosby, 1978.

Alexander, F. *Psychosomatic Medicine: Its Principles and Applications.* New York: W. W. Norton, 1950.

Caplan, G. *Principles of Preventive Psychiatry.* New York: Basic Books, 1964.

————. *Theory and Practice of Mental Health Consultation.* New York: Basic Books, 1970.

Gillum, R., and Barsky, A. "Diagnosis and Management of Patient Noncompliance." *Journal American Medical Association* 228 (1974): 1563–1567.

Holmes, T. H., and Rahe, R. H. "The Social Readjustment Scale." *Journal of Psychosomatic Research* 11 (1967): 213–218.

Jourard, S. *The Transparent Self.* New York: D. Van Nostrand, 1971.

Kübler-Ross, E. *On Death and Dying.* New York: Macmillan, 1969.

Lacey, J. I.; Bateman, D. E.; and Van Lehn, R. "Autonomic Response Specificity." *Psychosomatic Medicine* 15 (1953): 8.

Mahl, G. F. "Physiological Changes During Chronic Fear." *Annals of New York Academy of Science* 56 (1953): 240.

Mutter, A. Z., and Schleifer, M. "The Role of Psychological and Social Factors in the Onset of Somatic Illness in Children." *Psychosomatic Medicine* 28 (1966): 333–343.

Nelson, J., and Schilke, D. "The Evolution of Psychiatric Liaison Nursing." *Perspectives in Psychiatric Care* 14 (1976): 61–65.

Parsons, T. *The Social System.* New York: Free Press, 1951.

Rahe, R., and Arthur, R. "Life Change and Illness Studies: Past History and Future Directions." *Journal of Human Stress* 4 (March 1978): 3–15.

Sacher, E. J. "Current Status of Psychosomatic Medicine." In *Psychologic Care of the Medically Ill,* edited by J. Strain and S. Grossman, pp. 54–56. New York: Appleton-Century-Crofts, 1975.

Selye, H. *The Physiology and Pathology of Exposure to Stress.* Montreal: Acta Publishers, 1950.

Simonton, O., and Simonton, S. "Psychological Intervention in the Treatment of Cancer." *Psychosomatics* 21 (1980): 226–233.

Strauss, A. *Chronic Illness and the Quality of Life.* Saint Louis: C. V. Mosby, 1975.

Weisman, A. "The Dying Patient." In *Consultation-Liaison Psychiatry,* edited by R. Pasnau, pp. 237–244. New York: Grune and Stratton, 1975.

Zangari, M., and Duffy, P. "Contracting with Patients in Day to Day Practice." *American Journal of Nursing* (March 1980): 451–455.

Further Reading

Ballentine, R. *Diet and Nutrition: A Holistic Approach.* Honesdale, Pa.: Himalayan International Institute, 1978.

Carlson, C. E., and Blackwell, B. *Behavioral Concepts and Nursing Intervention.* Philadelphia: J. B. Lippincott, 1978.

Cheraskin, E., and Ringsdorf, W. *Psychodietetics.* New York: Bantam Books, 1974.

Chinn, P., ed. "Holistic Health." *Advances in Nursing Science* 2 (1980).

Cousins, N. *Anatomy of an Illness as Perceived by the Patient: Reflections on Healing and Regeneration.* New York: W. W. Norton, 1979.

Donavan, M. "Relaxation with Guided Imagery: A Useful Technique." *Cancer Nursing* 3 (February 1980): 27–32.

Fagerhaugh, S., and Strauss, A. *Politics of Pain Management: Staff-Patient Interaction.* Menlo Park, Calif.: Addison-Wesley, 1977.

Ferguson, M. *The Aquarian Conspiracy: Personal and Social Transformation in the 1980's.* Los Angeles: J. P. Tarcher, 1980.

Flynn, P. *Holistic Health: The Art and Science of Care.* Bowie, Md.: Robert Brady, 1980.

Fordyce, W. E. *Behavioral Methods for Chronic Pain and Illness.* St. Louis: C.V. Mosby, 1976.

Groves, J. "Taking Care of the Hateful Patient." *New England Journal of Medicine* 298 (1978): 883–887.

Hackett, T., and Cassem, N., eds. *Handbook of General Hospital Psychiatry.* St. Louis: C. V. Mosby, 1978.

Hackett, T.; Cassem, N. H.; and Wishnie, H. "The Coronary Care Unit, an Appraisal of Its Psychologic Hazards." *New England Journal of Medicine* 25 (1969): 1365–1370.

Hoff, L. *People in Crisis.* Menlo Park, Calif.: Addison-Wesley, 1978.

Jacobsen, E. *Anxiety and Tension Control.* Philadelphia: J. B. Lippincott, 1964.

Janken, J. "The Nurse in Crisis." *Nursing Clinics of North America,* March 1974, pp. 17–26.

Krieger, D. *Foundations for Holistic Health Nursing Practices.* Philadelphia: Lippincott, 1981.

Kuenzi, S. H., and Fenton, M. "Crisis Intervention in Acute Care Areas." *American Journal of Nursing* 75 (1975): 830–834.

Lambert, V., and Lambert, C. *The Impact of Physical Illness and Related Mental Health Concepts.* Englewood Cliffs, N.J.: Prentice-Hall, 1979.

Lipowski, Z. J. "Consultation Liaison Psychiatry: An Overview." *American Journal of Psychiatry* 31 (1974): 623–630.

Livsey, C. "Physical Illness and Family Dynamics." *Advances in Psychosomatic Medicine* 8 (1972): 237–251.

Mannino, F.; MacLennan, B.; and Shore, M. *The Practice of Mental Health Consultation.* DHEW Publication no. (ADM) 74–112. Washington D.C.: Government Printing Office, 1975.

Moos, R., ed. *Coping with Physical Illness.* New York: Plenum, 1971.

Murray, R. "Assessment of Psychologic Status in the Surgical ICU Patient." *Nursing Clinics of North America,* March 1975, pp. 69–81.

Pasnau, R., ed. *Consultation-Liaison Psychiatry.* New York: Grune and Stratton, 1975.

Pelletier, K. *Mind as Healer, Mind as Slayer.* New York: Dell Publishing, 1977.

————. *Holistic Medicine, from Stress to Optimum Health.* New York: Delacorte Press, 1979.

Peplau, H. "Psychiatric Nursing Skills and the General Hospital Patient." *Nursing Forum* 3 (1964): 28–37.

Perry, S., and Heidrich, G. "Placebo Response: Myth and Matter." *American Journal of Nursing* 81 (April 1981): 720–725.

Roberts, S. *Behavioral Concepts and the Critically Ill Patient.* Englewood Cliffs, N.J.: Prentice-Hall, 1976.

Robinson, L. *Liaison Nursing, Psychological Approach to Patient Care.* Philadelphia: F. A. Davis, 1974.

————. *Psychological Aspects of the Care of Hospitalized Patients.* Philadelphia: F. A. Davis, 1976.

Ryan, R. S., and Travis, J. W. *Wellness Workbook.* Berkeley, Calif.: Ten Speed Press, 1981.

Sandroff, R. "The Potent Placebo." *RN* 43 (April 1980): 35–96.

Schwartzman, S. "Anxiety and Depression in the Stroke Patient: A Nursing Challenge." *Journal of Psychiatric Nursing and Mental Health Services,* July 1976, pp. 13–17.

Simon, N., ed. *The Psychological Aspects of Intensive Care Unit Nursing.* Bowie, Md.: R. J. Brady, 1980.

Simonton, O., and Simonton, S. *Getting Well Again.* Los Angeles: J. P. Tarcher, 1979.

Totman, R. *Social Causes of Illness.* New York: Pantheon Books, 1979.

Williams, F. "The Crisis of Hospitalization." *Nursing Clinics of North America,* March 1974, pp. 37–45.

Zind, R. "Deterrents to Crisis Intervention in the Hospital Unit." *Nursing Clinics of North America,* March 1974, pp. 27–36.

25

Alternative Healing Therapies

by Joan Sayre

CHAPTER OUTLINE

Historical Roots of the Movement
    Cultural Change
    Humanistic and Existential Influences
    Psychotherapies as Social Indices
    Expanded Definitions of Psychiatric Treatment
Basic Premises of the New Therapies
    The Discovery of the Real Self
    Body–Mind Integration
    Self-regulation and Responsibility
Representative Alternative Healing Therapies
    Body Discipline and Body–Mind Awareness
    Therapies
    Psychological Growth Therapies
    Consciousness Development Therapies
Comparative Analysis
    General Themes
    The Therapeutic Problem
Relevance for Psychiatric Nursing
    The Shift from the Medical Model to a Social
    Model
    Frameworks for Assessing the New Therapies

Applying the New Therapies to Psychiatric
Nursing Practice
Key Nursing Concepts

LEARNING OBJECTIVES

After reading this chapter, students should be able to

- Identify the historical roots of the alternative therapies movement
- Discuss three basic themes of the new therapies
- Enumerate the therapeutic goals of representative alternative therapies
- Differentiate among the techniques of the alternative therapies
- Identify the risks faced by clients of the new therapies
- Analyze the new therapies in terms of their significance for clinical practice as well as for their effects on clients
- Discuss the movement from conventional medicine to holistic health as it parallels the change in nursing's approach to health problems based on a social model of emotional health

CHAPTER 25

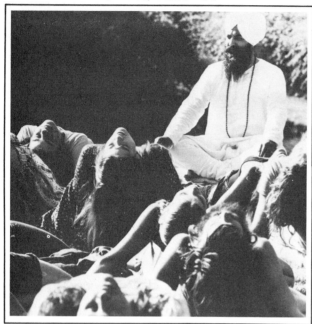

Traditional theory and practice in psychiatry are currently being challenged by concepts from other disciplines. These include sociology, religion, and philosophy. Critics claim that current practice is culture bound, limited to a medical, disease-oriented model, and lacking in historical or sociological perspective. Although psychiatric practice is changing as a result of these new perspectives, some critics feel that psychiatry is now a hopelessly anachronistic institution—one that actually oppresses people rather than treating them. These critics believe that a complete change in psychiatric practice is required in order for people to understand and deal with contemporary emotional difficulties.

The proliferation of naturalistic healing approaches reflects the belief that traditional psychiatry has little to offer modern humanity. These new therapies challenge traditional conceptions of the nature of human beings and their problems. Their originators claim that a new kind of therapy is required in postindustrial society. Decades of organized technology, labor, and mass advertising have deprived people of their freedom and creativity. Forced to conform to an increasingly complex and utilitarian society, people have lost their ability to experience the world for themselves. They have also become alienated from their natural bodily feelings as a result of the cultural overemphasis on intel-

lectual functioning. Average people use only a fraction of their capacity for creativity, emotionality, and experience. Today's materialistic culture has become a giant machine that exploits the ordinary person for the profit of the powerful few.

The new therapists of the holistic health movement reject psychiatry. In a deeper sense, they reject Western culture as well. Their goal is not merely to develop alternative therapies, but in many cases to eventually alter the very basis of the culture. They believe that only a complete change in the ways people view life will enable humanity to regain contact with itself and the fundamental energy of the cosmos. They teach people to overcome alienation by teaching them to purge themselves of destructive past influences caused by oversocialization.

HISTORICAL ROOTS OF THE MOVEMENT

Cultural Change

The alternative therapies movement developed along with the other important cultural changes of the sixties and seventies and continues to develop in the eighties. Some psychologists and psychiatrists began to criticize the medical model when they became aware that what is considered abnormal behavior is part of and reflects the specific culture (see Chapter 26). They gradually turned from examining the individual psyche to examining the environment with which the person interacted. They began to ask what behaviors were considered deviant, and how a person becomes known as abnormal. This sociological and political view of abnormal behavior was reinforced by the social concerns of the 1960s. Protests against oppression of minority groups, reaction against the Vietnam War, and struggle against an engulfing technology all dramatized the need to equalize power relationships in the society and to find alternative ways of solving human problems.

Gradual social change also resulted in the collapse of traditional American life-styles. Increase in production and expenditures raised the standard of living for wider segments of the middle class. More people had more opportunity to enjoy a materially satisfying, consumption-oriented life. Certain more fortunate citizens in the professional and white-collar classes had more leisure. But coupled with the advantages of a highly organized society were the disadvantages of the centralized bureaucratic structures necessary to administer that society. New industries of recreation, cultural activities, and mass communication standardized private life as well. Life became more meaningless as middle-class people lost the sense of being able to define their own goals. The decline in the authority of religious and educational institutions, which have traditionally provided meaning for the individual, compounded this dilemma.

One method of dealing with lack of meaning has been to engage in psychological explorations. The proliferation of workshops devoted to expanding the psyche and increasing sensory awareness is a reflection of this search for meaning. For most people with the psychological and financial resources, therapy and the search for self-knowledge have become ways of filling their leisure time and structuring their lives.

Humanistic and Existential Influences

Phenomenology and existentialism, with their emphasis on personal uniqueness and on the freedom to forge values, also influenced the rise of the alternative therapies movement. Humanistic and existential models emphasize the individual's capacity for full functioning as a human being. These models view illness as a failure to actualize the individual's tremendous potential. The purpose of therapy is not simply to treat disease, but to make personal growth possible. These models focus attention on improving the health of essentially well-adjusted people. Thus the basic problems psychiatry deals with have changed. The individual is no longer seen in isolation but as part of a complicated social network. Many problems believed to be individual in origin are now seen as social problems.

The medical model generally locates the cause of emotional problems within the individual's experience, while the social-political view focuses on the person's role in a historical and social context. An example of the difference between a medical orientation to a problem and a social and political one can be found in vary-

ing reactions to battered wives, wives who are assaulted and injured by their husbands.

The wife of a successful lawyer found that as her husband's work grew more demanding, he became more irritable. She was the outlet for his sense of frustration at work—after a difficult day in court, he would beat her. After numerous and progressively more violent encounters, she decided to consult a psychiatrist. He explained her situation on the basis of "female masochism" and urged her to explore her unconscious provocation of her husband, which he saw as the cause of the beatings. In the psychiatrist's view she needed to be punished and to submit to a male figure. A social-political viewpoint of the same situation would focus on women's basic oppression in society. It would explain a woman's powerlessness as arising from the fact that all conceptions of women and "women's nature" have been products of the dominant male frame of reference. Wife beating is a concrete expression of the prevailing myth of female inferiority. Men justify such assaults on the basis of a presumed need to discipline and guide women, since women want to be mastered. Women also accept the myth that women deserve to be, or even need to be, beaten, and that men have the right to beat them.

Psychotherapies as Social Indices

Perry London (1974) points out that in a sense psychotherapies are social indices, because psychology must treat the neuroses of the time. Changing fashions in psychotherapy reflect changing norms within the society. London outlines a theory of the social development of psychotherapy that explains the changes that have taken place in the practice of psychiatry. Psychoanalysis in the late nineteenth century was practiced in a dyadic model, as an interaction exclusively between the therapist and the client. Its purpose was to uncover symptoms that produced repression in the individual, a method appropriate to a moralistic Victorian society. Gradually, symptoms caused by repressed emotional conflicts were considered to be less of a problem.

By the period 1950–70, anxiety had become the important neurotic symptom. In the psychoanalytic period, feelings of anxiety were viewed as clues to the existence of unconscious problems. In newer psychological formulations, anxiety became the illness itself rather than the symptom of a more pervasive and hidden difficulty. Therapies such as T-groups, sensitivity groups, and crisis intervention mounted a direct attack on the anxiety rather than searching for repressed conflict. In the 1970s and the 1980s, psychoanalysis is concerned with ennui. This reflects the crucial change from the relief of specific forms of psychological suffering to a search for meaning in the face of a potentially meaningless existence. A more sophisticated awareness of life choices and the freedom from certain moral restraints have resulted in experimental life-styles.

The meaning of personal fulfillment is less related to the individual's ties with the community than in the past. People now are becoming more involved in their own individual needs and pleasures. According to London, the alternative therapies are part of a large therapeutic subculture that has developed to meet these needs. The alternative healing therapies reflect the shift from the treatment of symptoms toward the general improvement of mental health. This is achieved through techniques for enriching experience and facilitating human relationships. The latter techniques are particularly important in a mobile society, in which durable friendships and even family relationships have become difficult to achieve.

Expanded Definitions of Psychiatric Treatment

Because the emotional needs of people seeking therapy have changed, and because the number of potential clients has increased, the technical definitions of treatment have expanded. Effective therapy now includes such disciplines as transactional analysis and psychodrama. Critics have recently begun to question the value of traditional psychotherapy, since there are no scientific data to measure its effectiveness. This has intensified the debate over who is qualified to be a therapist. Each group trains its therapists according to its own standards for practice.

The trend toward viewing therapy as a part of ordinary life is removing some of the mystique from traditional psychiatric practice. Alternative therapies in general provide for a greater variety of psychological ideologies and methods. Traditionally, psychiatry has used the one-to-one therapist–client relationship in which exclusively verbal interaction took place. The new therapies have expanded this format to include groups of varying sizes. They also use a variety of verbal and nonverbal techniques, such as massage, meditation, and role playing.

BASIC PREMISES OF THE NEW THERAPIES

Each of the alternative healing therapies has its own definition of emotional health and has developed a unique method for achieving it. Some emphasize body–mind integration. Others use meditation and thought control to expand consciousness. Quite a few focus on providing catharsis for damaging experiences in the past. However, close examination of these theories and methods reveals three significant common areas:

1. The discovery of the real self through overcoming the intellect
2. Body–mind integration
3. Assumption of responsibility for the self and for the events in life

The Discovery of the Real Self

Liss's Theory   The new therapists emphasize the social repression in Western culture that prevents self-actualization. Most of them describe the distortions of the self that are caused by this repressive socialization. Jerome Liss's (1974) theory of the interrupted child is typical in this respect. According to Liss, young children still behave in a natural way. When they are hurt, they cry, when they are angry, they shout, and so on. Usually these strong expressions of feeling are not acceptable, and the child is squelched with threats of punishment or withdrawal of love. Thus the child is repeatedly interrupted in the expression of natural feelings. The energy behind the feeling the child is expressing gets "stuck."

Liss conceives of emotional energy as a fast flowing stream. When expression of feeling is blocked, emotional energy gets dammed up. Feelings continually press for expression, however. This increases the likelihood that new events will simply restimulate old feelings instead of evoking novel reactions. As natural feelings are continually interrupted, a person forms a collection of repressed feelings from the past. Finally all capacity to feel is lost. Instead, the person learns to intellectualize and substitutes the process of thinking for real experience, living in terms of beliefs, which are only distorted representations of the real world. Liss calls this condition "socially accepted insanity" and claims that most people suffer from it. In order to recover sanity, it is necessary to give up intellectual images and to live from complete feelings at each moment. Sane people, according to Liss, say and do exactly what they are feeling. Their lives are not centered on what they think they *should* do, but on what feels good to them from moment to moment.

Devaluation of the Intellect   Liss's theory epitomizes the criticism of the intellect that predominates in the alternative therapies. The main element of this criticism is that people repress their spontaneous feelings and learn to present a false picture to themselves and to the world. They act in terms of logic and abstract thinking in order to present a safe and acceptable personality to others. In so doing, they forfeit genuine experience. Their minds cannot deal with new events, and react only to the past. However, the past never conforms exactly to the present. For this reason the alternative healing therapies teach clients how to live fully in the present moment. They warn against analyzing experience. They teach people simply to let life be what it is—without holding any preconceived notions about it. This produces a true experience of the self in the world rather than the unreal life structure provided by the intellect.

New therapists call for an end to the dominance of rationality. This style of thinking, they claim, has limited human consciousness. New therapists claim that science has failed, citing as evidence humanity's alienation from itself and from its environment. Scientific knowledge has separated human beings from their individuality. Only phenomena that can be measured quantitatively are thought important, since scientific thought considers the subjective and irrational to be infantile forms of experience. The new therapists point to the increasing interest in mystical religion, ritual, occultism, and meditation as a reaction against the deficiencies of scientific thought.

The new therapists emphasize a duality between the objective and subjective modes of experience. They see reason as purely analytical, objective, and differential. They see subjectivity as intuitive, nonsystematic, and nondiscriminative. Reason predetermines a fragmented, incomplete experience. Intuition enables us to respond to the total event, because its processes are unencumbered by the rigid laws of logical thinking. Subjective consciousness, since it is holistic, cannot be adopted in part. A change to this mode involves a change from a focus on the quantity of phenomena to a focus on the quality of life. Value is not placed on production and achievement but on heightened sensory receptivity and a commitment to the immediate present.

Freeing yourself from the bonds of the past means more than nullifying the traumatic effects of the past. It means liberating the self from the very processes of logical thinking that produced repression and retention of the past. Life without logic will become the natural and simple process it was meant to be. People will live as small children do, unconcerned with all the dos and don'ts. Many new therapists assume that when clients have become healthy again, by ridding themselves of the destructive aspects of socialization, they will be able to live cooperatively with others. These therapists believe that people will then be able to meet their own needs without interfering with the rights of others.

Body–Mind Integration

A second basic theme of the new therapies is the need to reintegrate the body and the mind. New therapists attribute the body–mind split to the moralistic and restrictive socialization patterns in Western culture. People learn artificial standards of sexual propriety and avoid mentioning their unpleasant bodily functions. This adds to their sense of estrangement from their bodies. The way in which people often refer to "my body" expresses their degree of disidentification. According to some new therapists, the body–mind split is characteristic of the modern emphasis on intellectual capacity at the expense of sensuality and body awareness. This split permeates most people's consciousness and character style. Therapists such as Ida Rolf and Franz Alexander say that people need to reclaim their bodies and reeducate them to be responsive to pleasure.

The Aliveness of the Body   Body–mind therapists emphasize that current beliefs about the body are wrong. Supposedly the body is a solid and dense structure that does not change except through accidents and the slow deterioration of aging. Actually, these therapists say, the body is a flexible, fluid energy field that is continually changing. People who know this can experience the self in an entirely new way, with a subjective sense of energy and beauty.

Most people have never had this experience because they were programmed to use their bodies only in certain ways. For example, the male physical ideal in American culture is the extreme mesomorph with well-developed musculature, large shoulders, and slim hips. Because of cultural stereotypes, men are encouraged to develop a type of body structure that actually restricts effective physiological functioning. A tight, muscular chest inhibits the expansion of the lungs and heart, and rigidity of the connective tissues around the waist restricts the diaphragm, thus inhibiting the respiratory system. When the cardiovascular and respiratory systems are inhibited by a man's muscular overdevelopment, his cells are not fully oxygenated and the man does not feel as well as he would if his physique allowed free respiration and circulation.

Finally, a person's body is more than a mere physical structure. It stands for that person's unique life history. Physical and emotional events are recorded in posture and skin tone. Feelings and emotional conflicts are reflected in habitual postural modes. Body therapists emphasize that many physical traits are simply variables in personal history. People's bodies change constantly, and they can be released from damaging past influences. Thus one's present body is not inevitable.

Goals of the Body–Mind Therapies   One major goal of the body–mind therapies is to teach people to understand the body's role in creating and maintaining emotional problems. These problems are precipitated by past events that have not been fully experienced because of cultural prohibitions. The unexperienced event freezes in the body and is relived as the person futilely attempts to deal with it. The therapies that specifically emphasize reintegration of the body and mind stress the quick and forceful breaking of defensive barriers so that the self can be rid of past emotional conflicts. Body–mind therapists use various massage and exercise techniques to relax muscles and release trapped energy. These techniques provide for a catharsis of the damaging emotional memories that have been embodied in the form of muscle tension.

In order to prevent the self from experiencing emotional pain, the individual holds it back. This holding back results in the physical pain of muscle tension. Facing the pain results in an increase of energy for the individual, who no longer has to devote effort to controlling the expression of the pain. The process of becoming aware of pain is gradual and difficult. As we begin to become aware of our feelings, we experience a recurrence of the original emotional pain that was repressed.

Self-regulation and Responsibility

The importance of self-regulation and the assumption of complete responsibility for our own lives is a consistent theme in most of the new therapies. Apparently this self-regulation occurs most easily after we have purged the self of past problems. The new therapists emphasize that each child is born with an innate capacity to develop to his or her full potential. However, the child needs to be loved and allowed self-expression in order to grow. If these needs are not met, as they often are not, the child will not be psychologically whole. In order to develop, adults must take responsibility for making up in some way what they were deprived of in the past. We need to accept full responsibility for our present functioning by recognizing that our perceptions of the present are distorted by attitudes learned in the past. We must bear the fear and confusion involved in giving up an old frame of reference. Once we have accepted the finality of the past, we are free to recognize that the present and the future can be controlled.

The idea of accepting responsibility for the self seems to be based on the fact that we can choose how we view a given event. Our reactions to events, our feelings, and our opinions are all under our own control. Everything else, including material things (such as the natural world) and other people's opinions, is beyond our control. In order to be free, we must be concerned only with what is within our control. This means that we should only be concerned with changing our reactions and feelings. We should not try to change the material world or other people's personalities.

A deeper question involved in the issue of self-regulation concerns the nature of reality. According to the new therapists, reality consists of agreements among various people, usually the most powerful people, that certain things are so. These things, which exist by agreement, seem logical and fitting, but they are really illusions. Even the traditional ideas of physicalness—that objects have form, dimension, and existence in time—are erroneous. New therapists cite recent work in atomic physics, research into the psychology of perception, and linguistic analysis as evidence of current doubt about the validity of immediate perceptions and traditional notions of what is real. Physicists have shown that what we see as an apparently solid table is mostly empty space filled with countless particles moving at incredibly high velocities. Ideas are not real pictures of things out there but expressions of relationships among various events in the world. Ideas such as Marxism, capitalism, and Freudianism are not real things but relationships or agreements. They are true only insofar as they help people achieve certain goals and deal with the chaos of experience. According to est (one of the new therapies), when people accept the illusory character of what they had thought was real, they are liberated into an exciting world where they can find out for themselves what is really true. When people recognize that what is real is their own experience, they recognize that they can create the world they live in.

REPRESENTATIVE ALTERNATIVE HEALING THERAPIES

There are hundreds of alternative healing therapies currently being practiced in the United States, Canada, Western Europe, Africa, and India. Some, such as *est* and *Rolfing,* are prosperous and have large followings. Others, such as *Living Love,* and *Rebirthing,* are relatively obscure and localized. These therapies can be divided into three general categories:

1. Programs built around body discipline, health, and body–mind awareness
2. Programs built around psychological growth for people who want to make specific changes in their lives
3. Programs built around spiritual development and the attainment of altered consciousness

This section will explore representative therapies in each of these three categories. Our purpose is to clarify their common goals and to explore the variety of concepts and therapeutic strategies they use.

Body Discipline and Body–Mind Awareness Therapies

The new body–mind awareness therapies focus primarily on helping people express their intense and primitive feelings and heed the messages from their bodies. Cognitive processes are seen as distractions that inhibit awareness of emotions and bodily sensa-

tions. The goal in treatment is to reach the client's precognitive affect. This will enable the client to focus on the here and now.

Primal Scream Therapy   Arthur Janov (1970), the originator of primal scream therapy, treats what he calls "psychophysical illness." He believes that traditional psychotherapy is fragmented because it claims that emotional problems are caused by many factors. Janov thinks that emotional problems have only one cause—the failure to integrate feelings—and only one cure—primal scream therapy.

Emotional problems begin in early childhood. Healthy, innocent children become neurotic because their *primal needs* are not met. These primal needs include being fed when hungry, having physical closeness and sensory stimulation, being kept warm, and being allowed privacy and permission to develop our specific potential. When primal needs are denied, the result is primal pain. This early pain remains locked in the self and later causes neurotic behavior.

Adults act out this pain in a variety of ways—for example, in addictions and phobias. The severity of the neurosis depends on the amount of accumulated pain. Defending against this pain is a natural and necessary reaction designed to protect the integrity of the vulnerable child. However, adults do not need defenses, for their pain need not be devastating. The defenses must be dismantled step-by-step the way they were originally constructed. This eliminates blockages to the expression of feelings. Only in this way can the adult be cured. Unconscious feelings cannot be resolved simply by making them conscious. These feelings permeate the entire body and must be resolved organismically.

Liberation is achieved by reliving primal scenes—key scenes that represent the feelings involved in many similar events. Clients work through their fear of feeling so that they can let their feelings assume control of their personality. This process of emotional flooding permits the earliest memories to surface. Clients experience again their infantile anguish that their parents did not love them for what they were and that they were forced to conform to an ideal of what they "should" be. In this regressed state they express the anger and pain they never could admit. A primal experience is characterized by the use of childish language, the loss of time sense, and finally, a deep, retching scream. After a true primal, clients begin to see the futility of their lifelong struggle for approval and experience real and spontaneous feelings.

This intensive experiencing of primal pain is facilitated by the requirement that the first three weeks of therapy be devoted entirely to the primal process. The therapist works alone with one client during this time, attempting to break through defenses by engaging in verbal confrontation and encouraging early memory associations. The client then participates in a group therapy that emphasizes abreactive experience for an additional six to nine months. According to Janov, this therapy enables previously fragmented people to regain contact with their total selves.

Primal therapy is based on the belief that problems that derive from earliest experiences cannot be solved in the present. A woman with sexual dysfunction cannot be treated by examining the problems in her current relationships. The causal factors must be relived. Janov gives the example of a woman suffering from frigidity who, deep into a primal experience, took off her clothes and began to scream, "Daddy, I know you won't like me if I am a girl, but I have to be me!" She experienced again the full impact of her father's rejection of her sexuality. She was able to accept her primal pain that to be a girl was to be unloved. Eventually she recognized that she was frigid because each sexual experience reminded her that she was a girl. She did not want to be female because her father had taught her that it was better to be male. Her sexual problems were caused by this thwarting of her natural sexuality. According to Janov, only the living out of such early experiences resolves the problems that they cause in later life.

Rolfing   Rolfing, or structural integration, is based on the belief that psychological conflicts are recorded and perpetuated in the body. Ida Rolf (1977), the founder of this therapy, viewed the body as an area of energy within the earth's gravitational field. In order to function properly, a person must be in correct alignment with the forces of gravity. When the body is in an incorrect position, the myofascia or connective tissue that supports the body weight shortens and undergoes metabolic changes that decrease its energy and interfere with free movement.

Many people are not in proper relationship to the field of gravity because they have become alienated from their own bodily sensations. At different points in their development they have responded to inner and outer threats by turning off their responses. They have inhibited those responses by contracting the muscles that are related to the impulse that is being blocked. For example, if the impulse is aggressive they may

contract arm muscles. Repeated inhibition and the resulting muscular contractions produce chronically spastic muscles that inhibit motility. The musculature acts as a repository of stored feelings. Energy that would otherwise be available for conscious use is expended internally to keep these muscles tense.

As people age, their posture becomes a reflection of accumulated unresolved feelings. When people become aware of how they contract their muscles in traumatic situations, they can begin to take responsibility for their own physical structure by experimenting with alternative responses. Gracefulness and unitary movement are signs of personal integration. When a body is coordinated and balanced physically, there is a corresponding emotional balance.

Rolfing is a method of working with the body to achieve a realignment of the body structure. The basic therapy consists of ten one-hour sessions. The rolfer massages and manipulates the client's deep connective tissue. Once this tissue is freed, the body is able to realign itself with gravitational forces. The emotional release and physical healing that often accompany Rolfing are not the major goal of therapy. However, they are proof that emotional and physical problems are related to the body's misalignment. Many clients who have been rolfed report they have changed so much that they have difficulty relating to their past environment and must alter their work, interpersonal relationships, and values.

Bioenergetics   Alexander Lowen (1967, 1972), founder of the Institute for Bioenergetics, also emphasizes body work. Bioenergetics offers techniques for reducing muscular tension through the release of feelings. It makes less use of direct body contact (between client and therapist) than other body therapies, guiding the client instead through a series of exercises and verbal techniques. Stressor and releasor exercises are used to increase the client's awareness of body defenses. The exercises begin with deep breathing and progress to stretching and kicking the limbs. This enables the client to break through muscular rigidity and express feelings previously trapped in habitual postural modes. These modes, which are called *muscular armoring*, prevent the free flow of energy. The theory is comparable to that of other body–mind therapists.

If the body is relatively unalive, perceptions and responses are diminished. People in this situation are often depressed. According to Lowen, depressed people were denied the mother love they needed. Now they have no faith in themselves or in life. They cannot pursue the goals they really wish to achieve, and they are usually unaware of the reasons for their lifelessness. During bioenergetic therapy, these people are encouraged to make deep contact with their feelings of sadness. Lowen discusses a client with chronic depression who benefited by a session of screaming and kicking. Her depression lifted as she went through this series of exercises and was able to release her emotional controls. The intense energy that had previously been immobilized in depression became available to her. Lowen emphasizes that clients must break through frozen emotions by themselves and thus become able to care for themselves in the way their parents failed to do.

Lowen also thinks that the study of *auras*, or energy fields around the body, can be used to diagnose disturbances in body functioning. In the energy field of a person with Schizophrenia, for example, a trained observer can see characteristic alterations, such as interruptions of energy flow or color changes. Different parts of each person's body radiate different kinds of feelings. When chronic muscle tension blocks energy, negative feelings result. The head, neck, and shoulders can radiate openness and affirmation or express hostility and holding back. The belly can radiate pleasure and laughter or suffering. The legs can radiate security and balance or instability. When there are no constrictions that disturb energy flow, the feeling is positive, the personality is integrated, and the aura is bright and intense.

People excite and depress each other through their energy fields. People with strong energy fields influence others in a positive way. We are in touch with others only when our energy contacts and excites their energy. Bioenergetics attempts to facilitate this free flow of energy through exercises.

Gestalt Therapy   Gestalt therapy developed out of psychoanalysis. It was influenced to some extent by existentialism but primarily by the principles of gestalt psychology. Gestalt therapy teaches clients to develop an awareness of their own bodily processes as these affect the achievement of life goals and successful relationships.

Frederick Perls (1970, 1973), the originator of gestalt therapy, uses the term *gestalt* to refer to the person and what the person observes in the environment. A gestalt is a configuration consisting of ground—or general background—and figure—or what the perceiver observes as standing out from the background. The figure is the potential satisfier of a need. For example,

a man is walking down the street. He becomes hungry and begins to think about food. The street and the various stores on it are the ground. He sees a restaurant. The restaurant is the figure or the means of satisfying the man's need for food. The gestalt is the relationship between the man and the restaurant.

A gestalt may be open or closed. An open gestalt is a relationship between an individual and a figure that is not fulfilled, while a closed gestalt is a relationship that is fulfilled. An open gestalt is an incomplete situation in which unrecognized or unexpressed needs press for attention and prevent the formation of a new gestalt. A closed gestalt is a situation that is completed. The person is free to go on to another concern. If the man in the example passes by the restaurant, he leaves the gestalt open and still has the problem of satisfying his hunger. If he goes in and eats a meal, he closes the gestalt, and because he is no longer hungry, he can turn his attention to other matters.

People organize and regulate their actions through the process of gestalt formation and completion. Survival depends on being able to satisfy our needs while maintaining our individuality. Self-regulated people can choose what to take in from the environment and what to reject. They use sensory awareness to discriminate between choices. They use aggression to reject what is toxic to them, and they use digestion to assimilate what is nourishing. Taking in anything whole—whether food, beliefs, or role definitions—without chewing and assimilating it is called *introjection*. Introjection inhibits growth, because experiences are taken in without understanding them. Unassimilated personal qualities are unconscious characteristics (such as warmth, wariness, or generosity) that cannot be used in everyday life. The individual with unassimilated qualities is deprived of resources and is less inventive and flexible. Unassimilated personal qualities form the basis of a rigid and repetitive behavior that is unrelated to present needs.

Gestalt therapy is concerned with discovering and closing each long-standing, psychologically critical, open gestalt. This enables the client to move from neurosis to an authentic self. The therapist tries to help the client become aware of the process of self-regulation by bringing back into awareness the client's capacity for sensory experience and aggression. The therapist helps the client to regain touch with immediate experience by asking such questions as "What are you now aware of in your body?" In seeking to answer these questions, the client becomes more aware of previously blocked bodily feelings and also becomes more sensitive to the environment. This awareness is effective only when it is grounded in the client's immediate needs. It is not complete unless the client clearly recognizes the reality of the immediate situation and can effectively regulate his or her behavior in an intuitive way.

The therapist helps people without a fully functioning self to regulate their behavior. This is done by guiding the client through the layers of the neurosis until explosion is achieved. An *explosion* is an intense expression of feeling, usually related to unresolved grief, anger, joy, or orgasm. An explosion liberates the life energy. Clients who have experienced an explosion are then encouraged to focus awareness on situations in which they habitually feel "stuck."

Resolution of past experiences enables the individual to focus on the present. Unclosed gestalts from the past are dealt with through Perls's double chair technique. The client sits in one chair and fantasizes that a person significant to him or her is sitting in the other. The client is helped to conduct an imaginary conversation with this person. Then the client is taught to reverse roles, become the other person, and resume the dialogue. Unacknowledged feelings about the relationship will emerge, and the client works out the situation until the gestalt is closed. Dreams, current feelings, and body language are dealt with in a similar way, with the therapist encouraging descriptions of immediate perceptions. Gestalt therapy is unique in its focus on the resolution of specific experiences as they occur.

Orthomolecular Nutrition   The concept of orthomolecular nutrition was formulated by Linus Pauling. It involves treating mental disorders by providing the optimum molecular environment for the functioning of the brain (see Hoffer and Walker, 1978). Pauling believes that mental illness is one of the degenerative diseases produced by the Western diet, which is contaminated by additives such as salt, sugar, and chemicals, and lacking in sufficient raw, natural foods. Mental symptoms are thought to be manifestations of a central nervous system disorder caused by the resulting inadequate concentrations of necessary molecules. For instance, the mood alterations seen in the Depressive Disorders are explained on the basis of the client's excessive consumption of refined carbohydrates while Anxiety and Phobias are thought to be related to hypoglycemia. Chronic malnutrition is believed to cause visual and auditory misperceptions that result in hallucinations and delusions.

Orthomolecular psychiatry deals with such problems as Schizophrenia, drug addiction, and alcoholism with

various combinations of megavitamins, drugs, and a carefully controlled diet, although other standard psychiatric treatments are also used. All additives are removed from the client's diet, natural foods are restored, and megadoses of vitamins such as thiamine, riboflavin, and ascorbic acid are given, particularly for Schizophrenic Disorders. A basic concept of orthomolecular psychiatry is the biochemical individuality of each person—that is, everyone has unique dietary needs that vary widely from published norms. These dietary needs also change within the individual over time, and thus people must continually monitor themselves in order to maintain optimal health.

Therapeutic Touch   Therapeutic touch was developed by Dolores Krieger (1979). It is defined as the specific transfer of energy in a therapeutic manner in which some of the excess energies of the healer are directed to the client, or energy is transferred from one place to another within the body of the client. This technique is based on the concept of illness as an imbalance of energies in the body. *Prana* is the subsystem of energy which Krieger believes is the basis of the energy transfer in therapeutic touch. Normally healthy people have an excess of prana, and since each person is an open system, energy can be transferred to another person. This transfer of energy is not a cure but provides an infusion of energy for people depleted by struggles with illness until their own healing processes take over.

Therapeutic touch is a conscious, deliberate act whose steps correspond to the stages of assessment, diagnosis, intervention, and evaluation of the nursing process (see Chapter 4). The healer first prepares for the procedure through *centering,* the discovery of an inner physical and psychological stability in which the person achieves a sense that all facilities are under command. This gathers and focuses the healer's energies. The healer then *scans* the client without actually touching his or her body, attempting to sense temperature changes or feelings of pressure. These areas indicate a static condition or congestion in the client's energy field. Intervention consists of mobilizing these congested areas. The healer places his or her hands, with palms facing away from the client, in the area where pressure is felt and moves the hands away from the client's body in a sweeping gesture while consciously directing a flow of energy to the client. Therapists report relief of the sense of pressure they feel in problematic areas of the client's body and consider the treatment complete when they no longer perceive an imbalance in the person's symmetry.

Clients report a sense of relaxation and relief from pain. Krieger (1979) has demonstrated experimentally that therapeutic touch has produced a significant change in the hemoglobin component of red blood cells. Advocates of therapeutic touch have found that the freeing of bound energy is not long-lasting but that it does seem to facilitate the repatterning of energy necessary for healing.

Biofeedback   Biofeedback, or visceral learning, is a technique for gaining conscious control over unconscious body functions such as blood pressure and heartbeat. It has been demonstrated that people can voluntarily control some autonomic functions to a degree once thought impossible. This is done by using continuous feedback about the results of each consecutive attempt at control. In a typical session, a person might be given this feedback by equipment that amplifies body signals and translates them into a flashing light or a steady tone. Once people can "see" a heartbeat, for instance, and observe when it slows down or speeds up, they have the information they need to control their heart rate. They are instructed to change the signal as they observe it. They are not told to slow the heartbeat, but to slow the flashing light. If they can do this, their heart rate will be modified.

Biofeedback has proved successful in a variety of physical health problems that have a large psychological component. These include migraine headaches, insomnia, high blood pressure, gastric ulcers, and asthma. It has been shown, for instance, that migraine headaches can be relieved by increasing blood flow to the hands. Psychological states achieved through biofeedback can be beneficial in decreasing tension and reactions to stimuli.

Psychological Growth Therapies

A second group of alternative therapies emphasizes psychological growth for people who want to make specific changes in their work, life-style, or sexual functioning. In these therapies the client's presenting problem is often the focus for change. (In the traditional psychiatric model the presenting problem is considered to be a symptom, and the underlying cause is the focus for change.) They seek to help the client change ineffective behavior.

Transactional Analysis   Transactional analysis was originated by Eric Berne (1961, 1964, 1972). It is both a mode for understanding personality and a method of facilitating personal growth. The fundamentals of transactional analysis are discussed thoroughly in Chapter 6.

According to transactional analysis, people spend much of their time playing games. A *game* is an ongoing series of complementary ulterior transactions that progress to a well-defined, predictable outcome (Berne 1964, p. 48). Transactional analysis provides theories for the detailed analysis of many such games. Most of them provide negative satisfactions. The goal of transactional analysis is to teach the client to recognize and to stop playing games. Instead, the client seeks to attain *autonomy*, which is characterized by awareness, spontaneity, and intimacy (Berne 1964, p. 178).

Transactional analysis is usually conducted in a small group setting. It is contractual in nature. Clients are asked to define exactly what they are seeking in therapy and to make a contract to reach a certain goal. The therapist observes the transactions that take place among the group members' ego states and points out each client's characteristic way of transacting with others. Clients attempt to modify their transactions so that they will be more effective in reaching their goals. The basic belief is that clients can change if they are willing to give up the rewards of the negative games they have been playing. Transactional analysis is widely used in industry and management and in family and marital therapy (see Chapter 21). It is also used to treat special problems such as Schizophrenia, Alcoholism, and criminal behavior.

Encounter Marathon Groups   Encounter marathon groups are also used to improve interpersonal relationships. The term *encounter group* is a broad one, encompassing many types of group therapies variously known as sensitivity training, personal growth, and human potential therapies. Pioneered by Frederick Stoller, George Bach, William Schutz, and Elizabeth Mintz in the late 1960s, encounter groups were thought to facilitate the expression of feelings in a way mere verbalization could not accomplish (see Endore 1968). Early attempts at encounter groups originated from Moreno's psychodrama, T-groups or training groups for personnel management, and most notably groups run by the Esalen Institute in Big Sur, California.

The encounter marathon group consists of ten or fifteen people who meet together intensively for a few days or weeks. Marathon groups meet fairly continuously over a weekend, while mini-marathon groups meet for a day. The focus of these groups is the present experience. Members are encouraged to drop their inhibitions and allow other members to influence them emotionally. Nonverbal techniques are used to stimulate intense, honest, and highly personal communication. These techniques include dancing, touching, massage, and acting out dreams and fantasies.

One of the most important means of helping members of a group to relate to each other emotionally is through structured exercises. For example, participants may be asked to go around the room making eye contact with each member and holding that eye contact as long as they want to. They are then asked to tell the group how they felt about this experience. Problems are also acted out in the group setting. For example, a woman who was often rejected by others participated in an exercise in which all the group members locked hands in a circle, leaving her outside. She had to try to enter the circle and finally did so by taking the hands of members she felt close to. Her terror of being rejected from the group was then discussed, and the other members expressed their feelings about letting her into the circle.

The encounter experience provides feedback for each member's verbal and nonverbal behavior. Members are expected to put themselves voluntarily into the focus of the group's attention. Members are expected to be totally honest—to the point of brutal frankness if necessary. Giving advice, being vague or defensive, or talking about what "ought" to be done is attacked as evasive. Members are not allowed to make other members feel better in order to protect their self-concept, because this prevents them from standing up alone in front of the group as they must learn to do in everyday life. The encounter marathon group is designed to simulate the way in which the members relate to the important people in their lives and thus to reveal their core behavior patterns. Other group members' reactions give feedback on the effects of their behavior and enable them to experiment with more effective behavior. The encounter marathon also provides its members with a small group setting where they can express themselves and come to terms with common taboos about proper behavior.

Schutz and the Open Encounter Group
William Schutz (1967) has had a significant influence on the encounter movement through his work at the Esalen Institute, where he founded his open encounter therapy. Open encounter groups focus on helping clients know and like themselves. Schutz uses the concept of *naturalness,* by which he means the ability to develop normally after psychological blocks have been removed. Schutz views encounter as a way of life, because it offers an alternative to the usual devious ways

in which people relate to each other. He thinks that people should be able to be honest and open and emphasize their feelings in *every* relationship. Schutz has also been influenced by the body therapists. He believes that joy, the sign of the fully realized person, is achieved through developing one's physical structure as well as through one's personal functioning and interpersonal relationships. Blockages to the full flow of physical energy act as do psychological inhibitions—they limit the flow of energy and can eventually lead to illness. Encounter, as Schutz conceives it, is based on three interpersonal needs: the need to be important and worthwhile, the need to be competent in coping with the world, and the need to feel lovable (see FIRO theory in Chapter 18). Open encounter focuses on effective ways of meeting these needs.

Morita Therapy
Morita therapy was developed in 1920 by Masatake Morita (see Kora 1965). It is practiced primarily in Japan. It emphasizes the importance of action and the relative unimportance of thoughts and feelings. Clients are taught that the alleviation of symptoms is unessential, because symptoms do not necessarily interfere with goal-directed activity. According to Morita, this approach deals effectively with people's self-defeating preoccupation with their own behavior.

The treatment is limited to specific personality types—people who are suffering from depression, obsessive fears, and acute anxiety. Such people tend to criticize themselves severely for having these symptoms. The treatment begins with four to six days of bed rest in complete isolation. Clients cannot talk with others socially, read, or watch television. This isolation enables them to regain contact with their life goals and their need for help. During the second week clients attend group and individual therapy sessions in which they are encouraged to adopt other behaviors. The regime of stimulus deprivation is gradually relaxed to include reading, arts and crafts, and light work. During the third phase clients engage in heavy physical labor. During the last phase they are allowed to resume social relationships. Clients are told at this time that their proper role is to learn the principles of Morita therapy and then apply these principles to their lives.

Reality Therapy
William Glasser (1965) introduced reality therapy in 1964 and formed the Institute of Reality Therapy in 1969 to train professionals in the use of his techniques. Glasser stresses that the two major psychological needs are to love and be loved and to feel worthwhile to yourself and others. People who

cannot satisfy these two needs without harming others are irresponsible, not mentally ill. Such people will turn to delinquency and withdraw from society. This, in turn, causes a failure of identity. Glasser thinks that since about 1950 Americans have been living in a role-oriented society and have been concerned with finding a worthwhile identity. Reality therapy is designed to help irresponsible people do this.

According to Glasser, the most crucial element in finding an identity is a genuine and loving relationship with another person. The first step in treatment is to learn how to develop this kind of involvement, first with the therapist and then with others. The therapist relates warmly but professionally to the client. Often they do not discuss the client's specific problems. Instead they may discuss movies, books, current events, and life goals to develop the client's capacity for intellectual sharing. Glasser thinks that talking too much about problems only increases the client's feeling of failure and is also futile, since the past cannot be altered.

Identity is also formed by increasing the client's awareness of current behavior. Reality therapy focuses on what clients are *doing* rather than on what they are feeling, for Glasser thinks it is how people behave toward others that is crucial. Behaving in a responsible, competent way increases self-esteem. After clients become more aware of their behavior, they are helped to look at it critically in order to judge its effectiveness and social acceptability. Reality therapists think it is appropriate to involve themselves in discussions of what is morally right and wrong, although they do not specifically judge behavior. Clients are taught the limits of behavior, and reality is constantly emphasized.

After clients have constructed a reasonable plan to change behavior, they make a commitment to carry it out. The therapist never excuses a client from the responsibility of this commitment, but failure is not emphasized. The client is not allowed to offer rationalizations or intellectualizations but is simply given time until the pledge is fulfilled. When the client succeeds, praise is given to reinforce responsible behavior. Glasser has used principles of reality therapy successfully with delinquents and chronic psychotic clients.

Psychosynthesis Roberto Assagioli (1971) has developed a therapeutic system called psychosynthesis, which has been absorbed to some extent by the encounter movement. Assagioli stresses the arousal and development of the will, which, if successfully used, directs all other functions toward a deliberately chosen goal. This is achieved through teaching exercises to

develop the five phases of the will: motivation and deliberation, decision, affirmation, planning, and execution of the plan. Psychosynthesis focuses on the sublimation of sexual and aggressive energies into creative activities. It also provides for the practice of techniques that awaken superconscious spiritual energies. Assagioli emphasizes the importance of constructing meanings for life and developing clients' sense of responsibility for their decisions. Although he focuses on feelings of self-awareness and joy as well as on the suffering and loneliness inherent in life, his major concern is the conscious and planned reconstruction of the personality. The central purpose of psychosynthesis is the integration of all the qualities and functions of the individual.

Rational-Emotive Therapy Rational-emotive therapy was formulated by Albert Ellis (see Ellis and Harper 1975). Ellis defines beliefs as rational when they help the individual accept reality, live in intimate relationships with others, work productively, and enjoy recreational pursuits. Irrationality is self-destructive behavior. Rational-emotive therapy emphasizes human values as the important component of personality. Healthy functioning is possible only when the values we believe in are rational ones. Absolutist, perfectionist attitudes are irrational. Emotional reactions are not caused by events or by our emotional reaction to events but by belief systems. Being insulted, for instance, does not cause us to withdraw from others. Our *beliefs* about being insulted are what cause us to withdraw. Though it is rational to feel angry about insults, since they are destructive, withdrawal is irrational because it indicates that an individual has defined being insulted as a frightening event to be avoided. Both emotions and behavior depend on the cognitive mediating process that occurs in relation to every experience. Rational-emotive therapy helps people dispel their disturbing beliefs by explaining what irrational beliefs are and how they cause emotional difficulty. After they have logically analyzed their irrational beliefs, they see how unnecessary they are and eliminate them. The most common irrational belief is that a person must be competent and win the approval of others. People also feel that others must be kind and considerate, thus making their own lives easy and pleasant.

Rational-emotive therapy frequently uses reinforcing techniques to help people change. Clients are taught to reward themselves for working on self-defeating ideas and to penalize themselves if they do not. Ellis believes that group therapy and marathon encounters are most effective for this type of therapy. Clients are also shown how to speak and think more objectively and give up the use of vague terms and overgeneralizations in order to define their own problems in specific terms. For example, the client is shown that the statement "I have some characteristics that are irritating to others" is more precise than "I am an irritating person." Rational-emotive therapy teaches that people are worthy simply because they exist, and that it is futile to try to evaluate their total personality. Rational-emotive therapy narrows the focus for change to specific traits and behavior. Since people create most of their own psychological symptoms, they can eliminate these symptoms by changing their values.

Assertiveness Training   Assertiveness training has as its goal the reduction of anxiety in social settings and the development of effective social skills (also see Chapter 3). It teaches clients to recognize themselves as important beings who are entitled to an integrity and fulfillment that need not be sacrificed for anyone else. It classifies people in terms of a range of assertive behaviors. At one end are nonassertive people, who tend to suppress emotions, cannot resist manipulation by others, and cannot stand up for their own opinions and needs. At the other end are aggressive people, who meet their own needs at the expense of other people's self-respect and comfort. Both have problems in relationships. A basic goal of assertiveness training is to help clients to find a balance between these two extremes.

Clients are taught a list of behaviors they have a right to engage in—for example, changing their minds, refusing to offer reasons for their behavior, making mistakes, and admitting ignorance about something. They are then taught specific techniques for self-assertion. These include the role playing of such situations as coping effectively when someone is trying to change your mind, dealing with supervision, and working out compromises with peers. Heterogeneous group settings provide group support for new assertive behaviors. Generally groups meet weekly for six to twelve weeks, often with a male and a female therapist to expose the group to several assertive response styles. Role playing and the use of videotape and audio recorders are helpful in providing feedback to clients. Assertiveness training is currently most useful with adolescents, young adults, and women, because these groups are actively seeking more recognition and equality.

Sex Therapy   Masters and Johnson (1966) began studying human sexual response in the mid-1950s.

They conducted research into sexual physiology, sexual dysfunction, and homosexual response patterns. Current sex therapy is based on their findings.

Sex therapy is conducted by male and female cotherapists. The therapists alternate, one taking an active role in treatment while the other observes the interactions. Masters and Johnson rely on *reflective teaching*, in which they state objectively what they think the marital problem is and the ways in which the couple fail to communicate. They stress that since human sexuality is an inherent capacity, the goal of sex therapy is only to remove the barriers to full sexual functioning. It does this through a structured program of sexual encounters in an atmosphere in which performance and genital contact are not stressed. Masters and Johnson emphasize that a sexual problem in one of the partners is a shared problem. They stress the necessity for continual communication between the couple. Each partner is helped to become aware of what is erotically pleasing to the other. The greatest stress is on the closeness of the relationship, not on techniques per se. Sex therapy has had a high rate of success with such problems as impotence, premature ejaculation, orgasmic dysfunction in women, and vaginismus. A thorough treatment of this subject can be found in Chapter 12.

Addiction Group Therapy   Groups that deal with specific behavioral problems also include therapies for addictive behaviors. These groups resemble encounter groups in that they emphasize total honesty in the group encounter. Emphasis is also placed on present feelings, and rationalization or analysis is not permitted. Advocates feel that this type of "no crap" therapy clears away the evasions, politeness, and defenses that people use to hide their real selves.

One example is Synanon, a self-help community for ex-addicts founded in 1958 by Charles Dederich, a former alcoholic (see Yablonsky 1973). Dederich maintains that his special knowledge of therapy is gathered from a variety of sociological, religious, and literary sources. He says he is willing to use any ideas that will help him understand the human condition.

Synanon constitutes a new type of group therapy, since hostile confrontation between members is encouraged. This provides immediate catharsis for aggressive feelings. One of the most important aspects of this therapy is that sessions are conducted by a group of peers who themselves have suffered from problems with drugs. Synanon group therapy begins with conscious behavior in the present and "peels away" destructive aspects of the identity. Therapists justify the immediate attack on the defenses by the fact that clients addicted to drugs generally cannot endure the frustrations of long-term therapy. Dederich thinks that too much laxness in the beginning of therapy will only diminish the seriousness of the problem in the client's mind.

The major objective at Synanon is to make clients stop taking drugs. Then they can see what purpose drugs serve for them, so that they can develop the courage to deal with their problems in a direct and responsible way. Some therapists in Synanon do not consider what they do as group therapy in any traditional sense. They feel that they are engaged in a sport or a contest between clients and their addictions.

Daytop, an offshoot of Synanon, is another organization for ex-addicts.

Direct Decision Therapy   Direct decision therapy was founded by Harold Greenwald (1973). Its aim is to help the client make a specific decision to change some behavior and to implement this decision. The therapist points out the constant choices facing the client and the need to be aware of the continual choices one makes. Clients are helped to realize that they resist change because it involves the rigors of discipline and the renunciation of some advantages. Greenwald thinks that the therapist's role is to point out alternatives that the client may not be aware of, but he stresses that all decisions are made by the clients themselves.

Psycho-imagination Therapy   Psycho-imagination therapy was founded by Joseph Shorr (1972). It deals with the client's unique phenomenological world through the use of techniques that increase the client's awareness of conflicts. Major areas of internal conflict are brought to light by having clients imagine themselves in certain crucial situations and then discuss how they would feel and what they would do in these situations. For example, a client might be asked, "You are having a frightening dream about your parents. What would your mother do? Your father?" Or, "Imagine yourself as an infant again. How would you feel? How would your mother behave as she feeds you?" Through this type of exercise both client and therapist become more familiar with the client's inner world.

Schorr believes that clients must find their true identity. He believes that everyone has been assigned false identities by others. False identities are often unrealistically positive or negative. Helping clients to become familiar with their inner processes will gradually reveal to them their identity.

Confrontation Problem-solving Therapy   Confrontation problem-solving therapy was developed by Harry H. Garner (1971). This therapy teaches clients to rid themselves of learned behavior patterns that are irrelevant to the present. These patterns persist because responses that once met the client's needs for hunger, love, and mastery have become automatic processes and no longer require a process of problem solving. Problem solving is necessary to deal with any new situation in which not all the facts are known. People who fall back on automatic responses learned in the past cannot relate to the new aspects of current situations. In order to teach clients the necessity of problem solving, the therapist confronts them with their specific difficulties and asks them exactly how they are going to deal with these difficulties. Clients are thus compelled to assess their current situation, to speculate on various ways of dealing with it, and finally to choose the action most relevant to handle it.

Consciousness Development Therapies

A third group of alternative healing therapies focuses primarily on the attainment of a religious or spiritual orientation and the evolution to higher levels of consciousness. A higher level of consciousness is an awareness of the unity of the world and everything in it. These therapies use body–mind unification and specific psychological work, but most have as their primary goal an all-encompassing change in the way the client experiences life.

Arica   Arica, an offshoot of encounter group therapy, was developed in the late 1960s by a Bolivian, Oscar Ichazo (1977). Arica employs an eclectic group therapy approach, blending Eastern and Western disciplines to bring about the spiritual awakening that Ichazo believes is necessary to save Western culture from an otherwise inevitable decline. Ichazo believes that everyone begins as pure essence in loving and fearless unity with life. When the ego begins to develop, children imitate adults and lose their innocence. A contradiction develops between their inner feelings and social reality. They begin to lie and pretend in order to conform. This ego consciousness is a limited mode of awareness that separates children from reality. It leads to the formation of personality, which Ichazo thinks is a defensive layer over the pure essence. Ego consciousness leads to destructive feelings of fear and desire as individuals look away from their own essence to the world for completion.

Arica teaches clients to return to reality by overcoming societal conditioning. Higher states of consciousness then become possible, and life is easy and joyful as it was originally meant to be. Consciousness development is achieved through a series of mental processes that train clients to think with the total self rather than through the limited perspective of ego-dominated thoughts. Ichazo believes that as enough people are healed, the massive contradictions between reality and the intellect that presently characterize Western society will be overcome. To this end he has founded the Arica Institute and has organized training programs throughout the United States.

Living Love   The Living Love Way to Happiness and Higher Consciousness was developed by Kenneth Keyes (1977) in Berkeley, California, from the ideas of Christ, humanistic psychology, the Esalen Institute, Maslow, Lilly, Lorzyski, Ram Dass, and especially Buddha. Living Love defines itself as a science of happiness that has developed as part of the great consciousness awakening now taking place thoughout the world. Most people are still living at the level of consciousness appropriate to the time when survival in a physically dangerous world required domination of consciousness by the intellect. Personal development and the survival of civilization now depend on eliminating this lower consciousness, which is ego-directed, subject–object-oriented, and based on the survival needs of security, sensation, and power.

The client learns that consciousness consists of seven centers that act as filters of experience. The three lower centers permit people to experience only the concern with power and sensation. The middle center, that of *love,* permits them to accept everyone unconditionally. The center of *cornucopia* permits them to experience the friendly and perfect world we live in, and the center of *consciousness awareness* permits them to separate from the self. In this center they can observe social roles objectively. *Cosmic consciousness,* the final center, is attained by a very few. The person at this level transcends self-awareness and becomes a godlike being capable of pure awareness itself.

Erhard Seminar Training   Although Erhard Seminar Training, or est, does not claim any specific religious or spiritual orientation, its major goal is to effect a radical shift in the client's consciousness. Developed by Werner Erhard in 1971, est is a highly successful program for training clients to look at life from a holistic standpoint (see Porter and Taxson 1976). Erhard's synthesis of ideas and practices is taken from Zen, scientology, and the writings of Buckminster Fuller. Est is generally taught in highly structured weekend sessions. Lecture is combined with group participation and individual "mental exercises." Participants are challenged by the trainer to experience the world in a new way by taking total responsibility for their lives. They are taught that reality does not exist as an objective fact but only as a reflection of the individual's beliefs about what reality should be. The individual must learn to accept the responsibility of being the total creator of reality. Such consciousness can be achieved by an act of will. The individual is then able to see that life itself is a game with no inherent significance and that each person confers on life whatever importance and meaning it will have for that person.

Reasonableness, or looking for the causes of things, prevents people from living fully in the present. The mind limits learning because it strives to make life safe and consistent, and it cannot deal with new experience. The enlightened person recognizes that reason is only a reaction to the past and that life in the present does not conform to the belief system imposed on it by the mind. In order to live fully in the present, which is an important goal of est training, the individual has to relinquish thoughts of the past and assume responsibility for each moment as it comes. Even events we apparently had little influence on, such as finding ourselves in a sudden rainstorm without an umbrella, are situations for which we are responsible. Such events necessitate questioning ourselves about why we allowed this to happen. Estians believe that when individuals take such responsibility they begin to put themselves into successful situations.

Transcendental Meditation   Transcendental Meditation was founded by Maharishi Mahesh Yogi, who left an ascetic life in the Himalayas in 1958 to bring his spiritual message to the people of India, Europe, and the United States. The Transcendental Meditation program is the applied component of the Science of Creative Intelligence or SCI, the study of the levels of human consciousness. Maharishi reinterpreted the essence of Eastern thought to make it relevant to the modern world (Yogi 1963). He thought that a new Copernican revolution is about to produce a world in which consciousness itself will be valued in place of present-day materialism. Transcendental Meditation, or TM, will help humanity to raise its level of consciousness to bring about this new world. This will solve many urgent social problems. Maharishi organized a world plan to develop the full potential of the individual; to improve government, education, the environment, and the economic system; to eliminate crime; and to achieve his spiritual goals.

These changes will be based on the realization of what pure consciousness is. Pure consciousness is a state of contact with creative intelligence. Creative intelligence is an absolutely unchanging field of experience that is orderly, stable, and calm and that encompasses all possibility. Pure consciousness can only be contacted by transcending all experience through a process of meditation. In the TM technique this process begins on the surface level where we do all our thinking. Assisted by the repetition of a mantra (a special word selected to fit the individual meditator), the client experiences the "oncoming bubble" of deeper thought. Pure consciousness then begins to dominate awareness. The deeper clients go into this consciousness, the closer they are to the source of thought. The most refined level of thought is deeper than the awareness of personal existence and encompasses all experience. Achieving the level of pure creative intelligence can only be taught by people who have already achieved it themselves.

The state of meditation is equivalent to a state of deep rest. The heart rate slows, less oxygen is consumed, and blood lactate, a waste product of metabolism, decreases sharply. Meditation seems to have long-lasting effects as well. Stress-related problems such as insomnia, high blood pressure, and asthma diminish. Alpha waves, which characterize brain activity during states of calm alertness, increase. TM helps people decrease their consumption of food, alcohol, tobacco, and drugs. It seems to quiet the brain, as the person makes contact with more orderly and coherent levels of the mind. The left hemisphere, which is responsible for rational and logical thinking, comes into electrical balance with the underdeveloped right hemisphere, which modulates intuition, holistic comprehension, and artistic qualities. Psychological benefits reported include overflowing feelings of love, greater self-integration, and a sense of oneness with the universe.

Learning TM requires a systematic course of instruction. An introductory lecture explains the benefits of TM. This is followed by a preparatory lecture during which the mechanism of meditation is explained. Next comes an interview, to enable the client to ask questions about TM. Finally there is an hour of personal instruction when the client is given a suitable mantra and instructed in its proper use. The mantra is a sound that seems meaningless (such as *shyam* or *aing*), but

each mantra has been studied and its individual effects are known. Mantras are thought to help calm the central nervous system by activating the areas responsible for emotion and decision making while stimulating the centers responsible for maintaining consciousness itself. Later, three checking meetings are held to monitor progress in meditation and to answer questions. Once the TM method is learned, no more instruction is needed. It is recommended that a person meditate for twenty minutes a day. The longer one meditates, the more one is able to reside in a state of pure consciousness.

Silva Mind Control Silva Mind Control, also called *psychorientology*, is a state of meditation that is second in popularity only to TM. It was developed in the 1940s by José Silva, a Mexican-American from Texas, and it teaches methods of increasing concentration, imagination, and memory (see Silva and Miele 1977). During the four-day course offered at various growth centers, lectures are given on the characteristics of brain waves. According to Silva, most people are in *beta consciousness*, which subjects them to tensions caused by the physical world. One goal of the course is the achievement of *alpha consciousness*, which makes harmony with inner processes possible. Instruction is given in relaxation training, using classical conditioning and a mild form of hypnosis. Clients are taught how to count backward slowly to the accompaniment of mind control sound, which is a low repetitious beat. They are taught physical exercises to relax various muscle groups. During states of relaxation they are encouraged to repeat such sentences as "Every day in every way I am getting better and better" and "I have full control and complete dominion over my thoughts and senses."

Interspersed with relaxation conditioning are lectures on astrology, dreams, extrasensory perception, and auras, as well as discussions on how to solve problems by programming the mind for positive action. Clients are taught to resolve difficulties through dreams and visual exercises. For example, a woman might be instructed to reach alpha consciousness level and then to visualize a full-length mirror with a black frame. The woman next visualizes her problem written on the mirror. She studies the problem, removes it visually from the mirror, and changes the color of the frame from black to white. The solution to the problem will be visible in the white framed mirror. Clients are also taught to imagine advisors or assistants—historical or contemporary figures whom they can call on for assistance. Techniques of *effective sensory projection* enable clients to project themselves first into inanimate objects such as pieces of metal, then to animate objects such as trees and flowers, and finally into the bodies of other persons. The client can then diagnose illness and transmit positive energy to cure it. Mind control advocates claim that this method has cured cancer, blindness, and deafness. Clients are taught that they will eventually be able to project their consciousness to any point in the universe.

Eriksonian Hypnosis   Milton Erikson is generally recognized as a leading proponent of the use of hypnosis in medical and psychotherapeutic contexts (see Bandler and Grinder 1975). Erikson redefined hypnosis as an experience originating in the client in order to cope with a problem overwhelming to the conscious mind. Autohypnotic trance is an altered state of consciousness in which important internal emotional or cognitive processes block out everyday reality. This state of trance is used by the client and the therapist to maximize behavioral potential and treat organic and psychological problems. The relaxation and refocusing of attention on inner reality which occurs during trance can replace maladaptive views of reality.

Hypnotic induction techniques are a way of giving the client the advantage of spontaneous healing processes arising from the unconscious. Although therapists can assist in inducing trance, they do not control it and can only offer suggestions to the subject based on their knowledge of the client's difficulties. The conscious mind of the client cannot control the trance state either. The individual's conscious mind can only offer suggestions and cannot instruct the unconscious how to achieve the desired behavioral change. For instance, if clients use autohypnosis to relieve pain, they enter a trance with a general question for the unconscious such as, "How can I be free of pain?" They must relinquish the issues of how and when this pain relief will be achieved to the autonomous functioning of the unconscious.

Erikson believes that individuals do not operate directly on the world but act through a model or map of what they believe the world is like. As a result, some aspects of their experience are ignored or distorted, thus limiting possibilities for a full life. Individuals preoccupied with pain are distorting their view of the world and increasing their discomfort, because focusing attention on pain only sustains the sensation of having pain. Relieving this pain involves seeing it as only a part of total experience. In a trance state, pain

is separated from total experience and individuals reorient their focus to a state of relaxation and wellbeing. They "forget" about pain.

The purpose of autohypnosis is to create a receptive emotional state in clients, thus enabling them to recognize some of their unrealized or only partially realized potential for experience. It is based on the clients' feelings in the "here and now."

Neurolinguistic Programming (NLP)   NLP was formulated by Richard Bandler, a computer scientist, and John Grinder, a linguist (1979). It has many similarities to Ericksonian hypnosis, but in addition to bringing the client to a fuller awareness of reality, NLP also offers a new pattern of responses to use in dealing with the world. According to NLP, most people use the same three or four basic approaches to all life situations. To be flexible and meet events realistically, people need a dozen or more ways of relating. NLP is based on the idea that these new strategies can be learned by imitating the effective strategies of others. People who are unusually talented in any way can be studied in order to determine the structure of their talent. This structure can be quickly taught to others to give them the basis for that same behavior. Since NLP is based on the systematic structure of experience, it can be used for any desired behavioral change, such as the treatment of phobias; eliminating smoking, drinking, and insomnia; and treating many physical problems.

NLP emphasizes the differences in ways of thinking among individuals. These differences correspond to the three principles of kinesthetics: vision, hearing, and feelings. When therapists make an initial contact, clients will probably be thinking in terms of one of these three representational systems; that is, they will be generating visual images, concentrating on feelings, or focusing on sounds. To gain rapport with the client, therapists adjust their behavior to correspond to the client's representational system. For example, they would reply, "I hear what you are saying" to a client who is primarily oriented to sound. A purpose of therapy is to help clients become aware of their own frame of reference and then help them develop other systems so they can have a total sensory experience. In dealing with specific problems, intervention can be as simple as substituting one system for another in order to break up habitual behavioral patterns. For example, a client with a fear of heights discovered that every time she went to a window she had a visual picture of herself falling from the window. She was taught to substi-

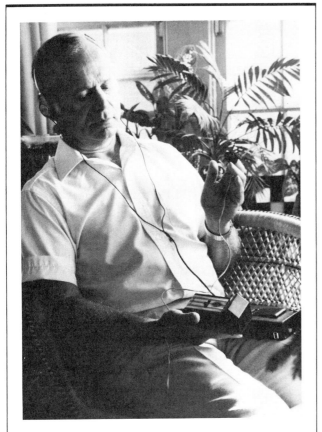

Biofeedback is a popular alternative healing therapy that represents a shift toward independence and away from professional control. This man uses biofeedback to reduce job-related stress and to improve his racquetball game.

tute an auditory experience for the visual one, that is, to go to the window singing loudly. This extinguished the phobic response.

Another technique of dealing with problems is to dissociate from the situation. According to NLP, one reason people feel guilty is because they imagine a look of displeasure on another person's face in response to something they have done, and then they feel guilty about it. When clients "step outside" the situation, they no longer feel guilty because they have a new perspective on the problem.

Other difficulties have their origins in systems that are not completely available to consciousness. People who are chronically depressed are the victims of unconscious images. They are conscious only of their feelings about the images and not the images themselves. One therapeutic technique is *reframing*, which is a specific way of contacting the portion of the person that is causing a certain behavior to occur. It is assumed that all behavior has a positive function in

some context. The purpose of reframing is to help clients discover a new, more acceptable behavior that satisfies the same intention. The therapist first helps clients distinguish between the behavior and the intention. For some people, headaches may be a way of asserting themselves in certain situations. Although the unconscious mind understands this, clients are not consciously aware of it. Therapists ally themselves with the clients' unconscious, help them identify the headache as the pattern to be changed, and then teach them to reframe the situation or create a new behavior, such as making their needs known verbally, rather than experiencing headaches.

NLP allows the therapist and client to determine exactly what changes in the client's experience are necessary to accomplish a given outcome. It is based on the idea that people already have the resources they need in order to change. NLP helps clients match the appropriate response to the appropriate context.

COMPARATIVE ANALYSIS

General Themes

The alternative healing therapies discussed above represent a sampling of approaches to the transformation of the self. A summary of their characteristics is given in Table 25–1. Some of these, such as Living Love, are therapeutic applications of ancient Eastern religions. Others, such as transactional analysis and gestalt therapy, are accepted in many traditional psychiatric circles. Some of these new therapies are shallow and opportunistic and will not endure. Others are thoughtful and responsible attempts to deal with human problems. All reflect an important movement toward alternatives to traditional psychiatric theory.

A general theme common to most of these therapies is that socialization destroys the inherently effective functioning of people's lives and accounts for their unhappiness. Each therapy offers its particular explanation of this phenomenon. While their methods differ, all involve stripping away the false overlay of the defenses of the personality in order to reach the real self. Some therapies define the effects of socialization in terms of the traditional concept of the repression of painful experience. These therapies include Primal Scream and Rolfing. Ida Rolf tried to strip clients of their muscular compensations for past injuries in order

Table 25-1 ALTERNATIVE HEALING THERAPIES

Therapy	Name of Originator	Therapeutic Goals	Central Techniques
Body discipline and body-mind awareness therapies			
Primal scream	Arthur Janov	To release primal pain caused by early frustration of need to be loved	Producing emotional flooding by breaking down personality defenses
Rolfing or structural integration	Ida Rolf	To realign body with gravitational forces, opening up chronic muscle blocks, which prevent free functioning	Massage and manipulation of deep connective tissues; encouraging expression of feelings about body and related experiences
Bioenergetics	Alexander Lowen	To reintegrate body and mind	Stressor and releasor exercises; emotional catharsis
Gestalt	Frederick Perls	To resolve significant emotional experiences and increase ability to choose experience	Fantasy; role playing; emotional catharsis; group work; discussing dreams and body language
Therapeutic touch	Dolores Krieger	To rebalance body energies	Deliberate transfer of energy from healer to healee through touch
Orthomolecular nutrition	Linus Pauling	To provide for ingestion of optimal levels of nutrients	Diet counseling; megadoses of vitamins
Biofeedback	Originated from work of Neal E. Miller	To gain conscious control over some autonomic functions such as heart rate and blood pressure	Mechanical feedback while client attempts to control autonomic function
Psychological growth therapies			
Transactional analysis	Eric Berne	To improve social interaction; to increase self-esteem and ability for intimacy	Analyzing components of interaction to recognize and eliminate destructive forms
Encounter marathon	Fred Stoller, George Bach, William Schutz, Elizabeth Mintz	To increase ability for intense and honest communication	Nonverbal techniques; structured interpersonal exercises to break down personality defenses
Esalen encounter ("open encounter")	William Schutz	To break through self-deception in order to know and like the self	Nonverbal techniques and structured interpersonal exercises
Morita therapy	Masatake Morita	To relieve depression, obsessive fears, and acute anxiety	Period of stimulus deprivation followed by specific instructions to behave in a nonneurotic way
Reality therapy	William Glasser	To satisfy needs for self-esteem and love in a responsible way	Involvement with the therapist leads to ability to care for others, increased awareness of effectiveness and social acceptability of personal current behavior
Psychosynthesis	Roberto Assagioli	To arouse and develop the will	Exercises to sublimate sexual and aggressive energies into creative activities
Rational-emotive therapy	Albert Ellis	To eliminate irrational beliefs; to change specific behavior	Explaining irrational beliefs; positive reinforcement of effective behavior; group marathon encounters

Table continues on next page

Table 25–1 continued

Therapy	Name of Originator	Therapeutic Goals	Central Techniques
Assertiveness training	Robert Alberti, Michael Emmons, Sherwin Cotler, etc.	To decrease anxiety in social settings; to develop effective social skills	Role playing in group settings; teaching basic human rights and social skills
Sex therapy	William Masters, Virginia Johnson	To remove inhibitions that produce sexual problems such as impotence, premature ejaculation, and orgasmic dysfunction	Process of reconditioning during which couple engage in gradual and nonthreatening sexual encounters
Synanon: addiction group therapy	Charles Dederich	To eliminate destructive aspects of identity to enable client to stop using drugs	Direct attack on defensive behavior in peer group setting
Direct decision therapy	Harold Greenwald	To make a specific decision to change a behavior	Exploring life choices and alternatives for action
Psycho-imagination therapy	Joseph Shorr	To find true identity	Role playing in imaginative situation; exploring subjective reactions
Confrontation problem-solving therapy	Harry Garner	To reconstruct past and current erroneous perceptions; to increase social responsiveness	Confronting problems; fostering reality testing
Consciousness development therapies			
Arica	Oscar Ichazo	To recover the true self lost through socialization	Eclectic blend of meditation and body awareness techniques
Living Love	Kenneth Keyes	To develop higher consciousness; to rid the self of desires	Instruction about levels of consciousness; reprogramming by mental exercises
Erhard Seminar Training (est)	Werner Erhard	To liberate the self from the fallacies of logical thinking; to accept total responsibility for life	Lecture; mental exercises; testimonials
Transcendental Meditation	Maharishi Mahesh Yogi	To make contact with the creative intelligence underlying existence; to relieve specific problems	Lecture; instruction in use of mantra and meditation techniques
Silva Mind Control	José Silva	To achieve alpha consciousness, which makes possible harmony with inner processes and gives ability to diagnose illness and solve emotional problems	Relaxation training; hypnosis; techniques of sensory projection
Eriksonian hypnosis	Milton Erikson	To maximize behavioral potential and treat organic and psychological problems	Autohypnosis
Neurolinquistic Programming	Richard Bandler and John Grinder	Enable client to learn new patterns of behavior	Imitative learning; reframing; dissociation from problem situations

to reach the hidden level of pain and achieve catharsis. This is not much different in principle from the traditional psychotherapeutic approach of helping clients relax their psychological defenses so they can face difficult emotional truths that have been distorting experience.

Other therapies, such as est and Living Love, make the more radical claim that it is the very structure of the mind in Western culture that is the cause of humanity's difficulties. According to this viewpoint, the programming of the culture, which becomes dominant in early childhood, takes over our perceptual apparatus and blinds us to the natural process that is the true source of our being. The disadvantages of urban-industrial culture, such as loneliness and alienation, are cited as illustrations of the limitations of socially acquired consciousness. Our defenses against emotional problems manifest themselves in different ways. According to structural integration, they are expressed in body tensions and distortions of posture. Gestalt therapy emphasizes the gaps in our experience of reality and the way we confuse our own feelings with the feelings of others because we cannot take the responsibility for our own experience. For estians, the analytical, logical intelligence is the frightened mind's defense against the unpredictability of the real world.

In yet other therapies, such as Arica, the ego itself is seen as a necessary but temporary phase in the evolution of consciousness. These therapies are based on the belief that the ego was once important in integrating individual experience, but that it has now become a handicap because it creates an artificial division between external and internal life. The next step in evolution will result in the freeing of the self from the prison of the ego and the attainment of the real self, which is one with the universe. The real self exists in an entirely different system in a space, beyond any particular concept or point of view. Problems are no longer areas to be worked on but are lived out effortlessly as we flow with the stream of life. The painfulness of desire is overcome once we recognize that since we are unified with all that exists, there is nothing to want.

The Therapeutic Problem

The therapeutic problem is to strip away or change the behavior structure to allow the natural life force to reassume control. The alternative healing therapies use a variety of procedures to achieve this. These procedures fall into four general categories of therapeutic approach.

Affective Education   The first approach sees therapy as *affective education*. Affective education breaks down the verbal and cerebral monopoly over the personality to allow the capacity for feeling to emerge. This is difficult in a society that punishes the expression of certain emotions and rewards conformity and role playing. Primal scream therapy seeks to unfreeze the anesthetized feelings that predominate in American culture. It emphasizes specific painful feelings toward significant others that have been repressed in childhood. This approach assumes that unfreezing feelings enables the individual to be fully alive in the present.

Living in the Present Moment   The second approach teaches clients to experience the present fully. It encourages them to be aware of and to overcome current emotional blocks, in order to lead more effective and enjoyable lives. Emotions are reshaped by focusing on interactions in the here and now. This approach is used in gestalt therapy, bioenergetics, psychosynthesis, psycho-imagination therapy, and encounter groups. These therapies consider the past to be unimportant, since it cannot be changed. Only feelings and immediate personal experience are thought to be valid, and the more intense the feeling or experience, the more therapeutic its expression is assumed to be.

Different therapies view this direct and personal experience in different ways. Bioenergetics emphasizes the experience of the truth of the body that occurs when clients are aware of bodily movement, impulses, and restraints. Encounter groups emphasize the experience of feelings in current interpersonal settings rather than through bodily sensations. The basic idea is that clients can develop an awareness of experience by increasing their awareness of other people's feelings.

Problem Solving   The third approach focuses on the problem-solving or life-coping processes rather than on individual emotional reactions. The major assumption of this approach is that a person who learns to think realistically and to handle problems effectively will be able to disregard or eliminate self-defeating emotions. This is the opposite assumption from that taken by the first two methodologies discussed, which claim that self-defeating emotions should be eliminated first, and then the individual will be able to live more effectively. The group of therapists who emphasize problem solving stress effective, rational behavior rather than the expression of emotions. Transactional analysis, reality therapy, and rational-emotive therapy all use this approach.

Each therapy has its own idea of what interferes with the problem-solving process. The rational-emotive therapists blame irrationality and unrealistic expectations. The reality therapists blame socially irresponsible behavior. Transactional analysis therapists believe that people make conscious life plans or *scripts* in childhood or early adolescence. These scripts make the rest of their lives predictable. Because scripts are based on consciously willed decisions, they can be revoked by similarly willed decisions. Although emotional insights are considered in this group of therapies, the focus is on intellectual understanding.

Generally these therapies also involve a contract between the therapist and the client. This contract preserves the client's self-determination. It also demonstrates that clients play an active role in decision-making about their own lives. These therapies assume that when clients make a decision to change based on accurate information about their situation, they will be able to change.

Transcendence into Higher Forms of Consciousness
The fourth approach does not teach clients to express emotion or to solve problems but to transcend the human condition. These therapies are meant as a means of evolutionary progression into higher forms of consciousness. Therapists concerned with transcendence conceive of human beings as unfinished and unable to realize themselves in the restricting circumstances of the world. They urge people to reclaim the human potential they have sacrificed in their scramble to control and develop the natural world. Some of these therapies are hybrids of Western psychology and Eastern religions. Others are eclectic blends of religious traditions. The introspective and visionary qualities of this group of therapies, which includes Arica, TM, and Living Love, represent attempts to go beyond the diminished human image produced by the past two centuries of industrialism. In the view of their proponents, modern psychology has underestimated human beings. In emphasizing their animal nature, it has denied their spiritual potential.

The goal of these disciplines is to release people from the suffering that the lower level of consciousness produces. They are not concerned with why people suffer or with their feelings about suffering, but only with how that suffering can be relieved. The way out of suffering is to recognize that the satisfaction of desire does not produce happiness. Transcendental Medi-

tation uses the mind's natural tendency to "wander in the search of happiness" to turn attention away from external objects and events to the inner source of true bliss.

RELEVANCE FOR PSYCHIATRIC NURSING

The Shift from the Medical Model to a Social Model

The growing variety and popularity of alternative therapies represents an important shift away from the medical and psychoanalytic models. These changes are affecting the context of psychiatric nursing theory and practice. Currently, the roles of therapist and client are structured according to the medical model. In this model, the physician determines the nature of the disease, which is presumed to have been produced by natural causes. Treatment and prognosis are specific to the diagnosis. Physicians treat clients and leave them under the care of the nurse. The client's role entails certain rights and duties. Clients are relieved of normal social responsibilities, are not blamed for their condition, and are entitled to special care. The client's duties are to seek help, to cooperate fully with that help, and to try to get well. The medical model is discontinuous, since it specifies a partial rather than a total view of the problem of emotional disturbance. It has only two goals: to treat the client and at the same time to accumulate medical knowledge.

The psychoanalytic model is continuous, since it attempts to explain the entire dynamic of a client's life. Psychoanalytic practice deals with the lifelong continuum of emotional problems. It stresses an etiology learned through the reconstruction of the client's past. The hidden forces that control the client's life can be understood only by an expert. The client has the right to compassion and the right not to be judged. As in the medical model, the client is expected to cooperate with therapy. There are important differences between the medical and psychoanalytic models, notably with respect to goals. The goal of the psychoanalytic model is broader: increased self-understanding rather than treatment of a specific disease (see Chapter 2).

Although the new therapies borrow elements from the medical and psychoanalytic models, they represent a general shift in the direction of a social model. The social model defines emotional difficulties as symptoms of a sick society. Treatment should consist of improving social conditions and can be carried out by a variety of people. Though the new therapies use parts of the social model, it is important to note that they use the model only to *define* the problem. In their formulation, the damaging effects of the culture are worked out only with respect to individual clients or small groups. None of these models offers a program for social change. It is assumed that once individuals change, a healthy culture will follow.

Evidence of the shift to a social model has already been observed in changes from institutional to community treatment settings; in the increasing acceptability of paraprofessionals as counselors; in the gradual replacement of the extended psychoanalytic model by briefer therapies; and in the growing tendency to treat families and groups rather than individuals (see Chapters 18 and 21). Therapies in which the removal of symptoms is an acceptable goal are increasing in prestige. Areas once considered mystical rather than scientific, such as meditation and hypnosis, are viewed with more respect. In general, mental health professions have become more aware of the various social, biological, and environmental factors that influence behavior. As the alternative therapies continue to proliferate, the medical model will be further undermined, and with it the assumption that only physicians can treat emotional difficulties.

Frameworks for Assessing the New Therapies

In order to take advantage of the opportunities for theoretical development and practice offered by the alternative healing therapies, the nurse must understand their social and psychological implications. Current opinion varies with respect to these therapies. Some see them as a profound regression, others as the forerunners of a consciousness revolution. The truth probably lies somewhere in between, and the nurse must be able to think through the various arguments carefully.

Criticism of Their Clientele   The clientele of the new therapies have been categorized as socially deprived, both of material commodities and of interpersonal gratification. Critics of the new therapies think that these people seek therapy because their lack of inner resources evokes a craving for social contact. Critics see the new therapies as repressive and inspirational approaches that fail to cure their clients' alien-ation because the goals of therapy are vaguely defined, and because their therapeutic techniques allow the release of hidden pathology that cannot be discussed and resolved. At their most harmless, these therapies serve as sheltered workshops for the socially inept.

Criticism of Their Therapeutic Techniques   According to critics, techniques that facilitate learning by emphasizing intense personal experience encourage the direct gratification of aggressive, sexual, and dependency wishes. This regression is masked by claims that it represents honesty and love. The physical contact in nonverbal exercises stimulates a superficial sense of intimacy with strangers, thus reactivating early experiences of maternal physical contact. This facilitates the acting out of infantile wishes without providing any insight into their origins. Experiences in the new therapy programs may have negative effects, particularly when the programs are conducted by inadequately trained leaders. While these groups may offer adventures for the emotionally jaded, they are dangerous for the seriously disturbed. People in real need of psychiatric treatment are deluded into denying the seriousness of their problems and are led to believe they can get help without the intervention of a professional. The concept of sickness is trivialized. New therapies teach clients that although everyone is sick, most people are not *very* sick. Clients are encouraged to seek ways to be happy with a minimum of effort and responsibility. Irrational solutions are fostered. So is intimate contact without the responsibilities of commitment.

A major focus of the new therapies is an exorcism of the superego. Inhibitions related to early problems in excretory and sexual development are attacked. This is particularly dangerous, because it mobilizes primitive drives that years of socialization have sought to suppress. Though the group can offer superficial support during the collapse of ego defenses, it cannot, being impermanent itself, offer a new social network to support the release of impulses. The new therapies are no more than radical and potentially dangerous experiments with feeling and behavior.

For those who, like Charles Fair (1970), view the self as the result of an arduous effort to gain control over primary process thinking, the antirationality of the new therapies represents a profound regression in ego capacity. Fair views the development of cognitive abilities that enable people to control their basic primitive reactiveness to stimuli as *the* significant step in achieving humanness. This control allows for flexible thought and action and enlarges the capacity for self-possession and planning. The self must be developed—it cannot be merely released, as the new therapies claim. Fair views the new therapies as a withdrawal from the responsibilities of adult existence and a return to a childlike state of omnipotence.

Criticism of Their Asocial Nature

Other critics feel that the new therapies may eventually destroy the culture. These critics point out that clients of the new therapies are urged to be concerned only with their own development and standards. They are told that no one is responsible for their lives but themselves. This viewpoint demonstrates a profound ignorance of the reciprocity between the self and the world. Personality is developed and maintained through one's relationships and activities in the world. The new therapies represent a trend toward narcissism and a denial of community and history. The consciousness-awakening movement in particular is an attempt to replace social institutions with the self. Its radical egotistic approach undermines the validity of interpersonal relationships.

Robert Lifton (1969) defines the "protean life style" of today as a continuous series of experiments with life in which new experience itself is the primary value. This produces people with undeveloped characters and little internalization of morals, people who define themselves only in terms of their roles in various social encounters. This life-style is directly destructive to the major function of the culture, which is to make the world consistent and meaningful. Doctrines that emphasize the release of feelings and impulses also disorganize the culture, since they destroy the necessity for any general rules about behavior. According to Phillip Reiff (1968), the purpose of the new therapies is simply the destruction of order.

Reiff believes that these therapies pander to the need for self-preservation in an era of instability by promising quick peace of mind and a sense of purpose. They naively assume that human nature is innately pleasant. This romantic idealization assumes that there is a normal condition in which people become happy and good simply by being true to their nature. This viewpoint completely ignores the tremendous influence of history and culture on the individual.

Criticism of Superficial Interpersonal Styles

The democratization of psychotherapy has resulted in what R. D. Rosen (1975) calls a proliferation of "psychobabble," or self-revelations couched in psychological language. "Get in touch with your feelings," "Be

yourself," and "Connect with others" are all examples of psychobabble. These stereotyped phrases seem on the surface to reflect a concern with insight into the self and honest communication with others. But discussing our personal lives with near-strangers is becoming a common social pattern, and new acquaintances may quickly find themselves talking not about work and hobbies but about their own alcoholism and impotence. However, much of this supposedly personal communication is stereotyped conversation that actually prevents real spontaneity and candor. People reveal the most private facts about themselves, but this type of interaction is only behavior meant to signal that they are "with it." It does not appease the real need for self-disclosure, because the intimate facts are separated from feelings. These people are not really revealing anything personal. In a sense, psychobabble can be seen as a way of manipulating others by demonstrating that they have positive social value and are a safe people to relate to. These superficial interpersonal styles are dangerous, because they blunt the impact of our deepest feelings and needs.

Extravagant Claims for the New Therapies

Extravagant claims for the new therapies are typified by Theodore Roszak's (1977) statement that they signal the dawning of an "Age of Aquarius." Roszak feels that a transformation of human personality of evolutionary proportions has begun. Meditation and the spiritual disciplines of the new therapies are rituals of rebirth, ways of purifying ourselves of the past so that we can achieve our true identity. Roszak thinks people will recognize their infinite potential when they understand their lives as a succession of experimental identities that change as self-knowledge increases. In the Age of Aquarius, a community of people striving for mutual enlightenment will replace the ineffective institutions of family and professions.

Effectiveness of the New Therapies

Other, more tentative, affirmations of the new therapies suggest that their rapid rise indicates the emergence of a new type of client in American society—a client with whom individual psychotherapy cannot cope. The isolation and conformity necessary in an industrialized society have produced a generation of lonely and passive people who cannot specifically formulate their problems but instead express a general sense of discontent. Traditional therapies often fail with this type of client because they are too structured to appeal to people who already feel severely restricted by society's conventions. The importance of getting in touch with feelings rather than intellectualizing about behavior appeals to alienated people who have difficulty relating to their emotions. Contemporary people who are characterized by a sense of powerlessness look to the therapist to give them direction and strength—and indeed, to formulate their problems.

The new therapies fill an important role in meeting the needs of this type of person. They provide opportunities for self-expression and the sharing of experience that contemporary society cannot offer. Groups in particular provide a sense of community in a society where relationships are fragmentary. The rapid intervention these therapies provide is also crucial in a fragmented and mobile society. Nonverbal techniques make unnecessary the often long and tedious process of talking things out. In a society in which the range of allowable physical contacts has been narrowed to a sexual context, they also meet an important need for the expression of nonsexual physical affection. Other techniques, such as meditation, may deal effectively with the stimulus overload of an intrusive technical world. Meditation develops the capacity to turn off responses to external signals in order to attend to the threatened inner life. This, too, is an important need.

Supporters of the new therapies point out that the domination of psychoanalysis has finally come to an end with the growth of a generation who does not feel the need to analyze the past. In any case, only a privileged few can afford the time and money required for this type of treatment. People who would like help with their problems find the new therapies more accessible. These therapies also offer a greater choice of structure and method and so can be more individualized. For example, some emotionally confused people cannot deal with problem-solving methodologies. Emotional reshaping may be more beneficial for this type of client. Others might find their emotional confusion increased by this technique. They would be more responsive to explicit instructions on how to form effective coping patterns. Repressed, well-controlled people would benefit most from therapy that enabled them to express their feelings. People who are well adjusted to the culture; but who wish to expand the limits of their experience, might prefer a growth-oriented encounter therapy.

The new therapies can also contribute to traditional psychotherapies. Traditional psychotherapies can adopt verbal and meditation techniques to facilitate long-term, verbally oriented therapy. The influence of the new therapies on traditional practice will result in a de-emphasis of past experience and new emphasis on the present. This is necessary to shorten the time required for therapy. Techniques that are primarily verbal will be used less often and will be replaced by more active techniques. These changes will enable traditional psychotherapists to be more flexible in dealing with various client problems.

Applying the New Therapies to Psychiatric Nursing Practice

The development of the alternative healing therapies offers several options for psychiatric nursing. Nurses can experiment with alternative healing therapies and examine ways of using some of these methodologies, as Dolores Krieger has done in therapeutic touch. Nurses can also incorporate procedures from the new therapies into their own practice—for example, teaching breathing and other relaxation exercises to clients. Techniques of abreaction or encounter can be used to supplement nursing practice if the therapist has gone through the training for these specific methodologies.

The change from conventional medicine to holistic medicine represented by the new therapies parallels changes in nursing's approach to health problems. The content of these therapies can be usefully incorporated into our thinking about holistic health. This holistic approach offers a greater range of practice for the nurse as the focus of responsibility shifts from the physician to a more equal partnership with the client and other health professionals. As clients seek more autonomy in health care, their changing needs will alter the practice of medicine and nursing. As consumers demand a holistic approach to health, the medical model will be increasingly seen as deficient in regard to: ethics; human relationships; and the interaction between body, mind, and environment—approaches that nursing has traditionally emphasized.

The new therapies highlight the importance of the connection between state of mind and state of health. As nurses become more sensitive to the effects of stressful emotion on the body and the subtle ways in which illness expresses emotional problems, we can develop more specific ways of preventing illness. The new therapies offer a concept of therapy as aiding natural healing processes, in which symptoms are not simply to be eliminated but studied as messages about the underlying distress of the client. An increasing emphasis on noninvasive techniques will prevent iatrogenic or physician-caused illness, such as the side effects of drugs and the debilitating influence of institutionalization, and will also give more opportunity to nurses to practice interpersonal interventions.

KEY NURSING CONCEPTS

✔ The new therapies challenge traditional psychiatry to diversify its mode of practice. They represent a shift away from the treatment of symptoms toward the general improvement of mental health.

✔ Alternative healing therapies emphasize intuitive and subjective experience. They can be viewed as a revolt against the scientific and materialistic aspects of American culture and provide low-cost, short-term alternatives to traditional psychotherapy.

✔ The new therapies offer an important means of exploring and questioning traditional psychiatric practice.

✔ Alternative healing therapies are numerous and diverse in their approach to emotional health. However, a general theme common to most new therapies is that socialization destroys the inherent effective functioning of people's lives and accounts for their suffering.

✔ Basic themes of the alternative therapies include emphasis on discovery of the real, subjective self by overcoming logical thinking; closer integration and functioning of the mind and body; and assumption of responsibility for one's life.

✔ A central belief inherent in the alternative therapies is that traditional therapy modes err by overemphasizing rationality, deemphasizing the body, concentrating on verbal methods of therapy, and conferring prestige and mystery that robs people of their capacity to deal with their own problems.

✔ For purposes of classification, alternative healing therapies may be divided into three groups: body–mind awareness therapies, psychological growth therapies, and consciousness development therapies built around spiritual development and the attainment of altered consciousness.

✔ The therapeutic problem for alternative healing therapies is to strip away or change the behavior structure to allow the natural life force to reassume control.

✔ Many of the new therapies' methods—such as abreaction, massage, exercise, meditation, role playing, lecture, encounter, and problem solving—emphasize overcoming faulty socialization, which they believe curtails the individual's view of life.

✔ Critics of the new therapies believe that clients risk uncovering emotional problems without adequate emotional support for working them through; that the therapies reinforce acting out a person's desires without recognizing social responsibilities; and that the techniques encourage superficial social relationships.

✔ Supporters of the new therapies believe that their diversity opens them to clients who cannot relate to more traditional therapy; that they offer a sense of community that traditional psychiatric treatment does not; and that they represent an evolutionary change to a more complete, holistic form of consciousness.

✔ The psychiatric nurse may use techniques of the alternative therapies to supplement nursing practice.

References

Applebaum, S. *Out in Inner Space: A Psychoanalyst Explores The New Therapies.* New York: Anchor Press, 1979.

Assagioli, R. *Psychosynthesis.* New York: Viking Press, 1971.

Bandler, R., and Grinder, J. *Frogs Into Princes: Neurolinguistic Programming.* Moab, Utah: Real People Press, 1979.

————. *Patterns of the Hypnotic Techniques of Milton H. Erikson.* Vol. I. Cupertino, Calif.: Meta Publications, 1975.

Berne, E. *Transactional Analysis in Psychotherapy.* New York: Grove Press, 1961.

————. *Games People Play.* New York: Grove Press, 1964.

————. *What Do You Say After You Say Hello?* New York: Grove Press, 1972.

Castaneda, C. *The Teachings of Don Juan: A Yaqui Way of Knowledge.* New York: Ballantine Books, 1968.

Ellis, A., and Harper, R. A. *A New Guide to Rational Living.* Englewood Cliffs, N.J.: Prentice-Hall, 1975.

Endore, G. *Synanon.* New York: Doubleday, 1968.

Fair, C. *The Dying Self.* New York: Doubleday Anchor Books, 1970.

Garner, H. H. *Psychotherapy and the Confrontation Problem-solving Technique.* St. Louis: Warren Green II, 1971.

Glasser, W. *Reality Therapy.* New York: Harper and Row, 1965.

Greenwald, H. *Decision Therapy.* New York: Wyden Books, 1973.

Hoffer, A., and Osmund, H. *How To Live with Schizophrenia.* New York: University Books, 1966.

Hoffer, A. and Walker, M. *Orthomolecular Nutrition.* New Canaan, Conn.: Keats Publishing, 1978.

Ichazo, O. *The Human Process for Enlightenment and Freedom.* New York: Simon and Schuster, 1977.

Janov, A. *The Primal Scream.* New York: G. P. Putnam, 1970.

Johnson, D. *The Protean Body.* New York: Harper and Row, 1977.

Keyes, K. *Handbook to Higher Consciousness.* 5th ed. St. Mary, Ky.: Living Love Consciousness Center, 1977.

Kora, T. "Morita Therapy." *International Journal of Psychiatry* 1 (1965): 611–645.

Kreiger, D. *The Therapeutic Touch.* Englewood Cliffs, N.J.: Prentice-Hall, 1979.

Lifton, R. *Boundaries.* New York: Simon and Schuster, 1969.

Liss, J. *Free to Feel.* New York: Praeger Publishers, 1974.

London, P. "The Psychology Boom." *Psychology Today,* June 1974, pp. 62–70.

Lowen, A. *The Betrayal of the Body.* New York: Macmillan, 1967.

————. *Depression and the Body.* Baltimore: Penguin Books, 1972.

Masters, W. F., and Johnson, V. E. *Human Sexual Response.* Boston: Little, Brown, 1966.

Perls, F. *The Gestalt Approach.* Palo Alto, Calif.: Science and Behavior Books, 1970.

————. *The Gestalt Therapy Book.* New York: Julian Press, 1973.

Porter, D., and Taxson, D. *The Est Experience.* New York: Aware Books, 1976.

Reiff, P. *The Triumph of the Therapeutic.* New York: Harper and Row, 1968.

Rolf, I. *Rolfing: The Structural Integration of Human Structure.* Boulder, Colo.: Rolf Institute, 1977.

Rosen, R. D. "Psychobabble." *New Times,* October 31, 1975, pp. 44–49.

Roszak, T. *Unfinished Animal.* New York: Harper and Row, 1977.

Schutz, W. *Joy: Expanding Human Awareness.* New York: Grove Press, 1967.

Shorr, J. *Psycho-Imagination Therapy.* New York: Intercontinental Medical Book, 1972.

Silva, J., and Miele, P. *The Silva Mind Control Method.* New York: Simon and Schuster, 1977.

Yablonsky, L. "Synanon." In *Direct Psychotherapy,* vol. 2, edited by R. R. M. Jurjevich. Coral Gables, Fla.: University of Miami Press, 1973.

Yogi, M. M. *The Science of Being and the Art of Living.* New York: Signet Books, 1963.

Further Reading

Abell, R. *Own Your Own Life.* New York: Bantam Books, 1976.

Alberti, R. E., and Emmons, M. L. *Your Perfect Right: A Guide to Assertive Behavior.* 2d ed. San Luis Obispo, Calif.: Impact Publishers, 1974.

Assagioli, R. *The Act of Will.* Baltimore: Penguin Books, 1974.

Back, K. *Beyond Words.* New York: Russell Sage Foundation, 1972.

Binder, V.; Binder, A.; and Rimland, B. *Modern Therapies.* Englewood Cliffs, N.J.: Prentice-Hall, 1976.

Bloomfield, H.; Cain, M.; Jaffe, P.; and Kory, R. *T.M.: Discovering Inner Energy and Overcoming Stress.* New York: Delacorte Press, 1975.

Casriel, D. *A Scream Away from Happiness.* New York: Grosset and Dunlap, 1972.

Cheraskin, E.; Ringsdorf, W. M.; and Brecher, A. *Psychodietetics.* New York: Bantam Books, 1976.

Downing, G. *Massage and Meditation.* New York: Random House, 1974.

Dychtwald, K. *Body–Mind.* New York: Pantheon Books, 1977.

Fenwich, S. *Getting It: The Psychology of Est.* New York: J. B. Lippincott, 1976.

Ferguson, M. *The Aquarian Conspiracy.* Los Angeles: J. P. Tarcher, 1980.

Frederick, C. *Est: Playing the Game the New Way.* New York: Dell Publishing, 1974.

Garfield, C., ed. *Rediscovery of the Body*. New York: Dell Publishing, 1977.

Glasser, W. *The Identity Society*. New York: Harper and Row, 1972.

————. *Positive Addiction*. New York: Harper and Row, 1976.

Goldberg, P. *The T.M. Program: The Way to Fulfillment*. New York: Holt, Rinehart and Winston, 1976.

Hampden-Turner, C. *Radical Man: The Process of Psychosocial Development*. New York: Doubleday Anchor Books, 1971.

Harper, R. *The New Psychotherapies*. Englewood Cliffs, N.J.: Prentice-Hall, 1975.

Harris, T. *I'm O.K.—You're O.K.* New York: Harper and Row, 1969.

Hart, J.; Corrieri, R.; and Binder, J. *Going Sane*. New York: Jason Aronson, 1975.

Howard, J. *Please Touch*. New York: McGraw-Hill, 1970.

Hunter, R. *The Storming of the Mind: Inside the Consciousness Revolution*. New York: Doubleday Anchor Books, 1972.

James, M., and Jongeward, D. *Born to Win*. Reading, Mass.: Addison-Wesley, 1971.

Janov, A. *The Anatomy of Mental Illness*. New York: G. P. Putnam, 1971.

————. *The Primal Revolution*. New York: Simon and Schuster, 1972.

Jonas, G. *Visceral Learning*. New York: Cornerstone Library, 1974.

Jones, F. *Body Awareness: A Study of the Alexander Technique in Action*. New York: Schocken Books, 1976.

Lankton, S. R. *Practical Magic: The Clinical Applications of Neurolinguistic Programming*. Cupertino, Calif.: Meta Publications, 1979.

Lowen, A., and Lowen, L. *The Way to Vibrant Health: A Manual of Bioenergetic Exercises*. New York: Harper and Row, 1977.

Maisel, E. *The Resurrection of the Body*. New York: Delta Books, 1974.

Masters, W. F., and Johnson, V. E. *Human Sexual Inadequacy*. Boston: Little, Brown, 1970.

Maultsby, M. C. *Help Yourself to Happiness*. Boston: Esplanade Publishers; New York: Institute for Rational Living, 1975.

Namikoshi, T. *Shaitsu Therapy: Theory and Practice*. Tokyo: Japan Publishers, 1974.

Needleman, J. *The New Religions*. New York: Pocket Books, 1974.

Newbold, H. L. *Mega-Nutrients for Your Nerves*, New York: Peter H. Wyden, 1975.

Olson, P. *Emotional Flooding*. Vol. 1. *New Directions in Psychotherapy*. New York: Human Sciences Press, 1976.

Ornstein, R. *The Psychology of Consciousness*. New York: Viking Press, 1972.

Perls, F. *Gestalt Therapy Verbatim*. Moab, Utah: Real People Press, 1967.

————. *Ego, Hunger, and Aggression*. New York: Vintage Books, 1969.

Phelps, S., and Austin, N. *The Assertive Woman*. San Luis Obispo, Calif.: Impact Publishers, 1975.

Rogers, C. *Carl Rogers on Encounter Groups*. New York: Harper and Row, 1970.

Rossi, E. L., ed. *The Collected Papers of Milton Erikson on Hypnosis in Four Volumes*. New York: John Wiley, 1980.

Roszak, T. *The Making of a Counterculture*. New York: Doubleday, 1968.

Ruitenbeek, H. *The New Group Therapies*. New York: Avon Books, 1970.

Tart, C., ed. *Transpersonal Psychologies*. New York: Harper and Row, 1977.

Torrey, E. F. *The Mind-Game*. New York: Emerson Hale, 1972.

Williams, R., and Kalita, D., eds. *A Physicians Handbook on Orthomolecular Medicine*. Elmsford, N.Y.: Pergamon Press, 1977.

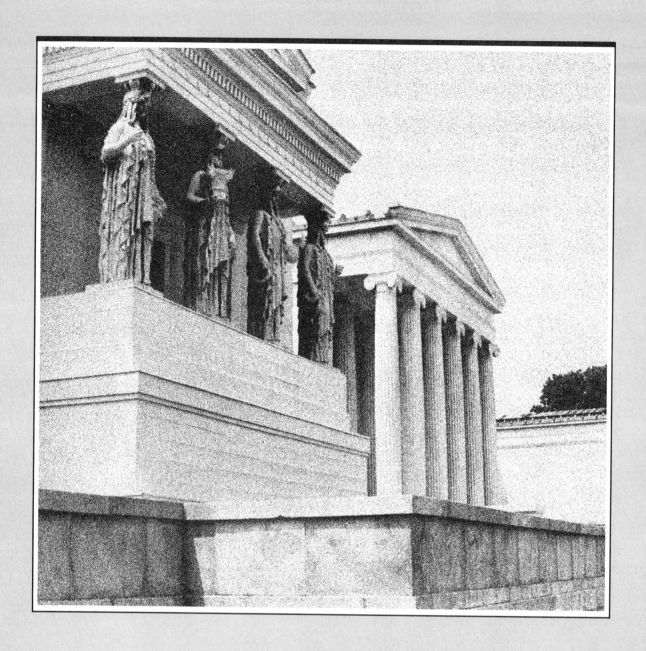

PART SIX

Social, Political, Cultural, and Economic Issues

THIS SECTION OF THE BOOK *brings together topics that have several commonalities. These topics expand the psychiatric nurse's scope of practice beyond the one-to-one relationship that has been its hallmark for decades. They require a knowledge base in politics, law, anthropology, and economics that only recently has become germane to nursing curricula. They reflect a philosophical perspective that considers the social context of psychiatric careers—both the client's and the psychiatric professional's.*

When psychiatric nursing emphasized the one-to-one relationship, becoming an expert clinician was a paramount goal. In contemporary society, an expert clinician also needs to be an astute politician, and sometimes even a diplomat, to be effective. Chapters 26, 27, and 28 are devoted to cultural considerations (including folk healing practices), legal and political issues, and a contemporary critique of the community mental health movement. These topics enable nursing students or practitioners to comprehend their role in the larger picture of the health care delivery system.

In planning care for clients, contemporary psychiatric nurses must take into account the multiplicity of human problems, their complexity, and their interrelationships. In this final section, we assist the practitioner to make sense of the complexities encountered when practice is moved outside the protective walls of the hospital, when nurses expand their professional role within the hospital, when old definitions of "illness" and "abnormality" are reconsidered, and when mental health problems are viewed as social and cultural as well as psychological and biochemical. In a changing field, this knowledge base is needed to foster the respect, caring, vision, and hope that characterize the professional nurse.

26

The Cultural Context of Psychiatric Nursing Practice

CHAPTER OUTLINE

Relevance of Culture for Psychiatric Nursing Practice

The Assumptive World

When Assumptive Worlds Differ

Cultural Complexity and Diversity

Dangers in Cultural Stereotyping

The YAVIS Syndrome in Mental Health Care

Biosocial Factors Influencing Diagnosis and Treatment

Ethnicity

Socioeconomic Class

Religious Beliefs

Age

Place of Residence

Sex and Marital Status

Analysis of Biosocial Factors

Oppression

Contemporary Sociopolitical Influences on Mental Health Care

The Feminist Movement

The Gay Rights Movement

The Gray Panther Movement

Religious Cults

Folk Beliefs and Healing Practices

The Folk Systems of Black Americans

The Folk Systems of Hispanic Americans

The Folk Systems of Asian Americans

The Folk Systems of American Indians

Culturally Aware Strategies for Nursing Intervention

Understanding Your Own Sociocultural Heritage

Incorporating Principles of Effective Communication

Becoming Familiar with and Using Folk Beliefs and Healing Practices

Using Counseling Techniques Specific to the Client's Distress

Key Nursing Concepts

LEARNING OBJECTIVES

After reading this chapter, students should be able to

- Demonstrate awareness of the relevance of sociocultural factors in psychiatric nursing practice

- Identify the inherent dangers in sociocultural stereotyping

- Discuss biosocial and sociopolitical forces that influence mental health

- Comprehend folk beliefs and healing practices and incorporate them in nursing care

- Analyze their own sociocultural heritage and its effect on the nurse–client relationship

- Develop culturally aware strategies for nursing intervention

CHAPTER 26

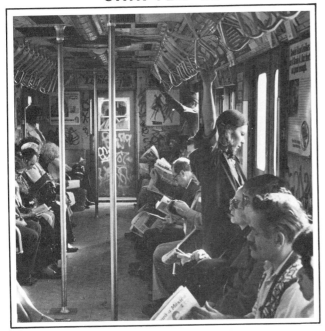

The 7,000 fans filing into the auditorium wear denim, big zippers, and black leather. Dave D. drove from his home 125 miles away from this decaying city to see and hear the Black Sabbath rock group in concert. "They're my favorite group," says Dave, "demonist, raunchy, drugs, sex, rock 'n roll. You know, heavy metal." He stands outside the auditorium in his Black Sabbath T-shirt with the skull and crossbones decal, crushing beer cans as fast as he drains them. Once in the auditorium the agitated crowd goes wild, flicking butane lighters in the air, waving black crosses, and jumping up and down. When the members of Black Sabbath form the symbol of devil horns with their fingers, their screaming fans return the signal. A security officer stationed in the corridor looks at the crowd, shakes his head, and rolls his eyes skyward. "It's going to be a fun night," he says.

In a remote Eskimo village, a thirty-four-year-old woman sits quietly, seemingly preoccupied with her own thoughts, in a trancelike state. Suddenly she leaps to her feet, throwing objects at the wall and heaping verbal abuse on her husband. His attempts to calm her do not work, and when he attempts to restrain her physically, she wrests herself from his grasp, tears off her clothing, and runs screaming out into the snow. Hearing her shrieks most of the adults of the village run after her across the snowfields. Although she initially outdistances them, she begins to tire, and the villagers finally catch up with her as she drops exhausted into the snow. They carry her back to her home where she falls into a deep

Subway riders in New York City may have little in common. Intervening humanistically with clients who hold different assumptive world views is a complex task for the psychiatric nurse.

sleep. When she awakens she recalls nothing of the episode. The people of the village are not surprised by her behavior. Pibloqtok *can happen to anyone. No treatment is necessary; on awakening the next day the person behaves as usual.*

On a busy downtown street walks a shy, introverted young Southeast Asian refugee, who has just been fired from his job as a restaurant dishwasher. The job was hard to come by in the first place, and now he and his family are faced with the discouraging prospect of trying to feed six people on the few dollars that remain from his last paycheck. At a crowded intersection the young man suddenly pulls a knife and begins to slash wildly at the startled people around him. He appears to be in a murderous rage and struggles with great strength, despite his small frame, against several people who are attempting to restrain and disarm him. A passing police cruiser picks him up and takes him to the police station. However, by this time he seems to be in a deep depression and fails to respond to their questions. The police take him to the community mental health center, where he is admitted to the inpatient unit and treated for depression. In Southeast Asia he would have been known as a victim of amok, *the condition on which the phrase "run amok" is based.*

RELEVANCE OF CULTURE FOR PSYCHIATRIC NURSING PRACTICE

The behavior of the Black Sabbath fans, the Eskimo woman, and the Southeast Asian refugee has deep meaning for them and for others interacting with them. For the working class fans attending the Black Sabbath concert it was "a chance to get blown away before going back to work tomorrow morning," a chance to party. For the police officer it was a night to ride herd on an unruly crowd who seemed bent on destroying themselves and one another with drugs, drinking, and sex. Some American mental health professionals might loosely (and consequently unreliably and probably invalidly) diagnose it a large-scale demonstration of Antisocial Personality Disorder.

In the Eskimo village, the hysterics of *pibloqtok* are a culturally sanctioned release in a society that stresses conformity and repression. In Western society, we might label the Eskimo woman as hysterical, sexually repressed, or acting out. In American psychiatric terminology she might be said to be suffering from a Dissociative Disorder.

In the sixteenth century in Southeast Asia, *amok* referred to the behavior of brave fighters who chose to die in battle rather than lose. Those who ran amok fighting colonial oppression were honored and treated with respect. Although no longer socially acceptable, the cultural tradition remains, and maladjusted persons who have been humiliated still occasionally run amok, although episodes of amok are becoming less frequent. Outdated diagnostic practices in psychiatry might have led to a diagnosis of paranoid schizophrenia, or manic-depressive psychosis in the pre-DSM-III days.

The commonality of these three case studies is that in all of them the culture has an idea of what insanity *should* be, and of the meaning of the behavior of its members. Culture shapes the very way we conceive of illness. Culture determines not only who is labeled mentally ill and under what circumstances (see Chapters 2, 5, and 10), but also the nature of the treatment and the identity of the helper. Therefore, a humanistic position in psychiatric nursing care must take account of culture and its influence on both client and nurse. This chapter pinpoints the relevance of culture for psychiatric nursing practice, discusses cultural complexity and diversity, biosocial factors and sociopolitical forces influencing mental health, oppression in contemporary society, folk beliefs and healing practices, the importance of cultural self-analysis for caregivers, culturally aware strategies for nursing intervention, and oppression counseling, blending insights from nursing, anthropology, sociology, and social psychology. It also explores the ways in which culture influences the perception, classification, process of labeling, explanation, symptoms, and treatment of what is called mental illness.

The Assumptive World

In order to make sense out of the world in which we live, we develop a set of assumptions based on our experiences. We use these assumptions to predict how others are likely to behave and what the effects of our own actions are likely to be. This set of assumptions has been termed the *assumptive world*, which is "a highly structured, complex, interacting set of values, expectations, and images of oneself and others, which guide and in turn are guided by a person's perceptions and behavior and which are closely related to his emotional states and his feelings of well-being" (Frank 1974, pp. 20–21). From all the stimuli reaching them, members of a culture select those that fit best with their assumptive worlds. It is reminiscent of the process of selective inattention described in Chapter 14.

People are not always clearly aware of their assumptions. For example, a nursing student may be aware of his assumptions about increased federal spending for defense, but unaware of his assumption that he views manipulation of others as the only means available to achieve success. The latter is probably more enduring and held with greater conviction because it is more intimately related to the nurse's sense of self-worth and feelings of well-being. The assumptive view about defense spending is more easily changed because it is influenced more by facts and logic. Enduring, unconscious assumptions are particularly important in psychiatric nursing, because they have the greatest effect on the behavior of both nurses and clients and resist change so strongly.

When Assumptive Worlds Differ

The assumptive world is formed during early life. Family and other groups in the neighborhood, school, church, or workplace transmit not only their own cultures, but also aspects of the larger culture of which they are a part. In well-knit or isolated cultures the assumptions are more highly shared than in the highly mobile industrial societies of the Western world. Members of a well-knit, isolated society like the Eskimo village discussed earlier will have more in common than the tenants of a multistory apartment building in New York City or Paris. This poses a complex task for the psychiatric nurse attempting to intervene humanistically with clients who hold different assumptive world views. Before intervening, the nurse must find out what cultural factors influence the behavior of clients and caregivers. Although this chapter discusses a number of cultural factors to help the nurse begin developing cultural awareness, the maintenance of cultural awareness is a life-long personal and professional task.

When people have similar assumptive systems, the interactions between them tend to be satisfying. When their assumptive worlds do not fit together their interactions are more likely to result in frustration and conflict.

Both Allison and Mary were staff members on a partial hospitalization unit of a community mental health center in a large metropolitan area. They were also members of a stress management group for mental health staff led by a psychiatric nursing consultant. In one of the early sessions Allison and Mary vented the frustration and anger they felt in their professional and citizen roles.

Allison, a social worker, lived in an upper-middle-class suburb. At a town meeting the night before she had attempted to persuade her neighbors and friends to approve a rezoning petition for a halfway house for mentally retarded adults on the residential street where she lived. She was both angered and hurt by the comments and behavior of her neighbors who hotly accused her of decreasing property values on their street by supporting the rezoning for the halfway house. She didn't understand why she was pointedly ignored after the meeting and left out of an invitation to have coffee and dessert with a neighbor across the street. Allison thought her neighbors' attitude toward the halfway house project was heartless and "redneck."

Mary's frustrations revolved around her continued but unsuccessful efforts to persuade Fatima, a client of the medication clinic at the mental health center, to agree to participate with her in one-to-one counseling. Fatima came to the attention of the emergency clinic after an unsuccessful suicide attempt with two bottles of baby aspirin. Fatima had received a prescription for antidepressant medication, but Mary had failed to persuade Fatima to agree to one-to-one counseling that she believed Fatima would find helpful. Fatima and her husband Saleh lived in a small Arab-American enclave in the center city. Saleh refused his wife permission to contract for one-to-one work, and Fatima would not consider going against her husband's wishes. Since Fatima and Saleh had no phone, Mary made three home visits when Saleh was at work to try to change Fatima's mind. Mary couldn't understand why Saleh refused his wife the opportunity Mary offered, or why Fatima, who had earlier expressed an interest in working with Mary, was now angry with her and refused to answer the door on her fourth visit.

It is tempting at times like these to think that an artificially forced fit might make things okay. It would be easy to ignore cultural differences in attitude, belief,

values, perceptions, or behavior. If we do, however, all we achieve is superficial agreement. Frustration and conflict will soon break through such an agreement.

Cultural Complexity and Diversity

The United States, Canada, and many other Western countries are multiethnic societies; that is, they are composed of many *ethnic groups*. Each ethnic group has a unique culture shared by its members. The culture is perpetuated when its members teach their children the norms, or rules and standards, of the group. These norms become the standard by which other ethnic groups are judged. The belief that your own ethnic group is superior to others, the one to which others should be compared, is called *ethnocentrism*. Health care workers and health care consumers are both subject to ethnocentrism.

Many of the European immigrants who arrived in the United States in the 1900s found that assimilation was not only helpful but sometimes necessary to achieve status and reap the financial rewards of their new country. If they maintained their ethnic identity and retained the dress, customs, language, and rituals of their ethnic group, they often found themselves part of an oppressed minority group. However, American society has regained its ethnic consciousness, and there is an increasing emphasis on the positive aspects of ethnic differences. We have become a culturally diverse society with a heightened sense of ethnic identification and ethnocentrism.

Dangers in Cultural Stereotyping

One person cannot be aware of all the cultural factors that should be taken into consideration in planning and implementing a particular psychiatric nursing intervention. A frequent solution to this dilemma is to go to the literature or the resource person likely to know the most about the culture in which we are interested. In doing so, however, we must put the data in the proper perspective. There is a danger of cultural stereotyping, that is, assuming that all members of one ethnic heritage are alike without taking steps to verify the assumption. The following case example dramatizes a health care team's experience of overenthusiasm for group data about Indian culture.*

*The quote on the following page is from J. Chapman and H. Chapman: *Psychology of Health Care: A Humanistic Perspective,* Monterey, Calif., Wadsworth Health Sciences, 1983.

Maria was brought to the medical center because she seemed to "not be learning right." As a result of an evaluation elsewhere—with which the parents were not happy—they became aware of her epilepsy and that her neurological difficulty was caused by a disease that would be fatal in several years, no matter what was done. The staff at our center immediately developed in their consideration of the family a high sensitivity to their being "special," since they were urban Navajo and had a child soon to die. The staff did not know much about the Navajo people and assumed that perhaps the other evaluation center had not fully appreciated that particular culture.

The staff became enthusiastic about formal review of the literature on the Navajo culture and a large workshop conference was held on religious medicine of the Indian culture in general and the practices of the Navajo in particular. Indian participants conferred with us, as did several staff members who had worked on an Arizona Navajo reservation. The in-service experience was excellent, and we *factually* learned much about the Navajo people.

It was a double-edged experience, however. Many assumptions we had made about this family went by the wayside, since we now "knew" about Navajos; yet it became clear as we talked enthusiastically about applying our new-found knowledge that we were making new assumptions that tended to lump them into a group like "all Navajos." We knew that we had not fallen into the trap of lumping them into Anglo culture. Neither did we feel that we were failing to be "culture conscious." But something was wrong.

Only after we reflected on what *they* had come to us for and began to struggle with what kinds of helping action *they* wanted did we realize that we did not have much detail about *these particular* parents' notion of help—regardless of culture. We retracked with them. Our first surprise was that although they originally came "from the reservation" they knew less about Navajo culture factually than we and experientially less than they both had wanted. They both had been separated from their parents at five years of age and spent most of their life in government schools. They related in an embarrassed fashion that they believed that they knew nothing that could be learned from either the Anglo or Navajo cultures. They were lost between two cultures.

They said that they knew that Maria was not going to live a long time. Their anxiety was long and deep and they had to live with that fact in their own way, but *right now* they could not live *with* her happily. She was an overactive, resistive, hard-to-manage child and would allow them to go nowhere without her. She was described as "ruling the roost." Yes, they wanted her to live and learn; but in the here and now they felt helpless and at a loss as to "how to raise her" or any other child whom they might have.

Our other surprise was that they trusted us more than we had assumed that they possibly could. We knew that they periodically used their medicine man when they went back home. We had assumed that they trusted him more and perhaps would not hear us. However, when asked, they stated that they would not have come to us if they did not think that we could help and that they could have gone back to the reservation for help anytime and chose not to with their immediate concerns.

In looking back on this, I sometimes wonder if we would not have saved a lot of time and been more effective if right at the beginning we had simply said to them: "We don't know anything about *you*; we are different; let us spend some time in finding out about each other."

The YAVIS Syndrome in Mental Health Care

In 1964 Schofield surveyed a random sample of 377 psychiatrists, social workers, and psychologists. He uncovered what he called "The YAVIS Syndrome," an overwhelming preference for Young, Attractive, Verbal, Intelligent, and Successful clients. If therapists followed their preference, they would exclude large numbers of people—the elderly, the unattractive, members of some minority groups, the mentally retarded, and the poor—from their case loads. In fact, the 1978 President's Commission on Mental Health identified people from these categories as members of "underserved populations." (See Chapter 28 for a discussion of the commission's report to the President.)

According to Redlich and Kellert (1978), many mental health agencies assign their less desirable clients to the most junior, least experienced, or least educated staff members, which usually means the nurse or the paraprofessional. In many instances they account for most of the referrals made to psychiatric nurse clinical specialists in private practice. Middle- and upper-class young adults are most likely to be treated by psychiatrists while middle-class adolescents get their counseling from social workers.

BIOSOCIAL FACTORS INFLUENCING DIAGNOSIS AND TREATMENT

Biosocial, or sociodemographic, factors are the characteristics that identify people by the roles they occupy in relation to other members of the larger society.

These characteristics include ethnicity, socioeconomic class, religious beliefs, age, place of residence, sex, and marital status. Remember that while research data provide guidelines for practice, a rigid interpretation of these data may result in cultural stereotyping rather than in truly individual, culturally aware nursing care. Confirming the precise relationship of these social circumstances to psychiatric conditions requires further research.

Ethnicity

In the research linking culture with mental disorder, schizophrenic symptomatology is viewed as an exaggeration of the usual coping behavior found within that culture. For example, in a study of hospitalized schizophrenic clients, Breen (1968) found that Jewish Americans were more likely to be diagnosed as having hebephrenic, simple, or catatonic schizophrenia, while Black Americans were more likely to be diagnosed as having paranoid schizophrenia. The diagnosis in Jewish Americans was linked with a cultural pattern of dependency in response to stress, which Breen called aggression-controlling. The diagnosis of paranoid schizophrenia in Black Americans was linked with aggression-expressing cultural behavior.

The effect that cultural difference and oppression have on assessment and diagnosis is less clear, since the inherent biases in traditional middle-class assessment techniques cast doubt on their utility in assessing the mental health of people who do not fit the middle-class stereotype. Although black people receive a higher proportion of schizophrenic diagnoses, they do not necessarily have a higher rate of this psychosis. A similar phenomenon is found in the psychiatric diagnosis of Chicanos. In comparing the clinical judgments of therapists working with black and Chicano clients, Florez (1975) found that the greater the cultural distance between therapist and client, the less accurate the diagnosis and the more likely that these differences will be seen as psychopathology. Language barriers also increase the difficulty. In one study, when Hispanic clients were interviewed in English, psychiatric ratings reflected significantly greater psychopathology than when they were interviewed in Spanish (Marcos et al. 1981). Dunham (1976) also found that failing to take culture into account may cause misdiagnosis. Assessment devices that define effective behaviors in terms of the ethnic group being assessed seem to assess minority clients more accurately (Smith et al. 1978), but there is some doubt whether mental health professionals with different backgrounds will be able to interpret such devices correctly.

In addition to questions of assessment and diagnosis, we must also consider the ways in which methods of treatment may be influenced by ethnic differences. For instance, Blacks may have unanticipated drug side effects when treated for Depression with tricyclics because of higher blood levels of nortriptyline (Ziegler and Biggs 1977). Another factor influencing treatment is the folk beliefs and healing practices of the client's cultural group. They may be more effective than conventional therapy and may heighten the effect of conventional therapy or help reduce resistance to it.

Socioeconomic Class

In general, the research reports that the highest overall rates of psychiatric disorder—especially Schizophrenia and Personality Disorders—are found in the lower socioeconomic groups. An interesting finding is that this is especially the case in studies conducted in urban settings (Dohrenwend 1975).

A thoughtful review of these studies and of the life circumstances of the poor, the unemployed, and the undereducated reveals greater exposure to stressful life events brought on by poverty, social failure in school or on the job, illness, and the absence of social resources. For example, Vaillant (1980) notes that chronic unemployment is correlated with chronic depression and emotional instability. Confirming the precise relationship of these social circumstances to psychiatric conditions requires further research.

Religious Beliefs

Religious beliefs strongly influence when, how, and why persons seek help for emotional dysfunction, and how others perceive their symptoms of emotional distress. For example, Matthenson (1975) reports instances of Haitian immigrants being diagnosed as schizophrenic because they heard voices, an experience that is valued in the Haitian folk religion. Another example reported in the literature is that of a young, male, Hassidic Jew whose repeated opening of his female counselor's office door was perceived as paranoid behavior. However, his behavior was prompted by the religious admonition against being alone behind closed doors with a woman who is not a family member (Hankoff, Blumenthal, and Borowick 1977). A more recent phenomenon involves the increasing participation of middle- and upper-class teenagers and young adults in extremist religious cults and their parents' frantic efforts to "deprogram" them. These religious factors are considered in a later portion of this chapter.

Age

Children and the elderly have been identified as underserved segments of the American population. Drug and alcohol abuse are increasing among the elderly, who experience sociocultural stress such as isolation and loss through retirement, the illness or death of family and friends, and change of residence. Organic brain dysfunction in the elderly is also more apt to occur during periods of sociocultural stress. While new symptoms of mental dysfunction increase in persons over the age of sixty-five, Butler and Lewis (1973) did not find a corresponding increase in the number of elderly persons receiving treatment. They suspect that lack of money, increasing dependence on other people, and negative caregiver attitudes may be responsible. These factors are more thoroughly discussed in Chapter 22.

Correspondingly, the overall rate of adolescent suicide has more than tripled since 1955. Teenage drug and alcohol abuse has also risen dramatically. These increases have been most dramatic among middle- and upper-class teens in response to pressure for academic and social achievement. The stresses and strains that children and adolescents face are detailed in Chapters 19 and 20.

Place of Residence

Where a person lives may also affect coping style. In urban settings, where the unexpected is the norm and threats to person, property, and self-view are prevalent, emotional disorders are often characterized by anxiety and antisocial responses (Kaplan 1982). Anxiety and antisocial behavior may be more adaptive for psychological survival in the alienated and isolated environment of the city. On the other hand, Depression may be a more functional response in rural areas where people tend to depend on one another more and to avoid overt hostile acts that disrupt the social equilibrium. Studies comparing the incidence of psychologic distress in urban and rural settings have found that Bipolar Affective Disorder is more common in

nonurban settings whereas Schizophrenia and Personality Disorder are more common in cities (Dohrenwend 1975).

Sex and Marital Status

The relationship of sex and marital status to psychologic disorder has also been a subject for study. In a review of seventeen studies, Gove and Tudor (1973) found higher rates of mental illness for females. Further, these rates were related to marital status in the following ways:

- Married women were more likely to have higher rates than married men (in all seventeen studies).
- Single men were more likely to have higher rates than single women (in seven of eleven studies).
- Single men were more likely to have higher rates than married men (in thirteen of fourteen studies).
- Married women were more likely to have higher rates than single women (in eleven of fourteen studies).

They concluded that being married produced greater stress for women while being single was more stressful for men. Higher rates were also found among persons of either sex who were divorced or widowed.

Other research reported that women were diagnosed more frequently with manic-depressive psychosis (Bipolar Affective Disorder in DSM-III) and with the old DSM-II categories of neurosis in which Depression was the presenting affect. Men, on the other hand, were more often diagnosed as having a Personality Disorder in which aggression is the presenting behavior. Thus, the behavior tolerated in women was socially unacceptable in men. Instead, men tended to cope through repression and suppression or aggression, behaviors traditionally viewed as masculine.

Analysis of Biosocial Factors

Since social scientists first discovered that some groups of people have a higher incidence of mental illness than certain other groups, they have been trying to uncover the reasons why this happens. An analysis of the biosocial factors discussed here reveals that stress appears to be a common denominator. Society expects people to relate in certain ways to one another and to the community at large. An individual's ability to meet these role expectations can be influenced by social forces such as poverty, prejudice, war or natural disasters, child-rearing practices, family relationships, education, population mobility, technology, and community support systems. When these forces thwart a person's attempts to fulfill social and cultural expectations, the person may adopt what society considers to be less healthy behavior. Higher rates of mental illness are found among groups experiencing more of these stresses.

Oppression

Historically, oppression is a process or relationship between and among persons that has been characterized by Somers (1977) as undesirable, depriving, and destructive. Rules and prescriptions are carried out by the power of one group over another less powerful group:

- adults over children
- one ethnic group over others
- men over women
- heterosexuals over homosexuals
- the young over the old
- the ablebodied over the handicapped
- the rich over the poor
- teachers over students
- gentiles over Jews
- health care professionals over clients

Regardless of the political–sociological sense of the word, oppression prevents the oppressed from using abilities to the fullest, making choices, and affirming the self. Further, the oppressor is deprived of the opportunity for full and open contact with the person or group being oppressed, and the relationship between them is rigid and stereotyped. Table 26–1 lists common feelings and behaviors related to differences in power. The movements discussed below are responses to the rigidities of systems that cause distress to less powerful people. Later in this chapter we will consider therapeutic strategies that may be helpful in working with people who have been distressed by such experiences.

CONTEMPORARY SOCIOPOLITICAL INFLUENCES ON MENTAL HEALTH CARE

Some recent sociopolitical movements have enriched our understanding of the human condition and expanded our opportunities for humanistic psychiatric nursing practice. The feminist, gay rights, patients' rights (see Chapter 5), and Gray Panther movements herald the new activism of oppressed groups in American society. The departure of thousands of young Americans from the mainstream of society and its established religions to dedicate themselves to new spiritual leaders and exotic cults has created new cultures and new sources of stress. A fifth significant force—the community mental health movement—is analyzed in Chapter 28.

The Feminist Movement

Some recent research suggests that, in little more than a decade, the feminist movement has already had a beneficial effect on the mental health of women. Improving the job market for women has led to greater equality, and therefore to increased self-esteem.

However, while sex is now rarely a factor in diagnosis or treatment goals (Zeldow 1978), sex-role stereotypes still influence both clients and mental health workers. For example, an advertisement in a recent issue of a prestigious medical journal shows a disheveled and harassed woman burdened by mops and brooms. The caption reads: "You can't set her free but you can help her feel less anxious." Our mental health journals continue to promote chemicals as the answer to oppression, and physicians are twice as likely to prescribe mood-altering drugs for women. The one-sided research into the effects of the Vietnam war on veterans is another example of persistent sexism. Until 1982, women veterans (mostly nurses and other medical personnel) were excluded from these studies, although the women reported experiences indicating that they, too, have experienced Post-traumatic Stress Disorder.

Women nurses have been active in the feminist movement. In 1973 the National Organization for Women organized Nurses NOW as a response to the difficulties of living as a woman and practicing as a nurse in a male-dominated society and health care system. Nurses NOW chapters across the country have worked to raise the consciousness of women nurses and clients. Other nurse's groups have addressed

---

Table 26-1   FREQUENTLY DESCRIBED FEELINGS AND BEHAVIORS RELATED TO DIFFERENCES IN POWER

View of the More Powerful	View of the Less Powerful
Feelings	
Having more comfort, more gratification.	Having less comfort, less gratification.
Feeling lucky, safe, and secure.	Feeling insecure, anxious.
Experiencing more pleasure, less pain.	Experiencing less pleasure, more pain.
Having less tendency to depression.	Having strong tendency to depression.
Feeling superior, masterful, entitled.	Feeling inferior, incompetent, deprived.
Feeling hopeful.	Feeling trapped, hopeless, helpless, with few choices.
Feeling anger at noncompliance in the less powerful.	Feeling anger at inconsiderate control by the powerful.
	Feeling anger at feelings of powerlessness.
Having fear of loss of power.	Having fear of abandonment by the powerful.
Having fear of the anger of the less powerful.	Having fear of the anger of the powerful.
Having fear of retaliation by the less powerful.	Having fear of own anger at the powerful.
Having guilt over injustices that result from power.	
Behavior	
Projecting onto the less powerful unacceptable attributes, such as being lazy, dirty, evil, sexual, and irresponsible, as justification for maintaining power and control.	Projecting onto the power group acceptable attributes, such as being smart, competent, and attractive.
Having distrust, being guarded and rigid due to vigilance needed to maintain power and control.	Having distrust, being guarded and sensitive to discrimination, often seeming paranoid to the power group.
Denying the more powerful position and its favorable effects on benefactors and unfavorable effects on victims.	Denying the less powerful position and its effects.
Displaying a paranoia resulting in delusions of superiority, grandiosity, unrealistic sense of entitlement, arrogant behavior, and tendency to distort reality with a consequent unreal assessment of the self and the less powerful.	Displaying a paranoia resulting in the acceptance of a dependent position, passivity, and the assumption of stereotypes, such as a physical or stud image, dumbness, delinquency, and addiction, with a consequent unreal assessment of oneself and the more powerful.

Table continues on next page

---

themselves to the problem of recruiting and retaining adequate numbers of nurses to staff hospitals. This problem has been traced to lack of autonomy and collaboration due to sex-role stereotyping (New York Times 1981). District 5 of the Georgia Nurses Association (1981) prepared an eight-question checklist in a consciousness-raising effort directed at physicians attending an annual meeting of the American College of Surgeons. Their questions to the doctors included:

• Are *you* a part of the hospital nursing shortage?

• Do you know there is a body of nursing knowledge and actions separate and different from (while complementary to) medical knowledge?

• Do you accept and encourage suggestions from nurses about client care in a spirit of collaboration and honest inquiry? Or do you discourage and ridicule attempts to communicate and collaborate?

• Do you write routine post-op nursing care orders instead of encouraging RNs to write their own?

• Do you believe nurses are there to serve you, or to serve clients?

View of the More Powerful	View of the Less Powerful
Isolating, avoiding, and distancing from the less powerful; taking comfort in sameness; becoming unable to tolerate differences in people; and lacking enriching cross-cultural experiences.	Isolating, avoiding, and distancing from the more powerful.
Displaying entitled, controlling, dominating behavior.	Utilizing autonomous, oppositional, manipulative, and passive-aggressive behavior as a defense against powerlessness.
Having a need for a victim, someone to scapegoat and control.	Striking out, becoming verbally or physically aggressive to ward off control.
Identifying with the aggressor, leading to justification for an exertion of power or violence, dehumanizing behavior, and pleasure at human suffering.	Identifying with the aggressor, leading to self-hatred, self-devaluation, aggressive violence, dehumanizing behavior, and pleasure at human suffering.
Identifying with the less powerful, leading to a wish to repudiate power.	
Projecting aggression outside the group onto the less powerful to enhance group cohesiveness and unity. (This behavior is assisted by a sense of entitlement.)	Projecting aggression outside the group onto the more powerful to enhance group cohesiveness and unity. (This behavior is reinforced by a sense of justice.)
	Directing aggression within the ethnic group, resulting in conflictual relationships that are destructive to group cohesiveness.
Experiencing conflict and confusion resulting from (1) a sense of injustice versus a need to hold on to the power and (2) a wish to share the power versus the fear of rejection by one's own ethnic group.	Experiencing conflict and confusion resulting from the need to function in two worlds: that of the under-powered and that of the powerful.
Developing a tolerance for conflict, ambivalence, and contradiction, which, when mastered, leads to flexibility, resourcefulness, creativity, and high self-esteem.	Developing a tolerance for conflict, ambivalence, and contradiction, which, when mastered, leads to flexibility, resourcefulness, creativity, and high self-esteem.
	Sublimating aggression in adaptive ways that lead to the ambition to achieve.

Source: E. B. Pinderhughes, "Teaching Empathy in Cross-Cultural Social Work." Copyright 1979, National Association of Social Workers, Inc. Reprinted with permission from *Social Work*, Vol. 24, No. 4, (July 1979), pp. 314–315, Table 1.

The efforts of this group and Nurses NOW demonstrate the increasing political awareness and activism of women nurses.

The Gay Rights Movement

As early as 1935 Margaret Mead concluded in her study of three New Guinea tribes that a society that disregards the totality of human potential and artificially connects gender with specific approved behaviors creates its own cultural deviants. According to Mead, an individual who is homosexual because of innate temperament may find it impossible to adjust to the accepted standards of a society in which heterosexuality is the only "normal" sexual orientation.

Almost forty years passed before the American Psychiatric Association (APA) voted in December 1973, amidst considerable controversy (Stoller et al. 1973), to eliminate homosexuality from its list of mental disorders. Later printings of DSM-II, the diagnostic and statistical manual in use at the time, showed homosexuality as a sexual deviation called sexual orientation disturbance. DSM-III, published in 1980, demonstrates a subsequent refinement of thinking and clarification of values by making it clear that homosexuality is a disorder of sexual functioning only when the individual views his or her homosexuality as an unwanted and persistent source of distress. This category, called Egodystonic Homosexuality (see Chapter 12), is culture bound, because its predisposing factors are:

- Internalized negative societal attitudes toward homosexuality
- Viewing a socially sanctioned, heterosexual, family life-style as desirable

Since this public statement of the powerful APA, public statements have been made by the national organizations representing the other traditional mental health disciplines—American Nurses Association, American Psychological Association, and National Association of Social Workers. The American Nurses Association made its first public statement in 1978.

What happened between 1935 and 1980 to make the APA accept Mead's early findings? An important force behind this startling reevaluation was the political and social activism of gay people themselves. A 1969 confrontation between police and homosexuals in New York's Stonewall Inn in Greenwich Village is regarded by the homosexual community as the beginning of the nationwide gay rights movement. "Gay Pride Week," an annual June event, commemorates the anniversary of the Stonewall riot with major demonstrations in large cities. In the late 1960s and early 1970s gay people formed groups such as Gay Liberation Front, Mattachine Society, and Daughters of Bilitis, not only for mutual support, but also to fight against social oppression and to dispel the stereotypes and myths associated with homosexuality. They succeeded, at least, in ridding themselves of an automatic diagnosis of mental illness. The gay rights movement seems now to be focusing its efforts on promoting legislation to protect the constitutional rights of homosexual persons.

The Gray Panther Movement

The Gray Panthers, a group of radical elders; the American Association of Retired Persons; and the National Council of Senior Citizens have helped dispel some of the stereotypes associated with aging by demonstrating that older people can be shakers and movers in society rather than placid inhabitants of rocking chairs. The increased numbers of aged people have affected every aspect of society—health care, leisure, housing, business, education. Older people have only recently begun to recognize themselves as a powerful force in society and to organize in order to recommend legislation to improve their status. There has been some dissent to their lobbying effort by those who believe services should be provided on the basis of need rather than age (Neugarten 1980).

The efforts of the Gray Panthers have gone a long way toward facilitating positive views of aging and self-determination for the elderly. The foundation in 1977 and rapid growth of the International Association for Humanistic Gerontology, a professional association concerned with humanistic and holistic approaches to aging and programs for the elderly (Dychtwald 1980), is another example of the increasing receptivity of the helping professions to the unique needs and potential of a continually expanding elderly population (see Chapter 22).

Religious Cults

In the late 1960s thousands of young Americans left the mainstream of our society and its established religions to dedicate themselves to new spiritual leaders and exotic cults.

Few people on the outside knew very much about these cults, and rumors began to spread. Soon there were many stories of strange activities among cultists: "brainwashing," people held against their will, perverse commands by cult leaders living in luxury, and followers dutifully carrying out the commands of the cult leader. Cultists, however, insisted that they had freely chosen a life-style in which they had found personal and spiritual fulfillment unavailable to them in society at large.

In November 1978 the events in Guyana confirmed the worst suspicions of the anticultists. Over 900 people participated in a mass suicide ordered by Jim Jones, the leader of the People's Temple. An American congressman, California's Leo J. Ryan, and members of the news team that accompanied him on his fact-finding trip were murdered. The Jonestown tragedy made the cult phenomenon a front page story. Before Jonestown, not many people were interested in cults or in the people who joined them. Shocked by the mass suicide, people became suspicious and wanted to know more about the People's Temple and groups like it. Mental health professionals had already begun to treat ex-cultists who were experiencing radical personality changes, affective and cognitive mental dysfunctions, and family schisms. Psychiatrist John G. Clark, Jr. and psychologist Michael Langone began a more rigorous and formal study of destructive conversions at Massachusetts General Hospital. Their interest formed the basis for the establishment of the Center on Destructive Cultism to provide a national focus for theoretical research, develop professional counseling expertise, and educate the public (Clark et al. 1981).

Cults have been called neoreligious movements; "disfavored" religions; nonconventional, nontraditional religions; and pseudoreligions. There are over 3,000 of them in America today. They are a product of the American tradition of religious diversity that extends back to the original colonization period, and they are protected by the First Amendment to the Constitution. Those whose members experience the problems identified earlier—radical personality change, affective and cognitive mental dysfunction, and family schism—are destructive. This chapter is concerned only with those cults that regularly cause distress to their members.

Characteristics of Destructive Cults
Destructive cults share several characteristics. They:

- Have charismatic leaders who demand total submission
- Have rigid belief systems
- Demand complete commitment to the cult as "family"
- Practice milieu control
- Actively recruit vulnerable people
- Deprive recruits and/or members of food, rest, and health care
- Place heavy emphasis on fund-raising

CHARISMATIC LEADERS Charisma is a special quality of leadership that inspires unswerving allegiance and devotion. The charismatic leader is self-assured and has purpose. He has the power and personal strength to transcend the problems of daily life and is perceived by his followers as a divine instrument chosen by some higher force. Therefore, his teachings and commands are to be obeyed at all costs. As with Charles Manson and Jim Jones, unquestioned authority can lead to tragedy. Passionate devotion to a living leader is one of the most dangerous aspects of cultism.

RIGID BELIEF SYSTEMS Almost all cults have an apocalyptic world view—that is, society is doomed, and Armageddon is at hand. However, they believe that cult members will be spared and, under the direction of the cult's leader, will become the controlling force in a new social order.

COMPLETE COMMITMENT The leader and his family live together, often in a communal life-style. A member's family of origin and other nonbelievers are perceived as negative forces, perhaps as instruments of Satan. Uniformity and agreement in the cult family are essential.

Kneisl (1981a) has used Irving Janis's work to help psychiatric nurses understand what goes on in destructive cults. Janis coined the term *groupthink* (discussed in Chapter 9) to refer to what goes on in highly cohesive groups in which uniformity and agreement are given such high priority that critical thinking is impossible or unacceptable. These groups have developed norms around the maintenance of unity and loyalty regardless of the cost. The eight main symptoms of groupthink are certainly relevant to understanding the dynamics that operate in cults and can be reviewed in Chapter 18.

MILIEU CONTROL Destructive cults discourage or prevent their members from maintaining ties with former friends and family. Members are often denied access to newspapers, radio, or TV, and the camp, training center, or headquarters of the cult may be geographically isolated. New recruits may have arrived at night in a car or van with obscured windows and may have little idea where they are or where the nearest city or town is.

RECRUITMENT OF VULNERABLE PEOPLE Many recruiters have been painstakingly trained to seek out certain types of individuals who might be inclined to join their group if approached in the right way. They look for prospects who are experiencing the difficult transition between childhood and maturity and are sensitive, idealistic, and searching for their place in the world.

For the most part, recruiters seek new members who are young, white, middle to upper class, and have some college education, although some high school students have been recruited. College freshmen, newly away from home, are typically disoriented, lonely, and unsure of themselves, and graduating seniors on the brink of leaving the familiar life pattern are also vulnerable. Besides college campuses, other popular recruiting grounds are transportation centers such as airports or bus terminals. Young people traveling alone with backpacks are prime targets.

Cult recruiters also tend to look for "loners," offering them peer affiliation and approval, or for persons temporarily depressed by a poor grade, or the breakup of a romance. Individuals who are not inner directed, or who are uncertain of their identity, may feel a sense of relief at having found an authority figure (Schwartz and Kaslow 1979).

Idealistic individuals are also vulnerable. The recruiter may offer the opportunity to work for a "cause"— the poor, the drug-addicted, or the disadvantaged— whether or not there is such a program. Today's cults also offer the opportunity to rebel against the hypocrisy of society just as the "hippies" and "flower children" did.

Recruiters approach potential members with some innocuous remark or offer some small item for sale. Then they strike up a brief conversation about their group or organization. Often the group is a "front" for one of the cults. Such deception is viewed as a legitimate way to win members for the cult. The Reverend Sun Myung Moon of the Unification Church calls it "heavenly deception." Recruiters may offer a hot meal, friendly conversation, or the opportunity to attend a lecture. If recruits accept the offer they are met with unconditional acceptance and flattery. This technique is known as "love-bombing." Members urge recruits to stay overnight, spend a weekend at the group's camp, or return tomorrow for fellowship and another lecture. They are made to feel that not to do so would violate the wishes of their new friends who think so highly of them.

PHYSIOLOGICAL DEPRIVATION   If recruits accept an offer to stay overnight or spend the weekend, they may be kept up late at night and awakened frequently, often to celebrate in joyous song during the middle of the night. One potential cult member told of being awakened after a long and exhausting day by the members urging him to join in a rendition of "You Are My Sunshine." Another told of being fed such spicy food that the recruits were awake all night with gastrointestinal distress and diarrhea. In a fatigued and weakened state the next day, they were even more vulnerable and suggestible. During the day members and recruits put in long hours in fund-raising activities, prayer, or lectures that drone on and on producing a trancelike state. Meals heavy on starches and low on protein may also be designed to produce lethargy.

Since symptoms of illness may be viewed as just punishment for past sins, members may not seek health care. Symptoms of mental ill health are often treated with the same benign neglect. In some cults nutrition is so poor that youths may be described as asexual, women may miss menstrual periods or cease

them altogether, and members exhibit other symptoms such as hair loss.

FUND RAISING   Cults raise funds by selling flowers or other small objects or requesting donations. Members may pledge to raise a certain amount each day and become carried away in zealous overbidding with their peers. They may have to spend the greater part of twenty-four hours attempting to meet their pledges. Some cults raise funds through business enterprises and own farms, fleets of fishing boats, incense and candle factories, bakeries, used clothing and furniture stores, and so on.

The cult leader often lives in far greater luxury than do his followers. Members believe that the "master" deserves a life of luxury because he is a very special person. The cult leader is referred to here as "he," because almost all cult leaders are men. In most destructive cults, women are relegated to a secondary status to cook and clean as well as praying and raising funds. They are rarely allowed the opportunity to participate in the decisions of the group.

Destructive Cults versus Other Religious Groups   Some people say that cults are really no different from other established or more traditional religions. It is important to recognize some essential differences, however.

- In traditional religions the leader is subject to the same laws as the followers. In fact, leaders serve as role models for their followers.

- Other religions do not practice physiological deprivation, although special diets may be followed.

- While most religions encourage contributions or tithing, the contributions in some cults approach 100 percent of earnings and are not used for the benefit of all. A large portion may find its way into the leader's pockets.

- Destructive cults often perceive themselves as above the laws of the land. They establish their own laws and feel free to disregard any other moral and legal laws.

- Other religious groups do not practice "heavenly deception;" they identify themselves from the outset.

Brainwashing   Destructive cults are often accused of having "brainwashed" the young persons who join them. *Brainwashing* or thought control is the alteration of personal conviction, belief, habits, and attitudes by means of intensive coercive indoctrination. The term brainwashing was first used in the 1950s to explain the psychological damage experienced by American soldiers who were held prisoner during the Korean War.

Critics contend that isolation, deprivation of sleep, protein-deficient diets, intense peer pressure, lengthy mandatory lectures, spiritual disciplines (such as meditation techniques and chanting), or exotic rituals that raise group emotions to intense peaks have resulted in "snapping." This is defined as an alteration of the mental state by the conversion experience, in which the new recruit is no longer in control. The results of these experiences and counseling strategies for cult members who have experienced them are discussed later in this chapter.

This whole issue of brainwashing has been brought to the attention of the courts, but because there is no clear evidence that cult members have indeed been brainwashed, it is insufficient to overcome the "freedom of religion" clause of the First Amendment. Recent headlines indicate just how much attention the courts are giving to this problem. The New York State Assembly has approved the first anticult bill in the nation. It will allow families of cult members to take legal custody of them for up to 90 days. Opponents say that the bill is so poorly written that it would allow the court-sanctioned kidnapping of people who belonged to established, organized religions. One assemblyman joked that the bill could even apply to the U.S. Navy. Minnesota has approved a similar law.

FOLK BELIEFS AND HEALING PRACTICES

Folk beliefs and healing practices are culture-specific ways of handling physical problems and emotional conflicts. For example, members of some cultural groups, such as Chicanos and Appalachian whites, believe that illnesses caused by witches' spells may not respond to drugs. This may account for a client's seeming noncompliance with a treatment plan. In some other ethnic groups, such as the Indians of North, Central, and South America; Chinese Americans; and Japanese Americans, herbal products are used to treat both physical and mental disorders. The culturally unaware mental health team member may not know that such herbs are being used or that they may produce both positive or negative interactions with medications.

Folk beliefs and healing practices reflect the assumptive world view of the particular culture. In most West-

ern societies disease is viewed as the result of such natural phenomena as microbes, viruses, chromosomal abnormality, or chemicals. Many Third World people, however, believe that supernatural forces cause illness, and cures can be effected by appealing to the supernatural force through witches or sorcerers or by controlling the force with magic.

As members of these ethnic groups become more middle class, they tend to abandon their folk healing practices. Recent studies indicate, however, that folk beliefs may persist longer. One study of 450 college students in the United States and Ireland found that about 70 percent of the students relied on such magic as carrying good luck charms to an exam, crossing their fingers, having a lucky number, or knocking on wood. Reliance on magic can be seen in even technologically advanced groups.

Being aware of folk health care systems will help the nurse provide better health care to particular groups of people. Culturally aware nurses will be able to devise more meaningful nursing care plans and perhaps, in the process, discover ways in which the middle-class Western system of health care can be humanized by incorporating folk beliefs and practices. The case study below demonstrates how an understanding of folk health care systems can be used to facilitate mental health treatment.

Henri, a twenty-one-year-old Haitian refugee, was brought by his family to the emergency room of a large general hospital in Miami. Family members believed Henri to be possessed by an evil spirit. They told the emergency room staff that they had been unable to control him for two days. He had been breaking dishes and glasses in the family's small apartment, shouting obscene curses in Creole at his mother, and attacking his brother on a number of occasions, screaming, "I am God the Son." Psychiatrists summoned by the ER staff noted that he was out of contact with reality, prescribed massive doses of tranquilizers, and arranged for his transfer to the inpatient psychiatric unit, where Henri remained for three more days with no decrease in his violent behavior. A surgical staff nurse who had been raised in Cuba and was familiar with Santeria (Cuba's folk blend of Catholicism and mysticism) heard of Henri's strange behavior. She suggested to one of her colleagues on the psychiatric unit that a voodoo practitioner might be helpful. After the psychiatric nurse confirmed that the family did believe in voodoo, she brought the suggestion to a team conference. After much heated discussion the team decided to try an exorcism by a voodoo priest if the family agreed. The exorcism was carried out at the

Table 26–2   SELECTED CHARACTERISTICS OF SIX AMERICAN ETHNIC GROUPS

Ethnic Group	Aproximate Time of United States Population Influx	Estimated Population (1979)	Traditional Family Structure	Expression of Pain	Folk Healers
Black Americans	1600s	25,000,000	Extended/ matriarchal and egalitarian	Open, public	Hoodoo men and ladies Root doctors Blood doctors
Mexican Americans	400 B.C.	7,000,000	Extended/ patriarchal	Open, public	Curanderos
Puerto Ricans	1900s	1,700,000	Extended/ patriarchal	Open, public	Espiritistas
American Indians	13000–18000 B.C.	900,000	Extended/ patriarchal and matriarchal	Closed, private	Medicine men
Chinese Americans	1700s	500,000	Extended/ patriarchal	Closed, private	Herbalists Herb pharmacists Acupuncturists
Japanese Americans	1800s	700,000	Extended/ patriarchal	Closed, private	Herbalists

Source: G. Henderson, and M. Primeaux, *Transcultural Health Care.* Menlo Park, Calif.: Addison-Wesley Publishing Co., 1981, p. 67.

offices of a community mental health outreach center in Miami's Little Haiti. The inpatient psychiatric staff who observed the exorcism ceremony found that their client became very quiet after it. Henri returned to their unit where traditional treatment was continued and he improved rapidly.

The unique aspect of this situation is that the psychiatric team was able to allow for a folk health care system that stood in opposition to the system of health care they espoused. There is a strong contradiction between traditional and folk health systems in terms of the relationship between practitioners and clients. In folk systems, both define the nature of illness and health, while in traditional systems practitioners are likely to have a monopoly on defining the nature of illness and health. The process of treatment is another basis for comparison. In folk systems, the process of treatment is a social act while in traditional systems it is a technological act. The folk systems of some specific groups—Black Americans, Hispanic Americans, Asian Americans, and American Indians—are dis-

cussed more thoroughly in the following sections. Their essential characteristics are outlined in Table 26–2.

The Folk Systems of Black Americans

It is not easy to categorize the folk systems and healing practices of Black Americans for a number of reasons. For one, the system is a unique blend of African folklore, fundamentalist Christianity, the Voodoo religion of the West Indies, and some tenets of both classic and modern medicine. For another, folk medicine is more likely to be important to Black Americans who live in the southern United States or rural areas or who are recent immigrants, because they are less likely to have been thoroughly assimilated into the larger culture. However, folk practices may also be important to Black Americans living in the urban Northeast and the West, and to other groups as diverse as the Pennsylvania Dutch, Appalachian Whites, Louisiana Cajuns, Puerto Ricans in New York, or Mexican Americans in San Antonio.

According to Snow (1981), who has studied the health beliefs and practices of low-income Black Americans, three major themes underlie their folk medical beliefs:

- The world is a hostile and dangerous place.
- The individual is subject to attack from external sources.
- The individual is helpless, without internal resources to combat such an attack, and must depend on outside aid.

Because the individual is a potential victim of attack, it is prudent to be suspicious of others, to beware of the effects of natural and supernatural forces, and to engage supernatural aid against these attacks.

Black people from Africa and the West Indies brought with them a belief in magic and witchcraft as the means of countering evil spells, harmful magic, or the punishment of a wrathful God. *Obeah*, or black magic, is still practiced in the southeastern United States. Originally from the West Indies, Obeah thrives among Bahamians and the Bahamian population in southern Florida. According to Scott (1981), there are several male and female Obeah practitioners in the Miami area who use plants, ground fibers, ground glass, and various herbs in the folk remedy mixtures they provide. These mixtures can also be used to put a hex, a fix, or a "mojo" on another. The witchcraft may be said to have been "put on," or "thrown at" the victim, who may actually be frightened to death by the knowledge of having been hexed. Root doctors, known as *Hoodoo men* or *Hoodoo ladies*, are also consulted for their ability either to neutralize or to cause a hex.

Voodoo, a West African word that means god or spirit, is sometimes confused with Obeah. According to Voodoo, a religion, the spirits of the dead can visit the world of the living to bless or curse people. In Haiti, a blend of Voodoo and Catholicism called *Vodun* is of prime importance in the religious life of Haitian peasants. Voodoo Priests (*Houngan*) or priestesses (*Mambo*) may exorcise evil spirits or may cause injury to an enemy by sticking pins into a wax image of the enemy. Voodoo and other forms of spiritualism are integral to the folk medicine of Black Americans.

The Folk Systems of Hispanic Americans

The Hispanic American population includes a number of diverse ethnic groups from Spanish-speaking countries in Central and South America and some Caribbean islands. According to Henderson and Primeaux (1981, p. 70) census projections anticipate that there will soon be more Hispanic Americans than Black Americans.

It would be an error to assume that all Spanish-speaking groups share the same beliefs. Some of the subcultural differences between Mexican Americans, Puerto Ricans, and Cubans, for example, are discussed below. Even the most apparent commonality, language, is not always shared, since there are a number of Spanish dialects spoken in the United States.

Common beliefs of Hispanic Americans about the causes of illness are:

- Illness is the result of *mal de ojo,* or evil eye.
- Illness is God's punishment for previous sins.
- A *hot–cold* (*caliente–frio*) imbalance of body humors is responsible for disease.

Mal de ojo is thought to be the result of a witch purposefully casting a spell or a person involuntarily injuring a child by looking admiringly at it. Magical amulets such as coral, jet, scapulars of the saints, and tiny bags of salt or garlic around the neck or wrist are used to help protect one from the evil eye. The fear of severe injury or death from the evil eye is so great that it may contribute to what Engel (1971) calls a *lethal life situation,* an otherwise sudden and unexplained rapid death under conditions of psychological stress.

Among Mexican Americans, Cubans, and Puerto Ricans the *espiritista* or spiritualist is believed to be capable of putting a person in touch with the dead. *Espiritismo,* a religious cult of European origin, is a way to counteract or prevent mal de ojo and is also concerned with moral behavior. In contrast to the espiritista, the Cuban *santero,* who is a practitioner of *Santeria* (the unique blend of Catholicism and mysticism referred to in the earlier case study involving Henri), is not concerned with the client's moral behavior. Both espiritistas and santeros prescribe folk remedies, such as teas, herbs, salves, and lotions, which may be purchased in a *botanica,* a store that sells these items along with religious articles such as statues and scapulars. The Mexican American family may see another type of healer called a *curandero* or *curandera* in order to nullify a fright (*susto*) thought to be associated with loss of the soul. Other strong emotional experiences that may cause physical results are more characteristic of Hispanic Americans than some of the other ethnic groups detailed in this chapter. They include sibling jealousy,

Table 26-3 HOT-COLD DISEASES OR CONDITIONS AND THEIR TREATMENT					
Hot Diseases or Conditions	**Cold Diseases or Conditions**	**Hot Foods**	**Cold Foods**	**Hot Medicines and Herbs**	**Cold Medicines and Herbs**
Infections	Cancer	Chocolate	Fresh vegetables	Penicillin	Bicarbonate of soda
Kidney diseases	Earache	Cheese	Tropical fruits	Aspirin	Milk of magnesia
Diarrhea	Rheumatism	Temperate-zone fruits	Dairy products	Castor oil	Sage
Rashes and other skin eruptions	Tuberculosis	Chilipeppers	Low-prestige meats (goat, fish, chicken)	Cod liver oil	Linden
Sore throat	Common cold	Cereal grains		Iron preparations	Orange flower water
Warts	Headache	Goat milk	Honey	Vitamins	
Constipation	Paralysis	High-prestige meats (beef, water fowl, mutton)	Raisins	Anise	
Ulcers	Stomach cramps		Bottled milk	Cinnamon	
Liver complaints	Teething	Oils	Barley water	Garlic	
	Menstrual period	Hard liquor	Cod	Mint	
	Joint pain	Aromatic beverages		Ginger root	
	Malaria	Coffee		Tobacco	
	Pneumonia	Onions			
		Peas			
		Eggs			

anger, shame or embarrassment, rejection, or sadness for example.

The hot–cold theory of disease espoused by many Hispanic Americans stems from the classic theory spelled out by Hippocrates, the father of medicine. In the Hippocratian theory, it is necessary to balance blood, phlegm, black bile, and yellow bile (the four body humors) in order to achieve or maintain health. In her discussion of the health care needs of Spanish-speaking clients, Murillo-Rohde (1981) identifies the characteristics of each of these body humors in relation to both temperature and moisture—blood is hot and wet, phlegm is cold and wet, black bile is cold and dry, and yellow bile is hot and dry. When the four humors are balanced and the body is warm and somewhat wet, the body is healthy. When the humors are not balanced and the body is very hot, cold, dry, wet, or any combination of these, the body may become diseased. Treatment by using the proper "hot" or "cold" foods, herbs, or medicines is thought to restore the body to its normal balance. Hot diseases are treated by cold foods, herbs, or medicines, and vice versa. Although hot and cold foods, illnesses, and treatments vary from ethnic group to ethnic group, Table 26–3

lists some of the major characteristics of hot–cold theory. It can be used as a general guide in considering both the Hispanic American population discussed here and the Asian American population discussed later in this chapter.

"Bad air" is another explanation for illness that seems to be related to the hot–cold theory of disease. "Bad air" is often night air, particularly cold air or a cold draft, that is thought to cause illnesses such as earache, rheumatism, facial paralysis, and tuberculosis. There is no simple explanation for "bad air," however, since it also seems to be connected to some extent with the belief that "aire" is an evil spirit, the result of witchcraft, or a dangerous emanation from a corpse or from the moon (moonlight).

The Folk Systems of Asian Americans

Persons whose ethnic heritage is identified with China, Japan, Korea, Southeast Asia, and such Pacific islands as Samoa, Guam, and the Philippines are identified as Asian American. According to Chang (1981), American nurses are more likely than ever before to have contact with clients from Asian backgrounds because of the recent influx of new immigrants from these countries. No one set of characteristics describes or categorizes Asian Americans, since there are similarities as well as differences among these various groups of people. Most of the specific examples in this section relate to Chinese Americans and Japanese Americans because together they comprise the largest Asian American population in the United States.

A strong Chinese influence pervades the folk systems of all Asian people. Traditional Chinese medicine is a well-organized system of medical theory with a strong philosophical character. It uses herbs, other flora, acupuncture, acupressure, massage, and nutrition principles, which all figure prominently in the holistic health movement as well. A resurgence of interest in traditional Chinese medicine in the People's Republic of China is resulting in the integration of these traditional forms of healing with Western biomedical science. "Barefoot doctors" in China are agricultural workers in rural communes who are chosen to receive special training as part-time medical workers to provide integrated health care (Weisberg and Graham, 1977). Unlike much of Western medicine, this form of health care focuses on preventing illness.

Chinese folk medicine evolved from a systems view of the universe. Each organism in the universe interacts with and is affected by all others in the universe. The system derives its energy from the Yin and the Yang, two opposing forces that must be in perfect balance in order for physical and mental health and social harmony to be maintained (Campbell and Chang 1981). The Yang is a positive force that produces light, warmth, and fullness, while the Yin is a negative force that produces darkness, cold, and emptiness. Figure 26–1 of the Yin and Yang symbol illustrates these two opposing forces. In Asian American folk systems some parts of the body are Yang and others are Yin. Yin and Yang are also symbols for hot and cold with Yin being a cold energy force and Yang a hot energy source. As in the caliente–frio theory, hot foods are used to treat Yin illnesses and cold to treat Yang illnesses. See Table 26–3 for a general guide to the hot–cold theory also espoused by many Hispanic Americans.

Asian American clients may go directly to an herb pharmacist to receive a prescription for their symptoms, or they may be diagnosed and treated by an herbalist or acupuncturist. Sometimes clients see a Western physician as well, shopping around for the best physician or healer and selecting a personal combination of herbs, pills, and food for treatment (Louie 1974).

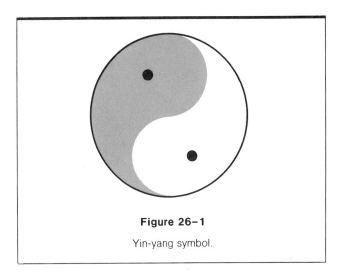

Figure 26–1

Yin-yang symbol.

The Folk Systems of American Indians

In American Indian culture, the word "medicine" can be equated with "mysterious." It is linked to the supernatural religious experience central to the existence of the American Indian. According to Primeaux and Henderson (1981, p. 244), it is impossible to separate Indian medicine and religion or to make distinctions between physical and mental illness.

The medicine man, or *shaman*, is the central healing figure. Because the Native American theory of disease includes physical, social, psychological, and environmental aspects, closely intertwined with spiritual and religious aspects, the germ theory is rejected. The medicine man conducts a tribal healing ceremony, a highly ritualized and religious way of coping with illness and death. The shaman may also involve family members in the healing ritual, because family members (including a large extended family of cousins, aunts, and uncles, etc.) are important sources of support during periods of crisis. It may be important to the family and to the client to have the healing ceremony carried out at the bedside of a hospitalized person. A medicine bundle containing charms or fetishes to ward off evil; a bag of herbs, plants, or roots to provide the curative aspect; a drum or rattle; and a special costume for the medicine man may all be integral parts of the healing ceremony. The rattle may be shaken, or the drum beaten, while the healer chants the remedies revealed to him by the spirits.

Foods have symbolic meaning as well as nutritional value to Native Americans. For example, before visitors enter a home, the occupants sprinkle cornmeal on their shoulders in order to prevent them from bringing illness inside. Cornmeal may also be sprinkled around the bed of a hospitalized person or directly on the client (Primeaux and Henderson 1981, p. 245).

CULTURALLY AWARE STRATEGIES FOR NURSING INTERVENTION

We have seen how cultural and social class differences between client and nurse may impede a nurse's best intentions. Some fundamental transcultural nursing premises (Henderson and Primeaux 1981) that will underscore this section are:

- Nurses cannot solve clients' problems, but they may be able to help clients solve their own problems.

- The easiest, least creative response to transcultural conflict is to pretend that it does not exist.

- Every client behaves according to unwritten ethnic customs and traditions.

- Every successful effort by nurses to teach clients the elements of scientific medicine alienates clients from relatives and friends who do not have this knowledge.

- Previous transcultural experience is a valuable asset when used as a general guide. However, such experience can be a liability if the nurse believes it provides the answer to every transcultural problem.

- We will make mistakes in transcultural interactions, but we should learn from our mistakes and not repeat them.

Understanding Your Own Sociocultural Heritage

Gaining awareness of sociocultural differences requires that nurses first come to understand their own backgrounds and the influence of that background on their practice. Chapter 3 explored some dimensions of self-knowledge through an examination of the concept of personal integration. This chapter urges nurses to acknowledge and explore their own sociocultural heritage. As with Allison, the social worker, and Mary, the nurse in an earlier case example, health workers may become angry with clients, families, or communities who they judge by their own standards. Nurses are better able to meet the socio-cultural needs of a client when they acknowledge that a culture and a society

influence their beliefs, values, attitudes, and behavior. The following questions are designed to facilitate acknowledgment of the nurse's own sociocultural heritage.

QUESTIONS THAT ACKNOWLEDGE SOCIOCULTURAL HERITAGE

- What ethnic group, socioeconomic class, religions, age group, and community do you belong to?
- What experiences have you had with people from ethnic groups, socioeconomic classes, religions, age groups, or communities different from your own?
- What were those experiences like? How did you feel about them?
- When you were growing up what did your parents and significant others say about people who were different from your family?
- What about your ethnic group, socioeconomic class, religion, age, or community do you find embarrassing or wish you could change? Why?
- What sociocultural factors in your background might contribute to being rejected by members of other cultures?
- What personal qualities do you have that will help you establish interpersonal relationships with persons from other cultural groups? What personal qualities may be detrimental?
- What assumptions do you hold about the people who populate our world?

Answering these questions honestly and completely is the important first step in self-awareness. The second step involves exploring beliefs and attitudes that may be different from or the same as those held by the client. Nurses might ponder the following statements (Henderson and Primeaux 1981, p. 55).

EXPLORING SPECIFIC SOCIOCULTURAL ATTITUDES

- I accept opinions different from my own
- I respond with compassion to poverty-stricken people
- I think interracial marriage is a good thing
- I would feel uncomfortable in a group in which I am the ethnic minority
- I consider failure a bad thing
- I invite people I don't like to my home
- I believe that the Ku Klux Klan has its good points
- I set realistic life goals
- I would enjoy serving as a juror in a rape case
- I am concerned about the treatment of minorities in employment and health care

- I feel uncomfortable in low-income neighborhoods
- I prefer to conform rather than disagree in public
- I value friendship more than money
- I maintain high ethical standards as a professional
- I would not object to premarital sex for my children
- I spend a lot of time worrying about social injustices without doing much about them
- I believe that almost anyone who really wants to can get a good job
- I have a close friend of another race
- I would rather attend a concert than an athletic contest

Incorporating Principles of Effective Communication

Language may be a barrier in working with culturally different clients. Both nurse and client may feel helpless and alienated from one another when they do not speak the same language. The client who does not understand what is happening may appear angry, noncompliant, or apathetic. It is crucial to assess the client's behavior as a response to the language barrier. However, there are certain measures that nurses can take to overcome this barrier if it exists. These measures, along with principles of effective communication with members of different cultures, are included in Table 26-4.

Becoming Familiar with and Using Folk Beliefs and Healing Practices

Deciding from whom and when health care will be sought is often a sociocultural matter. A client may have already consulted a mambo, espiritista, hoodoo man, or herbalist, and may continue to follow their suggestions, drink their teas, or apply their salves and poultices. Attempting to persuade clients to reject their folk beliefs and healing practices in favor of "orthodox scientific care" may result in their feeling increasingly alienated.

The nurse may be able to reinforce selected folk healing practices that will further enhance the client's feeling of well-being. For example, the hot–cold theory of disease illustrated in Table 26-3 may be included in the planning phase. Foods and medicines that support the hot–cold theory may be compatible with the client's health needs. Some healer treatments and medicines may help treat the client's difficulty. Folk healers can often be very supportive, and there is no valid reason not to allow or encourage their cooperation in

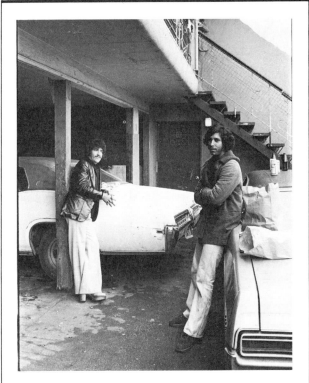

Folk beliefs and healing practices help to determine from whom and when health care will be sought. It would be a mistake to assume that all members of ethnic groups consult healers or psychics.

the treatment plan. The example of Henri's experience with a voodoo doctor shows that it can be beneficial. Curanderos often help clients overcome their reactions to frightening experiences (we might call them panic attacks). Cooperating with folk healers may help you develop a trusting relationship with clients and reduce their suspiciousness of orthodox psychiatric care. It is particularly important to avoid implied or direct ridicule. While you may not believe in "the evil eye," the client may. Rather than argue about what caused the client's hallucinations or depression, acknowledge the folk belief without necessarily accepting it. A statement like, "I have heard about the evil eye, but we think this is something else," may help you avoid an ongoing battle. An alternative may be to avoid discussions of etiology and focus on what is to be done.

Using Counseling Techniques Specific to the Client's Distress

Sociocultural factors must be considered before using any of the nursing interventions described in this text. The strategies listed thus far should facilitate most

Table 26-4   COMMUNICATING WITH CLIENTS FROM DIFFERENT CULTURES

Strategy	Rationale
1. If you don't speak the language of your client try the following:	
a. Enlist the aid of a family member or friend of the client.	Being able to help will increase the helper's self-esteem. Knowing that a concerned person is directly participating may help the client feel less anxious.
b. Seek out a bilingual staff member in the setting.	Larger institutions often have bilingual employees on their staffs. Smaller agencies often employ indigenous staff.
c. Ask another client to translate.	Another client can be helpful in translating cultural beliefs as well as language. Being able to help boosts self-esteem.
d. Use other agencies as resources.	Health and social services departments, international institutes, college language departments, neighborhood houses, or cultural centers will often know of people who are willing to volunteer as translators.
2. Select the words you use carefully, avoiding buzz words and jargon. Speak clearly, pacing yourself to be neither too fast nor too slow.	Words that are slurred, have many syllables in them, or are too technical make communication more difficult. Speaking too fast may overload the client and make it difficult for the client to follow. Speaking too slowly may lose the client's attention.
3. Select the gestures you use with care, using your nonverbal behavior to underscore your words and your actions.	The proper use of gestures can clarify a message, and drawings can sometimes be helpful. Be careful, however; not all gestures mean the same thing in all cultures.
4. Listen to your client's words and watch your client's gestures carefully. Do your best to understand and validate the meaning they have for you.	Listening carefully to the client will help you avoid focusing on what you will say or do next and will demonstrate your genuine concern for the client's distress.

nurse–client interactions. However, nurses must also make the effort to base plans of care on their clients' sociocultural backgrounds. Table 26–5 contains the guidelines for counseling Japanese Americans developed by Furuta. Nurses should develop similar guidelines for their work with clients from other cultures.

When Clients Need Help With Oppression Experiences   All people have been oppressed, at least to some extent, but some groups of people have experienced oppression more often and with greater intensity than others. Table 26–6 outlines the ways in which people cope with oppression.

The chronic effects of oppression can be physiologically, psychologically, and socially destructive to the individual. When people wish to gain further awareness of their oppression experiences and work on them, guiding questions, such as those that follow, often facilitate the working through of powerlessness, anger, guilt, demoralization, or other feelings that often result.

USEFUL QUESTIONS FOR COUNSELING ON OPPRESSION EXPERIENCES

- When did you last feel oppressed?
- What did it feel like? How was it for you? What did you think? And what did you do?
- Who has oppressed you the most? An individual? A group?
- How have other people reacted when you have expressed your oppression?
- What has been your typical reaction to your oppression?
- Try to remember your first memory of being oppressed?
- Scan, from your first memory forward, your experiences of being oppressed by (parents, whites, adults, men, anglos, etc.).
- Describe a time you felt good about what you did when you were oppressed.
- Who is your heroine, your hero, your model—someone whose coping with oppression you very much admire?

Table 26–5 ETHNIC IDENTITY GUIDE FOR COUNSELING JAPANESE AMERICANS		
	Acculturative Balance	
	Traditional Orientation (Japanese)	**Anglo Orientation (American)**
Client Dimensions		
Self-presentation	Interdependent, other-oriented	Independent, self-oriented
	Self-controlled	Self-expressive
	Self-effacing	Self-assertive
	Identifies self within familial context	Identifies self as an individual
Self-esteem determined by	Fulfilling family roles and obligations	Fulfilling own needs for mastery, self-actualization, "doing own thing"
	Bringing honor to family, "doing good"	Taking responsibility for own behavior
	Enduring under adversity	
Shame and/or guilt caused by	Bringing embarrassment, dishonor to family or group	Violating one's conscience
	Failing to fulfill family role and obligations	Failure to meet one's standards and expectations
Conflict and anxiety dealt with by	Internalizing, somatizing, withdrawal, depression, autism, or rarely, acting out	Various behaviors including acting out
Communication	Restrained, emotionally controlled, indirect, more nonverbal than verbal	Spontaneous, direct, verbal
Therapist ethnicity preference	Japanese American or nonethnic who is acculturated to Japanese American values and mores	Anglo or may have no preference
Counseling Considerations		
Goals	Interdependence, functioning within family (household) system	Individuation, autonomous functioning
	Mutually defined by client and therapist	Defined by therapist or client and therapist
	Rebalancing of intergenerational obligations	Alleviation of symptoms or actualization of individual potential
Preferred therapeutic modality	Preference for family, then individual therapy	Family, group and/or individual therapy as appropriate
Therapist role	Active participant, observation	Nondirective or directive intervention as appropriate
	Directive intervention	
Requirements of therapist	Understanding of Japanese popular culture (have consultant if necessary)	Understanding of Anglo popular culture
	Education and training in family and individual therapies	Education and training in therapies appropriate to clients; family, group, individual
	Bilingualism (if client is issei, older nisei, or kibei)	
Therapy site	Clients' home; community facility (nonpsychiatric)	Counseling or mental health facility
Duration and frequency	Preferably brief, 1 to 6 months Weekly	Variable according to therapist and client assessment of need

Source: B. S. Furuta, "Ethnic Identities of Japanese-American Families: Implications for Counseling," in: *Understanding the Family: Stress and Change in American Family Life*, edited by C. Getty and W. Humphreys. Norwalk, CT.: Appleton-Century-Crofts, 1981, pp. 226-227.

- What is stopping you *right now* from acting like your heroine or hero?
- What oppressions have you heard others talk about?
- In what ways have you experienced anything similar?
- What impact have other people's oppressions had on your life?
- If you were feeling strong, in charge of yourself, what would you be doing now about your and others' oppressions?

Source: B. J. Somers, "Working on Oppression: A New Therapeutic Strategy." California State University, Los Angeles, MS. 1977.

Table 26–6   DISTRESSED AND UNDISTRESSED INTERPERSONAL REACTIONS TO OPPRESSORS

Distressed	Undistressed
Away from Oppressor	
Victim	Detached
Powerlessness	Autonomous
Helplessness	Own life-style and
Numbness	culture
Demoralization	
Toward Oppressor	
Identification with	Loving
oppressor	Helping
Pseudointimacy	Caring
Pretense	Playful with oppressor's
Accommodation	actions
Passivity	
Servility	
Against Oppressor	
Displaced anger	Resisting
Dramatics	Interrupting
Delinquency	Collective action
Guilt-inducing	Teasing
Rebellion	

Source: B. J. Somers, "Working on Oppression: A New Therapeutic Strategy." California State University, Los Angeles, MS. 1977.

When Clients Need Help With Destructive Cult Experiences   How do cultists become ex-cultists? Some become disillusioned with cult life, find themselves incapable of submitting to the cult's demands, grow bitter about discrepancies they perceive between rhetoric and practice, and leave on their own or with the help of family or friends. Others (some 75 percent) leave cults through legal conservatorships granted to their parents, and still others are "rescued" by Ted Patrick or people like him. Patrick's highly controversial technique involves kidnapping cultists with their parents' help and deprogramming them. Some say he violates religious freedom.

Most parents who want to remove their adult offspring from a cult do so by seeking court appointment as conservators. While the grounds for doing so vary from state to state, for the most part the court must find the person "gravely disabled," that is, unable to manage personal property and finances or to provide for such personal needs as food, clothing, and shelter. Judges then set a date for a final hearing when the adult offspring can be present. In the meantime, parents attempt to effect a change of heart using persuasion, psychotherapy, deprogramming, or a combination of techniques. Elective or not, the days away from the cult atmosphere give cult members a chance to think, rest, and see friends and family.

Often cult members say they were hoping for rescue and were grateful for intervention. They had felt powerless to leave because of social and psychological pressure from other cult members. Many felt guilty about considering defecting and feared the cult's retaliation. In addition, they were uncertain of how they would manage in the outside world.

Other cult members, however, have not been talked out of their beliefs during the conservatorship hiatus. Their increasingly successful legal attack on such practices has been backed by the American Civil Liberties Union; the National Council of Churches; the Alliance for the Preservation of Religious Liberty (a San Diego-based antideprogramming group); and several associations of psychologists, philosophers, and theologians. They have asserted their constitutional right to practice their own religion, no matter how unacceptable it is to family and friends. The conservatorship actions, they say, violate federal civil rights laws that guarantee that courts and court officers cannot be used to deny an individual's basic rights to freedom of religion, speech, association, and privacy.

Most ex-cultists struggle at one time or another with some or all of the following difficulties and problems (Singer 1979) and report that it takes them from six to eighteen months to function in their lives at levels commensurate with their histories and talents.

- *Depression.* Without the cult's twenty-four-hour regime of ritual, work, worship, and community, ex-members often feel purposeless. Moreover, they discover that they must still deal with family and personal issues left unresolved at the time of their conversion. They must contend with a variety of new losses—lost years in the cult, being out of step and behind their peers in career and life pursuits, and a loss of self-esteem as they perceive themselves as deceived and used by the cult. Quite naturally, all these difficulties often produce profound Depression.

- *Loneliness.* Leaving a cult means leaving behind friends, shared purpose, brotherhood, and a sense of community. Regaining family and old friends often fails to make up for the resulting loneliness.

- *Sexual conflicts.* Struggles with issues of sexuality, dating, and marriage that most cultists experienced before joining the cult are reduced in most cults because of their strict rules. Others in orgiastic cults such as the Children of God undergo enforced sexuality rather than celibacy. In either case, sexual conflicts remain to be worked out.

- *Indecisiveness.* Because most cult groups prescribe virtually every activity, certain individuals find they are unable to make their own decisions. They cannot put together an organized plan for taking care of themselves, holding a job, going to school, or having a social life.

- *"Floating."* Such cult practices as long repetitive lectures, chanting while half-awake, meditating, and wearing headsets to bed that pipe the leader's sermons into their ears produce states of altered consciousness and suggestibility called "floating." Former cult members find that a variety of conditions, such as stress and conflict, a depressive low, or certain significant words or ideas, can trigger a return to the trancelike state they knew in cult days. Like the flashbacks of drug users, floating episodes are most frequent immediately after leaving the group, but in certain people they still occur weeks or months later. There are a few reports of episodes continuing to occur for up to two years in people who exhibited signs of pathology before entering the cult.

- *Blurring of mental acuity.* In most cults, members are cut off from anything but the simplest right–wrong notions and don't think and reason about contingencies. Subtle cognitive inefficiencies and changes may occur, and many former members have to take simple jobs until they regain former levels of competence.

- *Uncritical passivity.* Many ex-cultists cannot listen and judge; they listen, believe, and obey, taking the comments of others as commands. It takes time to regain former critical skills.

- *Fear of the cult.* When former cult members retain some belief in cult doctrine, warnings of heavenly damnation for themselves, their ancestors, and their children can be a terrible burden to bear. Efforts to get members back into the cult range from moderate harassment to the use of force.

- *The fishbowl effect.* The constant watchfulness of family and old friends and the curiosity of new acquaintances can be difficult to bear. Returnees may feel that others refuse to hear anything but the negative aspects of group life. If they talk of positive aspects the result is often increased watchfulness on the part of others.

- *The agonies of explaining.* Many people are still unfamiliar with cults, and returnees find it difficult to explain to such people why they joined in the first place, and why they were unable simply to walk away later.

- *Guilt.* Many ex-members feel great remorse over cult activities particularly in relation to fund raising and recruitment, and they worry about how to right these wrongs.

- *Perplexities about altruism.* Ex-cultists are often perplexed about how to select which of the many altruistic organizations will allow them to remain independent.

- *Money.* Many cult members have raised more money by fund raising on the streets than they will ever be able to earn in a job. Some skillful and dedicated solicitors can bring in as much as $1,500 day after day. One claimed to have raised $30,000 in a month by simply selling flowers.

- *No longer being elite.* One of the most poignant comedowns of postcult life is no longer to feel chosen, a member of an elite called out of the anonymous masses to save the earth.

Because of these difficulties and problems, ex-cultists and their families may seek help from mental health professionals. On the other hand, parents may seek information about a specific cult, advice about how to extricate their child from a cult, or professional help in deprogramming. Table 26–8 includes information about a number of anti-cult groups to which nurses can refer parents for support (Kneisl 1981b).

Table 26-8 ANTICULT GROUPS
American Family Foundation, Inc. Center on Destructive Cultism 89 State Street, Suite 300 Boston, Mass. 02109
Citizens Engaged in Freeing Minds P.O. Box 82664 Atlanta, Ga. 30354
Citizens Engaged in Reuniting Families Box 348 Harrison, N.Y. 10052

Citizens Freedom Foundation
Box 7000-89
1719 Via El Prado
Redondo Beach, Calif. 90277
  (New York City: 212-988-7875)
  (New Jersey: 201-836-5791)

Citizens United for Freedom Box 183 Boston, New York 14025
Committee Engaged in Freeing Minds Box 5084 Arlington, Texas 76011
Free Minds, Inc. Box 4216 Minneapolis, Minn. 55414
Individual Freedom Foundation Box 48 Ardmore, Pa. 19003
Texans United for Freedom P.O. Box 35912 Houston, Texas 77035

Source: C. R. Kneisl. "The Cult Phenomenon." Paper presented at Perspectives in Psychiatric Care '81: The Second Annual Psychiatric/Mental Health Nursing Conference, New York, 1981(b).

The American Family Foundation Center on Destructive Cultism serves as a national clearinghouse.

Deprogramming can fail and further alienate the convert from his parents. It can also cause psychological damage, especially if the deprogrammer is not sensitive to long-standing mental health problems. Parents should be aware of the legal risks as well and should be prepared to shoulder the cost—often more than $10,000 for deprogrammers, detectives, security, lodging, travel, and legal and mental health consultation. They should also know that problems may remain and that ex-cultists will require support during their return to mainstream society. Professionals have to consider the ethics and realize that they, too, may be the targets of lawsuits.

A thorough assessment is, of course, the prelude to treatment of cult converts. According to Clark and his associates (1981) it is important to:

- Evaluate current mental status and the nature of the developmental tasks confronting the client
- Identify the strengths and weaknesses of current and past family relationships
- Identify the existence of precult psychopathology, focusing on the six months preceding conversion
- Inquire into the nature of the cult environment
- Perform a thorough health assessment in order to determine any dietary or medical problems

Once the assessment has been completed, ex-cultists need help in coping with daily tasks. The nurse will find that being directive and making use of environmental resources will help ex-cultists face the crises of everyday life. However, in the interests of promoting decision-making skills former cultists should be encouraged to do as much for themselves as possible.

Because of the returnee's problems with "floating" episodes and cognitive inefficiencies and changes, techniques such as reflection, paraphrasing, and interpretation may be insufficient. This person needs information about the cult phenomenon and someone who can demonstrate or model commonsense analytical processes.

The nurse must help the ex-cultist member reconnect to the past by awakening old memories and bringing to the fore developmental tasks that were "placed on hold" during the person's stay in the cult. Nurses should be careful not to overwhelm returnees with anxiety but should get them working on reconnecting to the past and dealing with day-to-day crises very early in the counseling experience.

It is not as clear when we should elicit and confront the returnee's cult experience, however, because of the diversity in backgrounds and coping skills of former cult members. The pace and intensity should be that which can be handled by the client. Examining their conversion will help returnees understand their present difficulties, decrease their guilt and tendency to blame themselves for their conversion, identify the factors or dynamics that may have influenced their conversion or may be contributing to current distress. The client's coping skills will dictate how quickly these tasks can be undertaken.

The returnee and counselor should also explore the experience of love, friendship, and sense of purpose in the cult. Although ex-members may become acutely disillusioned when recognizing that these experiences were less solid than they seemed to be, the recognition helps diminish their guilt over leaving the cult. This analysis may cause both anger and grief. The nurse needs to help the ex-member identify and respond constructively to the various aspects of this mixture of emotions.

Counseling of current cult members proceeds more slowly. Nurses should direct their energies toward the development of rapport and should take care not to assault the convert's beliefs while simply presenting another way of looking at things. They can gently explore any doubts about the cult and stimulate critical faculties by encouraging clients to examine the pros and cons of each point of view. Supportiveness and a good sense of timing are important when working with cult members.

Counseling of parents should help them to reflect on their cult-related experience, articulate more accurately their thoughts and emotions about these experi-

ences, assess the validity of their insights into the cult phenomenon, deal constructively with the caretaker urge, promote the child's psychological development, and cope effectively with any of their own personal and marital problems, whether of recent or remote origin. The nurse should resist "diversions," e.g., the temptation to work on an "interesting" marital conflict or to escape the ambiguity of the cult counseling process by focusing on a problem that feels comfortable. Nevertheless, personal, marital, or family conflicts may sometimes be so severe as to sabotage any therapeutic strategy aimed at assisting the convert. Thus, from time to time it may be necessary to place a convert's problems "on the back burner," however risky this may be, in order to concentrate on serious problems within the family. Occasionally a convert's potential or actual return may be so disruptive to the family equilibrium that the clinician is faced with the prospect of breaking up the family while trying to "save" the convert. As with so many aspects of the cult phenomenon, there are no clear-cut guidelines about what to do in such situations.

KEY NURSING CONCEPTS

✔ Cultures define what "sanity" and "insanity" should be and therefore define the meaning of the behavior of their members.

✔ The "assumptive world" is a set of assumptions people make about their world. An individual's "assumptive world view" helps predict how others are likely to behave and the possible effects of one's actions on others.

✔ The assumptive world is formed during early family life experiences and in interactions with many other groups.

✔ When assumptive worlds of interacting people differ, their interactions are less likely to be satisfying.

✔ Sociocultural factors may inhibit or facilitate the delivery of humanistic psychiatric nursing.

✔ Multiethnic societies present a special challenge to the nurse attempting to communicate and interact across "assumptive world views."

✔ Some factors that may affect the provision of humanistic psychiatric nursing care include cultural complexity and diversity, cultural stereotyping, and the mental health professional's preference for the YAVIS client.

✔ Biosocial factors that influence mental health include ethnicity, socioeconomic class, religious beliefs, age, place of residence, sex, and marital status. Among these factors, stress appears to be a common denominator in the incidence of mental illness.

✔ Contemporary sociopolitical forces influencing mental health include civil rights movements for feminists, gays, clients, and elders; the development of new religious cults; and the community mental health movement.

✔ Contemporary sociopolitical movements may be viewed as responses to the rigidities of oppressive systems that cause distress to less powerful persons.

✔ Folk beliefs and healing practices are culture-specific ways of handling physical problems and emotional conflicts. They reflect the assumptive world view of the particular culture.

✔ In folk systems, the process of treatment is a social act rather than a technological act.

✔ Becoming familiar with and using folk beliefs and healing practices, and incorporating principles of effective communication, are essential to communicating with clients from different cultures.

✔ In counseling clients from different cultures, techniques need to be adapted to meet specific needs of the clients.

✔ It is important for the nurses to understand their own sociocultural heritage as well as those of the clients with whom they interact.

✔ The maintenance of a position of cultural awareness is a life-long personal and professional responsibility.

References

Albin, R. S. "Feminism: Mental Health Relation Seen." *Buffalo Courier Express,* 9 August 1981, pp. G4–G5.

Breen, M. "Culture and Schizophrenia: A Study of Negro and Jewish Schizophrenics." *International Journal of Social Psychiatry* 14 (1968): 282–289.

Butler, R., and Lewis, M. *Aging and Mental Health: Positive Psychosocial Approaches.* St. Louis: C. V. Mosby, 1981.

Campbell, T., and Chang, B. "Health Care of the Chinese in America." In *Transcultural Health Care,* edited by G. Henderson and M. Primeaux. pp. 162–171. Menlo Park, Calif.: Addison-Wesley, 1981.

Chang, B. "Asian-American Patient Care." In *Transcultural Health Care,* edited by G. Henderson and M. Primeaux, pp. 255–278. Menlo Park, Calif.: Addison-Wesley, 1981.

Chapman, J. and Chapman, H., *Psychology of Health Care: A Humanistic Perspective.* Monterey, Calif.: Wadsworth, 1983.

Clark, J. G.; Langone, M. D.; Daly, R. C. B.; and Schecter, R. E. *Destructive Cult Conversion: Theory, Research, and Treatment.* Boston: American Family Foundation, 1981.

Dohrenwend, B. P. "Sociocultural and Social–Psychological Factors in the Genesis of Mental Disorders." *Journal of Health and Social Behavior* 16 (1975): 365–392.

Dunham, H. W. "Society, Culture, and Mental Disorder." *Archives of General Psychiatry* 33 (1976): 147–156.

Dychtwald, K. "Humanistic Gerontology: A Positive Approach to Aging and Elder Care." *The Humanist* 40 (July-August 1980): 26–32.

Engel, G. "Sudden and Rapid Death During Psychological Stress: Folklore or Folk Wisdom?" *Annals of Internal Medicine* 74 (1971): 771–782.

Florez, R. M. F. "Differential Diagnosis of Caucasian, Black, and Chicano Patients in Mental Health Center." *Smith College Studies of Social World* 46 (1975): 57–58.

Frank, J. D. *Persuasion and Healing.* Rev. ed. New York: Schocken Books, 1974.

Georgia Nurses Association. *American Nurse,* April 1, 1981, p. 35.

Gmelch, G., and Felson, R. "Can a Lucky Charm Get You Through Organic Chemistry?" *Psychology Today* 13 (December 1980): 75–78.

Gove, W. R., and Tudor, J. F. "Adult Sex Roles and Mental Illness." *American Journal of Sociology* 78 (1973): 812–835.

Hankoff, I. D., Blumenthal, M., and Borowich, A. E. *Jewish Ethno-psychiatry.* New York: Federation of Jewish Philanthropies, 1977.

Henderson, G., and Primeaux, M. "The Importance of Folk Medicine." In *Transcultural Health Care,* pp. 59–77. Menlo Park, Calif.: Addison-Wesley, 1981.

Kaplan, H. B. "Sociodemographic Factors, Mental Health Status, and Mental Health Care." In *A Clinician's Manual of Mental Health Care: A Multidisciplinary Approach,* pp. 194–204. Menlo Park, Calif.: Addison-Wesley, 1982.

Kiev, A. *Magic, Faith, and Healing.* New York: Free Press, 1964.

Kneisl, C. R. "The Cult Phenomenon." Paper presented at Perspectives in Psychiatric Care '81: The Second Annual Psychiatric/Mental Health Nursing Conference, New York, May 24, 1981(a).

————. "Understanding Destructive Cults and Counseling Ex-Cultists." Paper presented at Third Southeastern Regional Conference of Clinical Specialists in Psychiatric-Mental Health Nursing. Virginia Beach, Virginia, September 24, 1981(b).

Louie, T. "Illness Concept and Management Among Chinese-Americans in San Francisco." Paper presented June 11, 1974, at the American Nurses Association Biennial Convention, San Francisco, California.

Marcos, L. R., Urcuyo, L., Kesselman, M., and Alpert, M. "The Language Barrier in Evaluating Spanish-American Patients." In *Transcultural Health Care,* edited by G. Henderson and M. Primeaux, pp. 38-48. Menlo Park, Calif.: Addison-Wesley, 1981.

Matthenson, M. A. "Is Crazy Anglo Crazy Haitian?" *Psychiatry Annals* 5 (1975): 79-83.

Mead, M. *Sex and Temperament in Three Primitive Societies.* New York: William Morrow, 1935.

Murillo-Rohde, I. "Hispanic American Patient Care." In *Transcultural Health Care,* edited by G. Henderson and M. Primeaux, pp. 224-238. Menlo Park, Calif.: Addison-Wesley, 1981.

Neugarten, B. (interviewed by E. Hall). "Acting One's Age: New Rules for Old." *Psychology Today* 13 (April 1980): 66-80.

"The Nurse's Discontent," *New York Times,* August 10, 1981, p. A. 14.

Primeaux, M., and Henderson, G. "American Indian Patient Care." In *Transcultural Health Care,* pp. 239-254. Menlo Park, Calif.: Addison-Wesley, 1981.

Redlich, F., and Kellert, S. "Trends in American Mental Health." *American Journal of Psychiatry* 135 (1978): 22-28.

Report to the President of the President's Commission on Mental Health. Vol. I. U.S. Government Printing Office: Washington, D.C., 1978.

Schofield, W. *Psychotherapy: The Purchase of Friendship.* Englewood Cliffs, N.J.: Prentice-Hall, 1964.

Schwartz, L. L., and Kaslow, F. W. "Religious Cults, the Individual and the Family." *Journal of Marital and Family Therapy* 5 (April 1979): 15-26.

Scott, C. S. "Health and Healing Practices Among Five Ethnic Groups in Miami, Florida." In *Transcultural Health Care,* edited by G. Henderson and M. Primeaux, pp. 102-114. Menlo Park, Calif.: Addison-Wesley, 1981.

Singer, M. R. "Coming Out of the Cults." *Psychology Today* 12 (January 1979): 72-80.

Smith, W. D., Burlew, A. K., Mosley, M. H., and Whitney, W. M. *Minority Issues in Mental Health.* Reading, Mass.: Addison-Wesley, 1978.

Snow, L. F. "Folk Medical Beliefs and Their Implications for the Care of Patients: A Review Based on Studies Among Black Americans." In *Transcultural Health Care,* edited by G. Henderson and M. Primeaux, pp. 78-101. Menlo Park, Calif.: Addison-Wesley, 1981.

————. "Sorcerers, Saints, and Charlatans: Black Folk Healers in Urban America." *Culture and Medical Psychiatry* 2 (1978): 87-91.

Somers, B. J. "Working on Oppression: A New Therapeutic Strategy." California State University, Los Angeles, MS 1977.

Stoller, R. J., et al. "A Symposium: Should Homosexuality Be in the A. P. A. Nomenclature?" *American Journal of Psychiatry* 130 (1973): 1207-1216.

Vaillant, G. "The Mental Health of the Unemployed." *Psychology Today* 13 (December 1980): 28-29.

Weisberg, M. D., and Graham, J. R. *A Barefoot Doctor's Manual.* Oceanside, N.Y.: Cloudburst Press of America, 1977.

Zeldow, P. "Sex Differences in Psychiatric Evaluation and Treatment." *Archives of General Psychiatry* 35 (1978): 89-93.

Ziegler, V., and Biggs, J. "Tricyclic Plasma Levels." *Journal of the American Medical Association* 238 (1977): 2167-2169.

Further Reading

Backup, R. "Implementing Quality Care for the American Indian Patient." *Washington State Journal of Nursing* (Special Supplement 1979): 20-24.

Baumli, F. "Men's and Women's Liberation: A Common Cause." *The Humanist* 40 (July-August 1980): 20-24.

Brodsky, A. M. "A Decade of Feminist Influence on Psychotherapy," *Psychology of Women* 4 (Spring 1980): 331-344.

Gove, W. R. "Mental Illness and Psychiatric Treatment Among Women." *Psychology of Women* 4 (Spring 1980): 345-362.

Hand, W. D. *American Folk Medicine.* Berkeley, Calif.: University of California Press, 1976.

Jameton, A. "The Nurse: When Roles and Rules Conflict." *Hastings Center Report* 7 (1977): 22-23.

Lantz, J. R., and Meyer, E. A. "The Dirty House." *Nursing Outlook* 27L (1979): 590-593.

Leininger, M. *Transcultural Nursing: Concepts, Theories, and Practices.* New York: John Wiley, 1978.

Martin, E. P., and Martin, J. M. *The Extended Black Family.* Chicago: University of Chicago Press, 1978.

Martinez, R. A. *Hispanic Culture and Health Care: Fact, Fiction, Folklore.* St. Louis: C. V. Mosby, 1978.

Meleis, A. I. "The Arab American in the Health Care System." *American Journal of Nursing* 81 (June 1981): 1180–1183.

Ramaekers, M. J. "Communication Blocks Revisited." *American Journal of Nursing* 79 (1979): 1079–1081.

Sorkin, A. *The Urban Indian.* Lexington, Mass.: Heath, 1978.

Sullivan, R. "Some Values, Beliefs, and Practices of the Elderly in the United States: Implications for Health and Nursing Care." *Transcultural Nursing Care* 2 (1977): 13–26.

Tripp-Reimer, T., and Friedl, M. "Appalachians: A Neglected Minority." *Nursing Clinics of North America* 12 (1977): 41–54.

Veith, I. *The Yellow Emperor's Classic of Internal Medicine.* Rev. ed. Berkeley, Calif.: University of California Press, 1972.

Warner, R. "Witchcraft and Soul Loss: Implications for Community Psychiatry." *Hospital and Community Psychiatry* 28 (1977): 686–690.

Legal Considerations in Psychiatric Nursing Practice

by Joanne Keglovits

CHAPTER OUTLINE

Madness and the Law—A Look at the Past
    Jewish Law—The Talmud
    Greek Law
    Roman Law
    The Visigothic Code
    Development of English Law
    Madness in the New World
Twentieth-Century Mental Hygiene Laws
    Model Legislation—The Draft Act
    Status of Legislation after the Draft Act
Some Recent Court Decisions
    Right to Treatment
    Commitment Procedures
    Civil Rights
    The Client–Therapist–Public Relationship
    Right to Refuse Treatment
Overview of Mental Hygiene Laws
    Admission
    Rights of Clients
    Participation in Legal Matters
    Separation from a Mental Institution

Two Current Mental Health Laws
    New York State's Mental Hygiene Law
    California's Mental Hygiene Law
The Implementation of Clients' Rights
    The Role of Care Givers
    Staff Knowledge and Attitudes
Key Nursing Concepts

LEARNING OBJECTIVES

After reading this chapter, students should be able to
- Describe the historical relationship between madness and the law
- Analyze key court decisions about mental health laws
- Identify the major components of mental health legislation
- Relate mental health legislation to humanistic psychiatric nursing practice
- Describe the relationship between the legal and civil rights of mental clients and humanistic psychiatric nursing practice

CHAPTER 27

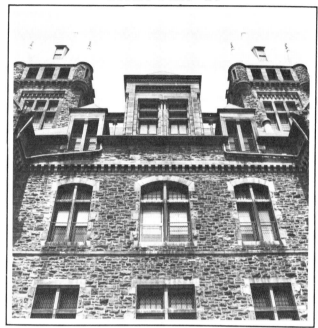

Before reviewing contemporary legal practices, this chapter takes a brief historical look at the relationship between madness and the law. A historical approach puts present-day practices into perspective and offers a sense of continuity.

MADNESS AND THE LAW—A LOOK AT THE PAST

Law develops in a social context, ideally in response to the problems and needs of the governed. Traditionally, mental disability has been considered a private matter, except where either public safety or legal issues (usually regarding property) were at stake. Only in the last few hundred years has society been seeking out its mentally disturbed members to do something for them.

Jewish Law—The Talmud

The Talmud, the authoritative body of Jewish law and tradition, mentions mental illness in relation to its legal implications. The insane were held to be mentally incompetent and therefore not legally responsible for their actions. Mentally disordered people were not held responsible for the harm they might cause. On the other side of the coin, a competent person was not held legally responsible for defaming a mentally disordered person. It was not possible for a mentally disordered person to validate a marriage or testify in court. If an individual was judged mentally incompetent, the court could appoint a guardian. A knowledge of the episodic nature of mental disorders is reflected in the Talmud, which reinstates full legal effectiveness to the person during any lucid periods.

The Talmud tries to come to grips with the problem of defining mental illness. It does so largely in behavioral terms. Wandering alone at night, tearing one's garments, and spending the night in a cemetery, if done at other than ritually "correct" times, might be

Mental illness affects the lives of many individuals in the United States. Statisticians predict that one out of every twelve Americans is likely to be hospitalized at some time for mental illness. Laws pertaining to mental illness assume major importance when viewed in terms of the vast number of people likely to be affected by them. Both the laws and their implementation concern psychiatric nurses.

The many civil and constitutional rights retained according to law by an individual hospitalized for mental disability are of little use unless the individual is aware of them. The full implementation of clients' rights is frequently the responsibility of psychiatric personnel, specifically psychiatric nurses. As treatment providers, these nurses have the legal responsibility to inform the people under their care of their legal rights. Nurses are often uniquely familiar with all phases of a client's treatment, since admission papers, consent forms, orders for medication, and restrictions pass through their hands. The psychiatric nurse who is not acquainted with the relevant law will not be able to act as an advocate for clients if infringements of their rights occur (see Chapter 5).

Psychiatric nurses may also feel a responsibility to influence the direction of mental health care in this country. To do this, they have to become involved in policy formation and the drafting of legislation. Familiarity with existing mental health legislation is a necessity if nurses are to become politically active.

considered irrational and call an individual's sanity into question. Admitting the lack of any effective treatment for mental disorders, the Talmud says little about this subject. It does, however, make the observation that old age and excessive grief can cause mental disorders.

Greek Law

On the whole, Greek law took account of mad people chiefly in relation to protection of the community and protection of the mad person's property. The *dike paranoias*—a legal procedure comparable to modern guardianship or conservatorship proceedings—was one instrument used in Athens to protect family property. It is the basis of this passage in Plato's "Laws" (*Dialogues* 1964, 11:929c):

> If disease, or old age, or evil disposition cause a man to go out of his mind, and he is ruining his house and property, and his sons doubt about indicting him for insanity, let him lay the case before the eldest guardians of the law, and consult with them. And if they advise him to proceed, and the father is decided to be imbecile, he shall have no more control over his property, but shall live henceforth like a child in the house.

Plato also indicates that the insane were generally not held responsible for criminal action. Referring to sacrilege, conspiracy, and treason, he says (*Dialogues* 1964, 11:834d):

> Any of these crimes may be committed by a person not in his right mind, or in the second childhood of old age. If this is proved to be the fact before the judges, the person in question shall not be punished further, unless he have on his hands the stain of blood. In this case he shall be exiled for a year, and if he returns before the expiration of the year, he shall be retained in the public prison two years.

Greece was a slave-owning society, and the law also dealt with defects in the bodies and minds of slaves put up for sale. According to the law, the seller was obliged to declare any known defects that were not self-evident to the prospective buyer. A seller who failed to do so was required to give a full refund. The defective slaves themselves were given little legal protection and were probably driven out to wander in the street and run the risk of being stoned. To safeguard against this, Plato proposed that a heavy fine be levied on anyone who had a mad slave and did not take care of him or her.

Plato also advocated keeping a mad person at home by any means possible. "If a man is mad," he said, "he shall not be at large in the city, but his relations shall keep him at home in any way they can; or if not, let them pay a penalty" (*Dialogues* 1964, 11:934d).

Roman Law

In dealing with the mentally disordered, Greek and Roman laws exhibit several similarities. The Romans appointed a curator to take charge of a mad person's property, and this resembles the procedure of dike paranoias employed by the Greeks. The oldest Roman law code—the Law of Twelve Tables—dating from the fifth century B.C., provided that, "If a person is insane authority over him and his property shall belong to his agnates, and in default of these to his clansman" (Johnson 1961, p. 9). A "furiosus" or mad person in Rome, as in Greece, lacked the capacity to effect a legal act. Any contract, including the marriage contract, was void—whether or not the other party was aware of the disturbed person's state. The mad person was not held liable for fines or damages for any wrongs committed, although historians believe this rule was acknowledged only reluctantly in the classical period. Curatorship or guardianship over property and legal incapacity in both Rome and Greece began with a person's madness and ended during lucid periods.

Initially, there was no Roman procedure by which a person might be declared officially insane. It is believed that the pronouncement of madness probably came from the family or clan. According to historians, the fundamental question—when a person was to be regarded as mad—was never discussed. This was considered a question of fact and was not subject to any rules of law. Guardianship or curatorship in Rome kept the mad person's property within the agnatic family, where only relationships through males were recognized. Initially, the guardian had full and complete power over the goods of the mad person, but, as the law developed, the guardian's jurisdiction over the property was limited to administrative matters. The guardian was also held accountable to the mad person if that person recovered.

The Visigothic Code

The successful invasion of Rome in the fifth century A.D. by the barbaric Germanic tribes ushered in what is commonly called the Dark Ages. The laws of the Germanic tribes supplanted Roman law in western Europe. The Visigothic Code, drafted between 466 and 485 A.D., and followed in France and Spain, showed the influence of Roman law. According to this code, any insane person, whether deranged from infancy or later in life, was not allowed to testify in court or enter into a contract while insane but could do so during any lucid period.

Development of English Law

In the reign of Henry I (1068–1135) a law made parents responsible for any insane offspring, specifying that care of the child had to be benevolent. The principle of diminished responsibility was often used in assessing the guilt of an insane person for criminal acts. Diminished responsibility means that the person lacks the capacity to form full intent to commit a criminal act. The person with diminished responsibility is usually held accountable on a lesser charge or receives a less severe sentence. Guardianship of a mentally disordered person and control of the person's property were assumed by the feudal lord in early England. After consolidation of the crown in the thirteenth century, this function was assumed by the king, who, as *parens patriae* (father of his country), was considered the protector of the personal and property interests of his subjects.

According to the statute of *De Praerogativa Regis*, enacted by Edward II sometime between 1255 and 1290, the mentally disordered were divided into two classes—idiots and lunatics. The term *idiot* was used for persons known to have had "no understanding" from birth. *Lunatic* applied to individuals known to have had "understanding" but for some reason unfortunate enough to have lost it. The king was required to use the profits from the disordered person's estate to provide for that person and to save any remaining profits from the estate in case the person became sane again and the guardianship ended. In the case of idiots, the crown was allowed to retain any excess profit from the estate. It was therefore more profitable for the crown to manage the estate of an idiot than that of a lunatic.

The insane were generally excluded from the community in a variety of ways. If violent, they were likely to be shackled in a prison. Toward the end of the fifteenth century, a likely fate might have been execution for being a witch. The Middle Ages are generally credited with driving out or excluding the insane from community life, while the Renaissance is noted for its methods of exclusion by confinement. Historians theorize that the switch occurred because of two events: (1) the closing of many monasteries that had fallen into

disrepute because of scandalous practices by the monks, and (2) a drastic decrease in the incidence of leprosy, which left thousands of leprosaria empty and ready to house the insane (see Chapter 1).

The priory of the Order of Saint Mary of Bethlehem was founded in London in 1247 and, by the fifteenth century, was providing for a small number of lunatics. By 1774, Bethlehem Hospital, or "Bedlam" as it is best known, was the largest hospital involved in housing the insane in England. A porter is reported to have absconded from Bethlehem Hospital in 1403 with an assortment of chains and irons, giving some idea of the type of treatment probably given to the inmates. Until the seventeenth century, patients, referred to as "Toms o' Bedlam," were given a recognizable badge licensing them to beg. In *King Lear* (act 3, scene 4) Shakespeare describes these wandering Toms o' Bedlam when he speaks of

> Poor Tom, that eats the swimming frog, the toad, the tadpole, the wall-newt in the water; that in the fury of his heart, when the foul fiend rages, eats cow-dung for salets; swallows the old rat and the ditch-dog; drinks the green mantle of the standing pool; who is whipped from tithing to tithing, and stock punished, and imprisoned.

Until the sixteenth century, the church was largely responsible for the poor. The Protestant Reformation, along with the dissolution of the monasteries, decreased the effectiveness of the church at a time when the number of poor people was increasing rapidly, due to many social and economic changes. High unemployment, poverty, vagabondage, begging, and thievery were a few of the social ills the populace looked to the crown to address. In 1536, Henry VIII tried to solve the problem by making paupers a charge of the local municipalities, towns, and parishes. The burden was too great, however, and in 1601 the overall responsibility was shifted from local to national authorities by the Poor Laws of Queen Elizabeth.

Under the Poor Laws, the poor and the destitute insane received the same treatment. They were either eligible for dole payments or hired out to farmers, who were to provide for them in exchange for their labor. Vagabondage was discouraged by requiring residence status to qualify a person for relief. Recipients under the Poor Laws were easily identified by a large red or blue P on their clothing. Abuses of the dole and the farming out system kept cropping up, and the controlled system of a workhouse was developed as a solution. The abandoned monasteries and leprosaria were ready for conversion to workhouses.

Madness in the New World

The American colonists brought to the New World not only their wordly possessions but also much of the culture and tradition of their mother countries. Their sparsely populated communities were predominantly agricultural and rural. Instances of mental illness that emerged were dealt with largely on an informal basis by either the family, the community, or both.

Mentally disordered people came to the attention of the authorities either through inability to provide and care for themselves or through unruly or violent behavior. To avoid assuming responsibility for such people as public charges, towns subjected unsightly or undesirable nonresidents to the settlement laws or customs, and, like other paupers, these unwanted people were "warned away." Disturbances caused by violent or irrational behavior were dealt with in a variety of ways. Incarceration was common if a jail existed. Simply whipping sometimes produced the desired effect.

The family had primary responsibility for the welfare of any member who became insane. However, local towns and communities were not against helping a family support an insane member. Many incidents are recorded in which local tax money was alloted to help maintain a mentally disordered person. For example, the Upland (Delaware County, Pennsylvania) County records for 1676 show that the court ordered a small block house to be built for a man who was described as "bereft of his natural senses," after his father complained to the court that he was too poor to provide for his son.

A special structure was ordered to be built in New York City in 1677 for the confinement of Peter Paull, a "lunatick." Until the completion of this one-man asylum, the court directed that Paull, "bee confined into prison in the hold." In 1677, Massachusetts passed a statute directing the selectmen of towns having any dangerously distracted persons to "take care of them so that they do not damify others." This Massachusetts statute provided the legal basis for the forcible restraint of the violent, and served as model legislation to other New England colonies.

On May 20, 1720, the mayor's court in New York directed the churchwarden to pay some four shillings a week for the support of a widow who was "non compos mentis" (Latin for "not having mastery of one's mind"). In some locales it was customary to house insane paupers in private dwellings at the public's expense. This task was usually taken on by local officials or clergy and apparently did not require any

judicial procedures. It was probably more a practical solution to a community problem than the legal precursor of "commitment" of a person to the custody of another.

The insane were among the patients of this country's first general hospital. Pennsylvania Hospital was opened through the efforts of the Quakers, Benjamin Franklin, and others in 1756. Treatment, rather than mere confinement of the mentally ill, was its stated goal for these patients, though the state of medical knowledge was such that treatment consisted of bleeding, blistering, and purging in the damp restraining cells of the hospital's cellar. There were no statutes governing commitment of the insane in colonial times, and any person, relative, friend, or enemy could apply to the manager of the hospital or a physician for an order of admission. As chains and irons were part of the environment, it was a simple task to subdue a protesting individual.

The first American hospital devoted exclusively to the care and treatment of the insane opened in Williamsburg, Virginia, in 1773. The only other colony to establish a hospital that accepted mentally ill patients in the eighteenth century was New York, which began building its first general hospital in 1774, with the intention of allotting the cellar of the north wing to the insane. The Revolutionary War and a fire delayed the opening until 1792. As promised, the cellar of New York Hospital received the insane.

The number of insane people residing in these early institutions never reached large proportions. In Philadelphia Hospital between 1752 and 1754, only 18 of the 117 patients admitted were reported insane. Even in 1784, Benjamin Rush reported that only 34 mental patients were in residence. In New York Hospital between 1792 and 1794 fewer than 10 cases had been admitted.

Mental illness was generally not recognized as a major medical problem or a pressing social concern in the United States in the seventeenth and eighteenth centuries. American society was still largely rural, and in most cases the insane could be dealt with in an informal manner. The few more populated urban areas, such as Philadelphia and New York, where informal means were no longer adequate, did move to establish hospitals to deal with problems associated with mental disorder. As early as 1724, Boston selectmen had considered adding a section to the almshouse, to separate the poor from the insane. But for various reasons it was not until 1818 that Massachusetts Asylum was opened.

The Growth of Mental Hospitals   The growth of the mental hospital in the early nineteenth century was not a chance occurrence but the result of numerous social factors. It arose from the general spirit of reform and humanitarianism permeating western Europe and the United States. Scientific and technological advances, coupled with the successful struggle for political democracy in the United States and France, were proof to many people that humanity could tackle and conquer any problem. Also, the Second Great Awakening, a religious movement that swept the United States between 1795 and about 1835, did much to weaken the Calvinistic notion that human nature was inherently depraved. The awakening emphasized religious beliefs more compatible with the philosophy of the Enlightenment. Ministers and laypeople alike began to work toward the "perfectibility" of the individual and society through social reform.

During the same period, news of Philippe Pinel's work with the insane in France (1806, reprint 1962) and William Tuke's in England (see Tuke, D., 1882; 1885) was reaching across the Atlantic. Because of the social changes accompanying the French Revolution, Pinel had the opportunity to put the theories inspired by his classic predecessors into practice at the Bicêtre and Salpêtrière in Paris. He abolished systematized brutality with chains and whips, which had made the fate of the insane worse than that of criminals. History reports that intelligent understanding replaced the chains, and many of the inmates improved dramatically. Meanwhile in England, Tuke, unhappy about the institutions available for mentally ill Quakers, was planning the York Retreat. The approach used by Pinel and Tuke was referred to as "moral treatment." In today's terminology it could be explained as the resocialization of the insane within an institutional setting where their physical and social environment could be completely and therapeutically restructured. Moral treatment, by providing an alternative to mere confinement of the insane, played a major role in the development of institutional care and treatment of the mentally ill in the United States.

Private philanthropy was largely responsible for the hospital movement in the early nineteenth century. In response to the needs brought on by increases in the population, hospitals were established in urban areas. These early corporate hospitals, such as McLean Asylum in Massachusetts (opened in 1818), Friend's Asylum in Frankfort, Pennsylvania (1817), Hartford Retreat in Connecticut (1824), and Bloomingdale Asylum in New York City (1818), were small and used "moral treatment" on a homogeneous population with an astounding degree of success. Dr. Eli Todd, superintendent of the Hartford Retreat, reported recovery in over 90 percent of the patients with mental illness of less than one year's duration. Even though these institutions were private, they were founded with the intention of meeting the needs of the entire community. They gradually redefined their purpose, however, and excluded almost all nonpaying patients. The success of these corporate hospitals, with their high rates of "cures," did much to convince the public of the humanitarian, medical, and economic benefits of institutional care and treatment.

An important legislative step in the gradual move toward public provision for the insane in New York was taken in 1809. This state passed the first legislation to deal with the insane as a distinct group, entitled to care and medical treatment in special hospitals. It mandated overseers of the poor to contract with the New York Hospital for the care of their insane paupers. In reality, the law did little to affect the institutional provisions for the insane pauper. The hospital's facilities were limited to some eighty beds, which were filled whenever possible with private, paying patients. In addition, local public overseers found it to the communities' economic advantage to keep the indigent insane in local poorhouses.

It became clear in the mid-1820s that the corporate mental hospitals would be unable to meet the needs of all those requiring services. Responsibility for the mentally ill, then, began gradually to shift away from the corporate hospitals (just as it had, to a certain extent, shifted away from the family and to the corporate hospital). It now moved to the new institution on the horizon—the public mental hospital.

The Growth of Public Mental Hospitals   A number of factors combined in the second quarter of the nineteenth century to make traditional and informal mechanisms ineffectual. It was a time of immigration of ethnic minorities, of rapid population growth, and of periodic economic depressions and unemployment. These factors taken together brought the problems associated with poverty and "dependence" to the fore. There was wide variation in opinion about the causes of poverty and dependence. According to their Puritan upbringing, most people saw these conditions as arising from a lack of "moral fiber." Others acknowledged contributory circumstances, such as illness, while still others attributed these conditions to the unequal social and economic order in society.

State governments began to reexamine their existing poor laws. In 1823, the New York legislature authorized a study by the secretary of state, John Yates. Yates's report was highly critical of the operation and effectiveness of the state's poor laws. According to him, dependence was being perpetuated and the needs of the insane and idiotic were being ignored. Yates's report and others like it fostered an increase in institutional care for dependent groups, with the care and treatment of the insane linked with welfare and dependence measures.

The public mental hospital movement also gained in momentum through the efforts of the "Bay State" activists. Reverend Louis Dwight, through activities in the Boston Prison Discipline Society, promoted his idea that mentally ill people belonged in hospitals. Appropriations for the erection of a 120-bed state mental hospital won the approval of the Massachusetts legislature under the guidance of Horace Mann. The first Massachusetts state hospital opened in Worcester in 1833 under the leadership of Samuel B. Woodward, and it gained a national reputation for recovery of 80 to 91 percent of its acute patients. *Acute patient* usually meant a person who had been mentally ill for less than six months. The example set by the citizens of Massachusetts became a model for other states. Dr. Woodward went on to be elected president of the newly formed Association of Medical Superintendents of American Institutions for the Insane, which changed its name to the American Psychiatric Association in 1923.

In New York, Governor Enos T. Throop, in his 1830 annual address to the legislature, called attention to the neglect suffered by the insane poor in almshouses and jails. The insane poor were still kept in jails, even though a law in 1827 had mandated that no lunatic could be confined in the same room with any person charged with a criminal offense. The insane individual was to be sent to the asylum in New York City, the county poorhouse, or the almshouse, and the family was to be responsible for the cost. The law went on to state that a lunatic could not be removed from the family's custody, if it "confined and maintained" the insane person in a manner approved of by the local town overseer. In response to Governor Throop's plea, the legislature appointed a committee to investigate the problem. In its report, the committee condemned the practice of confining the insane poor in county poorhouses, where they were either auctioned off as servants to the highest bidder or simply neglected. The committee recommended the erection of at least one state hospital. In 1836, appropriations were made for

the establishment of the New York State Lunatic Asylum, to be built in Utica. It opened, still unfinished, in January 1843. Because of their greater likelihood of recovery, paupers whose insanity was of recent origin were to be given preference over both paying patients and chronic cases.

The movement for state mental hospitals was also accelerated throughout the country by the crusade of Dorothea Dix. After teaching a Sunday school class of female convicts in an East Cambridge jail in Boston in 1841, Dix stumbled across a number of insane inmates confined in the prison. Horrified by what she saw, she went on to make a personal examination of the almshouses and jails in Massachusetts and reported her findings to the legislature in the form of a lengthy memorial. For three decades, Dix reported to state legislatures the often abominable conditions in the almshouses, jails, and mental hospitals in their states. After making her exposés, she insisted to legislators that the state had moral, humanitarian, and legal obligations

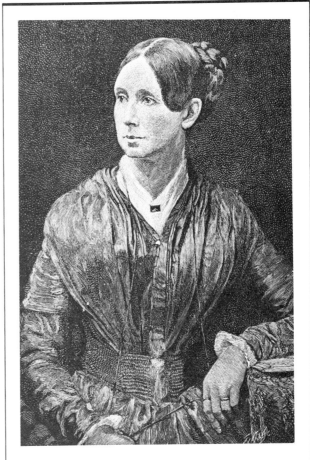

Dorothea Dix, humanitarian, activist, and crusader, is sometimes criticized as responsible for institutionalization becoming an end in itself.

toward the mentally ill. Dix's determination about this single issue gained her a broad base of support, and she was eventually responsible for founding or enlarging over thirty mental hospitals. It is suggested by J. Sanborn Bockoven (1956, p. 187), an authority on moral treatment, that Dix's reform movement, with its emphasis on bringing people into asylums without any planning for effective treatment, was responsible at least in part for the downfall of moral treatment in the United States.

Dix's memorial to the New York legislature in January 1844 was a biting indictment of the county poorhouses. It contained case after case of men and women chained in outhouses, unprotected against the cold, confined in dark cells with manacles, iron balls, and collars, and subjected to beating at the slightest provocation. Dix advocated the removal of all the insane from the poorhouses. She recommended that acute cases be sent to either the Utica State Asylum or the private Bloomingdale Asylum. In her estimations, four to six asylums were needed for the confinement of the chronic cases in New York State. In 1865, after much debate, and another survey of conditions of the insane in the poorhouses and county asylums by Dr. Sylvester D. Willard, secretary of the New York Medical Society, funds were finally allocated for the erection of an asylum for the chronic insane. Willard Asylum, with a capacity of 1,500, opened in 1869.

Institutionalization had become an end in itself. As a carryover from the high rate of "cures" effected by moral treatment, people believed that once insane persons were within the walls of an asylum, they were well on their way to recovery. The fact that asylums had less and less to offer in the form of treatment did not seem to matter in the public mind. The deterioration of asylums was often rationalized away with an attitude that the foreign insane paupers, who made up a large portion of the increasing patient population, would not appreciate nice things. American psychiatry provided another rationalization. Under the influence of Dr. John P. Gray, it began explaining mental illness in terms of physical lesions. Mental hospitals began to be organized to treat the mentally ill as the physically ill were treated. Rest and diet were considered important adjuncts to nature in curing the underlying physical disease thought to be present. Therefore, scientific psychiatry also provided an explanation for the futility of moral treatment, and replaced it with custodial care.

Early Commitment Cases Even though mental hospitals increased in size and number, commitment procedures continued to be easy and informal, without much concern for the individual's right to liberty. During the 1840s two lawsuits in particular captured the legal profession's, and to a certain extent the public's, attention regarding the problem of personal liberty and wrongful civil commitment. In 1845, Josiah Oakes, using the common law right of habeas corpus (a writ requiring the agency holding a person in custody to show that it is doing so legally and properly), successfully petitioned the Massachusetts Supreme Court for his release from McLean Asylum in Massachusetts on the grounds that he had been illegally committed by his family. In its decision, *Matter of Oakes,* 8 Law Rptr. 123 (Mass. Sup. Ct. 1845), the court first acknowledged the constitutional provision that no person should be deprived of life or liberty without due process of law, which in this case, according to the court, meant judgment of the individual by a jury of peers or the law of the land. The court also acknowledged that private institutions for the insane, such as McLean, had been in use and sanctioned by the law. The court went on to state:

> The right to restrain an insane person of his liberty is found in that great law of humanity which makes it necessary to confine those who, going at large, would be dangerous to themselves or others. In the delirium of a fever, or in the case of a person seized with a fit, unless this were the law, no one could be restrained against his will. And the necessity which creates the law creates the limitation of the law.
>
> The question must then arise in each particular case, whether a person's own safety, or that of others, requires that he should be restrained for a certain time, and whether restraint is necessary for his restoration, or will be conducive thereto. The restraint can continue as long as the necessity continues. This is the limitation, and the proper limitation. The physician of the asylum can only exercise the same power of restraint which has been laid down as competent, to be exercised by others in like cases. [Quoted in Ordronaux 1878, p. 52.]

This decision is said to have set a new precedent for the detention of the alleged insane. The old standard of "detention of the violent" was not applicable in this case. Oakes had been detained for "therapeutic reasons," because he was thought to suffer from hallucinations and was conducting his business affairs in an unsound manner. The charge grew out of the fact that Oakes, an elderly and generally judicious man, had become engaged to a woman of questionable character shortly after his wife's death.

The second case that drew attention, particularly from physicians and hospital employees who were regularly involved in commitment proceedings, was that of Hinchman (see Brakel and Rock 1970, p. 7; Deutsch 1949, p. 423). Hinchman, a patient at the Friends' Asylum in Philadelphia, instituted a civil suit for his wrongful detention. The suit was filed against his family, the physician, and the hospital employees involved in his commitment. In addition to regaining his freedom, he succeeded in obtaining damages. Isaac Ray (1871, p. 369), a noted physician, not at all pleased with the court's decision, voiced his opinion that the evidence showed beyond a doubt that Hinchman was violently and dangerously insane. Commitment legislation was seen as necessary not only to safeguard the prospective patient but also for the protection of hospital employees.

Dissatisfaction with Mental Hospitals and Commitment Procedures

With recovery rates declining and reports that a large number of insane persons were still in almshouses, despite the increase in the number and cost of asylums, mental hospitals came under attack. The publication of exposés by former mental patients added fuel to the fire of public mistrust of these hospitals. Charles Reade's very successful novel *Hard Cash*, which appeared in the United States in 1864, dramatized the dangers of the commitment laws to the general public. The story was built around the illegal commitment of a sane, young hero, through the conniving of some business associates. It was reportedly based on an actual incident in which Reade himself had been instrumental in the release of the young man wrongfully committed.

The exposés published by Mrs. E. P. W. Packard (1867, 1868, 1887), who charged that she had been unjustly committed to Illinois State Hospital for three years by her husband, also gained national attention. Under the 1851 commitment statute in effect in Illinois, a married woman could be detained in an asylum at her husband's request, without the evidence required in other cases. When she finally regained her freedom, Mrs. Packard traveled around the country addressing public meetings and legislatures on the need for more protective legislation to prevent the railroading of sane people into insane asylums. As a result of her efforts, several states changed their commitment laws to include procedural safeguards already present in the criminal law, such as:

- Notice of a pending commitment hearing
- A jury trial to determine the individual's sanity

The new Illinois commitment law, which had been known as Mrs. Packard's "personal liberty" bill, re-

quired a jury trial in every commitment proceeding. Ironically, Richard Dewey (1913), after examining old hospital records, contended that jury trials resulted in the commitment of a greater number of sane people than any other commitment proceeding. The Illinois compulsory jury trial law was repealed in 1893. However, the last state to eliminate the mandatory jury, Texas, did so only in 1953 by constitutional repeal.

Establishment of State Regulatory Agencies

In the later nineteenth century, some state legislatures once again authorized studies to look at their public policies. The result of most of these studies was the establishment of new state regulatory agencies. In New York, Governor Reuben E. Fenton's 1867 annual message urged the legislature to establish a central supervisory agency. Acting on the governor's proposal, the legislature passed a law creating the Board of State Commissioners of Public Charities. The act directed the commissioners to visit and inspect all charitable and correctional facilities. In 1873, the board's supervisory powers were expanded to include all public and private welfare institutions. The act also specifically authorized the board to visit and inspect all institutions for the care, treatment, or detention of the insane. A license was now required from the board for the establishment or operation of an asylum. A state commissioner on lunacy was appointed who was an ex-officio member of the board and reported directly to it. In response to the public outcry against "railroading," the commissioner was given broad investigatory powers to prevent abuses in commitment proceedings and mental care.

Lunacy Legislation in the 1870s

Much of the lunacy legislation enacted in the United States during the 1870s was in reaction to public distrust of mental hospitals. The emphasis in the legislation was on preventing the commitment of sane individuals. Once the question of sanity was settled, protective legislation usually ended. The model for lunacy legislation was the criminal law system, with its procedural safeguards of sworn complaints, open hearings, and jury trials. Unlike criminal sentences, however, commitments were for an indefinite period of time. Civil rights were automatically taken away during confinement.

Review of an 1874 act consolidating New York's state lunacy laws illustrates some of these points. Civil commitment to an institution in New York could be effected by the certification of two physicians, who said under oath that the person was insane. Yet the person could not remain confined in an asylum for more than five days, unless the certification was approved by a judge of the court of record from the county in which the alleged lunatic had resided. The judge had discretion to call a jury to settle the question of the individual's sanity.

An insane asylum was considered a judicial hospital, to which no one could be admitted without due process of law. Therefore, lunatics did not have the authority or the capacity of mind to commit themselves. They had to be committed by the court. The first voluntary admission law was passed in 1881 in Massachusetts and was at first limited to paying patients.

Remembering the decision in the Hinchman case, the New York statute provided some protection for the hospital superintendent, saying this official could not be held responsible for damage for false imprisonment of a sane person who had been legally committed as a lunatic, unless fraud and conspiracy could be proved. It is noteworthy that the 1874 statute addressed a question still unanswered today—must a lunatic be dangerous to justify confinement? The state reasoned that, just as the state may place restraints on certain individuals for the protection of the community, so society is bound to protect individuals from their own acts.

Mental disabilities took a heavy toll on an individual's civil rights in 1874. According to the law, a lunatic, legally speaking, had "no mind," and was held to be mentally incompetent. Thus, insane persons could not make a contract, engage in a partnership, or marry, although insanity after marriage did not constitute a ground for divorce. Lunatics could not be punished for crimes, but they could be sued for injuries done to others. Still, an unsound mind might serve as a good defense in mitigation of damages for slander or libel. The law also held that the custodian of a lunatic could, when all appeals to reason failed, use violence to restrain violence, without being held liable for assault.

The Rise of State Care   During the 1880s many states other than New York moved toward centralized control of welfare institutions. From the moment the new state boards were established, there was tension and conflict between them and hospital officials. The boards often admonished hospital administrators for extravagance or mismanagement, or disagreed with them over the hospital's role or policy. Although they differed from state to state, the issues boiled down to one—centralized versus decentralized control of state mental hospitals.

By 1881 there were six state hospitals for the insane in New York, two for chronic cases and four for acute

cases. Legislation had been passed in 1865 requiring all counties to send their chronic cases, formerly housed in local poorhouses, to the Willard Asylum. Willard, with a bed capacity for 1,500, was soon overcrowded, and certain counties were therefore allowed to care for their chronic insane in county asylums. They were required to follow the guidelines provided by the Board of State Commissioners of Public Charities, yet many welfare leaders felt that conditions in the county asylums and poorhouses were intolerable. These could be remedied, they argued, only by the state's full assumption of care for the insane—chronic and acute alike.

By 1890, a movement based on this belief had led to passage of the State Care Act. According to its provisions, the state was districted, and each state hospital was to be responsible for both the acute and chronic cases in its district. The cost of hospitalization for poor and indigent patients was to be borne by the state alone. Supervision of the care and treatment of the mentally ill was to rest in the hands of the State Commission on Lunacy. In 1921 this commission became the State Hospital Commission, and in 1927 it became known as the State Department of Mental Hygiene. The effects of New York's State Care Act spread beyond the boundaries of New York and prompted similar legislation in other states.

The die was cast: the structure and function of mental hospitals and the framework in which they were to operate had been institutionalized. Mental hospitals continued to grow. Mental illness continued to grow. Seven more state hospitals were established in New York in the decade following the State Care Act, and another seven have been added since the turn of the century. In the report of a commission established by Governor Thomas Dewey in 1944 to make an impartial survey of the operation of the Department of Mental Hygiene and the state hospitals, twenty civil mental hospitals were said to be caring for over 80,000 patients, along with six institutions for the mentally defective and epileptic with over 16,000 patients (Commission to Investigate 1944).

By 1955, the problems stemming from mental illness had become so vast that Congress endorsed establishment of a Joint Commission on Mental Illness and Health. The commission was to analyze the needs and resources of the mentally ill and make recommendations for a national policy. Its final report (Joint Commission 1961) opened with the strong and unequivocal assertion that the institutional system caring for the mentally ill in the United States was a dismal failure. "Viewed either historically or currently," it charged (p.

4), "the care of persons voluntarily admitted to public mental hospitals constitutes the great unfinished business of the mental health movement."

TWENTIETH-CENTURY MENTAL HYGIENE LAWS

Despite many advances in psychiatric theory and treatment, nineteenth-century legal practices remained on the statute books of most states well into the twentieth century. However, over the years commitment procedures lost many of their protective elements. After World War II, prominent psychiatrists and psychiatric organizations began attacking these commitment laws on the ground that they were hindering the delivery of good psychiatric care to the mentally ill. Words such as *escapee* and *parole* were believed to stigmatize the mentally ill, and jury trials instead of being helpful were said to be traumatizing. This reform movement in the late 1940s and early 1950s reasoned that "railroading" or wrongful commitment was a myth. Psychiatrists argued that mental hospitals were in fact too crowded to want to take in people who were not mentally ill. Because of this overcrowding, psychiatric decisions about who would get into a mental institution could be counted on to be correct.

Model Legislation—The Draft Act

One of the results of psychiatric dissatisfaction with the legal safeguards surrounding admission to mental hospitals was the publication in 1952 of the Draft Act Governing Hospitalization of the Mentally Ill, which was prepared by the National Institute of Mental Health. The Draft Act was to serve as a working model, to be adapted by state legislatures according to local needs and conditions. To broaden the access of the mentally ill to hospital facilities, it strongly advocated voluntary admission and made provisions for admission on medical certification. To avoid the "exposure of private troubles," it also included provisions for formal proceedings for indeterminate involuntary hospitalization. This eliminated most of the medically objectionable proceedings, including notice of a hearing, compulsory presence of the allegedly insane individual at the hearing, and jury trial. Legal safeguards were to be provided for the client to protest after confinement.

Status of Legislation after the Draft Act

After publication of the Draft Act, various states adopted new laws that not only updated their terminology (substituting the terms *mentally ill* for *insane* and *certification* for *commitment*) but also adopted the Draft Act's recommendation of medical certification and nonjudicial procedures for involuntary hospitalization. Even in states where judicial commitment procedures remained, they were found to have deteriorated largely into unrestrained medical admissions. For example, before the 1964 revision of New York's Mental Hygiene Law, most prospective clients in New York State went through certification or commitment to a mental hospital. According to the statute, individuals had a right to a hearing before certification to determine whether they needed care and treatment in an institution. However, notice of the right to a hearing could be waived if it could be shown that notice would be either useless or harmful to the client. When a special committee of the New York Bar Association studied the operation of the Mental Hygiene Law from 1960 to 1962, it found that in practice fewer than 10 percent of the clients committed throughout the state had had a hearing and that clients generally did not receive notice of their right to one (Special Committee 1962). The few hearings that were held were limited almost exclusively to the New York City area and were found to be brief, informal, and lacking in any organized presentation of the client's side. When no hearing was held, the judge usually signed the court commitment on the basis of the petition for hospitalization and the report of two physicians. Although the existing statute did allow for voluntary admissions, the committee found that they made up only one-fifth of admissions. Even so, Albert Deutsch (1961, p. 43) in his testimony before the Subcommittee on the Constitutional Rights of the Mentally Ill in 1961, cited New York, with 20 percent of its clients admitted voluntarily, as one of the most advanced in the movement toward voluntary admission. In its report the committee recommended that voluntary admission be encouraged, that the need for initial hospitalization be decided by doctors, and that there be adequate safeguards for the protection of the civil rights of clients immediately after admission. To ensure that the procedural rights of involuntary clients were enforced the committee recommended the establishment of a new statewide agency, the Mental Health Review Service. In October 1980 the Mental Health Systems Act was signed into law by President Carter. It is credited with being the first to include sections on mental health rights and advocacy for the mentally ill. The Mental Health Systems Act provides some direction for states to review and revise their mental health laws to ensure that clients receive the protection and services they require.

SOME RECENT COURT DECISIONS

The courts have traditionally been concerned with the possibility of wrongful commitment. Little attention was paid to the restrictions placed on the legal and civil rights of an individual, once hospitalized. In recent years, however, the courts have become more concerned with the substantive rights of a hospitalized individual, including the right to treatment, the right not to perform institutional labor, and retention of civil rights such as the rights to communication, visitation, religious activities, and medical self-determination. Even though most court cases have been decided at the local or federal district court level, some have been appealed all the way to the United States Supreme Court, where decisions affect the law throughout the country. The following is a summary of some of the most significant cases, grouped around five mental health areas: (1) the right to treatment, (2) commitment procedures, (3) civil rights of clients, and (4) the client–therapist–public relationship, and (5) the emerging and controversial right to refuse treatment.

Right to Treatment

The first argument for a right to treatment for involuntarily committed individuals came from Morton Birnbaum, a lawyer and a physician, in an article published in 1960. However, the ground-breaking cases did not come from the familiar circles of civil commitment but rather from individuals who had been sidetracked from the prison system into hospitals.

Rouse v. Cameron   The first case to address the right to treatment issue directly and gain national attention was *Rouse v. Cameron,* 373 F.2d 451 (D.C. Cir. 1966). In 1962, Charles Rouse had been brought to trial for carrying a dangerous weapon, which is a misdemeanor in the District of Columbia, and carries a maximum sentence of one year. Instead of being convicted and sent to trial, Rouse pleaded "not guilty by reason of insanity," and was sent to the maximum security pavilion at Saint Elizabeth's Hospital for treatment.

Four years later, Rouse questioned his detention by means of a writ of habeas corpus on the ground that he had not received any psychiatric treatment. His lawyer argued that this was the quid pro quo to which he was entitled—that is, treatment in exchange for loss of liberty. Under District of Columbia law the plea of insanity takes away criminal responsibility and subjects the defendant to an automatic involuntary commitment. State laws vary tremendously on how the committed person obtains release. Some state statutes require the person to remain committed until pardoned by the governor. Others require the person to meet the same criteria for discharge as any other civilly committed individual.

Judge David Bazelon, speaking for the United States Court of Appeals for the District of Columbia, stated that involuntary commitment is imposed because it is assumed that the criminal offender needs treatment for a mental condition. If treatment is not given, as in Rouse's case, the court held, the offender is deprived of basic rights. Although Judge Bazelon said Rouse was entitled to treatment on the basis of the present District of Columbia statute, he indicated that there might be a constitutional basis for the right as well. Whenever possible, however, courts will base their decisions on statutory rather than constitutional grounds.

Nason v. Bridgewater   Another important decision was the Supreme Judicial Court of Massachusetts ruling in *Nason v. Bridgewater,* 233 N.E.2d 908 (Mass. 1968). John Nason, a man indicted for murder, had been sent to Bridgewater State Hospital, because he was found incompetent to stand trial. After spending five years at Bridgewater, the Massachusetts facility for the dangerously insane, he filed a writ of habeas corpus for his release on the ground that he was not receiving adequate treatment, and he requested transfer to another facility. Through expert testimony, Nason's attorneys were able to show that staffing at Bridgewater was so grossly inadequate that Nason was simply receiving custodial care. The court acknowledged the existence of a constitutional right to treatment, at least for incompetent people awaiting trial, and even went on to suggest what a proper treatment plan for Nason would be.

While *Rouse* and *Nason* may have had little impact on the actual delivery of care in most institutions around the country, they did articulate the right to treatment and provided a statutory and tentative constitutional rationale for that right.

Wyatt v. Stickney (Wyatt v. Aderholt)   The next step in the move to establish a right to treatment through the court system was taken in Alabama in 1970, with the filing of *Wyatt v. Stickney*, 344 F. Supp. 373 (M.D. Ala. 1972). It was the first class suit successfully brought against a state's entire mental health system. The issue was detention without treatment of individuals committed civilly and involuntarily. The court established that involuntary clients have a constitutional right to individualized treatment that will give each of them a realistic chance to be cured or at least improve. The court found that the treatment program in Alabama state institutions was deficient in three fundamental areas. It did not provide:

1. A humane psychological and physical environment
2. Qualified staff to administer adequate treatment
3. Individualized treatment plans

To remedy these defects, the court promulgated a lengthy and detailed set of standards, including:

- Provisions against institutional peonage
- A number of protections to ensure a humane psychological and safe physical environment
- Minimum staffing requirements
- Establishment of a human rights committee at each institution
- A requirement that every client have a right to the least restrictive setting necessary for treatment

If the standards could not be met and clients were denied adequate treatment, the court stated, they had to be released from custody. In the words of Judge Johnson, "to deprive any citizen of his or her liberty upon the altruistic theory that confinement is for humane therapeutic reasons and then fail to provide adequate treatment violates the very fundamentals of due process" (*Wyatt v. Stickney*, 325 F. Supp. 781, 785 [M.D. Ala. 1971]).

For a time there was some question whether the *Wyatt* ruling, recognizing the constitutional basis for the right to treatment, would be upheld in subsequent decisions. In 1972, a neighboring federal district court in Georgia held that there was no constitutionally guaranteed right to treatment (*Burnham v. Georgia*, 349 F. Supp. 1335 [M.D. Ga. 1972]). But since then, the *Wyatt* decision has been affirmed by the federal court of appeals (503 F.2d 1305 [5th Cir. 1974]).

Donaldson v. O'Connor   Another important development in the constitutional right to treatment controversy was *Donaldson v. O'Connor*, 493 F.2d 507 (5th Cir. 1974). Kenneth Donaldson, an involuntary patient in a Florida mental hospital for over fourteen years, brought suit against the hospital superintendent, alleging that the superintendent had maliciously deprived him of his constitutional right to liberty. At trial, the jury found that (1) Donaldson had received not merely inadequate treatment but no treatment at all, (2) he was not dangerous, (3) acceptable community alternatives were in fact available for Donaldson, and (4) the doctor, knowing all this, had "maliciously" refused to release him.

On appeal, the federal court of appeals held that there is a constitutional right to treatment, and it awarded $38,000 in compensatory and punitive damages to Donaldson. However, the United States Supreme Court declined to affirm the court of appeals finding of constitutional right to treatment. The Court said that the case raised a single question concerning every person's constitutional right to liberty—that is: Does one have the right to be discharged from custodial care if not dangerous to self or others, the right not to receive treatment if one can survive safely in freedom? The unanimous answer was yes (*O'Connor v. Donaldson*, 43 U.S.L.W. 4929 [1975]).

This precedent-setting decision in June 1975 did not decide the damage issue in the case, however. The Supreme Court remanded that issue for reconsideration by the lower court in light of the decision in another case dealing with the liability of a civil service employee. In February 1977, at the age of sixty-seven, Kenneth Donaldson was awarded $20,000 from two defendant psychiatrists. Donaldson's lawsuit had been undertaken in the public interest by the American Civil Liberties Union and the Mental Health Law Project, and a ruling in early May 1977 entitled Donaldson to recover reasonable attorneys' fees. Donaldson has written a book about his confinement, *Insanity Inside Out* (1976), and is reported to spend much of his time now lecturing and writing.

Commitment Procedures

Within the last few years lawsuits have dealt with the procedural rights of mental patients. This is in character, as wrongful commitment has traditionally found redress in the courts. However, with recent rulings overthrowing the commitment statutes in several states, the courts have become an important factor in shaping mental health legislation.

Lessard v. Schmidt, 349 F. Supp. 1078, 1092 (E.D. Wis. 1972), a class action suit decided by a federal district court, provided the precedent for overthrowing several outmoded commitment statutes. Before October 17, 1972, an individual in Wisconsin could be committed if the court was satisfied that the person had a mental disease to such an extent that care and treatment was required for his or her own welfare or that of the community.

After the decision in *Lessard,* commitment could be made only if there was an extreme likelihood that the person would do immediate harm to self or others unless confined. Not only were the commitment critieria more stringent but the mechanism of commitment also became tighter. The court ruled that, under the due process provisions of the Constitution, individuals facing involuntary commitment were entitled to the same procedural safeguards present in criminal proceedings. The safeguards were to include:

- A hearing within forty-eight hours after detention
- Court-appointed counsel if the individual was unable to afford a private attorney
- The right of the individual to be present and heard
- Notification to the person's family about the proceedings
- Proof beyond a reasonable doubt that the person was dangerous and imminently harmful to self or others
- The right of the person to remain silent to avoid self-incrimination
- Consideration of a less restrictive alternative

While the *Lessard* decision was applauded by civil libertarians, it appalled others and evoked articles citing cases of individuals who were felt to have "died with their rights on" as a result of the court's ruling. Although the *Lessard* decision was vacated twice by the Supreme Court, the decision eventually was reinstated by the federal district court and continues to influence other courts and commitment legislation.

Of additional relevance is the provision for conservators (legally appointed guardians) for persons judged incapable of managing themselves and/or their property. Most recently, Michigan and New York, among other states, have legislated conservatorship laws to provide the opportunity to remove persons from cults to which they belong so that they may be deprogrammed or receive physical and/or mental health care. The forced removal of persons from cults through conservatorships is discussed more fully in Chapter 26.

Civil Rights

The mentally disabled have traditionally been denied many of the basic civil and personal rights taken for granted by most Americans. (For a patient's bill of rights, see Chapter 5.) With the mobilization of patients' rights groups and the attention given to this subject by the civil liberties union, lawsuits have been brought about issues such as wages, education, living arrangements, and discrimination.

In 1973, a federal district court ruled in *Souder v. Brennan,* 367 F. Supp. 808 (D.D.C. 1973), that patient-workers are covered by the provisions of the Fair Labor Standards Act and entitled to be paid a minimum wage for their work. The court refuted the argument that "therapeutic work" need not be reimbursed. Because this was a class action suit, the decision applied not only in the District of Columbia where the case was decided, but also in state and private facilities throughout the country.

The *Souder* ruling generated a great deal of attention, because it required the Department of Labor to act as a supervisor in hospitals across the country. Even so, improvement did not occur in all cases. Some hospitals dropped their "work therapy" programs altogether, and clients found themselves even less active than before.

The Client–Therapist–Public Relationship

In recent years, with pressures from government, courts, and insurance companies, the concept of the client–therapist relationship has had to expand to include the public. Areas of litigation include such issues as the right of informed consent, confidentiality of client records, and the involvement of third-party payors in treatment programs. A recent California Supreme Court decision illustrates the competition between two responsibilities of the mental health professional:

1. Confidentiality to the client
2. Protection of the public from the "violent" client

The court's ruling underlines the therapist's responsibility to balance the two.

In *Tarasoff v. Regents of the University of California,* 13 Cal. 3d 177, 529 P. 2d 553, 118 Cal. Rptr. 129

(1974), the parents of Tatiana Tarasoff successfully sued the University of California, claiming that a psychotherapist on the staff of the university's student counseling center had a responsibility to warn their daughter that his client, Prosenjit Poddar, had threatened to kill her when she returned from a trip abroad. At the time, the psychologist did notify campus security officers that he believed his client was dangerous and should be involuntarily committed for observation and treatment. However, Poddar appeared rational to the police and promised them he would stay away from Ms. Tarasoff. Poddar terminated treatment, and two months later killed Tatiana Tarasoff.

The suit was brought on two accounts: (1) failure to warn Tarasoff, and (2) failure to detain Poddar for treatment. Although the suit was dismissed by the lower courts, on appeal the California Supreme Court reversed the dismissal, saying that, despite the unsuccessful attempt to confine Poddar, the therapist knew that Poddar was at large and dangerous and had a duty to warn Tarasoff of the danger. The court recognized the patient's right to confidentiality but said this must be weighed against the public's need for safety against violent assault, especially when an individual in danger can be identified.

The *Tarasoff* decision raises significant problems for the clinician, especially since the majority of expert opinions and research data indicate that neither psychiatrists nor anyone else can reliably predict the future violence of a mentally disordered person. The Tarasoff concept was recently reaffirmed in a New Jersey decision, *Mackintosh v. Milano* 168 N.J. Super. 466 (Law Div. 1979).

Right to Refuse Treatment

The courts articulated a committed client's right to treatment over a decade ago. In the last few years, the courts have also been asked to rule on whether the client in a mental institution has the right to refuse treatment. Refusing treatment usually means refusing medication, since most other forms of therapy cannot be forced on a person. For example a client cannot be forced to talk in individual or group therapy, and treatment with recognized potential harm such as electroconvulsive therapy (ECT) requires informed written consent.

Rennie v. Klein   One of the first cases to address the right to refuse treatment (medication) was *Rennie v. Klein*, 462 F. Supp. 1131, 1145 (1978). It was initiated in December 1977 by John Rennie, an involuntarily

committed patient at a New Jersey state hospital who claimed that the hospital and the New Jersey Department of Human Services were violating his constitutional rights by forcibly administering medication. Mr. Rennie had objected to the side effects produced by Thorazine and lithium carbonate.

Judge Stanley Brotman ruled that involuntarily committed clients have a qualified right to refuse psychotropic medication. Involuntary clients were addressed because New Jersey statutes already stated that voluntary clients have an absolute right to reject medication. His decision was based on the constitutional right to protect their mental processes from governmental interference. Judge Brotman, impressed by the side effects of psychotropic medication, stated, "Individual autonomy demands that the person subjected to the harsh side effects of psychotropic drugs have control over their administration" (*Rennie v. Klein* 462 F. Supp at 1145).

Judge Brotman did qualify the right to refuse, listing four factors to be considered in overriding a client's objection:

1. Safety. Is the client a physical threat to other clients or staff?
2. Competency. Is the client competent to make treatment decisions?
3. Less restrictive means. Do less restrictive means of treatment exist, and are they available?
4. Risk versus benefit. What are the risks of permanent side effects from the proposed treatment?

In 1979 Mr. Rennie's complaint was amended to include class action allegations, and the court went on to add more specific steps to be followed in implementing an involuntarily committed client's qualified right to refuse treatment. These included

- Notify clients that they have a right to refuse medication.
- Provide clients with information regarding potential side effects from the medication
- Obtain written consent prior to initiation of medication.

If written consent is withheld by a client already declared "legally incompetent" by the court or certified "functionally incompetent" by a treating psychiatrist, the decision to medicate forcibly would be referred to a "client advocate." It would be at the client advocate's discretion to request a hearing before an inde-

Table 27–1 REVIEW OF COURT DECISIONS		
Case	**Date**	**Subject**
Rouse v. Cameron	1966	Lack of psychiatric treatment
Nason v. Bridgewater	1968	Lack of psychiatric treatment with request of transfer to another facility
Wyatt v. Stickney (class action)	1970–74	Detention without treatment of involuntarily committed individuals
Donaldson v. O'Connor	1974–77	Right to liberty in the absence of treatment
Lessard v. Schmidt (class action)	1972–74	Constitutionality of Wisconsin's commitment statute
Souder v. Brennan (class action)	1973	Minimum wages for working clients
Tarasoff v. Regents of University of California	1974–76	Confidentiality versus the duty to warn
Rennie v. Klein (amended to class action 1979)	1977–79	Qualified right to refuse medication
Roger v. Okin (class action)	1975–79	Absolute right to refuse medication in nonemergency situations

pendent psychiatrist, who would base a decision on the four factors mentioned above. In the case of a competent though involuntarily hospitalized person, a hearing before an independent psychiatrist would be required at which the client would have the right to legal counsel. The commissioner of the Department of Human Services would be the person responsible for appointing client advocates and independent psychiatrists.

Rogers v. Okin   Another important case in the establishment of a client's right to refuse medication is *Rogers v. Okin*, 478 F. Supp. (D. Mass. 1979). In 1975 a class action suit was initiated by clients at Boston State Hospital who contended that their constitutional

rights were being violated by the hospital's practice of using forced seclusion and medication in nonemergency situations. Judge Joseph Tauro issued a temporary restraining order against the use of seclusion and medication without the client's informed consent. In the case of a person declared incompetent by the court, informed consent would need to be elicited from the client's guardian. This restraining order applied to both voluntary and involuntary clients. In 1979, after a lengthy trial, the court made the temporary restraining order permanent.

Judge Tauro based his decision on the constitutional right to privacy (right to be left alone) and the first amendment right to freedom of thought. While Judge Tauro recognized that safety considerations might necessitate forcible administration of medication, he allowed much less discretion on the part of the hospital staff than did Judge Brotman in *Rennie*. Only in emergencies that create a substantial likelihood of physical harm to the client or others could medication be forcibly administered. Judge Tauro did not include a set of procedures to be followed in the case of client refusal, as had been done in *Rennie*. Instead, hospital staff were directed to apply to the court for a competency hearing and subsequent appointment of a guardian for clients they believed were incompetent to make treatment decisions. The decision in *Rogers* is considered to be more far reaching than that in *Rennie*, since it grants competent clients and guardians of incompetent clients an absolute right to refuse medication in nonemergency situations.

These recent court decisions are summarized in Table 27–1.

OVERVIEW OF MENTAL HYGIENE LAWS

Each state has statutes spelling out procedures for admission to, and discharge from, mental hospitals. Some states also have statutes on the medical and legal rights of individuals once they are in the hospital.

Admission

The two major categories of hospitalization are voluntary and involuntary. Admission and release procedures differ between them.

Voluntary   All states now have some provision for *voluntary admission*. Basically, voluntary admission comes about by written application for admission by prospective clients, or by someone acting in their behalf, such as a parent or guardian. As the word *voluntary* implies, the client has a right to demand and obtain release. However, all but two states have what is called a "grace period" in which the client agrees to give notice, usually in writing, of an intention to leave. Depending on the statute, this grace period can last from forty-eight hours (in Alaska) to fifteen days (in New Hampshire). It is justified on the ground that the hospital staff needs time to examine the client to determine whether a change to involuntary status is indicated. The extra time also gives family and staff the opportunity to try to persuade the client to remain voluntarily. This "conditional provision" is seen by Bruce Ennis (1972), Thomas Szasz (1963), and others as a covert form of involuntary hospitalization.

There are few statutory assurances in most states that voluntary clients must be adequately informed of their rights and status. Only nine states specifically require a voluntary client to be advised of the right to request release.

Informal voluntary admission, an alternative to the structure and personal concessions required in voluntary admission, is an option in at least ten states, including New York, Pennsylvania, and Connecticut. This procedure is akin to that required in a medical admission. The prospective patient verbally requests admission and is free to leave the institution at any time. Informal voluntary admission procedures are more likely to be an option in general and private facilities than in state institutions.

Involuntary The state's ability to hospitalize or commit an individual involuntarily is sanctioned by one of two state powers:

1. Police power, which enables the state to hospitalize people who, because of their illness, are considered dangerous to others
2. Parens patriae power, which enables the state to take on the role of protector and assume responsibility for people considered dangerous to themselves or, because of a mental disability, unable to care for themselves and in a potentially dangerous situation

Most states provide for more than one involuntary hospitalization procedure. Involuntary hospitalization can come about if the designated body, such as a court, an administrative tribunal, or the required number of physicians, find that the prospective client's mental state meets the statutory criteria for involuntary admission. The criteria vary from state to state. In a few states involuntary admission is justified only if the individual is dangerous to self or others as a result of a mental disorder. Most states augment this, however, by stating that the client's need for care and treatment may also justify commitment. Six states do not specify dangerousness as a ground, and the need for care and treatment is sufficient cause for involuntary commitment in those states. Involuntary hospitalization can be divided into three categories: (1) emergency, (2) temporary or observational, and (3) extended or indeterminate.

EMERGENCY Emergency involuntary hospitalization is available in thirty-nine states. It is a temporary measure with limited short-range goals, and it deals largely with the prevention of behavior likely to create a "clear and present" danger to the client or others. Under common law, any official or private person has the right to detain a dangerous mentally disordered person.

To initiate emergency detention, some formal application is required. In some states any citizen may make the application. In others it is limited to police officers, health officers, and physicians. Fourteen states require judicial approval before hospitalization. Because this type of involuntary admission is an emergency measure and warranted only until the appropriate legal steps can be taken, the statutes limit the amount of time an individual can be detained. The limits range from twenty-four hours (in Colorado) to sixty days (in Ohio). The usual practice is to allow detention for a five- to ten-day period.

TEMPORARY OR OBSERVATIONAL Provisions for temporary or observational involuntary hospitalization started appearing in the statute books in the late 1940s. This detention can be described as the involuntary commitment of an allegedly mentally deranged individual for a specified period of time to allow for adequate observation so that a diagnosis can be made and treatment instituted. The actual time period varies. It can be as short as seventy-two hours (in California) and as long as six months (in Florida).

Application for the temporary hospitalization of a person in need of aid can be made by any citizen in some states. Others require a family member or guardian, a health or welfare officer, or a physician to apply. Temporary hospitalization may be brought about by the medical certification of one or two physicians or may require further approval by a judge, justice, or district attorney in some jurisdictions.

At the end of the observation period, several options are available. The treating physician may (1) discharge the client, (2) have the client stay voluntarily, or (3) file an application for extended hospitalization. In at least nine states, observational hospitalization is mandatory before a court ruling in favor of extended hospitalization.

EXTENDED OR INDETERMINATE Indeterminate or extended involuntary hospitalization can come about through either judicial or nonjudicial procedures. *Judicial* hospitalization procedures require that a judge or jury determine whether the person is mentally ill to a degree that requires extended hospitalization. If so, the court orders the client hospitalized for an extended period (60 to 180 days) or an indeterminate time.

Although at least forty-two states have judicial hospitalization procedures, they vary widely from state to state. They range from those that require a full-dress judicial hearing and determination to those that eliminate the courts from the initial decision but permit court review of it.

Proceedings are usually initiated by an application for hospitalization of an allegedly mentally ill person. A few states permit any person or citizen to make or swear to the application. Others allow only one or more of the following groups: relatives, public officers, physicians, and hospital superintendents. Supporting

medical evidence may or may not be required at the time of application.

Most states having judicial hospitalization procedures make some provision for a prehearing medical examination in addition to the medical certification required to support the application. Usually the examination is conducted by two examiners. Three states require the examination to be done by a committee consisting of two medical and one nonmedical members.

In twenty-six of the forty-two jurisdictions having judicial hospitalization procedures, it is mandatory to notify the person sought to be hospitalized of the proposed hearing. In nine other states this right is waived if it would be harmful to the client's condition. Some states make notice of the hearing optional, and still others have no statutory provisions on the subject. Few states specify when a client should be given notice of the upcoming hearing. Without sufficient notice it is unlikely that a person can prepare an adequate defense. While most of the states contend that the person facing a commitment hearing has a right to legal counsel, only twenty-four have provisions for court-appointed counsel for the person who has none.

A hearing is mandatory in most states, although a few states leave it to the client to request it. While the client's presence is required at the hearing in a few states, most states merely permit attendance if it is not thought to be harmful to the client's condition or if the client in fact demands it. Few states require the hear-

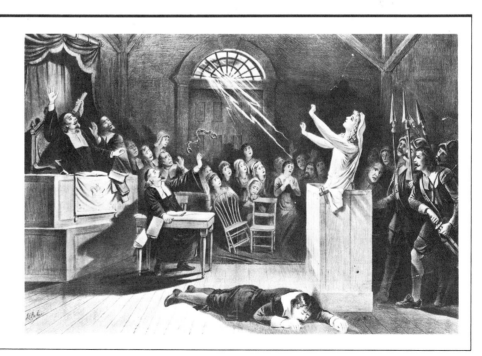

This early lithograph of a witch in court is reminiscent of the judicial commitment procedures for involuntary hospitalization that still exist in some states.

Table 27–2 VOLUNTARY AND INVOLUNTARY HOSPITALIZATION COMPARED				
	Voluntary Admission		**Involuntary Admission**	
	Informal	*Voluntary*	*Emergency*	*Temporary*	*Extended*
Release	Anytime	Usually conditional	Average after 5 to 10 days	After a range from 72 hours to 60 days	After a range from 60 to 180 days or after an indeterminate time
Use	Limited	Increasing	Increasing	Increasing	Decreasing
Criteria for admission	Client request	Client request	Usually client dangerousness	Client dangerousness and/or need of care and treatment	Client dangerousness and/or need of care and treatment

ing to be held in a courtroom. Most say the place is entirely discretionary.

Jury trials are no longer mandatory in any state, but sixteen states still have provisions for the use of a jury to decide the question of hospitalization. However, only in Michigan and Oklahoma are jury trials mandatory if demanded by clients or someone acting in their behalf. In other states it is left to the court's discretion.

Nonjudicial procedures for extended or indeterminate involuntary hospitalization include both administrative and medical certification. Ten states have provisions for *administrative* hospitalization procedures. Extended hospitalization is brought about by an administrative board, which basically follows the same procedures used in judicial hospitalization. However, as a rule, administrative hearings and investigations are less formal than court proceedings. Most statutes provide for the administrative board to be composed of physicians. A few allow a judge or attorney to be a member.

Involuntary hospitalization by *medical certification*, an alternative to the more traditional judicial commitment, is available in thirty-one states. It is usually advocated for clients who are incapable of consenting to voluntary treatment, although they do not protest hospitalization. These individuals are generally called "nonprotesting" clients. The need for hospitalization is usually determined by an examination by one or more physicians and documented by a medical certificate. Most states require that the certification be presented to a judge. The judge does not review the actual merits of the commitment but merely verifies the genuineness of the signature and the qualifications of the physician. All states having medical certification provide either for judicial proceedings if the client contests the hospitalization at any time after certification or for expanded habeas corpus proceedings.

A comparison of voluntary and involuntary admissions is presented in Table 27–2.

Rights of Clients

Communication All but ten states have some statutory provisions on client correspondence. The basis for laws granting communication rights is that such communication can expose cases of wrongful hospitalization. Generally communication is unrestricted or guaranteed to named public officials or the central hospital agency for the state. Eighteen states extend this guarantee to include correspondence with attorneys. Most states require that any correspondence limitation be part of the client's clinical record. Fifteen states require that writing materials be furnished. A few states require that stamps and a mailbox also be available to clients.

Half the states have some statutory provisions concerning visitation. However, hospital authorities are generally given broad discretionary powers in curtailing this right.

Mechanical Restraints Though improvements in treatment have decreased the use of mechanical restraints, such restraints still play a role in some treatment programs (see Appendix E). Only about half the states have attempted to regulate their use by statute. These provisions generally specify that restraints be used only under the following conditions:

- When their use is necessary to meet the client's medical needs
- When they are ordered by a physician
- When their use is made part of the client's medical record

Statutes seldom differentiate among the many types of physical restraints—muffs, leather straps, belts, straitjackets, dry packs, among others—or the length of time a restraint may be used.

Psychosurgery and Electroconvulsive Therapy   Only a small number of states have statutes specifically governing psychosurgery and electroconvulsive therapy (see Chapter 23). Generally, the consent of the client is required, or the consent of a relative or guardian if the client is incompetent. California does not mention consent, but simply states that every client has the right to refuse shock treatments or lobotomy. New York State requires "informed" consent, which necessitates that the client be told that shock treatment entails risk of serious injury or death. In the cases that have been brought before the courts, physicians have rarely been held liable for physical injuries to clients as the result of shock treatment.

Periodic Review   Half the states have some provision for periodic review of involuntary clients. Periodic review provides some protection for the individual against spending more time than necessary in the hospital. Review is required every six months in some states, or every year in others. A few states require review "as frequently as necessary," or "from time to time." The actual scope of the review is usually not governed by statute. The trend in recent years has been away from hospitalization for indeterminate periods of time. In New York and California, short-term commitment is the rule, and court review is necessary to extend commitment for another short period.

Participation in Legal Matters

Contracts   Generally, clients committed to a mental hospital maintain their right to make a valid contract, unless they have also been judged incompetent. In most states commitment proceedings are separate from those for competence. Therefore, an individual who is "legally incompetent" is not necessarily subject to commitment, and an individual committed to an institution is not automatically legally incompetent. Even

though the issue of contracts may seem clear-cut, in reality, a client's right to contract may be restricted by the administrative regulations of hospitals and state mental health agencies. A contested contract would most likely be a matter for the court to decide.

Wills   In order to make a valid will an individual must

- Be aware of making a will
- Be familiar with the property being disposed of
- Know the names, identities, and relationship of the people named in the will

An individual labeled with a psychiatric diagnosis, whether in or out of the hospital, can make a valid will as long as these requirements are met. Psychosis with accompanying delusions does not in and of itself negate a valid will. The delusions have to produce a significant distortion of the person's perception of the property, family, or personal relationships to invalidate the will.

Marriage and Divorce   According to statute and common law, a valid marriage contract hinges on the individual's possession of sufficient mental capacity to give consent. Sufficient mental capacity implies that the person

- Understands the nature of the marriage relationship
- Knows the duties and obligations involved

The statutes of a small number of states prohibit marriage by mentally disordered persons because they are believed to be incapable of making a contract. More states, however, prohibit marriage by the mentally disordered on the grounds that they are "insane" or "of unsound mind," without specifically defining these terms. Despite these prohibiting statutes, few states even try to enforce the prohibition outside mental institutions.

Most states have provisions for annulment or divorce on the ground of prenuptial mental disability. Within the last twenty years, divorce on the grounds of postnuptial mental disability has been incorporated in the statutes of most states.

Voting   The majority of states do not actually prohibit hospitalized persons from voting. In fact, in some, legislation specifically preserves this right. The institutionalized are eligible to register to vote in twelve states. In eighteen others the ability to vote depends on a hospitalized client's legal competence. Only in Kentucky, Missouri, and Oklahoma are individuals confined to an institution ineligible to vote. All states except Louisiana allow absentee voting by disabled persons. The hospitalized client's right to vote is probably more restricted by caretaker and community apathy than it is by statute.

Right to Drive   Statutes on driving privileges are difficult to interpret. Most states will not issue a driver's license to mentally disturbed persons. In some states this restriction also applies to epileptics, drug addicts, and alcoholics. Several states suspend a person's driver's license as soon as the individual enters a mental institution. Other jurisdictions limit the restriction to individuals admitted involuntarily, while still others base suspension on legal competence.

Right to Practice a Profession   The ability of a hospitalized client to practice a profession is usually impaired simply by the physical confinement. However, the majority of states have some statutes prohibiting the practice of a profession by a mentally disturbed person. The vagueness of the statutes many times makes it difficult to know when they are applicable. As a rule it is up to the professional licensing board to suspend or revoke the license of a member who is believed to be too mentally incapacitated to practice a profession safely, even though not hospitalized.

Separation from a Mental Institution

A client can separate from a mental institution in one of three ways: (1) death, (2) escape, and (3) discharge.

Death   The death rate in mental institutions is considerably higher than that encountered in the general population. In 1969, death accounted for roughly 7 percent of the separations from mental institutions. The use of mental institutions as the last resting place for many unclaimed elderly people, and the advanced age of the institutionalized, "backward," often lobotomized clients of twenty or thirty years ago, may account in part for this high mortality rate.

Escape   A client may take the initiative and decide to terminate relationship with the institution by informally leaving the hospital grounds. This is commonly referred to as escape, elopement, or being AWOL (ab-

sent without leave). Generally, voluntary clients cannot be returned to the hospital against their will. However, involuntarily committed clients may be brought back to the hospital against their will with the assistance of the police, if necessary.

Discharge   Like admission, discharge from a mental hospital can have various layers of complexity. Discharges occur in one of two ways—conditionally or absolutely.

CONDITIONAL   As implied by the word *conditional,* complete discharge in this situation depends on whether the person fulfills certain conditions over a specified period of time, usually six months to a year. Compliance with outpatient care, demonstrated ability and willingness to take medications, and ability to meet the needs of daily living are a few of the many possible prerequisites. An individual who is unable to meet the specified conditions can be reinstitutionalized without going through any legal admission procedure. An individual committed for an extended or indeterminate time is more likely to be a candidate for conditional than absolute discharge.

ABSOLUTE   The legal relationship between the institution and the client is terminated by an absolute discharge. If the client should require readmission to the hospital at any time, even a few hours after discharge, a new hospitalization proceeding would be required.

An absolute discharge can be brought about in three ways:

1. An administrative discharge is issued by the hospital officials
2. A judicial discharge is ordered by the courts
3. A writ of habeas corpus is ordered by the courts on the client's application

As a rule, the authority for discharging involuntary clients rests in the hands of the hospital superintendent, and they are given administrative discharges. However, a few statutes extend this power to the central agency responsible for supervising mental institutions in the state, such as the Department of Mental Hygiene. The client has no formal method of initiating an administrative discharge.

The majority of states also provide for a *judicial* discharge, which is initiated by an application to the court by the client, the client's family, or any citizen who is in disagreement with hospital authorities over the client's need to be hospitalized. A few states require the application to be accompanied by a medical certificate attesting to the client's competence. Nineteen of the thirty-five states that provide for judicial discharge require a medical examination by a person independent of the hospital staff. On the whole, most state statutes do not require that parties having an interest in the outcome of the case be given an opportunity to appear in court and present their views. In many states judicial discharge does not depend on complete recovery. A degree of improvement may be sufficient. Massachusetts, Michigan, and Rhode Island specifically allow for the discharge of unimproved clients, provided they are not currently dangerous to themselves or others. Twenty states guard against frequent applications for discharge by the same clients by imposing a six-month to one-year waiting period between requests.

All states recognize the right of clients, or persons acting in their behalf, to question their detention in a mental hospital by means of a *writ of habeas corpus*. This writ, dating back to English common law, is available not only to mental clients but also to any person deprived of liberty through illegal detention. In thirty-five states the writ is used only to test the legality of the original detention. The question of the need for continued confinement of the client is not addressed by habeas corpus. In the last few years, some courts have expanded the writ to include an examination of the client's mental status at the time of the proceedings. In these cases the basic criterion for further detention or release is the client's present mental status. This expanded use of the writ is reflected in the statutes of at least sixteen states.

TWO CURRENT MENTAL HEALTH LAWS

So far we have examined mental health legislation in a piecemeal overview. While it is impossible to describe the mental health laws of every state, an in-depth analysis of two existing state statutes presents the general picture.

New York State's Mental Hygiene Law

The New York State Mental Hygiene Law is some five hundred pages long. However, for our purposes it is sufficient to discuss only selected sections, such as those dealing with the relationship of the Department of Mental Hygiene to the hospitalization of individuals. When the law was revised in 1964, the New York Bar Association's recommendation for a mental health review or information service was included. The Mental Health Information Service is required to study and review the retention of all hospitalized clients. It must provide information to clients about their rights to a judicial hearing and review and to be represented by legal counsel. The service must seek independent medical opinion, and, if a court hearing is requested, assemble information about the client for the court.

The Mental Hygiene Law was recodified (a restructuring more complex than revising) in 1973. At that time the New York State Nurses Association and an ad hoc group of psychiatric nurses prepared a *Position Statement on the Proposed Recodification of the Mental Hygiene Law* (1970), pointing out not only those areas of the proposed legislation that were unclear but also those believed to be in violation of clients' rights. While specific recommendations of the group were modified, the overall impact was substantial.

Article 33 of the law deals with clients' rights. It begins with a declaration:

Notwithstanding any other provision of law, no person shall be deprived of any civil right, if in all other respects qualified and eligible, solely by reason of receipt of services for a mental disability nor shall the receipt of such services modify or vary any civil right of any such person, including but not limited to civil service ranking and appointment, the right to register for and to vote in elections, or rights relating to the granting, forfeiture, or denial of a license, permit, privilege, or benefit pursuant to any law [McKinney's 1979, 34A:33.01].

The Department of Mental Hygiene points out, in an explanation of this "bill of rights" for clients, that the mere fact of mental disorder does not in itself deprive a person of the right to own land, marry, make a will, or generally enter into contractual arrangements. Only if clients are judicially declared incompetent, and a committee has been duly appointed for them, may they be barred from entering into contractual agreements except through that committee.

The law also states that "a person receiving services for a mental disability shall receive care and treatment that is suited to his needs and skillfully, safely, and humanely administered with full respect for his dignity and personal integrity" (McKinney's 1978, 34A:33.03). It goes on to specify the minimum requirements to assure the protection of clients in their care and treatment. These include individualized treatment plans, periodic review, physical examinations, and client consent to any surgery, shock treatments, major medical treatments, or the use of experimental drugs or procedures. All of these must be recorded in the client's chart. Regulations by the Department of Mental Hygiene elaborate on the general items set down in the statutes. For example, they call for client participation to the fullest extent possible in the establishment and revision of an individual service plan.

Consent   According to the Department of Mental Hygiene regulations, all clients have a right to object to any form of care and treatment and to appeal decisions with which they disagree. Voluntary and informally admitted clients may not be treated over their objections. If the client objects to all recommended treatment, the regulations suggest that the client should, after notification, be discharged from the facility. If appropriate, the facility director can convert the client's status to "involuntary." Involuntary clients can be treated over their objections after a court order is obtained authorizing their retention and the treatment is reviewed by the head of the service.

Communication   The recodified Mental Hygiene Law ensures each client the right to communicate freely and privately with people outside the institution. This right may be limited only to protect the client's safety or to avoid serious harassment of others by the client. Correspondence with public officials, attorneys, clergy, and the Mental Health Information Service must not be restricted and must be forwarded without being opened. Clients must have access to telephones and stationery and must be given frequent and convenient opportunities to meet visitors. Each client also has the right to refuse visitors.

Confidentiality   The clinical record must contain all matters relating to the admission, legal status, care, and treatment of the client. Information may be released by the Department of Mental Hygiene, with the consent of the client, to physicians, to social and welfare services involved in the care and treatment of the client, and to other persons who obtain consent. Information reported to the Department of Mental Hygiene and clinical records should not be public records and should not be released without the consent of the client, except by a court order or to the Mental Health Information Service or to attorneys representing clients in proceedings in which involuntary hospitalization is at issue.

Admission   A person may be admitted to an institution either voluntarily or involuntarily. Voluntary admission can occur in one of two ways: with or without formal, written application. An informally admitted client may leave the facility at any time after admission. However, for voluntary clients to effect release, they must give written notice of the desire to leave. After receiving such notice, the physician must either discharge the client or apply to the court within seventy-two hours for an order authorizing the involuntary retention of the client.

An individual may be involuntarily presented to a psychiatric hospital in one of three ways: by a peace officer, by the judiciary, or by the director of a community service or the director's psychiatric designee. Emergency commitment may be effected for a person "alleged to have a mental illness for which immediate observation, care, and treatment in a hospital is appropriate *and* which is likely to result in serious harm to himself or others" (McKinney's 1978, 34A:9.39). The alleged dangerous and mentally disturbed person may be detained for a forty-eight-hour period on the examination of a staff physician. If the staff physician's findings are confirmed by the examination of a psychiatrist on the staff of the hospital, the person may then be held for up to fifteen days.

Certain designated persons may apply for the admission of a person alleged to be mentally ill and in need of involuntary care and treatment. The director of a hospital may receive and retain such a person for up to sixty days on certification of two examining physicians. Commitment may be extended with judicial approval in consecutive six-month, one-year, and two-year increments thereafter. A person retained in a facility, or a relative or friend in behalf of the client, is entitled to a writ of habeas corpus to question the cause and legality of the detention. Before the 1964 revision of the Mental Hygiene Law, which provided for periodic review of involuntary clients, involuntary commitment was for an indefinite period, and application for a writ of habeas corpus was the usual manner in which a case was reviewed after the initial admission.

California's Mental Hygiene Law

The Community Mental Health Services Act went into effect in California in July 1969. The law is comprised of two acts; the Lanterman-Petris-Short Act, and a revised version of the Short-Doyle Act of 1957. The Short-Doyle Act deals with the administration of largely state-supported community mental health services, while the Lanterman-Petris-Short Act (LPS) is primarily concerned with the involuntary treatment of mentally disordered, alcoholic, and drug-addicted persons.

Emergency Commitment   Under LPS, an individual is eligible for involuntary detention if considered a danger to others or self, or too gravely disabled to provide for basic needs of food, clothing, and shelter. Emergency commitment for involuntary evaluation and treatment can be accomplished for a seventy-two-hour period with or without a court order.

NONJUDICIAL EVALUATION   An individual believed to be in need of involuntary detention can be brought to a mental health clinic for evaluation by a peace officer or other designated professional person, such as a physician, psychologist, social worker, professional nurse, or member of the clergy. The person requesting the individual's admission is then required to submit in writing a statement that, based on personal observation, he or she believes the individual to be a danger to self or others or gravely disabled. The individual may not be required to stay for the full seventy-two hours if a less restrictive treatment, such as crisis intervention or outpatient care, is applicable and available, according to the evaluation of the facility's staff.

JUDICIAL OR COURT-ORDERED EVALUATION   Before LPS, court commitment was initiated by a petition to the court requesting hospitalization on the ground that an individual was "mentally disordered." A medical certification, though not necessarily by a psychiatrist, usually had to accompany the petition. LPS modifies this procedure by requiring screening by a multidisciplinary outreach team before any court action is taken on a petition. If the team finds that the individual meets the legal requirements for involuntary admission and that hospitalization is the only feasible alternative, this recommendation is communicated to the court. The court then orders the individual into a hospital for a seventy-two-hour evaluation period.

Decision after Evaluation Period   Some time before the end of the seventy-two-hour period, the professional staff of the inpatient facility must choose one of the four possible alternatives for the involuntarily detained individual:

1. Release without further treatment
2. Treatment undertaken voluntarily

3. Certification for fourteen days of intensive treatment
4. Recommendation for conservatorship

Extended Treatment   If an individual involuntarily committed for evaluation is not released after seventy-two hours, the psychiatrist must certify in writing that the individual needs further treatment. Court intervention is not required at this time, but according to the statute clients have a right to judicial review of their cases and must be granted a hearing by writ of habeas corpus.

At the end of the fourteen-day intensive treatment period a number of options are again available to the professional staff. The person in charge of the facility may recommend that the individual be:

• Released
• Certified for an additional fourteen-day period if believed to be an active suicide risk
• Recommended for ninety-day postcertification treatment if considered imminently dangerous
• Recommended for conservatorship

The suicidal individual detained for an additional fourteen days must be released at the end of that period. Therefore, the law allows a maximum of thirty-one days of involuntary hospitalization for high-risk suicidal individuals.

Postcertification   There are stringent time limits on the postcertification procedure. The petition for ninety-day postcertification treatment must be filed with the court by the twelfth day of hospitalization, to enable the hearing to be held on the fourteenth day of the intensive treatment period. Postcertification is an adversary process and therefore requires testimony, cross-examination, and factual evidence that the individual is dangerous and requires additional treatment. Clients have the right during the hearing to request a jury trial to decide whether they are dangerous. This ninety-day postcertification procedure is rarely used, according to reports.

Conservatorship   The head of an inpatient facility can recommend conservatorship for individuals believed to be gravely disabled as a result of a mental disorder or impaired by chronic alcoholism. The request goes to the officer providing conservatorship investigation in the county. This officer then makes a recommendation to the superior court, after examining all available alternatives. The officer recommending conservatorship also submits a list of the most likely person, state or local agency, or county officer to act as conservator for the disabled individual.

All conservatees have the right to jury trial to determine whether they are gravely disabled. Once the conservatorship is made final, the court may selectively impose restrictions on the disabled individual's civil rights, such as the right to drive a car, possess firearms, or enter into certain types of contracts. Conservatorship terminates after one year, but it may be renewed by the court on the petition of two physicians or licensed psychologists. Conservatees may petition the supreme court every six months for a rehearing on their conservator status.

Legal and Civil Rights of Hospitalized Clients   California law requires the following list of rights to be prominently posted in both English and Spanish in every inpatient facility and brought to the attention of every new client:

- The right to wear your own clothes, to keep and use personal possessions, including toilet articles, and to keep a reasonable sum of money for small purchases while in the hospital
- The right to have individual storage space for private use
- The right to see visitors daily
- The right to have reasonable access to telephones where confidential conversations are possible
- The right to receive unopened correspondence and to have stationery, stamps, and access to a mailbox
- The right to refuse shock treatments
- The right to refuse lobotomy

In 1978 the legislature explicity stated that persons hospitalized for mental illness are guaranteed the same legal rights and responsibilities of other citizens, including the following:

- A right to treatment services that take place in the least restrictive setting in order to maximize independent functioning
- A right to dignity, privacy, and humane care
- A right to "freedom from," which includes excessive or unnecessary use of restraints, seclusion, medica-

tion, abuse, or neglect. Specifically, medication should not be used as punishment or for staff convenience or as a substitute for other programs
- A right to prompt medical care and treatment
- A right to religious expression
- A right to participate in appropriate publicly funded educational programs and community activities
- A right to physical exercise and recreation
- A right to be free from dangerous procedures

Any of these rights may be denied by the professional person in charge of the facility. However, information about the denial of a client's rights must be made part of the client's clinical record. Confidentiality of the client's record is also guaranteed by statute. In fact, any willful and knowing release of confidential information subjects the offender to a suit for $500.

THE IMPLEMENTATION OF CLIENTS' RIGHTS

This chapter has reviewed some of the recent court decisions increasing the procedural and substantive rights of mental hospital clients, along with the current mental hygiene laws in New York and California. However, the rights mental clients have in theory and in practice often differ. Richard Price and Bruce Denner (1973, p. 7) aptly comment on this phenomenon:

> Although Pinel was able to remove the chains from the inmates of the Bicêtre by declaring that they were mentally ill, today many people lose a substantial portion of their human and civil rights when the same declaration is made about them.

The discrepancy between rights in theory and in practice is often cited, but it has received little systematic attention. The ethical dilemmas that nurses face in relation to client's rights are analyzed in Chapter 5.

The Role of Care Givers

Arthur Cohen, testifying before the Senate Subcommittee on the Constitutional Rights of the Mentally Ill (1970), speculated that psychiatric personnel are reluctant to enforce the legal rights of clients because they believe these rights make their own jobs harder. Another possibility is suggested by Thomas Szasz (1963) and others, who contend that lack of enforcement is a result of the "medical model" approach to mental disability. Within the medical model, an individual is labeled "mentally ill" because of certain behavior or "symptoms." The label bears the connotation that sickness will prevent clients from knowing what is good in the way of treatment.

Realizing that the legal rights of committed individuals can be hollow unless clients are given some assistance to make those rights meaningful, New York has provided for the Mental Health Information Service. Even though the service is notified of each involuntary admission, a representative does not see each client routinely. Usually only when the client contacts the service or requests a hearing, does a representative act. In three out of the four Mental Health Information Service departments in New York State, a hospital staff member is responsible for providing clients with written and verbal notice of their admission, their rights under the applicable section, and a description of the Mental Health Information Service. In addition, the service is available only during business hours, nine to five, Monday through Friday. Therefore, clients must depend on the caretakers around them to offer accurate information about their legal rights.

Often, truly effective implementation—practices that allow clients to exercise the rights to which they are theoretically entitled—depends on the attitude of the psychiatric personnel working with the clients. Clients' rights are bound to remain empty legal concepts if professionals and paraprofessionals show scorn for them or implement them in an outwardly hostile or perfunctory manner.

In the public mental hospital system, the community, not the client alone, is the primary consumer. The hospitalized person, who lacks a power base from which to operate, is more often considered a "product to be mended" than an actual consumer. Psychiatrist Toaru Ishiyama (1970) believes it is sheer folly to depend on psychiatric personnel for commitment to significant upgrading of the service system with the client's needs and rights in mind. Their commitment is doomed to a short life. He suggests that systematized demands for improvement be built into the mental hospital, with the client encouraged by an advocate to negotiate for services as a consumer.

Staff Knowledge and Attitudes

Noting that the protection of clients' rights in a mental hospital depends to a great extent on the psychiatric

personnel's awareness of legal safeguards, Laurence Tancredi and Diane Clark (1972) carried out a small study to assess the knowledge of psychiatric personnel about the legal rights of mental clients. Psychiatrists, social workers, and nurses involved in admissions at a New England medical center were interviewed and asked questions derived from the statutes of the state in which the institution was located. The investigators reported that psychiatric personnel were generally unaware of clients' legal rights at the time of admission and during hospitalization. To sensitize psychiatric personnel to the legal rights of mental clients, the investigators suggested educational programs focusing on the practical features of clients' rights in a clinical setting.

Also noting the discrepancy between legal rights in theory and in practice, Rona Laves and Allen Cohen (1972) hypothesized that these rights were not being enforced because either (1) psychiatric personnel were not well informed about the relevant laws and therefore could not effectively implement them, or (2) psychiatric personnel were well informed but disinclined to support or actively implement clients' rights because they did not agree with them. To assess staff knowledge of and attitudes toward the legal rights of mental clients, Laves and Cohen constructed cognitive, attitudinal, and behavioral questionnaires based on the New Jersey statutes and the United States Constitution. Close to 500 questionnaires were distributed to psychiatric personnel in the New Jersey area. While the attitudes of all groups of psychiatric personnel were found to be generally favorable to civil rights for clients, respondents were reported to be functioning under a serious deficiency of knowledge about the legal rights of clients.

A recent study by Paul Freddolino (1980) found that support for clients' rights among state hospital personnel (psychiatrists, psychologists, social workers, nurses, and therapy aides) was affected most strongly by (1) the person's power or level of responsibility; (2) the prestige of the person's profession; (3) socioeconomic factors, such as sex, race, and education, which are linked to power in our society; and (4) the extent of direct client contact. Direct care providers, of which nurses were a large number, were found to be least supportive of extending clients' rights. Freddolino hypothesized that this was because extension of clients' rights is perceived as threatening to staff responsible for both maintaining order and dealing directly with clients who often are angry over their involuntary confinement. Any extension of the client's rights has the greatest impact on the jobs of direct care providers. Freddolino urges administrators, legislators, and judges to provide some outside mechanism of enforcement when changes in the area of clients' rights are considered, and not simply to rely on institutions to implement a pro-clients' rights philosophy in actual practice.

KEY NURSING CONCEPTS

✔ Law develops in a social context—ideally in response to the problems and needs of the governed.

✔ Factors influencing the development of laws about the rights of mentally disturbed persons include the state of medical knowledge, the community's acceptance of some responsibility, and the legal profession's sensitivity to the social and civil liabilities that befall the mentally disturbed.

✔ Knowledge of existing mental health legislation is essential for nurses to become politically active and protect the legal rights of individuals using mental health services.

✔ Not until communities started to offer treatment that necessitated confinement did laws become concerned with the insane person's loss of freedom and basic civil rights.

✔ Early commitment procedures were easy and informal without much concern for the rights of the individual.

✔ Because of dissatisfaction with mental hospital and commitment procedures, state regulatory agencies began to be established in the latter part of the nineteenth century.

✔ Mental health legislation varies considerably from state to state. In every state mental hygiene laws identify procedures for admission to and discharge from mental hospitals, but only some states deal with the medical and legal rights of hospitalized persons.

✔ The Mental Health Systems Act of 1980 provides some direction for states to review and revise their mental health laws to ensure that clients receive the protection and services they require.

✔ Members of the health professions are being held increasingly accountable for their behavior. They need to become familiar with the state laws that govern their responsibilties and actions.

✔ Contemporary issues concerning rights of hospitalized clients include access to communication, use of mechanical restraints, use of psychosurgery and electroconvulsive therapy, and provision for periodic review of involuntary clients.

✔ Contemporary forensic considerations important in humanistic psychiatric nursing practice include involuntary admission criteria, the right to treatment, civil rights of hospitalized persons, client–therapist relations, and the controversial right to refuse treatment.

✔ Theory about rights of mental clients often is not reflected in practice.

✔ Effective implementation of client's rights frequently depends on awareness, support, and advocacy by the psychiatric nurse.

References

Birnbaum, M. "The Right to Treatment." *American Bar Association Journal* 46 (1960): 499–505.

Bockoven, J. S. "Moral Treatment in American Psychia-try." *Journal of Nervous and Mental Disease* 125 (1956): 167–194, 292–321.

Brakel, S., and Rock, R. *The Mentally Disabled and the Law.* Chicago: University of Chicago Press, 1970.

Cohen, A. *Constitutional Rights of the Mentally Ill.* Hearings of the Senate Subcommittee on Constitutional Rights of the Committee on the Judiciary, 91st Congress, 1st and 2nd Sessions, November 4, 5, 12, 13, 18, 19, 1969, and August 12, 1970, p. 227. Washington, D.C.: Government Printing Office, 1970.

Commission to Investigate the Management and Affairs of the Department of Mental Hygiene of the State of New York. *The Care of the Mentally Ill in the State of New York.* New York: Government Press, 1944.

Deutsch, A. *The Mentally Ill in America.* New York: Columbia University Press, 1949.

—————. *Constitutional Rights of the Mentally Ill.* Hearings of the Senate Subcommittee on Constitutional Rights of the Committee on the Judiciary, 87th Congress, 1st Session, March 28, 1961, p. 43, Washington, D.C.: Government Printing Office, 1961.

Dewey, R., "The Jury Law for Commitment of the Insane in Illinois." *American Journal of Insanity* 69 (1913): 571–584.

Dialogues of Plato. 4th ed. Translated by B. Jowett. Oxford: Clarendon Press, 1964.

Donaldson, K. *Insanity Inside Out.* New York: Crown Publishers, 1976.

Ennis, B. *Prisoners of Psychiatry.* New York: Avon Books, 1972.

Freddolino, P. "Factors Affecting the Patients' Rights Ideology of Mental Hospital Personnel." In *New Directions In Psycholegal Research,* edited by P. Lipsitt and B. Sales, pp. 293–326. New York: Van Nostrand Reinhold, 1980.

Ishiyama, T. "The Mental Hospital Patient-Consumer as a Determinant of Services." *Mental Hygiene* 54 (1970): 221–229.

Johnson, C. A. *Ancient Roman Statutes.* Austin: University of Texas Press, 1961.

Joint Commission on Mental Illness and Health. *Action for Mental Health.* New York: Basic Books, 1961.

Laves, R., and Cohen, A. "A Preliminary Investigation into the Knowledge of and Attitudes toward the Legal Rights of Mental Patients." *Journal of Psychiatry and Law,* June 1972, pp. 49–78.

McKinney's Consolidated Laws of New York. Vol. 34A, *Mental Hygiene Law.* St. Paul: West Publishing, 1978.

"Mental Health Sytems Act: Summary and Analysis." *Mental Disability Law Reporter* 4 (1980): 383–390.

National Institute of Mental Health, Federal Security Agency. *A Draft Act Governing Hospitalization of the Mentally Ill.* Public Health Service Publication no. 51. Washington, D.C.: Government Printing Office, 1952.

New York State Nurses' Association. *Position Statement on the Proposed Recodification of the Mental Hygiene Law.* Presented to the Joint Legislative Committee on Mental

and Physical Handicaps at Public Hearing, New York, November 12, 1970.

Ordronaux, J. *Commentaries on the Lunacy Laws of New York.* New York: John D. Parsons, 1878.

Packard, Mrs. E. P. W. *Mrs. Packard's Prison Life.* Chicago: Published by the author, 1867.

—————. *The Prisoner's Hidden Life, or Insane Asylums Unveiled.* Chicago: Published by the author, 1868.

—————. *Modern Persecution.* Hartford, Conn.: Published by the author, 1887.

Pinel, P. *A Treatise on Insanity.* 1806; reprint edition, New York: Hafner Press, 1962.

Price, R., and Denner, B., Eds. *The Making of a Mental Patient.* New York: Holt, Rinehart and Winston, 1973.

Ray, I. *Medical Jurisprudence of Insanity.* 5th ed. Boston: Little, Brown, 1871, p. 369.

Reade, C. *Hard Cash.* London: Chatto and Windus, 1895.

Special Committee of the Association of the Bar of the City of New York. *Mental Illness and Due Process.* Ithaca, N.Y.: Cornell University Press, 1962.

Szasz, T. *Law, Liberty and Psychiatry.* New York: Macmillan, 1963.

Tancredi, L., and Clark, D. "Psychiatry and the Legal Rights of Patients." *American Journal of Psychiatry* 129 (1972): 328–330.

Tuke, D. *Chapters in the History of the Insane in the British Isles.* London: Kegan Paul, Trench, 1882.

—————. *The Insane in the United States and Canada.* London: H. K. Lewis, 1885.

West's Annotated Welfare and Institutions Code of California. Vol. 73A. St. Paul, Minn.: West Publishing, 1981.

Willard, S. *Report on the Condition of the Insane Poor in the County Poorhouses of New York.* Report to the New York State Legislature, January 13, 1865.

Further Reading

Appelbaum, P., and Gutheil, T. " 'Rotting With Their Rights On': Constitutional Theory and Clinical Reality in Drug Refusal by Psychiatric Patients." *Bulletin of the American Academy of Psychiatry and Law* 7 (1979): 306–315.

Birnbaum, M. "The Right to Treatment: Some Comment on Its Development." In *Medical, Moral and Legal Issues in Mental Health Care,* edited by F. Ayd, pp. 97–141. Baltimore: Williams and Wilkins, 1974.

Brooks, A. *Law, Psychiatry and the Mental Health System: 1980 Supplement.* Boston: Little, Brown, 1980.

Chamberlin, Judi. *On Our Own: Patient-Controlled Alter-*

natives to the Mental Health System. New York: Hawthorn Books, 1978.

Cohrssen, J., and Kopolow, L. *Court Screening and Patient Advocacy: A Handbook of Principles for Community Mental Health Centers.* Rockville, Md.: National Institute of Mental Health, 1979.

Dreher, R. "Origin, Development and Present Status of Insanity as a Defense to Criminal Responsibility in the Common Law." *Journal of the History of the Behavioral Sciences,* January 1967, pp. 47-57.

Ennis, B., and Siegel, L. *The Rights of Mental Patients.* New York: Avon Books, 1973.

Ettlinger, R. A. "Advocate Informs Patients of Rights and Responsibilities." *Hospital and Community Psychiatry* 24 (1973): 465-470.

Ford, M. "The Psychiatrist's Double Bind: The Right to Refuse Medication." *American Journal of Psychiatry* 137 (1980): 332-339.

Freidman, P. *Legal Rights of Mentally Disabled Persons.* Washington, D.C.: Mental Health Law Project, 1979.

Golann, S., and Fremouw, W. *The Right to Treatment for Mental Patients.* New York: John Wiley, 1976.

Greenblatt, M. "The Class Action Suits and the Rights of Patients." In *Psychopolitics,* pp. 73-96. New York: Grune and Stratton, 1978.

Kahle, R., and Sales, B. "Due Process of Law and the Attitudes of Professionals toward Involuntary Civil Commitment." In *New Directions In Psycholegal Research,* pp. 265-292. New York: Van Nostrand Reinhold, 1980.

Kittrie, N. N. *The Right to Be Different.* Baltimore: Penguin Books, 1971.

————. "The Flowering and Decline of the Therapeutic State?" In *Medical, Moral and Legal Issues in Mental Health Care,* edited by F. Ayd, pp. 81-96. Baltimore: Williams and Wilkins, 1974.

Kopolow, L., and Bloom, H. *Mental Health Advocacy: An Emerging Force In Consumers' Rights.* Rockville, Md.: National Institute of Mental Health, 1977.

Kramer, K. "The Subtle Subversion of Patients' Rights by Hospital Staff Members." *Hospital and Community Psychiatry* 25 (1974): 475-476.

Litwack, T. R., and Ennis, B. "Psychiatry and the Presumption of Expertise: Flipping Coins in the Courtroom." *California Law Review* 62 (1974): 693-752.

Mayo, C., and Havelock, R. "Attitudes toward Mental Illness among Mental Hospital Personnel and Patients." *Journal of Psychiatric Research* 7 (1970): 296-300.

Palmer, A., and Wohl, J. "Voluntary Admission Forms: Does the Patient Know What He's Signing?" *Hospital and Community Psychiatry* 23 (1972): 250-252.

Pfohl, S. *Predicting Dangerousness: The Social Construction of Psychiatric Reality.* Lexington, Mass.: D. C. Heath, 1978.

Roth, L. "Mental Health Commitment: The State of the Debate, 1980." *Hospital and Community Psychiatry* 31 (1980): 385-396.

Roth, L., and Meisel, A. "Dangerousness, Confidentiality and the Duty to Warn." *American Journal of Psychiatry* 134 (1977): 508-511.

Rubin, J. "The Mentally Disabled and the Courts." In *Economics, Mental Health and the Law,* pp. 32-62. Lexington, Mass.: D. C. Heath, 1978.

Slovenko, R., and Luby, E. "From Moral Treatment to Railroading Out of the Mental Hospital." *Bulletin of the American Academy of Psychiatry and the Law* 11 (1974): 223-236.

Spensley, J.; Barter, J.; and Werme, P. "Involuntary Hospitalization—What For and How Long?" *American Journal of Psychiatry* 131 (1974): 219-223.

Stone, A. "Overview: The Right to Treatment—Comments on the Law and Its Impact." *American Journal of Psychiatry* 132 (1975): 1125-1134.

————. *Mental Health and Law: A System in Transition.* New York: Jason Aronson, 1976.

————. "Recent Mental Health Litigation: A Critical Perspective." *American Journal of Psychiatry* 134 (1977): 273-279.

Suchotliff, L.; Steinfeld, G.; and Tolchin, G. "The Struggle for Patients' Rights in a State Hospital." *Mental Hygiene* 54 (1970): 230-240.

Szasz, T., and Alexander, G. "Law, Property and Psychiatry." *American Journal of Orthopsychiatry* 42 (1972): 610-622.

Tancredi, L. "The Right to Refuse Psychiatric Treatment: Some Legal and Ethical Considerations." *Journal of Health, Politics, Policy and Law* 5 (1980): 514-522.

Tancredi, L.; Leib, J.; and Slaby, A. *Legal Issues in Psychiatric Care.* New York: Harper and Row, 1975.

Treffert, D. "The Practical Limits of Patients' Rights." *Psychiatric Annals,* April 1975, 158-161.

Urmer, A. "Implications of California's New Mental Health Law." *American Journal of Psychiatry* 132 (1975): 2152-2153.

Warren, C. A. B. "Involuntary Commitment for Mental Disorder: The Application of California's Lanterman-Petris-Short Act." *Law and Society Review* 11 (1977): 395-426.

Wexler, David B. *Mental Health Law—Major Issues.* New York: Plenum Press, 1981.

Zusman, J., and Carnahan, W. *Mental Health New York Law and Practice.* New York: Matthew Bender, 1975.

28

Community Mental Health

CHAPTER OUTLINE

Turning Points in Psychiatric Care
Emergence of the Community Mental Health
Movement
    The 1960s: A Bold New Approach
    The 1970s: Realistic Problems
    The 1980s: Dismal Prospects
Underlying Concepts
    Systems Perspective
    Levels of Prevention
    Interdisciplinary Collaboration
    Consumer Participation and Control
    Comprehensive Services
    Continuity of Care
Nursing Roles in Community Mental Health
    Applying the ANA Standards
    Levels of Community Mental Health Nursing
    Primary, Secondary, and Tertiary Prevention
Critique of Community Mental Health
and the Deinstitutionalization Movement
    Lack of True Innovation
    Conceptual Confusion
Deinstitutionalized Alternatives
    The Soteria House Approach
    Self-care Nursing for True Chronic Clients
Emerging Networks
Key Nursing Concepts

LEARNING OBJECTIVES

After reading this chapter, students should be able to

- Identify the social conditions that led to the development of the community mental health movement
- Discuss the impact of legislation on community mental health
- Explain the six concepts basic to community mental health philosophy
- Relate the ANA Psychiatric-Mental Health Nursing Standards of practice and professional performance to community mental health nursing
- Identify community mental health nursing roles appropriate to the educational preparation, skills, and experience of the individual nurse
- Describe community mental health nursing roles and functions in terms of primary, secondary, and tertiary levels of prevention
- Evaluate the problems of the community mental health and deinstitutionalization movements
- Discuss two examples of residential innovations in community care of the severely and chronically mentally disordered

CHAPTER 28

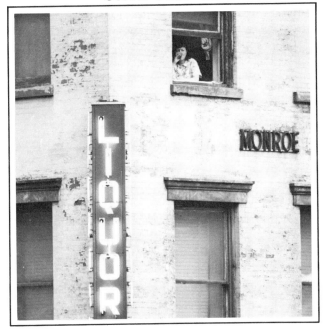

In the cavernous interior of a large railroad terminal, a thirty-nine-year-old woman actually makes her home on an old wooden bench, surrounded by three large plastic bags that hold all her earthly possessions. She is one of an estimated 18,000 homeless men and women in New York City thought by various observers to be former residents of state psychiatric hospitals. In another city a twenty-four-year-old community college student attends classes during the day and lives, along with six other young adults, in a well-kept house on a quiet residential street staffed by mental health counselors and community volunteers. In yet another metropolitan area, a sixty-two-year-old man walks to a storefront clinic in his neighborhood where he tells the receptionist in his native Italian that his pill bottle is empty and he needs another prescription.

What these three people have in common are their experiences with a system for delivery of mental health services called community mental health. This chapter explores the dimensions of their experience in which the locus of care has shifted in two decades from large, often isolated, state institutions to the community itself.

Advocates of the community mental health movement establish clinics in urban areas to better reach and serve severely disordered and lonely people. Some critics of this movement believe that clients are better treated in state mental hospitals.

TURNING POINTS IN PSYCHIATRIC CARE

Psychiatric professionals are fond of calling the turning points that have occurred in psychiatric care "revolutions." The community mental health movement is often referred to as the third revolution in psychiatry (the first was the provision of treatment for, rather than incarceration of, the mentally ill; the second was the emphasis on intrapsychic causes, an outgrowth of psychoanalysis). However, a number of other turning points have been responsible for creating the social conditions that led to the development of the community mental health movement:

- In the late 1700s Philippe Pinel of Paris cast off the chains and irons that bound mentally disordered persons and ushered in the era of moral management and mental institutions (the first revolution).

- At the turn of this century Sigmund Freud of Vienna developed a method of investigation, therapeutic technique, and body of scientific concepts and propositions called psychoanalysis (the second revolution).

- During World War II almost 2,000,000 late adolescent and young adult men were found unfit for military service because of psychiatric and neurological findings, and large numbers of military personnel and veterans required psychiatric treatment and hospitalization.

- The National Institute for Mental Health was created in 1946, heralding the beginning of a new federalism in the provision of mental health services.

- Drug treatment for mental illness began in the early 1950s.

- In 1955 the National Mental Health Study Act established the Joint Commission on Mental Illness.

- In his 1963 message to Congress, President John F. Kennedy called for a "bold, new approach" to the problems of mental illness and mental retardation.

The first five turning points have been discussed in other chapters (1, 2, 5, 11, 16, 27). This chapter is concerned with the events that began in 1955 and shaped the social movement that we know as community mental health.

EMERGENCE OF THE COMMUNITY MENTAL HEALTH MOVEMENT

- In the ten years following the end of World War II, the inpatient population of state psychiatric institutions grew from 450,000 to 550,000. New institutions were built and old ones became more crowded. This had a profound impact on the economic health of many states and drew the attention and concern of politicians at local, state, and national levels. They were the moving force responsible in 1955 for legislating the National Mental Health Study Act that established the Joint Commission on Mental Illness and Health. This group was charged with the responsibility of studying the mental health needs of the nation and making recommendations for a national mental health program.

- Psychotropic drugs, especially tranquilizers such as Thorazine, were being used more and more. They helped staff members manage large numbers of clients in crowded conditions. Research into chemotherapy and the etiology of mental illness seemed to promise an answer or cure that could be discovered at any time. One contemporary psychiatric nursing leader tells of being discouraged by other nurses and physicians from becoming a psychiatric nurse when she graduated from a diploma nursing program in 1958. They predicted that research would discover a chemical basis for mental illness within one to two years. Treatment would become a question simply of administering the right pill, thus making psychiatric nurses and mental hospitals obsolete. When the cause and the cure hadn't been found six years later this leader finally enrolled in a graduate program in psychiatric-mental health nursing. A quarter of a century has now passed since she first heard the cause/cure prediction of her colleagues.

- Group therapy and short-term or brief (five to six sessions) individual psychotherapy instituted to treat large numbers of military personnel began to be used for other segments of the population. Mental health professionals began to consider options other than costly long-term individual psychotherapy or long-term hospitalization.

- Milieu therapy, sometimes called sociotherapy, began to develop based on the efforts of Maxwell Jones, who established therapeutic communities in English hospital settings (1953), and Alfred Stanton and Morris Schwartz (1949) and Milton Greenblatt, Richard H. York, and Esther Lucille Brown (1955), who studied milieus in the United States.

The 1960s: A Bold New Approach

By 1961, the Joint Commission on Mental Illness and Health had presented its report, *Action for Mental Health*, to Congress. The report concluded that psychiatric services in this country were woefully inadequate. The landmark recommendations of the group called for a shift from institutional to community-based care; a more equitable distribution of mental health services; preventive services; consumer participation in both the planning and delivery of mental health services; the hiring and training of citizens in the community as nonprofessional mental health workers; the education of increased numbers of mental health professionals; publicly supported research; and shared federal, state, and local funding for the construction and operation of a system of community-based care through community mental health centers.

President Kennedy appointed a cabinet-level committee to study the Joint Commission's recommendations and on February 5, 1963, he delivered the first presidential message concerned with the mental health of the nation. In it President Kennedy called for "a bold new approach" in which mental health services would be integrated with community life (Kennedy 1963). Congress responded by passing legislation to implement the president's proposal in the form of the Mental Retardation Facilities and Community Mental Health Centers Construction Act (P.L. 88–164; frequently referred to as the Community Mental Health Centers Act) before the end of the year. This legislation authorized 150 million dollars in federal funds to be matched by state funds over three years in the construction of comprehensive community mental health centers. In order to qualify for federal funding, the five essential services outlined in Table 28–1 had to be offered.

A center could continue to receive federal support in decreasing proportions for an eight-year period. It was expected that after this time centers would be able to operate on state and local funds and fees re-

Table 28-1 ESSENTIAL COMMUNITY MENTAL HEALTH SERVICES		
1963	**1975**	**1981**
Inpatient care. 24-hour hospitalization for any person in the community requiring around-the-clock care. Outpatient care. Psychiatric treatment for clients living at home. Partial hospitalization. Treatment programs for clients not requiring around-the-clock care. Day treatment programs allow clients to return home at night. Night treatment programs allow clients to maintain jobs during the day and return to the hospital at night. Emergency care. 24-hour emergency services. Consultation and education. To professionals or community groups in schools, health clinics, churches, courts, law enforcement agencies, etc.	Five essential services mandated in 1963 plus: Follow-up care. On-going programs for community residents after discharge from a mental health facility. Transitional services. Living arrangements for persons unable to live on their own but not requiring hospitalization, or newly discharged from a mental health facility and requiring assistance in adjusting to living on their own. Services for children and adolescents. Mental health diagnostic treatment, liaison, and follow-up services for children and adolescents. Services for elderly. Mental health diagnostic, treatment, liaison, and follow-up services for the elderly. Screening services. Assistance to courts and other agencies to screen persons referred to mental health agencies. Alcohol abuse services. Programs geared toward prevention, treatment, and follow-up in alcohol abuse. Drug abuse services. Programs geared toward prevention, treatment, and follow-up in drug abuse.	Outpatient care Partial hospitalization 24-hour hospitalization and emergency care Consultation and education Screening services

ceived from services. In 1965 legislation extended federal funding for community mental health services through 1968, and the program was extended once again in 1970. At this time funding for services to children and adolescents was specifically provided in response to the 1969 report of the Joint Commission on the Mental Health of Children which cited inadequate programs for young people. This amendment also provided for service provision to drug and alcohol abusers, and for mental health consultation.

The 1970s: Realistic Problems

Unfortunately the Community Mental Health Centers Act program often did not work as planned. Some states and local municipalities did not have funds to match those available at the federal level. Some centers, especially those in poverty areas or predominant-

ly rural areas, were unable to generate sufficient revenue through fees. Services that generated little or no income, such as public education and mental health consultation, began to suffer.

The 1975 amendments to the 1963 law (Community Mental Health Center Amendment P.L. 94–63) not only reemphasized the goals of the 1963 legislation, but also required that each center provide the seven additional mental health services outlined in Table 28–1. This requirement meant that in order to receive funds, a community mental health center might have to provide services not necessarily needed by the population it served.

The next major assessment of the mental health needs of the nation began in 1977 when President Carter established a twenty-member President's Commission on Mental Health. Unlike the Joint Commission of 1955, which was dominated by physicians, this group included a nurse, Martha Mitchell, the chairperson of the ANA Division on Psychiatric and Mental Health Nursing Practice. Three other professional nurses served on adjunct committees. *Report to the President of the President's Commission on Mental Health* (1978) focused on the following major areas:

- Providing community-based services as the keystone of the mental health system
- Improving community support systems and networks among families, neighbors, community organizations, and existing service components
- Establishing national health insurance that would include coverage for mental health care
- Encouraging mental health coverage (including outpatient) in all health insurance plans
- Continuing the phaseout of large public mental hospitals and improving services in the remainder
- Providing funding to increase the number of mental health professionals, especially those working with minorities, children, and the aged
- Establishing a center with a strong emphasis on primary prevention within the National Institute for Mental Health
- Protecting the human rights of persons in need of mental health care
- Improving the delivery of services to underserved populations and high-risk populations, such as minorities and the chronically ill, through a new federal program
- Developing an advocacy program for the chronically mentally ill
- Increasing support for research related to mental health and illness
- Providing health education to the public and increasing the public understanding of mental health problems
- Centralizing the evaluation efforts of governmental agencies concerned with mental health

The commission's report had special significance for psychiatric nurses. It was hailed as the first official high-level document to give visibility to the professional competence of nurses in mental health care (Hadley 1978). The document specifically mentioned nurses in sections concerned with manpower shortages, training and education for primary care practitioners, and mental health care providers whose services should be reimbursed by insurance companies.

The 1980s: Dismal Prospects

The Community Mental Health Systems Act of 1980 was a major achievement of the outgoing Carter administration. It was designed to implement the recommendations made by the president's commission authorizing the funding of community mental health centers, services to high-risk populations, ambulatory mental health care centers, a prevention unit and associate director for minority concerns at NIMH, rape research and services, and recommending a model mental health patient's bill of rights. Its basic task was to coordinate the two-tiered system of mental health care that had evolved since President Kennedy's 1963 efforts. The severely mentally ill continued to inhabit state institutions, and those with less acute problems used the services of federally funded community mental health centers. Unfortunately, there was little coordination between these two systems. Clients discharged from state institutions often failed to receive follow-up services, and certain populations—the chronically mentally ill, the elderly, and youth—fell between the two systems. This act was intended to coordinate federal and state efforts.

Before the programs authorized by this legislation to start in 1982 could get off the ground the political climate changed and significantly altered the role of the federal government in the nation's mental health. The 1980 Community Mental Health Systems Act was essentially repealed in 1981 when the 97th Congress passed the new Reagan administration's Omnibus Budget Reconciliation Act (P.L. 97–35). The new budget placed the mental health services programs formerly administered by NIMH into an alcohol, drug abuse, and mental health services block grant, shifting the decision-making about allocation of funds to the states and decreasing the federal role in coordination.

The decrease in the federal budget has had and will continue to have far-ranging effects on the community mental health movement. It cuts funding for community mental health centers and other mental health care delivery programs. Community mental health centers will cease to be funded after 1984, but funding reductions will be felt as early as 1983. Mandated services have been reduced from twelve to five (see Table 28–1) and their continuing existence and quality will depend on state support, private funding, and earned revenue. Legislative impact on the community mental health movement is outlined in Table 28–2. Budget reductions have already resulted in a decrease in staff at NIMH, which has lost a number of key people. For example, the deputy director of NIMH until 1981 was

Table 28-2   LEGISLATIVE IMPACT ON THE COMMUNITY MENTAL HEALTH MOVEMENT

1955	National Mental Health Study Act (P. L. 840-182) establishes the Joint Commission on Mental Illness and Health.
1961	Joint Commission on Mental Illness and Health presents its report *Action for Mental Health* to Congress.
1963	President John F. Kennedy's special message to Congress on mental illness and mental retardation advocates federal participation in mental health programs.
	Mental Retardation Facilities and Community Mental Health Centers Construction Act (P. L. 88-164) provides matching funds of $150 million for construction of community mental health centers and mandates five essential mental health services.
1965	Funding for community mental health centers extended through 1968.
1969	Joint Commission on the Mental Health of Children report, *Crisis in Child Mental Health: Challenge for the 1970s* addresses the problems of inadequate mental health services for children and adolescents.
1970	Amendment to 1963 Community Mental Health Centers (CMHC) Act extends program funding and increases service provision to include children, drug and alcohol abusers, and consultation.
	National Institute for Drug Abuse and National Institute for Alcoholism and Alcohol Abuse established.
1975	Community Mental Health Centers Amendments, Title III (P. L. 94-63) extends services of CMHC to include specific underserved groups, etc., and increases mandated essential services to twelve.
1977	President Jimmy Carter establishes President's Commission on Mental Health to identify the mental health needs of the nation.
1978	*Report to the President from the President's Commission on Mental Health* published in April.
1980	Mental Health Systems Act to coordinate services between state institutions and community mental health centers passed.
1981	Omnibus Budget Reconciliation Act (P. L. 97-35) of new Reagan administration and 97th Congress requires drastic federal funding cuts. Alcohol, drug abuse, and mental health services put under block grant under state control. Essential services reduced to five.
1982-1983	States begin to apportion funding for mental health services under block grant.
1984	Termination of funding for community mental health under terms of 1981 Budget Act.

a nurse, Rhetaugh Dumas, who had also served as chief of the Psychiatric Nursing Education Branch and deputy director of the Division of Manpower and Training Programs. Discouraged by the budget cuts, the policy shift away from federal involvement in mental health programs, and the decision to phase out clinical training programs for mental health professionals and paraprofessionals (most of which prepared people to work with underserved populations and encouraged the entry of minorities into the field), Dr. Dumas left government service in 1981 to become Dean of the School of Nursing at the University of Michigan (Dumas 1981).

The federal budget for 1983 is constructed to continue support for mental health research and for the training of mental health researchers. According to Department of Health and Human Services Secretary Richard Schweiker, there is more hope in research than in the provision of services (Washington Report on Medicine and Health 1982). However, the changing shape of the research efforts themselves has alarmed many people concerned with (1) the present burgeoning mental health problems in this country, and (2) the large numbers of homeless people on the streets who have "fallen between the cracks" of our two-tiered system of mental health care. The administration has asked that only research devoted to the neurosciences be supported and that social research support be eliminated. While Congress has not thus far honored this specific request, current research support appears to be headed in that direction.

What do these events mean for clients, communities, and mental health professionals in the rest of the eighties? Most observers take a rather dismal view of the future, predicting increased racial tension, crime, and drug and alcohol abuse; poorer mental health care; more homeless and chronically mentally ill people causing greater community distress; and an increase in stress-precipitated problems such as anxiety, family violence, and divorce (Winslow 1982). There is growing concern over the enlarging population of young adult chronic clients in the community who are likely, some observers feel, to suffer most from cuts in clinical programs (Pepper, Kirshner, and Ryglewicz 1981). Most critics await the demise of community mental health programs and their desertion by psychiatric nurses, psychologists, psychiatrists, and social workers. Desertion by psychiatrists has already begun. The economic conditions of the 1980s provide the greatest threat yet to the community mental health movement.

UNDERLYING CONCEPTS

The basic philosophy of the community mental health movement is that health care is a right and, therefore, mental health services should be available to all people. The six concepts basic to community mental health are discussed below.

Systems Perspective

The systems perspective provides a holistic view of people and their environment and has already been described in Chapters 2 and 21. Basic to community mental health is the notion that people constantly interact with the environment. A systems perspective requires broadening the scope of mental health care beyond the individual to the system (community) as a whole with holistic awareness of the biological, psychological, and sociocultural forces that influence interacting systems.

Levels of Prevention

Since its early origins, the community mental health movement has emphasized prevention. Initially, Gerald Caplan (1964) adapted the concepts of preventive medicine for application to psychiatry in general and to community mental health in particular. The levels of prevention in mental health care are:

- Primary prevention—reducing the incidence of mental disorders of all types in a community by preventing potentially harmful social conditions or by directly intervening to alter them if they do exist

- Secondary prevention—identifying disorders that do occur and treating them as early and as quickly as possible, thereby reducing their duration and returning the client to participation in the community as soon as possible

- Tertiary prevention—reducing the impairment that may result from the disorders that do occur by instituting early rehabilitation programs

This concept is the foundation for the nursing role in community mental health, which is described later in this chapter.

Interdisciplinary Collaboration

The essential services of community mental health cannot be totally provided by the members of any one discipline or paraprofessional group. Blurring of roles between and among mental health professionals is even more apparent in community mental health programs. It can be traced to the 1961 report of the Joint Commission on Mental Illness and Health that recommended that nurses provide brief, short-term psychotherapy to psychiatric clients. While some nurses in some sections of the country were already doing so, it further legitimated their psychotherapy role. The 1963 legislation funded graduate level clinical specialist programs to prepare nurses at the psychotherapist level. The lines between psychiatric nursing and the other mental health professions became even more indistinct and even psychiatric nurses have experienced difficulty in defining what is unique to nursing. Fortunately, increased nursing research and the development of nursing theories have helped define this area for psychiatric nurses. Interdisciplinary collaboration among mental health team members, the nature of their relationships, and the consequences of role blurring are taken up in Chapter 3. How the development of nursing theories and nursing research have helped to define the unique aspects of the nursing role is the major focus of Chapter 4. Also see Appendix E.

Interdisciplinary collaboration is also influenced by the setting in which the community mental health nurse practices. The following settings (Leininger 1969) also influence practice today:

- Undifferentiated. In these settings the roles of mental health professionals are flexible. They are based on the individual's abilities, experience, and interests. It is difficult to distinguish the professional disciplines to which members belong. These settings are most common in multiservice agencies and community mental health centers.

- Traditional. Traditionally based roles are determined primarily by the profession to which each individual member belongs. Each profession makes its own contributions. The setting is often a traditional hospital-based program.
- Ambivalent. These are settings characterized by confusion and uncertainty over who should do what. In actual practice vacillation occurs between the undifferentiated and traditional roles.

The challenge in mental health team work is to balance flexible role boundaries with areas of unique expertise in order to deliver more effective and higher quality mental health care.

Consumer Participation and Control

Consumer participation and control is another outgrowth of the 1960s era. Although the 1961 Joint Commission report recommended community involvement and it was supported by the subsequent legislation, the practical aspects were not clear. In many instances citizen participation continued as it had in the past; socially prominent citizens, wealthy contributors, and health care providers continued to serve on the governing bodies of mental health agencies. The 1975 amendments provided clarifying guidelines for citizen participation by requiring governing bodies of new community mental health centers to be composed of people living in the area served by the community mental health center, at least half of whom should not be health care providers. In addition, it required that centers in operation before 1975 appoint community members in an advisory capacity to their governing boards. This legislation aimed to ensure that the services provided by community mental health centers would respond to the needs of the citizens. This demonstrated both the philosophical and policy commitment to a decision-making role for the citizens of a given community.

Members of the community also participate in other ways. Large numbers of indigenous nonprofessionals have been employed by community mental health programs as human service workers. Because they understand the problems of the community and the language and customs of ethnic groups specific to that community, they have been quite successful in delivering personalized mental health services. Chapter 3 describes the characteristics of these mental health workers.

Comprehensive Services

The community mental health philosophy is committed to providing a full range of comprehensive services to all the members of a community. These services are described throughout this chapter and are outlined in Table 28-1. The foundation for the provision of comprehensive services rests on a holistic approach to the community as client.

The community as client is defined in terms of *catchment areas*, geographically circumscribed areas comprising a city, or several rural communities, with from 75,000 to 200,000 residents. This effectively divides a population into segments whose mental health needs can be met by a specifically designed system of services. Optimally, the segments are small enough to promote collaborative relationships within the system of services.

Continuity of Care

Continuity of care means that, while providing comprehensive services to clients, caregivers also assume the responsibility of monitoring or assisting clients in their move from one program to another. In traditional mental health care systems, separate programs rarely interface, and clients may feel that they have been shuttled from one mental health agency to another. In some instances, clients become discouraged or embarrassed about obtaining needed services. Others are unable to be persistent or seek help in the first place. The continuity of care concept in community mental health was intended to correct these problems. Unfortunately, the community mental health movement has not fulfilled its promise in relation to the concept.

NURSING ROLES IN COMMUNITY MENTAL HEALTH

Community mental health nursing roles consist of a wide scope of activities from the maintenance of mental health and prevention of illness to treatment and rehabilitation. In the broadest sense of the words, the community is the client. Since people are constantly interacting with the environment, when community mental health nurses provide direct services to individual clients, they also direct attention toward the client's community.

Applying the ANA Standards

One of the ANA Psychiatric Nursing Professional Performance Standards (see Appendix A for the complete list of the recently revised standards) provides an umbrella for community mental health nursing practice at the clinical specialist level:

> **Standard 10: Utilization of Community Health Systems** The nurse participates with other members of the community in assessing, planning, implementing, and evaluating mental health services and community systems that include the promotion of the broad continuum of primary, secondary, and tertiary prevention of mental illness.

While demonstrating competence in meeting Standard 10 has been determined by the ANA to be in the province of the specialist, the community mental health nurse generalist uses all the other standards as guidelines for practice.

Levels of Community Mental Health Nursing

There is no one set of skills, educational preparation, or nursing experience that determines who is and who is not a community mental health nurse. Both generalists and specialists practice in community settings. They are identified by their commitment to the philosophy and concepts presented earlier in this chapter. However, their roles do vary according to the educational preparation, skills, and experience they possess. Table 28–3 identifies three different levels of community mental health nursing in regard to education and experience, professional responsibilities, licensure and certification, and employment settings.

Primary, Secondary, and Tertiary Prevention

Community mental health nurses hold the principles of primary, secondary, and tertiary prevention as central to their clinical work. In primary prevention, the nurse is concerned with preventing new cases of mental disorder by counteracting harmful stressors. Nursing activities are directed toward fostering mental well-being and identifying potential stressors and segments of the population that may be at high risk. In secondary prevention, the nurse attempts to shorten the duration of

a mental disorder through early case-finding and treatment and to reduce its prevalence in a given segment of the population. In tertiary prevention, the nurse implements treatments and rehabilitative services for clients who have been diagnosed as mentally disordered. Table 28–4 gives specific examples of community mental health nursing roles and functions in all three levels of prevention.

CRITIQUE OF COMMUNITY MENTAL HEALTH AND THE DEINSTITUTIONALIZATION MOVEMENT*

Lest the following critique be used to justify a further medicalization of mental health problems and a retreat from the principles of community psychiatry, we have tried to make the apparent criticisms understandable in light of the circumstances. Leaving aside these contextual considerations makes it easier to find community mental health's deficiencies sufficient to conclude the whole thing was a mistake. This conclusion is particularly tempting at a time when we are witnessing a swing of the pendulum of opinion away from a social conception of the cause and treatment of mental disorders to a much more biologically oriented one. Our point is not that the old state hospital system is preferable to community health systems, but that a system originally set up as a competitive alternative to the state hospital has done so little to define the breadth and limitations of possible alternatives to hospitalization and to promote the goal of deinstitutionalization for clients.

Lack of True Innovation

The community mental health movement represents the essence of the new hospital psychiatry. Its purposes are to:

- Deemphasize long-term hospitalization.
- Institute the notion of brief hospitalization for the stabilization of acute crises.
- Develop community resources to treat and support the mentally ill person without resorting to institutionalization.

*Adapted by permission from Holly Skodol Wilson, *Deinstitutionalized Residential Care for the Mentally Disordered: The Soteria House Approach.* New York: Grune and Stratton (1982).

Practitioner	Community Mental Health Nurse I	Community Mental Health Nurse II	Clinical Nurse Specialist in Community Mental Health
Table 28–3 LEVELS OF COMMUNITY MENTAL HEALTH NURSING			
Education and experience	Nursing diploma or associate degree with minimum one year of psychiatric nursing experience Baccalaureate degree graduate	Baccalaureate degree plus two years of clinical experience	Master's degree in psychiatric/mental health nursing
Professional responsibilities	Interviewing techniques, interpersonal relationship skills, basic knowledge of prevention, assess client's level of functioning, observations/data collection, facilitate and use community resources	Mental health education, supportive therapy, behavioral management of psychiatric disorders, therapeutic one-to-one relationship, crisis intervention technique, assessment of client's functioning, knowledge of family theory, group dynamics, personality development, sociopsychological principles, theories, methods of mental health treatment	Insight oriented psychotherapy, family therapy, group therapy, psychoanalytic theory, psychopathology, diagnostic evaluation, community organization, mental health consultation, supervision, eclectic approach to mental health and treatment
Licensure and certification	Professional licensure by state	Professional licensure by state, American Nurses' Association Certification as Psychiatric and Mental Health Nurse	Professional licensure by state, after two years of clinical experience: eligible for American Nurses' Association Certification in Psychiatric and Mental Health Nursing; clinical specialist in psychiatric and mental health nursing—adult or children and adolescent
Employment settings	Community mental health centers, community nurse for psychiatric inpatient setting, preventive programs	Community mental health centers, crisis intervention teams, high risk populations—child abuse, rape, drug abuse, preventive programs	Community mental health centers, crisis intervention multiservice center, mental health consultant and/or supervisor, private mental health facilities, individual private practice, administration, teaching, research

Source: J. S. Berns, and M. S. Hamilton, "Nursing Role in Community Mental Health," in L. L. Jarvis, *Community Health Nursing: Keeping the Public Healthy.* Philadelphia: F. A. Davis, 1981, p. 328.

Table 28–4 COMMUNITY MENTAL HEALTH NURSING ROLES AND FUNCTIONS		
Primary Prevention	**Secondary Prevention**	**Tertiary Prevention**
Identifying potentially stressful conditions in the community and high-risk populations	Providing brief psychotherapy to individuals, groups, and families	Helping to plan for a client's discharge from the hospital
Holding effective parenting classes for adolescent parents, at day-care centers, in schools	Suicide prevention hot line counseling and staffing crisis intervention programs	Coordinating and monitoring follow-up care in home, halfway house, foster care home, or other transitional service
Holding divorce therapy groups for couples, families, and individuals	Providing counseling to victims of violence and their significant others	Teaching clients self-care activities before discharge from the hospital
Providing mental health consultation to health care providers	Holding stress reduction groups for health care providers	Serving as a client advocate
Providing mental health education to members of the community	Case-finding and referring clients in need of treatment	Providing individual, group, and family psychotherapy
Consulting with self-help groups	Providing emergency mental health services	Referring clients to self-help groups or after-care services
Being politically active in relation to mental health issues	Intake, screening, and assessment of clients	Staffing partial hospitalization programs

The psychiatric hospital is no longer viewed as the end point in the lives of psychiatric clients but as a turning point at which clients and their social network reintegrate in order to carry on the struggle of community life.

Regardless of their list of essential services, community mental health programs as developed in the United States have two essential features:

1. The establishment, in the community, of psychiatric services for the mentally ill, which would have previously been part of the state hospital program.

2. The establishment of services for clients who formerly would not have been considered in need of psychiatric care. The emphasis here is on indirect consultation and education in the hope of preventing "breakdowns" under stress.

Coupled with the emphasis on community treatment and evolving as well from a dissatisfaction with custodial care, humanitarian concerns for the mentally ill have precipitated legislation in most states geared to securing certain civil liberties and legal rights for clients. These mental health laws discussed in Chapter 27 have stipulated procedures to be followed in order to hospitalize individuals with or without their consent, criteria for hospitalization, and regulations about con-

tinuing care and discharge. In the view of some mental health professionals, these changes have brought significant economic and legal forces into the context of contemporary psychiatric treatment. Government planners and managers now set health policy and establish priorities. The demands made by these new systems of monitoring and control have substantially altered the practice of psychiatric care leading to the development of complicated mechanisms for processing clients through treatment. These new processes are designed to negotiate a complex maze of nonclinical considerations peripheral to the actual treatment programs themselves.

In short, conventional treatment in the community mental health system has become a highly prescriptive, elaborately formal structure of policy, regulations, and standards. Complying with these procedures demands increasing attention from mental health professionals. The old state hospital warehouse has been replaced by a similarly bureaucratized clearinghouse where care and treatment consist primarily of an institutionalizing dispatching process that denies self-care, self-determination, and a self-control to clients. Instead, they are held, screened, patched together, stamped with a diagnostic label, sorted into a legal category, and returned to an unwelcoming community placement (Wilson 1982).

Inpatient hospital units under the community mental health system must fill the social control gap left by the closing of traditional state hospitals. Mental health clinicians in such settings must become agents of the community; regardless of how much the community may desire successful treatment and rehabilitation of the mentally disordered, it demands safe custody of those individuals it rejects. Viewed in this light, the community mental health inpatient psychiatric facility must respond to multiple and contradictory messages. It stands at the intersection of community care and traditional institutionalism with its emphasis on isolation and custodialism. It must protect the community but at the same time guarantee the client's rights. It must provide for custodial needs of individuals whom society rejects and yet facilitate return as quickly as possible to the rejecting community.

Conceptual Confusion

Between 1955 and 1975 the new term "deinstitutionalization" was introduced into the writing and practice of American psychiatric professionals. Under the banner of deinstitutionalization the census of resident clients in American state mental hospitals decreased from 559,000 to 193,900 or approximately 60 percent. The quantitative goal set for the deinstitutionalization movement was a 50 percent reduction in the client population of state hospitals for the mentally ill within two decades (Minkoff 1978).

One might expect that a concept with the apparent power and impact of deinstitutionalization would have considerable consensus of meaning for its advocates and users. On the contrary, deinstitutionalization is surrounded with definitional disorder. The boundaries imputed to the term change from writer to writer, and variations exist in language as well as meaning.

The language used to explain deinstitutionalization reveals a crowded assortment of uneasy cohabitants: reintegration, native communities, natural caregivers, bold new approach, crisis-oriented services, social reform, humanization, community mental health centers, civil liberties, self-care, dumping, revolving door, trans-institutionalization, continuity of care, treatment alternatives, rehabilitation, support system, psychiatric chronicity, and cost effectiveness. This lexicon of diverse terminology adds to the difficulties of studying and assessing the practices of deinstitutionalization.

Variations in the meaning or intent of the term's users are similarly broad. According to Bachrach (1978), deinstitutionalization is simultaneously a fact, a

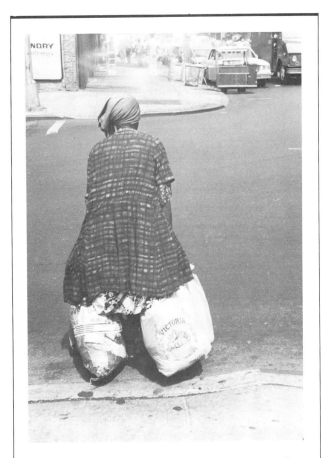

This "bag lady" carries all her earthly possessions with her. She is one of the homeless.

philosophy, and a process. The well-known fact is that the resident population of state hospitals has decreased from about half a million to about 190,000 or about 66 percent. The philosophy represents an expression of civil libertarian emphasis on rights of individuals and modification of environments as the primary avenue of social change. The process refers to the avoidance of traditional hospital settings for treatment of the mentally ill and the concurrent expansion of community-based facilities.

Bassuk and Gerson (1978) equate the nature of deinstitutionalization with a massive reform movement in the delivery of mental health services parading under the banner of community mental health. But they raise questions about whether deinstitutionalization represents an enlightened revolution or an abdication of responsibility. Due to shortcomings in legislation, lack of funding, and the unanticipated impact of discharged clients on communities, the dual promise of an extensive support system of comprehensive, coordinated community care and prevention programs has never been fulfilled. Instead, according to these critics, hospitalized clients have been released haphazardly to a nonsystem of aftercare that has meant real hardship and even tragedy. Roughly half of the homeless men and women are former residents of state psychiatric hospitals. Critics of the deinstitutionalization movement cite inadequate discharge planning, weak follow-up efforts, scarce supportive housing, rampant inflation, rising rents, fixed subsistence income, and a shrinking supply of low-income dwellings as reasons for the swelling ranks of the homeless. Most of the discharged clients whose releases from hospitals were to "unknown" living arrangements had unknown destinations because they had no place to go. Critics argue that basic human needs for shelter and food must be satisfied before more sophisticated therapeutic measures can have any chance of success. Others challenge that the aims of social reform and effective treatment have become entangled and that while social justice may be a necessary condition for successful treatment, it is not a sufficient one.

Klerman (1979) views deinstitutionalization as primarily a shift from a state owned and operated monopoly to a pluralistic and diversified system of services that resulted from a short-lived consensus between lawyers interested in civil rights, budget advisors pressured by economic forces who viewed deinstitutionalization as an opportunity to shift mental health financing from state to national levels, and theorists and researchers in social psychiatry. In this view, deinstitutionalization is first and foremost a shift in location and funding arrangements.

Talbott (1979) calls deinstitutionalization a misnomer and substitutes his own terminology, including "transinstitutionalization," a circumstance in which chronically mentally ill clients have been shifted from a single lousy institution to multiple wretched ones, a shuffle to despair and a national tragedy. He characterizes the outcomes of the deinstitutionalization movement as:

• The dramatic appearance of large numbers of dirty, hallucinating, strange faces on city streets, in low-cost ghettos, and deteriorating neighborhoods, in his terms "naked men dancing on Broadway and bag ladies on Park Avenue"

• Transfer of thousands more clients to nursing homes

• Mental health service patterns of use characterized by falling between the cracks, a total lack of

follow-up, and the revolving door of continued readmissions

• Demoralization, demedicalization, and deterioration within remaining state hospitals

Stern and Minkoff (1979) identify six paradoxes of value that in their view have led to ineffective and inefficient deinstitutionalization programs. The ultimate of these is the community mental health paradox in which the stronger the commitment of community caregivers to community mental health ideals of primary prevention and consultation, the greater the stress when the ideals don't work. As a result, we're tempted to conclude that if chronic clients don't do well under community programs, the life in old state hospitals may be better for them.

Fink and Weinstein (1979) remind us that some see community mental health centers as agencies to rid the community of the causes of mental illness—poverty, racism, unemployment, poor housing, crime, riots, etc. In their view, the fatal flaw of deinstitutionalization has been this attempt to make community mental health programs responsible for the quality of life rather than for the treatment and prevention of mental illness.

Overall, the literature on deinstitutionalization despite its variations yields one clear area of agreement among users of the term. The shift of care and funding arrangements for the chronically and severely mentally ill from single-purpose, custodial state hospitals to multipurpose services based near clients' families and communities has not solved the problems of at least several populations of clients.

DEINSTITUTIONALIZED ALTERNATIVES

Deinstitutionalization is one of the most important developments in the history of psychiatry, yet the well-intentioned reform movement has from its beginning been plagued by a variety of problems. In addition to the *revolving door syndrome* (i.e., short stay with rapid turnover and eventual repeated readmissions to the hospital), large numbers of discharged former clients who are still disturbed live bleak lives in board and care homes, in nursing homes, and on skid row. The problem rests with the erroneous notion that institutionalization is merely a matter of the location and funding arrangements of psychiatric care and the widespread devaluation of any form of long-term residential care for anyone. However, if we view institutionalization as the process by which an individual is denied self-care and self-determination to the point of exchanging personal independence for institutional control and decision-making, the shortest possible hospitalization need not be the crucial goal. Instead, mental health professionals can begin to define and study the full range of possible innovative alternatives to institutionalizing modes of care—alternatives specifically directed toward relinquishing institutional dependency and control and fostering self-care and self-control. Our disenchantment with deinstitutionalization should be used to rethink the concept from its origins. The following list of proposals offers a starting point:

- We must continue to pursue the goals of deinstitutionalization, confused as they might be. We must remember that just as institutionalization was both a process and an effect, deinstitutionalization is also both a process and an effect

- The most significant problem in the contemporary American mental health care system is dealing effectively with psychiatric chronicity

- We need sustained, and not merely transitional, life support settings for many chronic clients: alternative living situations that balance the restriction of clients' freedom with protection for the client and the community

- Key processes in such settings include training in self-care and community living skills, improvement of employability, incentives for taking increasing responsibility, development of social skills, and provision of leisure time activities

- A successful program for deinstitutionalization would be enhanced by the contributions of a cadre of specialists for chronic clients

Nurses have always had the primary responsibility for creating an environment for client care. Therefore, nurses are a likely source of the cadre of specialists in residential alternatives where chronic clients can be taught and supported in developing skills of self-care and self-determination (see Chapter 16).

The Soteria House Approach

In their comprehensive review of research on the treatment of the chronic client, Test and Stein (1978) describe Soteria House, an experimental residence in San Jose, California, as "a residential setting with a permissive unstructured milieu staffed by paraprofessionals who attempt to guide resident clients through their psychoses." Their description was confirmed in Wilson's (1982) study of how some degree of social order was possible in such a permissive, unstructured milieu. Findings from the Soteria studies indicated that the improvised, self-regulating system of *Infracontrol* at Soteria House yielded a marked increase in self-determination and self-control of staff members and resident clients alike. Some critics argue that Soteria House is merely a small isolated island of innovation that self-selects the least entrenched and most hopeful psychiatric clients, is surrounded by ideological zealots, and produces a sizable Hawthorne effect (see Chapter 9). In short, that it is merely part of an uncoordinated nonsystem of pilot projects without a broader systems perspective or the necessary conditions or principles for expanding itself into a viable system for effective care.

Key Processes Observations of day-to-day life in the natural setting at Soteria House revealed an alternative residential care setting for diagnosed schizophrenics where conventional psychiatric arrangements for social control are muted and denied. There are no locked doors, medications, formal therapies, rigid schedules, or rules to control the behavior of young, first-break (but likely to become chronic) clients who live there. Similarly, there are no orientation programs, job descriptions, task assignments, or hierarchy of differentiated roles to provide the specially selected nonprofessional staff members with guidelines for their work. Finally, there are no guarded gates and no official immunity to keep Soteria from the control of outside licensing, funding, and regulatory agencies.

Soteria was modeled after its English prototype Kingsley Hall. Both settings advocate a view of Schizophrenia as a crisis in living with unique potential for reintegration and growth if it is not forced into some premature interruption through the use of psychotropic medicines and other conventional control measures. Staff members in both settings think of themselves as LSD-type guides with an ideology of freedom and nonintervention. In short, Soteria is set up both structurally and idologically as a noncontrol system.

Infracontrol A conceptual explanatory scheme called "Infracontrolling" conveys the basic social process of interaction in the Soteria setting. It explains how resident clients, staff members, and outsiders maintain social order under conditions of espoused freedom and nonintervention. Infracontrolling is comprised of three main subprocesses:

1. "Presencing," a strategy whereby the mere physical presence of sufficient numbers of other people provides tacit control capability for residents, fosters expectations for their own self-control, and redefines client behavior to some variation of normal

2. "Fairing," for solving staff work problems by "estimating one's fair share," and shared community ethics that discourage being unfair

3. "Limiting intrusion," a process that includes minimizing approachability, situational positioning, limiting and contouring disclosures, and avoiding incidents to deflect and disengage external control agents from impinging on Soteria's autonomy

Institutionalization, once believed to be a consequence of living one's life within the requirements of an impersonal, controlling, bureaucratic state hospital, is clearer if we view it as a process of care and effects on the minds and behavior of people rather than a quality of location. Through the processes of infracontrolling, Soteria has enhanced self-determination, self-care, and self-control for at least a limited group of mentally disordered young adults diagnosed as schizophrenic. As Mosher and Menn (1978) found, the young diagnosed schizophrenic subjects at Soteria House recovered and attained a better psychosocial adjustment after two years in its nurturant, supportive, and deinstitutionalizing psychosocial environment.

Although Soteria House has survived economically for ten years with the support of a web of research and staffing grant funds, most of contemporary public urban psychiatry emphasizes an eclectic, pragmatic approach that has yielded a vast array of institutional and practice approaches capable of handling a large and diversified caseload with efficiency. Psychiatric professionals have come to understand their work in terms of intake, screening, referrals, discharge, rates of turnover, budgets, facilities, and staffing. Soteria House by contrast is an experimental approach on an extremely small scale. It continues to be highly selective of both clients and staff members. Although infracontrolling may prove adequate in preserving social order under Soteria's unique conditions, its inability to handle large numbers of diversified clients may limit its applicability within the broader movement. In order to constitute any real competitive force the Soteria House approach will have to be generalized and perhaps transformed. Nevertheless, mental health professionals should select from this approach properties and processes of care, management, and organizational principles that might effectively be generalized or integrated into established models, particularly those directed to the growing population of new young chronic clients.

Self-care Nursing for True Chronic Clients

Clinical observations, the psychiatric literature, and most recently the diagnostic categories of the DSM-III (see Chapter 8) raise the possibility that there are some chronic clients for whom the Soteria House approach is unrealistic. These people are described as the "true chronics" by Goldman (1981). True chronics are clients who suffer severe and persistent mental or emotional disorders that interfere and substantially limit primary aspects of daily life, such as personal self-care, interpersonal relationships, work, or schooling. Such prolonged functional disability caused or aggravated by severe mental disorders has now become the chief distinguishing characteristic of this population of chronic clients. These are the people who have required institutional care for an extended duration and have become institutionalized.

Despite our recognition that such clients exist, it is not as easy to identify them as Goldman's reference might suggest. The general definition of chronic disease established by the Commission on Chronic Illness is:

All impairments or deviations from normal which have one or more of the following characteristics: Are permanent; Leave residual disability; Are caused by nonreversible pathological alterations; Require special training of the patient for rehabilitation; May be expected to require a long period of supervision, observation, or care.

The American Psychiatric Association Conference on the chronic mental client used the following general definition by Bachrach (1979): "Those individuals who are, have been, or might have been but for the deinstitutionalization movement on the rolls of the long-term mental institutions, especially state hospitals." Bachrach has attempted to define chronic clients by location. She identified five subgroups of the population that at one time would have been the residents of state hospitals. In the community are clients released from the hospital and clients who have never been hospitalized. (Soteria House focused on the latter group.) In hospitals are old long-term clients, recent short-term clients, and finally new long-term clients who probably will not be discharged. Minkoff (1978) refined Bachrach's general definition by distinguishing three separate but overlapping chronic populations:

1. The chronic mentally ill—people who are continuously ill for two years according to DSM-III.

2. The chronic mentally disabled—subgroup of the chronic mentally ill characterized by partial or total impairment of instrumental role performance.

3. Chronic mental clients—people who have continuously and/or for a long duration been hospitalized or received mental health services.

However we define chronic clients, they have certain identified needs or services. These needs include material resources, such as food, clothing, decent housing, medical and psychiatric care, transportation, and money; vocational rehabilitation resulting in marketable skills and job opportunities; and less tangible needs such as resocialization, day-to-day coping skills, reduction of bizarre behavior, motivation to remain involved with life and a source of nurturing, affirming, and helpful interpersonal alliances. The Functional Adaptation Model or the Self-care Approach describes psychiatric nursing's approach for meeting these needs of chronic psychiatric clients (Underwood 1978).

Self-care Model of Nursing* Nursing education for psychiatric nurses has for the past few decades emphasized psychotherapeutic and psychological models (see Chapter 2) rather than nursing models (see Chapter 4), thus raising questions about the potential for any unique nursing contribution to the mental health team. Psychiatric nurses need a model of nursing in order to make a unique and valued contribution to the mental health services team beyond services in areas where roles are blurred. The Self-care Model offers a clearer picture of the nature of nursing and nursing's valuable part in the community mental health movement. It draws heavily from existing knowledge and skills in nursing and organizes them to guide the client care offered by psychiatric nurses. Nursing evolves out of a tradition and present day pattern that emphasizes a twenty-four-hour, seven-day-a-week commitment to client care, a holistic view of mind-body relations, an emphasis on care rather than cure, and a focus on

*This section is based on the current clinical and research work of Patricia R. Underwood. Summarized with permission.

client strengths. Nursing also includes knowledge about mental disorder, chronicity, institutionalizing processes, and effective approaches to clients in residential settings. The processes or skills nurses use include problem-solving, decision-making, health teaching and interpersonal communication (Chapter 4).

In brief, the Self-care Model originated by Orem (1980) and adapted to psychiatric clients by Underwood (in press) guides nurses in using nursing processes to help clients establish, maintain, or increase self-care and self-determination in day-to-day living (see Chapter 4). Using this approach, the psychiatric nurse can minimize the institutionalizing effects of psychiatric care and psychiatric disabilities and thus help the client avoid a life-style of institutionalized psychiatric chronicity and dependency.

Orem defines self-care as the practice of activities that individuals initiate and perform on their own behalf to maintain life, health, and well-being. Self-care activities produce conditions that support the individual in development and maturation. Underwood (1978) operationalizes the following five universal self-care requisites from Orem's eight original self-care requisites.

- Air, food, and fluid
- Elimination
- Body temperature and personal hygiene
- Rest and activity
- Solitude and social interaction

Nursing action meets self-care needs in a therapeutic way when it supports life processes and promotes normal functioning; maintains normal growth, development, and maturation; prevents, controls, or cures disease and injuries; and prevents or compensates for disability.

Nursing actions according to Orem (1971) include:

- Acting or doing for clients when they are critically ill, unconscious, or unable to participate in decision making.
- Guiding clients when they require direction or supervision to make choices or take action.
- Supporting clients by acting as an advocate in their attempts to obtain resources essential to life, health, and well-being. Support may be offered by a look, a touch, or simple physical presence, as well as verbal exchange.

- Providing an environment that promotes personal development in relation to meeting present and future demands for action and provides respect for human beings and the use of their actualized potential.
- Teaching clients by helping them obtain knowledge or skill essential to a particular series of acts.

All of these nursing actions may be used in a *wholly compensatory, partially compensatory,* or *supportive, educative nursing system of care.* Depending on the client's assessed self-care level, however, each has as its goal establishing, maintaining, or increasing the client's ability for self-care and self-determination in day-to-day living.

The categories of universal self-care requisites, therapeutic self-care demands, helping methods, and types of nursing care systems have been implemented and studied by Underwood since 1975 on six inpatient psychiatric wards. The implementation of the Self-care Model has emphasized creating an environment that supports the acquisition of community living skills rather than hospital adjustment. Underwood's nursing approach, further outlined in Chapter 16, includes:

- Systematic and regular assessment of each client into levels of self-care and adaptive functioning
- Systematic and regular assessment of self-care activities in each of the categories
- Nursing care plans and specific nursing orders that address problems of self-care identified through the assessment process
- Integration of the nursing approach into all interdisciplinary team treatment plans

Preliminary findings of a pilot study of Underwood's approach indicate that implementation of self-care produced a nursing care delivery system that encouraged program clarity, clear communication, group cohesiveness, and increased time for staff and clients to interact. Such an environment had a demonstrable positive impact on clients' ability to be helpful and supportive with each other, to focus on and prepare for community living, and to be self-sufficient, responsible, and independent in their personal self-care.

The generalizability of self-care, the concept of widespread nurse-run centers as part of genuine innovation in deinstitutionalization, and the psychiatric nurse's unique contribution to mental health services as teachers of self-care are all intriguing questions for future research.

Table 28–5   TYPES OF ALTERNATIVE SETTINGS

Approach	Example
Shape-up and ship out	"Pathroads," Utah
Quasi-religious	"The Farm," Tennessee
Supportive family self-care	William Ware Residence, Oregon

Emerging Networks

Wilson's study (1982) of Soteria illustrated one residential setting that emphasized a sanctuary for expression of feelings and "journey through madness." The Self-care Nursing Model is a residential approach emphasizing a practical orientation and the teaching of community survival skills to chronic clients. Recognizing that these two examples might represent nodes in an expanding network of community-based residential healing communities, the Center for Schizophrenia Studies at NIMH attempted to compile a preliminary directory of nontraditional residential psychiatric settings. The directory constituted a description of what appears to be an evolving social movement undergoing rapid change, reorganization, reformation, and growth. In the 1978 directory were a total of sixty such settings located in twenty-four states. Most were in California (eight) and Minnesota (five). A secondary comparative analysis among categories of client population, staff characteristics, philosophy and treatment approach, and major problems reflects an array and diversity that is quite unanticipated. However, Table 28–5 shows the major types into which the treatment settings can be categorized.

Is is hoped that future research on the short- and long-term impact of psychosocial milieus on the chronically and severely mentally disordered will answer at least the following questions:

- Can major typologies of milieus be constructed based on ideological and operational variables?
- What are the structural features characterizing such settings?
- What sociopsychological processes represent the dominant mode of interaction?
- What diagnostic categories of clients appear to benefit from nonmedical, nonhospital, residential treatment?

- What roles do professional mental health personnel assume in these settings, particularly nurses? What are the characteristics of nonprofessional staff?

- How do such settings compare to conventional, hospital-based modalities in terms of cost-effectiveness and client outcome?

- What linkages or relationships exist between the alternative settings and the general community mental health system?

Answers to these and other critical questions raised by the contemporary community mental health movement will be essential to those who plan mental health interventions and follow-up care and support in the community. As policy, deinstitutionalization had little research to support it prior to implementation. Innovations in community alternatives require the leverage of research to avoid pitfalls of the recent past.

KEY NURSING CONCEPTS

✔ The community mental health movement (known as "the third revolution" in psychiatry) is a social movement as well as a system for the delivery of community-based mental health services.

✔ Landmark recommendations made in 1961 by the Joint Commission on Mental Illness and Health drew the attention and concern of politicians and mental health professionals toward the woefully inadequate psychiatric services in the country.

✔ Millions of dollars of federal funding were provided for the construction of comprehensive community mental health centers, mental health research, and training programs for mental health care providers.

✔ Other major studies, such as the 1978 report of the President's Commission on Mental Health, gave visibility to the professional competence of nurses in mental health care and made significant recommendations toward coordinating the two-tiered system of mental health care that had evolved.

✔ In the two-tiered system of mental health care the severely mentally ill continued to inhabit state institutions, and those with less acute problems used the services of community mental health centers. Certain populations (recently discharged clients, the chronically mentally ill, the elderly, youth, and minority groups, for example) by necessity fell in between.

✔ The 1980 Community Mental Health Systems Act (which was intended to coordinate the two-tiered system) could not be implemented without a change in the political and economic climate. In addition, decreases in the federal budget caused increasing concern over the possible demise of community mental health programs.

✔ The basic philosophy of the community mental health movement is that health care is a right and, therefore, mental health services should be available to all people.

✔ Six concepts central to community mental health are (1) a systems perspective; (2) an emphasis on prevention; (3) interdisciplinary collaboration, balancing flexible role boundaries with unique areas of expertise; (4) consumer participation and control; (5) the provision of comprehensive services to the community as client as defined by geographical catchment areas; and (6) continuity of care for clients in their movement from one program to another.

✔ Community mental health nursing roles include such diverse activities as effective parenting classes; divorce therapy groups; suicide prevention counseling; case-finding; planning for a client's discharge; teaching self-care activities; staffing partial hospitalization programs; and providing individual, group, and family psychotherapy.

✔ The ANA Standards provide guidelines for both nursing generalists and specialists who practice in community settings.

✔ Conventional treatment under the community mental health system has become a highly prescriptive, elaborately formal structure of policy, regulations, and standards in which the old state hospital warehouse has been replaced by a similarly bureaucratic clearing house.

✔ Part of the community mental health systems' dilemma is that it must protect the community and, at the same time, guarantee the client's rights.

✔ Deinstitutionalization is simultaneously the *fact* that the resident population of state hospitals has decreased about 66 per cent, and a *philosophy* of civil-libertarian emphasis on clients' rights and expanded-care services based in the clients' communities.

✔ Shifting the location and funding arrangements for the chronically and severely mentally disordered has not solved their problems.

✔ Genuine innovation is needed in devising residential alternative-care approaches, particularly for the severely and chronically mentally disordered.

References

Bachrach, L. L. "A Conceptual Approach to Deinstitutionalization." *Hospital and Community Psychiatry* 29 (1978): 573–578.

————. "Planning Mental Health Services for the Chronic Patient." *Hospital and Community Psychiatry* 30 (1979): 387–392.

Bassuk, E. L., and Gerson, S. "Deinstitutionalization and Mental Health Services." *Scientific American* 238 (1978): 46–53.

Berns, J. S., and Hamilton, M. S. "Nursing Role in Community Mental Health." In *Community Health Nursing: Keeping the Public Healthy*, edited by L. L. Jarvis, pp. 319–353. Philadelphia: F. A. Davis, 1981.

Caplan, G. *Principles of Preventive Psychiatry.* New York: Basic Books, 1964.

Dumas, R. G. "The Psychiatric-Mental Health Clinical Nurse Specialist: A Future View." Keynote address at the Third Southeastern Regional Conference of Clinical Specialists in Psychiatric Nursing, September 24, 1981, Virginia Beach, Virginia.

Fink, P., and Weinstein, S. P. "Whatever Happened to Psychiatry? The Deprofessionalization of Community Mental Health Centers." *American Journal of Psychiatry* 136 (1979): 406–409.

Goldman, H. H. "Defining and Counting the Chronically Mentally Ill." *Hospital and Community Psychiatry* 32 (1981): 21–27.

Greenblatt, M.; York, R. H.; and Brown, E. L. *From Custodial to Therapeutic Patient Care in Mental Hospitals.* New York: Russell Sage Foundation, 1955.

Hadley, R. "President's Commission Sets National Mental Health Goals." *The American Nurse* 10 (1978): 1.

Joint Commission on Mental Health of Children. *Crisis in Child Mental Health: Challenge for the 1970s.* New York: Harper and Row, 1969.

Jones, M. *The Therapeutic Community.* New York: Basic Books, 1953.

Kennedy, J. F. "Mental Illness and Mental Retardation." Presented at the 88th Congress, 1st Session. House of Representatives Document 58. Washington, D.C., 1963.

Klerman, G. L. "National Trends in Hospitalization." *Hospital and Community Psychiatry* 30 (1979): 110–113.

Leininger, M. "Community Psychiatric Nursing: Trends, Issues, and Problems." *Perspectives in Psychiatric Care* 7 (1969): 11.

Minkoff, K. "A Map of Chronic Mental Patients." In *The Chronic Mental Patient*, edited by J. Talbott, pp. 11–37. Washington, D.C.: American Psychiatric Association, 1978.

Mosher, L. R., and Menn, A. Z. "Community Residential Treatment for Schizophrenia: Two Year Follow-Up." *Hospital and Community Psychiatry* 29 (1978): 715–723.

Orem, D. *Nursing Concepts of Practice*, 2d ed. New York: McGraw-Hill, 1980.

Pepper, B.; Kirshner, M. C.; and Ryglewicz, H. "The Young Adult Chronic Patient: Overview of a Population." *Hospital and Community Psychiatry* 32 (1981): 463–469.

Report to the President of the President's Commission on Mental Health. Vol. I. Washington, D.C.: U.S. Government Printing Office, 1978.

Stanton, A., and Schwartz, M. "The Management of a Type of Institutional Participation in Mental Illness," *Psychiatry* 12 (1949): 13–26.

Stern, R., and Minkoff, K. "Paradoxes in Programming for Chronic Patients in a Community Clinic." *Hospital and Community Psychiatry* 30 (1979): 613–617.

Talbott, J. A. "Deinstitutionalization: Avoiding the Disasters of the Past." *Hospital and Community Psychiatry* 30 (1979): 621–624.

Test, M. A., and Stern, L. I. "Community Treatment of the Chronic Patient: Research Overview." *Schizophrenia Bulletin* 14 (1978): 350–364.

Underwood, P. R. *Nursing Care as a Determinant in the Development of Self-Care Behavior by Hospitalized Adult Schizophrenics,* DSN dissertation, University of California, San Francisco, 1978.

————. *Self-Care Nursing Model for the Chronically Mentally Ill Adult* (in press).

Washington Report on Medicine and Health, "The Changing Mission of ADAMHA", January 11, 1982.

Wilson, H. S. *Deinstitutionalized Residential Alternatives for the Severely Mentally Disordered: The Soteria House Approach.* New York: Grune and Stratton, 1982.

Winslow, W. W. "Changing Trends in CMHCs: Keys to Survival in the Eighties." *Hospital and Community Psychiatry* 33 (1982): 273–277.

Further Reading

Adelson, P. Y. "The Back Ward Dilemma." *American Journal of Nursing* 80 (1980): 422–425.

Clark, C. C. *Mental Health Aspects of Community Health Nursing.* New York: McGraw-Hill, 1978.

Craig, A. E., and Hyatt, B. A. "Chronicity in Mental Illness: A Theory of the Role of Change." *Perspectives in Psychiatric Care* 26 (1978): 139–154.

Davis, A. J., and Underwood, P. "Role Function and Decision Making in Community Mental Health." *Nursing Research* 25 (1976): 256–258.

Krauss, J. B. "The Chronic Psychiatric Patient in the Community: A Model of Care." *Nursing Outlook* 28 (1980): 308–314.

Langsley, D. G. "The Community Mental Health Center: Does It Treat Patients?" *Hospital and Community Psychiatry* 31 (1980): 815–819.

Perls, S. R.; Winslow, W. W.; and Pathak, D. R. "Staffing Patterns in Community Mental Health Centers." *Hospital and Community Psychiatry* 31 (1980): 119–121.

Wing, J. K. "From Institutional to Community Care." *Psychiatric Quarterly* 53 (1981): 139–152.

1982 ANA Standards of Psychiatric and Mental Health Nursing Practice

PROFESSIONAL PRACTICE STANDARDS

Standard I THEORY

The nurse applies appropriate theory that is scientifically sound as a basis for decisions regarding nursing practice.

Standard 2 DATA COLLECTION

The nurse continuously collects data that are comprehensive, accurate, and systematic.

Standard 3 DIAGNOSIS

The nurse utilizes nursing diagnoses and/or standard classification of mental disorders to express conclusions supported by recorded assessment data and current scientific premises.

Standard 4 PLANNING

The nurse develops a nursing care plan with specific goals and interventions delineating nursing actions unique to each client's needs.

Standard 5 INTERVENTION

The nurse intervenes as guided by the nursing care plan to implement nursing actions that promote, maintain, or restore physical and mental health, prevent illness, and effect rehabilitation.

Standard 5A PSYCHOTHERAPEUTIC INTERVENTIONS

The nurse uses psychotherapeutic interventions to assist clients in regaining or improving their previous coping abilities and to prevent further disability.

Standard 5B HEALTH TEACHING

The nurse assists clients, families, and groups to achieve satisfying and productive patterns of living through health teaching.

Standard 5C ACTIVITIES OF DAILY LIVING

The nurse uses the activities of daily living in a goal-directed way to foster adequate self-care and physical and mental well-being of clients.

Standard 5D SOMATIC THERAPIES

The nurse uses knowledge of somatic therapies and applies related clinical skills in working with clients.

Standard 5E THERAPEUTIC ENVIRONMENT

The nurse provides, structures, and maintains a therapeutic environment in collaboration with the client and other health care providers.

Standard 5F PSYCHOTHERAPY

The nurse utilizes advanced clinical expertise in individual, group, and family psychotherapy, child psychotherapy, and other treatment modalities to function as a psychotherapist, and recognizes professional accountability for nursing practice.

Standard 6 EVALUATION

The nurse evaluates client responses to nursing action in order to revise the data base, nursing diagnoses, and nursing care plan.

Reprinted by permission from the American Nurses' Association, 2420 Pershing Road, Kansas City, Mo.

PROFESSIONAL PERFORMANCE STANDARDS

Standard 7   PEER REVIEW

The nurse participates in peer review and other means of evaluation to assure quality of nursing care provided for clients.

Standard 8   CONTINUING EDUCATION

The nurse assumes responsibility for continuing education and professional development and contributes to the professional growth of others.

Standard 9   INTERDISCIPLINARY COLLABORATION

The nurse collaborates with other health care providers in assessing, planning, implementing, and evaluating programs and other mental health activities.

Standard 10   UTILIZATION OF COMMUNITY HEALTH SYSTEMS

The nurse participates with other members of the community in assessing, planning, implementing, and evaluating mental health services and community systems that include the promotion of the broad continuum of primary, secondary, and tertiary prevention of mental illness.

Standard 11   RESEARCH

The nurse contributes to nursing and the mental health field through innovations in theory and practice and participation in research.

DSM-III Classification
Axis I-V

All official DSM-III codes and terms are included in ICD-9-CM. However, in order to differentiate those DSM-III categories that use the same ICD-9-CM codes, unofficial non-ICD-9-CM codes are provided in parentheses for use when greater specificity is necessary.

The long dashes indicate the need for a fifth-digit subtype or other qualifying term.

AXES I AND II:
CATEGORIES AND CODES

Disorders Usually First Evident in Infancy, Childhood or Adolescence

Mental Retardation   (Code in fifth digit: 1 = with other behavioral symptoms [requiring attention or treatment and that are not part of another disorder], 0˙ = without other behavioral symptoms.)

317.0(x)   Mild Mental Retardation, ———
318.0(x)   Moderate Mental Retardation, ———
318.1(x)   Severe Mental Retardation, ———
318.2(x)   Profound Mental Retardation, ———
319.0(x)   Unspecified Mental Retardation, ———

Attention Deficit Disorder
314.01   with Hyperactivity
314.00   without Hyperactivity
314.80   Residual Type

Conduct Disorder
312.00   Undersocialized, Aggressive

Source: The American Psychiatric Association, Diagnostic and Statistical Manual of Mental Disorders, Third Edition, Washington, D.C., APA 1980. Reprinted by permission.

312.10   Undersocialized, Nonaggressive
312.23   Socialized, Aggressive
312.21   Socialized, Nonaggressive
312.90   Atypical

Anxiety Disorders of Childhood or Adolescence
309.21   Separation Anxiety Disorder
313.21   Avoidant Disorder of Childhood or Adolescence
313.00   Overanxious Disorder

Other Disorders of Infancy, Childhood, or Adolescence
313.89   Reactive Attachment Disorder of Infancy
313.22   Schizoid Disorder of Childhood or Adolescence
313.23   Elective Mutism
313.81   Oppositional Disorder
313.82   Identity Disorder

Eating Disorders
307.10   Anorexia Nervosa
307.51   Bulimia
307.52   Pica
307.53   Rumination Disorder of Infancy
307.50   Atypical Eating Disorder

Stereotyped Movement Disorders
307.21   Transient Tic Disorder
307.22   Chronic Motor Tic Disorder
307.23   Tourette's Disorder
307.20   Atypical Tic Disorder

307.30 Atypical Stereotyped Movement Disorder

Other Disorders with Physical Manifestations

307.00 Stuttering

307.60 Functional Enuresis

307.70 Functional Encopresis

307.46 Sleepwalking Disorder

307.46 Sleep Terror Disorder (307.49)

Pervasive Developmental Disorders   Code in fifth digit: 0 = Full Syndrome Present, 1 = Residual State.

299.0x Infantile Autism, _____

299.9x Childhood Onset Pervasive Developmental Disorder, _____

299.8x Atypical, _____

Specific developmental disorders
Note: These are coded on Axis II.

315.00 Developmental Reading Disorder

315.10 Developmental Arithmetic Disorder

315.31 Developmental Language Disorder

315.39 Developmental Articulation Disorder

315.50 Mixed Specific Developmental Disorder

315.90 Atypical Specific Developmental Disorder

Organic Mental Disorders

Section 1. Organic Mental Disorders whose etiology or pathophysiological process is listed below (taken from the mental disorders section of ICD-9-CM).

Dementias Arising in the Senium and Presenium
Primary Degenerative Dementia, Senile Onset,

290.30 with Delirium

290.20 with Delusions

290.21 with Depression

290.00 Uncomplicated

Code in fifth digit:
1 = with Delirium, 2 = with Delusions, 3 = with Depression, 0 = Uncomplicated.

290.1x Primary Degenerative Dementia, Presenile Onset, _____

290.4x Multi-infarct Dementia, _____

Substance-induced

ALCOHOL

303.00 Intoxication

291.40 Idiosyncratic Intoxication

291.80 Withdrawal

291.00 Withdrawal Delirium

291.30 Hallucinosis

291.10 Amnestic Disorder

Code severity of Dementia in fifth digit: 1 = Mild, 2 = Moderate, 3 = Severe, 0 = Unspecified.

291.2x Dementia Associated with Alcoholism, _____

BARBITURATE OR SIMILARLY ACTING
SEDATIVE OR HYPNOTIC

305.40 Intoxication (327.00)

292.00 Withdrawal (327.01)

292.00 Withdrawal Delirium (327.02)

292.83 Amnestic Disorder (327.04)

OPIOID

305.50 Intoxication (327.10)

292.00 Withdrawal (327.11)

COCAINE

305.60 Intoxication (327.20)

AMPHETAMINE OR SIMILARLY ACTING SYMPATHOMIMETIC

305.70 Intoxication (327.30)

292.81 Delirium (327.32)

292.11 Delusional Disorder (327.35)

292.00 Withdrawal (327.31)

PHENCYCLIDINE (PCP) OR SIMILARLY ACTING
ARYLCYCLOHEXYLAMINE

305.90 Intoxication (327.40)

292.81 Delirium (327.42)

292.90 Mixed Organic Mental Disorder (327.49)

HALLUCINOGEN

305.30 Hallucinosis (327.56)

292.11 Delusional Disorder (327.55)

292.84 Affective Disorder (327.57)

CANNABIS

305.20 Intoxication (327.60)

292.11 Delusional Disorder (327.65)

TOBACCO

292.00 Withdrawal (327.71)

CAFFEINE

305.90 Intoxication (327.80)

OTHER OR UNSPECIFIED SUBSTANCE

305.90 Intoxication (327.90)

292.00 Withdrawal (327.91)

292.81 Delirium (327.92)

292.82 Dementia (327.93)

292.83 Amnestic Disorder (327.94)

292.11 Delusional Disorder (327.95)

292.12 Hallucinosis (327.96)

292.84 Affective Disorder (327.97)

292.89 Personality Disorder (327.98)

292.90 Atypical or Mixed Organic Mental Disorder (327.99)

Section 2. Organic Brain Syndromes whose etiology or pathophysiological process is either noted as an additional diagnosis from outside the mental disorders section of ICD-9-CM or is unknown.

293.00 Delirium

294.10 Dementia

294.00 Amnestic Syndrome

293.81 Organic Delusional Syndrome

293.82 Organic Hallucinosis

293.83 Organic Affective Syndrome

310.10 Organic Personality Syndrome

294.80 Atypical or Mixed Organic Brain Syndrome

Substance Use Disorders

Code in fifth digit: 1 = Continuous, 2 = Episodic, 3 = in Remission, 0 = Unspecified

305.0x Alcohol Abuse, _____

303.9x Alcohol Dependence (Alcoholism), _____

305.4x Barbiturate or similarly acting sedative or hypnotic Abuse,

304.1x Barbiturate or similarly acting sedative or hypnotic Dependence, _____

305.5x Opioid Abuse, _____

304.0x Opioid Dependence, _____

305.6x Cocaine Abuse, _____

305.7x Amphetamine or similarly acting sympathomimetic Abuse, _____

304.4x Amphetamine or similarly acting sympathomimetic Dependence, _____

305.9x Phencyclidine (PCP) or similarly acting arylcyclohexylamine Abuse, _____ (328.4x)

305.3x Hallucinogen Abuse, _____

305.2x Cannabis Abuse, _____

304.3x Cannabis Dependence, _____

305.1x Tobacco Dependence, _____

305.9x Other, mixed or unspecified Substance Abuse, _____

304.6x Other Specified Substance Dependence, _____

304.9x Unspecified Substance Dependence, _____

304.7x Dependence on Combination of Opiod and other Nonalcoholic Substance, _____

304.8x Dependence on Combination of Substances, excluding opioids and alcohol, _____

Schizophrenic Disorders

Code in fifth digit: 1 = Subchronic, 2 = Chronic, 3 = Subchronic with Acute Exacerbation, 4 = Chronic with Acute Exacerbation, 5 = in Remission, 0 = Unspecified.

SCHIZOPHRENIA

295.1x Disorganized, _____

295.2x Catatonic, _____

295.3x Paranoid, _____

295.9x Undifferentiated, _____

295.6x Residual, _____

Paranoid Disorders

297.10 Paranoia

297.30 Shared Paranoid Disorder

298.30 Acute Paranoid Disorder

297.90 Atypical Paranoid Disorder

Psychotic Disorders Not Elsewhere Classified

295.40 Schizophreniform Disorder

298.80 Brief Reactive Psychosis

295.70 Schizoaffective Disorder

298.90 Atypical Psychosis

Neurotic Disorders

These are included in Affective, Anxiety, Somatoform, Dissociative, and Psychosexual Disorders. In order to facilitate the identification of the categories that in DSM-II were grouped together in the class of Neuroses, the DSM-II terms are included separately in parentheses after the corresponding categories. These DSM-II terms are included in ICD-9-CM and therefore are acceptable as alternatives to the recommended DSM-III terms that precede them.

Affective Disorders

Major Affective Disorders Code Major Depressive Episode in fifth digit: 6 = in Remission, 4 = with Psychotic Features (the unofficial non-ICD-9-CM fifth digit 7 may be used instead to indicate that the psychotic features are mood-incongruent), 3 = with Melancholia, 2 = without Melancholia, 0 = Unspecified.

Code Manic Episode in fifth digit: 6 = in Remission, 4 = with Psychotic Features (the unofficial non-ICD-9-CM fifth digit 7 may be used instead to indicate that the psychotic features are mood-incongruent), 2 = without Psychotic Features, 0 = Unspecified.

BIPOLAR DISORDER

296.6x Mixed, _____

296.4x Manic, _____

296.5x Depressed, _____

MAJOR DEPRESSION

296.2x Single Episode, _____

296.3x Recurrent, _____

Other Specific Affective Disorders

301.13 Cyclothymic Disorder

300.40 Dysthymic Disorder (or Depressive Neurosis)

Atypical Affective Disorders

296.70 Atypical Bipolar Disorder

296.82 Atypical Depression

Anxiety Disorders

PHOBIC DISORDERS (OR PHOBIC NEUROSES)

300.21 Agoraphobia with Panic Attacks

300.22 Agoraphobia without Panic Attacks

300.23 Social Phobia

300.29 Simple Phobia

ANXIETY STATES (OR ANXIETY NEUROSES)

300.01 Panic Disorder

300.02 Generalized Anxiety Disorder

300.30 Obsessive Compulsive Disorder (or Obsessive Compulsive Neurosis)

POST-TRAUMATIC STRESS DISORDER

308.30 Acute

309.81 Chronic or Delayed

300.00 Atypical Anxiety Disorder

Somatoform Disorders

300.81 Somatization Disorder

300.11 Conversion Disorder (or Hysterical Neurosis, Conversion Type)

307.80 Psychogenic Pain Disorder

300.70 Hypochondriasis (or Hypochondriacal Neurosis)

300.70 Atypical Somatoform Disorder (300.71)

Dissociative Disorders (or Hysterical Neuroses, Dissociative Type)

300.12 Psychogenic Amnesia

300.13 Psychogenic Fugue

300.14 Multiple Personality

300.60 Depersonalization Disorder (or Depersonalization Neurosis)

300.15 Atypical Dissociative Disorder

Psychosexual Disorders

Gender Identity Disorders   Indicate sexual history in the fifth digit of Transsexualism code: 1 = Asexual, 2 = Homosexual, 3 = Heterosexual, 0 = Unspecified.

302.5x Transsexualism, _____

302.60 Gender Identity Disorder of Childhood

302.85 Atypical Gender Identity Disorder

Paraphilias

302.81 Fetishism

302.30 Transvestism

302.10 Zoophilia

302.20 Pedophilia

302.40 Exhibitionism

302.82 Voyeurism

302.83 Sexual Masochism

302.84 Sexual Sadism

302.90 Atypical Paraphilia

Psychosexual Dysfunctions

302.71 Inhibited Sexual Desire

302.72 Inhibited Sexual Excitement

302.73 Inhibited Female Orgasm

302.74 Inhibited Male Orgasm

302.75 Premature Ejaculation

302.76 Functional Dyspareunia

302.51 Functional Vaginismus

302.70 Atypical Psychosexual Dysfunction

Other Psychosexual Disorders

302.00 Ego-dystonic Homosexuality

302.89 Psychosexual Disorder not elsewhere classified

Factitious Disorders

300.16 Factitious Disorder with Psychological Symptoms

301.51 Chronic Factitious Disorder with Physical Symptoms

300.19 Atypical Factitious Disorder with Physical Symptoms

Disorders of Impulse Control Not Elsewhere Classified

312.31 Pathological Gambling

312.32 Kleptomania

312.33 Pyromania

312.34 Intermittent Explosive Disorder

312.35 Isolated Explosive Disorder
312.39 Atypical Impulse Control Disorder

Adjustment Disorder

309.00 with Depressed Mood
309.24 with Anxious Mood
309.28 with Mixed Emotional Features
309.30 with Disturbance of Conduct
309.40 with Mixed Disturbance of Emotions and Conduct
309.23 with Work (or Academic) Inhibition
309.83 with Withdrawal
309.90 with Atypical Features

Psychological Factors Affecting Physical Condition

Specify physical condition on Axis III.
316.00 Psychological Factors Affecting Physical Condition

PERSONALITY DISORDERS
Note: These are coded on Axis II.
301.00 Paranoid
301.20 Schizoid
301.22 Schizotypal
301.50 Histrionic
301.81 Narcissistic
301.70 Antisocial
301.83 Borderline
301.82 Avoidant
301.60 Dependent
301.40 Compulsive
301.84 Passive-Aggressive
301.89 Atypical, Mixed or other Personality Disorder

V Codes for Conditions Not Attributable to a Mental Disorder That Are a Focus of Attention or Treatment

V65.20 Malingering
V62.89 Borderline Intellectual Functioning (V62.88)
V71.01 Adult Antisocial Behavior
V71.02 Childhood or Adolescent Antisocial Behavior
V62.30 Academic Problem
V62.20 Occupational Problem
V62.82 Uncomplicated Bereavement
V15.81 Noncompliance with Medical Treatment
V62.89 Phase of Life Problem or Other Life Circumstance Problem

V61.10 Marital Problem
V61.20 Parent-Child Problem
V61.80 Other Specified Family Circumstances
V62.81 Other Interpersonal Problem

Additional Codes

300.90 Unspecified Mental Disorder (Nonpsychotic)
V71.09 No Diagnosis or Condition on Axis I
799.90 Diagnosis or Condition Deferred on Axis I

V71.09 No Diagnosis on Axis II
799.90 Diagnosis Deferred on Axis II

AXIS III: PHYSICAL DISORDERS OR CONDITIONS

Axis III permits the clinician to indicate any current physical disorder or condition that is potentially relevant to the understanding or management of the client. These are the conditions exclusive of the "mental disorders section" of ICD-9-CM. (The 9th edition of the International Classification of Diseases.) In some instances the condition may be etiologically significant; in other instances the physical disorder is important to the overall management of the client. In yet other instances, the clinician may wish to note the presence of other significant associated physical assessment findings, such as "soft neurological signs." Multiple diagnoses are permitted on this axis.

AXIS IV: SEVERITY OF PSYCHOSOCIAL STRESSORS			
Code	Term	Adult Examples	Child or Adolescent Examples
1	None	No apparent psychosocial stressor	No apparent psychosocial stressor
2	Minimal	Minor violation of the law; small bank loan	Vacation with family
3	Mild	Argument with neighbor; change in work hours	Change in schoolteacher; new school year

4	Moderate	New career; death of close friend; pregnancy	Chronic parental fighting; change to new school; illness of close relative; birth of sibling
5	Severe	Serious illness in self or family; major financial loss; marital separation; birth of child	Death of peer; divorce of parents; arrest; hospitalization; persistent and harsh parental discipline
6	Extreme	Death of close relative; divorce	Death of parent or sibling; repeated physical or sexual abuse
7	Catastrophic	Concentration camp experience; devastating natural disaster	Multiple family deaths
0	Unspecified	No information, or not applicable	No information, or not applicable

AXIS V: HIGHEST LEVEL OF ADAPTIVE FUNCTIONING PAST YEAR

Levels	Adult Examples	Child or Adolescent Examples
1 SUPERIOR Unusually effective functioning in social relations, occupational functioning, and use of leisure time.	Single parent living in deteriorating neighborhood takes excellent care of children and home, has warm relations with friends, and finds time for pursuit of hobby.	A 12-year-old girl gets superior grades in school, is extremely popular among her peers, and excels in many sports. She does all of this with apparent ease and comfort.
2 VERY GOOD Better than average functioning in social relations, occupational functioning, and use of leisure time.	A 65-year-old retired widower does some volunteer work, often sees old friends, and pursues hobbies.	An adolescent boy gets excellent grades, works part-time, has several close friends, and plays banjo in a jazz band. He admits to some distress in "keeping up with everything."
3 GOOD No more than slight impairment in either social or occupational functioning.	A woman with many friends functions extremely well at a difficult job, but says "the strain is too much."	An 8-year-old boy does well in school, has several friends, but bullies younger children.
4 FAIR Moderate impairment in either social relations or occupational functioning, or some impairment in both.	A lawyer has trouble carrying through assignments; has several acquaintances, but hardly any close friends.	A 10-year-old girl does poorly in school, but has adequate peer and family relations.
5 POOR Marked impairment in either social relations or occupational functioning, or moderate impairment in both.	A man with one or two friends has trouble keeping a job for more than a few weeks.	A 14-year-old boy almost fails in school and has trouble getting along with his peers.
6 VERY POOR Marked impairment in both social relations and occupational functioning.	A woman is unable to do any of her housework and has violent outbursts toward family and neighbors.	A 6-year-old girl needs special help in all subjects and has virtually no peer relationships.
7 GROSSLY IMPAIRED Gross impairment in virtually all areas of functioning.	An elderly man needs supervision to maintain minimal personal hygiene and is usually incoherent.	A 4-year-old boy needs constant restraint to avoid hurting himself and is almost totally lacking in skills.
0 UNSPECIFIED	No information.	No information.

APPENDIX C

Comprehensive
Mental Health Assessment

Erie County Department of Mental Health

Completion of the forms on pp. 854–860 follows the "Initial Contact" (Figure 8-1, p. 186) and provides more detailed demographic and client information. It may take anywhere from one to several contacts with the client in order to complete all the relevant items on these forms.

RATING SCALES

The rating scales are designed to provide a more objective picture of an individual's level of function or dysfunction by rating the person in ten Life Areas and six areas called Signals of Distress on a 5-point scale with standard definitions ascribed to each scale. Crises or mental health problems arise from broken life attachments in one of the ten life areas. Such broken attachments are also often manifested by signals of distress. The assessment rating scales enable workers to describe and evaluate individuals in a sufficiently comprehensive way so that specific service goals can be identified.

Since assessment is an *ongoing process* over time, these forms should assist the worker in recording changes in a client's level of functioning, which then has implications for revising the service contract.

Initial Assessment Phases

During the Initial Assessment Phase, the worker records a composite of several viewpoints or perspectives (Worker [W], Client [C], and Significant Other [O]) in relation to each life function or signal of distress. During or after the clinical interview(s), the worker should decide on a rating for the sixteen items. This decision is based on his/her observation and interviewing skills. Assessment can be further expanded by asking the client and/or significant others to rate the client's level of functioning. All the areas may not be assessed at any one time, but should be completed prior to completion of the service contract.

Working Phase

Reassessment may be done at any time during the service interval if the worker finds significant life changes or progress made on goals to *warrant* an interim assessment.

Termination Phase

At the completion of the service contract, when the client and counselor have worked toward termination, a final assessment is done to (a) suggest whether the level of func-

Source: L. A. Hoff, *People in Crisis* (Menlo Park, Calif.: Addison-Wesley Publishing Co., 1978), pp. 295–318, 320–24. Reproduced by permission of the Erie County Department of Mental Health; Mental Health Services, Erie County, Corporation IV, South East Corporation V, and Lakeshore Corporation VI.

The form and specifications were developed by a Task Force of workers representing Corporation IV, South East Corporation V, Lakeshore Corporation VI, and the Erie County Department of Mental Health. Members: Marsha Aitken, Maureen Becker (Chairperson), Barbara Bernardis, George Deitz, Lee Ann Hoff, Elizabeth Keller.

For samples of forms not included here and for complete specifications for use of these forms, the reader is referred to Erie County Department of Mental Health, 95 Franklin Street, Buffalo, New York 14202.

tioning desired has been achieved, and (b) make a comparison between the initial and termination functional levels.

Follow-up

After termination of service, the person should be contacted periodically to ascertain whether any further service is needed or desired. The follow-up contact should be negotiated as part of the service contract and carried out unless the person states that he or she does not wish to be contacted after termination of service. Follow-up contacts are particularly important for the person who finds it very difficult to ask for and use help during early stages of a problem before a serious crisis develops.

ASSESSMENT RATING SCALE DESCRIPTIONS AND DEFINITIONS

Rating scale descriptions and definitions are intended to provide the worker with a more comprehensive understanding of the meaning of each assessment area. The examples cited in the definitions of each scale are just that, examples. The worker should recognize that there will be numerous other examples of real-life situations which will be analogous to those provided. Also, while no rating of a person can be *completely* objective, the scale definitions provide a framework for eliminating subjective assessment as much as possible.

A. LIFE FUNCTIONS

1. Physical Health

Description   This scale is intended to focus on a person's physical health needs as well as ability to identify, regulate, anticipate, and seek treatment for those needs. Physical illness refers to symptoms, whether real or imagined. Ratings should be made considering severity of illness and need for an immediate medical response. Considerations include: sleeping, eating, drinking, alcohol and drug use/abuse, weight, posture, motor mannerisms, physical complaints, general nutrition, personal hygiene, dental hygiene, activity level, medication, physical impairments/disabilities.

Ratings

1. *High:* Person is involved in pursuit of physical health as a part of living. Is aware of and follows through on physi-

cal health problems when they occur. Enjoys good physical health with no present need for medical services.

2. *Moderate High:* Person has health problems and can identify, regulate, and anticipate them.

3. *Moderate:* Person has physical problems and can identify them; however, is inconsistent in seeking medical attention; e.g., sees physician for prescription, but self-medicates.

4. *Low/Moderate:* Person has physical symptoms that indicate medical attention is needed. Has knowledge that a problem exists but is not making an effort to seek assistance. Person requires regulation by others and reminders that physical needs are important.

5. *Low Functioning:* Person has physical symptoms that require immediate medical attention and are potentially life threatening (malnutrition, heart pain, dehydration, excessive obesity). The person is not concerned about the problem and is not making any efforts to seek medical treatment.

2. Self-acceptance/Self-esteem

Description   This scale is intended to assess an individual's feelings towards the self as a person—the degree to which he or she feels capable, adequate, and valuable as a person.

Ratings

1. *High Functioning:* Individuals are enthusiastic about life and confident of their resources and capacities for personal adjustment. They employ a realistic standard of self-appraisal based upon awareness of both positive and negative traits. While not viewing themselves as perfect, they see themselves as capable and adequate. Their goals are realistically based upon their capacity for achievement and they choose appropriate means for goal solutions. They are capable of feeling guilt and anxiety when they have violated their own internalized standard of personal conduct. Their aspirations are consistent with their capacity and are organized within a systematic life-style that permeates the past, present, and future. Failure can be accepted without damaging their basic sense of personal adequacy. They adjust relatively easily to frustrations of daily life and can change their goals consistent with personal and/or situational changes. Since they feel basically adequate, they are capable of total personality development and can creatively actualize the full range of their inner potential. Basic self-acceptance translates into basic acceptance of others and allows them to freely enjoy social interactions. It is important to distinguish those individuals with a genuine positive self-regard from those who practice denial of negative self-regard.

2. *High/Moderate:* Individuals are usually productively involved in many areas of life. Their expectations are realistic and they usually set goals consistent with their ability. Since they realistically accept having some negative traits, they are relatively free from anxiety, guilt, and blame. They are committed to the development of their potential and usually view themselves as being in relative control of their life situation. They accept frustration as a fact of life and adjust their goals accordingly. Under extreme stress they may question their ability and self-worthy and many experience a minor and temporary decline in functioning. They rarely have feelings of depression and they advance beyond personal responsibility to being able to assume responsibility in relationships with others.

3. *Moderate Functioning:* These individuals characterize the majority of the population. Their sense of adequacy and competence is sufficiently strong to allow self-management and responsibility to others within the context of their daily lives. While there is awareness of both negative and positive traits, there may be some distortion of either. They may have some difficulty in accepting failure and may rely upon support from others in dealing with frustration. At times, they protect themselves through falsification of their own ability or the circumstances relating to failure of goal achievement. With sufficient stress they may temporarily underaspire or overaspire to goals and may engage in self-depreciation and/or blaming of others. Guilt and anxiety are determined by an appropriate internalized standard of personal conduct, but at times they may accept responsibility for events over which they lack control. Some negative traits may be denied and some positive traits exaggerated. While being reasonably self-confident, they may become defensive when their behavior or accomplishments are challenged. Their means-goals relationships are appropriate and usually consistent with their capacity, although they usually do not develop their full potential. At times they may experience mild depression and have fleeting fantasies of suicide which are not acted out in actual behavior. They usually have a few close friendships and are capable of interpersonal relationships based upon the acceptance of others.

4. *Low/Moderate:* Individuals are inconsistent in their self-evaluations. While usually feeling inadequate in managing their problems, they have sporadic periods of renewed confidence in their coping ability. They basically feel inadequate, guilty and self-condemning with frequent fantasies of suicide and possible attempts. While they are cognitively aware of some positive traits, they generally feel negatively toward themselves and act accordingly. Periods of positive mood are reactions to situational determinants rather than to positive self-regard which may also represent attempts to overcome unwanted depression. They experience their daily life as stressful and feel unable to manage ordinary problems.

5. *Low Functioning:* Individuals are preoccupied with a sense of personal failure and guilt. They generally feel inadequate and incompetent and characteristically focus upon their negative traits and are unaware of and deny having positive traits. The tendency to condemn themselves is overt and prominent to the extent of self-punishment, including frequent suicide ideation or actual attempts. There is obvious defenselessness and open admission of worthlessness. Frustration tolerance is weak with a lack of capacity for coping with stress resulting from personal and situational changes. There is a pronounced inability to plan objectives realistically. Individuals may underaspire or overaspire to goal achievements which lead to actual failure due to their unrealistic standard of self-expectation. There is a sense of hopelessness, pessimism, self-doubt, and acute depression. Unfavorable comparison with others often leads to social withdrawal. These people cannot accept responsibility for themselves or for others. Basic self-rejection usually results in a critical and condemning attitude toward others.

3. Vocational/Occupational

Description   This area focuses on the person's present employment/vocational role in terms of

- Extent to which it meets his or her financial needs.
- Individual's degree of satisfaction with present employment or role, e.g., Are you working to your level of capacity—or above it? If unemployed, do you have any job skills or education that could be developed? If unemployed, ascertain the degree of activity around job search. e.g. What have you done to find a job? Are you working two jobs which interfere with family life?

Occupation refers to: student, homemaker, retired, as well as usual occupations.

Ratings

1. *High:* Person is employed and working at full capacity. Person expresses satisfaction with job or retirement.

2. *Moderate/High:* Person is employed. Satisfied with job, not actively seeking for better paid work, but says, "I wish I could make more." Or, person is retired and quite satisfied with self-support.

3. *Moderate:* Person is employed but expresses dissatisfaction with present job in terms of (a) pay, (b) advancement, (c) hours, and/or; (d) nature of work. Has fairly stable job history and can get and keep jobs. Is aware of skills, but does not show much activity around changing jobs for self-betterment. Person is only moderately happy with retirement role and lacks options for use of time.

4. *Low/Moderate:* Person is unemployed at present, has worked in past, but work history is sporadic. Takes job when he or she can get them, but leaves, gets fired, or laid off. Has some skills but is not aware of them. Is retired and has few options for satisfying use of time.

5. *Low:* Person is unemployed. Has no vocational goals. Cannot assess self in terms of future employment. No skills. Is retired and has no satisfying outlets.

4. Immediate Family

Description   This scale is intended to assess the ability of family members to provide support and problem-solving assistance during crisis as well as on a day-to-day basis.

Ratings

1. *High:* Person is able to rely on the family as a unit during times of emotional crisis as well as on a day-to-day basis. Family is usually always able to meet the person's needs and can offer both positive as well as negative feedback in a constructive way.

2. *Moderate/High:* Person relies on family members in times of crisis; however, family members are not always able to respond completely or in a consistently constructive way.

3. *Moderate:* Person relies on at least two family members and can depend on them in times of need. Person has no real sense that these people would help for extensive periods of time.

4. *Low/Moderate:* Person has one family member that he or she talks to; however, does not rely on them except in extreme cases. Feels family doesn't care about him or her.

5. *Low:* Person feels like family is never around when needed—acts as if he or she were not a member of the family. Person depends on nonfamily members when in trouble. Person is isolated and does not have a regular support system.

5. Intimate Relationships

Description   Intimate relationship is defined as "a close, familiar, and usually affectionate or loving relationship" which is usually limited to one or a few people. This rating measures the extent to which a person can have such a relationship in which there is mutual sharing of positive/negative feelings. Such relationships are often characterized by a sense of openness, honesty, and feelings of support. Although sexual intimacy may also be an important part of this relationship, the scale is intended to emphasize social or psychological intimacy even when a sexual relationship may not exist, e.g. a close brother-sister relationship.

Ratings

1. *High:* Person has intimate contact with a few others and the intimacy is acknowledged by all. There is a strong sense of permanency and future interactions are seen as important to maintain. Relationships are relaxed, open, and mutual understanding exists through honest interaction. Time is spent together by choice and significant moments are treasured.

2. *Moderate/High:* Person has intimate contact with (at least) a few others and the feeling of closeness is shared by both. The relationship has permanent qualities and though it may be closed in some areas, time is spent together by choice and for extended periods.

3. *Moderate:* Person can identify a close relationship in which there is intimacy and an honest sharing of feelings. A sense of permanence has existed or does exist, at least potentially, and some time is spent together.

4. *Low/Moderate:* Person has or had some marginal intimate relationships that were seen as somewhat supportive. These relationships may be strained, but feelings about the other can be discussed and there is a possibility for developing a relationship.

5. *Low:* Person has no intimate contacts with others, real or fancied. Is closed, defensive, and resistant to talking about feelings for others at present or in the past.

6. Residential Situation

Description   This area refers to a person's basic shelter needs, how he or she meets those needs, and the degree of satisfaction the person expresses about his or her residence; e.g., How do you judge your housing situation?

   Is the person concerned about poor housing or is there little awareness that housing is substandard: e.g., If living situation is poor, what are you doing to improve your living situation? Does your living situation contribute to other problems, or (if the situation is good), does it improve your functioning? Is there overcrowding, rent too high, safety hazards, adequate heat and plumbing, lead paint, etc.?

Ratings

1. *High:* Living conditions are more than adequate. Owns home or lives in excellent surroundings. Person expresses satisfaction with present living situation and privacy is available at any time. Living situation is stable.

2. *Moderate/High:* Living conditions are adequate in terms of size and state of repair, with some degree of privacy, but not entirely satisfactory to the person. Is actively searching for better housing that is affordable. May include a transitional living situation that is adequate but temporary.

4. *Moderate:* Living conditions are adequate, but premises need repair or lack the degree of privacy that would be considered appropriate. Person expresses dissatisfaction, but is not actively looking for alternatives or is complaining about the state of disrepair of an unsafe neighborhood; does not do anything to correct the situation.

4. *Low/Moderate:* Living conditions are below standard, with no activity around improvement; or person is being evicted, not actively searching for other placement. Eviction due to nonpayment of rent or other problems is viewed as the landlord's fault. Feels there is not much that can be done about living conditions.

5. *Low:* Currently has no place to live, is living in temporary housing, or is living in conditions which require a change due to health problems. There is a definite need to provide alternative housing immediately. Living conditions are unstable.

7. Financial

Description This area includes:

- Extent to which a person's financial needs are met; e.g., Do you make enough money to comfortably support yourself?
- Source of income. If unemployed or retired: Are you on welfare? Social Security? Veteran's benefits?
- Ability of the person to budget the money which he or she does have.

Ratings

1. *High:* Person has a sufficient source of income and moderate to extensive savings. Anyone would be willing to lend him or her $500 without concern. Has excellent credit rating. Has some potential for finding other sources of income if current job was terminated. Budgets income well and is capable of making good investments.

2. *Moderate/High:* Person has a good source of income and perhaps some savings or investments to fall back on if income were suddenly discontinued. Has some friends/family or a good credit rating which could be drawn upon if necessary.

3. *Moderate:* Person has a fixed source of income or a job which permits basic needs to be met, but requires some careful budgeting in order to purchase desired "extras." Has limited borrowing power from a few friends or other resources. Is generally able to budget funds but would be hard pressed if income were suddenly terminated.

4. *Low/Moderate:* Person has income either through public assistance or from a job, but it meets only the most basic needs. Person may or may not be able to meet the stringent budgeting required for living on a fixed income.

5. *Low:* Person has no source of income at present. May also owe money on some/several debts. There is no money to cover the coming week's expenses. His or her credit rating is nil and person has no one whom he or she could borrow from. Must have immediate assistance in order to cover basic living costs.

8. Decision-Making Ability

Description The purpose of this scale is to assess the strategy, process, and effectiveness of the person's decision-making and problem-solving performance relative to goals and actual outcomes. Emphasis should be focused upon the person's cognitive functioning with less attention paid to emotional factors that are involved in the decision-making process.

Ratings

1. *High:* Individual is very task oriented and sets realistic goals consistent with ability. He or she thinks before acting and shows evidence of logical thought process in goals-means-ends relationships. Individual feels basically secure and self-confident as decision maker. He or she approaches problem-oriented situations with necessary emotional detachment—appropriately scanning the field; collecting relevant information, while holding extraneous factors constant; reviewing alternative solutions to the problem; and considering consequences of each alternative before implementing actions. If the choice is incorrect, the person shifts to a more appropriate alternative rather than clinging compulsively to the original one, and he or she accepts responsibility for the decisions.

2. *High/Moderate:* The individual enjoys a full emotional life but is quite capable of task orientation when making decisions. There is usually no apparent emotional interference with the continuity and logic of thought process, except when numerous problems occur simultaneously or when individual problems have severe consequences. The belief in oneself as decision maker is stable, and the person more often than not accepts the consequences of his or her decisions, even during those infrequent times of acting impulsively. The individual sometimes chooses a particular course prematurely; considers consequences of alternative solutions before acting, sometimes acting impulsively; usually shifts to a more appropriate alternative if actual experience shows original alternative to be incorrect; and usually accepts responsibility for decisions, although sometimes he or she will blame the situation or other people for mistakes. At times feelings may confuse thought processes and the person may either temporarily withdraw or rely upon others for help in problem situations.

3. *Moderate:* Individual shows a blending of task- and self-orientation. At times, goal priorities may be in mutual conflict or goals-means relationships may be inconsistent. Nevertheless, the person is reasonably capable of making effective decisions most of the time. He or she collects relevant information, sometimes scanning either too narrowly or broadly; reviews alternative solutions, sometimes choosing a particular one prematurely; and considers consequences of alternative solutions before acting, sometimes acting impulsively. The person usually shifts to a more appropriate alternative if actual experience shows the original alternative to be incorrect; and usually accepts responsibility for his or her decisions, although sometimes either blaming the situation or other people for personal mistakes. At times feelings may confuse thought processes, and the person may either temporarily withdraw or rely upon others for help in problem situations.

4. *Low/Moderate:* Individual is mainly self-preoccupied and is unable to concentrate for the necessary period of time to arrive at a problem solution. Thought processes are scattered and shifting; and impulsively arrived at solutions are implemented without considering alternatives. There is a noticeable degree of compulsive clinging to alternatives in spite of their ineffectiveness in actual experience. The person will quite desperately accept advice from others and will doubt his or her own capacity for decision making. Beliefs are often without foundation in reality and the person frequently thinks in a fatalistic way that he or she is incapable of altering surrounding situations.

5. *Low:* Individual is quite disorganized and reveals an obvious emotional interference with thought processes. He or she is self-preoccupied, impulsive, inconsistent, and distracted. When faced with a problem situation, the person becomes frightened and withdrawn and may either seek support and advice from others, or avoid social contact altogether. Solutions to problems are impulsive and later regretted and disowned. Goals are inconsistent and unrealistic and means-goals relationships are inappropriate. Thought processes are scattered with considerable distractedness and shifting. Beliefs may take the form of compulsions and delusions and, at times, hallucinations may be present. Events taking place in the person's life appear to have no order or purpose and seem to be outside the individual's control.

9. Life Philosophy

Description   This area examines the extent to which a person has life goals and a system of values. One's values guide a person in determining the "rightness" or "wrongness" of an idea or action. It is essential to assess whether there exists a system of values upon which goals and actions follow; not whether a person's value system is consistent with and/or acceptable to society's view of life. Certain life styles have special ritual/taboos or "laws"/guidelines/norms which are consciously followed or ignored. A client's ability to "judge" a certain situation or to have a sense of a "good" or "bad" conscience are indicators of the existence of a value system. The person's value system forms the basis for various life goals and aspirations.

Children and those persons with certain mental handicaps (e.g., mental retardation or psychosis) will tend to utilize their parents' or significant other's value system to guide their behaviors and attitudes.

Ratings

1. *High:* A system of values exists that reflects the origins of "right" and "wrong" judgments. This system can be described by the person and is used as a guide for goals and behaviors in ambiguous or ill defined situations of varying kinds. The person's behavior reflects actions that are consistent with this value system. The person has set meaningful goals and has achieved them to his or her satisfaction.

2. *Moderate/High:* Person is in the process of defining his or her own value system and goals, and recognizes the need for same. Is usually satisfied with knowing "right" from "wrong." Experiences occasional confusion or ambivalence when facing complex situations involving "ethical" issues or decisions which are neither "black" nor "white" but in "gray" areas. May also be confused occasionally about what he or she wants out of life.

3. *Moderate:* A hierarchy or degrees of "rightness"/"wrongness" exists with some things being considered "forbidden." Behaviors are not entirely consistent with these judgments. Person can acknowledge the existence of a value system but it is "imposed" or "inherited" from others rather than truly integrated and acknowledged as one's own. Goals very often are those set for the sake of others or in response to pressure rather than for self. The value systems of most children would fall into this category.

4. *Low/Moderate:* Person has a value system which allows individual actions to be labeled as "right" or "wrong." There is no underlying scheme, so behaviors may not always be consistent. Similar situations can produce unexpected or different reactions. Person has poorly defined life goals and is generally frustrated in his or her attempts to achieve goals.

5. *Low:* Has no value scheme that expresses itself in a consistent pattern of behavior. Actions and decisions appear inconsistent and haphazard. Person appears at times to have "no conscience at all," and is generally directionless.

10. Leisure Time Use/Community Involvement

Description   This area refers to how a person uses leisure time and the degree of satisfaction that he or she obtains from it. Leisure time can be monitored by the extent the person uses available community resources appropriately and the extent to which these resources are sought out. Community involvement is determined by the extent the person participates in the community outside of his or her home. Leisure time is any time when the person is not at place of employment or not occupied with child-rearing and/or other housekeeping activities. It would include going to the movies, the pool hall, playgrounds, etc. Is a person's leisure time so limited that there is no time for self, significant other, or family relationships to develop (as in the case of the person who works two jobs)? Does a person have too much leisure time (as in the case of being unemployed or retired)? For example, Do you have ample leisure time which helps you function in other life areas? Is leisure time a burden? A lonely period? A real bore?

Ratings

1. *High:* Feels comfortable with amount of leisure time. Realizes the necessity for leisure and uses this time for constructive projects, meetings, and recreational activities. Does not become over-involved. Regulates leisure time use very well. Is quite aware of community resources and actively involves self in several community activities. Has some sense of responsibility to his or her community.

2. *Moderate/High:* Has definite ideas about how to use leisure time and is aware of the need for it. Expresses satisfaction, but sees room for improvement and actively pursues it. Has knowledge of his or her community and becomes involved in the community on occasion.

3. *Moderate:* Recognizes the need for leisure time and has some available. Tends to become over-involved on occasion, but does not recognize this as a pattern. Has difficulty in regulating use of leisure time. Only occasionally will the person seek community activities or involvement due to some limited social skill or lack of transportation to community resources/activities.

4. *Low/Moderate:* Uses leisure time inappropriately. Is interested in some activities, but is inconsistent in pursuing them. Wants to do something, but doesn't know what. Has a talent or interest but cannot bring self to pursue it. Participates in community activities if encouraged, but would not initiate such activities for him/herself. Depends almost totally on others for knowledge of community resources.

5. *Low:* Never has any time to relax. Never knows what to do with leisure time. Sits and ruminates, feels like nobody cares. Not interested in anything outside of home. May engage largely in passive activities; e.g., watching television. Has never developed or engaged in outside interests, or did so only in the distant past. Person is almost totally unaware of potential community resources.

11. Feeling Management

Description   The intent of this rating is to measure the person's awareness of feelings and ability to appropriately use and manage feelings in various situations. This rating concerns the way in which a person's defense mechanisms protect him or her against problems in living; the person's ability to regulate impulsive behavior; the person's ability to control or work through painful feelings, e.g., How would you judge your ability to handle your feelings?; or your ability to accept and value positive feelings?

Ratings

1. *High:* Person is aware of feelings, can express them at will, and can take appropriate action to discharge or regulate them. Person can effectively acknowledge and appreciate the value of both negative and positive feelings which can lead to the "actualizing" state of living.

2. *Moderate/High:* Person can generally express and regulate feelings in all but a few situations. Can discriminate between positive and negative feelings most of the time.

3. *Moderate:* Person has an awareness of feelings that can be expressed and behavior is usually appropriate to the feelings, but mechanisms for working out feelings are not generally available.

4. *Low/Moderate:* Self-corrective and control capacities are limited to survival activities on a physical level. Person is a "victim" of feeling states. Cannot regulate actions in accordance with appropriateness of acts, but responds to feelings in a reactive way. Tends to be able to identify only strong negative feelings, for example, anger.

5. *Low:* Has no self-corrective or control capacity and requires structure and control to be imposed upon him or her from others. Has no awareness of feelings that can be expressed. Feelings tend to "erupt" and tend to be quite destructive to the individual or to others. Behavior tends to be incongruent with feelings after inappropriate over-/under-reactions.

B. SIGNALS OF DISTRESS

12. Lethality Toward Self

Description   This scale is intended as a guide to assess the suicide potential of a particular individual at the time of assessment. Specific signs (based on the study of completed suicides) are applied to the individual in an effort to predict as accurately as possible whether or not a person is likely to commit suicide. The person should be assessed as to

- *Suicide Plan:* a person with a well-thought-out plan including specific time, place, circumstances (e.g., excluding possible rescue) with a readily available high lethal method (gun, jumping, carbon monoxide poisoning, barbiturates, hanging, car crash) is a high risk for suicide; e.g., How are you planning to kill yourself? Do you have a gun? Do you have pills? What kind? How many?

- *History of Suicide Attempts:* a person who has made previous high lethal attempts or changes plan from low lethal to high lethal is a higher risk than a person with history of low lethal or no attempts.

- *Resources and Communication with Significant Other:* any person with poor coping ability and loss of interpersonal support system or inability to maintain communication with existing resources is a high risk; e.g., Is there anyone you feel you can turn to when you're really down? Does _____ know that you're feeling like killing yourself? What is _____'s response to your threat, plan, etc.? This last question is included because significant others may, in fact, encourage would-be attempters by not caring or, in fact, telling them to go ahead.

- *Age, Sex, Race:* suicide risk increases with age for white males. More white males than females commit suicide. Among racial minority persons, there are more suicides under the age of forty than among older persons.

- *Marital Status:* more divorced, separated, and single persons commit suicide than married persons.

- *Physical Illness:* presence of physical illness increases suicide risk.

- *Drinking and Drug Abuse:* drinking or other drug abuse, accompanying impulsiveness, and loss of control increase suicide risk, especially in the presence of available high lethal methods. In addition, use of either legal or illegal drugs such as barbiturates, sleeping medications, or LSD may also raise impulsiveness and cause loss of control.

- *Recent Loss:* personal loss or threat of loss such as of a spouse, parent, status, money, or job increases suicide risk. In some situations a job promotion may actually be perceived as a loss because the individual feels he or she no longer has the capabilities to handle the situation, or the supports to carry through.

- *Unexplained Change in Behavior:* e.g., sudden reckless driving and drinking by a previously careful, sober driver can be an indicator of suicide danger. Another unexplained behavioral change to look for is the giving away of valued possessions suddenly, making a will, or purchasing a large life insurance policy.

- *Isolation:* a person who is isolated both emotionally and physically is at greater risk than a nonisolated person. This may sometimes be a sudden and unexplained withdrawal or self-imposed isolation.

- *Depression:* signs include sleeplessness, early wakening, weight loss, anorexia, amenorrhea, sexual dysfunction, crying, agitation, hopelessness: e.g. How is your appetite? Do you sleep well? Have you lost weight lately? Depression is not *universally* present in all high lethal persons.

- *Critical Life Event:* a person experiencing the stress of a life crisis situation who lacks internal/external resources for satisfactory resolution of the crisis is a greater risk for suicide than others.

Explicit, direct questions must be asked of the person regarding all these signs if the information is not already available through other assessment data.

Ratings

1. *High Functioning:* No predictable risk of suicide now. No suicidal ideation or history of attempts, has satisfactory social support system, and is in close contact with significant others.

2. *High/Moderate:* Low risk of suicide now. Person has suicidal ideation with low lethal method, no history of attempts, or recent serious loss. Has satisfactory social support system.

3. *Moderate Function:* Moderate risk of suicide now. Has suicidal ideation with high lethal method but no plan, or threats. Has plan with low lethal method, history of low lethal attempts: e.g., employed female, age 35, divorced, with tumultuous family history.

4. *Low/Moderate:* High risk of suicide now. Has current high lethal plan, obtainable means, history of previous attempts, is unable to communicate with a significant other; e.g., female, age 50, living alone, with drinking history; or black male, age 29, unemployed, and has lost his lover.

5. *Low Functioning:* Very high risk of suicide now. Has current lethal plan with available means, history of suicide attempts, is cut off from resources; e.g., white male, over 40, physically ill and depressed, wife threatening divorce, is unemployed.

13. Lethality Toward Quality

Description   This scale is intended as a guide to assess the homicide potential or danger of assault by a particular individual at the time of assessment. The following signs are applied to the potentially homicidal individual:

- *Homicide Plan:* the person with a high lethal specific plan and available means for homicide is a high risk; e.g., Do you ever get so angry that you feel like killing? How do you plan to do it? Do you have a gun?

- *History of Homicide, Impulsive Acting Out, or Homicide Attempts:* for example, Have you ever felt like hurting anyone before? Did you carry out your urge to kill someone? If so, what happened? Did someone stop you? Were you able to stop your self? Do you ever feel like you are losing control of yourself? What do you usually do when you feel you are losing control?

- *Resources and Communications with Significant Other(s):* most homicides occur within family units between/ among individuals previously acquainted; e.g., How do you usually express your anger toward someone close to you? Is there someone you feel you want to get even with? Are you open to exploring other more constructive ways of expressing your anger?

- *Drinking/Drug Use/Abuse:* a person who drinks frequently and also has a history of impulsive acting out behavior is a higher risk for homicide or assault than a non-drinker. Drinking and accompanying impulsivity and loss of control through substance use and abuse may also raise homicidal lethality, especially in the presence of available high lethal methods.

- *Other Criteria:* the person who is suicidal as well as homicidal is an even higher risk because the consequential effects of homicide are not possible deterrent. In the event that homicidal threats or references are made, however trivial these may seem, such references should be thoroughly checked out.

Ratings

1. *High Functioning:* No predictable risk of assault or homicide now; e.g., no homicidal ideation, urges, or history of same; basically satisfactory support system, social drinker only.

2. *High/Moderate:* Low risk of homicide now; e.g., has occasional assault or homicidal ideation with some urges to kill, no history of impulsive acting out or homicidal attempts, occasional drinking bouts, basically satisfactory social support system.

3. *Moderate Functioning:* Moderate risk of homicide now; e.g., has frequent homicidal ideation and urges to kill, no specific plan; history of impulsive acting out, but no homicide attempts; episodic drinking bouts; stormy relationships with significant other with periodic high tension arguments.

4. *Low/Moderate:* High risk of homicide now; e.g., has homicidal plan; obtainable means; drinking history; history of impulsive acting out, but no homicide attempts; stormy relationships and much verbal plus occasional physical fighting with significant others.

5. *Low Functioning:* Very high risk of homicide now; e.g., has current high lethal plan; available means; history of homicide attempts or impulsive acting out and feels a strong urge to "get even" with a significant other; history of drinking with possibly also high lethal suicide risk.

---

14. Substance Use

Description   This area refers to use and abuse of prescription or nonprescription drugs of all kinds (e.g., heroin, methadone, hallucinogens, amphetamines, barbiturates, tranquilizers, antidepressants, LSD) and alcohol.

The emphasis is on the person's ability to control consumption of drugs (social drinking and prescription diet pills can be examples of controlled consumption). When the controls break down, use changes to abuse. Abuse can be measured by how and to what degree it is self-destructive, the potential lethality (e.g., alcohol and barbiturates—high lethal combination), the degree to which use interferes with usual everyday functioning, or actually prevents the person from functioning.

This area also considers the person's awareness of drug use as a potential problem, current abuse as a problem, and the person's level of activity around alleviating or changing the self-destructive behavior.

Ratings

1. *High:* Never a problem. All substance use is constructive and controlled.

2. *High/Moderate:* Rarely a problem. Usually drinks or takes drugs within socially acceptable limits or on prescription, but feels a need every now and then to get drunk or high. However, this generally does not interfere with his or her social and family network or normal functioning.

3. *Moderate:* Some problems. An occasional "drunk," or periodic consistent drug intake. Drug use sporadic and can be traced to a precipitating event, e.e., "I got depressed because . . ." Person realizes danger of becoming potential substance abuser and shows some activity around preventing this.

4. *Low/Moderate:* Frequent problems. Usually drinks or takes drugs "to get/keep going." Frequently the pattern gets out of control; person goes on binges or has "weekend highs." Constantly promising to improve. Social and family network weak, but intact. Tends to be cyclical. Potential danger not perceived because person is always "starting over."

5. *Low:* Constant problems. Currently abusing drugs/alcohol to the extend that it has caused a breakdown in social and family network; actual or threatened loss of employment due to absences; financial problems. Person denies problem with abuse, little activity around changing or alleviating situation, *even though situation is perceived as stressful.* There is an expression of "no hope."

15. Legal Problems

Description   This area focuses on the *degree* to which the person's current legal involvement is a problem which interferes with everyday functioning, and the *nature* of the legal involvement.

On the "degree of involvement" continuum, how do his or her legal problems interfere with

* Job possibilities
* Mental health
* Physical health

Under "kind of involvement," assaultive behavior toward others is included, as well as differentiation between crimes against persons vs. crimes against property, or both.

If the arrests and charges concern driving while intoxicated, or include other drug involvement, the degree of substance use needs to be better assessed.

The person's concern or lack of concern about the consequences of his or her actions should be taken into consideration and should be related to a homicide/suicide lethality assessment.

Also, a clear picture should be obtained of what charges are pending against the person, and the severity of those changes, i.e., violations, misdemeanors, or felonies.

Divorce action generally does not include a legal problem.

Ratings

1. *High:* Has never been arrested, convicted, or charged with any misdemeanor or felony, or has never been to family court. Is about to retain an attorney if he or she needs one, or knows how to obtain one through Legal Aid or the Public Defender's Office.

2. *High/Moderate:* Has been arrested or fined or charged with a family (civil) and/or criminal offense once, but has had no subsequent arrests or problems with the law. The person has or knows of an attorney to handle legal problems.

3. *Moderate:* Person has been arrested or fined or charged with a family offense or a criminal offense but did not serve time. May be on probation, but accepts responsibility of probation.

4. *Low/Moderate:* Person has a history of offenses, has served time, and when on probation/parole goes to probation/parole officer only when he or she feels like it.

5. *Low:* Has presently pending charges and is awaiting court hearing or trial. Is currently on probation, parole, or both, and may have to serve time if convicted of present charge.

16. Agency Use

Description   This area refers to the person's ability to negotiate with helping systems in the community in order to obtain his or her goals for service. Assessment should consider

* Individual's degree of knowledge about existing services; e.g. Do you know where to get the help you need?
* Ability to contact agency.
* Ability to follow through with contacts.
* Ability to insure that he or she gets the service from the agency or goes to a more appropriate agency; e.g., When you don't get help you need, what do you usually do?

Agencies are defined as service clusters that exist in the community or within reachable distance, e.g., lawyers, doctors, and welfare system.

Ratings

1. *High:* Always successful. Has knowledge of agencies and is able to contact the appropriate agency to fill need. Follows through on contacts. Is able to find out about new agencies and use them appropriately. Expresses satisfaction with agencies. Can relate to the agency as a whole.

2. *High/Moderate:* Usually successful. Has good knowledge of agencies. Is able to contact agencies and follow through. Usually contacts agencies appropriate to needs. Has had favorable experience with some agencies, but not with others. Does not understand that requests for services may be inappropriate to a particular agency. Feels it depends on the person you contact whether or not you get services.

3. *Moderate:* Sometimes successful. Has fair knowledge of resources and contacts agencies for help. Follows through only if agency follows up or contacts person after "dropping out." Feels like he or she doesn't "want to bother anyone" with problems.

4. *Low/Moderate:* Seldom successful. Has limited knowledge of resources. Has understanding of needs, but cannot select appropriate agency. Contacts agencies but does not follow through: "agency shopped." Feels "nobody really understands" his or her problem.

5. *Low:* Never successful. Has no knowledge of existing services. Does not understand own needs or how an agency can meet them. Feels no one can help, no one can do anything about his or her problems.

COMPREHENSIVE MENTAL HEALTH ASSESSMENT

ID # _____

Name _____
          First   Middle   Last

Assessment Date _____ Time _____ AM   Place of Assessment _____ _____
                                                        PM

RATING SCALE

1	2	3	4	5
High Functioning	High/Moderate Functioning	Moderate Functioning	Low/Moderate Functioning	Low Functioning

(W = Worker; C = Client; O = Other)

A. LIFE FUNCTIONS
1. __Physical Health__   -Medical Information (Include relevant items; eg. illnesses, surgery, physical impairment, allergies, pregnancy, birth defects)

Current medical care   Yes___ No___
Family Physician or Medical Clinic(s) NAME _____
Address _____ Last time seen _____
Phone _____

Medication Use	Name	Dosage	Duration	Physician/Clinic
1.				
2.				
3.				
4.				
5.				

Comments:

W   C   O
__   __   __

2. __Self-Acceptance/Self-Esteem__

Comments:

W   C   O
__   __   __

3. __Vocational/Occupational___Employed___Homemaker___Student___Other _____
Employer/School
Name _____ Job Title (Functional) _____
Address _____ How long? _____
Phone # _____ Unemployed _____ How long? _____
(Optional) Education/Training _____

Comments:

W   C   O
__   __   __

MH-2

4. Immediate Family   Parental Status-

        Children? Yes____No____How many? _____

Comments:

                                          W   C   O

                                          — — —

(Refer to Child Screening Checklist if appropriate)

5. Intimate Relationships   Marital Status-

Never
Married _____ Married _____ Widowed ____Divorced _____ Separated ___Living Together ____ How Long ____

    Comments:

                                          W   C   O

                                          — — —

6. Residential   Living situation-

    Lives alone ___Lives with family ___Other ___ (specify)_____

Comments:

                                          W   C   O

                                          — — —

SIGNIFICANT OTHER INFORMATION

Name	Nature of Relationship	Age	Grade *	Within Household	Outside Household Address	Phone

*Special Class Placement   **MH-2A**

COMPREHENSIVE MENTAL HEALTH ASSESSMENT (con't.)

Name _____   ID# _____

RATING SCALE

1	2	3	4	5	
High Functioning	High/Moderate Functioning	Moderate Functioning	Low/Moderate Functioning	Low Functioning	W = Worker C = Client O = Other

7. Financial   Source of income _____

   Comments:

                                                            W   C   O

                                                            __   __   __

8. Decision Making/Cognitive Functions

   Comments:

                                                            W   C   O

                                                            __   __   __

9. Life Philosophy/Goals

   What are your life goals?   1 _____
                                      2 _____
   Comments: 3 _____

                                                            W   C   O

                                                            __   __   __

10. Leisure Time/Community Involvement

    Comments:

                                                            W   C   O

                                                            __   __   __

11. Feeling Management

    Comments:

                                                            W   C   O

                                                            __   __   __

MH-3

B. SIGNALS OF DISTRESS

12.   Lethality-Self   History of Self-Injury-
                                Method _____ _____   Outcome

_____ within last month   _____ Medical Treatment Only
_____ within last 6 months   _____ High Lethal   _____ Hosp. Intensive Care
_____ within last year   _____ Low Lethal   _____ Hosp. Psychiatric
_____ over 1 year ago   _____ Out-pt. Follow-up
                                                                                 _____ No Treatment

        Total number of suicide attempts _____ Date of last attempt ___ _____

        Comments: (include ideation and threats)

                                                                            W   C   O

                                                                           ___   ___   ___

13.   Lethality-Other
             History of Injury to Other   Client Outcome   Victim
Date   Method _____   _____ Medical Treatment Only   _____
_____ within last month   _____ Hosp. Intensive Care   _____
_____ within last 6 months   _____ High Lethal   _____ Hosp. Psychiatric   _____
_____ within last year   _____ Low Lethal   _____ Out-pt. Follow-Up   _____
_____ over 1 year   _____ No Treatment   _____
        Total number of assaults___ _____ Date of last assault _____ _____ Other (_____)   _____

        Comments: (include ideation and threats)

                                                                            W   C   O

                                                                           ___   ___   ___

14.   Substance Use-Drug and/or Alcohol
      Other Drug Use (include alcohol use)
                        Type   Present Use   Past Use   Duration
1. _____
2. _____
3. _____
4. _____
5. _____
6. _____

                                                                            W   C   O

                                                                           ___   ___   ___

15.   Legal

        a.   Pending Court Action   Yes _____   No _____   Where _____
        b.   On Probation   Yes _____   No _____   When _____
        c.   On Parole   Yes _____   No _____   Probation Officer _____
        d.   Conditional Discharge   Yes _____   No _____   Parole Officer _____
      Comments: Judge _____

                                                                            W   C   O

                                                                           ___   ___   ___
                                                                                  MH-3A

COMPREHENSIVE MENTAL HEALTH ASSESSMENT (cont.)

Name _____ ID# _____

		RATING SCALE		(W = Worker; C = Client; O = Other)
1	2	3	4	5
High Functioning	High/Moderate Functioning	Moderate Functioning	Low/Moderate Functioning	Low Functioning

16. <u>Agency Use</u>

Previous Mental Health Service Contacts

Outcare: Name of Agency _____ Phone # _____
          Contact Person _____ Date of last Contact _____
          Address _____

Incare: Name of Agency _____ Phone # _____
         Contact Person _____
         Address _____ Date of last Hosp. _____
         Reason for Admission _____
         How often _____ How long _____ Avg. length of stay _____

Comments:

                                                                          W   C   O

                                                                          —   —   —

<u>Optional Information</u>

        Religious Concerns ___ Yes ___ No ___ What _____
        Ethnic Cultural Background Problems Yes ___ No ___ What _____

<u>Narrative Summary of Assessment</u>:

Assessed by _____ Date _____ **MH-4**

COMPREHENSIVE MENTAL HEALTH ASSESSMENT

Client Self-Assessment Worksheet

Date _____ Name _____

1. Physical Health

    How is your health?

    Comments: _____

    _____

    _____

    _____

Circle one for each question.

Excellent
Good
Fair
Poor
Very Poor

2. Self-Acceptance/Self-Esteem
    How do you feel about yourself as a person ?

    Comments: _____

    _____

    _____

    _____

Excellent
Good
Fair
Poor
Very Poor

3. Vocational/Occupational

    (Includes student & homemaker)
    How would you judge your work/school situation?

    Comments:

    _____

Excellent
Good
Fair
Poor
Very Poor

4. Immediate Family

    How are your relationships with your family and/or
    spouse?

    Comments: _____

    _____

Excellent
Good
Fair
Poor
Very Poor

5. Intimate Relationship(s)

    Is there anyone you feel really close to and can rely on?

    Comments: _____

    _____

    _____

Always
Usually
Sometimes
Rarely
Never

6. Residential

    How do you judge your housing situation?
    Comments: _____

    _____

    _____

    _____

Excellent
Good
Fair
Poor
Very Poor

7. Financial

    How would you describe your financial situation?

    Comments: _____

    _____

    _____

    _____

Excellent
Good
Fair
Poor
Very Poor

8. Decision Making ability
    How satisfied are you with your ability to make life decisions?
    Comments: _____

    _____

    _____

Always Very Satisfied
Almost Always Satisfied
Occasionally Dissatisfied
Almost Always Dissatisfied
Always Very Dissatisfied

MH-6

Circle one for each question.

9. Life Philosophy

How satisfied are you with how your life goals are working for you?

Comments:_____

_____

_____

Always Very Satisfied
Almost Always Satisfied
Occasionally Dissatified
Almost Always Dissatisfied
Always Very Dissatisfied

10. Leisure Time/Community Involvement

How satisfied are you with your use of free time?

Comments:_____

_____

_____

Always Very Satisfied
Almost Always Satisfied
Occasionally Dissatisfied
Almost Always Dissatisfied
Always Very Dissatisfied

11. Feeling Management

How comfortable are you with your feelings?

Comments:_____

_____

_____

_____

Always Very Comfortable
Almost Always Comfortable
Occasionally Uncomfortable
Almost Always Uncomfortable
Always Very Uncomfortable

12. Lethality (self)

Is there any current risk of suicide for you?

Comments:_____

_____

_____

No Predictable Risk of Suicide Now
Low Risk of Suicide Now
Moderate Risk of Suicide Now
High Risk of Suicide Now
Very High Risk of Suicide Now

13. Lethality (other)

Is there any risk that you might physically harm someone?

Comments:_____

_____

_____

No Predictable Risk of Assualt Now
Low Risk of Assault Now
Moderate Risk of Assault Now
High Risk of Assault Now
Very High Risk of Assault Now

14. Substance Use (Drug and/or Alcohol)

Does use of drugs/alcohol interfere with performing your responsibilities?

Comments:_____

_____

_____

Never Interferes
Rarely Interferes
Sometimes Interferes
Frequently Intereferes
Constantly Interferes

15. Legal

What is your tendency to get in trouble with the law?

Comments:_____

_____

_____

No Tendency
Slight Tendency
Moderate Tendency
Great Tendency
Very Great Tendency

16. Agency Use

How successful are you with at getting help from agencies (or doctors) when you need it?

Comments:_____

_____

Always Successful
Usually Successful
Moderately Successful
Seldom Successful
Never Successful

Any additional comments?

MH-6A

Mental Health Resources*

Addicts Anonymous
Box 2000
Lexington, Kentucky 40501
A self-help organization concerned with narcotics addiction.

Alcoholics Anonymous
(World Services)
Box 459
Grand Central Station
New York, New York 10017
A self-help organization concerned with alcoholism; Al-anon is concerned with the spouse of the alcoholic; Al-ateen is concerned with the children of the alcoholic.

Alzheimer's Disease and Related Disorders
     Association
32 Broadway
New York, New York 10004
This group has banded together to provide support, to develop and disseminate helpful information, and to encourage research on Alzheimer's disease.

Anorexia Nervosa and Associated Disorders
Suite 2020
550 Frontage Road
Northfield, Illinois 60693
This self-help organization for persons with anorexia nervosa, bulimia, and related disorders was founded by Vivian Meehan, a nurse, who now serves as its president.

Association for Humanistic Gerontology
1711 Solano Avenue
Berkeley, California 94707
A professional association, international resource-sharing network, and an information clearing-house concerned with humanistic and holistic approaches to aging and programs for the elderly. Sponsors a news magazine, conferences, and training seminars.

*Self-help organizations must rely on donations. If you write, please don't forget to include a long, stamped, self-addressed envelope.

Epilepsy Foundation of America
1828 L Street, N.W., Suite 406
Washington, D.C. 20036
A voluntary agency concerned with epilepsy.

Family Service Association of America, Inc.
44 East 23rd Street
New York, New York 10010
A social work organization providing mental health services to families under stress and information and research on family living.

Florence Crittenton Association of America
608 South Dearborn Street
Chicago, Illinois 60605
An organization concerned with unmarried mothers and adolescent girls having problems in adjustment.

Friends for Sobriety
American Humanist Association
7 Harwood Drive
Amherst, New York 14226
A humanist organization of men and women dedicated to helping each other maintain a sober, productive, and happy way of life through achieving sobriety.

National Association for Mental Health
1800 North Kent Street
Arlington, Virginia 22209
A voluntary agency concerned with mental health.

National Association for Retarded Citizens
2501 Avenue J
Arlington, Texas 76010
A voluntary agency concerned with the retarded.

National Clearinghouse for Drug Abuse
     Information
Box 1701
Washington, D.C. 20013
An organization that disseminates drug abuse information.

National Committee for Prevention of Child Abuse
Box 2866
Chicago, Illinois 60690
An organization concerned with physically and emotionally abused and neglected children.

National Council on Alcoholism
2 Park Avenue
New York, New York 10016
A voluntary agency concerned with alcoholism.

National Society for Autistic Children
401 East 65th Street
New York, New York 10021
A self-help organization for parents of autistic children.

Neurotics Anonymous International
Room 1426, Colorado Building
1341 G Street
Washington, D.C. 20005
A self-help organization concerned with neuroses.

Overeaters Anonymous
Box 6190
Torrance, California 90504
A self-help group concerned with obesity that provides information and addresses of local chapters.

Parents Anonymous
(National Office)
Phone only (toll-free number)
(800) 352-0386
A self-help organization for parents who abuse their children.

Parents without Partners, Inc.
80 Fifth Avenue
New York, New York 10011
A self-help organization concerned with single, widowed, or divorced parents and their children.

Parents United
P. O. Box 84353
Los Angeles, California 90073
A self-help group concerned with child molestation, and particularly incest, providing protection for children and support for families and affiliated with a professional therapy program. Daughters/Sons United chapters also exist.

President's Committee on Mental Retardation
ROB #3
Seventh and D Streets, S. W.
Washington, D.C. 20201
An organization concerned with mental retardation.

Recovery, Inc.: The Association of Nervous and Former Mental Patients
116 South Michigan Avenue
Chicago, Illinois 60603
A self-help organization for persons with mental problems and former mental patients.

Stepfamily Foundation, Inc.
333 West End Avenue
New York, New York 10023
Offers a newsletter, awareness workshops, telephone counseling, private and group counseling for stepparents, and complex households with children of both spouses.

Straight Partners
P. O. Box 1603
Hyattsville, Maryland 20788
An organization for straights who have married homosexuals (both gays and lesbians) providing a network of emotional support and help in learning how to cope with the situation.

Toughlove
Community Service Foundation
P. O. Box 70
Sellersville, Pennsylvania 18960
A parent support group for parents whose children are in trouble.

Valium Anonymous
Box 404
Altoona, Iowa 50009
Founded in 1978, this self-help group for persons hooked on Valium has chapters springing up all over the country.

U.S. Department of Health, Education, and Welfare Alcohol, Drug Abuse, and Mental Health Administration (ADAMHA)
5600 Fishers Lane
Rockville, Maryland 20852
The federal office of HEW concerned with alcohol and drug abuse and mental health.

APPENDIX E

Annotated Psychiatric Nursing Research Studies

In an attempt to add to the cumulative knowledge of research findings on which clinicians might base practice, the following selective contemporary annotations have been compiled. The studies included in this resource were published in one of the established research journals* between 1980–1982 or identified in the cumulative index to nursing literature as "Psychiatric Nursing (research)" and published by a nurse author during the same recent period. All annotations here were also selected by O'Toole[†] in her comprehensive review of seventy-one studies for their reflection "on the state of research and theory development in psychiatric nursing over the last ten years." Educational studies and studies that emphasize psychosocial aspects of general health were excluded by O'Toole and also by us. Furthermore, articles that use clinical vignettes and nonsystematic case studies or fail to report the research methodology used to generate findings were not included. Like O'Toole, we do not claim that this resource is reflective of all important psychiatric nursing research in the recent past. We do believe, however, that this sample underscores the practice implications of research findings and illustrates the emerging empirical basis for clinical practice decisions in our field. Undoubtedly this compendium offers students and clinicians a beginning to which they may continue to add.

Ellison, E. S. "Social Behavior and Psychosocial Adjustment of Single and Two-Parent Children." *Western Journal of Nursing Research.* Vol. 3, No. 3 (1981): 283–301.

Acknowledging that most research of the past has been conducted with the assumption that single parenthood is a deviant form of family life, this study attempts to fill a gap in the literature on the possible differences in psychosocial adjustment between single and two-parent children from an essentially well sample of nineteen children between 8 and 11 years of age enrolled in an elementary school noted for its innovative teaching methods. Data collection procedures consisted of observations of classroom behaviors using an observation schedule especially designed for the study and assessment of the children's psychosocial adjustment, using the Louisville School Behavior Checklist Form A for ages 7-13. The children of single versus two-parent families were compared on these two measures using appropriate statistical tools. The most striking finding of this study is that although lower academic achievement was noted consistently in single-parent children by teachers, few differences were noted in classroom behavior or on teacher ratings of psychosocial adjustment, aside from their ratings of academics. Relating to peers seemed particularly important to single-parent children. One limitation of the study was that information of the children's actual academic performance was not available.

The following implications for nurse counseling and client/family education were offered by the nurse who conducted this research:

1. Peer associations play a central role in socialization of school-aged, single-parent children. Consequently, parent education programs for divorced, separated, and widowed parents should include information regarding the importance of good peer relationships to psychosocial development.

2. Nurses need to share information with teachers about assessing and facilitating communication skills for children, particularly with single-parent children whose relationships with peers emerged as critical to their good adjustment.

---

* *Western Journal of Nursing Research, Journal of Psychiatric Nursing and Mental Health Services* (currently the *Journal of Psychosocial Nursing), Nursing Research, Research in Nursing and Health, Journal of Advanced Nursing.*

† A. W. O'Toole, "When the Practical Becomes Theoretical." Journal of Psychiatric Nursing and Mental Health Services. Vol. 18, No. 3 (December 1981): 11-19.

Ernst, C.; Vanderzyl, S.; and Salinger, R. "Preparation of Psychiatric Inpatients for Group Therapy." *Journal of Psychiatric Nursing/Mental Health Services.* Vol. 19, No. 7 (July 1982): 28–33.

The purpose of this study was to investigate whether a preparatory session for psychiatric inpatients entering group therapy would promote more realistic client role expectations of the group therapy experience. The sample for this research consisted of thirty volunteer psychiatric inpatients from a large V.A. hospital. The clients were randomly assigned to two experimental conditions—(1) the film "Turning Point" and literature about group therapy, and (2) a neutral film and neutral written information. Subsequently, both groups were evaluated on a thirty-item self-report inventory called the PEI-R. A two-tailed test of the mean scores for the two groups resulted in a nonstatistically significant trend in favor of the preparation for group therapy received by the first group. This group was less approval- and advice-seeking. The fact that the trend was not statistically significant was attributed to the small sample size and limitations of the PEI-R instrument, which was originally designed to measure a client's expectations of individual therapy, not group therapy. Implications for nursing practice encourage the development of methods to prepare clients for effective and realistic expectations for group therapy and continued research into their effectiveness.

Flaskerud, J. H. "Perceptions of Problematic Behavior by Appalachians, Mental Health Professionals, and Lay Non-Appalachians." *Nursing Research.* Vol. 29, No. 3, (May-June 1980): 140–148.

This study was based on the ideas that the culture of a group influences the labels that group places on people's behavior, particularly when the issue involves labeling problematic behaviors as "mental illness." In it, three groups of randomly selected respondents representing the Appalachian culture (N = 50) and the American culture (54 mental health professionals and 50 lay persons) were interviewed to compare the labels placed on problematic behavior described in vignettes. Data were analyzed using a one-way analysis of variance as well as qualitative analysis of interview data. No significant differences were found between the two subgroups of non-Appalachians, but significant differences between each of these groups and the Appalachians were established. Behaviors that Appalachians labeled as lazy, mean, immoral, criminal, or psychic were labeled as mental illnesses by mental health professionals and lay persons. Furthermore, while the non-Appalachians recommended some type of psychiatric management of these behaviors, Appalachians recommended either tolerance or punishment through the social or legal system. Implications for psychiatric nursing underscore the

importance of considering cultural diversity when labeling client behavior and deciding on appropriate goals.

Giberson, D. and Larson, E. "Factors that Affect Patient Compliance with Psychiatric Follow-up Therapy After Hospital Discharge." *Nursing Research.* Vol. 31, No. 1, (January/February 1982): 373–375.

This investigation evaluated clients who attended their first follow-up appointments, based on demographic factors. This study examined the importance of clients meeting with their future outpatient therapists prior to hospital discharge, as well as the clients' perception of a change in the severity of their illness and their level of satisfaction with inpatient care. Based on a review of their clinical records and telephone interviews with 117 clients discharged from an eighteen-bed psychiatric unit in a teaching hospital over a three-month period, findings indicated that follow-up attendance/posthospital discharge was significantly greater among clients who met with their referral therapist beforehand irrespective of other variables, such as discharge diagnosis and medication regimen. Such findings support a practice of predischarge appointments in discharge planning for clients who make the transition from inpatient to outpatient therapy.

Gibson, D. E. "Reminiscence, Self-Esteem and Self-Other Satisfaction in Adult Male Alcoholics." *Journal of Psychiatric Nursing and Mental Health Services.* Vol. 18, No. 3 (March 1980): 7–11.

The research problem in this study was to determine if there were differences in self-esteem and satisfaction with that self-esteem in adult male alcoholics who did not participate in a Reminiscence Group when compared with a similar group who did. Sixty-one adult male alcoholics were selected as a convenience sample from a southwestern city detoxification center. Half the sample participated in a series of three Reminiscence Group sessions over a three-day period, and half of the sample did not. When the two groups were compared on mean scores of a Self-Esteem Questionnaire a near significant trend toward lower scores for the reminiscing group members was revealed. Such findings even in the absence of random assignment to control and experimental groups suggest that reminiscence should be used with caution with this population, according to the investigator at least.

Hardin, S. B. "Comparative Analysis of Nonverbal Interpersonal Communication of Schizophrenics and Normals." *Research in Nursing and Health.* Vol. 3, (1980): 57–68.

Nonverbal communications of schizophrenics and normals in a dyadic interaction were analyzed and compared in this nursing study. Twelve purposively (not randomly) selected women were videotaped in normal-normal, normal-schizophrenic, and schizophrenic-schizophrenic communication acts for thirty minutes, using a PLATO IV computer program and a modified Kendon Kinesic Notation System. Sets of nonverbal behaviors were recorded at one-second intervals; the frequency and duration scores for these sets of nonverbal behaviors with corresponding communication meanings were totaled. Using an analysis of variance statistical operation, the three groups differed significantly at the p .05 level in engagement and defensiveness, and normal interactors were the least imitative of the three comparative groups. Analysis of the patterns of nonverbal communication also revealed differences among the groups lending support to the theory that schizophrenics communicate in disjunctive ways. However, implications for clinical practice from this study urge the encouragement of schizophrenic-schizophrenic communication in small groups of dyads without such dilutants as cards, T.V., games, and even therapists. Limitations in the methodology of the study were also identified.

Hinds, P. "Music: A Milieu Factor with Implications for the Nurse-Therapist." *Journal of Psychiatric Nursing and Mental Health Services.* Vol. 18, No. 6 (June 1980): 28-33.

This study investigated the effects of one type of music on the social interactions observed in group play therapy with ten male children, ages 8 to 10. A behavioral checklist was developed by the researcher to measure five outcome behaviors: verbalization, proximity with group cotherapists, proximity with other group members, involvement in toy exchanges, and involvement in acts of physical aggression. Using a Pearson-Product Moment Coefficient statistic, the investigator established a high association of these target behaviors to one another. Subsequent analysis established that the first four behaviors showed a significant association with the presence of music. The clinical importance of this study's findings rests with the notion that it may be possible to influence children's observable behaviors through manipulation of environmental facts, such as the presence of music in a group therapy session. Generalizations from this study are limited by its small sample size and lack of a control group with randomly assigned subjects.

Karshmer, J. F.; Kornfeld, J.; and Carr, A. "Causal Attribution: Bias in the Nurse-Patient Relationship." *Journal of Psychiatric Nursing and Mental Health Services.* Vol. 18, No. 5, (May 1980): 25-30.

This study of twenty nurses and twenty patients in a small inpatient psychiatric unit of a general hospital focused on attribution—the process of judging the causes of behaviors and events encountered in social situations. Of

particular interest was delineating whether or not nurses and clients differ in their tendency to name external pressures in the environment or internal factors when observing behavior. In short, the role of the observer was the independent variable in this study, and the locus of causes attributed to behaviors was the dependent variable. Findings indicated that both nurses and clients chose internal explanations for clients' behavior. When sorting cards describing nurse behaviors, however, clients made equal internal and external attributions, even though nurses themselves attributed this second set of behaviors to internal causes. The clinical implication of these findings is that nurses by virtue of theoretical perspective, habit, or intuition favor internal over situational causation in seeking explanations for client behavior and that these biases may influence accurate assessment of maladaptive behavior.

Navin, H. L., and Welson, J. "Caffeine Consumption and Sleep Disturbance in Acutely Ill Psychiatric Inpatients." *Journal of Psychiatric Nursing and Mental Health Services.* Vol. 18, No. 3 (March 1980): 37-42.

The purpose of this study was to determine the relationship between caffeine consumption and sleep disturbances in a population of acutely ill psychiatric inpatients. A convenience sample of eighty-two clients—aged 18 to 65, diagnosed as schizoprenic or having an Affective Disorder, able to speak and read English, legally competent and in contact with reality, but able to leave the ward only with an escort—were rated using a Sleep Pattern checklist during a period of four months in which regular and decaffeinated coffee were alternately served according to a "blind" design. Contrary to the expected results, clients exhibited more sleeplessness and symptoms of anxiety during the period that they were drinking decaffeinated coffee. Regular coffee drinking was associated with going to sleep later but with sleeping more hours, at least in this particular study. The increased sleeplessness and need for PRN medication during the decaffeinated coffee period might be attributed to symptoms of caffeine addiction and, if so, suggests implications for health teaching regarding substance use by clients.

Papa, L. L. "Responses to Life Events as Predictors of Suicidal Behavior." *Nursing Research.* Vol. 29, No. 6 (November-December 1980): 362-369.

This study considered the interaction of a complex of predictor variables—including hopelessness, locus of control, preference for inclusion, control, affection, and stress from life events—in relation to degree of suicide intent. Using statistical methods (including multiple regression), hopelessness was the only variable significantly related to suicide intent. The sample for this study was obtained from sixty consecutive suicide attempters who entered a

Texas hospital for treatment after unsuccessful attempts. Intent Scale for Suicide Attempters was divided in two parts: Circumstances Related to Suicide Attempt and Self-Report. Validity and reliability for this measure had been reported. While the investigator suggests that understanding the relationship between hopelessness, preference for affection, locus of control, and suicide intent would contribute to suicide prevention, assessment, and treatment, she cautions clinicians about formulating implications for practice until her study is replicated.

Savedra, M. and Tesler, M. "Coping Strategies of Hospitalized School-Age Children." *Western Journal of Nursing Research.* Vol. 3, No. 4, (1981): 371–384.

To plan and implement care for children who must be hospitalized, nurses need to understand the strategies used by school-age children to deal with the stresses of the experience. This exploratory study addressed two questions: (1) What strategies does the 6-12-year-old child hospitalized for surgery use to cope with the experience? (2) Can parents provide information on admission to the hospital that will help nurses predict what strategies a child will use? Data were collected from thirty-three children (eighteen boys and fifteen girls), 6-12-years-old, who were admitted to a university hospital for elective procedures and accompanied by one or both parents. Observations of the children were made using a direct-coping adaptation protocol and occurred at specific stress points and times during their hospitalization. A questionnaire developed by the nurse researcher was administered to parents asking for the child's usual responses in situations, including exposure to new experiences, people, and fear. Data were analyzed and indicated that children's predominant behavior before surgery was precoping or orienting—demonstrating the need for nursing interventions that enable a hospitalized child to get the needed information to be comfortable in the patient role. All children except one attempted to control behaviors postsurgery and some presurgery as well. Thus, while viewed as resistive by some nurses, it needs to be redefined as the healthy response of a child who is working at regulating the amount of adaptation to be made on an already compromised position. Diminished child verbalization and parents' view of their children's emotional status as overly positive also have implications for a liaison psychiatric nursing care plan for hospitalized children.

Savitz, J., and Friedman, M. I. "Diagnosing Boredom and Confusion." *Nursing Research.* Col. 30, No. 1 (January-February 1981): 16–19.

An interview schedule to determine whether clients could be diagnosed psychologically as being in a bored, confused, or adaptive state of mind was constructed and tested with a total of seventy-nine clients over 15-years-old in a middle-class rural community. The six-question interview schedule that resulted proved to be objective, reliable, and reasonably valid. Limitations acknowledge the need to replicate the study across more diverse populations and to account for the effects of drugs on the diagnosis. Clinical practice implications underscore the value of planning interventions with bored people that assist them to seek greater variety and novelty in their lives. Confused clients, on the other hand, can benefit by seeking greater familiarity, simplicity, and regularity in their lives. The key explanatory variable in this study was the balance of predictability in clients' lives. Adaptive individuals were characterized in an optimally predictable situation.

Schoffstall, D. "Concerns of Students Nurses Prior to Psychiatric Nursing Experience: An Assessment and Intervention Technique." *Journal of Psychiatric Nursing Mental Health Services.* Vol. 19, No. 11, (November 1981): 11–14.

This study recognized that stereotypes associated with clients and psychiatric hospitals can have a powerful impact on students' abilities to learn. Therefore, the author attempted to identify a method that can be used preclinically in the classroom setting to assess and reduce the anxiety of students who are about to begin their clinical experience in psychiatric nursing. She designed a "fantasy exercise" to identify student concerns and anxieties, to identify factors that influence the nurse-client relationship, to provide information, and to create discussion about subjective experiences related to hospitalization and psychiatric diagnoses. The seventy-three responses from three classes were categorized into several broadly defined categories of concern that include

1. Students' fears that they might influence clients in some special, unique, and irrevocable way during their experience.

2. Students' expectations for personal growth and insight.

3. Students' concerns about lacking sufficient therapeutic skills.

4. Students' fear of danger—physical or emotional.

5. Students' concerns about meeting or encountering the bizarre.

6. Students' fear of the fine line between themselves and the clients and the possibility of becoming emotionally disturbed themselves.

Implications drawn by the author encourage the use of her fantasy exercise assessment technique to reduce student anxiety about the psychiatric nursing experience, although her study did not actually address testing the effectiveness of the approach.

Traver, T., and Moss, A. V. "Psychiatric Patient's Opinions of Nurses Ceasing to Wear Uniform." *Journal of Advanced Nursing.* Vol. 5, (1980): 47–53.

Psychiatric clients at two general hospitals were asked whether they felt that nurses on their ward should wear uniforms or ordinary clothes. In one of the hospitals the procedure was repeated immediately after the nurses changed from uniforms to ordinary clothes and again at five and seven month intervals. The results showed a general preference among clients for nurses to wear uniforms. There was no clear trend for increased acceptance of ordinary clothes on the experimenting wards. The tendency was that older clients preferred uniforms and clients under 29 years had a preference for ordinary clothes. Because of the small sample size and the short fourteen-month time span the authors of this study suggest that its results be interpreted with caution. Despite their own findings, they continue to suggest that style of dress is relevant to the creation of an informal therapeutic environment.

Whaley, M. S., and Ramirez, L. F. "The Use of Seclusion Rooms and Physical Restraints in the Treatment of Psychiatric Patients." *Journal of Psychiatric Nursing and Mental Health Services.* Vol. 18, No. 1, (January 1980): 13–16.

In an attempt to develop an assessment tool (checklist) to guide the rational use of locked-door seclusion rooms and/or physical restraints, a three-question questionnaire was administered to mental health professionals at a V.A. hospital. The questions were

1. Why do you think clients have to go in seclusion or restraints?
2. How do you determine when clients are ready to come out of seclusion or restraints?
3. In order of importance state the reasons you've listed above.

Findings from the 100 respondents to these questions yielded the following conclusions:

1. The use of seclusion rooms and/or restraints is highly emotional for clients and staff. There are only vague and subjective guidelines to regulate such use.
2. Most indications for use of seclusion and restraints center around issues of violence, destructive behavior, protection of the client reduction of stimuli, and the client's own request.

The decision to terminate seclusion or restraints is made in relation to the above behaviors being reduced and the increased ability of the client to exercise self-control. Implications for practice that may be derived from this essentially self-report study include use of the "Indications for Placing a Patient in Seclusion" form published by the authors of this article.

GLOSSARY

Abreaction A process by which repressed material, particularly a painful experience or conflict, is brought back to a person's consciousness. The person then not only recalls but also relives the repressed material, which is accompanied by affective response.

Accenting Nonverbal cues that emphasize verbal ones; for example, holding a finger in front of pursed lips to emphasize the verbal command "Shhh!"

Accommodation Adjustment of the individual to the object in the environment; incorporation of an experience as it actually is.

Acting in The expression of certain kinds of unconscious conflicts through behavior directly within the therapeutic session, although the unconscious impulse is not verbalized or remembered. It is a more subtle form of resistance than acting out. Postural acts or body movements, such as a client's seductive pose in front of the therapist, are examples.

Acting out The expression of certain kinds of unconscious conflicts through behavior, although the unconscious impulse is not verbalized or remembered.

Action language Movements as statements mediated primarily through the central nervous system.

Active listening Attentive involvement with the client; a therapist's ability to hear the client without interpreting along the lines of the therapist's own experiences or problems.

Adaptation Modification of an individual, as a result of an interchange between individual and environment, that enhances the possibilities for further interchange. It involves the components of assimilation and accommodation, which operate simultaneously in mutual adaptation between individual and environment.

Addicted life styles Disruptive life-style having complex physiological, psychological, and sociological dimensions. In DSM-III categorized as a Personality Disorder on Axis II.

Addiction Strong dependence, both physiological and emotional, on alcohol or some other drug. The term *drug dependence* is gradually replacing *drug addiction.*

Adjustment The process by which and success with which an individual copes with life in the culture.

Adolescence The period of considerable physical and psychosocial human development between the ages of twelve and twenty. It is frequently accompanied by conflicting ideas and feelings as the individual moves between the docility of latency and the acclimatization of adulthood.

Adult ego state In transactional analysis theory, the ego state responsible for the objective appraisal of reality and the capacity to process data.

Affect Emotion or feeling; the tone of one's reaction to persons and events.

Affection need The interpersonal need to establish and maintain a satisfactory relation between self and other people with regard to intimacy and liking.

Affective Disorder Disturbed personal coping pattern in which the client feels extreme sadness, withdraws socially, often feels guilty, and expresses self-deprecatory thoughts or experiences an elevated expansive mood with hyperactivity, pressure of speech, inflated self-esteem, decreased need for sleep.

Aggression Forceful, goal-directed behavior that may be physical or verbal.

Akathesia A reversible extrapyramidal syndrome characterized by motor restlessness experienced by the client as an urge to pace, a need to shift weight from one foot to the other, or an inability to sit or stand still. Responds well to oral antiparkinsonian agents.

Alcoholic In popular usage, a term for those whose continued or excessive drinking results in impairment of personal health, disruption of family and social relationships, and loss of economic security.

Algorithms Behavioral steps, or step-by-step procedures, for the management of common problems to provide structured, standardized guidelines for decision making.

Alternative family A group of persons, with or without blood or marriage ties, who live and interact together in order to achieve common goals.

Alzheimer's disease A progressive brain atrophy, usually fatal within a few years; may be known as *presenile dementia.* With the progression of the condition there is often memory and judgment loss, loss of interest, and carelessness. Symptoms worsen until disorientation, epileptiform attacks, and contractures are evident. The cause of this rare disease is unknown, and there is no known treatment.

Ambivalence Simultaneous conflicting feelings or attitudes toward a person or object; the subjective state of simultaneously loving and hating an object.

Amnesia Sudden and total loss of memory for events of a period of time; the period may range from a few hours to a lifetime.

Anaclitic Characterized by excessive dependence. Often said of children who depend too much on one parent. *Anaclitic depression* is a depressed state in a child that is associated with loss of a parent.

Anticipatory guidance A process that aims to help persons cope with a crisis by discussing the details of the impending difficulty and problem solving before the event occurs.

Antidepressant drug A medication used to treat severe depression. Antidepressants are divided into two principal categories, the tricyclic compounds and the monoamine oxidase inhibitors.

Antipsychotic drug A medication used to control certain psychotic symptoms, notably disordered thinking, agitation, and excitement. The principal classes of antipsychotics are phenothiazines, thioxanthenes, butyrophenones, and rauwolfias.

Anxiety A diffuse feeling of dread, apprehension, or unexplained discomfort; a subjectively painful warning of impending danger that motivates the individual to take corrective action in order to relieve this unpleasant feeling.

Anxiety Disorder Disturbed personal coping pattern in which anxiety is either the predominant disturbance or a secondary disturbance that is confronted if the primary symptom is taken away.

Apathy Lack of feeling, interest, concern, or emotion.

Artifacts Items in contact with interacting persons that may act as nonverbal stimuli. Examples are jewelry, clothing, cosmetics, and perfumes.

Assertiveness Asking for what one wants or acting to get what one wants in a way that respects the other person.

Assertiveness training An alternative therapy that is usually accomplished in groups to help people who tend either to be passive and discount themselves or to be too aggressive. Assertiveness techniques and exercises are designed to teach individuals to ask for what they want and to refuse requests from others without feeling guilty.

Assimilation Adaptation of the environment to oneself; taking in experience only to the extent one can integrate it.

Assumptive world view A set of more or less implicit assumptions a person constructs about self and the nature of the world enabling the person to predict the behavior of others and the outcome of his or her own actions.

Asyndetic communication A form of interpersonal interaction in which elements in the statements of one speaker function as unrelated cues for the next speaker. Connecting links between the statements are not clear, and, to the listener, the conversation seems disjointed.

Attachment An interactive process in which two individuals commit themselves together. The term commonly refers to an infant's ties to a parent.

Autism Living within oneself; a process of subjective, introspective thinking often rich in fantasy.

Autistic Relating to private, individual affects and ideas that are derived from internal drives, hopes, and wishes. Most commonly refers to the private reality of persons labeled schizophrenic as opposed to the shared reality of the external world.

Autonomy Independence or self-governance.

Bad trip An acute anxiety and panic reaction by a user of psychedelic drugs who is not prepared for the physical and psychological sensations associated with drug use.

Barometric events The actions of the unconflicted members of a group (catalysts), which serve to move the group forward into the next phase of group work.

Basic human needs theory A life theory developed by Abraham Maslow that provides a framework for viewing physical and emotional needs in a hierarchical order.

Behavior Any human activity, either mental or physical. Some behavior can be observed, but other behavior can only be inferred. For example, an observer can infer from physical activity that mental behavior has taken place.

Behaviorist model of psychiatry A model, based on the research of Ivan Pavlov and J. B. Watson, that is sometimes called *stimulus-response learning* or *behavioral conditioning*. It assumes that symptoms associated with neurosis and psychosis are clusters of learned behaviors that persist because they are rewarding to the individual.

Behavior modification A method of reeducation or treatment mode based on the principles of Pavlovian conditioning and further developed by B. F. Skinner; an effort to change "disturbed" or "disordered" behavior patterns through modification techniques.

Bestiality Engaging in sexual relations with animals; also referred to as *zoophilia*.

Bioethics A recently developed field that applies ethical reasoning to issues and dilemmas in the area of health care.

Biofeedback Also called visceral learning, this alternative healing therapy posits a technique for gaining conscious control over unconscious body functions by using continuous feedback about the results of each consecutive attempt at control.

Biological therapies   The treatment of emotionally disturbed or incapacitated clients by physiological means. Also called somatotherapies.

Bisexuality   Engaging in sexual relations with individuals of both sexes.

Blended family   The joining of two nuclear families that have missing adult members to form a new nucleus.

Blind spot (psychological)   An area of someone's personality that the person is totally unaware of. Unperceived areas are often hidden by repression so that the individual can avoid painful emotions.

Blocking   Stopping the expression of a thought.

Blotting paper syndrome   A countertransference phenomenon in which staff members unconsciously begin to act out a feeling that a client is unable to express or experience. Commonly found in relation to symptoms.

Body image   An individual's concept of the shape, size, and mass of his or her body and its parts; the internalized picture that a person has of the physical appearance of his or her body.

Bonding   An interactive process in which two individuals commit themselves together. The term commonly refers to a parent's ties to an infant.

Brainwashing   The alteration of personal conviction, belief, habits, and attitudes by means of intensive coercive indoctrination.

Burnout   A condition in which health professionals lose their concern and feeling for the clients they work with and begin to treat them in detached or dehumanized ways. It is an attempt to cope with the intense stress of interpersonal work by distancing.

Castration complex   Fear of the loss of or injury to the genitals.

Catalysts   Unconflicted members of a group who are able to move the group on to the next phase of group work.

Catatonic state (catatonia)   A state characterized by muscular rigidity and immobility, usually associated with Schizophrenia.

Catchment area   A geographically circumscribed area comprising a city, or several rural communities, with 75,000 to 200,000 residents.

Catharsis   A basic process in psychotherapy, in which the client freely puts personal feelings, thoughts, daydreams, and interpersonal problems into words. The process usually produces a feeling of relief.

Cathexis   In psychoanalysis, the attachment of emotion to an object, person, or idea. It may be positive or negative emotion (love or hate).

Cerea flexibilitas   See *Waxy flexibility*.

Change agent   An outside force or person acting for another in a deliberate effort to improve a situation.

Character   The enduring attitudes an individual develops toward the self and the world.

Checking perceptions   A communication skill in which the therapist shares how he or she perceives and hears the client and asks the client to verify these perceptions. Perception checks are used to make sure that one person understands the other.

Child ego state   In transactional analysis theory, the ego state that represents the archaic relics of early childhood.

Circumstantiality   A disturbance in associative thought processes in which a person digresses into unnecessary details and inappropriate thoughts before communicating the central idea.

Client   A consumer of health services. This term is used instead of *patient* by some mental health professionals who oppose the medical model of mental disorder.

Clinical psychologist   A psychologist specially educated and trained in the area of mental health. Certification is at the doctoral level after the candidate has completed a one-year internship at an approved facility. Clinical psychologists perform psychotherapy, plan and implement programs of behavior modification, and select, administer, and interpret psychological tests.

Coercive power   The power a person has to deliver negative consequences or remove positive ones in response to the behavior of group members.

Cognitive   Relating to the mental processes of thought, memory, comprehension, and reasoning.

Cognitive function theory   A life theory that emphasizes the importance of communicative and exploratory or problem-solving behaviors, especially use of language and the thought processes in the development and functioning of the personality.

Cohesiveness   A sense of belonging; the result of all the forces acting on members to remain in a group.

Commitment   The legal process by which a person is confined to a mental hospital. It may be voluntary or involuntary. Also a sense of dedication and responsibility.

Communal family   A group of many persons living together who have negotiated the privileges and responsibilities associated with their roles, material possessions, economic concerns, sexual expressions, and parenting activities.

Communication   An ongoing, dynamic, and ever-changing series of events in which one event affects all the others. Responding with *meaning* is the essence of effective communication. Meaning must be mutually negotiated between persons.

Community mental health   A system for the delivery of mental health services based on a shift from institutional to community-based care in which primary, secondary, and tertiary prevention are emphasized.

Community mental health center   The executive locus

for applying community psychiatry concepts. Centers include inpatient (twenty-four-hour) facilities, partial hospitalization facilities (such as day, night, and weekend hospitals), outpatient departments, emergency services, consultation services, and education programs.

Complementary message   A nonverbal message that adds to or modifies a verbal message.

Complementary relationships   Relationships based on the enjoyment of differences and interdependence. They may deteriorate when one partner controls what the complementarity is and how it is maintained.

Compulsion   An uncontrollable persistent urge to perform an act repetitively in an attempt to relieve anxiety.

Compulsive life-styles   Disruptive life-styles characterized by excessive conformity and conscientiousness.

Concreteness (concrete thinking)   A primitive type of thinking that assumes a literal, superficial meaning of ideas. It is characteristic of children, retarded individuals, and schizophrenics.

Conditioning   Learning that occurs through reinforcement, in which behaviors are rewarded and persist.

Confabulation   The unconscious filling of gaps in memory by imagining experiences that have no basis in fact.

Confirmation   A communication by one person that agrees with or ratifies the other's view of self.

Conflict   A clash between opposing forces. It may be conscious or unconscious, intrapersonal or interpersonal.

Conflicted member   A member of a group whose posture toward authority or intimacy is inflexible, rigid, or compulsive.

Confrontation   A communication that deliberately invites another to self-examine some aspect of behavior in which there is a discrepancy between what the person says and does.

Connotative meaning   A meaning for a word or term that comes from a person's own experience.

Contract   A plan of action and goals mutually negotiated between client and mental health professional. Can be compared to the *nursing care plan* used in more tradition settings but the contract focuses more on client input and therapist/staff accountability.

Contradicting message   Nonverbal behavior that conveys the opposite meaning of a verbal message.

Control need   The interpersonal need to establish and maintain a satisfactory relation between self and others with regard to power and influence.

Conversion reaction   Pre-DSM-III term for a disturbed personal coping pattern in which an anxiety-provoking impulse is converted into somatic symptoms.

Convulsion   A violent involuntary contraction of some or all of the muscles.

Cooperator   In game theory, a person interested in helping both self and partner. (See *Maximizer* and *Rivalist*.)

Coping mechanisms   Operations outside a person's awareness that protect the person against anxiety; defense mechanisms.

Coping skill   An adaptive method or capacity developed by a person to deal with or overcome a psychological or social problem.

Coprolalia   Sexual pleasure obtained from using obscene language.

Coprophagia   Sexual pleasure associated with eating feces.

Coprophilia   Sexual pleasure involving a desire to defecate on or be defecated on by a partner.

Corrective emotional experience   Reexposure under favorable circumstances to an emotional situation that a client could not handle in the past.

Counterpersonal   Expending great amounts of energy to avoid intimacy and to maintain distance.

Countertransference   Sigmund Freud's term for irrational attitudes taken by an analyst toward a patient. It may create problems in psychotherapeutic work. The therapist needs to become aware of countertransference and seek consistent supervision to intervene when it occurs.

Couples therapy   An extension of the more traditional marital therapy to the therapy of interactional dyads when difficulties between the partners are specific to their relationship.

Covert   Covered or sheltered; concealed or disguised; not openly acknowledged.

Covert rehearsal   A stage in communication in which a person moves to make sense of the input received and develops and organizes a message *before* generating it.

Creative arts therapist   A therapist who uses the media of art, music, dance, or poetry to facilitate clients' personal experiences and increase their social responses and self-esteem.

Creativity   A form of thinking, closely linked with problem solving, in which the individual establishes new relationships, solves problems, behaves in an innovative or inventive manner, or produces new artistic or literary products.

Crisis   A situation in which customary problem-solving or decision-making methods are no longer adequate; a state of psychological disequilibrium. A crisis may be a turning point in a person's life.

Crisis counseling   A counseling strategy designed to be brief (five to six sessions) and issue-oriented. It may be individual, group, or family therapy.

Crisis intervention   An intervention process aimed at reestablishing the client's functioning at a level equal to or better than the precrisis level.

Crisis sequence Three sequential time periods—precrisis, crisis, and postcrisis—identified in the crisis model of mental health delivery.

Culture An organized set of beliefs, values, and ideas held by a group of people.

Cunnilingus Mouth to vulva sexual activity; oral stimulation of the female genitals.

Cyclothymic life-style A disruptive life-style characterized by recurring episodes of high and low moods.

Cyclothymic reaction See *Manic-depressive reaction.*

Decompensation Disorganization of a previously stable emotional adjustment or defensive system.

Defense mechanisms Operations outside of a person's awareness that the ego calls into play to protect against anxiety; the psychoanalytic term for coping mechanisms; also called mental mechanism.

Deinstitutionalization The shift of care and funding arrangements for the chronically and severely mentally ill from single-purpose, custodial state hospitals to multipurpose services based near clients' families and communities.

Déjà vu An illusion of visual recognition in which a new situation is incorrectly regarded as a repetition of a previous experience. This phenomenon occurs occasionally in everyone's life, but the schizophrenic is likely to report it with great frequency.

Delirium Confusion in thinking often accompanied by fear. It stems from an acute organic reaction and is characterized by restlessness, confusion, disorientation, bewilderment, agitation, and affective lability.

Delirium tremens (DTs) An acute psychotic state usually occurring after a prolonged and copious intake of alcohol.

Delusion An important personal belief that is almost certainly not true and is resistant to modification.

Delusions of grandeur An individual's belief that he or she has a special relationship to the world, for example, that he or she is a prominent person, living or dead, or is related to such a person.

Delusions of persecution An individual's belief that he or she is harassed, in danger, under investigation, and/or at the mercy of some powerful force.

Dementia praecox An obsolete medical model term that preceded the term *Schizophrenia.*

Denial A defense mechanism, or coping mechanism, by which the mind refuses to acknowledge a thought, feeling, wish, need, or reality factor.

Denotative meaning A meaning that is in general use by most persons who share a common language.

Dependent life-styles Disruptive life style having the common characteristic of fearfulness. In DSM-III includes Avoidant, Dependent, and Passive-Aggressive Personalities.

Depersonalization A dissociative phenomenon characterized by feeling of strangeness or unreality of the self or the environment.

Desensitization A process in which a person is exposed serially to a predetermined list of anxiety-provoking situations graded in a hierarchy from the least to the most frightening, with the goal of reducing the anxiety these situations cause.

Detached concern The ability to distance oneself in order to help others. Regarded as an essential personal quality in avoiding burnout, in values clarification, in ethical dilemmas, in using appropriate assertiveness, and in maintaining empathic abilities.

Detachment A behavior pattern characterized by general aloofness in interpersonal contact. manifestations may include intellectualization, denial, and superficiality.

Development The orderly and systematic unfolding of human potential in the growth of the organism, resulting from both inborn, hereditary, maturational factors and environmental influences.

Developmental crisis A crisis that occurs in response to the unique stress common to all persons in a particular period of human maturation and transition.

Developmental stages A series of normative conflicts or specific psychosocial tasks with which every person must deal. Developmental stages are a kind of timetable for personality development specifying the desirable rate of growth or accomplishment and favoring certain aspects of development at the expense of others.

Deviance Behavior characterized by marked differences in actions, morals, and attitudes from the usual social standards.

Digital language Verbal or discursive language; spoken words.

Disconfirmation A communication by one individual that rejects the other's view of self.

Disengaged families Families in which there is apathy, unresponsiveness, and a lack of relationship or connection among members.

Disintegrative life pattern A category of behavior traditionally called psychosis in psychiatric terminology. It is a life pattern characterized by disturbances in verbal and motor behavior that reflect disintegration of perception, thought, affect, and motivation.

Disorientation Impairment in the understanding of temporal, spatial, or personal relationships. Lack of awareness of the correct time, place, or person.

Displacement A defense or coping mechanism in which a person discharges pent-up feelings on persons less threatening than those who initially aroused the emotion.

Disqualification A communication that invalidates one's own communications or those of the other.

Disruptive life-styles (disruptive coping styles) Categories of behavior traditionally called *personality disorders, character disorders,* and *personality trait disturbances* in psychiatric terminology. The individual exhibiting this behavior is often society's "troublesome" member and is relatively free from the experience of anxiety or stress. In DSM-III includes eccentric or odd, dramatic or emotional, and anxious or fearful Axis II Disorders.

Dissociation   A coping mechanism that protects the self from a threatening awareness of uncomfortable feelings by denying their existence in awareness.

Dissociative coping patterns   Somewhat uncommon and bizarre responses to stress. They include Psychogenic Amnesia, Sleepwalking and Depersonalization Disorders, Psychogenic Fugue, and Multiple Personality.

Disturbed personal coping pattern   A category of behavior traditionally called *psychoneurosis* in psychiatric terminology. It is characterized by loss of ability to make choices, conflict, repetition, rigidity, ineffective solutions, alienation, feelings of being troubled and distressed, and secondary gain. In DSM-III includes the syndromes of Anxiety Disorders, Dissociative Disorders, Somatoform Disorders, and Affective Disorders.

Dominant emotional themes   Emotional themes that are repetitive. An individual who responds to many situations with the same feeling is narrowing his or her range of potential feelings.

Double bind   Two conflicting communications from someone who is crucial for a person's survival. One message is usually verbal and the other nonverbal.

Down's syndrome (mongolism)   A type of developmental disability with a complex of congenital deformities, including defective brain development and mental deficiency. It is characterized by an oriental appearance to the face, which gave rise to the name *mongolism.*

Drive   In psychoanalytic theory, an impulse to action arising in the id from the organism's biological and physiological needs and experienced in consciousness as a feeling, a fantasy, or a need to act. The libidinal and the aggressive drives are those primarily involved in psychological conflict. Personality theory uses the term *motivation.*

Drug abuse   A value-laden term; generally drug use that can cause legal, social, and medical problems.

Drug addiction   A state of chronic intoxication that is detrimental to an individual and that is produced by repeated consumption of a drug. The condition is characterized by (1) an overpowering need to take the drug, (2) a willingness to obtain the drug by any means including illegal ones, (3) a tendency to increase the dose, and (4) dependence on the affects of the drug.

Drug- and alcohol-dependent life-style   A disruptive life-style characterized by continued use of alcohol and drugs to the impairment of physical health, social relationships, and economic security.

Drug dependence   A condition in which a person (1) requires a certain drug to maintain his or her functioning, (2) develops a tolerance for it requiring increased doses, (3) develops physical withdrawal symptoms if the drug is stopped, and (4) psychologically feels that it is impossible to get along without the drug.

Drug use   Ingestion in any manner of a chemical that has an effect on the body.

DSM-III   Abbreviation for the 3rd edition of the Diagnostic and Statistical Manual of Mental Disorders published by the American Psychiatric Association in 1980.

Dualistic view of mind-body relations   A philosophical view that mind and body are separate phenomena that may be (1) causally interrelated, (2) parallel but independent, or (3) unrelated. This view is contrasted with the monistic view.

Dynamics   An explanation of forces (usually unconscious) that are presumed to be at work in a client and that result in the particular symptoms or manifestations observed.

Dystonic reactions   An early, dramatic, extrapyramidal reaction to treatment with antipsychotic medication occurring in the first days of treatment characterized by bizarre and severe muscle contractions usually of the face, tongue, or extraoccular muscles, producing torticollis, opisthotonas, and occulogyric crises. Readily reversible with the use of antiparkinsonian agents.

Eccentric life-styles   A disruptive life-style in which there is severe impairment in normal functioning. Includes Paranoid, Schizoid, and Schizotypal Personality Disorders.

Echolalia   Repetition of another person's words or phrases. Most frequently seen in Schizophrenia, particularly the catatonic types.

Echopraxia   Imitation of another person's movements. Most frequently seen in catatonic schizophrenia.

ECT (electroconvulsive therapy)   A treatment, generally for depression, that uses electric current to induce unconsciousness and convulsive seizures. It is a controversial treatment that raises ethical issues.

EEG (electroencephalogram)   A method of tracing and recording the electrical activity of the brain.

Ego   A theoretical construct of the organized part of the personality structure that includes defensive, perceptual, intellectual-cognitive, and executive functions. Conscious awareness resides in the ego, although not all operations of the ego are conscious.

Egocentric   Self-centered; preoccupied with one's own needs, and lacking in interest in others.

Ego-dystonic   Distressing to the individual. For example, disturbed coping patterns are said to be Ego-dystonic.

Ego functions   The functions of self-regulation, balance maintenance, and integrity preservation. They include perception, control of voluntary movement, management of memory, production of adaptive delay between perception and action, choice between "fight" or "flight," selection of needs to be gratified, judging and evaluating internal and external conditions, problem solving, learning, and reality testing.

Ego psychology A personality theory that places conscious emphasis on adaptation to external reality and enhanced understanding and knowledge of object relations, role performance, and interpersonal transactional relationships.

Ego-syntonic Not at odds with one's sense of self. For example, disruptive coping patterns are said to be ego-syntonic.

Electra complex Erotic attachment of a female child to her father.

Electrosleep therapy A treatment mode for schizophrenic, anxious, or depressed persons, in which low milliamperage, pulsed, unidirectional current is passed through electrodes placed over the orbits and mastoid processes. Sleep does not actually occur. Treatments are aimed at relieving anxiety, insomnia, and depression.

Elopement The departure or flight of a patient from a client psychiatric hospital without the consent of the staff.

Emotion See *Affect*.

Empathy The ability to feel the feelings of other people so that one can respond to and understand their experiences on their terms. It is differentiated from sympathy in that empathy does not contain elements of condolence, agreement, or pity.

Encounter group A form of sensitivity training that emphasizes experiencing individual relationships within the group and that minimizes intellectual and didactic input. The focus is on the present rather than the past or outside problems of group members.

Enmeshed families Families in which interactions are intense and focus on power conflicts rather than affection. The mother tends to be overcontrolling in such families.

Ennui A feeling of weariness and discontent resulting from satiety or lack of interest.

Epigenetic principle A concept adapted from embryology by Erik Erikson; the belief that physical and psychosocial growth are regulated innately in the capacities of the individual and arise in relation to others through social expectations.

Epilepsy A disorder characterized by periodic, recurring, short-lived disturbances of consciousness. It may have no apparent organic basis or it may be due to organic lesions.

Esalen encounter group An alternative therapy that emphasizes sensory awareness. Groups do structured exercises and focus on experiencing and deepening interpersonal relations. Members are encouraged to break free from social and muscular inhibitions, to experience their bodies in a different, richer sense, to emphasize doing, and to de-emphasize intellectual integration of experience.

est (Erhard seminar training) An alternative therapy in which clients are treated to a "standard training" seminar lasting from fifteen to eighteen hours each day for two consecutive weekends. Werner Erhard, its founder, describes the purpose of the training as transforming an individual's ability to experience living so that "situations you have been trying to change or have been putting up with clear up just in the process of life itself."

Ethics The principles of morality; the rules of conduct recognized in respect to a particular class of human actions.

Ethnic group A group of individuals who share an unique culture based on commonly accepted norms, standards or rules.

Ethnocentrism The belief that your own ethnic group is superior to others and is the one to which others should be compared.

Euthanasia The intentional termination of a life of such poor quality that it is considered not worth living.

Etiology Cause.

Exhibitionist A person who exposes his or her sexual organs to the opposite sex in situations where exposure is socially defined as inappropriate, for the purpose of his or her own sexual arousal.

Existential psychotherapy A type of therapy that emphasizes confrontation, primarily in the here-and-now interaction, and focuses on feeling experiences rather than rational thinking.

Expert power The power a person possesses as a result of having some special skill or knowledge.

Extended family All persons related by birth, marriage, or adoption to the nuclear family.

External crises Difficult situational events that may or may not be anticipated.

Facilitative communication Communication that aims at initiating, building, and maintaining fulfilling and trusting relationships with other persons.

Fairing Managing staff members' tasks by estimating one's fair share, a concept developed in Wilson's research at Soteria House.

Family boundaries The limits that define who participates in the family system and how.

Family life chronology The equivalent of a family system's psychosocial history.

Family life-style A family's biased perception of the outside world and its automated means of coping with this world, designed to uphold particular images of the family.

Family myths A series of fairly well integrated beliefs shared by all family members, concerning each other and their positions in the family, that go unchallenged despite their distortions of reality.

Family themes A family's perceptions of its history and origins.

Family therapy Psychotherapy in which all, or almost all, members of a family system participate at once.

Family time line A family genealogy or tracing that serves as a limited means for understanding a family's roots.

Fantasy A defense mechanism that is a sequence of mental images, like a daydream. It may be conscious or unconscious. It is considered by some to be an individual's attempt to resolve an emotional conflict.

Feedback The process by which performance is checked and malfunctions corrected; a regulatory function in the communication process, requiring two persons—one to give it and one to receive it.

Fellatio Mouth to penis sexual activity; oral stimulation of the male genitals.

Fetish A material object that embodies special meaning or mysterious and awesome qualities for a person, often linked with feelings of pleasure.

Fixation The arrest of psychosexual development at any stage before complete maturation; Sigmund Freud's term for a person's overemphasis or dependence on a childish tendency.

Flashbacks Either visual distortions (intense colors, trails, seeing geometric forms in objects), or an experience of reliving intense emotions that occurred during a previous drug experience, while under the effects of a hallucinogenic drug.

Flatness of affect A dull or blunt emotional tone attached to an object, idea, or thought. It is most frequently observed in schizophrenic disorders.

Flight of ideas A state in which thoughts come so quickly and bring so many associations that no single thought can be clearly expressed. The person's ideas occur in a rapid and endless variety, with only a single, slim thread connecting them.

Flow chart A diagrammatic way of illustrating the occurrence of and relationships among different events in a system. It is used with the problem-oriented medical recording system to highlight recurring events.

Folie à deux A condition in which two closely related people exhibit nearly identical psychopathological conditions.

Forensic psychiatry The branch of psychiatry that deals with the legal aspects of psychiatric disorders.

Free association A psychoanalytic technique whereby a patient says whatever comes to mind.

Fugue A state in which the individual completely forgets past life and associations but is unaware of this and may wander far from home for days at a time.

Functional Having a psychological rather than an organic (physical) cause.

Functional Adaptation/Self-Care Model of Nursing A nursing model, originated by Orem (1971) and adapted for psychiatric clients by Underwood (in press), that guides nurses in using nursing processes to help clients establish, maintain, or increase self-care and self-determination in day-to-day living. Useful in helping the nurse minimize the institutionalizing effects of psychiatric care and psychiatric disability.

Gender identity The psychological state in which a person comes to believe "I am female" or "I am male"; the first stage in gender development.

Gender role The socially accepted characteristics and behaviors for a given biological gender to learn and perform.

General Adaptation Syndrome (GAS) The objectively measurable structural and chemical changes produced in the body when stress affects the whole body. The GAS occurs in three stages: (1) alarm, (2) resistance, and (3) exhaustion.

General systems theory A conceptual framework that can be applied to living systems or people and that integrates the biological and social sciences logically with the physical sciences.

Genuineness The ability to be real or honest with another; closely related to respect.

Gestalt therapy A type of psychotherapy that emphasizes treatment of the person as a whole—biological component parts and their organic functioning, perceptual configuration, and interrelationships with the outside world. Focuses on sensory awareness of here-and-now experiences rather than on past recollections or future expectations.

Goblet issues Issues of minor importance to a group but that serve the important function of helping members get to know each other and test one another out. They constitute a vehicle for "sizing up" people.

Grand mal epilepsy A seizure disorder characterized by tonic-clonic seizures with loss of consciousness. It may be preceded by an "aura" or special signs and sensations that signal a forthcoming seizure.

Grief work The work of mourning that can be identified as emancipation from bondage to the deceased, readjustment to the environment in which the deceased is missing, and formation of new relationships.

Grieving The process of separating from a highly valued person, place, object, or ideal. Successful grieving consists of three phases: shock and disbelief, developing awareness, and restitution or resolution.

Group Any two or more persons who are set off from others, either temporarily or permanently, by a special type of association.

Group psychotherapy Psychotherapy of several clients at the same time in the same session. It may emphasize examination of the interpersonal relationships of members of the group to see how they usually interact with others.

Groupthink The mode of thinking engaged in by persons who are members of a highly cohesive in-group in which uniformity and agreement are given such priority that critical thinking is impossible or unacceptable; term coined by Irving Janis.

Guilt An affect associated with self-reproach.

Hallucination A sensory impression in the absence of external stimuli that occurs during the waking state.

Hallucinogen A chemical that can produce delirium and defects in perception in human beings.

Hawthorne effect The phenomenon discovered from industrial psychology studies at a Western Electric plant in the 1920s that workers tend to respond with increased production to any kind of environmental change, even a change back to a former state that had a lower production rate.

Here-and-now approach A technique that focuses on understanding interpersonal and intrapersonal responses and reactions as they occur in the therapy session. There is little or no emphasis on past history and experiences.

Hidden agenda A personal goal, unknown to others, that is at cross-purposes with dominant group goals.

High-level wellness A condition characterized by energy, vitality, and zest for life. More than the absence of disease, high-level wellness is a state of complete physical, mental, and social well-being.

Holistic view The view that the "whole" is inextricably related and linked to each part. In psychiatric nursing, a holistic approach views a client as a complex organic whole with physical, mental, emotional, social, and cultural dimensions. Holistic life theory explains the life process as a total field of events in which the individual and the environment are engaged in a constantly changing interaction.

Homeostasis The principle that all organisms react to changing conditions in an effort to maintain a relatively constant internal environment.

Homosexual A person who engages in sexual relations with members of the same sex.

Hostility (aggressivity) Actual or threatened aggressive contact. It is generally differentiated from anger in that hostility is considered to be destructive in intent while anger may be a constructive expression.

Hot line A telephone crisis counseling service often used in crisis intervention centers to provide immediate contact between a person in crisis and a counselor.

Humanism A view of human beings that values the individual's freedom of choice. In psychiatric nursing practice, a philosophy of devotion to the interests of human beings wherever they live and whatever their status. It reaffirms the spirit of compassion and caring for others and constructively and wholeheartedly affirms the joys, beauties, and values of human living.

Humanistic symbolic interactionism A view of human beings founded on belief in the inherent value of the individual's freedom of choice and having as basic premises that (1) human beings act toward things on the basis of the meaning that the things have for them. (2) the meaning of things in life is derived from or arises out of the social interaction a person has with others, and (3) meanings are handled in and modified through an interpretive process by the person in dealing with the things he or she encounters.

Hyperactivity A state of increased rate of activity. It may include emotional lability and flight of ideas.

Hypochondriasis Exaggerated concern with one's physical health, not based on organic pathology.

Hystrionic life-style A disruptive life-style characterized by excitability, emotional instability, and self-dramatization. The individual seeks attention and frequently engages in superficial, seductive behavior.

Id A psychoanalytic construct: a completely unorganized reservoir of energy derived from a person's drives and instincts.

Ideas of reference A state in which a person believes that certain events, situations, or interactions are directly related to him or her.

Identification A defense mechanism in which a person incorporates the mental picture of an object and then patterns the self after that object.

Identity The "whole" of self-awareness, made up of experiences, memory, perceptions, emotions, and sensory input.

Identity confirmation The process of nurse–client interaction in which there is continuous mutual reassessment of the other. In social interactionist theory, personal identity is not considered a fixed product, but rather an entity that is constantly confirmed through interaction with others.

Illusions Misperceptions and misinterpretations of externally real stimuli. Visual and auditory illusions are much more common than tactile, olfactory, and gustatory illusions.

Immediacy A communication skill in which the nurse responds to what is happening between the client and the nurse in the here-and-now.

Imparting information A communication skill in which the nurse makes statements that give needed data to the client and therefore encourages further clarification based on additional input.

Impulsive behavior Behavior that appears to be unpredictable and unmotivated by observable events, situations, or interactions. The individual behaving impulsively is unable to exert socially expected controls and may be verbally or physically destructive, aggressive, or violent.

Impulsive life-style A disruptive life-style characterized by behavior patterns that are in conflict with society, frequently including criminal or violent acts.

Incest Sexual relations between blood relatives or members of same socialization unit other than husband and wife.

Inclusion need The interpersonal need to establish and maintain relationships with others with respect to interaction and association.

Incorporation A coping defense mechanism in which a person symbolically takes within the self the attributes of another person.

Individuation The developmental process whereby a person becomes aware of his or her uniqueness and distinctions from others.

Informational power The power a person possesses when group members believe he or she has access to information not available elsewhere that will be useful in accomplishing the group's goal.

Infracontrol Wilson's conceptual explanatory scheme conveying the basic social process of interaction that maintain social control in the Soteria House setting.

Inkblot test See *Rorschach test.*

Input One phase of a symbolic interactionist model of communication, in which a person is motivated through some stimulus, either external or internal, toward some goal that requires him or her to engage in a social relationship with another.

Insanity An obsolete medical term for psychosis or mental illness. It continues to be used in legal terminology.

Insight The ability to understand one's own motives, psychodynamics, and behavior.

Insulin therapy A treatment for schizophrenia, introduced by Manfred Sakel, now no longer used in major psychiatric hospitals. It consists of the production of coma, with or without convulsions, through the intra-muscular administration of insulin.

Intellectualization A defense mechanism in which intellectual processes are overused to avoid closeness or affective experience and expression. It is closely related to rationalization.

Intelligence The capacity to deal effectively with one's environment. It includes the ability to learn, to remember what is learned, to be flexible in applying previous learning to new situations, to think logically, and to reason abstractly.

Intelligence tests Instruments designed to measure intelligence. They may provide useful information particularly in evaluating the presence and degree of mental retardation. Commonly used intelligence tests include the Stanford-Binet test, the Wechsler Adult Intelligence Scale, and the Wechsler Intelligence Scale for Children.

Interaction process analysis (IPA) A verbatim and progressive recording of the verbal and nonverbal interactions between client and nurse within a given period of time.

Internal crises The anticipated crises of human development and maturation.

Interpersonal communication Communication that takes place between two persons and in small groups; person-to-person communication.

Interpersonal theory of psychiatry Harry Stack Sullivan's theory that the aim of psychiatry is to understand and correct a client's disturbed communication process in the context of a client–therapist relationship based on a reciprocal learning situation.

Intrapersonal communication A level of communication that occurs within the self, involving perceptions of self and others. It is primary to other levels of communication.

Intrapsychic Arising within the self; also referred to as *intrapersonal.*

Introjection A defense or coping mechanism in which one individual accepts another's values and opinions as his or her own.

Involuntary commitment The legal process by which a person is confined, without consent, to a mental hospital. There are three categories: (1) emergency, (2) temporary or observational, and (3) extended or indeterminate. Criteria vary from state to state.

Involutional psychosis Pre-DSM-III medical model diagnostic term for a disorder commonly characterized by insomnia, anxiety, depression, and sometimes paranoid ideas. It is generally first seen in individuals over forty-five years of age with no history of previous mental disorder, and it may be associated with menopause in women and climacteric in men.

Jacksonian epilepsy A seizure disorder characterized by focal or partial motor seizures. The seizure begins with twitching of a muscle group, often fingers, and progresses upward to the arm, neck, and head, often becoming a generalized seizure.

Johari Window A theoretical tool used to represent the total person in relation to other persons; a graphic model of awareness in interpersonal relations.

Judgment The capacity to anticipate the consequences of one's behavior and to eliminate behaviors that are ineffective. It involves the ability to behave appropriately in terms of external reality and is closely linked with reality testing.

Kinesics The study of body movement (for example, facial expressions, gestures, and eye movements) as a form of nonverbal communication.

Labeling A process of categorizing nonconforming behavior with a name that then serves to reinforce and stabilize that behavior. In Thomas Scheff's societal-reaction theory, mental illness is believed to be a label given to diverse forms of deviance that do not fit under any other explicit label, such as delinquency. Mental illness is thus viewed as a form of residual deviance, and labeling enters a person into the deviant role of mental client.

Labile   Unstable; characterized by rapid change. It is often used with reference to emotions.

Latent   Unconscious or unrevealed; below the surface but potentially able to achieve expression.

Learned helplessness (excessive dependence)   A condition in which a person attempts to establish and maintain contact with another by adopting a helpless, powerless stance.

Legacies   Tangible and intangible personal assets that give life substance and meaning.

Legitimate power   The power a person possesses when group members believe he or she has a right to have influence over them because of that person's position in the group or organization.

Lesbian   A female homosexual.

Lethality assessment   An attempt to predict the likelihood of suicide, in order to guide the helping person's behavior. It may be used to decide whether to hospitalize a suicidal person and what alternatives the person has other than suicide.

Libido   In psychoanalytic theory, the sexual drive.

Life cycle   According to Erikson, stages through which each individual must progress in the attempt to attain psychosocial maturity.

Life review   A process of reviewing painful and disappointing life events, ventilating feelings, sharing another's perspective, and modifying self-perception. Frequently used in mental health counseling with the aged.

Life script   An unconscious life plan; term coined by Eric Berne.

Life-style   An enduring pattern of perceiving and functioning.

Limiting intrusion   Strategies for preventing problems with outsiders, discovered in Wilson's research at Soteria House.

Linking   A communication skill in which the nurse responds to the client in a way that ties together two events, experiences, feelings, or persons. It may be useful in connecting the past with current behaviors.

Lithium therapy   The treatment of manic or hypomanic states with lithium salts.

Local Adaptation Syndrome (LAS)   The manifestation of stress in a limited part of the body (for example, the body tissues that are directly subjected to stress in an infected wound).

Looseness of association   A phenomenon commonly observed in schizophrenic disorders whereby an apparent-ly unrelated experience or idea reminds a person of some other experience or idea.

Magical thinking   The belief that merely thinking about an event in the external world can cause it to occur. It is the consequence of regression to an early phase of development.

Manic-depressive Disorder   Medical model diagnostic term for a group of disintegrative reactions whose chief characteristic is mood swings, ranging from profound depression to acute mania, with periods of relative normality between psychotic episodes. Called Bipolar Affective Disorder in DSM-III.

Manipulation   A behavior pattern characterized by attempts to exploit, or actual exploitation of interpersonal contact.

MAO inhibitor (Monoamine oxidase inhibitor)   An agent that inhibits the enzyme monoamine oxidase (MAO), which oxidizes such monoamines as norepinephrine and serotonin. Some MAO inhibitors are highly effective as antidepressants.

Marital therapy   See *Couples therapy.*

Masochism   The derivation of erotic gratification from experiencing physical or mental pain.

Masturbation   Sexual gratification derived by oneself, usually by stimulation of one's own genitalia.

Maturational crises   Developmental crises; predictable life events or turning points that occur in most individual's lives.

Maximizer   In game theory, a person interested only in his or her own gain. (See *Cooperator* and *Rivalist.*)

Medical-biological model of psychiatry   A model based on classification that emphasizes systematic observation, naming, and classification of symptoms, and views emotional-behavioral disturbances as diseases like any other disease. Abnormal behavior is assumed to be directly attributable to a disease introduced from outside the body or an internally developed toxic biochemical.

Medical model approach to mental illness   The view of madness as an illness or disease process requiring treatment by medical personnel. This approach frequently is criticized for not taking into account the social, behavioral, economic, and cultural aspects of client and environment.

Megavitamin therapy   See *Orthomolecular medicine.*

Mental disorder   In DSM-III, conceptualized as a behavioral or psychological pattern that occurs in an individual and is associated with either a painful symptom (distress) or impairment in important areas of functioning (disability).

Mental health/human service worker   The newest addition to the roster of persons on the psychiatric team. Also known as "indigenous nonprofessionals" recruited in an attempt to bridge the gap between middle-class-oriented professionals and clients from lower socioeconomic or otherwise disadvantaged populations.

Mental mechanisms   See *Coping mechanisms.*

Mental Retardation   A developmental disability resulting in subnormal general intellectual functioning that may be evident at birth or may develop during childhood. Learning, social adjustment, and maturation are impaired, and emotional disturbance may be present.

Mental status examination   Usually a standardized procedure with the primary purpose of gathering data to determine etiology, diagnosis, prognosis, and treatment.

Metacommunication   A communication *about* a communication; the second level of communication—the relationship level—which says something about the relationship between the participants.

Mid-life crisis   The set of problems that arises when people discover visible signs that they are aging and become preoccupied with the notion of their own mortality. It frequently occurs between thirty-five and forty-five years of age. It is sometimes called an *authenticity crisis.*

Milieu   The social and cultural aspects of an environment that can influence the behavior of the persons in it.

Milieu therapy   Treatment that emphasizes appropriate socioenvironmental manipulation for the benefit of the client.

M'Naghten rules   The legal rules used in most English-speaking courts to determine whether a psychiatrically ill person is responsible for a criminal act he or she committed. It is based mainly on whether the person knew the "nature and quality" of the act and that doing it was "wrong."

Modeling   Setting a living example for a learner to follow; a way of transmitting values.

Mongolism   See *Down's syndrome.*

Monistic view of mind-body relations   The philosophical view that mind and body are one. It contrasts with the dualistic and the humanistic interactionist views.

Mourning   See *Grieving.*

Multiple personality   A dissociative pattern in which the person is dominated by two or more distinct personalities, each of which determines the person's behavior and attitudes during the period that it is uppermost in "consciousness."

Narcosynthesis   The interpretations or other psychotherapeutic interventions a therapist makes in narcotherapy while the client is under drug influence and may be more available for insight.

Narcotherapy   The use of intravenous barbiturates and stimulants to facilitate a client's expression of highly charged feelings.

Necrophilia   Having sexual relations with a corpse.

Neologism   A private, unshared meaning of a word or term. Neologisms are frequently characteristic of the language of schizophrenic individuals.

Networking   The use of any number of services and individuals to meet a person's needs.

Neurosis   A pre-DSM-III mental disorder characterized by anxiety. *(See Psychoneurosis.)*

Niacin Therapy   See *Orthomolecular medicine.*

Nonverbal communication   Communication between two or more people without the use of words. Facial expressions, gestures, and body postures are examples.

Norms   The set of unwritten rules of conduct or prescriptions of behavior established by members of a group.

Nosology   The study of diseases, particularly classification of diseases.

Nuclear family   A two-parent, time-limited, two-generation family, consisting of a married couple and their children by birth or adoption.

Nursing care plan   A means of providing nursing personnel with information about the needs and therapeutic strategy for each client. It may provide an ongoing, up-to-date record of goal-directed individual nursing care, when source-oriented recording methods are used. When problem-oriented recording methods are used, the nursing plan may be an outgrowth of the record.

Nursing diagnosis   The conceptualization of a client's need, problem, or situation from the unique perspective of the theoretical constructs in the discipline of nursing.

Nursing history   The foremost method of collecting data from the primary source (the client). Differs from medical or psychiatric histories in that they focus on client's perception and explanation related to their illness, hospitalization and care.

Nursing process   The conscious, systematic set of cognitive behavioral steps that comprise the clinical act in nursing practice.

Object language   Messages conveyed intentionally and unintentionally by the display of material things, such as the clothing and jewelry a person wears.

Object relation   The emotional attachment one person has for another as opposed to feelings for oneself.

Obsession   A persistent idea, thought, or impulse that cannot be eliminated from consciousness by logical effort.

Obsessive-compulsive life-style   A disruptive life-style characterized by overconscientious, overmeticulous concern. The individual is exceedingly conformist, is rigid in viewpoint, adheres to strict standards, and is prone to self-doubt.

Occupational therapist   In mental health settings, a professional who uses manual and creative techniques to achieve desired interpersonal and intrapsychic responses from clients.

Oedipus complex   In psychoanalytic theory, a distinct group of associated ideas, aims, instinctual drives, and fears generally observed in children three to six years of age. The child's sexual interest is attached chiefly to the parent of the opposite sex and is accompanied by aggressive wishes and feelings for the parent of the same sex.

One-to-one relationship A mutually defined, collaborative, goal-directed client-therapist relationship for the purpose of crisis intervention, counseling, or individual pyschotherapy.

Ontological security A satisfactory development of "consciousness of the self"; similar to personal integration.

Oppression A destructive, depriving relationship or process among persons of unequal power.

Organicity Indicative of organic changes in the brain; for example, errors of judgment and memory, loss of coordination.

Orthomolecular nutrition (megavitamin therapy or niacin therapy) A popular approach to the treatment of schizophrenia, in which large doses of niacin (vitamin B_3, nicotinic acid) are administered to clients.

Overload In communication theory, sensory input that exceeds a person's tolerance level or capacity.

Overpersonal group members Persons who direct their efforts toward reaching a high degree of intimacy with all other group members.

Overt Open to view or knowledge; not concealed or secret.

Panic An acute, intense attack of anxiety associated with personality disorganization.

Paralanguage (paralinguistics) Aspects of verbal communication beyond or in addition to language itself, such as voice quality (pitch and range) and noises without linguistic structure (sobbing, groaning, laughing).

Paranoid life-style A disruptive life-style characterized by hypersensitivity, rigidity, suspiciousness, jealous envy, and self-importance. The individual tends to blame others and feel they have a malevolent intent. He or she feels mistreated and misjudged.

Paraphrasing An activity or communication skill in which the nurse restates what she or he has heard the client communicating. It offers an opportunity to test the nurse's understanding of what the client is attempting to communicate.

Parent ego state In transactional analysis theory, the ego state that incorporates the feelings and behaviors learned from parents or authority figures.

Parkinsonian syndrome A syndrome that may occur after a week or two of antipsychotic medication therapy characterized by masklike faces, resting tremor, general rigidity of posture with slow voluntary movement, and a shuffling gait. Treatable with an antiparkinsonian agent.

Passive-aggressive life-style A disruptive life-style characterized by use of passive behavior to express hostility. The behavior includes obstructionism, pouting, procrastination, stubbornness, and intentional inefficiency.

Patient Medical model term for a consumer of health services (See *Client*).

Patient stripping The procedures often accompanying admission to a hospital unit, in which clients are stripped not only of their customary roles and of the control of their own fates but of many of their personal possessions as well.

Pedophilia Sexual satisfaction gained by an adult from engaging in sexual activities with immature children.

Perception The experience of sensing, interpreting, and comprehending the world; a highly personal and internal act.

Perseveration A pattern of repeating the same words or movements despite apparent efforts to make a new response.

Personal change groups Groups that focus on helping members to develop more satisfying and adaptive life-styles and relationships. They emphasize the psychological and social content and the dynamics of interpersonal behavior.

Personality The accumulated, characteristic behaviors and thoughts unique to each individual. (See *Character*)

Personality Disorders Medical model diagnostic classification for patterns of chronic lifelong maladaptive behavior and occasional symptoms of psychotic or psychoneurotic disorders. (See *Disruptive life-styles*.)

Personality tests Instruments designed to measure personality characteristics. Many are called *projective tests*, because they evoke projection in the responses of the person being tested. Commonly used personality tests include the Rorschach test, the Thematic Apperception test (TAT), the Minnesota Multiphasic Personality Inventory (MMPI), the Draw-a-Person test, the Sentence Completion test, and the Bender-Gestalt test.

Personal space The "invisible bubble" of territory around a person's body into which intruders may not come.

Petit mal epilepsy A seizure disorder that originates in childhood, rarely having onset after the age of twenty. It is characterized by lapses of consciousness with twitching of facial muscles, lapses of consciousness with myoclonic twitches, and episodes of sudden loss of consciousness and muscle tone.

Phallic symbol Anything that represents the penis. Common phallic symbols include spears, knives, guns, mushrooms, and the Washington Monument.

Phantom experience The sensation of feeling a part of the body that is no longer there.

Phantom pain Perception of pain in a body part that has been surgically or accidentally separated from the body.

Phenothiazine derivative A compound derived from phenothiazine that is particularly known for its antipsychotic property. Phenothiazine derivatives are among the most widely used drugs in medical practice, particularly in psychiatry.

Phobia An intense fear of some situation not ordinarily associated with danger. The phobia causes the person to avoid the situation.

Play therapy Therapy used with children, usually of preschool and early latency ages. The child reveals problems on a fantasy level with dolls, toys, and clay. The therapist may intervene with explanations about the child's responses and behavior in language geared to the child's comprehension.

Pleasure principle In psychoanalytic theory, the tendency for the id to seek pleasure and avoid pain. The demands of the pleasure principle become modified by the reality principle and the individual thereby develops the capacity to delay immediate release of tension or achievement of pleasure.

Pointing A communication skill that calls attention to certain kinds of statements and relationships.

Pornography Commercial sexual depictions or live sexual displays.

Pragmatics of human communication The behavioral effects of human interaction; the interpersonal relation between communicators—a reciprocal process.

Preconscious In psychoanalytic theory, the mental events that can be brought into conscious awareness through an act of attention.

Premature ejaculation The condition in which a man ejaculates before the woman who is his sexual partner reaches orgasm.

Prescencing An infracontrol strategy whereby the presence of sufficient numbers of people provides tacit control capability, fosters expectations for self-control, and redefines behavior to some variation of normal, developed in Wilson's research at Soteria House.

Primary gain Gain a person derives from the function of a symptom itself. For example, a hysterical paralysis may provide primary gain to an individual who seeks punishment for unconscious misdeeds.

Primary impotence The condition of a man who has never been able to maintain an erection sufficiently to accomplish sexual intercourse.

Primary orgasmic dysfunction The condition of a woman who has never had an orgasm by any method.

Primary prevention Elimination of factors that cause or contribute to the development of disease.

Primary process thinking In psychoanalytic theory, a type of autistic mentation characteristic of dreams, psychosis, and early stages of life, in which logical thought processes, reality, and the restrictions of time and space are ignored.

Private meanings Word meanings that can be used to communicate with others only when agreement on what the word means is negotiated. The private meaning then becomes a shared meaning. Schizophrenic speech, for example, is often characterized by private, unshared language. (See *Neologism*.)

Problem-oriented recording A system of recording that organizes the same raw data as source-oriented recording into a comprehensive whole that can be used for assessment, planning, evaluation, research, and health care audit. It includes four elements: data base, problem list, initial plans, and progress notes. It is considered by many mental health professionals to be an improvement over the traditional source-oriented system.

Problem solving A specific form of intellectual activity used when an individual faces a situation he or she is unable to handle in terms of past learning. Problem-solving strategies are considered crucial in any psychotherapeutic endeavor. They consist of the following sequential steps: observation, definition, preparation, analysis, ideation, incubation, synthesis, evaluation, and development.

Process illumination Recognition, examination, and understanding of the here-and-now transactions between people.

Processing A complex and sophisticated communication skill in which direct attention is given to the interpersonal dynamics of the nurse-client experience. Process comments focus on the content, feelings, and behavior experienced within the nurse-client relationships.

Projection A defense or coping mechanism in which a person's own unacceptable feelings and thoughts are attributed to others.

Propinquity Geographical nearness; proximity.

Prostitution The sale of sexual services, most commonly by women to men.

Proxemics The study of the space relationships maintained by persons in social interaction, including the dimensions of territoriality and personal space.

Pseudomutuality An "as if" condition in which a family behaves as if it were a close and happy family, although the members do not form intimate bonds with one another as individuals.

Psychiatric aide A paraprofessional who provides much of the direct service to hospitalized persons. Paraprofessionals are also being trained for and used in community mental health settings. Most receive in-service training, although community college programs for mental health workers have recently been established.

Psychiatric audit A means of appraising the quality of care received by clients of mental health services. The client's chart may be reviewed and the quality of care required may be compared with actual practice.

Psychiatric clinical nurse specialist A graduate of a master's program providing specialization in the clinical area of psychiatric/mental health nursing. Clinical specialists in psychiatric settings provide individual, family, and group psychotherapy in inpatient, outpatient, community mental health, and private practice milieus. They also teach, consult, administer programs, and conduct research. Certification programs are established in New York and New Jersey and on the national level, through the American Nurses' Association.

Pyschiatric history   A traditional record, oriented to the medical model, designed to elicit information about an individual's previous psychiatric experiences and encounters. Information may be provided by family, friends, and others about the client, resulting in a variety of perceptions, which may differ greatly from those of the client.

Psychiatric nursing   A specialty within the nursing profession in which the nurse directs efforts toward the promotion of mental health, the prevention of mental disturbance, early identification of and intervention in emotional problems, and follow-up care to minimize long-term effects of mental disturbance.

Psychiatric nurse   According to the American Nurses' Association, a registered nurse in a psychiatric setting who possesses a minimum of a bachelor's degree.

Psychiatric social worker   A graduate of a two-year master's program in social work with an emphasis in the field of psychiatry. This professional's roles include counseling and psychotherapeutic work as well as dealing with the full range of social problems that clients and their families present.

Psychiatrist   A physician whose specialty is mental disorders or mental diseases. Certification in psychiarty is provided by the American Board of Psychiatry and Neurology. Generally, psychiatrists are responsible for diagnosis and treatment. They may be oriented to somatotherapy, psychotherapy, or community psychiatry.

Psychic determinism   In psychoanalytic theory, the tenet that none of human behavior is accidental, that emotional and behavioral events do not happen randomly or by chance. Each psychic event is believed to be determined by the ones that preceded it.

Psychoanalysis   A theory of human development and of human behavior, and a form of psychotherapy developed by Sigmund Freud and his followers. It is a form of insight therapy that relies on the technique of free association to explore the dynamic, psychogenic, and transference aspects of a client's personality.

Psychoanalyst   A physician who has undergone psychoanalytic training. Psychoanalysts are found primarily in private practice in large urban settings.

Psychoanalytic model of psychiatry   An approach founded by Sigmund Freud, holding that all psychological and emotional events are understandable. The meanings behind behavior are sought from childhood experiences that are believed to cause adult neurosis. Therapy in this model consists of clarifying the psychological meanings of events, feelings, and behavior and thereby gaining insight

about them. Psychoanalysis has emerged as a method of investigation, a therapeutic technique, and a body of scientific concepts and propositions.

Psychodrama   A form of group psychotherapy, developed by Jacob Moreno, that uses dramatic techniques and the language and setting of theatrical productions to achieve psychotherapeutic goals.

Psychogenic   Originating from psychological mechanisms, without an organic pathological condition.

Psychological tests   Tests that are generally administered and interpreted by clinical psychologists. There are two types: intelligence tests and personality tests.

Psychoneurosis (neurosis)   Traditional term for a psychological disorder in which maladaptive behavior patterns produce psychiatric distress for the individual. In DSM-III the neurotic disorders are included in Effective, Anxiety, Somatoform, Dissociative, and Psychosexual Disorders.

Psychopathic   In outdated medical model terminology, having an impulsive life-style.

Psychophysiological disorder   A physical illness that is strongly influenced by pyschological problems; called a *psychosomatic disorder* in earlier medical model terminology.

Psychosis   A state in which a person's mental capacity to recognize reality, communicate, and relate to others is impaired, thus interfering with the person's capacity to deal with life demands. (*See Disintegravtive life pattern.*)

Psychosocial assessment   A dynamic process that begins in the initial contact with the client and continues throughout the nurse-client experience. Its focus is on assessing the social and psychodynamic data gathered from interaction with the client rather than formulating a psychiatric diagnosis. Instead of adopting a medical model orientation, the psychosocial assessment is directed toward assessing the client's difficulties in living.

Psychosurgery   Surgical removal or distruction of brain tissue with the intent of altering behavior, even though there may be no direct evidence of structural disease or damage in the brain. Marked controversy about ethical and legal questions surrounds the use of this extreme method of treatment.

Psychotherapy   In a medical model framework, a form of treatment for psychiatric disorders characterized by a special relationship between the patient and a professional whose goal is to modify particular symptoms or patterns of behavior that are considered maladaptive by the client. In a humanistic framework, a special relationship between client and therapist through which they mutually define problem areas and negotiate goals for the client in an effort to increase the client's satisfaction in living

Psychotropic   Having an effect on the mind.

Public communication   Communication between a person and several other people, such as a public speech or communication through the mass media.

Questioning A very direct communication activity that may be useful when the nurse needs specific information from the client. There are two types: (1) open-ended questioning focuses on the topic but allows freedom of response, (2) closed-ended questioning limits the client's responses to yes or no. When used to excess, questioning acts to control the nature and extent of the client's responses.

Rape Forced sexual intercourse without the partner's consent. The legal definition of rape as a crime varies from state to state. A distinction is made between statutory rape, involving the seduction of a minor, and forcible rape, in which the victim is over eighteen years of age.

Rationalization A defense or coping mechanism in which a person falsifies experience by constructing logical or socially approved explanations of behavior.

Reaction formation A defense or coping mechanism in which unacceptable feelings are disguised by repression of the real feeling and reinforcement of the opposite feeling.

Reality principle In psychoanalytic theory, largely a learned ego function whereby people develop the capacity to delay immediate release of tension or achievement of pleasure. This is Sigmund Freud's term for the practical demands of society, which are often in conflict with the individual's own wishes.

Reality testing The ability to differentiate one's thoughts and feelings from the outside world. Psychological introspection is considered a sophisticated form of reality testing. Imparied reality testing results in opinions that are based not on validated experience but on emotional needs that block accurate perception of reality.

Reciprocal inhibition The technique of paring an anxiety-provoking stimulus with another stimulus that is associated with a feeling of opposite quality strong enough to suppress the anxiety.

Recreational therapist A health care worker who plans and guides recreational activities to provide socialization, healthful recreation, and desirable interpersonal and intrapsychic experiences.

Reductionism The belief that everything can be explained in terms of simple components; a psychological theory that reduces the scope of interest to atomistic phenomena; the opposite of a holistic approach.

Referent power The power a person has when other group members identify or want to be like him or her.

Reflecting A communication skill in which the nurse reiterates either the content or the feeling message of the client. In *content* reflection, the nurse repeats basically the same statement as the client. In *feeling* reflection, the nurse verbalizes what seems to be implied about feelings in the client's comment.

Registered nurse in psychiatric setting A registered nurse who may have received basic preparation in a diploma, associate degree, or baccalaureate program, who is a generalist, and who works in the specialized psychiatric setting. This nurse frequently provides the bulk of the nursing care to clients in inpatient settings.

Regression A coping mechanism whereby the individual reverts to earlier patterns of behavior.

Relating and regulating messages Nonverbal cues that tell others when to stop, start, revise, or limit an act.

Repeating messages Nonverbal cues that say the same thing as a verbal cue but in a different way; a gesture that repeats or accentuates a spoken idea.

Repression A coping mechanism in which unacceptable feelings were kept out of awareness.

Requesting illustration A communication skill in which the client is asked to give an example to clarify a meaning in order to help the nurse understand better.

Resistance All the phenomena that interfere with and distrupt the smooth flow of feelings, memories, and thoughts. In the traditional psychoanalytic sense, anything that inhibits the patient from producing material from the unconscious. Resistance is often cited by psychotherapists to "explain" unsuccessful treatment of a client.

Retardation of thought A condition in which thoughts come very slowly and are difficult to express. There may be such a dearth of thought that communications are monosyllabic. Mutism may be observed in severe retardation of thought.

Reversal A coping mechanism in which the person manifests an instinctual wish by the opposite action thought, or feeling; inversion.

Revolving door syndrome A term describing a pattern of short stay with rapid turnover and eventual repeated readmissions to a hospital under the community mental health movement.

Reward power The power an individual has if he or she can deliver positive consequences or remove negative ones in response to other members of a group.

Rivalist In game theory, a person interested only in defeating his or her partner. (See *Cooperator* and *Maximizer*.)

Role A pattern of behavior expected of an individual within a group.

Role playing A technique in family therapy or group therapy in which members act out the parts of other members.

Rorschach test (inkblot test) A personality test in which a person says whatever comes to mind as he or she looks at a series of ten standardized cards with inkblots on them. It is believed to reveal many aspects of the individual's personality structure and emotional functioning.

Sadism Sexual pleasure or erotic gratification derived from inflicting physical or mental pain.

Scapegoating The process in which one member of a family or group is blamed for misfortunes and problems.

The scapegoat is given the role of whipping post, draining off the family or group system's feelings of guilt and inadequacy.

Schema The internal representation of some specific action. Operational schema are mental structures of a high order. People do not usually acquire them until adolescence, when they become capable of abstract thinking.

Schismatic families Families involved in chronic strife and controversy, particularly between the parents.

Schizoid life-style A disruptive life-style characterized by withdrawal, daydreaming, and detachment. The individual appears shy, seclusive, solitary, and sensitive. Such a person is usually viewed by others as eccentric.

Schizophrenia Medical model diagnostic term for a disintegrative life pattern characterized by thinking disorder, withdrawal from reality, regressive behavior, poor communication, and impaired interpersonal relationships. Four symptoms ("the four A's") are considered classic: (1) disturbances in association, (2) flattened affect, (3) ambivalence, and (4) autism. The term is criticized by some mental health professionals as a "label" that tends to elicit the disturbed functioning from an individual over time.

Sculpting Building a living sculpture of a family based on a member's perceptions. The actual physical placement of members in postures and locations is used.

Secondary gain The social and psychological uses a client may make of symptoms, for example, gaining sympathy, psychological support, financial advantages, or special treatment by virtue of being labeled ill.

Secondary impotence A current inability to maintain or achieve an erection by a man with a history of past successful entries.

Secondary prevention The early detection and treatment of disease.

Security operation An interpersonal theory, a behavior that is used to avoid or lessen anxiety; analogous to *coping mechanism* and *defense mechanism*.

Selective inattention A filtering out of stimuli under conditions of moderate and severe anxiety.

Self-actualizing Defined by Abraham Maslow as making full use of one's talents and potentials; doing the best one is capable of doing.

Self-awareness A sense of knowing what one is experiencing. It is a major goal of all therapy, individual and group.

Self-concept A person's image of self, usually the conscious image.

Self-esteem The degree to which one feels valued, worthwhile, or competent.

Self-fulfilling prophecy A phenomenon in which an individual, through selective inattention, distorts his or her perceptions of another and then gradually develops man-

nerisms and behavioral traits that cause the other to relate to him or her as expected. The interpersonal distortion thus becomes self-perpetuating.

Self-system (self-dynamism) One of Harry Stack Sullivan's central concepts—that the self is a construct built out of the child's experience. It is made up of "reflected appraisals" learned in contacts with other significant people.

Senile Relating to, characterized by, or manifesting old age.

Separation anxiety An infant or child's fear and apprehension upon being removed from the parent figure. A parallel process occurs in the termination phase of a nurse-client therapeutic relationship, as the client relives the anxiety associated with childhood loss of the supportive figure.

Sex therapy The active treatment of sexual dysfunctions by a qualified therapist.

Shaping An intervention designed to change behavior emitted by a client.

Should system The proscriptions that are handed down to each individual, usually by parent figures. Examples are: "You should not talk back to your elders," "Girls should be neat and tidy," "Big boys don't cry." A person with a strong "should system" is likely to be anxious, rigid, and cautious in relationships with others.

Sibling rivalry Competition between brothers and sisters for parental affection.

Sick role An identity adopted by an individual as a "patient" that specifies a set of expected behaviors, usually of a dependent nature.

Significant Others Persons who are important to the client. They may be part of the client's support system and may be useful in time of stress.

Sign language Formalized gestures used to convey meaning.

Single parent family A two-generation family consisting of one parent and his or her offspring living together.

Situational crisis A crisis that occurs in response to stressful or traumatic external events.

Situational disorders Medical model classification for transient mental health disturbances that are not psychotic in nature. These disturbed reactions are considered to result from "overwhelming" environmental stress, although what is overwhelming may differ greatly from one individual to another. (Called Post Traumatic Stress Disorder in DSM-II)

Situational orgasmic dysfunction A condition in which a woman is able to have orgasms under certain conditions and at certain times but not others.

Skewed families Families who seem peaceful on the outside but maintain this peace because the parents have somehow reached a compromise concerning a serious personality problem in one of them. Children in these families may have to escape a world of insoluble conflicts.

SOAP   The style of narrative notes written in a problem-oriented system of recording; an acronym for *subjective* (the problem as perceived by the client), *objective* (clinical findings or observations), *assessment* (what the analysis and synthesis of the subjective and objective data suggest), and *plan* (proposed solutions for the identified problems).

Social-interpersonal model of psychiatry   A model of psychiatry whose advocates believe that crucial social processes are involved in the development and resolution of disturbed behavior. It focuses on the larger and more general context of deviant behavior and on the processes by which an individual comes to be labeled or identified as deviant.

Socialization   A complex process by which an individual acquires the skills to adapt to the demands and restrictions of society.

Social network   The natural social relationships that people have, in addition to the family, that can be mobilized as their support systems.

Social network therapy   An extended group therapy that brings together the friends, neighbors, relatives, fellow workers, etc., in a family's community.

Societal reaction theory   Thomas Scheff's theory that mental illness is a label given to certain behaviors that violate the rules of conduct imposed by various significant others. The focus for psychiatry, then, is on the interplay between the deviant and the audience—the person and the social context.

Sociodrama   An experiential technique in which a person acts out specific situations in a drama. Emphasis is on the commonalities in the social roles of people.

Sociopathic   Having an impulsive life-style. In medical model terminology, psychopathic.

Sociotherapy   A treatment mode emphasizing environmental, social, and interpersonal factors rather than intrapsychic factors.

Sodomy   Any sex act other than face-to-face coitus between a man and woman. The legal meaning varies from state to state.

Somatic delusion   The belief that one's body is changing and responding in some unusual way.

Somatic language   Statements mediated through the autonomic nervous system.

Somatoform Disorders   Disturbed personal coping pattern characterized by physical symptoms suggesting physical disorders for which there is no positive evidence of organic or physiological causes.

Somatotherapy   The treatment of emotionally disturbed or incapacitated clients by physiological means. (See *Biological therapies*.)

Somnambulism   Sleepwalking; a dissociated or fugue-like state in which the person moves about but appears to be asleep.

Source-oriented recording   A traditional method of recording health care data, consisting of a clinical record or chart with chronological notations made by individual health team members. This method is becoming less common with the increase in use of problem-oriented methods of recording.

Split personality   A condition in which a person shows two or more kinds of behavior; multiple personality; inaccurately used by laypeople to refer to schizophrenia.

Stanford-Binet Scale   A commonly used intelligence test for children, consisting of a series of tasks of increasing difficulty.

Stigma   A mark of disgrace; a stain or reproach. Often attached to persons known to have been treated for a mental disorder.

Stress   Stress or tension experienced by a person in a situation.

Stress-adaptation theory   A framework for understanding how individuals react to stress. Stressors may be physical, chemical, physiological, developmental, or emotional. Life itself is stressful in that it involves a process of adaptation to continual change. Though adaptation is stressful it is not necessarily harmful and can be exciting and rewarding.

Structuring   A communication skill directed toward creating order or evolving guidelines. A nurse may structure content or structure the parameters of the nurse-client relationship.

Sublimation   A coping mechanism in which unacceptable drives are diverted into personally and socially acceptable channels.

Substituting   In communication theory, use of nonverbal cues in place of words; for example, the award of a bouquet or roses to a performer to convey audience appreciation.

Substitution   A coping mechanism in which a person replaces an unacceptable wish, desire, emotion, or goal with one that is more acceptable.

Suicide   The taking of one's own life. It is considered destructive aggression turned inward.

Summarizing   A communication skill in which main ideas are highlighted. Summarizing reviews for client and nurse what the main themes of the conversation were. It is useful in helping the client to focus thinking.

Superego   A theoretical construct comprised of that organized part of the personality structure, mainly unconscious, that includes one's ego ideals and the "conscience" that criticizes and prohibits one's drives, fantasies, feelings, and actions.

Superficiality   Shallowness of contact, commonly considered a form of resistance against interpersonal intimacy.

Support system Elements in the environment that the client depends on in time of stress. They may be individuals (significant others) or material objects (such as home, financial assets, employment).

Suppression A defense or coping mechanism in which unacceptable feelings and thoughts are consciously kept out of awareness.

Symbolic interactionism A distinctive approach to the study of human conduct based on the premises that 1) human beings act toward things on the basis of the meaning that the things have for them, 2) the meaning of things in life is derived from the social interactions a person has with others, and 3) people handle and modify the meanings of the things they encounter through an interpretive process.

Symmetrical relationships Relationships based on maintaining equality between members. They allow for respect and trust but may deteriorate into competition.

System An identifiable set of components characterized by a boundary, with interaction and interrelationship among the components. Anything that affects one part of the system affects every other part and the system as a whole. The combined interrelationships constitute a meaningful whole, and the system is greater than the sum of its parts.

Tangential response An inappropriate response to a statement in which the content of the statement is disregarded. The reply is directed toward either an incidental aspect of the initial statement, the type of language used, the emotions of the sender, or another facet of the same topic.

Tardive dyskinesia A disorder characterized by involuntary movements of the face, jaw, and tongue, resulting in bizarre grimacing, lip smacking, and protrusion of the tongue. The syndrome frequently occurs after years of antipsychotic drug treatment.

Task-oriented groups Groups created to achieve specific ends or resolve specific problems. They emphasize substantive rather than affective content.

Territoriality The assumption of a proprietary attitude toward a geographic area by a person or a group.

Tertiary prevention The elimination or reduction of residual disability following illness.

Therapeutic Acting to heal or to cure; considered "good" for the client. In psychiatric settings, traditionally the staff, therapist, or agency has decided what is considered "good." In humanistic approaches this is negotiated between client and mental health worker.

Therapeutic alliance A conscious relationship between a helping person and a client in which each implicitly

agrees that they need to work together to help the client with personal problems and concerns.

Therapeutic communication A theory developed by Jurgen Ruesch, defining communication as all the processes by which one individual influences another.

Therapeutic intimacy A therapeutic communication requiring high involvement and commitment in which the participants move beyond superficial social responses into meaningful areas of concern for the client. A major focus is the developing relationship between nurse and client.

Thought disorder A condition in which associations tend to lose their continuity so that thinking becomes confused, bizarre, incorrect, and abrupt.

Time line A visual representation of the family as a dynamic system of interrelationships. Family therapists use time lines in the assessment of families to communicate the impact of events on the family system.

Tranquilizing drug A drug that depresses central nervous system function in a highly selective manner, exerting a calming effect without appreciably impairing the person's level of awareness. *Major tranquilizer* is synonymous with *antipsychotic drug.*

Transactional analysis (TA) A system introduced by Eric Berne that has four components: (1) structural analysis of intrapsychic phenomena, (2) transactional analysis proper, (3) game analysis, and (4) script analysis. TA is used in both individual and group psychotherapy.

Transcendental Meditation (TM) A learned meditation technique originally stimulated by the Maharishi Mahesh Yogi. In TM a person may sit with eyes closed for two twenty-minute sessions every day, concentrating on a *mantra.* The objective is to relieve tension and to improve bodily feeling and interpersonal relationships.

Transference In psychoanalytic theory, considered an unconscious phenomenon in which feelings, attitudes, and wishes originally linked with significant figures in one's early life are projected onto others who have come to represent these figures in one's current life.

Transsexual An individual who engages in sexual relationships with members of the same biological sex and who feels he or she is trapped in the body of the wrong sex.

Transvestite An individual who dresses in the clothes of the opposite sex.

Trauma Injury; in psychiatric terms, a noxious state of any duration in which a person feels overwhelmed with stimuli that he or she cannot master and control.

Triangle An interpersonal interaction involving three people, diagrammed as the points of a geometric triangle.

Triangulation A process in which two of the three individuals in a triangle are in a close, cozy relationship while the third is kept at a distance or left out. Triangulation is dysfunctional, because interpersonal issues are "solved" by shifting the closeness or distance among members rather than by working the problem out.

Tricyclics The most commonly used class of antidepressant drugs. Tricyclics are close in chemical structure to the phenothiazines and have many similar side effects, but they have profoundly different effects on mood, behavior, and cognition. They are not antipsychotic when given to Schizophrenic clients and may aggravate a psychosis.

Unconflicted member (independent member) A group member who is able to assess situations and alter roles or behavior appropriately.

Unconscious In psychoanalytic theory, mental processes of which the individual is unaware.

Underload In communication theory, insufficient information, which interferes with an individual's ability to comprehend the message of the other.

Undoing A compulsive act that is performed in an attempt to prevent or counteract the consequences that the client irrationally anticipates from a frightening obsessional thought or impulse.

Vaginismus An involuntary tightening or spasm that occurs in the outer third of the vagina. It can be severe enough to make sexual intercourse impossible.

Values Concepts of the desirable; what is of worth to an individual. Values influence the way people behave.

Values clarification A systematic method of teaching the process of valuing. Its strategies and exercises engage the learner in becoming aware of personal beliefs and values, choosing among alternatives, and matching stated beliefs with actions.

Verbal communication The sharing of thoughts, feelings, and attitudes with others through speech.

Voluntary commitment The legal process by which a person chooses to be admitted to a mental hospital. It requires written application by the person or by someone acting in his or her behalf, such as a parent or guardian.

Voyeur An individual who receives principle erotic gratification from clandestine peeping.

Waxy flexibility (cerea flexibilitas) A condition in which a person tends to hold for long periods of time any anatomical position in which he or she is placed. Most frequently seen in catatonic schizophrenics, withdrawn subtype.

Wernicke-Korsakoff syndrome A syndrome usually associated with alcoholism and characterized by confusion, disorientation, and amnesia with confabulation.

Withdrawal A behavior pattern characterized by avoidance of contact. It may be functional or dysfunctional in nature. Withdrawal may be avoidance of interpersonal relationships and/or of a sense of reality.

YAVIS syndrome An acronym describing therapist's documented preference for *young, attractive, verbal, intelligent* and *successful* clients.

Zoophilia See *Bestiality*.

INDEX

Abdellah, Faye, 75, 76
Abstract thinking, mental status
    examination and, 190
Abuse, of aged, 643-44
Accentuation, in communication, 112
Acceptance
    psychiatric nursing practice and, 51-52
    in treating disturbed children, 545-46
Accommodation, in Piagetian theory,
    241-42
Accountability, autonomy and, 85
Acetaminophen, interactions with alcohol,
    656
Acetohexamide, interactions with alcohol,
    656
Acetylcholine, psychotic conditions and,
    424
Ackerman, Nathan, 12, 612, 615
Act, communication as, 107
Acting in, therapeutic relationship and,
    167-68
Acting out
    adolescent, 578
    sexual, consultation and, 720-21
    therapeutic relationship and, 166-67
Action language, 113
Active euthanasia, 92
Active values, 47
Acupressure, 775
Acupuncture, 775
    for psychogenic pain, 368
Acute catatonic excitements,
    electroconvulsive therapy and, 692
Acute dystonic reactions, antipsychotic
    drugs and, 673
Acute intermittent porphyria, organic
    brain syndromes and, 485
Adaptation
    health as, 248
    in Piagetian theory, 241
    stress, 239-40
Adaptation theory, 78
Adaptive functioning, rating scale of,
    202-3
Addicted life-style, 381, 386-94
Addiction, stereotyping and, 91
Addiction group therapy, 740-41
Addison's disease, 468
    organic brain syndromes and, 483,
    485-86
    recent weight loss and, 191
Adjustment disorder, treatment of, 679
Adler, Alfred, 11, 28, 29, 33, 36, 216

Adolescence
    acting out in, 578
    authority figures and, 5
    definition of, 566
    developmental theories of,
    568-72
    emotional development in, 568
    identity formation in, 569-70
    mental development in, 567
    normative process of, 566-68
    Oedipal conflict in, 568-69
    physical and sexual development in,
    566-67
    psychosocial development of,
    comparative chart of, 573
    satisfactory genital activity and, 572
    social development in, 567-68
    suicide in, rate of, 764
Adolescent
    anger and hostility of, 583-85
    anxiety and resistance of, 581-83
    nursing care plan for, 583
    communication with, 580
    dietary problems of, 589
    drug use and abuse by, 589-91
    homosexuality v. heterosexuality and,
    587-89
    hospitalization of, 574-79
    juvenile delinquency and, 591-92
    outpatient treatment of, 573-74
    scapegoating and, 585
    nursing care plan and, 586
    sexual behavior of, 579-80, 585-89
    suicide and, 592-600
    testing of limits by, 580-81
    nursing care plan and, 582
    in therapeutic communities, 577-78
Adolescent parents, 331-32
Adoptive parents, 326-27
Adrenal corticosteroids, arthritis and,
    463
Adrenocorticotrophic hormone, alarm
    reactions and, 258
Adulthood
    consolidation in, 240
    mid-life crisis and, 262-64
Advocacy, symbolic interactionism and,
    6-7
Affect
    assessment of, 160-61
    disintegration of, 407, 411
    interventions in, 438-40
    mental status examination and, 188

Affection
    interpersonal needs and, 503-4
    sex and, 317
Affective disorders, 369-77 (See also
    Bipolar affective disorder)
    biochemistry and, 20
    diagnosis of, social class and, 90
    electroconvulsive therapy and, 692
    mental status examination and,
    192-93
    organic, 484
    sex and, 317
    treatment of, 688-90
Affective education, 748
Affiliation, for depressed clients, 372-76
Age
    assessing lethality in suicide and, 291
    diagnosis and treatment and, 764
Aged (See also Old age)
    attitudes toward, 638-39
    sources of, 639
    care of, intervention in, 652-62
    habits and strengths of, 635
    needs of, 635-36
    Maslow's hierarchy and, 637
    personal revelation promotion among,
    639
    psychic distress of, 649-51
    family reactions to, 651-52
Aggressivity, intervention in, 170-71
Aggressor, 224
Aging
    developmental tasks of, 636-38
    disorders of, genetic factors in, 20
    fear of, 640
    physical and neural changes in, 635
    problems of, reactions to, 644-49
    sex and, 317
    stresses of, 640-44
Agitation, akathisia v., 673-74
Agoraphobia, 360
Agranulocytosis, antipsychotic drugs and,
    675
Aguilera, D., 704
Aid to Families with Dependent Children
    (AFDC), 325, 328
Akathisia, 673-74
    agitation or psychotic relapse v., 674
Akineton (See Biperiden)
Al-anon, 519
Alarm reaction, general adaptation
    syndrome and, 258-59
Al-a-teen, 519

Alcohol
  acute intermittent porphyria and, 485
  adolescent abuse of, 589-90
  drug interactions with, 656-57, 678
  effects of, 593-94
  Korsakoff's syndrome and, 488
  organic brain syndromes and, 484
  Wernicke's encephalopathy and, 491
Alcohol addiction, 386-90 (See also
    Alcoholism)
Alcohol detoxification, antianxiety drugs
    in, 690
Alcoholic cirrhosis, organic brain
    syndromes and, 487
Alcoholics, personality traits of, 388
Alcoholics Anonymous, 390
Alcohol intoxication, unsteady gait and,
    191
Alcoholism
  aged and, 651
  erection difficulties and, 299
  incest and, 310
  intervention in, 388-90
  oral fixation and, 25
  orthomolecular psychiatry and, 736
  self-help groups for, 519
  sex and, 317
  transactional analysis and, 737
Aldosterone, alarm reactions and, 258
Alertness, paranoid personality and, 399
Alexander, Franz, 15, 459, 700, 701,
    731
Algorithms, 207
  for depression, 372, 373-76
  suicide intervention and, 291
Alien control, delusions of, mental status
    examination and, 188
Alienation
  disconfirmation and, 116
  medieval, 8-9
Aliphatics, 670
Allergy
  antidepressant drugs and, 680
  antipsychotic drugs and, 675
  interventions in, 469
  psychophysiological, 463-64
Alliance for the Preservation of Religious
    Liberty, 780
Allport, G. W., 585
Alpha consciousness, 743
Alternative family, 607-8
Alternative therapies
  addiction group, 740-41
  Arica, 741-42
  assertiveness training, 740
  assessment of, 750-52
  bioenergetics, 734-35
  biofeedback, 737
  body-mind integration in, 731-32
  comparative analysis of, 745-50
  confrontation problem-solving, 741
  devaluation of intellect in, 731
  direct decision, 741
  discovery of real self in, 730-31
  effectiveness of, 751-52
  encounter marathon groups, 737-38

Alternative therapies (continued)
  Erhard Seminar Training (est), 742
  Eriksonian hypnosis, 744
  gestalt, 735-36
  Living Love, 742
  Morita, 738
  neurolinguistic programming, 744-45
  open encounter groups, 738
  orthomolecular nutrition, 736
  premises of, 730-33
  primal scream, 733-34
  psycho-imagination, 741
  psychosynthesis, 739
  rational-emotive, 739-40
  reality, 738-39
  relevance of, 749-52
  Rolfing, 734
  self-regulation and responsibility in,
    732-33
  sex, 740
  Silva Mind Control, 743-44
  therapeutic touch, 736-37
  Transactional Analysis, 737
  Transcendental Meditation, 742-43
Alternative therapies movement
  humanistic and existentialist influences
    on, 729
  social change and, 728-29
Altshul, A., 144
Alzheimer's disease, 648
  organic brain syndromes and, 490
Ambivalence
  disintegration of motivation and, 413,
    442
American Association of Mental
    Deficiency, 471
American Civil Liberties Union, 780
American Family Foundation of
    Destructive Cultism, 782
American Group Psychotherapy
    Association, 216
American Indians, folk systems of, 775-76
American Nurses' Association, 55, 65,
    141, 709, 768, 820
  standards of, 66-73, 824, 836-37
American Psychiatric Association, 10, 19,
    140, 197, 313, 345, 411, 471, 533,
    534, 535, 767, 793
  Diagnostic and Statistical Manual of
    (See DSM-III)
American Psychological Association, 768
American Society of Group
    Psychotherapy and Psychodrama,
    216
Amini, F., 577, 580
Aminoaciduria, 471, 472
Amitriptyline
  for anxiety attacks, 684
  for depression, 678, 680
  interactions with alcohol, 656
Amnesia
  postconcussional, differentiation of,
    366
  psychogenic, 364
    differentiation of, 366
Amnestic disorder, alcohol-induced, 488

Amnestic syndrome, organic, 484
Amobarbital
  effects of, 595
  narcotherapy and, 694
Amphetamines, 394
  effects of, 594-95
  for depression, 677, 679, 684
  for hyperactivity, 684
  interactions with alcohol, 657
  organic brain syndromes and, 484
Amputation clubs, 519
Amputees, phantom experiences and,
    283
Amyotrophic lateral sclerosis, organic
    brain syndromes and, 486
Amytal (See Amobarbital)
ANA Standards, 836-37
  community mental health and, 824
Anaclitic depression, hospitalized child
    and, 555
Anaclitic therapy, 575
Anal intercourse, 307
Anal sadism, 26
Anal stage
  in childhood development, 529
  psychoanalytic theory and, 25-26
Analgesics, interactions with alcohol, 656
Analysis, problem solving and, 162
Analytic group psychotherapy, 518
Andry, R. G., 572
Anencephaly, 474
Anesthesia
  antipsychotic drug interactions with,
    678
  perinatal retardation and, 475
Anesthetics, interactions with alcohol, 656
Anger, adolescent, 583-85
Angina pectoris, 462
Anima/animus, Jungian theory and, 12
Anorexia nervosa, 465-66, 589
  nursing care plan for, 590-91
Anthony, E. J., 216
Antialcohol preparations, interactions with
    alcohol, 656
Antianginal drugs, interactions with
    alcohol, 656
Antianxiety drugs, 688-90
  antipsychotic drugs v., 688
  effects of, 688-89
Anticipatory guidance
  body image crises and, 283
  post-traumatic stress disorder and, 287
Anticonvulsants
  antipsychotic drug interactions with,
    678
  interactions with alcohol, 656
Anticult groups, 782
Antidepressant drugs, 14, 676-84
  antipsychotic drug interactions with,
    678
  clinical considerations and, 677
  for depression, 424
  interactions with alcohol, 656
  overdose and, 680
  side effects of, 681
  tricyclics, 677-82

Antidepressant drugs (continued)
  dosages of, 678-80
  side effects of, 680-82
Antidiabetic agents, interactions with
    alcohol, 656
Antihistamines
  for anxiety, 689-90
  interactions with alcohol, 656
Antihypertensives, interactions with
    alcohol, 656
Anti-infective agents, interactions with
    alcohol, 656
Antimania drug (*See* Lithium carbonate)
Antimicrobial agents, interactions with
    alcohol, 656
Antiparkinsonian drugs, 673
  for acute dystonic reactions, 673
Antipsychotic drugs, 14, 669-76
  allergic effects of, 675
  antianxiety drugs v., 688
  autonomic nervous system effects of,
    672-73
  blood, skin, and eye effects of, 675
  choice of, 669-71
  dopaminergic receptors and, 20
  dosage of, 670-71
  drug interactions with, 678
  endocrine effects of, 675
  extrapyramidal effects of, 673-74
  major effects of, 669
  for schizophrenia, 669, 671-72
  side effects of, 677
Antisocial life-style, 381
Anxiety
  adolescent, 581-83
    nursing care plan for, 583
  aged and, 649
  castration, 27
  change and, 250
  conflict and, 349
  conversion disorder and, 366-67
  cues to, 350
  degrees of, 349-50
  disorders associated with, 191
  disturbed coping patterns and, 349-51
  fear v., 350
  inappropriateness and, 266
  intellectualization and, 257
  operational definition of, 351
  phobic disorders and, 360
  separation, hospitalized child and, 555-56
  sources of, 351
  specificity model of, 700-1
  thought disintegration and, 407
  treatment of, 688-90
Anxiety attacks, treatment of, 684
Anxiety disorders
  childhood, 534-35
  intervention in, 356-59
  nursing care plan for, 359
  symptomatology of, 357
Apollonian principles, 650
Appearance
  diagnostic implications of, 191
  in mental status examination, 187

Approach-avoidance conflict, 348
Appropriateness, in communication,
    113-14
Areiti, S., 165
Argyle, Michael, 111
Arica, 741-42, 748
Arica Institute, 742
Aristotle, 86
Aroskar, Mila A., 85, 86
Artane (*See* Trihexyphenidyl)
Arthritis
  interventions in, 469
  psychophysiological, 463
Arthur, R., 702
Artifacts, communication and, 112
Art therapy, 551-52
Art therapy groups, 521
Asceticism, in adolescence, 569
Asian Americans
  counseling of, ethnic identity guide for,
    779
  folk systems of, 774-75
Aspirin, interactions with alcohol, 656
Assagioli, Roberto, 739
Assertiveness, 49
Assertiveness training, 740
Assessment, 160-61
  of affective disorders, 372-76
  behavioral, 161
  of childhood emotional disturbances,
    540-44
  cognitive, 161
  emotive, 160-61
  in family therapy, 617-20
  of manic behavior, 376-77
  neurological, 191
  nursing process and, 66-67
  of organic brain syndromes, 482
  of parent-child fit, 338-39
  of parenting skills, 334-36
  physiological, 190-91
  psychosocial, 185, 204-5
  sex counseling and, 318
  of small groups, 510
Assimilation, in Piagetian theory, 241
Association of Medical Superintendents of
    American Institutions for the Insane,
    793
Assumptive world, 760
Asthma, psychophysiological, 463
Asymmetry, diagnostic implications of,
    191
Atarax (*See* Hydroxyzine)
Atherosclerosis, organic brain syndromes
    and, 486-87
Atopic dermatitis, psychophysiological,
    463
Attachment, 323
Attention deficit disorders
  with hyperactivity, 534
  treatment of, 684
Attitude, definition of, 46
Attitudes, toward aged, 638-39
Attneave, L., 612
Attraction, group cohesion and, 228

Auras, 735
Authenticity, one-to-one relationships and,
    142-43
Authority
  decision making and, 225
  destructive obedience to, 233-34
  difficulty with, phallic stage of
    development and, 27
  group analysis and, 504-7
Authority figures, adolescent hostility
    toward, 5
Autism
  characteristics of, 531
  etiology of, 531-32
  nursing care plan for, 537-39
  schizophrenia and, 418
Autistic thought, 407
Autoimmune disease, organic brain
    syndromes and, 486-87
Autonomic nervous system
  antipsychotic drugs and, 672-73
  organs innervated by, 352
  responses to anxiety, 351
Autonomy
  development of, in adolescence, 570
  developmental life phases theory and,
    242
  professional accountability and, 85
  in transactional analysis, 737
Availability, psychiatric nursing practice
    and, 51
Aventyl (*See* Nortriptyline)
Avoidance
  phobic disorders and, 360
  stress and, 353
Avoidance-avoidance conflict, 349
Avoidant disorders, childhood, 534
Avoidant life-style, 381
Awareness, grieving process and, 279-80

Bach, George, 737
Bachrach, L. L., 13, 827, 830
Bacterial infections, organic brain
    syndromes and, 486
Bad trips, 394-95
Baez, Joan, 313
Bandler, R., 744
Barbiturates, 394, 692
  acute intermittent porphyria and, 485
  antipsychotic drug interactions with,
    678
  cerebral functioning in the aged and,
    672
  effects of, 595
  for insomnia, 691
  interactions with alcohol, 656
  organic brain syndromes and, 483, 484
Barns, E., 658
Barometric events, group analysis and,
    507
Barsky, A., 721, 722
Bartholin's glands, 297
Basque, L., 170
Bassuk, E. L., 827
Batemen, D. E., 701

Bates, B., 193
Bateson, Gregory, 12, 427, 612, 616
Battered women, 284-85
Bay of Pigs, 230
Bazelon, David, 798
Beavin, J., 115, 116, 611
Becker, Howard, 32, 266, 392
Bedlam, 790
Bedwetting, 533
Beers, Clifford W., 11
Behavior
    developmental model of, 265-66
    disturbed, aged and, 644-45
    family, 610-11
    impulsive, disintegration of motivation
        and, 412, 442-44
    in mental status examination, 187
    ritualistic, autism and, 531
    unexplained change in, risk of suicide
        and, 291
    violent, disintegration of motivation
        and, 442-44
Behavior modification, 89
    for disturbed children, 553-54
    for eating disorders, 469
    for psychogenic pain, 368
    for psychophysiological allergy, 469
Behavior patterns, intervention strategies
        in, 168-75
    summary of, 176-80
Behavior theory, psychosis and, 426-27
Behavioral assessment, 161
Behavioral disorders, in childhood,
        533-34
Behaviorism, family therapy and, 612
Behaviorist model
    assumptions of, 30-31
    critique of, 32
    psychiatric nursing practice and, 31-32
Beliefs
    about mental illness, 46
    types of, 45
Bell, John, 12
Bell, Norman W., 616
Belli, Melvin, 638
Belmaker, R. H., 418, 420
Benadryl (*See* Diphenhydramine)
Bender-Gestalt Test, 197, 198, 477
Benedict, Ruth, 12
Benfer, B., 165
Bennis, Warren, 504-5, 507, 516
Benzedrine (*See also* Amphetamines)
    effects of, 594
Benzodiazepine agents, for
        psychophysiological cardiovascular
        disorders, 469
Benzodiazepines, 692
    for alcohol detoxification, 690
    for anxiety, 689-90
    cerebral functioning in the aged and,
        672
    for insomnia, 690-91
    interactions with alcohol, 657
Benztropine, 673
    for acute dystonic reactions, 673

Berkman, L., 659
Berman, Ellen M., 628
Berne, Eric, 116, 117, 737
Bestiality, 310
Beta consciousness, 743
Bethlehem Hospital, 790
Betrayal funnel, 400
Betts, V., 73
Bibliotherapy groups, 521
Bicêtre, 10
Bierer, J., 216
Biggs, J., 763
Bilateral oophorectomy, sexual difficulties
        associated with, 315
Biochemistry, psychiatric, 20
Bioenergetics, 734-35, 748
Bioethics, principles of, 87, 88
Biofeedback, 737
Biofeedback training, for
        psychophysiological allergy, 469
Biological imperative, gender identity and,
        308
Bioperiodicities, 20, 21
Biorhythms, 20-21
    restlessness and, 21, 22
    spectrum of, 21
Biperiden, 673
Bipolar affective disorder, 376-77, 420-23
    characteristics of, 419
    demographics of, 764
    development of, 425-26
    differentiation of, 371
    dynamic formulation of, 426
    electroconvulsive therapy and, 692
    manic episode of, diagnostic criteria for,
        422
    patterns of, 688
    treatment of, 427-29
Birch, H., 338
Birnbaum, Morton, 798
Birth
    adjustments caused by, 262
    separation anxiety and, neurosis and,
        12
Birth order, effects on children, 262-63
Bisexuality, 313
Black, K., 623
Black Americans, folk systems of, 772-73
Black magic (Obeah), 773
Blacky Test, 198
Blended family, 606, 607
Bleuler, D., 418
Bleuler, Eugene, 11
Block, M., 643
Blocker, 224
Blocking, mental status examination and,
        187-88
Bloodletting, early psychotherapy and, 10
Bloomingdale Asylum, 792, 794
Blotting paper syndrome, 175
Blumenthal, M., 763
Blumer, Herbert, 4
Boatman, M. J., 531
Body discipline therapies, 733-37
Body humors, madness and, 8

Body image, alteration of, 281-83
Body-mind awareness therapies, 733-37
Body-mind integration, in alternative
        therapies, 731-32
Body transcendence, aging and, 636
Boerhaave, Hermann, 10
Bolman, William M., 626
Bonding, 323-24
Borderline life-style, 381
Boredom, aged and, 649-50
Borowich, A. E., 763
Boston Dispensary, 215
Boston Prison Discipline Society, 793
Boszormenyi-Nagi, I., 612
Boundaries, in family systems, 609
Bowel disorders
    interventions in, 469
    psychophysiological, 461-62
Bowen, M., 612
Bower, F., 71, 73
Bowie, David, 313
Bowlby, John, 104, 114, 323, 555
Bradykinin, headache and, 466
Brain abscess, organic brain syndromes
        and, 483, 486
Brain damage, obesity and, 464
Brainwashing, cults and, 770-71
Breastfeeding, self-help groups for, 519
Breasts
    female sexual response and, 301-2
    male sexual response and, 303
    sexual arousal and, 306
Breech presentation, perinatal retardation
        and, 475
Breen, M., 763
Breuer, Josef, 364
Brief therapy, for disturbed children,
        552-53
Brink, T., 652
Brodsky, A., 98
Bromley, D. B., 264
Brotman, Stanley., 801
Brown, Esther Lucille, 416, 575, 818
Brucellosis, organic brain syndromes and,
        486
Bulimia, 464-65
Burke, E. L., 577, 580
Burnout
    cues to, 54
    detached concern and, 42
    empathy and, 54
    reducing, 54-55
Burnside, I., 654
Burrows, T., 216
Burton, Pamela, 321, 525
Butler, R. N., 644, 645, 659, 764
Butyrophenones, 670

Caesarian section, perinatal retardation
        and, 475
Caffeine, 394
    interactions with alcohol, 657
    organic brain syndromes and, 484
Calcium lactate, for organic brain
        syndrome, 489

California's Mental Health Services Act, 809-11

Campbell, C., 579

Cannabis, organic brain syndromes and, 484

Caplan, Gerald, 273, 280, 281, 705, 706, 709, 822

Caplow, Theodore, 614

Carcinomatosis, recent weight loss and, 191

Cardiac arrhythmias, 462

Cardiac neurosis, 357, 462

Cardiovascular disorders
interventions in, 469
psychophysiologica, 462-63

Caretaker role, therapist role v., 144

Carkhuff, R., 144

Carlson, Bonnie E., 285

Carlsson, A., 20

Carp, A., 645

Carp, F., 645

Carter, E., 622

Carter, Jimmy, 796, 819

Castaneda, Carlos, 46

Castration anxiety, 27

Castration complex, psychoanalytic theory and, 26

Castration fantasies, 557
psychoanalytic theory and, 26

Castro, Fidel, 230

Catalysts, group analysis and, 507

Catania, J., 642

Catatonic schizophrenia, 11

Catatonic withdrawal, electroconvulsive therapy and, 692

Catecholamines
depression and, 20
headache and, 466
psychotic conditions and, 424
schizophrenia and, 20

Catharsis
ancient psychotherapeutic intervention and, 8
Freudian theory and, 11

Cathexis, psychoanalytic theory and, 25

Caudill, William, 575

Cavenar, J., 650

Centering, in therapeutic touch, 736

Central nervous system disease, properties of, 369

Central nervous system stimulants, 394

Cephalopelvic disproportion, perinatal retardation and, 475

Cerebral disorders, behavior change induced by, mechanisms of, 492

Cerebral palsy, mental retardation and, 475

Cerebral vascular disease, organic brain syndromes and, 486-87

Certification
of clinical specialists, 56
of psychiatrists, 56

Cervix, 298

Chamberlain, Neville, 230

Chang, B., 774

Change, anxiety and, 250

Chaplin, Charlie, 111

Character, anal stage of development and, 26

Charisma, cults and, 769

Chelating drugs, for Wilson's disease, 491

Chesler, Phyllis, 29, 98-99

Chess, S., 338

Chessick, R., 164

Chestnut Lodge, 14, 28, 432, 575

Chicago Psychoanalytic Institute, 28

Child abuse, 332-34
pattern of, 333-34
self-help groups for, 519

Child Abuse Listening Mediation Inc., 519

Child care
single parents and, 325
working parents and, 328

Child guidance center, 547

Child guidance movement, 611

Childhood
comparative ideas about, 241
development in, 240-45
development of self in, symbolic interactionism and, 244-45
schizoid disorder of, 536

Childishness, conversion disorder and, 367

Child molesting, 308-9

Child neglect, 332

Child psychiatry
levels of prevention in, 526-27
need for, 526

Children
birth order and, 262-63
hospitalized, 555-57
nursing care plans for, 558-62

Chloral hydrate, 13, 692
addictive doses of, 393
interactions with alcohol, 657
use of, 691

Chloramphenicol, interactions with alcohol, 656

Chlordiazepoxide
addictive doses of, 393
for alcohol detoxification, 690
for anxiety, 689-90

Chlorpromazine, 17, 416
for acute intermittent porphyria, 485
cholestatic jaundice and, 675
dopaminergic receptors and, 20
dosages of, 670-71
for children, 672
route of administration of, 671
for schizophrenia, 669
side effects of, 677

Chlorpropamide, interactions with alcohol, 656

Chlorprothixene, 670

Cholestatic jaundice, chlorpromazine and, 675

Chorea, anxiety and, 191

Chromosomal abnormalities, mental retardation and, 471-72

Chronic obstructive pulmonary disease, organic brain syndromes and, 483

Chronopsychophysiology, 20

Chum relationship, 571

Churchill, Winston, 638

Circadian biorhythms, 20-21

Circularity, in families, 611

Circumstantiality, mental status examination and, 187

Cirrhosis, organic brain syndromes and, 487

Civil rights, of mentally disabled, 800

Clark, Diane, 812

Clark, John G. Jr., 769, 782

Client advocacy, 667-68
need for, 667

Client-centered case consultation, 707

Clients
abilities of, therapeutic effectiveness and, 145
adolescent, families of, 601-2
engaging collaboration of, 61
privacy of, confidentiality and, 95-98
psychotic
contemporary services for, 432
nursing approach to, 429-45
rights of, 430, 805-6
implementation of, 811-13
suicidal, crisis intervention and, 291-92

Client-therapist-public relationship, 800-1

Clinical psychologist, 57

Clitoral orgasm, 304

Clitoris, 297
female sexual response and, 301, 302

Closed question, facilitative communication and, 127

Cloud, E., 148

Coalitions, family, 614

Cobb, S., 273, 278

Cocaine, 394
effects of, 596
organic brain syndromes and, 484

Cocaine bugs, 394

Codification, communication and, 113

Coercive power, 232

Cogentin (See Benztropine)

Cognition
aging and, 646-48
definition of, 407

Cognitive assessment, 161

Cognitive development theory, 241-42

Cognitive switch, gender identity and, 308

Cognitive values, 47

Cohen, Allen, 812

Cohen, Arthur, 811

Cohesion
assessment of, 229
group dynamics and, 228-32

Coital positions, 306-7

Coles, R., 569, 570

Colic, 533

Collaboration
engaging client in, 61
on mental health team, 60-61
one-to-one relationship work and, 139

Collaborative therapy, for couples, 628
Collagen vascular disease, organic brain syndromes and, 486-87
Color, environmental, group dynamics and, 223
Colostomy clubs, 519
Coma therapy, 666
Combat, general adaptation syndrome and, 258-59
Commitment
  cults and, 769
  one-to-one relationships and, 142
  procedures for, 799-800
Communal family, 606, 607-8
Communal parents, 327-28
Communication
  as an act, 107
  adolescent styles of, 580
  client's rights and, 805
  with culturally different clients, 777
  definition of, 104
  disturbances in, 116
  with disturbed children, 544-45
  effective, skills fostering, 125-28
  ego states and, 116-21
  facilitative, 121-25
  ineffective, 128-29
  as an interaction, 107
  interaction process analysis of, 129-32
  levels of, 106-7
  models of, 107-10
    symbolic interactionist, 108-10
  modes of, 110-12
  New York State Mental Hygiene Law and, 809
  nonverbal, 110-12
  pathology by developmental age level, 114-15
  pragmatics of, 115-16
  process of, 104-7
  therapeutic, 112-15
  as a transaction, 108-10
  variables influencing, 104-6
  verbal, 110
    autism and, 531
    nonverbal v., 112
Community client groups, 522
Community Health Centers Act (1963), 14
Community health nurse, adolescents and, 572-74
Community mental health movement, emergence of, 817-22
Community mental health services, 417
  consumer participation in, 823
  deinstitutionalization movement and, 824-28
  interdisciplinary collaboration in, 822-23
  levels of prevention in, 822
  nursing roles in, 823-24
Community Mental Health Systems Act, 820
Community psychiatry, 34
Companionship, single parents and, 326

Competition, on mental health team, 60
Complaint, in psychiatric history, 187
Complementarity
  in communication, 115-16
  homeodynamics and, 77-78
Complementary transactions, 118
Complementation, in communication, 112
Compliance, client reasons for, 667
Comprehensive Community Mental Health Act (1963), 141
Compromiser, 224
Compton, B. R., 204, 205, 510, 617
Compulsions
  definition of, 361
  mental status examination and, 189
Compulsive life-style, 381, 395-98
  intervention in, 398
  paranoid personality v., 400
Concurrent therapy, for couples, 628
Conditioned reflex, 30
Conditioning, behavioral theory and, 30-31
Conduct disorders, in childhood, 533-34
Confabulation, aged and, 648
Confidants, for the aged, 659
Confidentiality
  client privacy and, 95-98
  group therapy and, 515
  interaction process analysis and, 211
  New York State Mental Hygiene Law and, 809
  therapeutic relationship and, 148
Confinement, Classical Age and, 9
Conflict
  anxiety and, 349
  approach-avoidance, 348
  avoidance-avoidance, 349
  disruptive life-styles and, 380
  disturbed coping patterns and, 355
  as a stressor, 348
Conformity
  adolescence and, 566
  excessive, in childhood, 534
Confrontation, facilitative communication and, 123, 127-28
Confrontation problem-solving therapy, 741
Confusion, in the aged, 647
Conjoint therapy, for couples, 628
Conjugal family, 606
Conscience, impulsive life-styles and, 384-85
Consciousness
  Freudian theory and, 11
  language and, 43
  of meaning, 43
Consciousness awareness, 742
Consciousness development therapies, 741-45
Consensus, decision making and, 225
Consent
  New York State Mental Hygiene Law and, 809
  sex and, 308-10
Conservatorship, 810-11

Consolidation, in adulthood and middle age, 240
Constipation
  in children, 533
  depressed clients and, 372
Consultant, qualifications for, 709-10
Consultation
  building relationships in, 710-11
  client in intensive care and, 719-20
  client-centered, 707
  client in pain and, 714-15
  client's family and, 717-18
  consultee-centered case, 708-9
  contract negotiation in, 711-13
  demanding client and, 713-14
  dependent client and, 715-17
  dying client and, 723
  guidelines for, 709
  in hospital setting, 706
  noncompliant client and, 721-23
  preventive aspects of, 705-6
  program-centered, 707-8
  sexual acting out and, 720-21
  types of, 706-9
Consultation-liaison psychiatry, 706
Consultee-centered administrative consultation, 708-9
Consultee-centered case consultation, 708
Contact
  establishment, in therapeutic relationships, 146
  termination of, in therapeutic relationships, 156-57
Content level, in communication, 115
Contracts
  client's rights and, 806
  consultation, 711-13
  in family therapy, 620
  in group analysis, 515-16
  noncompliance and, 722-23
Contradiction, in communication, 112
Control
  ego and, 347
  interpersonal needs and, 502-4
Conversion disorder, 366 (See also Somatoform disorders)
Cooper, David, 29
Cooperation, on mental health team, 60
Coordinator, 224
Coping mechanism, suicide as, 288-93
Coping patterns, disturbed (See Disturbed coping patterns)
Coping strategies, 352-53
  of the aged, 659
Coprolalia, 314
Coprophagia, 314
Coprophilia, 314
Cornelison, A., 615
Cornucopia, 742
Corona, 299
Corpora cavernosa, 298
Corpus spongiosum, 298
Correctness assumption, 90
Corticosteroids, arthritis and, 463

Cortisol, alarm reactions and, 258
Cortisone, alarm reactions and, 258
Cosberg, J., 643
Cosmic consciousness, 742
Cotherapy
    egalitarian, advantages/disadvantages
      of, 513
    group analysis and, 511-12
Counterdependent personality, group
    analysis and, 506
Counterpersonal personality, group
    analysis and, 506
Countertransference, 41, 163-65
    in child psychiatry, 547
    mental retardation and, 479
    unanalyzed, 175
Couples therapy, 626-29
    focus of, 629
    types of, 628
Covert rehearsal, in communication, 109
COYOTE, 311
Crasis, 8
Creative arts therapist, 60
Creativity, Rankian theory and, 12
Criminal behavior, genetic factors in, 20
Crisis (*See also* Mid-life crisis)
    definition of, 271
    development of, stress and, 271-73
    developmental, 276-78
    sequence of, 274-75
      diagram of, 276
    situational, 278-83
    typology of, 272
    victim, 283-88
Crisis intervention, 730 (*See also*
    Intervention)
    for the aged, 653
    emergence of, 273-74
    family violence and, 285
    psychotherapy v., 275
    suicidal clients and, 291-92
    as therapeutic strategy, 274
Crisis management, of disaster victims,
    288
Crisis theory, 273-74, 704-5
Critical distance, 159
Cronbach, L., 142
Crossed transactions, 118
CT scan, organic brain syndromes and,
    481
Cullen, William, 10
Cults, 607, 768-71
    characteristics of, 769-70
    clients with experiences of, counseling
      of, 780-83
    religious groups v., 770
Cultural background, group dynamics
    and, 222
Cultural stereotyping, dangers of, 761-62
Culture
    communication and, 106
    psychiatric nursing practice and,
      759-65
Cultures, complexity and diversity of, 761
Cummings, E., 637
Cunnilingus, 306

Cushing's syndrome, 468
    organic brain syndromes and, 483, 487
Cyclothymic disorders, 376
Cytomegalic inclusion disease, maternal,
    mental retardation and, 473

Dali, Salvador, 255
Dalmane (*See* Flurazepam)
Dance therapy groups, 521
Darwin, Charles, 240
Data collection, initial interview and,
    159-60
Daughters of Bilitis, 519, 768
Davis, Anne J., 85, 86, 87
Day care treatment centers, 548
Daydreams, mental status examination
    and, 189
Daytop, 519, 741
Deadline decade, 276
Death
    grief reactions to, 278-81
    single parent role and, 325
Decision making
    compulsiveness and, 397-98
    group dynamics and, 224-27
    methods of, 225
      strengths and limitations of, 226-27
    symbolic interactionism and, 6
Dederich, Charles, 740-41
Deep sleep therapy, 140
Defense mechanisms, 251-57
    life-style and, 382
    psychoanalytic theory and, 24
Defense-oriented reactions, 251-52
Deficiency states, organic brain
    syndromes and, 483
Definition, problem solving and, 161-62
Deinstitutionalization
    alternatives to, 828-33
    dimensions of, 13
Deinstitutionalization movement,
    community mental health and,
    824-28
Delirium
    mental status examination and, 192-93
    organic, 484
Delirium tremens, 387-88
Delusions, 9
    definition of, 407
    mental status examination and, 188-89
Dementia
    mental status examination and, 192-93
    organic, 484
    primary degenerative, aged and, 646,
      648
Dementia praecox, 11
Denial
    as a defense mechanism, 254-55
    intervention strategies in, 173
Denner, Bruce, 811
Deontology, 86-87
Department of Health and Human
    Services, 417
Dependency
    asthma and, 463
    conversion disorder and, 367

Dependency (continued)
    disturbed coping patterns and, 355
    excessive, intervention strategies in,
      173-74
    group analysis and, 504-7
    obsessive-compulsive disorders and,
      363
Dependent life-style, 381, 398-99
Depersonalization disorder, 364
Depression, 9
    aged and, 645-46, 650
    algorithm for, 372, 373-76
    anaclitic, hospitalized child and, 555
    antidepressant drugs for, 676-84
    assessing lethality in suicide and, 291
    biochemistry and, 20
    bioenergetics and, 734-35
    clinical features of, 371-72
    decision-making sequence for, 74
    demographics of, 764
    effects of drugs on, 668
    electroconvulsive therapy and, 692
    factors related to, 371
    holistic approach to, 239
    hospitalization and treatment for,
      changes in, 415
    indicated treatments for, 679
    mental status examination and, 192-93
    mid-life crisis and, 264
    negative transference responses in, 165
    recent weight loss and, 191
    treatment of, 428
    in women, 99
Depressive disorders
    differentiation of, 371
    dynamics of, 370-71
    features of, 370
    intervention in, 372-76
Deprivation, cults and, 770
Dereistic thought, 407
Desensitization
    behavioral theory and, 31
    for phobic disorders, 360
Desertion, single parent role and, 325
Desipramine
    for depression, 678, 680
    interactions with alcohol, 656
Desoxycorticosterone, alarm reactions
    and, 258
Despair, hospitalized child and, 556
Detached concern, 42
Detachment
    empathy and, 53
    hospitalized child and, 556
    intervention strategies in, 172-73
Detoxification, for alcoholics, 389-90
Deutsch, Albert, 796
Deutsch, D., 613
Deutsch, Helene, 12, 29
Deutsch, Morton, 227
Development
    adolescent, 566-68
    adulthood and, 262-64
    cognitive theory of, 241-42
    crises of, 276-78
    direction of, 246

Development (continued)
  genetic and environmental influences
    on, 245-46
  historical perspectives on, 240-45
  holistic approach to, 239-40
  middle age and, 264-65
  normal progession of, 528-31
  postadolescent, 261-62
  problem solving and, 162-63
  of self, symbolic interactionism and,
    244-45
  self-realization and, 249-50
  social interactionism and, 266
  stages of, 246
  standard path of, 265
  theories of, 260-65
Developmental anomalies, mental
  retardation and, 473
Developmental disorders, 535
Developmental life phases theory, 242-43
Deviance
  residual, mental illness as, 33
  social function of, 267
  society and, 266-67
Deviant identity, development of, 266-68
  class differences in, 267-68
Dewey, John, 240
Dewey, Richard, 795
Dewey, Thomas, 796
Dexedrine (See Dextroamphetamine)
Dextroamphetamine
  for depression, 680
  effects of, 595
Diabetes mellitus, 468
  erection difficulties and, 299
  mental retardation and, 473
  organic brain syndromes and, 487
Diagnosis
  biosocial factors in, 762-65
  criteria for manic episodes, 422
  criteria for schizophrenia, 421
  criteria for schizophreniform disorders,
    421
  mental status examination and, 187-90
  moral responsibility and, 91-92
  nursing, 67-70
  psychiatric history and, 187
  sociocultural influences on, 90-91
  stereotypes and, 91
  stigma of, 88-90
Diagnostic and Statistical Manual (See
  DSM-III)
Diazepam
  addictive doses of, 393
  for anxiety, 689-90
  interactions with alcohol, 657
Dibenzazepines, for depression, 680
Dibenzocycloheptenes, for depression,
  680
Dibenzoxazepines, 670
Dickson, W. J., 222
Diener, C., 173
Diet therapy, introduction of, 11
Diet workshop, 519
Diets, fad, 589
Diffuse brain disease, unsteady gait and, 191

Digital language, 113
Digitalis intoxication, 191
Dignity, shared, 142
Dihydroindolones, 670
Dihydroxyphenylalanine, psychotic
  conditions and, 424
Dike paranoias, 789
Dillon, K., 159
Dionysian principles, 650
Diphenhydramine, 673
  for acute dystonic reactions, 673
  for anxiety, 689-90
  interactions with alcohol, 656
Direct decision therapy, 741
Disaster response, phases in, 287
Disaster victims, 285-88
  crisis management of, 288
Disbelief, grieving process and, 278-80
Disengagement
  in families, 615
  family therapy and, 612
Disharmony, mental status examination
  and, 188
Disintegrative life patterns
  aged and, 646
  behavior associated with, 405-7
  contemporary nursing approaches to,
    429-44
  contemporary study and treatment of,
    417-29
  definition of, 407-14
  early study and treatment of, 415-17
  examples of, 414-15
Disorientation, in the aged, 647-48
Displacement
  as a defense mechanism, 256-57
  phobic disorders and, 360
Disqualifications, 116
Disruptive life patterns, aged and,
  645-46
Disruptive life-styles
  addicted, 386-95
  compulsive, 395-98
  development of, 382-83
  eccentric, 399-402
  impulsive, 383-86
  types of, 380-82
Dissociation
  anxiety and, 350
  as a defense mechanism, 252
  mental status examination and, 188
Dissociative disorders, 363-64
  forms of, 364
  intervention in, 364
  nursing care plan for, 365
Disturbed coping patterns (See also
    specific disorder)
  construction of, 355
  holistic view of, 346
  humanistic interactionist approach to,
    346-77
  intervention in, 355-77
  neurotic v. psychotic, 354
  properties of, 354-55
  recognition of, 354
  sex and, 317

Disulfiram, interactions with alcohol, 656
Divine Command Theory, 87
Divorce
  client's rights and, 806
  single parent role and, 325
Dix, Dorothea, 10, 793, 794
DMPEA, schizophrenia and, 20
Docherty, John P., 418
Doctor-Nurse game, 61
Dogmatism, 45-46
Dohrenwend, B. P., 763, 764
Domestic Violence Project, 284
Dominator, 224
Don Juan, 46
Donaldson, Kenneth, 799
Donaldson v. O'Connor, 799
Dopamine, 20
  psychotic conditions and, 424
  schizophrenia and, 676
Dopaminergic blockers, for schizophrenia,
  424
Dopaminergic receptors, antipsychotic
  agents and, 20
Dopaminergic system, schizophrenia and,
  424
Doriden (See Glutethimide)
Double-bind phenomenon, 427
  in families, 616
Doubt, developmental life phases theory
  and, 242
Douglas, William O., 638
Down's syndrome, mental retardation
  and, 471-72
Doxepin, for anxiety attacks, 684
Draft Act Governing Hospitalization of the
  Mentally Ill, 796
Draw-a-Person Test, 196-97
Dream interpretation
  ancient psychotherapeutic intervention
    and, 8
  Freudian theory and, 11
  psychoanalytic theory and, 23-24
Drinking, assessing lethality in suicide
  and, 291
Drives, psychoanalytic theory and, 25
Driving, client's rights and, 807
Drug abuse
  adolescent, 589-91
  assessing lethality in suicide and, 291
  definition of, 392
Drug addiction
  oral fixation and, 25
  orthomolecular psychiatry and, 736
  self-help groups for, 519
Drug dependence, 391-95
  definition of, 392
  intervention in, 395-96
Drug intoxication, unsteady gait and,
  191
Drug use
  adolescent, 589-91
  definition of, 392
Drugs
  alcohol interactions with, 656-57
  commonly abused, 394
  perinatal retardation and, 475

DSM-III, 19, 89, 197-204, 271, 287, 354, 364, 368, 380, 383, 384, 386, 398, 400, 411, 420, 427, 838-43
  Axes I and II, 200-1, 838-42
    multiaxial evaluation on, 201
  Axis III, 201, 842
    multiaxial evaluation on, 201
  Axis IV, 201-2, 348, 842-43
  Axis V, 202-3, 843
  classification of disruptive life-styles, 381
  diagnostic classifications of, 838-43
  diagnostic criteria for hyperactivity, 534
  diagnostic criteria for manic episodes, 422
  diagnostic criteria for mental retardation, 471
  diagnostic criteria for organic brain syndromes, 483-84
  diagnostic criteria for psychophysiological disorders, 459-60
  diagnostic criteria for psychotic disorders, 405
  diagnostic criteria for schizophrenia, 421
  diagnostic criteria for schizophreniform disorder, 421
  ego-dystonic homosexuality, 767-68
  multiaxial system of, 199-200
  paranoid life-style v. paranoid disorder, 400
  psychiatric diagnosis and, 23
  psychiatric-mental health nursing and, 203-4
  V-codes of, 91
Dualism, 6
Duffy, P., 722
Dumas, Rhetaugh, 821
Dunham, H. W., 763
Dunlap, M. J., 287
Dunn, Halbert, 247-48
Duodenal ulcer, psychophysiological, 460-61
Duval, Evelyn, 608
Dweck, C., 173
Dwight, Louis, 793
Dyads, family, 614
Dychtwald, K., 768
Dying client
  consultation and, 723
  support of, 660-62
Dysthymic disorders, 678
Dystonic reactions, antipsychotic drugs and, 673

Eating disorders (*See also* Anorexia nervosa; Bulimia; Obesity)
  interventions in, 469
  psychophysiological, 464-66
Ebersole, Priscilla, 633, 641, 650
Eccentric life-style, 399-402
Ectomorphs, 464
Edward II, 790
Effective sensory projection, Silva mind control and, 744

Efficiency, in communication, 113
Effigies, treatment of mental illness and, 8
Egalitarianism, in group therapy, 512
Ego
  control and, 347
  orality and, 25
  psychoanalytic theory and, 24-25
Ego defense mechanisms, 12
Ego-dystonic homosexuality, 91
Ego identity, aging and, 637-38
Ego psychology, 12
Ego states
  in wellness/illness, 117-18
  transactional analysis of, 121
Ego syntonic behavior, 380
Ego theory, 34
Ego transcendence, aging and, 638
Ehmann, V. E., 52
Einstein, Albert, 638
Ejaculation, 298-99
  orgasm v., 300
Ejaculatory duct, 299
Ekman, P., 112
Elaborator, 224
Elavil (*See* Amitriptyline)
Elder, J., 121
Electra conflict, 26-27
Electroconvulsive therapy (ECT), 19, 23, 666, 691-93
  client's rights and, 806
  complications of, 693
  course of treatment in, 693
  for depression, 679, 684
  indications for, 692
  procedure of, 692-93
Electrolyte imbalance, organic brain syndromes and, 483
Electroshock therapy, 14, 140
  introduction of, 11
Ellis, Albert, 739
Emotional abuse, of children, 332
Emotional disturbances (*See also specific disorder*)
  adolescent, family and, 601-2
  childhood, 527-39
    definition of, 527-31
    intervention in, 540-55
    treatment modes for, 547-55
Emotional health, characteristics of, 248-49
Emotional state, mental status examination and, 188
Emotionalism, conversion disorder and, 367
Emotive assessment, 160-61
Empathic resonance, 175
Empathy
  burnout and, 54
  definition of, 52
  detached concern and, 42
  facilitative communication and, 123
  psychiatric concepts of, 52-53
  for psychotic clients, 431
  self-awareness and, 44
  therapeutic use of, 53
  value of, 52
Empty nest syndrome, 276-77

Encephalitis, organic brain syndromes and, 486
Encopresis, 533
Encounter groups, 737-38, 748
Encounter marathon groups, 737-38
Encourager, 224
Endocrine disorders
  organic brain syndromes and, 483
  psychophysiological, 466-67
Endocrine function
  disease-induced alterations in, 468
  normal developmental alterations in, 467
Endocrinopathies, interventions in, 470
Engel, George L., 278, 773
English law, mental illness and, 790
Enmeshment
  in families, 615
  family therapy and, 612
Ennis, Bruce, 803
Enuresis, 533
Environment
  autism and, 531-32
  developmental process and, 245-46
  group dynamics and, 220-23
  mental health and, 249
  stress from, combating, 100
Environmental event, in communication, 109
Epididymis, 298, 299
Epigenetic principle, 242
Epilepsy, 9
  management of, 691
  mental retardation and, 475
  organic brain syndromes and, 490
  types of, 490
Epiloia, 491
Epoch of enlightenment, treatment of mental illness and, 10
Equal Rights Amendment (ERA), 308
Equanil (*See* Meprobamate)
Ergasia, 11
Ergasiatry, 11
Erhard, Werner, 742
Erhard Seminar Training (est), 742
Erikson, Erik, 12, 28, 29, 242-43, 245, 261, 264, 274, 425, 527, 566, 569-70, 572, 636
Erikson, Kai, 32, 88
Erikson, Milton, 744
Eriksonian hypnosis, 744
Esalen Institute, 737
Eskalith (*See* Lithium carbonate)
Espiritismo, 773
Essential hypertension, 462
est, 742
Estrogen, 298
Ethchlorvynol, 692
  use of, 691
Ethical dilemmas, 87-101
Ethical issues, analyzing, 85-86
Ethical perspectives, 86-87
  egoism, 86
  deontology, 86
  ideal observer theory, 87
  justice as fairness, 87

Ethical perspectives (continued)
theory of obligation, 87
utilitarianism, 87
Ethnic groups, characteristics of, 772
Ethnicity, diagnosis and treatment and,
763
Ethnocentrism, 761
Euthanasia, 92-93
Evaluation
nursing process and, 71-73
one-to-one relationship work and,
165-66
problem solving and, 162
Evil eye (mal de ojo), 773
Excessive conformity, in childhood, 534
Excessive dependence, intervention
strategies in, 173-74
Excessive fears, in childhood, 534-35
Exclusion, paranoid personality and,
400-1
Exercise
for depressed clients, 372
for manic clients, 377
stress and, 353
Exhaustion, general adaptation syndrome
and, 259
Exhibitionism, 311
conversion disorder and, 367
Existentialism, alternative therapies
movement and, 729
Exorcism, treatment of mental illness and,
7
Expectations, anxiety and, 351
Expert power, 232
Extended family, 606-7
Eye contact, 111

Facilitation, therapeutic effectiveness and,
144
Facilitative communication, 121-29
Facilitative intimacy, social superficiality v.,
121
Factitious disorders, 368
Fad diets, 589
Fagin, C., 141
Fair, Charles, 750
Fair Labor Standards Act, 800
Fallopian tubes, 298
Family
alternative, 607-8
blended, 606, 607
characteristics and dynamics of, 609-11
communal, 606
communicational/relational aspects in,
612-16
conjugal, 606
decline of, 322-23
developmental tasks, 608-9
disturbed adolescents and, 601-2
extended, 606-7
preventive psychiatry for, 626
approaches in, 627-28
schizophrenogenic, 427
single parent, 607
as system, 609
traditional nuclear, 606-7

Family constellation theory, 618-19
Family healer, 616
Family history, in psychiatric history, 187
Family homeostasis, 609
Family life chronology, 618, 619
Family life-style, 613-14
Family myths, 613-14
Family persecutor, 616
Family support groups, aged and, 654-55
Family support therapy, for the aged,
652-53
Family themes, 613-14
Family therapist, 553
qualifications of, 612
role of, 621-22
Family therapy, 23
adolescents and, 574
approaches to, 612
components of, 617-23
criteria for terminating, 623
definition of, 611
for disturbed children, 553
goal negotiation in, 620
intervention in, 621-23
for psychophysiological allergy, 469
schizophrenia and, 12
transactional analysis and, 737
treatment setting for, 616-17
Family violence, 284-85
Fantasy
as a defense mechanism, 255
castration, 557
masturbation and, 305-6
mental status examination and, 189
mutilation, 557
care plan for child with, 558
Fasting, neurosis and, 465
Fathering (See also Parenting)
role definition of, 324
Fatties Anonymous, 519
Fear
of aging, 640
anxiety v., 350
data indicating, 350-51
excessive, in childhood, 534-35
thought disintegration and, 407
Fearfulness, dependency and, 398
Federal Aid to Dependent Children, 329
Feedback
in communication, 114-15
in families, 611
nonthreatening, characteristics of, 125
self-disclosure and, 123
Feelings
disapproved, 45
self-awareness of, 44
submerged, 44-45
Fellatio, 306
Felsenfeld, N., 585
Female genitals, 297-98
Female masturbation, 304
Female orgasm, 300-4
psychoanalytic theory and, 28
Female sexual response, physiology of,
301-2
Femininity, body image alteration and, 282

Feminism
psychoanalytic theory and, 28-29
psychotherapy and, 98
Feminist movement, mental health care
and, 765-67
Fenichel, O., 163
Fenton, Reuben E., 795
Ferenczi, Sandor, 12, 459
Ferreira, Antonio J., 613
Fetal alcohol syndrome, 594
Fetishism, 314
Figes, Eva, 29
Finch, S. M., 600
Fink, P., 828
Firestone, Shulamith, 28
Five-Day Plan, 519
Flattening of affect, mental status
examination and, 188
Flavell, J. H., 567
Fleck, S., 615
Flexibility, in communication, 114
Fliedner, Friedericke, 13
Fliedner, Theodor, 13
Flight of ideas, mental status examination
and, 187
Florez, R. M. F., 763
Fluphenazine, 17, 670
route of administration of, 672
Flurazepam, 692
for insomnia, 691
Folie a deux, 9
Folk beliefs
black magic, 773
curandero, 773
evil eye (mal de ojo), 773
healing practices and, 771-76
hot-cold diseases (caliente-frio), 773-74
intervention and, 777
medicine man (shaman), 775
Folk systems
of American Indians, 775-76
of Asian Americans, 774-75
of Black Americans, 772-73
of Hispanic Americans, 773-74
Follower, 224
Food fads, 589
Food stamps, 329
Force, sex and, 310-11
Forcible rape, 310
Foreskin, 299
Formality, one-to-one relationship and,
137-38
Forman, J. B. W., 200
Foster parents, 327
Foucault, Michel, 9
Foulkes, S. H., 216
Framo, J., 612
Frank, J. D., 760
Franklin, Benjamin, 791
Freddolino, Paul, 812
Fredlund, D., 574
Free association, psychoanalytic theory
and, 24
Freedman, A. M., 419, 427
Freedom, control of, 92-94
Frenulum, 299

Freud, Anna, 12, 568
Freud, Sigmund, 11-12, 23-29, 142, 216, 239, 240, 243, 296, 304, 307, 364, 366, 425, 458, 566, 568-69, 572, 611, 817
Friedan, Betty, 29
Friedman, M., 459
Friend's Asylum, 792
Fromm, Erich, 33, 36
Fromm-Reichmann, Frieda, 575
Frustration, ulcer formation and, 460
Fugue, psychogenic, 364 (*See also* Dissociative disorders)
Fuller, Buckminster, 742
Functional vaginismus, interventions for, 316
Fundamental Interpersonal Relationship Orientation, 502-4
Furazolidone, interactions with alcohol, 656
Furuta, B. S., 778, 779

Gait, diagnostic implications of, 191
Galactosemia, 472
Galaway, B., 204, 205, 510, 617
Gambling, self-help groups for, 519
    Gam-Anon, 519
    Gamblers Anonymous, 519
Games
    in family therapy, 623
    in transactional analysis, 118-21
Garner, Harry H., 741
Gasoline, inhalation of, effects of, 596
Gastrointestinal disease, recent weight loss and, 191
Gaucher's disease, 472
Gay Liberation Front, 768
Gay rights movement, 767-68
Gazda, G. M., 128
Gebbie, K. M., 67
Geller, A., 144
Gender identity, 307-8 (*See also* Sexual identity)
    development of, 308
General adaptation syndrome, 258-59
General systems theory, 34
Generalized anxiety disorders
    intervention in, 356
    symptomatology of, 357
    treatment of, 689
Genetics, psychiatric, 20
Genital activity, puberty and, 572
Genital stage, psychoanalytic theory and, 27-28
Genitals
    female, 297-98
    male, 298-300
Genuineness, facilitative communication and, 123-24
Georgia Nurses Association, 766
German measles (*See* Rubella)
Gerson, S., 827
Gesell, A., 527
Gesell Developmental Schedules, 194
Gestalt therapy, 735-36, 748
Ghandi, Mahatma, 638

Gillum, R., 721, 722
Glans clitoris, 297
Glans penis, 298-99
Glaser, B. G., 281
Glaser, Kurt, 600
Glasser, William, 738-39
Glaucoma, antidepressant drugs and, 680
Glick, Paul, 607
Glue, inhalation of, effects of, 596
Glueck, E. and S., 572
Glutethimide, 692
    addictive doses of, 393
    use of, 691
Glycogen storage disease, 472
Goal direction, one-to-one relationship work and, 139
Goal response, in communication, 109
Goals, in family therapy, 620
Goblet issues, 504
Goffman, Erving, 89, 111, 400, 410, 416, 575
Goldman, H. H., 830
Gong, Joseph K., 618
Gove, W. R., 764
Graham, J. R., 775
Grandeur, delusions of, mental status examination and, 189
Gratification, oral stage of development and, 25
Gray, John P., 794
Gray Panthers, 768
Greek law, mental illness and, 789
Greenblatt, Milton, 416, 575, 818
Greenburg, Dan, 616
Greenwald, Harold, 741
Greer, Germaine, 29
Grief
    depressive disorders and, 372
    in old age, 661
    pathological, treatment of, 679
Grief reactions, 278-81
    morbid, 279
    symptomatology of, 279
    treatment of, 679
Grief work, 278
Grieving client, support of, 660-62
Griffith, A., 143
Grinder, J., 744
Griseofulvin, interactions with alcohol, 656
Group analysis (*See* Group therapy)
Group development
    phase I of, 505
    phase II of, 506-7
Group dynamics, 216-20
Group expert, decision making and, 225
Group norms, 228-30
Group observer, 224
Group therapists, qualifications for, 511
Group therapy, 23, 818
    activity therapies in, 521
    adolescents and, 574
    analytic, 518
    authority relations/personal relations approach in, 504-7
    client government in, 520-21

Group therapy (continued)
    couples, 628
    curative factors of, 511, 512
    disturbed adolescents and, 577-78
    disturbed children and, 549-51
    group contract in, 515-16
    here-and-now emphasis in, 516-18
    historical beginnings of, 215-16
    interactional, 510-18
    interpersonal needs approach in, 502-4
    Johari Window and, 499-502
    leaderless approach in, 512-14
    leadership in, 511-14
    medical-surgical patients and, 521-22
    member behaviors in, 517
    member selection in, 514
        interview and, 514-15
    multiple family, 519
    psychodrama in, 518
    self-help, 519
    small groups and, 510
    sociodrama in, 518
    stages in development of, 516
    therapeutic problem approach in, 507-10
Group work, aged and, 654
Groups
    effective, characteristics of, 220, 221
    encounter, 737-38
    forces acting on, 220-34
    ineffective, characteristics of, 221
    leadership in, 511-14
    remotivation and reeducation, 519-20
    self-help, 519
    varieties of, 216-19
Groupthink, 230-32, 769
    preventing, 233
Growth
    crisis resolution and, 271
    holistic approach to, 239-40
    process of, 246
    recapitulation theory of, 240
    theories of, 260-65
Growth hormone, arthritis and, 463
Grunebaum, Henry, 617
Guanethidine
    antipsychotic drug interactions with, 678
    interactions with alcohol, 656
Guilt, child abuse and, 333
Guttentag, Marcia, 98
Gynecomastia, antipsychotic drugs and, 675

Hackett, T. P., 281
Haldol (*See* Haloperidol)
Haley, J., 611, 612
Hall, E., 159, 222
Hall, G. Stanley, 240
Hall, Lydia, 75
Halleck, Seymour, 92, 100
Hallucinations
    definition of, 406
    mental status examination and, 189
Hallucinogens, 393-95
    effects of, 596-97
    organic brain syndromes and, 484

Hallucinosis, organic, 484
Haloperidol, 17, 670
  geriatric dosages of, 672
  side effects of, 677
Hammer, M., 428
Handel, G., 609, 613
Hankoff, I. D., 763
Hansell, Norris, 274
Hargreaves, W., 143
Harmonizer, 224
Harper, R. A., 739
Harris, L., 640
Hartford Retreat, 792
Haven, C., 659
Hawthorne effect, 223
Head trauma, mental retardation and, 475
Headache
  interventions in, 470
  psychophysiological, 466
Health
  as an adaptive process, 248
  emotional, characteristics of, 248-49
Health-illness continuum, 347
Heart attack, stress and, 272
Heart disease, predisposing factors in, 462
Heavy metals, organic brain syndromes and, 483
Hebephrenic schizophrenia, 11
Helicy, homeodynamics and, 77-78
Heller's disease, mental retardation and, 475
Hematoma, organic brain syndromes and, 483, 490-91
Hemorrhage, organic brain syndromes and, 486-87
Henderson, G., 773, 775, 776
Henderson, Virginia, 75, 76
Henry, W., 637
Henry I, 790
Hepatic encephalopathy, organic brain syndromes and, 487
Hepatic failure, organic brain syndromes and, 483
Hepatitis, organic brain syndromes and, 487
Heredity
  autism and, 532
  developmental process and, 245-46
  psychosis and, 423-24
Heroin, effects of, 598
Heroin addiction, 414
Herron, W. G., 419
Hess, Patricia, 641, 650
Hess, R. D., 609, 613
Heterophilic relationships, early adolescence and, 571-72
Heterosexuality, adolescent, 588
Hidden agendas, 230
  dealing with, 231
Hill, William F., 508-10, 516
Hinckley, John Jr., 190
Hippel-Lindau disease, 474
Hippocrates, 8, 700
Hispanic Americans, folk systems of, 773-74

Histamine, headache and, 466
History taking, 191
Histrionic life-style, 381
Hoff, Lee Ann, 288, 290, 291
Hoffer, A., 736
Holistic medicine (*See also* Alternative therapies movement)
  concepts of, 703-4
  individual response specificity model in, 701-2
  mind-body relations in, 6
  multicausation in, 702-3
  nonspecific stress model in, 701
  specificity model in, 700-1
Holistic nursing, 75
Hollingshead, A. B., 19
Hollister, L. E., 668
Holmes, T. H., 272, 273, 649, 702
Home crisis visits, 293
Homeodynamics, 77-78
Homeostasis, 347-48
  biorhythms and, 20
  family, 609
  general systems theory and, 34
Homosexual family, 607-8
Homosexuality
  in adolescence, 587-88
  deviance and, 266-67
  DSM-III classification of, 767-68
  ego-dystonic, 91, 768
  as expression of hostility, nursing care plan for, 588
  gender identity and, 307
  latency stage of development and, 27
  male, 313
    genetic factors in, 20
  paranoia and, 12
  phallic stage of development and, 27
  self-help groups for, 519
  as sickness, 313
  stereotyping and, 91
Hoodoo, 773
Hook, L. H., 223
Hope, psychiatric nursing practice and, 51
Hormones, adaptive, 258
Horney, Karen, 12, 28, 29, 33, 36
Hospital General (Paris), 9
Hospitalization
  admission and, 802-5
    involuntary, 803-5
    voluntary, 802
  of children, 555-56
    nursing care plan for, 561
  of infants, 557
    nursing care plan for, 559
  in psychiatric history, 187
  of toddlers, 556
    nursing care plan and, 560
Hostility
  adolescent, 583-85
    authority figures and, 5
    homosexuality and, 588
    intervention strategies in, 170-71
Hot lines, crisis, 274
Hughes, Howard, 360

Hulett, J. E. Jr., 108
Human behavior, individual meaning and, 4
Human potential movement, 41
Humanism (*See also* Symbolic interactionism)
  alternative therapies movement and, 729
  behaviorism and, 32
  nursing education and, 143
  one-to-one relationship work and, 142-43
  premises of, 5-6
  psychiatric nursing and, 6-7
Humanistic nursing, 75
Humphreys, L., 312
Hunger, hypothalamic control of, 464
Huntington's chorea, organic brain syndromes and, 487-88
Hurler's syndrome, 472
Hyde, R. W., 520
Hydralazine
  antipsychotic drug interactions with, 678
  interactions with alcohol, 656
Hydranencephaly, 474
Hydrocephalus, 474
  organic brain syndromes and, 483
Hydrochlorthiazide, antipsychotic drug interactions with, 678
Hydromorphone, interactions with alcohol, 657
Hydrotherapy, 14, 19
  introduction of, 11
  for psychotic conditions, 429
Hydroxydopamine, schizophrenia and, 20
Hydroxyzine, for anxiety, 690
Hygiene
  depressed clients and, 372
  diagnostic implications of, 191
Hymen, 297
Hyperactivity
  attention deficit disorder with, 534
  disintegration of motivation and, 412-13, 444-45
  treatment of, 684
Hyperhidrosis, psychophysiological, 463
Hyperparathyroidism, organic brain syndromes and, 489
Hypersensitivity, paranoid personality and, 399
Hypertension
  essential, 462
  organic brain syndromes and, 483, 486-87
Hypertensive crises, monoamine oxidase inhibitors and, 682
Hyperthyroidism, 468
  anxiety and, 191
  organic brain syndromes and, 488
Hypnosis
  Eriksonian, 744
  for psychogenic pain, 368
  for psychophysiological allergy, 469
Hypnotherapy, psychoanalytic theory and, 24

Hypnotic drugs, 690-92
Hypnotism, Freudian theory and, 11
Hypochondria, aged and, 651-52
Hypochondriasis, 366
Hypoglycemia, 467-68
  organic brain syndromes and, 483, 488
Hypoglycemic agents, interactions with
  alcohol, 656
Hypoparathyroidism, organic brain
  syndromes and, 489
Hypothyroidism, 468
  organic brain syndromes and, 488
Hypsarrhythmia, mental retardation and,
  475
Hysteria, 9
  Freudian theory and, 11

Ichazo, Oscar, 741
Id, psychoanalytic theory and, 24-25
Ideas of reference, paranoid personality
  and, 400-1
Ideation, problem solving and, 162
Identification
  as a defense mechanism, 253
  empathy and, 53
Identity (See also Deviant identity)
  adolescent, 569-70
  deviant, development of, 266-68
Identity confirmation, 143
Identity formation
  in adolescence, 570
  women and, 261
Idiopathic hypercalcemia, 472
Idiopathic spontaneous hypoglycemia,
  organic brain syndromes and, 488
Illich, Ivan, 247, 248
Illness
  assessing lethality in suicide and, 291
  holistic concept of, 700-3
  multicausational concept of, 702-3
Illusions, definition of, 406
Imipramine
  for depression, 678, 680
  for panic attacks, 684
Imitation, identification v., 253
Immediacy, facilitative communication
  and, 124
Impact, in disaster response, 287
Impotence
  antipsychotic drugs and, 675
  interventions for, 316
Impulsive behavior
  disintegration of motivation and, 412,
  442-44
Impulsive life-style, 383-86
  common features of, 384-85
  development of, 383-84
  intervention in, 385-86
Impulsivity, hyperactivity and, 534
Inadequacy, latency stage of development
  and, 27
Inappropriate antidiuretic hormone,
  organic brain syndromes and, 483
Inappropriateness, anxiety and, 266

Inattention
  compulsiveness and, 396-97
  hyperactivity and, 534
  selective, 350
Incantation, treatment of mental illness
  and, 7
Incest, 310
Inclusion, interpersonal needs and, 502-4
Incorporation, empathy and, 53
Incubation, problem solving and, 162
Indecisiveness, group decision making
  and, 226-27
Inderal (See Propranolol)
Individual freedom, control of, 92-94
Individual response specificity model,
  701-2
Individuals, social good v., 100-1
Indoleamine, psychotic conditions and,
  424
Industry, development of, in adolescence,
  570
Infancy, reactive attachment disorder of,
  532
Infection
  mental retardation and, 475
  organic brain syndromes and, 483
Influence, group dynamics and, 232-34
Informality, one-to-one relationship and,
  137-38
Information, facilitative communication
  and, 126
Information giver, 224
Information seeker, 224
Informational confrontation, 123
Informational power, 232
Infradian biorhythms, 20, 21
Ingham, Harry, 47, 499
Inhalants, abuse of, 395
Initial contact form, 185, 186
Initial interview, 159-60
Initiative, development of, in adolescence,
  570
Input, in communication, 108-9
Insight evaluation, mental status
  examination and, 190
Insight therapy, for psychotic conditions,
  429
Insincerity, impulsive life-styles and, 385
Insomnia, treatment of, 690-91
Instinct, 34
Institutionalization
  crisis intervention v., 275
  mentally retarded and, 480
  psychotherapy v., 275
  for psychotic conditions, 416
  of social rules, 260
Insulin coma, 14
Insulin coma therapy, 695
Insulin shock, 19
Insulin shock therapy, 140
Intellect
  devaluation of, in alternative therapies,
  731
  in mental status examination, 187

Intellectual level, mental status
  examination and, 190
Intellectualization
  in adolescence, 569
  as a defense mechanism, 257
  intervention strategies in, 173
Intelligence, 470-71
  assessment of, 161
  development of
  abnormal, 470-71
  Piaget's theory of, 242, 470
Intelligence tests, 194 (See also specific
  test)
Intensive care syndrome, 719
Interaction, communication as, 107
Interaction process, meaning formation
  and, 4
Interaction process analysis, 129-32,
  207-11
  confidentiality and comprehensiveness
  of, 211
  methods of, 207-11
  purposes of, 207
Interactional group therapy, 510-18
Interactionism
  family therapy and, 612
  symbolic (See Symbolic interactionism)
Interdependence
  adaptation and, 78
  group analysis and, 504-7
International Association for Humanistic
  Gerontology, 768
Interpersonal communication, 106-7
Interpersonal intimacy, need for, in
  adolescence, 571-72
Interpersonal needs, group interactions
  and, 502-4
Interpersonal relationships
  in adolescence, therapy and, 575
  emotional health and, 249
Interpersonal skills, in therapeutic
  relationships, 143-45
Interpretive confrontation, 123
Interrelationships, group analysis and,
  509
Intervention
  in affective disorders, 372-76
  in alcoholism, 388-90
  in anxiety disorders, 356-60
  in care of the aged, 652-62
  in childhood anxiety disorders, 535
  in childhood emotional disturbances,
  540-55
  in compulsive life-styles, 398
  culturally aware strategies for, 776-83
  in dependent life-styles, 398-99
  in disintegration of affect, 438-40
  in disintegration of motivation, 440-45
  in disintegration of perception, 433-35
  in disintegration of thought, 435-38
  in dissociative disorders, 364
  in disturbed coping patterns, 355-77
  in drug dependency, 395-96
  in family therapy, 621-23

Intervention (continued)
in impulsive life-styles, 385-86
in manic behavior, 376-77
in mental retardation, 477-80
in obsessive-compulsive disorders, 362
in organic brain syndromes, 491-93
in paranoid life-styles, 401
in parenting, 340
in phobic disorders, 360
in psychogenic pain, 368
in psychophysiological disorders, 467-70
in schizoid/schizotypal life-styles, 402
in somatoform disorders, 368-69
Intimacy
facilitative, superficiality v., 121
need for, in adolescence, 571-72
in postadolescence, 261-62
therapeutic, continuum of, 124
Intoxication, unsteady gait and, 191
Intrapersonal communication, 106
Introjection, as a defense mechanism, 253-54
Involutional psychosis, genetic factors in, 20
Involvement, lack of, autism and, 531
Invulnerability, groupthink and, 230
Iproniazid, 682
IQ (See Intelligence)
Ishiyama, Toaru, 812
Isocarboxazid, for depression, 680
Isolated nuclear family, 607
Isolation
assessing lethality in suicide and, 291
obsessive-compulsive disorders and, 361-62
in postadolescence, 261-62
Isoniazid, interactions with alcohol, 656

Jackson, Don D., 12, 115, 116, 609, 610, 611, 612, 629
Jacob-Crutzfeldt disease, organic brain syndromes and, 488
Jaffee, A. C., 333
Jameton, A., 85
Janis, Irving, 230, 231
Janov, Arthur, 733-34
Jansson, D., 143
Japanese Americans, counseling of, ethnic identity guide for, 779
Jarvik, L., 649
Jersild, A. T., 585
Jewish law, mental illness and, 788-89
Johari Window, 47-49, 499-502, 638
Johns Hopkins University, 11
Johnson, Lyndon B., 230
Johnson, Virginia, 28, 300, 304, 315, 740
Johnson-Soderberg, Sherry, 615
Joint Commission on Mental Health of Children, 329, 330, 526, 527, 819
Joint Commission on Mental Illness and Health, 12, 15, 141, 274, 796, 817, 818

Jones, Ernest, 12
Jones, Jim, 768, 769
Jones, Maxwell, 576, 818
Jones, S. L., 612, 616
Jourard, S., 723
Judgment
impulsive life-styles and, 384
mental status examination and, 190
Jung, Carl, 12, 636
Juvenile delinquency, 591-92

Kadushin, C., 267
Kahn-Goldfarb mental status questionnaire, 647-48
Kallmann, Franz, 20, 424
Kanner, L., 531
Kansas Boys Industrial School, 578-79
Kant, Immanuel, 79, 87, 345
Kantor, R. E., 419
Kaplan, H. I., 191, 419, 427, 764
Karasu, T. B., 92
Kaslow, F. W., 770
Keaton, Buster, 111
Keglovits, Joanne, 787
Keller, Helen, 43
Kellert, S., 762
Kemadrin (See Procyclidine)
Kennedy, John F., 230, 280, 817, 818, 820
Kennedy, Robert, 280
Kennell, J., 323
Kernicterus, perinatal retardation and, 475
Kesey, Ken, 100, 667
Kety, Seymour, 20
Keyes, Kenneth, 742
Kibbutzim, 607
Kimmel, H. E., 230
Kinesics, 111
King, Billie Jean, 313
King, Imogene M., 78
Kingsley Hall, 432, 829
Kinsey, A. C., 310, 313
Kirshner, M. C., 822
Klaus, M., 323
Klein, Norma, 337
Klerman, G. L., 828
Kneisl, C. R., 367, 518, 769
Kogan, N., 225
Kora, T., 738
Korsakoff's syndrome, organic brain syndromes and, 488
Kovel, Joel A., 346, 352
Kraemer, Heinrich, 9
Kraepelin, Emil, 11, 18, 19, 20
Krieger, Dolores, 736-37, 752
Kubler-Ross, E., 661, 723

Labeling
gender identity and, 308
need for, 89
process of, 89-90
self-fulfilling, 90

Labia majora/minora, 297
female sexual response and, 301, 302
Lacey, J. I., 701
Lactation, antipsychotic drugs and, 675
Laing, R. D., 29, 50, 408-9, 427, 429, 619
La Leche League, 519
Lamont, C., 6
Langfield, G., 419
Langley Porter Psychiatric Institute, 577, 579, 581, 589
Language, consciousness and, 43
Lanterman-Petris-Short Act, 809, 809-10
Laryngectomy clubs, 519
Latency stage
in childhood development, 530
psychoanalytic theory and, 27
regression of sexual development in, 568
Lathrop, V., 171
Lau, E., 643
Laves, Rona, 812
Lavin, M. A., 67
Law
mental hygiene, twentieth-century, 797-98
mental illness and, 788-97
Lawrence, D. H., 296
Lay analyst, 57
Lazarus, R. S., 260
Lazell, E. W., 215
Lead poisoning, mental retardation and, 475
Leadership, group dynamics and, 223-24, 511-14
Leaman, K., 332
Learned helplessness, intervention strategies in, 173-74
Legitimate power, 232
Lego, S., 140-41, 145
Leininger, M., 822
Lemert, Edwin, 33
Lenefsky, B., 171
Lesbianism, 313
Lessard v. Schmidt, 800
Lethality assessment, suicide and, 290-91
Lettieri, D. J., 589
Leukemia, priapism and, 299
Levine, James, 607, 610
Levine, Myra E., 78
Levinson, Daniel, 262
Levodopa, antipsychotic drug interactions with, 678
Lewin, K., 224
Lewis, M. I., 644, 645, 764
Libido, psychoanalytic theory and, 25
Librium (See Chlordiazepoxide)
Lidz, Theodore, 612, 615
Lief, Harold I., 628
Life change scale, 273
Life change units, 272
Life changes, stress and, 272-73
Life cycle
developmental phases of, 242-43

Life cycle (continued)
  Erikson's theory of, 569-70
  marital, tasks and stages in, 629
  phases of, 260-65
  self-realization in, 249-50
Life review therapy, for the aged, 659-60
Life scripts, self-fulfilling prophecy and, 613
Life-style (*See also* Disruptive life-styles)
  changes in, adulthood and, 262
  concept of, 380
  family, 613-14
  phobic disorders and, 360
  retirement and, 278
Life theory, holistic approach to, 239-40
Lifton, Robert, 751
Limbic system, psychosurgery and, 694
Limits, setting of
  in adolescence, 580-81
  in child psychiatry, 546-47
Lindemann, Erich, 273, 278
Lindemann, K., 661
Lindesmith, A., 392
Lindqvist, M., 20
Lindsey, K., 608
Linking, facilitative communication and, 127
Lipowski, Z. L., 484
Lippitt, R., 224
Liss, Jerome, 730-31
Lithane (*See* Lithium carbonate)
Lithium carbonate
  clients on, nursing care plan for, 686
  for depression, 678
  dosage of, 684-85
  for mania, 377, 424, 428, 684-87
  prophylactic uses of, 687
  for psychotic conditions, 428
  side effects of, 685-87
Living Love Way to Happiness and Higher Consciousness, 742
Lobotomy, 94 (*See also* Psychosurgery)
Local adaptation syndrome, 259
Locke, John, 240
Loeb Center for Rehabilitation, 75
London, Perry, 100, 729, 730
Loneliness, aging and, 640
Loss
  aging and, 640
  assessing lethality in suicide and, 291
  depressive disorders and, 370
  disturbed coping patterns and, 355
  grief reactions and, 278-81
Lou Gehrig's disease, 486
Louie, T., 775
Love, Freudian definition of, 572
Lowen, Alexander, 734-35
Lowenthal, M., 659
Loxipine, 670
  side effects of, 677
Loxitane (*See* Loxipine)
LSD, 393-94 (*See also* Hallucinogens)
  effects of, 597
Luft, Joseph, 47, 499
Lundeman, K., 642
Lying, impulsive life-styles and, 385

Macdonald, G., 643
Mackintosh v. Milano, 801
MacLennan, B. W., 585
Magical ritual, treatment of mental illness and, 7
Magical thinking, obsessive-compulsive disorders and, 362
Maharishi Mahesh Yogi, 742
Mahl, Gustav, 701
Maintenance roles, leadership and, 224
Majority vote, decision making and, 225
Male genitals, 298-300
Male homosexuality, 313
Male masturbation, 304
Male orgasm, 300
Male sexual response, physiology of, 303-4
Malinowski, Bronislav, 29
Malnutrition, mental retardation and, 473
Manaser, J. C., 351
Mania, 414
  hospitalization and treatment for, changes in, 415
  mental status examination and, 192-93
  treatment of, 684-88
Manic-depression, 11
  development of, 425-26
  diagnosis of, sex and, 764
  genetic factors in, 20
  heredity and, 423-24
  hospitalization and treatment for, changes in, 415
Manic disorders, 376-77
Manic episodes, diagnostic criteria for, 422
Manipulation, 171-72
  conversion disorder and, 367
  intervention strategies in, 172
Mann, Horace, 793
Mannes, Marya, 629
Manson, Charles, 6-7, 769
Maple syrup urine disease, 472
Mapping, family therapy and, 619
Marceau, Marcel, 111
Marchiafava's disease, 490
Marcos, L. R., 763
Marfan's syndrome, 474
Marijuana, 392-93 (*See also* Cannabis)
  adolescent abuse of, 591
  effects of, 599
Marital life cycle, tasks and stages in, 629
Marital status, diagnosis and treatment and, 764
Marital therapy (*See* Couples therapy)
Marriage, client's rights and, 806
Marsh, L. C., 216
Marsilid (*See* Iproniazid)
Martin, E. A. Jr., 508-10, 516
Marx, Groucho, 638
Masculinity, body image alteration and, 282
Maslach, C., 54
Maslow, Abraham, 76, 239, 247, 248, 274, 637, 638

Masochism
  sexual, 310
  women and, 12
Massachusetts Asylum, 791
Massachusetts General Hospital, 769
Massage therapy, introduction of, 11
Mastectomy clubs, 519
Masters, William, 28, 300, 304, 315, 740
Masturbation, 304-6
  adolescent, 586-87
  female, 304
  male, 304
  sexual fantasies and, 305-6
Maternal infections, mental retardation and, 473
Maternity, role requirements of, women and, 262
Mattachine Society, 519, 768
Matthenson, M. A., 763
McArdle, K., 146
McCann, J., 156
McLean Asylum, 792, 794
McLean Hospital, 13
Mead, George Herbert, 53, 215
Mead, Margaret, 12, 29, 767, 768
Meaninglessness, aging and, 640
Meanings, private v. shared, 110
Mechanic, David, 19
Medical-biological model, 18-23
  assumptions of, 18-19
  critique of, 21-23
  medical nomenclature and, 19-21
  psychiatric nursing practice and, 19
Medical nomenclature, 19-21
Medication, abuse of, aged and, 651
Medicine man, 775
Medicopsychiatric conditions (*See specific condition*)
Meditation, 752
Melancholia, 677
  electroconvulsive therapy and, 692
  treatment of, 679
Mellaril (*See* Thioridazine)
Mellow, J., 141, 165
Memory, mental status examination and, 189
Men, empty nest syndrome and, 276-77
Menarche, 566
Meningiti, organic brain syndromes and, 486
Meningoencephalitis, organic brain syndromes and, 483
Menn, A. Z., 830
Menninger, Karl, 34, 345
Menninger, W. C., 575
Menninger Clinic, 14, 575
Mental disorders, DSM-III differentiation of, 200-1, 354
Mental health
  environment and, 249
  interactionist approach to, 4
  old age and, 634-35
  self-actualization and, 247
  stress management and, 249
  traditional view of, 4
  of women, 98-99

Mental health care
  feminist movement and, 765-67
  gay rights movement and, 767-68
  Gray Panther movement and, 768
  YAVIS syndrome in, 762
Mental health consultation (*See* Consultation)
Mental health/human service worker, 57
Mental health laws
  California's, 809-11
  New York State's, 808-9
Mental health resources, 861-62
Mental Health Study Act (1955), 12
Mental Health Systems Act, 796-96
Mental health team
  collaborating on, 60-61
  members of, 55-57
Mental hospitals
  early American, 791
  establishment of, 10-11
  growth of, 792-94
  separation from, 807-8
Mental hygiene laws, 802-8
  twentieth-century, 797-98
Mental hygiene movement, 11
Mental illness
  assessing lethality in suicide and, 291
  beliefs about, 46
  contemporary developments and, 12-13
  era of alienation and, 8-9
  era of confinement and, 9
  era of magico-religious explanations and, 7-8
  era of mental hospitals and, 10-11
  era of moral treatment and, 10
  era of organic explanations and, 8
  era of psychoanalysis and, 11-12
  era of reason and observation and, 9-10
  era of ritualized social exclusion and, 9
  historical definitions of, 7-13
  interactionist approach to, 4
  law and, 788-97
  psychoanalysis and, 11-12
  responsibility and, 22-23
  self-help groups for, 519
  symbolic interactionist view of, 6
  Szasz's view of, 21-23
  traditional view of, 4
Mental Patient's Bill of Rights, 96
Mental retardation, 457, 470-80, 535-36
  (*See also* Mentally retarded)
  due to autosomal dominant inheritance, 474
  categories of, 471
  definitions of, 471
  diagnostic evaluation of, 477
  intervention in, 477-80
  level of, characteristic behavior at, 481
  mental status examination and, 192-93
  metabolic disorders associated with, 472
  perinatal causes of, 473-74
  postnatal causes of, 475
  prenatal causes of, 471-73

Mental retardation (continued)
  due to recessive/unknown inheritance patterns, 474
  sex and, 317
  sociocultural factors in, 475-76
Mental Retardation Facilities and Community Health Centers Act, 818
Mental status examination, 187-90
  differentiation of findings in, 192-93
  organic brain syndromes and, 482
Mentally retarded
  emotional vulnerability of, 476-77
  nursing care plan for, 479
  psychopathology of, 477
Meperidine
  antipsychotic drug interactions with, 678
  interactions with alcohol, 657
Meprobamate
  addictive doses of, 393
  for anxiety, 689-90
  interactions with alcohol, 657
Merhige, J., 170
Mescaline, 20, 394
  effects of, 597
Message generation, in communication, 109
Messick, J., 704
Metabolic disorders
  mental retardation and, 471, 472
  organic brain syndromes and, 483
  treatment approach in, 473
Metacommunication, 113, 115
Metatheory, 78
Methamphetamine, for depression, 680
Methaqualone, 692
  addictive doses of, 393
  for anxiety, 690
Methedrine, effects of, 595
Methyldopa, interactions with alcohol, 656
Methylphenidate
  for depression, 677, 680, 684
  for hyperactivity, 684
  narcotherapy and, 694
Methyprylon, 692
  use of, 691
Metronidazole, interactions with alcohol, 656
Meyer, Adolf, 11, 33
Meyers, J., 273
Microcephaly, 474
Middle age
  consolidation in, 240
  development in, 264-65
  generativity v. stagnation in, 264
  productivity of, 264-65
Mid-life crisis, 276-77
  adulthood and, 262-64
  characteristics of, 263-64
Midtown Manhattan Project, 459
Migraine, psychophysiological, 466
Milgram, Stanley, 233
Milieu therapy, 14, 23, 34, 89, 818
  for disturbed children, 532, 554-55
Miller, Henry, 296

Miller, T., 144
Millett, Kate, 29, 313
Miltown (*See* Meprobamate)
Mind-body relations, holistic view of, 6
Mindguards, groupthink and, 231
Minkoff, K., 827, 828, 831
Minnesota Multiphasic Personality Inventory (MMPI), 196, 198
Minority control, decision making and, 225
Mintz, Elizabeth, 737
Mintz, N., 223
Minuchin, Salvador, 612, 615
Mitchell, Martha, 820
Moban (*See* Molindone)
Modeling, learning of values and, 47
Models
  definition of, 78-79
  social psychiatric, 100
Molindone, 670
  side effects of, 677
Mongolism (*See* Down's syndrome)
Monism, 6
Monoamine oxidase inhibitors
  for depression, 428, 679, 680, 682-83
  hypertensive crises and, 682
  interactions with alcohol, 656
Monroe, Ruth, 35-36
Mons veneris, 297
Montessori, Maria, 240
Moore, J., 170
Morality
  groupthink and, 231
  impulsive life-styles and, 384-85
Moralizing, learning of values and, 47
Moreno, J. W., 205
Moreno, Jacob L., 216
Morgan, A. J., 205
Morita, Masatake, 738
Morita therapy, 738
Morphine, interactions with alcohol, 657
Morris, Jan, 307
Moscato, B., 61, 136
Mosher, L. R., 830
Mothering (*See also* Parenting)
  role definition of, 324
Motivation, disintegration of, 407, 412-13
  interventions in, 440-45
Mourning, stages of, 278-81
Moustakas, C., 640
Multiple orgasms, 304
Multiple personality, 364
Multiple sclerosis, 368
  organic brain syndromes and, 488
Munsadis, I., 144
Murillo-Rohde, I., 774
Murray, H. A., 196
Music therapy groups, 521
Mutilation fantasy, 557
  care plan for child with, 558
Mutism
  intervention strategies in, 170
  mental status examination and, 187
Mutter, A. Z., 702
Myocardial infarction, 462

Myoclonic seizures of infancy, mental
    retardation and, 475
Myotonia
    female sexual response and, 301, 302
    male sexual response and, 303, 304
Myths, family, 613-14

Nail biting, oral fixation and, 25
Narcissism
    conversion disorder and, 367
    oral fixation and, 25
Narcissistic life-style, 381
Narcotherapy, 694
Narcotics, interactions with alcohol, 657
Nardil (*See* Phenelzine)
Nason, John, 798
Nason v. Bridgewater, 798
National Association of Social Workers,
    768
National Council of Churches, 780
National Council of Senior Citizens, 768
National Institute of Mental Health, 12,
    287, 428, 817
    establishment of, 14, 140
National Mental Health Act (1946), 140
National Mental Health Study Act, 817,
    818
National Organization for Women,
    284-85, 308, 765-67
National Working Conference on
    Graduate Education in Psychiatric
    Nursing, 141
Naturalness, open encounter groups and,
    738
Navane (*See* Thiothixene)
Necrophilia, 310
Needs, Maslow's hierarchy of, 247
Negative reinforcement, behavioral theory
    and, 31
Negative transference, 174
Neglect, aged and, 643-44
Negotiated reality, 43-44
Negotiation
    one-to-one relationships and, 142
    symbolic interactionism and, 6-7
Nembutal (*See* Sodium pentobarbital)
Neologisms, 110
Neonatal sepsis, perinatal retardation and,
    475
Neoplasms, organic brain syndromes and,
    488-89
Network Against Psychiatric Assault, 408
Networking, aged and, 655-59
Neugarten, B., 768
Neurofibromatosis, 474
    organic brain syndromes and, 489
Neuroleptic agents
    for psychotic conditions, 428
    for schizophrenia, 424
Neurolinguistic programming, 744-45
Neurological assessment, 191
Neurosis, 10
    cardiac, 357
    diagnosis of, social class and, 19
    genetic factors in, 20
    psychosis v., 19
    separation anxiety and, 12

Neurotic behavior, behavioral definition
    of, 31
Neurotic conflict, psychoanalytic theory
    and, 24
Neurotransmitters, effects of drugs on,
    668
New England Hospital for Women, 13
New York Hospital, 791, 792
    Pathological Institute of, 11
New York Medical Society, 794
New York Society for the Prevention of
    Cruelty to Children, 284
New York State Care Act, 796
New York State Lunatic Asylum, 793
New York State Nurses' Association,
    808
New York State's Mental Hygiene Law,
    808-9
Nicotine, 394
Nicotinic acid, for organic brain
    syndrome, 489
Nightingale, Florence, 13
Nihilistic delusions, mental status
    examination and, 188-89
Nitroglycerin, interactions with alcohol,
    656
Noble savage, 240
Noctec (*See* Chloral hydrate)
Nocturnal emission, 587
Noise, environmental, group dynamics
    and, 223
Noludar (*See* Methyprylon)
Noncompliance, 721-23
    client's reasons for, 667
    contracting and, 722-23
    factors in, 722
Nonspecific stress model, 701
Nonverbal communication, 110-12
    verbal v., 112
Norepinephrine
    antidepressant drugs and, 684
    depression and, 20
    psychotic conditions and, 424
    secretion of, effects of drugs on, 668
Normality, optimal wellness and, 246-47
Norms, group, 228-30
Norpramin (*See* Amitriptyline)
Norris, Catherine, 21
Nortriptyline, for depression, 678, 680
Nosologies, psychiatric, 345
Nuclear family, 606-7
Nurse-client relationships (*See*
    Relationships)
Nurse-counselor, adolescents and, 574
Nursing care plan, 70-71, 206-7
    implementation of, 71
    properties of, 71
Nursing diagnosis, 67-70
Nursing history guide, 68-70
Nursing process, 65-74
Nursing standards, of American Nurses'
    Association, 836-37
Nursing theory, 75-80
    applications to practice, 80
    evaluating, 78-80
    historical antecedents of, 75
    overview of, 75-78

Nutrition
    for depressed clients, 372
    mental retardation and, 475
    orthomolecular, 736

Oakes, Josiah, 794
Obedience, destructive, authority and,
    233-34
Obesity, 464-65
    adolescent, 589
    oral fixation and, 25
    self-help groups for, 519
Object language, 113
Object love, in adolescence, 569
Obscenity, adolescent communication
    and, 580
Observation
    one-to-one relationship work and,
        158-59
    physiological assessment and, 191
    problem solving and, 161
    steps in, 158
Obsessions
    definition of, 361
    mental status examination and, 189
Obsessive-compulsive disorders, 361-63
    definition of, 361
    intervention in, 362-63
    psychodynamics of, 361-62
    sociocultural dynamics in, 362
Occupational therapist, 57
Oculogyric crisis, antipsychotic drugs and,
    673
Oedipal conflict, 12, 26-27
    adolescence and, 568-69
Oedipal stage, in childhood development,
    529-30
Old age (*See also* Aged)
    grief in, 661
    mental health and, 634-35
Omnibus Budget Reconciliation Act, 820
Ontological security, 43
Oophorectomy, sexual difficulties
    associated with, 315
Open encounter groups, 738
Open-ended question, facilitative
    communication and, 127
Openness, one-to-one relationships and,
    142
Operant conditioning, 31
Opinion, definition of, 46
Opinion giver, 224
Opinion seeker, 224
Opioids, organic brain syndromes and,
    484
Opisthotonos, antipsychotic drugs and,
    673
Oppositional disorders, in childhood, 533
Oppression, 765
Oppression experiences, counseling of
    clients with, 778-80
Optimal wellness, 246-49
    theories of, 248
Oral aggressive stage, 25
Oral fixation, 25
Oral sadistic stage, 25
Oral sex, 306

Oral stage
  in childhood development, 528
  psychoanalytic theory and, 25
Orality, ego development and, 25
Order of Saint Mary of Bethlehem, 790
Orem, Dorothea E., 76, 831
Organ language, 353
Organic affective syndrome, 484
Organic brain disease
  characteristic symptoms of, 191
  mental status examination and, 187
Organic brain syndromes, 457, 480-93
  alcohol abuse and, 387
  classification of, 483-84
  global, clinical features of, 485
  intervention in, 491-93
  mental status examination and, 192-93
  misdiagnosis of in the aged, 650
  psychiatric symptoms of, 481-82
  sex and, 317
Organic delusional syndrome, 484
Organic mental syndrome
  in the aged, antipsychotic medications
    and, 672
  electroconvulsive therapy and, 692
  narcotherapy for, 694
Organic personality syndrome, 484
Orgasm
  clitoral v. vaginal, 304
  female, 300-4
  male, 300
Orgasmic dysfunction, female,
  interventions for, 316
Orientation, mental status examination
  and, 189
Orlando, Ida Jean, 78, 141
Orsolits, M., 144
Orthomolecular nutrition, 736
Orwell, George, 230
Osmund, H., 736
Ostomies, sexual difficulties associated
  with, 316
Ovaries, 298
Overanxious disorders, childhood, 534
Overdose, of antidepressant drugs, 680
Overload
  aged and, 649
  in communication, 114

Packard, E. P. W., 795
Pain, psychogenic, 367-68
Panic, 350
Panic attacks, treatment of, 684, 689
Panic disorders
  intervention in, 356-58
  nursing care plan for, 358
  treatment of, 689
Papp, P., 622
Parad, Howard J., 274
Paradox, in families, 616
Paralanguage, 111
Paraldehyde, 13
Paralytic ileus, antipsychotic drugs and,
  672
Paranoia, 89
  aged and, 646
  homosexuality and, 12

Paranoia (continued)
  negative transference responses in,
    165
  stereotyping and, 91
Paranoid life-style, 381
Paranoid personality, 399-401
  characteristics of, 399-401
  compulsive life-style v., 400
  intervention and, 401
Paranoid reactions, 9
Paranoid schizophrenia, 11
Paraphilias, 308-14 (See also specific
  type)
Paraphrasing, facilitative communication
  and, 126
Parathormone, for organic brain
  syndrome, 489
Parathyroid disease, organic brain
  syndromes and, 483
Parathyroid hyperfunction, organic brain
  syndromes and, 489
Parent-child fit, 338-39
Parenting
  different structures of, 325-28
  process of, 322-24
  stress and, 329-34
Parents
  adolescent, 331-32
  adoptive, 326-27
  battering, 332-34
  communal, 327-28
  counseling, 334-40
  emotional support for, 323
  foster, 327
  single, 325-26
  step-, 327
  stress and, 329-34
  working, 328
Parents Anonymous, 519
Parkinson's disease, 673
  anxiety and, 191
Parkinsonian syndrome, 673
Parks, S., 159
Parnate (See Tranylcypromine)
Parsons, T., 704
Passive-aggressive life-style, 381
Passive euthanasia, 92
Passivity, women and, 12
Pathological grief, treatment of, 679
Pathological Institute of New York
  Hospital, 11
Patrick, Ted, 780
Patterson, Gerald, 612
Pattison, M. E., 428
Pattison, M. L., 428
Pauling, Linus, 736
Paull, Peter, 791
Pavlov, Ivan, 29-30
PCP (phencyclidine), 484
Peace Corps, 274
Pearl Harbor, 230
Peck, R., 636
Pedophilia, 308
Peer approval, adolescence and, 566
Peitchinis, J., 144
Pellagra, organic brain syndromes and,
  489

Penis, 298-99
  male sexual response and, 303
Penis envy, 27, 29
Pennsylvania Hospital, 10, 791
Pentobarbital (See Sodium pentobarbital)
People's Temple, 768
Peplau, Hildegard, 75, 76, 140, 141,
  158, 359
Pepper, B., 822
Peptic ulcer
  formation of, 461-62
  psychophysiological, 460-61
  theories explaining, 702
Perception
  communication and, 104-6
  disintegration of, 405-7
    interventions in, 433-35
  facilitative communication and, 126
Periarteritis nodosa, organic brain
  syndromes and, 487
Perineal prostatectomy, sexual difficulties
  associated with, 315
Perls, Frederick, 735-36
Pernicious anemia, organic brain
  syndromes and, 483
Perphenazine, 670
  for anxiety attacks, 684
Perseveration, mental status examination
  and, 187
Persona, Jungian theory and, 12
Personal fulfillment, meaning of, 730
Personal history, in psychiatric history,
  187
Personal relations, group analysis and,
  504-7
Personal space, 111
  group dynamics and, 220-22
Personality
  childhood experiences and, 240
  developmental life phases theory and,
    242-43
  paranoid, 399-401
  in psychiatric history, 187
  schizoid/schizotypal, 401-2
  type A, 459
    heart disease and, 462
Personality disorders, demographics of,
  764
Personality tests, 194-97
Personality theory, psychosis and, 424-26
Pertofran (See Amitriptyline)
Pervasive developmental disorder,
  childhood-onset, 532
Peyote, effects of, 597
Phallic stage, psychoanalytic theory and,
  26-27
Phantom experience, amputees and, 283
Phencyclidine, organic brain syndromes
  and, 484
Phenelzine, 682
  for depression, 680
Phenobarbital, effects of, 595
Phenomenology, formation of self and,
  243-45
Phenothiazines, 14, 17, 89, 670
  for depression, 684
  interactions with alcohol, 657

Phenothiazines (continued)
for organic brain syndrome in the aged, 672
Phenylketonuria, 471, 472
Phenytoin, interactions with alcohol, 656
Pheochromocytoma, organic brain syndromes and, 489
Phillips, L., 647
Philosophy, relevance of, 5
Phobic disorders, 360-61
intervention in, 360-61
life-style consequences of, 360
types of, 360
Phoenix House, 519
Photostudy, in family therapy, 622-23
Physical abuse, of children, 332
Physical aggressivity, intervention strategies in, 171
Physical deterioration, aging and, 640-41
Physical exertion, stress and, 353
Physical withdrawal, intervention strategies in, 169-70
Physiological assessment, 190-91
Physiological needs, adaptation and, 78
Physostigmine, for antidepressant drug overdose, 680
Piaget, Jean, 241-42, 243, 245, 470, 567
Picasso, Pablo, 255
Pierce, R., 144, 145
Pinel, Philippe, 10, 792, 817
Pinpointing, facilitative communication and, 127
Piperadines, 670
Piperazines, 670
Pituitary hyperfunction/hypofunction, organic brain syndromes and, 489
Placidyl (See Ethchlorvynol)
Plath, Sylvia, 86
Plato, 86, 789
Plawecki, H. and J., 639
Play, functions of, 548
Play acting, mental status examination and, 188
Play therapist, role of, 549
Play therapy, 548-49
Playboy, 224
Pleasure principle, psychoanalytic theory and, 25
Poetry therapy groups, 521
Poisons, organic brain syndromes and, 483
Poor Laws, 790
Porencephaly, 474
Pornography, 311-12
Porter, D., 742
Positive reinforcement, behavioral theory and, 31
Postadolescence
intimacy v. isolation in, 261-62
psychosocial moratorium and, 261-62
resolution in, 261
Postconcussional amnesia, differentiation of, 366
Postnatal counseling, 336-38
Post-traumatic stress disorder, 287
Postural hypotension, antipsychotic drugs and, 673

Poverty
cycle of, 329
factors associated with, 330
intervention in, 330
racism and, 329
Power
feelings and behaviors related to, 766-67
in families, 610
group dynamics and, 232-34
sources of, 232
Poznanski, E. O., 600
Pragmatics, communication and, 115-16
Prana, 736
Pratt, Joseph Hersey, 215
Preadolescence, 571
homosexuality and, 587
Preconscious, 24
Predictive principles, 71
Pregnancy
adolescent, 588-89
maternal infections during, mental retardation and, 473
Premature ejaculation, interventions for, 316
Prematurity
factors in, 474
mental retardation and, 474-75
Premortem dying, 281
Prenatal counseling, 334-36
Preoccupations
autism and, 531
mental status examination and, 188-89
Preparation, problem solving and, 162
President's Commission on Mental Health, 762
Pressure, groupthink and, 231
Pretexts, paranoid personality and, 400
Preventive psychiatry, 626, 705-6
Priapism, 299
Price, Richard, 811
Primal needs, 733
Primal scream therapy, 733-34, 748
Primary degenerative dementia
aged and, 646, 648
organic brain syndromes and, 490
Primary gain, disturbed coping patterns and, 355
Primary impotence, interventions for, 316
Primary orgasmic dysfunction, interventions for, 316
Primary prevention, 705
in community mental health, 824
Primary process thinking, 17
Primeaux, M., 773, 775, 776
Privacy, confidentiality and, 95-98
Problem-oriented recording, 206, 210
Problem solving, in alternative therapies, 748-49
Procedural technician, 224
Processing, facilitative communication and, 127
Process schizophrenia, 419-20
Procyclidine, 673
Profanity, adolescent communication and, 580

Professionalism, one-to-one relationships and, 139-40
Progesterone, 298
Program-centered case consultation, 708-9
Progress notes, problem-oriented, 206, 210
Proinflammatory hormones, alarm reactions and, 258
Projection
as a defense mechanism, 254
paranoid personality and, 399-401
Projective tests, 194-97
Prolixin (See Fluphenazine)
Propanediols, for anxiety, 690
Propoxyphene, interactions with alcohol, 657
Propranolol, for anxiety, 690
Prostaglandins, headache and, 466
Prostatectomy, sexual difficulties associated with, 315
Prostitution, 311
Protest, hospitalized child and, 556
Protriptyline, for depression, 678, 680
Proxemics, 111
Pruritis, psychophysiological, 463
Pseudohostility, in families, 614-15
Pseudomutuality, in families, 614-15
Psilocybin, 394 (See also Hallucinogens)
effects of, 597
Psychiatric aide, 57
Psychiatric attendant, 57
Psychiatric audits, 207
Psychiatric biochemistry, 20
Psychiatric diagnosis, DSM-III and, 23
Psychiatric genetics, 20
Psychiatric history, 187
Psychiatric jargon, avoidance of, 205-6
Psychiatric nurse, therapeutic effectiveness of, 143
Psychiatric nursing
behaviorist model for, 29-32
humanism and, 6-7
medical-biological model for, 18-23
psychoanalytic model for, 23-29
social-interpersonal model for, 32-36
symbolic interactionism and, 4-5
Psychiatric nursing clinical specialist, 56
Psychiatric nursing practice, culture and, 759-65
Psychiatric social worker, 57
Psychiatric technician, 57
Psychiatric treatment
expanded definitions of, 730
right to, 798-99
right to refuse, 801-2
Psychiatrist, 56
Psychiatry
history of ideas in, 7-13
medical model of, psychiatric nursing practice and, 3
Psychic determinism, psychoanalytic theory and, 23-24
Psychoactive drugs
for psychotic conditions, 416-17, 428

Psychoanalysis, 24
    family therapy and, 612
    treatment of mental illness and, 11-12
Psychoanalyst, 57
Psychoanalytic model
    assumptions of, 23-28
    critique of, 28-29
    psychiatric nursing practice and, 28
Psychobabble, 206, 751
Psychodrama, 216, 518, 730
Psychogenic amnesia, 364
    differentiation of, 366
Psychogenic fugue, 364
Psychogenic pain, 367-68
Psychogenic pain disorder, 366
Psycho-imagination therapy, 741, 748
Psychological growth therapies, 737-41
Psychological testing, 191-97
Psychomotor epilepsy, organic brain
        syndromes and, 490
Psychophysiological disorders, 458-70;
        see also specific disorder
Psychorientology, 743-44
Psychosexual development
    anal stage of, 25-26
    genital stage of, 27-28
    latency stage of, 27
    oral stage of, 25
    phallic stage of, 26-27
    psychoanalytic theory and, 25-28
Psychosexual disorders (See specific type)
Psychosis (See also specific type)
    diagnosis of, social class and, 19, 90
    mental status examination and, 192-93
    neurosis v., 19
Psychosocial assessment, 185, 204-5
Psychosocial moratorium,
        postadolescence and, 261-62
Psychosocial stressors, severity of, 202
Psychosocial therapy, for psychotic
        conditions, 428
Psychosomatic disorders, 458-60
Psychosomatic medicine, Alfred Adler
        and, 11-12
Psychosurgery, 140, 694-95
    client's rights and, 806
    ethics of, 94
    sites of, 695
Psychosynthesis, 739, 748
Psychotherapy, 23
    for the aged, 653
    analytic group, 518
    for bedwetting, 533
    crisis intervention v., 275
    for crisis situations, 274
    democratization of, 751
    for depression, 679
    for dissociative disorders, 364
    effectiveness of, supervision and,
        165-66
    feminism and, 98
    for grieving client, 661
    for obsessive-compulsive disorders,
        362-63
    one-to-one relationship in, 138
    for psychogenic pain, 368

Psychotherapy (continued)
    for psychophysiological allergy, 469
    for psychophysiological arthritis, 469
    for psychophysiological disorders, 458
    for psychophysiological headache, 470
    for psychotic conditions, 428
    for severely disturbed children, 532
    as a social index, 729-30
    use of antipsychotics and, 671
Psychotic conditions
    behavior theory and, 426-27
    biological factors in, 423-24
    community mental health and, 417
    descriptions of, 418-19
    institutionalization and, 416
    past history and, 419-23
    personality theory and, 424-26
    psychoactive drugs and, 416-17
    psychological factors in, 424-27
    social factors in, 427
    treatment of, 427-29
Psychotic relapse, akathisia v., 673-74
Psychotic syndrome, medical illnesses
        presenting, 669
Psychotic transference, 174-75
Psychotropic drugs, 668-91
    care of the aged and, 653-54
        administration guidelines for, 655
    early use of, 818
    for psychophysiological allergy, 469
    use of, ethics of, 94-95
Puberty
    genital activity and, 572
    Oedipal conflict and, 568-69
    suicide and, 592
Public communication, 107
Purgatives, early psychotherapy and, 10
Purging, ancient psychotherapeutic
        intervention and,

Quaalude (See Methaqualone)
Quakers, 791, 792
Quality of life, compulsive life-style and,
        397-98
Questioning, facilitative communication
        and, 127
Quinacrine, interactions with alcohol, 656

Race, assessing lethality in suicide and,
        291
Racism
    intervention in, 330
    poverty and, 329
Rahe, H., 649
Rahe, R. H., 272, 273, 702
Rank, Otto, 12
Rape, 308, 310
Rational-emotive therapy, 739-40
Rationalization
    as a defense mechanism, 255-56
    groupthink and, 230-31
Reaction formation
    as a defense mechanism, 256
    obsessive-compulsive disorders and,
        362
    repression and, 256

Reactive attachment disorder of infancy,
        532
Reactive schizophrenia, 419-20
Reade, Charles, 795
Reagan, Ronald, 820
Reality
    definition of, 406
    negotiated, 43-44
Reality distortion, paranoid personality
        and, 399
Reality orientation, for the aged, 658
Reality principle, psychoanalytic theory
        and, 25
Reality therapy, 738-39
Reasoning, mental status examination
        and, 190
Rebelliousness, in childhood, 533
Recall, mental status examination and,
        189
Reciprocal inhibition, for phobic
        disorders, 360
Recognition seeker, 224
Recoil, in disaster response, 287
Recording, systems of, 205-11
Recovery Incorporated, 216, 519
Recreational sex, 296
Recreational therapist, 60
Redl, F., 572
Redlich, F. C., 19, 762
Reeducation groups, 519-20
Referent power, 232
Reflected appraisals, organization of
        behavior and, 33
Reflection, facilitative communication and,
        126
Registered nurse, in psychiatric settings, 56
Regression
    in childhood, 535
    disintegration of motivation and, 412
    psychoanalytic theory and, 24
Regulating, in communication, 112
Reich, S., 144
Reich, Wilhelm, 29
Reiff, Phillip, 751
Reifler, B., 652
Reinforcement, behavioral theory and, 30
Relating, in communication, 112
Relational sex, 296
Relationship level, in communication, 115
Relationships
    client-therapist-public, 800-1
    in early adolescence, 571-72
    one-to-one
        characteristics of, 137-40
        history of, 140-42
        humanism and, 142-43
        informal v. formal, 137-38
        philosophical framework for, 142-43
    in preadolescence, 571
    professional v. social, 139
    therapeutic
        interpersonal skills in, 143-45
        phases of, 145-57
        processes in, 157-66
        resistance in, 166-68
    therapeutic v. social, 123

Religious beliefs, diagnosis and treatment and, 763-64
Religious cults, 607, 768-71
    characteristics of, 769-70
    clients with experiences of, counseling of, 780-83
Religious groups, destructive cults v., 770
Reliving, psychoanalytic theory and, 24
Remembering, psychoanalytic theory and, 24
Reminiscence, for the aged, 659-60
Remotivation, for the aged, 658
Remotivation groups, 519-20
Renal failure, organic brain syndromes and, 483
Rennie, John, 801
Rennie v. Klein, 801-2
Repetition, in communication, 112
Repression
    as a defense mechanism, 252
    psychoanalytic theory and, 24
    reaction formation and, 256
Repressive treatments, ethics of, 94-95
Reserpine, 191
    interactions with alcohol, 656
Residential treatment centers, 548
    milieu therapy in, 548
Residential treatment programs, for disturbed adolescents, 578-79
Residual deviance, mental illness as, 33
Resistance
    adolescent, 581-83
        nursing care plan for, 583
    general adaptation syndrome and, 259
    intervention strategies in, 168
    in therapeutic relationships, 166-68
Resnik, Harvey L. P., 274
Resocialization, for the aged, 658
Resolution, in postadolescence, 261
Resonancy, homeodynamics and, 77-78
Respect
    facilitative communication and, 123
    on mental health team, 60-61
    psychiatric nursing practice and, 51
Responsibility
    in alternative therapies, 732-33
    disease and, 22-23
    one-to-one relationships and, 142
Rest, for depressed clients, 372
Restitution, grieving process and, 280-81
Restlessness, biorhythmicity and, 20, 21
Restraints
    client's rights and, 805-6
    use of, ethics of, 95
Retention, mental status examination and, 189
Retirement, 277-78
Reverberation, empathy and, 53
Reward power, 232
Rexford, E., 338
Rh factor incompatibility, perinatal retardation and, 475
Rheumatoid arthritis, psychophysiological, 463
Richards, Linda, 13, 55
Richards, Renee, 307

Rigidity
    compulsiveness and, 395-96
    paranoid personality and, 399
Risk taking, group decisions and, 225-26
Risky shift, 225
Ritalin (See also Methylphenidate)
    for attention deficit disorder with hyperactivity, 534
Ritual purification, ancient psychotherapeutic intervention, 8
Ritualistic behavior, autism and, 531
Ritualized social exclusion, Middle Ages and, 9
Roethlisberger, F. J., 222
Rogers, Martha E., 77-78
Rogers v. Okin, 802
Role function, adaptation and, 78
Role playing, in family therapy, 623
Roles
    caretaker v. therapist, 144
    family, 610
    leadership and, 224
    sex, 308
Rolf, Ida, 731, 734, 745
Rolfing, 734
Roman law, mental illness and, 789
Rorschach, Hermann, 194
Rorschach Test, 194-96, 198
Rosen, R. D., 206, 751
Rosenman, R. H., 459
Roszak, Theodore, 751
Rouse, Charles, 798
Rouse v. Cameron, 798
Rousseau, Jean-Jacques, 240
Roy, Callista, 78
Rubella, maternal, mental retardation and, 473
Rubin, L., 276
Ruesch, Jurgen, 112-13
Runyon, N., 143
Rush, Benjamin, 10, 791
Russell, D., 649
Ryan, Leo J., 768
Ryglewicz, H., 822

Sacher, E. J., 701
Sack, A., 658
Sadism
    anal, 26
    sexual, 310
Sadock, B., 191, 419, 427
Sadomasochism, 310
Safety, for depressed clients, 372
Saint Elizabeth's Hospital, 798
Sakel, Manfred, 695
Salasnek, S., 577, 580
Salpêtrière, 10, 792
Sander, L., 338
Satir, Virginia, 607, 612, 614, 617, 618, 621, 623
Scapegoating
    in adolescence, 585
        nursing care plan for, 586
    in families, 615-16
Schedule of recent experience, 273
Scheff, Thomas, 19, 33, 410
Schema, in Piagetian theory, 241

Schismatic families, 615
Schizoid disorder of childhood, 536
Schizoid personality, characteristics of, 401-2
Schizophrenia, 11, 17, 23, 89, 408-9, 414
    antipsychotic drugs for, 669, 671-72
    biochemical factors in, 424
    biochemistry and, 20
    body image distortion in, 282
    characteristics of, 418-19
    communication and, 116
    demographics of, 764
    developmental process of, 425
    diagnosis of
        cultural differences in, 90
        ethnicity and, 763
        socioeconomic class and, 763
    diagnostic criteria for, 421
    dopamine and, 676
    dynamic formulation of, 426
    electroconvulsive therapy and, 692-93
    family double binds and, 616
    family therapy and, 12
    in female children, marital schism and, 615
    generational transmission of, 618
    genetic factors in, 20
    heredity and, 423-24
    hospitalization and treatment for, changes in, 415
    insulin coma therapy and, 695
    in male children, skewed marriages and, 615
    mental status examination and, 192-93
    orthomolecular psychiatry and, 736
    past history and, 419-20
    process, 419-20
    psychosurgery and, 694
    reactive, 419-20
    recent weight loss and, 191
    schizophrenogenic family and, 427
    serotonin metabolism and, 20
Schizophreniform disorder, diagnostic criteria for, 421
Schizophrenogenic family, 427
Schizotypal life-style, 381
Schizotypal personality, characteristics of, 401-2
Schleifer, M., 702
Schofield, W., 762
School phobia, 535
Schuable, P., 144, 145
Schuham, A. I., 616
Schutz, William C., 502, 504, 516, 737, 738
Schwartz, L. L., 770
Schwartz, Morris, 575, 818
Schweiker, Richard, 821
Scott, C. S., 773
Scripts, in transactional analysis, 749
Scrotum, 299
    male sexual response and, 303
Sculpting, in family therapy, 622
Secobarbital (See Sodium secobarbital)
Seconal (See Sodium secobarbital)
Second Great Awakening, 792

Secondary gain, disturbed coping patterns and, 355
Secondary impotence, interventions for, 316
Secondary prevention, 705
 in community mental health, 824
Sedative-hypnotics, 394
 addictive doses of, 393
Sedgwick, Rae, 622, 623
Seductive behavior, dealing with, 172
Seductiveness
 conversion disorder and, 367
 disturbed adolescents and, 579-80
Seghers, C. E., 223
Selective inattention, anxiety and, 350
Self
 emergence of, 42-49
 formation of, symbolic interactionism and, 243-45
 Jungian theory and, 12
 taking care of, 49-50
 therapeutic use of, 145
Self-abuse, aged and, 643
Self-actualization, 247
 Western culture and, 730-31
Self-awareness
 cognitive framework for, 47-49
 empathy and, 44
 establishment of trust and, 147
 of feelings, 44
Self-care deficit theory, 76-77
Self-censorship, groupthink and, 231
Self-centeredness, disturbed coping patterns and, 355
Self-concept
 adaptation and, 78
 dissociation and, 252
 repression and, 252
 stress management and, 250
Self-confessor, 224
Self-confidence, anal fixation and, 26
Self-consciousness, behavioral theory and, 32
Self-depreciation, delusions of, mental status examination and, 189
Self-destructiveness, 289 (*See also* Suicide)
Self-discipline, coping strategies and, 352-53
Self-disclosure, feedback and, 123
Self-dramatization, conversion disorder and, 367
Self-dynamism, organization of behavior and, 33
Self-esteem
 aged and, 659
 child abuse and, 333
 depression and, 371
 emotional health and, 248-49
 mid-life crisis and, 264
 posture and, 23
Self-fulfilling prophecy, life scripts and, 613
Self-help groups, 519
Self-image
 identity development and, 569
 significant others and, 42-43

Self-knowledge
 emotional health and, 248-49
 nursing profession and, 41-42
Self-neglect, aged and, 643
Self-realization, 249-50
Self-regulation, in alternative therapies, 732-33
Self-righteousness, anal fixation and, 26
Self-serving roles, leadership and, 224
Self-system, organization of behavior and, 33
Selye, Hans, 239, 257-60, 459, 701
Semen, composition of, 300
Senate Subcommittee on the Constitutional Rights of the Mentally Ill, 811
Sensitivity, psychiatric nursing practice and, 52
Sensitivity groups, 730
Sensorium
 assessment of, 161
 in mental status examination, 187, 189
Sentence Completion Test, 196, 198
Separation, marital, single parent role and, 325
Separation anxiety
 in childhood, 534-35
 hospitalized child and, 555-56
 neurosis and, 12
Serotonin
 antidepressant drugs and, 684
 headache and, 466
 metabolism of, schizophrenia and, 20
 psychotic conditions and, 424
Severe catatonic withdrawal, electroconvulsive therapy and, 692
Sex
 assessing lethality in suicide and, 291
 coping problems and, 317
 diagnosis and treatment and, 764
 oral, 306
 social problems and, 308-12
 violence and, 310-11
Sex education, for adolescent clients, 587
Sex flush
 female sexual response and, 301, 302
 male sexual response and, 303, 304
Sex hormones, arthritis and, 463
Sex roles, 308
Sex therapy, 314-18, 740
 assessment interview in, 318
Sexism, parenting and, 330-31
Sexual abuse, of children, 332
Sexual acting out, consultation and, 720-21
Sexual arousal
 intercourse and, 304
 techniques of, 306
Sexual behavior, adolescent, 585-89
Sexual fantasy, masturbation and, 305-6
Sexual identity (*See also* Gender identity)
 adolescent communication and, 580
 obesity and, 589
 phallic stage of development and, 27
 psychoanalytic theory and, 26-27
 social assignation of, 245

Sexual intercourse
 anal, 307
 arousal and, 304
 positions, 307
Sexual masochism, 310
Sexual object choice, gender identity v., 307
Sexual problems
 interventions for, 316
  Hegar dilators, 316
 treatment of, 314-18
Sexual response
 female, 301-2
 male, 303-4
 phases of, 300
 physiology of, 300-4
Sexual sadism, 310
Sexual sublimation, latency stage of development and, 27
Sexuality
 aging and, 642
 alternative, 312-14
 body image alteration and, 282
 normal v. abnormal, 296
 physiological, 297-7
 psychological, 307-8
 sociological, 308-12
Shadow, Jungian theory and, 12
Shallowness of affect, mental status examination and, 188
Shaman, 775
Shame, developmental life phases theory and, 242
Shands, Harley, 7
Shaping, behavioral theory and, 31
Shapiro, David, 144, 383, 396
Shapiro, T., 338
Shared dignity, 142
Sheehy, Gail, 261, 262, 264, 276, 277
Shepard, Herbert A., 504-5, 507, 516
Sheppard and Enoch Pratt Hospital, 14, 575
Sheresky, Norman, 629
Ship of Fools, 9
Shock, grieving process and, 278-80
Shore, H., 658
Shorr, Joseph, 741
Short-Doyle Act, 809
Sick role, 704
Sickle cell disease, priapism and, 299
Sign language, 113
Significant others
 assessing lethality in suicide and, 291
 developmental life phases theory and, 243
 self-image and, 42-43
Silva, Jose, 743
Silva Mind Control, 743-44
Silverstein, O., 622
Simmel, Ernst, 575
Simmonds' disease, 489
Simonton, O., 703
Simonton, S., 703
Simple phobia, 360
Simulation, mental status examination and, 188
Sinequan (*See* Doxepin)

Singer, M. R., 780
Single parents, 325-26
Sinnott, J., 643
Ska Children's Village, 601
Skewed families, 615
Skinner, B. F., 31
Skodol, A. E., 92, 199, 367
Slavson, S. R., 216
Sleeper, Frances, 140
Sleeping disturbances, infant, 533
Sleepwalking disorder, 364
Small, S. M., 187, 189
Smith, Janet, 667
Smith, W. D., 763
Smoke Watchers Anonymous, 519
Smoking
    oral fixation and, 25
    self-help groups for, 519
Snow, L. F., 773
Social change, alternative therapies
        movement and, 729
Social class
    development of deviant identity and,
        267-68
    psychiatric diagnosis and, 19
Social control, violence v., 92-94
Social exclusion, Middle Ages and, 9
Social good, individuals v., 100-1
Social-interpersonal model
    assumptions of, 32-34
    critique of, 35-36
    psychiatric nursing practice and, 34-35
Social interactionism, theories of
        development and, 266
Socialization, childhood development
        and, 240
Social learning, gender identity and, 308
Social networks, family therapy and, 612
Social phobia, 360
Social problems, sex and, 308-12
Social psychiatric model, 100
Social psychiatry, 34
Social Security, 329
Sociodrama, 518
Socioeconomic class, diagnosis and
        treatment and, 763
Sociopathy, 89
Sociotherapy, 818
Socrates, 86
Sodium pentobarbital, 692
    addictive doses of, 393
    effects of, 595
    interactions with alcohol, 656
Sodium pentothal (See Thiopental
        sodium)
Sodium secobarbital, 692
    addictive doses of, 393
    effects of, 595
    for insomnia, 691
    interactions with alcohol, 656
Solomon, H. C., 520
Solvents, inhalation of, effects of, 596
Somatic delusions, mental status
        examination and, 189
Somatic language, 113
Somatization disorder, 366

Somatizing, stress and, 353
Somatoform disorders, 364-69
    behavioral characteristics of, 366-67
    definition of, 366
    differentiation of, 368
    intervention in, 368-69
    nursing care plan for, 370
    pain and, 367-68
    properties of, 369
Somatotherapies, 19
    for psychotic conditions, 428
Somatotrophic hormones, alarm reactions
        and, 258
Somers, B. J., 765
Sommer, R., 222
Sopor (See Methaqualone)
Soteria House, 13, 432, 576, 671,
        829-30
Souder v. Brennan, 800
Source-oriented recording, 206
Spatial arrangements, group dynamics
        and, 223
Specificity model of illness, 700-1
Speck, R. V., 612
Speech, characteristics of, mental status
        examination and, 187
Spermatozoa, 299
Spire, Richard H., 282
Spitz, R., 555
Spitzer, R. L., 199, 200, 460
Spock, Benjamin, 336
Spontaneity, psychiatric nursing practice
        and, 51
Sprenger, Johann, 9
Srole, L., 459
St. Thomas Hospital (London), 13
Stagner, R., 649
Standard setter, 224
Stanford-Binet Intelligence Quotient, 470
Stanford-Binet Test, 194, 199
Stanton, Alfred, 575, 818
Stastny, J., 146
Status epilepticus, management of, 689
Statutory rape, 310
Stein, L., 20, 61, 829
Steiner, Claude, 613
Steinzor, Bernard, 223
Stelazine (See Trifluoperazine)
Stepparents, 327
Stereotypes
    battered women and, 284-85
    cultural, 761-62
    diagnosis and, 91
    group analysis and, 508-9
    groupthink and, 231
Sterilization, sexual difficulties associated
        with, 315
Stern, R., 828
Stever, J., 650
Steward, A., 171
Stewart, Isobel, 72
Stimulants
    abuse of, 394
    interactions with alcohol, 657
Stoller, Frederick, 737
Strauss, A., 281, 722

Stress
    adaptation to, 239-40
    adolescent parents and, 331
    aging and, 640-44
    alcoholism and, 386
    anxiety disorders and, 356-60
    arthritis and, 463
    behavioral change and, 250
    biorhythmicity and, 20
    coping strategies and, 352-53
    crisis development and, 271-73
    defense-oriented reactions to, 251-52
    disturbed children and, 544
    disturbed coping patterns and, 348-49
    environmental, combating, 100
    families and, 610
    general adaptation syndrome and,
        258-59
    headache and, 466
    heart attack and, 272
    interventions for, 259-60
    life changes and, 272-73
    local adaptation syndrome and, 259
    management of, mental health and,
        249
    parenting and, 329-34
    personal integration and, 50
    psychophysiological disorders and,
        467-69
    sex and, 317
    task-oriented reactions to, 251-52
    thought disintegration and, 407
    ulcer formation and, 460
Stress-adaptation theory, 257-60
Stress anxiety, aged and, 649
Stressors
    conflicts as, 348
    psychosocial, severity of, 202
    stress-adaptation theory and, 239
Strodtbeck, F. L., 223
Structural analysis, communication and,
        116-17
Structural integration, 734, 748
Structuring, facilitative communication
        and, 127
Sturge-Weber disease, 474
Stuttering, 353
Subdural hematoma, organic brain
        syndromes and, 490-91
Substance abuse, 386-87
    aged and, 651
Substance abuse disorders, 387-95
    in adolescence, 589-91
    alcohol addiction, 387-91
    drug dependence, 391-95
Substance dependence, 386-87
Substitution, in communication, 112
Succinylcholine, electroconvulsive therapy
        and, 692
Suggestibility, conversion disorder and,
        367
Suicide
    adolescent, 592-600
        rate of, 764
    aged and, 651
    assessing lethality in, 290-91

Suicide (continued)
  clinical variables in, 290
  clues in, 290
  as a coping mechanism, 288-93
  crisis intervention and, 291-92
  demographic variables in, 289-90
  depressive disorders and, 372
  ethics of, 92-94
  myths and realities of, 289
  social variables in, 289
Sulfa drugs, acute intermittent porphyria
    and, 485
Sullivan, Harry Stack, 12, 29, 33, 35-36,
    140, 243, 425, 429, 566, 571-72,
    575
Summarizing, facilitative communication
    and, 128
Sun Myung Moon, 770
Superego, psychoanalytic theory and,
    24-25
Superficiality
  facilitative intimacy v., 121
  intervention strategies in, 173
Supervision, therapeutic effectiveness
    and, 165-66
Suppression, as a defense mechanism,
    252-53
Suspicious thinking, paranoid personality
    and, 399
Sydenham's chorea, organic brain
    syndromes and, 491
Symbolic interactionism, 666
  abnormal v. normal in, 245
  communication model of, 108-10
  formation of self and, 243-45
  one-to-one relationship work and, 143
  premises of, 4
    implications for psychiatric nursing,
    4-5
Symbolic substitution, stress and, 353
Symbolization, phobic disorders and, 360
Syme, L., 659
Symmetry, in communication, 115-16
Sympathy, empathy and, 53
Symptomatology
  of alcohol withdrawal, 388
  of conversion disorder, 366
  definition of mental health/illness and,
    4, 6
  of generalized anxiety disorders, 357
  of grief reactions, 279
  life changes and, 273
  of mania, 419
  medical-biological model and, 21-22
  of organic brain syndromes, 481-82
  in psychiatric history, 187
  of schizophrenia, 418-19
Synanon, 740-41
Synergy, in families, 610-11
Synthesis, problem solving and, 162
Syphilis
  maternal, mental retardation and, 473
  organic brain syndromes and, 483,
    486
Systemic lupus erythematosus, organic
    brain syndromes and, 483, 487

Szasz, Thomas, 21-23, 29, 36, 88, 89,
    92, 94, 100, 408-9, 803, 811

Talbott, J. A., 13, 828
Talmud, mental illness and, 788-89
Tancredi, Larence, 812
Taractan (See Chlorprothixene)
Tarasoff, Tatiana, 801
Tarasoff v. Regents of University of
    California, 800-1
Taraxein, schizophrenia and, 20
Tardive dyskinesia, 674
  symptoms of, 674
Task roles, leadership and, 224
Task-oriented reactions, 251-52
Tauro, Joseph, 802
Taxson, D., 742
Tay-Sachs disease, 472
Tegel Sanitarium, 575
Telephone counseling, suicide prevention
    and, 293
Telescoping, phantom experiences and,
    283
Temple, Shirley, 283
Teresa, Mother, 638
Territoriality, 111
  group dynamics and, 220
Tertiary prevention, 705
  in community mental health, 824
Tertiary syphilis, organic brain syndromes
    and, 483
Test, M. A., 829
Testes, 299
  male sexual response and, 303
Testosterone, 299
T-groups, 730
THC, 394 (See also Hallucinogens)
Thematic Apperception Test, 196, 199
Therapeutic alliance, 145
  with battering parents, 334
  psychoanalytic theory and, 24
Therapeutic community, 574-78
  development of, 576-77
  value of, 575-76
Therapeutic contract, 148
  elements of, 150
  sample, 151
Therapeutic counseling, sexual problems
    and, 315-18
Therapeutic intervention; see Intervention
Therapeutic models
  behaviorist, 29-32
  medical-biological, 18-23
  psychoanalytic, 23-29
  social-interpersonal, 32-36
Therapeutic touch, 736-37
Therapist role, caretaker role v., 144
Therapy (See also specific type)
  anaclitic, 575
  for disturbed children, 548-55
  individual v. group, 511
Thiamine
  for Korsakoff's syndrome, 488
  for Wernicke's encephalopathy, 491
Thiopental sodium, narcotherapy and,
    694

Thioridazine, 670
  dosages for children, 672
  interactions with alcohol, 657
  side effects of, 677
Thiothixene, 670
  side effects of, 677
Thioxanthenes, 670
Thomas, A., 338
Thompson, Clara, 29
Thorazine (See Chlorpromazine)
Thought, disintegration of, 407-10
  interventions in, 435-38
Thought content
  assessment of, 161
  disturbances in, 161
Threats, intervention strategies in, 171
Thrombosis, organic brain syndromes
    and, 486-87
Throop, Enos T., 793
Thyroid disease, organic brain syndromes
    and, 483
Thyroid hormone, arthritis and, 463
Tillelli, J. A., 333
Time line, family therapy and, 618-19
Tobacco
  antipsychotic drug interactions with,
    678
  organic brain syndromes and, 484
Todd, B., 654
Todd, Eli, 792
Tofranil (See Imipramine)
Toilet training, 26
Tolazamide, interactions with alcohol,
    656
Tolbutamide, interactions with alcohol,
    656
Toman, Walter, 618
Tomlin, Lily, 313
Topographic theory, 24
T.O.P.S., 519
Torticollis, antipsychotic drugs and, 673
Touch, communication and, 111-12
Toxemia of pregnancy, mental retardation
    and, 473
Toxic organic brain syndrome, 9
Toxoplasmosis, maternal, mental
    retardation and, 473
Traditional nuclear family, 606-7
Tranquilizers
  for anxiety, 688-90
  erection difficulties and, 299
  interactions with alcohol, 657
Transaction, communication as, 108-10
Transactional Analysis (TA), 730, 737
  communication and, 116, 118-21
  scripts in, 749
Transcendence, aging and, 636, 638
Transcendental Meditation (TM), 742-43,
    749
Transference, 163-65, 174-75
  negative, 174
  psychoanalytic theory and, 24
  psychotic, 174-75
Transient ischemic attacks, 648
Transitional transactions, 121
Translocation shock, 643

Transsexualism, 313-14
    phallic stage of development and, 27
    urological timetable for management
        of, 314
Transvestism, 313-14
Tranylcypromine, for depression, 680
Trauma, disturbed coping patterns and,
    355
Traumatic disorders, organic brain
    syndromes and, 483
Traumatic experience, psychoanalytic
    theory and, 24
Triangles, family, 614
Triangulation, in families, 614
Triavil, for anxiety attacks, 684
Tricyclic antidepressants, 428
Tricyclics, 677-82
    antipsychotic drug interactions with,
        678
    for depression, 679
    dosages of, 678-80
    interactions with alcohol, 656
    side effects of, 680-82
Trifluoperazine, 670
    dosages for children, 672
    geriatric dosages of, 672
    side effects of, 677
Trihexyphenidyl, 673
Trilafon (See Perphenazine)
Trisomy 21 (See Down's syndrome)
Trogdon, K., 143
Truax, C., 144
Trumbull, Robert, 93
Trust
    development of, in adolescence, 569
    difficulty with, oral fixation and, 25
    group dynamics and, 227-28
    therapeutic relationship and, 147-48
Tuberculosis, organic brain syndromes
    and, 486
Tuberous sclerosis, 474
    organic brain syndromes and, 491
Tudor, Gwen, 402, 576
Tudor, J. F., 764
Tuinal (See Sodium secobarbital)
Tuke, William, 792
Turek, D., 333
Tyhurst, James S., 273, 287
Type A personality, 459
    heart disease and, 462

Ulcer
    interventions in, 469
    psychophysiological, 460-61
Ulcerative colitis, psychophysiological,
    461-62
Ulterior transactions, 118-21
Ultradian biorhythms, 20, 21
Unanimity, groupthink and, 231
Unconscious, psychoanalytic theory and,
    24
Underload, in communication, 114
Underwood, P. R., 831, 832
Undoing, obsessive-compulsive disorders
    and, 362
Unemployment compensation, 329
Unification Church, 770

Unipolar affective disorder
    electroconvulsive therapy and, 692
    patterns of, 688
Urinary meatus, female, 297
Urolangia, 314
Urticaria, psychophysiological, 463
Uterus, 298
    female sexual response and, 301, 302
Utica State Asylum, 794

Vagina, 298
    female sexual response and, 301, 302
Vaginal orgasm, 304
Vaginismus, interventions for, 316
Valium (See Diazepam)
Valliant, G., socioeconomic class and, 763
Values
    communication and, 106
    learning of, 46-47
    middle age and, 265
    types of, 45
Values clarification
    detached concern and, 42
    learning of values and, 47
Van Buren, Abigail, 222
Van Lehn, R., 701
Van Praag, H. M., 418, 420
Vas deferens, 298, 299
Vascular disorders, organic brain
    syndromes and, 483
Vascular headache, psychophysiological,
    466
Vasodilators, interactions with alcohol,
    656
V-codes (See DMS-III)
Vennen, M., 156
Verbal communication, 110
    lack of, autism and, 531
    nonverbal v., 112
Verbal threats, intervention strategies and,
    171
Verbal withdrawal, intervention in, 170
Vestibule, 297
Victim crises, 283-88
Victomology, 284
Vineland Social Maturity Scale, 194
Violence
    continuum of, 286
    family, 284-85
    sex and, 310-11
    social control v., 92-94
Visigothic code, mental illness and,
    789-90
Vision, psychiatric nursing practice and,
    52
Vistaril (See Hydroxyzine)
Vital balance, 348
Vitamin B12, for organic brain syndrome,
    490
Vitamin D, for organic brain syndrome,
    489
Vivactyl (See Protriptyline)
Vodun, 773
Vogel, Ezra F., 616
von Recklinghausen's disease, 474
    organic brain syndromes and, 489
von Sacher-Masoch, Leopold, 310

Voodoo (Houngan/Mambo), 773
Voting, client's rights and, 806-7
Voyeurism, 311, 414
Vulva, 297

Wallach, M. S., 225
Walsh, M., 71
Warmth, facilitative communication and,
    125
Watson, J., 653
Watzlawick, P., 115, 116, 611, 619
Wechsler Adult Intelligence Scale, 194,
    199
Wechsler Intelligence Scale for Children,
    194, 199
Wechsler Memory Scale, 199
Weight loss, diagnostic implications of,
    191
Weight Watchers, 519
Weinstein, S. P., 828
Weisberg, M. D., 775
Weisman, Avery D., 281, 723
Weissman, M., 98
Wellness
    high-level, 247-48
    optimal, 246-49
    theories of, 248
Wellness/illness, ego states in, 117-18
Wells, L., 643
Werner, A. M., 351
Wernicke's encephalopathy, organic brain
    syndromes and, 491
Wernicke-Korsakoff's syndrome, organic
    brain syndromes and, 483
Weyer, Johann, 9
White, C., 642
White, R. K., 224
White, William Alanson, 28, 33
White House Conference on the Family,
    606
Whitehead, Alfred North, 85
Whitley, M. P., 318
Wholeness, in families, 609
Wiedenbach, Ernestine, 78
Willard, Sylvester D., 794
Willard Asylum, 794, 796
Williams, C. C., 273
Williams, J. B. W., 197, 199, 200, 203
Willingham, D., 318
Wills, client's rights and, 806
Wilmer, Harry, 576
Wilson, H. S., 13, 197, 200, 203, 367,
    576, 826, 829, 832
Wilson's disease, 472
    organic brain syndromes and, 483, 491
Winslow, W. W., 822
Wise, C. D., 20
Witchcraft, 9
Withdrawal
    alcohol, 387
        antianxiety agents and, 690
        symptoms of, 388
    amphetamine, 394
    in childhood, 535
    disintegration of motivation and, 412,
        442
    intervention in, 169-70

Withdrawal (continued)
  stress and, 353
Wolanin, M., 647
Wolberg, L., 146, 160
Wolff, A., 216
Wolpe, Joseph, 31
Women
  battered, 284-85
  depression and, 99
  empty nest syndrome and, 276-77
  identity formation and, 261
  mental health of, 98-99
  mid-life crisis and, 276-77
  role requirements of maternity and, 262

Woodward, Samuel B., 793
Worcester State Hospital, 11
Word Association Test, 199
Word-building, 35
Working parents, 328
World Health Organization, 197, 411
Wyatt v. Stickney, 799
Wynne, Lyman, 614-15

Yablonsky, L., 740
Yalom, Irvin, 510, 516-17
Yang, 775
Yates, John, 793
YAVIS syndrome, 762

Yin, 775
Yogi, Maharishi Mahesh, 742
York, Richard H., 416, 575, 818
York Retreat, 10, 792
Yura, H., 71

Zangari, M., 722
Zeldow, P., 765
Ziegler, V., 763
Zilberg, N. J., 577
Zoophilia, 310
Zung, W., 650
Zung depression scale, 650